HANDBOOK OF MEDICAL-SURGICAL NURSING

SECOND EDITION

HANDBOOK OF MEDICAL-SURGICAL NURSING

SECOND EDITION

Springhouse Corporation
Springhouse, Pennsylvania

Staff

Senior Publisher
Matthew Cahill

Art Director
John Hubbard

Managing Editor
David Moreau

Senior Editor
Naina Chohan

Acquisitions Editors
Patricia Kardish Fischer, RN, BSN; Louise Quinn

Clinical Consultants
Maryann Foley, RN, BSN; Collette Hendler, RN, CCRN

Copy Editors
Cynthia C. Breuninger (manager), Karen Comerford, Brenna Mayer, Pamela Wingrod

Designers
Arlene Putterman (associate art director), Susan Hopkins Rodzewich, Jeff Sklarow

Typography
Diane Paluba (manager), Joyce Rossi Biletz, Phyllis Marron, Valerie Rosenberger

Manufacturing
Deborah Meiris (director), Pat Dorshaw (manager), T. A. Landis, Otto Mezei

Production Coordinator
Margaret A. Rastiello

Editorial Assistants
Beverly Lane, Mary Madden

The clinical procedures described and recommended in this publication are based on research and consultation with nursing, medical, and legal authorities. To the best of our knowledge, these procedures reflect currently accepted practice; nevertheless, they can't be considered absolute and universal recommendations. For individual application, all recommendations must be considered in light of the patient's clinical condition and, before administration of new or infrequently used drugs, in light of the latest package-insert information. The authors and the publisher disclaim responsibility for any adverse effects resulting directly or indirectly from the suggested procedures, from any undetected errors, or from the reader's misunderstanding of the text.

Printed in the United States of America.
HMSN-021198

 A member of the Reed Elsevier plc group

Library of Congress Cataloging-in-Publication Data

Handbook of medical-surgical nursing.—2nd ed.
p. cm.
Includes bibliographical references and index.
1. Nursing—Handbooks, manuals, etc.
2. Surgical nursing—Handbooks, manuals, etc.
I. Springhouse Corporation.
[DNLM: 1. Perioperative Nursing—handbooks. WY 49 H2357 1997]
RT51.H352 1997
610.73—dc21
DNLM/DLC 97-20429
ISBN 0-87434-877-3 (alk. paper) CIP

Contents

Contributors and consultants

Susan C. Baltrus, RN,C, MSN
Senior Level Coordinator
Central Maine Medical Center
Lewiston

Sally A. Brozenec, RN, PhD
Assistant Professor
Rush University College of Nursing
Chicago

Mary Ann Cali-Ascani, RN, MSN, OCN
Oncology Nurse Manager
Oncology Clinical Nurse Specialist
Easton (Pa.) Hospital

Marilyn A. Folcik, RN, MPH, ONC
Assistant Director, Department of Surgery
Hartford (Conn.) Hospital

Ellie Franges, MSN, CNRN, CCRN
Director, Neuroscience Services
Sacred Heart Hospital
Allentown, Pa.

Lori Gibson, RN, MS, CNS
Medical Case Manager
Clinical Nurse Specialist
Del E. Webb Memorial Hospital
Sun City West, Ariz.

Lisa K. Hansen, RN, MS, AOCN
Clinical Program Specialist
Autologous Bone Marrow Transplantation
Legacy Good Samaritan Hospital
Portland, Ore.

Linda Hoebler, RN, MSN
GYN Oncology Clinical Nurse Specialist
Allegheny General Hospital
Pittsburgh

Joyce Young Johnson, RN, PhD, CCRN
Assistant Professor
Georgia State University School of Nursing
Atlanta

Chris Platt Moldovanyi, RN, MSN
Registered Nurse Medical Consultant
Phillips and Mille
Middlebury Heights, Ohio

Nancy J. Reilly, RN, MSN, CRNP, CURN
Urologic Nurse Practitioner
Toms River, N.J.

Nancy V. Runta, RN,C, BSN, CCRN
Medical Surgical Staff Development
Educator
North Penn Hospital
Lansdale, Pa.

We extend special thanks to the following, who contributed to the first edition:

Marjorie L. Beck, RN
Linda M. Carney, RN, CNOR, ONC
Paulette Dorney, RN, MSN, CCRN
Susan Ezzone, RN, MS, OCN
Jeanne Hess, RN, CNOR
Christine A. Quigel, RN
Michelle C. Quigel, RN,BSN, CETN
Eileen Suida, RN
Naomi Walpert, RN, MS, CDE
Elaine G. Warner, RN, MS, CCRN, CS

Foreword

Since the publication of the first edition of the *Handbook of Medical-Surgical Nursing* in 1994, medical-surgical nursing has undergone an exciting transformation. Advances in technology, nursing science, the scope of nursing practice, and patient care delivery systems have all contributed to this phenomenon. Consequently, medical-surgical nurses have more opportunities than ever before to use their special skills. Demand for medical-surgical nurses remains high in hospitals, inpatient units, and acute care units as patient acuity rises and length of stay decreases. In addition, more medical-surgical nurses are venturing into nontraditional settings such as home care, long-term care, subacute care, case management, outcomes care, alternative care, wellness education, consulting, and informatics. Our broad knowledge base and skills, combined with our focus on caring, make us particularly well-suited for an ever-evolving health care environment.

The second edition of the *Handbook of Medical-Surgical Nursing* is uniquely designed to accommodate these rapid advances and changes in this nursing practice. Because of its contemporary approach, the *Handbook* provides a firm foundation for nursing students and beginning medical-surgical nurses as well as a valuable reference source for advanced practice nurses and nurses continuing their education.

The organizational strengths of the first edition have been retained. Patient care disorders are arranged alphabetically for easy accessibility and all disorders are comprehensively addressed using an easy-to-follow format, which includes a brief introduction to the disorder, its *causes,* and *complications;* pertinent health history and physical *assessment* techniques; common *diagnostic tests* and *treatment* strategies; *key nursing diagnoses, patient outcomes,* and related *nursing interventions* including *monitoring* and *patient teaching.* Throughout, numerous logos (for example, *life-threatening complications, nursing alert, checklists),* charts, and illustrations highlight and summarize critical information. Finally, selected references and an index are included.

Several features have been added or updated in this second edition to keep pace with changes in medical-surgical nursing. **New topics** include two newly emerging disorders – *Ebola* virus and hantavirus syndrome – and new entries on cryptosporidiosis, thalassemia, granulocytopenia and lymphocytopenia, and necrotizing fasciitis. **Updated NANDA taxonomy** is used for each disorder to demonstrate the interrelationship of assessment data, nursing diagnoses, and nursing interventions. **New logos** have been added, specifically *nursing priority flow charts* (graphically appealing algorithms designed to guide you through the clinical decision-making process by evaluating assessment findings, formulating nursing diagnoses, performing interventions, and evaluating results); *expert geriatric care* (addressing physiologic and psychosocial considerations specifically for geriatric patients with certain disorders and treatments); and *health promotion pointers* (focused on helping patients prevent illness or live better with the consequences of illness).

Medical-surgical nursing practice in an evolving health care environment requires versatile nurses who are able to plan activities that promote health; use advanced assessment, clinical decision-making, and diagnostic skills; and direct and coordinate therapeutic interventions. This second edition of *Handbook of Medical-Surgical Nursing* illustrates the scope and responsibilities of today's medical-surgical nurse in a readable and informative format. By including the latest information and building on the strengths of the first edition, this handbook enables us to deliver the best possible care to our medical-surgical patients.

Joyce K. Keithley, RN, DNSc, FAAN
Practitioner-Teacher and Professor
Department of Medical-Surgical Nursing
Rush University College of Nursing
Chicago

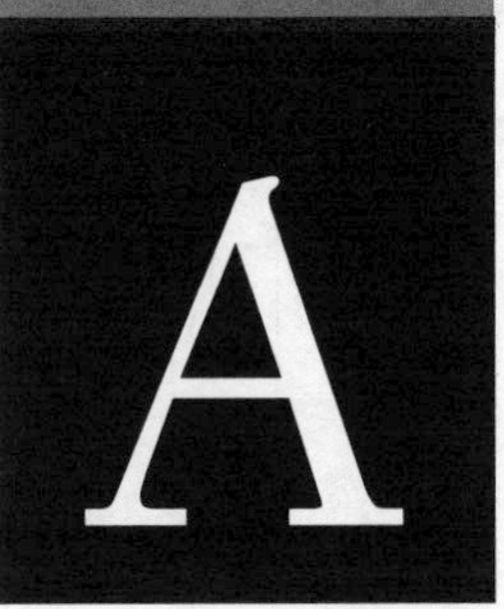

Abdominal aneurysm

An abnormal dilation in the arterial wall, an abdominal aneurysm typically occurs in the aorta between the renal arteries and the iliac branches. These aneurysms can be fusiform (spindle shaped) or saccular (pouchlike), and they develop slowly.

First, a focal weakness in the muscular layer of the aorta (tunica media), caused by degenerative changes, allows the inner layer (tunica intima) and outer layer (tunica adventitia) to stretch outward. Blood pressure within the aorta progressively weakens the vessel walls and enlarges the aneurysm.

Abdominal aneurysms occur most commonly in hypertensive white men ages 50 to 80.

Causes

About 95% of abdominal aortic aneurysms result from arteriosclerosis or atherosclerosis; the rest, from cystic medial necrosis, trauma, syphilis, and other infections.

Complications

More than 50% of all patients with untreated abdominal aneurysms die of hemorrhage and shock from aneurysmal rupture within 2 years of diagnosis. More than 85% die within 5 years.

Assessment

Most patients with abdominal aneurysms are asymptomatic until the aneurysm enlarges and compresses surrounding tissue. A large aneurysm may produce signs and symptoms that mimic renal calculi, lumbar disk disease, and duodenal compression.

The patient may complain of gnawing, generalized, steady abdominal pain, or low back pain that's unaffected by movement. He may have a sensation of gastric or abdominal fullness caused by pressure on the GI structures.

Sudden onset of severe abdominal pain or lumbar pain that radiates to the flank and groin from pressure on lumbar nerves may signify enlargement and imminent rupture. If the aneurysm ruptures into the peritoneal cavity, severe and persistent abdominal and back pain, mimicking renal or ureteral colic, occurs. If it ruptures into the duodenum, GI bleeding occurs with massive hematemesis and melena.

Inspection of the patient with an intact abdominal aneurysm usually reveals no significant findings. However, if the person is not obese, you may note a pulsating mass in the periumbilical area. Auscultation of the abdomen may reveal a systolic bruit over the aorta caused by turbulent blood flow in the widened arterial segment. Hypotension occurs with aneurysm rupture.

Palpation of the abdomen may disclose some tenderness over the affected area. A pulsatile mass may be felt; however, avoid

EXPERT GERIATRIC CARE

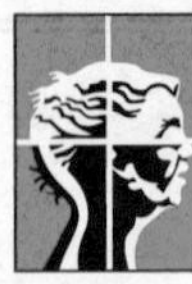

Aneurysms and the elderly

Because of the normal age-related changes in the elderly patient's vasculature, all patients over age 65 should be assessed for aneurysms. Most abdominal aneurysms occur between ages 60 and 90. Rupture is more common if the patient also has hypertension or if the aneurysm is larger than 6 cm.

deep palpation to locate the mass because this may cause the aneurysm to rupture. (See *Aneurysms and the elderly.*)

Diagnostic tests

Because an abdominal aneurysm seldom produces symptoms, it's typically detected inadvertently on a routine X-ray or during a physical examination. Several tests can confirm suspected abdominal aneurysm.

- *Abdominal ultrasonography* or *echocardiography* can determine the size, shape, and location of the aneurysm.
- *Anteroposterior* and *lateral X-rays* of the abdomen can detect aortic calcification.
- *Computed tomography scan* can note the aneurysm's effect on nearby organs.

Treatment

Usually, abdominal aneurysm requires resection of the aneurysm and Dacron graft replacement of the aortic section. If the aneurysm is small and produces no symptoms, surgery may be delayed, with regular physical examination and ultrasonography performed to monitor its progression. Large or symptomatic aneurysms risk rupture and need immediate repair.

In acute dissection, emergency treatment before surgery includes resuscitation with fluid and blood replacement, I.V. propranolol to reduce myocardial contractility, I.V. nitroprusside to reduce and maintain blood pressure to 100 to 120 mm Hg systolic, and analgesics to relieve pain. An arterial line and indwelling urinary catheter will monitor the patient's condition.

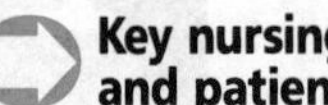

Key nursing diagnoses and patient outcomes

Anxiety related to possible aneurysm rupture. Based on this nursing diagnosis, you'll establish these patient outcomes. The patient will:

- state feelings of anxiety
- use support systems and perform stress-reduction techniques to assist with coping
- show abated physical signs of anxiety.

Risk for injury related to possible aneurysm rupture. Based on this nursing diagnosis, you'll establish these patient outcomes. The patient will:

- avoid activities that increase risk of rupture
- identify the signs of aneurysm rupture and what emergency measures to take
- understand the prescribed medical regimen and importance of follow-up care.

Fluid volume deficit related to hemorrhage caused by aneurysm rupture. Based on this nursing diagnosis, you'll establish these patient outcomes. The patient will:

- have his changed condition identified quickly and treated promptly
- regain and maintain a normal fluid and blood volume, evidenced by stable vital signs.

Nursing interventions

- Allow the patient to express his fears and concerns about the diagnosis.
- Offer the patient and his family psychological support.
- If the patient's condition is or becomes acute, expect him to be admitted to the intensive care unit (ICU).
- Administer ordered medications to control aneurysm progression. Provide analgesics to relieve pain, if present.
- Prepare the patient for elective surgery, as indicated, or emergency surgery, if rup-

ture occurs. In an emergency, a pneumatic antishock garment may be used while transporting him to surgery.

Monitoring

- Assess the patient's vital signs, especially blood pressure, every 4 hours or more frequently, depending on the severity of his condition.
- Evaluate kidney function by obtaining blood samples for blood urea nitrogen, creatinine, and electrolyte levels. Measure his intake and output.
- Monitor complete blood count for evidence of blood loss, reflected in decreased hemoglobin, hematocrit, and red blood cell count.
- If the patient's condition is acute, obtain an arterial sample for arterial blood gas analysis, as ordered, and monitor cardiac rhythm. Insert an arterial line to allow for continuous blood pressure monitoring. Assist with insertion of a pulmonary artery line to assess hemodynamic balance.
- Observe the patient for signs of rupture, which may be immediately fatal. Watch closely for any signs of acute blood loss: decreasing blood pressure; increasing pulse and respiratory rates; cool, clammy skin; restlessness; and decreased sensorium.

Patient teaching

- Provide psychological support for the patient and his family. If he is being admitted to the ICU, help ease their fears about this type of care, the threat of impending rupture, and any planned surgery. Take time to provide appropriate explanations and answer all questions.
- Explain the surgical procedure and the expected postoperative care in the ICU for patients undergoing complex abdominal surgery (I.V. lines, endotracheal and nasogastric intubation, mechanical ventilation).
- Instruct the patient to take all medications as prescribed and to carry a list of them at all times, in case of an emergency.
- Tell the patient not to push, pull, or lift heavy objects until the doctor allows.

Acquired immunodeficiency syndrome

Incurable and progressive, acquired immunodeficiency syndrome (AIDS) is marked by gradual destruction of CD4 + T cells by the human immunodeficiency virus (HIV). The resulting immunodeficiency predisposes the patient to opportunistic infections, unusual cancers, and other distinctive abnormalities.

Virtually any cell that has the CD4 + molecule on its surface may be infected by HIV. These include monocytes, macrophages, bone marrow progenitors, and glial, gut, and epithelial cells. Such infections can cause dementia, wasting syndrome, and hematologic abnormalities.

AIDS was first described by the Centers for Disease Control and Prevention (CDC) in 1981. Since then, the CDC has issued a case surveillance definition for AIDS and has modified it several times, most recently in 1993. (See *Classifying HIV infection and AIDS,* pages 4 and 5.)

In the United States, AIDS occurs most commonly in homosexual and bisexual men, I.V. drug users, neonates of HIV-infected women, recipients of contaminated blood or blood products (although the risk of receiving contaminated blood has been drastically reduced since 1985), and heterosexual partners of those in high-risk groups. Because of similar routes of transmission, AIDS shares epidemiologic patterns with other sexually transmitted diseases and hepatitis B.

Although the prevalence of HIV infection is unknown, it is estimated that more than 1 million people in the United States alone have the infection; more than 242,146 Americans had developed AIDS as of September 1992. The average duration between HIV exposure and diagnosis is 8 to 10 years, although the incubation period can vary.

Classifying HIV infection and AIDS

In 1993, the CDC revised its classification system for HIV infection and expanded its surveillance case definition for AIDS. The new classification groups HIV-infected patients according to three ranges of CD4+ T-cell counts and three clinical categories, which includes three new AIDS-indicator conditions. The following chart shows the nine mutually exclusive subgroups.

CD4+ T-cell categories	**Clinical categories**		
	A **Asymptomatic, acute (primary) HIV, or PGL**	**B** **Symptomatic, but not A or C conditions**	**C** **AIDS-indicator conditions**
≥500/μL	A1	B1	C1
200 to 499/μL	A2	B2	C2
<200/μL AIDS-indicator cell count	A3	B3	C3

CD4+ T-cell categories

These CD4+ T-cell ranges are considered positive markers for HIV infection:

- *Category 1:* 500 or more cells/μL of blood
- *Category 2:* 200 to 499 cells/μL of blood
- *Category 3:* less than 200 cells/μL of blood

Disease categories

The CDC defines three related disease categories as follows:

- *Category A:* Patients without symptoms, with persistent generalized lymphadenopathy (PGL), or with acute primary HIV infection. Conditions in categories B and C must not have occurred.

The course of AIDS can vary, but the syndrome usually results in death from opportunistic infections. Antiretroviral therapy—with zidovudine, for instance—and prophylaxis and treatment for common opportunistic infections can delay but not stop the progression. Most experts believe that virtually everyone infected with HIV will develop AIDS.

Causes

AIDS results from a human retrovirus that's classified as either HIV-1 or HIV-2. The most common cause of AIDS throughout the world is HIV-1. Less common, HIV-2 has been predominantly identified in western Africa and is thought to be less pathogenic than HIV-1. Both HIV-1 and HIV-2 destroy CD4+ T cells, the essential regulators and effectors of the normal immune response. HIV is transmitted by contact with infected blood or body fluids. Transmission results from such high-risk behaviors as sharing a contaminated needle or having unprotected sexual contact, especially anal intercourse, which results in mucosal trauma. Transmission may also occur through transfusion of contaminated blood or blood products. What's more, the virus can pass from an infected mother to the fetus through cervical or blood contact at delivery or to an infant through breast milk. HIV isn't transmitted by everyday household or social contact.

- *Category B:* HIV-infected patients with symptoms or diseases not included in category C, such as bacillary angiomatosis, oropharyngeal or persistent vulvovaginal candidiasis, fever or diarrhea lasting over 1 month, idiopathic thrombocytopenic purpura, pelvic inflammatory disease (particularly if complicated by tubo-ovarian abscess), and peripheral neuropathy.
- *Category C:* HIV-infected patients with disorders defined by the CDC as AIDS-indicator conditions.

AIDS-indicator conditions

The CDC recognizes the following AIDS-indicator conditions:

- Candidiasis of the bronchi, trachea, or lungs
- Candidiasis of the esophagus
- Cervical cancer, invasive
- Coccidioidomycosis, disseminated or extrapulmonary
- Cryptococcosis, extrapulmonary
- Cryptosporidiosis, chronic intestinal (persisting over 1 month)
- Cytomegalovirus (CMV) disease affecting organs other than the liver, spleen, or lymph nodes
- CMV retinitis with vision loss
- Encephalopathy related to HIV
- Herpes simplex, involving chronic ulcers (persisting over 1 month) or herpetic bronchitis, pneumonitis, or esophagitis
- Histoplasmosis, disseminated or extrapulmonary
- Isosporiasis, chronic intestinal (persisting over 1 month)
- Kaposi's sarcoma
- Lymphoma, Burkitt's (or its equivalent)
- Lymphoma, immunoblastic (or its equivalent)
- Lymphoma of the brain, primary
- *Mycobacterium avium* complex or *M. kansasii,* disseminated or extrapulmonary
- *M. tuberculosis* at any site (pulmonary or extrapulmonary)
- *Mycobacterium,* any other species, disseminated or extrapulmonary
- *Pneumocystis carinii* pneumonia
- Pneumonia, recurrent
- Progressive multifocal leukoencephalopathy
- *Salmonella* septicemia, recurrent
- Toxoplasmosis of the brain
- Wasting syndrome caused by HIV.

Complications

Repeated opportunistic infections eventually overwhelm the body's compromised immune defenses. These infections invade every body system, including the lungs, bone marrow, and brain. Neuropathy (HIV encephalopathy) occurs in 40% to 60% of infected patients.

Assessment

After initial exposure, the infected person may have no recognizable signs or may experience a mononucleosis-like syndrome for 3 to 6 weeks and then remain asymptomatic for years. His history usually suggests exposure to HIV – most often through unprotected sexual relations with an infected partner or sharing of I.V. needles.

The patient's initial complaints include fever, rigors, arthralgia, myalgia, maculopapular rash, urticaria, abdominal cramps, and diarrhea. Symptoms of aseptic meningitis, such as severe headache and stiff neck, may also occur. As the syndrome progresses, the patient may experience neurologic symptoms of HIV encephalopathy, an opportunistic infection, or cancer.

Your assessment may disclose palpable lymph nodes in two or more extrainguinal sites, a sign of lymphadenopathy. You may also observe behavioral, cognitive, and motor changes associated with progressive dementia, which occurs in about 30% of patients.

In children, the incubation time averages 17 months. A child's signs and symptoms resemble those of an adult, except that he's more likely to have a history of bacterial infections, such as otitis media, pneumonias other than that caused by *Pneumocystis carinii,* sepsis, chronic salivary gland enlargement, and lymphoid interstitial pneumonia.

Diagnostic tests

The CDC defines AIDS as an illness characterized by laboratory evidence of HIV infection and severe immunosuppression coexisting with one or more indicator conditions.

Patients ages 13 or over with repeatedly reactive screening tests for the HIV-1 antibody (enzyme-linked immunosorbent assay) who also have the HIV-1 antibody identified by supplemental tests (Western blot, immunofluorescence assay) are considered to be infected. Other methods for the diagnosis of HIV-1 may include direct identification of the virus in host tissues by virus isolation, antigen detection, and detection of HIV genetic material (deoxyribonucleic acid or ribonucleic acid) by polymerase chain reaction.

A CD4 + T-cell count is used to measure the severity of immunosuppression in a HIV-positive patient. An absolute CD4 + T-cell count of less than 200 cells/μl indicates severe immunosuppression. If the absolute count is unavailable, the percentage of CD4 + cells in total T cells may also be used; a percentage of less than 14 indicates severe immunosuppression. Because it consistently correlates with HIV-related immune dysfunction and disease progression, the CD4 + T-cell count is important in determining appropriate medical management of patients with AIDS.

Other markers of immune status, such as serum neopterin, beta-2 microglobulin, HIV p24 antigen, soluble interleukin-2 receptors, immunoglobulin A, and delayed type hypersensitivity (DTH) skin-test reactions, may be useful in the evaluation of individual patients. However, these tests aren't as strong predictors of disease progression or as specific for HIV-related immunosuppression as CD4 + T-cell counts. DTH skin-test reactions are often used in conjunction with the Mantoux tuberculin skin test to evaluate HIV-infected patients for tuberculosis infection and anergy.

Because many opportunistic infections are reactivations of previous infections, patients also commonly receive testing for syphilis, hepatitis B, tuberculosis (as mentioned above), toxoplasmosis and, in some geographic areas, histoplasmosis.

Treatment

No cure has yet been found for AIDS. However, several antiretroviral treatments can slow the progression of HIV or temporarily inactivate the virus. Also, immunomodulatory drugs strengthen the immune system, and anti-infective and antineoplastic drugs combat opportunistic infections and associated cancers. Some anti-infectives also serve as prophylaxis against opportunistic infections. New protocols combine two or more of these drugs to produce the maximum benefit with the fewest adverse reactions. Combination therapy also helps inhibit the production of mutant HIV strains resistant to a particular drug.

Although many opportunistic infections respond to anti-infective drugs, they tend to recur after treatment. Because of this, the patient usually requires continued prophylaxis until the drug loses its effectiveness or can no longer be tolerated.

Zidovudine, the most commonly used antiretroviral, effectively slows the progress of HIV infection, decreasing the number of opportunistic infections, prolonging survival, and curbing the progress of associated dementia.

Because of the significant risk of toxicity, only symptomatic patients or patients with a CD4 + T-cell count of 200 cells/μl or less receive the higher-dose regimen.

Asymptomatic patients with a CD4+ T-cell count at or below 500 cells/μl can receive the lower-dose regimen to help prolong the asymptomatic phase.

Didanosine, another antiretroviral drug, treats advanced HIV infection in adult patients and in pediatric patients over age 6 months. It can be used in adult patients with advanced HIV infection who've already received prolonged treatment with zidovudine.

Supportive treatment helps maintain nutrition and relieve pain and other distressing symptoms.

Key nursing diagnoses and patient outcomes

Anticipatory grieving related to the incurable, progressive nature of AIDS. Based on this nursing diagnosis, you'll establish these patient outcomes. The patient will:

- identify and express feelings about potential losses
- accept feelings and behavior brought on by potential losses
- use appropriate coping mechanisms to deal with potential losses and contact support groups, as needed.

Risk for infection related to frequent opportunistic infections. Based on this nursing diagnosis, you'll establish these patient outcomes. The patient will:

- maintain a normal temperature and white blood cell count and differential; cultures won't exhibit pathogen growth
- remain free of signs of infection
- demonstrate appropriate personal and oral hygiene and take appropriate daily precautions to prevent infection.

Social isolation related to misunderstanding of AIDS transmission and social stigma. Based on this nursing diagnosis, you'll establish these patient outcomes. The patient will:

- express his feelings about lack of supportive relationships
- identify and contact available resources to establish supportive relationships
- participate in social activity, as his health permits.

Nursing interventions

- To help prevent AIDS transmission, follow standard precautions.
- Treat infections as ordered.
- Provide the patient with 0.9% sodium chloride or bicarbonate mouthwash for daily oral rinsing. Avoid glycerin swabs, which dry the mucous membranes.
- Record the patient's caloric intake. He may need total parenteral nutrition, although this treatment creates a potential route for infection.
- Ensure adequate fluids during episodes of diarrhea.
- Provide meticulous skin care, especially in the debilitated patient.
- Encourage the patient to maintain as much physical activity as he can tolerate.
- Recognize that a diagnosis of AIDS has a devastating impact on the patient, his socioeconomic status, and his family relationships. Help him cope with an altered body image and the emotional burden of serious illness and the threat of death.

Monitoring

- Monitor the patient for fever and signs of infection, such as skin breakdown, cough, sore throat, and diarrhea. Assess for swollen, tender lymph nodes, and check laboratory values regularly.
- If the patient develops Kaposi's sarcoma, monitor the progression of the lesions.
- Watch for opportunistic infections or signs of disease progression.

Patient teaching

- Teach the patient and his family, sexual partners, and friends about AIDS and its transmission. Tell him not to donate blood, blood products, organs, tissue, or sperm.
- Urge the patient to inform potential sexual partners and health care workers that he has HIV infection.
- If the patient uses I.V. drugs, caution him not to share needles.
- Inform the patient that high-risk sexual practices for AIDS transmission are those that exchange body fluids, such as inter-

HEALTH PROMOTION POINTERS

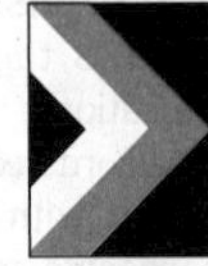

Using a condom

To help ensure that your patient who has HIV infection practices safe sex, make sure that he knows how to use a condom.

- Teach the patient how to apply it over his erect penis.
- Make sure the patient understands that he should apply the condom before entering his partner.
- Suggest using additional water-based lubricants, such as K-Y jelly (and not petroleum jelly), if necessary.
- Advise the patient to firmly hold the edges of the condom as he withdraws from his partner to reduce the risk of spillage.
- Teach him how to remove the condom by pinching the tip with one hand and unrolling it off with the other hand.
- Warn the patient not to store a condom for more than 1 year or to keep it in a wallet or near heat; these actions may cause the condom to break or develop holes when used.

course without a condom. (See *Using a condom.*) Discuss safe sexual practices, such as hugging, mutual masturbation, and protected sexual intercourse.

- Advise the female patient of childbearing age to avoid pregnancy. Explain that an infant may become infected before birth, during delivery, or during breast-feeding.
- Teach the patient to identify the signs of infection, and stress the importance of seeking immediate medical attention.
- Involve the patient with hospice care early in treatment so he can establish a relationship. If he develops AIDS dementia in stages, help him understand the progression of this symptom.

Acute respiratory failure

When the lungs can't adequately maintain arterial oxygenation or eliminate carbon dioxide (CO_2), acute respiratory failure results. Unchecked and untreated, the condition leads to tissue hypoxia. In patients with essentially normal lung tissue, acute respiratory failure usually produces a partial pressure of carbon dioxide in arterial blood ($Paco_2$) above 50 mm Hg and a partial pressure of oxygen in arterial blood (Pao_2) below 50 mm Hg.

These limits, however, don't apply to patients with chronic obstructive pulmonary disease (COPD). These patients consistently have a high $Paco_2$ (hypercapnia) and a low Pao_2 (hypoxemia) level. So for them, only acute deterioration in arterial blood gas (ABG) values – and corresponding clinical deterioration – signals acute respiratory failure.

Causes

Acute respiratory failure may develop from any condition that increases the work of breathing and decreases the respiratory drive. These conditions may result from respiratory tract infection (such as bronchitis or pneumonia), bronchospasm, or accumulated secretions secondary to cough suppression. Other common causes are related to ventilatory failure, in which the brain fails to direct respiration, and gas exchange failure, in which respiratory structures fail to function properly.

Complications

Tissue hypoxia, metabolic acidosis, and respiratory and cardiac arrest are among possible complications.

Assessment

Because acute respiratory failure is life-threatening, you probably won't have time to conduct an in-depth patient interview. Instead, you'll rely on family members or the patient's medical records to discover the precipitating incident.

On inspection, you'll note cyanosis of the oral mucosa, lips, and nail beds; nasal flaring; and ashen skin. You may observe the patient yawning and using accessory muscles to breathe. He may appear restless, anxious, depressed, lethargic, agitated, or confused. Additionally, he usually exhibits tachypnea, which signals impending respiratory failure.

Palpation may reveal cold, clammy skin and asymmetrical chest movement, which suggests pneumothorax. If tactile fremitus is present, you'll notice that it decreases over an obstructed bronchi or pleural effusion but increases over consolidated lung tissue.

Percussion – especially in patients with COPD – reveals hyperresonance. If acute respiratory failure results from atelectasis or pneumonia, percussion usually produces a dull or flat sound.

Auscultation typically discloses diminished breath sounds. In patients with pneumothorax, breath sounds may be absent. In other cases of respiratory failure, you may hear such adventitious breath sounds as wheezes (in asthma) and rhonchi (in bronchitis). If you hear crackles, suspect pulmonary edema as the cause of respiratory failure.

Diagnostic tests

- *ABG analysis* is the key to diagnosis (and subsequent treatment) of acute respiratory failure. Progressively deteriorating ABG values and pH – compared with the patient's "normal" values – strongly suggest acute respiratory failure. In patients with essentially normal lung tissue, a pH below 7.35 usually indicates acute respiratory failure. In patients with COPD, the pH deviation from the normal value is even lower.
- *Chest X-rays* identify underlying pulmonary diseases or conditions, such as emphysema, atelectasis, lesions, pneumothorax, infiltrates, and effusions.
- *Electrocardiography (ECG)* can demonstrate arrhythmias. Common ECG patterns point to cor pulmonale and myocardial hypoxia.
- *Pulse oximetry* reveals decreasing arterial oxygen saturation.
- *Blood tests,* such as an elevated white blood cell count, can indicate infection. Abnormally low hematocrit and hemoglobin levels signal blood loss, which indicates decreased oxygen-carrying capacity.
- *Serum electrolyte findings* vary. Hypokalemia may result from compensatory hyperventilation, the body's attempt to correct alkalosis; hypochloremia usually occurs in metabolic alkalosis.
- *Pulmonary artery catheterization* helps to distinguish pulmonary and cardiovascular causes of acute respiratory failure and monitors hemodynamic pressures.

Additional tests, such as a blood culture, Gram stain, and sputum culture, may identify the pathogen.

Treatment

Acute respiratory failure constitutes an emergency. The patient will need cautious oxygen therapy (nasal prongs, a nonrebreather mask, or a Venturi mask) to raise his PaO_2. If significant respiratory acidosis persists, mechanical ventilation with an endotracheal or a tracheostomy tube may be necessary. High-frequency ventilation may be initiated if the patient doesn't respond to conventional mechanical ventilation. Treatment routinely includes antibiotics (for infection), bronchodilators and, possibly, corticosteroids.

If the patient also has cor pulmonale and decreased cardiac output, fluid restriction and administration of positive inotropic agents, vasopressors, and diuretics may be ordered.

Key nursing diagnoses and patient outcomes

Impaired gas exchange related to altered oxygen supply caused by the underlying pulmonary condition. Based on this nursing diagnosis, you'll establish these patient outcomes. The patient will:

- exhibit Pa_{O_2} and breath sounds that return to baseline
- not experience dyspnea
- use correct bronchial hygiene to keep airways clear, which enhances oxygenation.

Ineffective airway clearance related to decreased energy, fatigue, or presence of tracheobronchial secretions. Based on this nursing diagnosis, you'll establish these patient outcomes. The patient will:

- cough and deep-breathe adequately to expectorate secretions
- demonstrate skill in conserving energy while attempting to clear airway
- maintain a patent airway.

Ineffective breathing pattern related to decreased energy or fatigue caused by underlying pulmonary condition or metabolic acidosis. Based on this nursing diagnosis, you'll establish these patient outcomes. The patient will:

- achieve maximum lung expansion with adequate ventilation
- demonstrate skill in conserving energy while carrying out activities of daily living
- exhibit a respiratory rate and pattern and ABG values that return to baseline and remain within this normal range.

Nursing interventions

- Orient the patient to the treatment unit. Most patients with acute respiratory failure receive intensive care. Acquainting the patient with procedures, sounds, and sights helps to minimize his anxiety.
- To reverse hypoxemia, administer oxygen at appropriate concentrations to maintain Pa_{O_2} at a minimum pressure range of 50 to 60 mm Hg. The patient with COPD usually requires only small amounts of supplemental oxygen.
- Maintain a patent airway. If your patient retains CO_2, encourage him to cough and breathe deeply with pursed lips. If he's alert, have him use an incentive spirometer. If he's intubated and lethargic, reposition him every 1 to 2 hours. Use postural drainage and chest physiotherapy to help clear secretions.
- Perform oral hygiene measures frequently.
- Apply soft wrist restraints for the confused patient, as ordered. This will prevent him from disconnecting the oxygen setup. However, remember that these restraints can increase anxiety, fear, and agitation. Check restraints and release every 1 to 2 hours.
- Position the patient for comfort and optimal gas exchange. Place the call button within the patient's reach.
- Maintain the patient in a normothermic state to reduce his body's demand for oxygen.
- Pace patient care activities to maximize the patient's energy level and provide needed rest.

If the patient requires *mechanical ventilation:*

- Check ventilator settings, cuff pressures, oximetry, and capnometry values often and ABG values as clinically indicated to ensure correct fraction of inspired oxygen (FI_{O_2}) settings.
- Suction the trachea as needed after hyperoxygenation. Provide humidification to liquefy secretions.
- Prevent infection by using sterile technique while suctioning and by changing ventilator tubing every 24 hours.
- Prevent tracheal erosion that can result from an overinflated artificial airway cuff compressing the tracheal wall's vasculature. Use the minimal-leak technique and a cuffed tube with high residual volume (low-pressure cuff), a foam cuff, or a pressure-regulating valve on the cuff. Measure cuff pressure every 8 hours.
- Implement measures to prevent nasal tissue necrosis. Position and maintain the nasotracheal tube midline within the nostrils, and provide meticulous care. Periodically, loosen the tape securing the tube to prevent skin breakdown. Avoid excessive movement of any tubes, and make sure

that the ventilator tubing has adequate support.
• Help the patient communicate without words. Offer him a pen and tablet, a word chart, or an alphabet board.

Monitoring

• Monitor the patient for a positive response to oxygen therapy, such as improved breathing, color, and oximetry and ABG values.
• Observe the patient closely for respiratory arrest. Auscultate chest sounds. Report any changes in ABG values immediately. Notify the doctor of any deterioration in oxygen saturation levels as detected by pulse oximetry. (See *Identifying respiratory failure.*)
• Watch for treatment complications, especially oxygen toxicity and adult respiratory distress syndrome.
• Frequently assess vital signs. Note and report an increasing pulse rate, rising or falling respiratory rate, declining blood pressure, or febrile state.
• Follow serum electrolyte levels carefully and take steps to correct imbalances. Monitor fluid balance by recording the patient's intake and output and daily weight.
• Check the cardiac monitor for arrhythmias.

If the patient requires *mechanical ventilation:*
• Monitor changes in oximetry or capnometry values after each change in the FIO_2 setting. Perform ABG analysis as clinically indicated.
• When suctioning the patient, check for any changes in sputum quality, consistency, odor, or color.
• Watch for complications of mechanical ventilation, such as reduced cardiac output, pneumothorax or other barotrauma, increased pulmonary vascular resistance, diminished urine output, increased intracranial pressure, and GI bleeding.
• Routinely assess endotracheal (ET) tube position and patency. Make sure the tube is placed properly and taped securely. Immediately after intubation, auscultate the lung fields to check for accidental intubation of the esophagus or the mainstem bronchus, which may have occurred during ET tube insertion. Also be alert for transtracheal or laryngeal perforation, aspiration, broken teeth, nosebleeds, vagal reflexes such as bradycardia, arrhythmias, and hypertension.
• After tube placement, watch for complications, such as tube displacement, herniation of the tube's cuff, respiratory infection, and tracheal malacia and stenosis.
• Monitor for signs of stress ulcers, which are common in intubated patients, especially those in the intensive care unit. Inspect gastric secretions for blood, especially if the patient has a nasogastric tube or reports epigastric tenderness, nausea, or vomiting. Also monitor hemoglobin and hematocrit levels, and check all stools for blood.

CHECKLIST

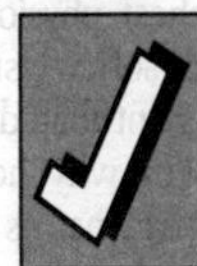

Identifying respiratory failure

Use the following measurements to identify respiratory failure:

- ☐ vital capacity less than 15 cc/kg
- ☐ tidal volume less than 3 cc/kg
- ☐ negative inspiratory force under -25 cm H_2O
- ☐ respiratory rate more than twice the normal rate
- ☐ diminished PaO_2 despite increased FIO_2
- ☐ elevated $PaCO_2$ with pH lower than 7.25.

Patient teaching

• Describe all tests and procedures to the patient and his family. Discuss the reasons

for suctioning, chest physiotherapy, blood tests and, if used, soft wrist restraints.
• If the patient is intubated or has a tracheostomy, explain why he can't speak. Suggest alternative means of communication.
• Identify reportable signs of respiratory infection.
• If applicable, teach the patient about the effects of smoking. Provide resources to help him stop smoking.

Acute tubular necrosis

The most common cause of acute renal failure in critically ill patients, acute tubular necrosis accounts for about 75% of all cases of acute renal failure. Also called acute tubulointerstitial nephritis, this disorder injures the tubular segment of the nephron, causing renal failure and uremic syndrome. Mortality can be as high as 70%, depending on complications from underlying diseases. Nonoliguric forms of acute tubular necrosis have a better prognosis.

Causes

Acute tubular necrosis results from ischemic or nephrotoxic injury, most commonly in debilitated patients. In ischemic injury, disrupted blood flow to the kidneys may result from circulatory collapse, severe hypotension, trauma, hemorrhage, dehydration, cardiogenic or septic shock, surgery, anesthetics, or transfusion reactions. Nephrotoxic injury may follow ingestion or inhalation of certain chemicals, such as aminoglycoside antibiotics and radiographic contrast agents, or may result from renal hypersensitivity.

Specifically, acute tubular necrosis can result from any of the following:
• diseased tubular epithelium that allows leakage of glomerular filtrate across the membranes and reabsorption of filtrate into the blood
• obstructed urine flow from the collection of damaged cells, casts, red blood cells (RBCs), and other cellular debris within the tubular walls
• ischemic injury to glomerular epithelial cells, resulting in cellular collapse and decreased glomerular capillary permeability
• ischemic injury to vascular endothelium, eventually resulting in cellular swelling, sludging, and tubular obstruction.

Complications

Nephrotoxic acute tubular necrosis doesn't damage the basement membrane of the nephron, so it's potentially reversible. However, ischemic acute tubular necrosis can damage the epithelial and basement membranes and can cause lesions in the renal interstitium. Infections (frequently septicemia) can complicate up to 70% of all cases and are the leading cause of death. GI hemorrhage, fluid and electrolyte imbalances, and cardiovascular dysfunction may occur during the acute phase or in the recovery phase. Neurologic complications occur commonly in elderly patients and occasionally in younger ones. Hypercalcemia may occur during the recovery phase.

Assessment

The patient's history may include an ischemic or a nephrotoxic injury that can cause acute tubular necrosis. The signs of acute tubular necrosis may be obscured by the patient's primary disease.

You may first note that the patient's urine output may be oliguric (less than 400 ml/24 hours); occasionally, in severe cases, urine output may be less than 100 ml/24 hours for several days.

Inspection may reveal evidence of bleeding abnormalities such as petechiae and ecchymoses. Hematemesis may occur. The skin may be dry and pruritic and, rarely, a uremic frost may be present. Mucous membranes may be dry, and the breath may have a uremic odor.

The patient may exhibit evidence of central nervous system involvement, such as lethargy, somnolence, confusion, disorientation, asterixis, agitation, myoclonic muscle twitching and, possibly, seizures.

Auscultation may reveal tachycardia and, possibly, an irregular rhythm. Rarely, a pericardial friction rub can be heard, indicating pericarditis. Bibasilar crackles may occur if congestive heart failure (CHF) is present. Palpation and percussion may reveal abdominal pain, if pancreatitis or peritonitis occurs, and peripheral edema, if CHF is present.

Fever and chills can signal the onset of infection.

Diagnostic tests

Diagnosis usually can't be made until the disorder becomes advanced. The most significant laboratory findings are urine sediment, containing RBCs and casts, and dilute urine with a low specific gravity (1.010), a high sodium level (40 to 60 mEq/liter), and a low osmolality (less than 400 mOsm/kg).

Blood studies reveal elevated blood urea nitrogen and serum creatinine levels, decreased serum protein levels, anemia, defects in platelet adherence, metabolic acidosis, and hyperkalemia.

Treatment

The disorder requires vigorous supportive measures during the acute phase until normal renal function resumes. Initial treatment may include administration of diuretics and infusion of a large volume of fluids to flush tubules of cellular casts and debris and to replace fluid loss. This treatment carries a risk of fluid overload. Long-term fluid management requires daily replacement of projected and calculated losses (including insensible loss).

Other appropriate measures to control complications include transfusion of packed RBCs for anemia and administration of antibiotics for infection. A patient with hyperkalemia may require emergency I.V. administration of 50% glucose, regular insulin, and sodium bicarbonate. Sodium polystyrene sulfonate may be given by mouth or by enema to reduce extracellular potassium levels. Peritoneal dialysis or hemodialysis may be needed for a catabolic patient.

Key nursing diagnoses and patient outcomes

Altered urinary elimination related to injury to the nephron's tubular segment. Based on this nursing diagnosis, you'll establish these patient outcomes. The patient will:

- demonstrate normal urine output
- not develop complications that can further damage the nephron, such as hypotension or infection
- have a normal urinalysis.

Fatigue related to anemia. Based on this nursing diagnosis, you'll establish these patient outcomes. The patient will:

- identify measures to prevent or relieve fatigue when performing daily activities
- plan rest periods throughout the day and obtain at least 8 hours sleep a night if possible
- exhibit normal hemoglobin levels and hematocrit.

Fluid volume excess related to compromised renal regulatory mechanisms. Based on this nursing diagnosis, you'll establish these patient outcomes. The patient will:

- maintain fluid intake and output within established limits
- not exhibit signs of fluid overload, such as elevated blood pressure, edema, crackles during lung auscultation, shortness of breath, and distended neck veins
- maintain a low-sodium diet and adhere to a fluid schedule.

Nursing interventions

- Administer fluids as needed to maintain fluid balance.
- Maintain electrolyte balance. Restrict foods that contain sodium and potassium,

such as bananas, prunes, orange juice, and baked potatoes. Check for potassium content in prescribed medications.
• Provide adequate calories and essential amino acids while restricting protein intake to maintain an anabolic state. Total parenteral nutrition (TPN) may be indicated for a severely debilitated or catabolic patient. If the patient is receiving TPN, keep his skin meticulously clean.
• Use aseptic technique, particularly when handling catheters, because the debilitated patient is vulnerable to infection. Immediately report fever, chills, delayed wound healing, or flank pain if the patient has an indwelling urinary catheter.
• If anemia worsens, transfuse blood as ordered. Use fresh packed cells instead of whole blood, especially in an elderly patient, to prevent fluid overload and CHF.
• If the patient develops acidosis, give sodium bicarbonate or, in severe cases, assist with dialysis.
• Perform passive range-of-motion exercises. Provide good skin care, and apply lotion or bath oil to prevent dry skin. Help the patient walk as soon as possible, but make sure he doesn't become exhausted.
• To prevent acute tubular necrosis, make sure every patient is well hydrated before surgery or after X-ray procedures that use a contrast medium. Administer mannitol, as ordered, to a high-risk patient before and during these procedures.
• Provide emotional support to the patient and his family. Encourage the patient to express his concerns about his inability to perform his expected role. Assure him that activity restrictions are temporary.

Monitoring

• Monitor the patient's vital signs, especially blood pressure, because hypotension diminishes renal perfusion and urine output.
• Check the patient frequently for fluid overload, a common complication of therapy. Accurately record intake and output, including wound drainage, nasogastric tube output, and peritoneal dialysis and hemodialysis balances. Weigh the patient at the same time every day. Also monitor him for other complications, such as anemia, acidosis, or hypercalcemia.
• Check the patient's hemoglobin, hematocrit, and electrolyte levels as ordered, and report imbalances.
• Carefully monitor a patient receiving a blood transfusion. Immediately discontinue the transfusion if early signs of transfusion reaction (fever, rash, and chills) occur.
• Watch for signs and symptoms of infection, such as fever, chills, malaise, or dysuria.

Patient teaching

• Teach the patient the signs of infection, and tell him to report them to the doctor immediately. Remind him to stay away from crowds and any infected person.
• Review the prescribed diet, including dietary restrictions, and stress the importance of adhering to it.
• Teach the patient how to cough and perform deep breathing to prevent pulmonary complications.
• Fully explain each procedure to the patient and his family as often as necessary, and help them set realistic goals.

Adenoviral infections

Adenoviruses cause acute, self-limiting, febrile infections, with inflammation of the respiratory or ocular mucous membranes or both. Thirty-five serotypes are known. These viruses produce five major infections, all of which occur in epidemics. They are common in all age-groups and may remain latent for years.

Adenoviruses affect almost everyone early in life, although maternal antibodies offer some protection during the first 6 months.

Reviewing major adenoviral infections

Infection	Age-group	Clinical features
Acute febrile respiratory illness	Children	Nonspecific coldlike signs, similar to those of other viral respiratory illnesses: fever, pharyngitis, tracheitis, bronchitis, pneumonitis
Acute respiratory disease	Adults (usually military recruits)	Malaise, fever, chills, headache, pharyngitis, hoarseness, and dry cough
Viral pneumonia	Children and adults	Sudden onset of high fever, rapid infection of upper and lower respiratory tracts, rash, diarrhea, intestinal intussusception
Acute pharyngoconjunctival fever	Children (particularly after swimming in pools or lakes)	Spiking fever lasting for several days, headache, pharyngitis, conjunctivitis, rhinitis, cervical adenitis
Acute follicular conjunctivitis	Adults	Unilateral tearing and mucoid discharge; later, milder symptoms in other eye
Epidemic keratoconjunctivitis	Adults	Unilateral or bilateral ocular redness and edema, periorbital swelling, local discomfort, superficial opacity of the cornea without ulceration

Causes
Transmission occurs by direct inoculation into the eye, by fecal-oral contamination (adenoviruses may persist in the GI tract for years after infection), or by inhalation of an infected droplet. The incubation period usually is less than 1 week. Although the acute illness lasts less than 5 days, it may be followed by prolonged asymptomatic reinfection.

Complications
Acute conjunctivitis, sinusitis, pharyngitis, and pneumonia can occur.

Assessment
Clinical features vary with the type of infection. (See *Reviewing major adenoviral infections.*)

Diagnostic tests
Definitive diagnosis requires isolation of the virus from respiratory or ocular secretions or from fecal smears. During epidemics, typical symptoms alone allow the doctor to make a diagnosis. Because adenoviral infections resolve quickly, serum antibody titers aren't useful for diagnosis. Blood tests show lymphocytosis in children. A chest X-ray may show pneumonitis when a respiratory disorder is present.

Treatment
No specific drugs are effective against adenoviruses, so treatment is mainly supportive. Ocular infections may require corticosteroids and direct supervision by an ophthalmologist. Infants with pneumonia should be hospitalized to monitor for and treat dangerous symptoms; adults with keratoconjunctivitis require hospitalization to treat symptoms that can cause

blindness. An experimental treatment, enteric-coated oral vaccines, has been used successfully in military recruits. Parenteral vaccines, which were used previously, aren't recommended because they caused a hybrid virus.

Key nursing diagnoses and patient outcomes

High risk for fluid volume deficit related to fever, diarrhea, or decreased oral intake. Based on this nursing diagnosis, you'll establish these patient outcomes. The patient will:
- maintain adequate fluid volume, as evidenced by stable vital signs
- identify signs of an adenoviral infection that can precipitate fluid volume deficit
- express an understanding of self-care measures to prevent fluid volume deficit.

Hyperthermia related to fever. Based on this nursing diagnosis, you'll establish these patient outcomes. The patient will:
- exhibit no fever
- express how to reduce his temperature.

Pain related to the effects of adenoviral infection. Based on this nursing diagnosis, you'll establish these patient outcomes. The patient will:
- state and carry out appropriate interventions for pain relief
- express a feeling of comfort and relief from pain.

Nursing interventions

- Provide respiratory care for the infant hospitalized with pneumonia.
- Plan care to provide rest periods.
- Ensure adequate fluids and nutrition.
- Give ordered drugs to relieve symptoms.

Monitoring

- Monitor the patient's vital signs, especially temperature.
- During the acute stage, monitor the patient's respiratory status and intake and output.
- Regularly assess the patient's eyes for redness, itching, and drainage.

Patient teaching

- Explain supportive measures, such as bed rest, adequate fluid intake, analgesics, and antipyretics.
- To help minimize the incidence of adenoviral infection, teach the patient proper hand-washing techniques to reduce fecal-oral transmission.
- Inform the patient that keratoconjunctivitis can be prevented by avoiding swimming pools during epidemics of keratoconjunctivitis and by adequately chlorinating swimming pools.

Adrenalectomy

The surgical resection or removal of one or both adrenal glands, adrenalectomy is the treatment of choice for adrenal hyperfunction and hyperaldosteronism. It's also used to treat benign and malignant adrenal tumors and as a secondary treatment of neoplasms elsewhere in the body that are dependent on adrenal hormonal secretions, such as cancers of the prostate and breast.

Because excessive levels of adrenal hormones can also stem from pituitary oversecretion of corticotropin, an adrenalectomy may be performed if primary treatment of the pituitary condition is unsuccessful in controlling the amount of corticotropin being secreted.

Procedure

After the patient is anesthetized, the surgeon will begin by using either an anterior (transperitoneal) or a posterior (lumbar) approach. The anterior approach gives the better view of both glands. In a unilateral adrenalectomy, the surgeon first identifies the gland, then dissects it free from the upper pole of the kidney. Wound closure follows. In a bilateral adrenalectomy, the surgeon identifies and dissects each gland separately, then closes the wound.

If the adrenalectomy is being performed because of a tumor, the surgeon will first explore the glands. If he finds a tumor, he either resects it or removes one or both glands, depending on the extent of involvement. To remove a pheochromocytoma, the surgeon carefully excises the affected adrenal gland and palpates the abdominal organs for other tumors.

Complications

Because the adrenal glands help maintain homeostasis and facilitate the body's stress response, adrenalectomy carries a high risk of postoperative complications, including life-threatening acute adrenal crisis. (See *Managing acute adrenal crisis,* pages 18 and 19.) Other complications include hemorrhage, poor wound healing, hypoglycemia, electrolyte disturbances, pancreatic injury, and hypotension (with removal of the gland) or hypertension (after manipulation of the gland, which may trigger a sudden release of catecholamines, especially if a pheochromocytoma is present).

Key nursing diagnoses and patient outcomes

Altered protection related to inability to produce adrenal hormones. Based on this nursing diagnosis, you'll establish these patient outcomes. The patient will:

- not experience hypotension, tachycardia, nausea and vomiting, restlessness, or other signs of acute adrenal crisis
- demonstrate protective measures, including compliance with adrenocorticoid replacement therapy, use of stress-reduction techniques, and early recognition and treatment of adrenal insufficiency.

Risk for infection related to suppressed inflammatory response caused by high adrenocorticoid levels preoperatively and use of adrenocorticoid replacement postoperatively. Based on this nursing diagnosis, you'll establish these patient outcomes. The patient will:

- maintain a normal temperature and white blood cell count and differential postoperatively
- have an incision that will appear clean, pink, and free of purulent drainage
- remain free of all other signs of infection.

Risk for injury related to dramatic fluctuations in blood pressure caused by sudden changes in adrenocorticoid or catecholamine levels or both. Based on this nursing diagnosis, you'll establish these patient outcomes. The patient will:

- maintain a normal blood pressure
- not experience the severe headaches, palpitations, or visual disturbances characteristic of hypertension or the light-headedness, pallor, or fainting characteristic of hypotension.

Nursing interventions

Expect to intervene as follows.

Before surgery

- Explain the procedure and its preparation to the patient and his family.
- If the patient has adrenal hyperfunction, provide support and a controlled environment to offset his emotional lability.
- As needed, obtain an order for a sedative to help him rest. Expect to administer medications to control his hypertension, edema, diabetes, cardiovascular symptoms, and increased risk of infection. Give glucocorticoids on the morning of surgery to prevent adrenal insufficiency during the operation.
- If the patient has hyperaldosteronism, draw a blood sample as ordered for laboratory evaluation. Expect to give oral or I.V. potassium supplements to correct low serum potassium levels. Monitor for muscle twitching and a positive Chvostek's sign (indications of tetany). Keep the patient on a low-sodium, high-potassium diet, as ordered, to help correct hypernatremia and hypokalemia. Give aldosterone antagonists for blood pressure control.
- If the patient has a pheochromocytoma, monitor his blood pressure carefully. Also watch closely for paroxysmal attacks of hypertension (sudden increase in blood pres-

(Text continues on page 20.)

LIFE-THREATENING COMPLICATIONS

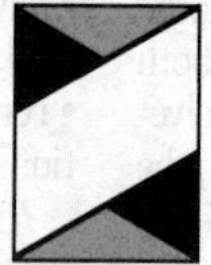

Managing acute adrenal crisis

After an adrenalectomy, especially a bilateral one, you'll need to be alert for signs and symptoms of acute adrenal crisis. Prompt emergency treatment is essential for this life-threatening complication, which results from a rapid decline in the level of adrenocorticoid hormones.

The patient is most prone to acute adrenal crisis during the first 24 to 48 hours after surgery, with the 9th to 12th hour postoperatively being the most common time of onset. If the patient has undergone bilateral adrenalectomy, he is at lifelong risk for this complication.

Warn the patient that the crisis may occur if he experiences marked stress without adjusting his glucocorticoid replacement therapy or if he abruptly stops his glucocorticoid therapy. If untreated, acute adrenal crisis can ultimately cause vascular collapse, renal shutdown, coma, and death.

Signs and symptoms

Watch for the following signs and symptoms: profound weakness, fatigue, nausea, vomiting, hypoglycemia, hypotension, dehydration and, occasionally, high fever followed by hypothermia.

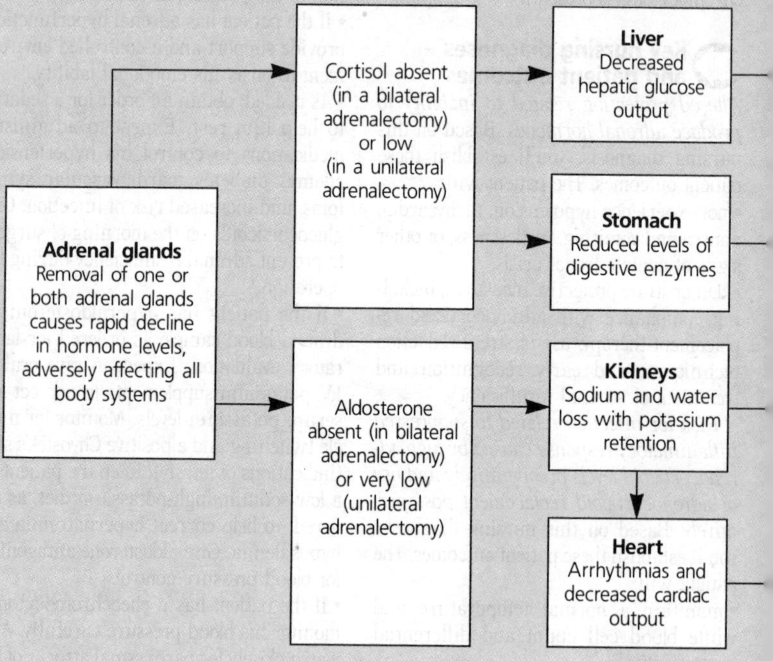

Adrenal glands
Removal of one or both adrenal glands causes rapid decline in hormone levels, adversely affecting all body systems

Cortisol absent (in a bilateral adrenalectomy) or low (in a unilateral adrenalectomy)

Aldosterone absent (in bilateral adrenalectomy) or very low (unilateral adrenalectomy)

Liver
Decreased hepatic glucose output

Stomach
Reduced levels of digestive enzymes

Kidneys
Sodium and water loss with potassium retention

Heart
Arrhythmias and decreased cardiac output

Emergency interventions

- Notify the doctor immediately.
- Expect to administer a bolus dose of hydrocortisone I.V., followed by subsequent doses every 6 to 8 hours until the patient's condition stabilizes; then taper the dose as ordered.
- Be prepared to administer fluids rapidly I.V. Vasopressors, in dosages titrated according to the patient's blood pressure, may be required.
- Closely monitor vital functions, such as vital signs, intake and output, electrocardiogram, blood glucose levels, and electrolytes.
- If fever persists despite hydrocortisone therapy, expect to administer an antipyretic agent and initiate cooling procedures.
- As ordered, insert a nasogastric tube to prevent aspiration if the patient is vomiting but not awake and alert.
- If hypoglycemia becomes profound or persists despite hydrocortisone therapy, expect to administer I.V. glucose.

The flowchart below summarizes what happens in adrenal crisis and pinpoints its warning signs and symptoms.

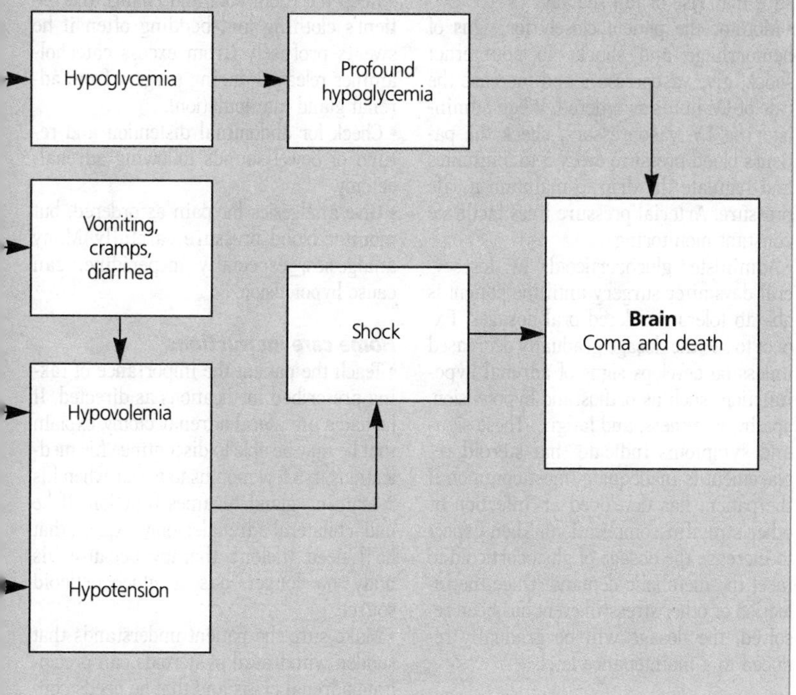

sure, severe headache, palpitations or tachycardia, diaphoresis, nausea, vomiting, and visual disturbances). If these occur, notify the doctor, keep the patient in bed with his head elevated 45 degrees, and monitor his vital signs closely.

• Before surgery for a pheochromocytoma, expect to administer long-acting agents to help control blood pressure. For 1 to 2 weeks before surgery, the doctor may prescribe catecholamine-synthesis blockers, such as metyrosine, and medications to control hypertension and tachycardia, such as phenoxybenzamine and propranolol. If so, check with the patient to make sure he has taken his medications correctly.

After surgery

• The first 24 to 48 hours after surgery are especially critical. Monitor urine output, and check vital signs closely—blood pressure may rise or fall sharply.

• Monitor the patient closely for signs of hemorrhage and shock. To counteract shock, give vasopressors and increase the rate of I.V. fluids as ordered. When administering I.V. vasopressors, check the patient's blood pressure every 3 to 5 minutes and regulate the drip to maintain a safe pressure. Arterial pressure lines facilitate constant monitoring.

• Administer glucocorticoids I.V. for several days after surgery until the patient is able to tolerate ordered oral dosages. Expect to see the dosage gradually decreased unless he develops signs of adrenal hypofunction, such as orthostatic hypotension, apathy, weakness, and fatigue. These signs and symptoms indicate that steroid replacement is inadequate (most common if the patient has developed an infection or other stressful complication). Then expect to increase the dosage of glucocorticoid to meet the metabolic demand. Once the infection or other stressful event has been resolved, the dosage will be gradually reduced to a maintenance level.

• Assess and document the presence or absence of signs of acute adrenal crisis every hour for the first 24 hours (most common 9 to 12 hours after surgery). Notify the doctor immediately if signs occur. Be prepared to administer additional doses of glucocorticoids I.V.

• Monitor the patient closely, and check laboratory reports for hypoglycemia because adrenalectomy removes the body's source of cortisol, which helps to regulate blood glucose levels. As ordered, also monitor the patient's sodium and potassium levels for alterations. Monitoring of serum potassium levels is especially important if the patient had primary aldosteronism before surgery or if he's receiving spironolactone, a potassium-sparing diuretic, for control of postoperative hypertension.

• Use aseptic technique when changing dressings to minimize the risk of infection.

• Keep the room cool and change the patient's clothing and bedding often if he sweats profusely (from excess catecholamines released during surgery from adrenal gland manipulation).

• Check for abdominal distention and return of bowel sounds following adrenalectomy.

• Give analgesics for pain as ordered, but monitor blood pressure carefully. Many analgesics, especially meperidine, can cause hypotension.

Home care instructions

• Teach the patient the importance of taking prescribed medications as directed. If he had a unilateral adrenalectomy, explain that he may be able to discontinue his medications in a few months to a year when his remaining gland resumes function. If he had a bilateral adrenalectomy, explain that he'll need lifelong therapy because his body no longer has a glucocorticoid source.

• Make sure the patient understands that sudden withdrawal of steroids can precipitate adrenal crisis and that he needs continued medical follow-up to adjust his steroid dosage appropriately during stress or illness.

- Teach the patient the signs of adrenal insufficiency, and make sure he understands how this can progress to adrenal crisis if not treated. Urge him to consult his doctor if he develops adverse reactions, such as weight gain, acne, headaches, fatigue, and increased urinary frequency (possible signs of overmedication). Advise him to take his steroids with meals or antacids to minimize gastric irritation.
- If the patient had adrenal hyperfunction, explain that he'll see a reversal of the physical characteristics of his disease within a few months. However, caution him that his improved physical appearance doesn't mean he can stop his medications.
- If the patient's incision isn't completely healed, provide wound care instructions. Advise him to keep the incision clean, to avoid wearing clothing that may irritate the incision, and to follow his doctor's instructions for applying ointments or dressings. Tell him to report signs of infection.
- Teach the patient how to reduce stress, if appropriate.
- Advise wearing a medical identification bracelet to help ensure adequate care in an emergency.

Adrenal hypofunction

Also called adrenal insufficiency, this disorder has primary and secondary forms. Primary adrenal hypofunction (Addison's disease) originates within the adrenal gland itself and is characterized by decreased mineralocorticoid, glucocorticoid, and androgen secretion. A relatively uncommon disorder, Addison's disease occurs in people of all ages and both sexes.

Adrenal hypofunction can also occur secondary to a disorder outside the gland (such as pituitary tumor with corticotropin deficiency), but aldosterone secretion may continue intact. With early diagnosis and adequate replacement therapy, the prognosis for both primary and secondary adrenal hypofunction is good.

Causes

Addison's disease occurs when more than 90% of the adrenal gland is destroyed. Such massive destruction usually results from an autoimmune process in which circulating antibodies react specifically against the adrenal tissue.

Other causes include tuberculosis, bilateral adrenalectomy, hemorrhage into the adrenal gland, metastatic tumors such as lung and breast carcinoma, infections such as histoplasmosis, human immunodeficiency virus, cytomegalovirus and, rarely, a familial tendency toward autoimmune disease.

Secondary adrenal hypofunction that results in glucocorticoid deficiency can stem from hypopituitarism (causing decreased corticotropin secretion), from abrupt withdrawal of long-term corticosteroid therapy (long-term exogenous corticosteroid stimulation suppresses pituitary corticotropin secretion and causes adrenal gland atrophy), or from removal of a nonendocrine, corticotropin-secreting tumor.

Adrenal crisis occurs in a patient with adrenal hypofunction when trauma, surgery, or other physiologic stress exhausts his body's stores of glucocorticoids.

Complications

Adrenal crisis, a critical deficiency of mineralocorticoids and glucocorticoids, is the most serious complication. It requires immediate, vigorous treatment.

Assessment

Assessment of patient history for adrenal hypofunction may reveal synthetic steroid use, adrenal surgery, or recent infection. The patient may complain of muscle weakness, fatigue, light-headedness when rising from a chair or bed, weight loss, cravings for salty food, decreased tolerance for even minor stress, and various GI disturbances, such as nausea, vomiting, anorexia, and chronic diarrhea. He may also complain of anxiety, irritability, and confusion. Reduced urine output and other symptoms of dehydration may occur. Women may have decreased libido due to reduced androgen production, and amenorrhea.

Inspection may detect poor coordination, dry skin and mucous membranes related to dehydration, and decreased axillary and pubic hair in women. The patient with Addison's disease typically has a conspicuous bronze coloration of the skin that resembles a deep suntan, especially in the creases of the hands and over the metacarpophalangeal joints, elbows, and knees. He may also exhibit a darkening of scars, areas of vitiligo (absence of pigmentation), and increased pigmentation of the mucous membranes, especially the buccal mucosa.

This abnormal coloration results from decreased secretion of cortisol (one of the glucocorticoids), which causes the pituitary gland to simultaneously secrete excessive amounts of melanocyte-stimulating hormone (MSH) and corticotropin. Secondary adrenal hypofunction doesn't cause hyperpigmentation because corticotropin and MSH levels are low.

Palpation may disclose a weak, irregular pulse, and auscultation of blood pressure reveals hypotension.

Diagnostic tests

Diagnosis requires demonstration of decreased corticosteroid concentrations in plasma or urine and an accurate classification of adrenal hypofunction as primary or secondary. After baseline plasma and urine steroid testing, these tests follow:

- *Metyrapone test* can confirm secondary adrenal hypofunction. It requires oral or I.V. administration of metyrapone, which blocks cortisol production and should stimulate the release of corticotropin from the hypothalamic-pituitary system. In Addison's disease, the hypothalamic-pituitary system responds normally and plasma reveals high levels of corticotropin; however, plasma levels of cortisol precursor and urine concentrations of 17-hydroxycorticosteroid don't rise.
- *Corticotropin stimulation test* is done if either primary or secondary adrenal hypofunction is suspected. This involves I.V. administration of corticotropin over 6 to 8 hours after samples have been obtained to determine baseline plasma cortisol and 24-hour urine cortisol levels. In Addison's disease, plasma and urine cortisol levels fail to rise normally in response to corticotropin; in secondary disease, repeated doses of corticotropin over successive days produce a gradual increase in cortisol levels until normal values are reached.
- *Rapid corticotropin test* demonstrates plasma cortisol response to corticotropin. After obtaining plasma cortisol samples, an I.M. injection of cosyntropin is given. Plasma samples are taken 45 minutes after administration. If plasma cortisol doesn't rise, adrenal insufficiency is suspected.

In a patient with typical symptoms of Addison's disease, the following laboratory findings strongly suggest acute adrenal insufficiency:

- decreased cortisol levels in plasma (under 10 mcg/dl in the morning, with lower levels in the evening); because this test is time-consuming, crisis therapy shouldn't be delayed for results
- reduced serum sodium and fasting blood glucose levels
- increased serum potassium, serum calcium, and blood urea nitrogen levels
- elevated hematocrit and elevated lymphocyte and eosinophil counts.

In addition, X-rays may show a small heart and adrenal calcification.

Treatment

Lifelong corticosteroid replacement is the main treatment for all patients with primary or secondary adrenal hypofunction. In general, cortisone or hydrocortisone (which have a mineralocorticoid effect) are given. Patients with Addison's disease may also need fludrocortisone to prevent dangerous dehydration and hypotension. Women with Addison's disease who have muscle weakness and decreased libido may benefit from testosterone injections but risk unfortunate masculinizing effects.

Treatment for adrenal crisis is prompt I.V. bolus administration of 100 mg of hydrocortisone, followed by hydrocortisone diluted with dextrose in 0.9% sodium chloride solution or dextrose 5% in saline solution and given I.V. until the patient's condition stabilizes. Up to 300 mg/day of hydrocortisone and 3 to 5 liters of I.V. 0.9% sodium chloride solution may be required during the acute stage. With proper treatment, the crisis usually subsides quickly, with blood pressure stabilizing and water and sodium levels returning to normal. After the crisis, maintenance doses of hydrocortisone preserve physiologic stability.

Key nursing diagnoses and patient outcomes

Altered protection related to decreased ability to produce and release adrenocorticoid hormones as needed. Based on this nursing diagnosis, you'll establish these patient outcomes. The patient will:
- not experience hypotension, tachycardia, nausea and vomiting, restlessness, or other signs of adrenal crisis
- demonstrate protective measures, including compliance with adrenocorticoid replacement therapy, use of stress-reduction techniques, and early recognition and treatment of adrenal insufficiency.

Risk for infection related to suppressed inflammatory response caused by steroid therapy. Based on this nursing diagnosis, you'll establish these patient outcomes. The patient will:
- maintain a normal temperature and white blood cell count and differential
- remain free of infection
- take precautions to avoid or decrease the risk of infection.

Knowledge deficit related to inadequate understanding of adrenal hypofunction and steroid therapy. Based on this nursing diagnosis, you'll establish these patient outcomes. The patient will:
- express a need to know about adrenal hypofunction and steroid therapy
- express an understanding of what he has learned about adrenal hypofunction and steroid therapy
- state his intentions to seek help from health professionals, when needed, and adhere to the prescribed medical treatment.

Nursing interventions

- Administer a corticosteroid as ordered. Until the onset of the mineralocorticoid effect, force fluids to replace excessive fluid loss.
- Control the patient's environment to prevent stress. Encourage him to use relaxation techniques. Plan periods of rest during the day, and gradually increase activities, depending on the patient's tolerance.
- Encourage the patient to dress in layers to retain body heat, and adjust room temperature if possible.
- Provide good skin care. Use alcohol-free skin care products and an emollient lotion after bathing. Turn and reposition the bedridden patient every 2 hours. Avoid pressure over bony prominences.
- Use protective measures to minimize the risk of infection. Provide the patient with a private room and reverse isolation if necessary. Limit visitors, especially those with infectious conditions. Use meticulous hand-washing technique.
- Consult a dietitian to plan a diet that maintains sodium and potassium balances and provides adequate proteins and carbohydrates. If the patient is anorexic, suggest six small meals a day to increase calorie intake. Keep a late-morning and evening snack available in case he becomes hypoglycemic.

• Encourage the patient to verbalize his feelings about body image changes and sexual dysfunction. Discuss fear of rejection by others, and offer emotional support. Help him to develop coping strategies. Refer him to a mental health professional for additional counseling if necessary.

Monitoring

• If the patient also has diabetes mellitus, check blood glucose levels periodically because steroid replacement may necessitate adjustment of the insulin dosage.
• Observe the patient for cushingoid signs, such as fluid retention around the eyes and face. Check fluid and electrolyte balance, especially if he is receiving mineralocorticoids. Monitor weight, blood pressure, and intake and output to assess body fluid status. Remember, steroids administered in the late afternoon or evening may cause central nervous system stimulation and insomnia in some patients. Check for petechiae because the patient may bruise easily.
• If the patient receives only glucocorticoids, observe for orthostatic hypotension or electrolyte abnormalities, which may indicate a need for mineralocorticoid therapy.
• In women receiving testosterone injections, watch for and report facial hair growth and other signs of masculinization. A dosage adjustment may be necessary.
• In adrenal crisis, monitor vital signs carefully, especially for hypotension, volume depletion, and other signs of shock. Check for decreased level of consciousness and reduced urine output, which may also signal shock. Monitor for hyperkalemia before treatment and for hypokalemia afterward (from excessive mineralocorticoid effect). Check for cardiac arrhythmias.

Patient teaching

• Explain that lifelong steroid therapy is necessary. Teach the patient and his family to identify and report signs and symptoms of drug overdose (weight gain and edema) or underdose (fatigue, weakness, and dizziness).
• Advise the patient that he may need to increase the dosage during times of stress (when he has a cold, for example). Warn that infection, injury, or profuse sweating in hot weather may precipitate adrenal crisis. Caution him not to withdraw the medication suddenly because this may also cause adrenal crisis.
• Instruct the patient always to carry a medical identification card stating that he takes a steroid and giving the name and dosage of the drug. Teach him and his family how to give an injection of hydrocortisone, and advise them to keep an emergency kit available containing a prepared syringe of hydrocortisone for use in times of stress.
• Instruct the patient to take steroids with antacids or meals to minimize gastric irritation. Suggest taking two-thirds of the dosage in the morning and the remaining one-third in the early afternoon to mimic diurnal adrenal secretion.
• Inform the patient and his family that the disease causes mood swings and changes in mental status, which steroid replacement therapy can correct.
• Review protective measures to decrease stress and help prevent infections. For example, the patient should get adequate rest, avoid fatigue, eat a balanced diet, and avoid people with infectious conditions. Also provide instructions for stress management and relaxation techniques.

Adrenogenital syndrome

Excessive production of adrenal androgens causes adrenogenital syndrome, resulting in masculinization, virilization, and hermaphrodism. In true hermaphrodism the person has both ovarian and testicular tissues, a uterus, and ambiguous gonads distributed in various patterns. Adrenogenital syndrome may be inherited (congenital adrenal hyperplasia [CAH]) or acquired (adrenal virilism), usually as a result of an adrenal tumor.

CAH is the most common adrenal disorder in infants and children; simple virilizing CAH and salt-losing CAH are the most common forms. Adrenal virilism is rare and affects females twice as often as males.

Causes

CAH is transmitted as an autosomal recessive trait that causes deficiencies in the enzymes needed for adrenocortical secretion of cortisol and, possibly, aldosterone. Compensatory secretion of corticotropin produces varying degrees of adrenal hyperplasia.

In simple virilizing CAH, deficiency of the enzyme 21-hydroxylase results in underproduction of cortisol. In turn, this cortisol deficiency stimulates increased secretion of corticotropin, producing large amounts of cortisol precursors and androgens that don't require 21-hydroxylase for synthesis.

In salt-losing CAH, 21-hydroxylase is almost completely absent. Corticotropin secretion increases, causing excessive production of cortisol precursors, including salt-wasting compounds. However, plasma cortisol levels and aldosterone – both dependent on 21-hydroxylase – fall precipitously and, in combination with the excessive production of salt-wasting compounds, expedite acute adrenal crisis. Corticotropin hypersecretion stimulates adrenal androgens, possibly even more than in simple virilizing CAH, and produces masculinization.

Other rare CAH enzyme deficiencies exist and lead to increased or decreased production of affected hormones.

Complications

Unless salt-losing CAH is treated promptly, dehydration and hyperkalemia may lead to cardiovascular collapse and cardiac arrest in neonates. Other complications of adrenogenital syndrome include hypertension, infertility, adrenal tumor, and the tendency to develop adrenal crisis in times of stress.

Assessment

Assessment findings depend on the disorder's cause and the patient's age and sex. Suspect CAH in infants hospitalized for failure to thrive, dehydration, or diarrhea as well as in tall, sturdy-looking children with a history of episodic illnesses.

Inspection of the female neonate with simple virilizing CAH finds ambiguous genitalia (enlarged clitoris with urethral opening at the base and some labioscrotal fusion) but a normal genital tract and gonads. Inspection of an older female child with simple virilizing CAH reveals signs of progressive virilization: early appearance of pubic and axillary hair, deep voice, acne, and facial hair. Patient history notes failure to begin menstruation.

On inspection, the male neonate with simple virilizing CAH has no obvious abnormalities. However, at prepuberty, the child shows accentuated masculine characteristics, such as a deepened voice, an enlarged phallus, and frequent erections.

At puberty, the males have small testes. Both males and females with this condition may be taller than other children their age due to rapid bone and muscle growth. But because excessive androgen levels hasten epiphyseal closure, they may exhibit abnormally short adult stature.

Parents of an infant with salt-losing CAH may disclose that the child is apathetic, fails to eat, and has diarrhea. Without prompt treatment, the infant may develop fatal adrenal crisis in the first week of life (vomiting, dehydration from hyponatremia, and hyperkalemia).

Inspection of the older female with salt-losing CAH finds more complete virilization than in the simple form, even the development of male external genitalia without testes. The male child with this condition has no external genital abnormalities.

Diagnostic tests

Although ambiguous external genitalia suggest hermaphrodism, a gonadal biopsy and chromosomal studies are needed to confirm it just as the following test findings are needed to confirm adrenogenital syndrome:

- elevated levels of urine 17-ketosteroids (17-KS), which can be suppressed by administering oral dexamethasone
- increased urine metabolites of hormones, particularly pregnanediol
- elevated levels of plasma 17-hydroxyprogesterone
- normal or decreased urine levels of 17-hydroxycorticosteroids
- hyperkalemia, hyponatremia, and hypochloremia in the presence of excessive urine 17-KS and pregnanediol, and decreased urine aldosterone levels, which confirm salt-losing CAH in infants with symptoms of adrenal hypofunction or adrenal crisis in the first week of life.

Treatment

Simple virilizing CAH requires correction of the cortisol deficiency and inhibition of excessive pituitary corticotropin production by daily administration of cortisone or hydrocortisone. Such treatment returns androgen production to normal levels. Measurement of urine 17-KS determines the initial dose of cortisone or hydrocortisone; this dose is usually large and is given I.M. Subsequent dosage is modified according to decreasing urine 17-KS levels. Infants must continue to receive I.M. cortisone or hydrocortisone until age 18 months; after that, they may take the drug orally.

The infant with salt-losing CAH in adrenal crisis requires immediate I.V. 0.9% sodium chloride and glucose infusion to maintain fluid and electrolyte balance and to stabilize vital signs. If this treatment doesn't control symptoms while diagnosis is being established, I.M. and, occasionally, I.V. hydrocortisone may be necessary. Later, maintenance therapy includes adrenocorticoid replacement. Close monitoring of fluid balance and serum electrolytes is necessary.

Based on the anatomy of the external genitalia and chromosomal evaluation, sexual assignment and reconstructive surgery may be recommended. For example, the female with masculine external genitalia requires reconstructive surgery, such as correction of the labial fusion and of the urogenital sinus. Such surgery is usually scheduled between ages 1 and 3 after the effect of cortisone therapy has been assessed.

Key nursing diagnoses and patient outcomes

Altered protection related to increased risk of adrenal crisis during times of stress caused by underproduction of cortisol and possibly aldosterone. Based on this nursing diagnosis, you'll establish these patient outcomes. The patient will:

- not experience hypotension, tachycardia, nausea and vomiting, restlessness, or other signs of adrenal crisis
- demonstrate or provide protective measures, including compliance with adrenocorticoid replacement therapy, use of stress-reduction techniques, and early recognition and treatment of adrenal insufficency.

Body image disturbance related to masculinization, virilization, and hermaphrodism caused by excessive production of adrenal androgens. Based on this nursing diagnosis, you'll establish these patient outcomes. The patient will:

- communicate feelings about change in body image
- express positive feelings about himself
- demonstrate two new coping behaviors.

Knowledge deficit related to inadequate understanding of adrenogenital syndrome and steroid therapy. Based on this nursing

diagnosis, you'll establish these patient outcomes. The patient or caregiver will:
- indicate a need to know about adrenogenital syndrome and steroid therapy
- express an understanding of adrenogenital syndrome and steroid therapy
- state an intention to follow ordered medical therapy, including seeking help from health care professionals when needed.

Nursing interventions

- Administer steroid replacement therapy, as ordered.
- When caring for an infant with adrenal crisis, keep the I.V. line patent, infuse fluids, and give steroids, as ordered.
- Provide protective measures to minimize external stress. Limit visitors, provide a private room, and decrease environmental stimuli.
- Encourage the parents and the older child to verbalize their feelings about altered body image and fear of rejection by others. Offer a positive but realistic assessment of the patient's condition. Assist the parents and child to identify strengths and use them to develop coping strategies. Refer the family to a mental health counselor if necessary.

Monitoring

- When caring for an infant with adrenal crisis, monitor body weight, vital signs, respiratory status, urine output, and serum electrolyte levels.
- Monitor the patient receiving desoxycorticosterone for edema, weakness, and hypertension. Be alert for significant weight gain and rapid changes in height because normal growth is an important indicator of adequate therapy.

Patient teaching

- If reconstructive surgery is indicated for a child with CAH, explain what type of surgery will be performed and what type of care the patient will need preoperatively and postoperatively. Provide reassurance to the parents and child, and clear up any misconceptions they might have about the surgical procedure.
- Teach the parents of an infant with adrenogenital syndrome about normal growth and development and how their child may differ. Correct misconceptions about the disorder, and explain treatment options. Explain how the choice of sexual assignment is made and how abnormalities are surgically corrected. Refer the family to a genetic specialist for counseling.
- Advise the parents and the child that long-term steroid therapy is necessary. Warn them not to discontinue steroids abruptly to prevent potentially fatal adrenal insufficiency.
- Teach the patient and the family to identify and report signs of drug overdose and underdose, stress, and infection, which may require altered steroid dosages.
- Instruct the patient to wear a medical identification bracelet indicating that she's receiving prolonged steroid therapy and providing information about dosage.
- Stress the importance of continued medical follow-up throughout the patient's life.

Adult respiratory distress syndrome

A form of pulmonary edema, adult respiratory distress syndrome (ARDS) can quickly lead to acute respiratory failure. Also known as shock, stiff, white, wet, or Da Nang lung, ARDS may follow direct or indirect lung injury.

Increased permeability of the alveolocapillary membranes allows fluid to accumulate in the lung interstitium, alveolar spaces, and small airways, causing the lung to stiffen. This impairs ventilation, reducing oxygenation of pulmonary capillary blood. Difficult to recognize, the disorder can prove fatal within 48 hours of onset if not promptly diagnosed and treated.

Although this four-stage syndrome can progress to intractable and fatal hypoxemia, patients who recover may have little or no permanent lung damage.

In some patients, the syndrome may coexist with disseminated intravascular coagulation (DIC). Whether ARDS stems from DIC or develops independently remains unclear. Patients with three concurrent ARDS risk factors have an 85% probability of developing ARDS.

Causes

Trauma is the most common cause of ARDS, possibly because trauma-related factors, such as fat emboli, sepsis, shock, pulmonary contusions, and multiple transfusions, increase the likelihood that microemboli will develop.

Other common causes of ARDS include anaphylaxis, aspiration of gastric contents, diffuse pneumonia (especially viral), drug overdose (for example, heroin, aspirin, and ethchlorvynol), idiosyncratic drug reaction (to ampicillin and hydrochlorothiazide), inhalation of noxious gases (such as nitrous oxide, ammonia, and chlorine), near-drowning, and oxygen toxicity.

Less common causes of ARDS include coronary artery bypass grafting, hemodialysis, leukemia, acute miliary tuberculosis, pancreatitis, thrombotic thrombocytopenic purpura, uremia, and venous air embolism.

Complications

Severe ARDS can lead to metabolic and respiratory acidosis and ensuing cardiac arrest.

Assessment

As you conduct your assessment, be alert for rapid, shallow breathing; dyspnea; tachycardia; hypoxemia; intercostal and suprasternal retractions; crackles and rhonci; restlessness; apprehension; mental sluggishness; and motor dysfunction. ARDS is staged from I to IV, and each stage has typical signs. (See *Recognizing ARDS stages.*)

Diagnostic tests

- *Arterial blood gas (ABG) analysis* (with the patient breathing room air) initially shows a reduced partial pressure of oxygen in arterial blood, or $Pa{O_2}$ (less than 60 mm Hg), and a decreased partial pressure of carbon dioxide in arterial blood, or $Pa{CO_2}$ (less than 35 mm Hg). Hypoxemia despite increased supplemental oxygen is the hallmark of ARDS. The resulting blood pH usually reflects respiratory alkalosis. As ARDS worsens, ABG values show respiratory acidosis (increasing $Pa{CO_2}$ [more than 45 mm Hg]) and metabolic acidosis (decreasing bicarbonate levels [less than 22 mEq/liter]) and declining $Pa{O_2}$ despite oxygen therapy.
- *Pulmonary artery catheterization* helps identify the cause of pulmonary edema by measuring pulmonary capillary wedge pressure (PCWP). This procedure also allows collection of samples of pulmonary artery and mixed venous blood that show decreased oxygen saturation, reflecting tissue hypoxia. Normal PCWP values in ARDS are 12 mm Hg or less.
- *Serial chest X-rays* in early stages show bilateral infiltrates. In later stages, findings demonstrate lung fields with a ground-glass appearance and, eventually (with irreversible hypoxemia), "whiteouts" of both lung fields.

Differential diagnosis must rule out cardiogenic pulmonary edema, pulmonary vasculitis, and diffuse pulmonary hemorrhage. Etiologic tests may involve sputum analyses (including Gram stain and culture and sensitivity); blood cultures (to identify infectious organisms); toxicology tests (to screen for drug ingestion); and various serum amylase tests (to rule out pancreatitis).

Treatment

Therapy focuses on correcting the cause of the syndrome if possible and preventing progression of life-threatening hypoxemia and respiratory acidosis. Supportive care consists of administering humidified oxygen by a tight-fitting mask, which facilitates the use of continuous positive airway pressure (CPAP). However, this therapy alone seldom fulfills the ARDS patient's ventilatory requirements. If the patient's hypoxemia doesn't subside with this treatment, he may require intubation, mechanical ventilation, and positive end-expiratory pressure (PEEP). Other supportive measures include fluid restriction, diuretic therapy, and correction of electrolyte and acid-base imbalances.

When a patient with ARDS needs mechanical ventilation, sedatives, narcotics, or neuromuscular blocking agents (such as vecuronium) may be ordered to minimize restlessness (and thereby oxygen consumption and carbon dioxide production) and to facilitate ventilation.

When ARDS results from fatty emboli or a chemical injury, a short course of high-dose corticosteroids may help if given early. Treatment with sodium bicarbonate may be necessary to reverse severe metabolic acidosis. Fluids and vasopressors may be needed to maintain blood pressure. Nonviral infections require treatment with antimicrobial drugs.

Key nursing diagnoses and patient outcomes

Anxiety related to potential for ARDS to develop into acute respiratory failure and possible death. Based on this nursing diagnosis, you'll establish these patient outcomes. The patient will:

- state or write down feelings of anxiety about his condition and death
- use support systems to assist with coping
- demonstrate diminished physical symptoms of anxiety.

Impaired gas exchange related to direct or indirect lung injury. Based on this nursing diagnosis, you'll establish these patient outcomes. The patient will:

Recognizing ARDS stages

ARDS is staged from I to IV as follows:

Stage I
In this first stage, the patient may complain of dyspnea, especially on exertion. Respiratory and pulse rates are normal to high. Auscultation may reveal diminished breath sounds.

Stage II
Respiratory distress becomes more apparent in Stage II. The patient may use accessory muscles to breathe and appear pallid, anxious, and restless. He may have a dry cough with thick, frothy sputum and bloody, sticky secretions. Palpation may disclose cool, clammy skin. Tachycardia and tachypnea may accompany elevated blood pressure. Auscultation may detect basilar crackles. (Stage II signs and symptoms may be incorrectly attributed to other causes, such as multiple trauma.)

Stage III
The patient may struggle to breathe if he's in Stage III. A vital-signs check reveals tachypnea (more than 30 breaths/minute), tachycardia with arrhythmias (usually premature ventricular contractions), and a labile blood pressure. Inspection may reveal a productive cough and pale, cyanotic skin. Auscultation may disclose crackles and rhonchi. The patient will need intubation and ventilation.

Stage IV
At this late stage, the patient has acute respiratory failure with severe hypoxia. His mental status is deteriorating, and he may become comatose. His skin appears pale and cyanotic. Spontaneous respirations are not evident. Bradycardia with arrhythmias accompanies hypotension. Metabolic and respiratory acidosis develop. When ARDS reaches this stage, the patient is at high risk for fibrosis. Pulmonary damage becomes life-threatening.

• demonstrate adequate gas exchange with therapy, evidenced by ABG values that return to normal and restoration of normal respiratory function
• recover from ARDS with no residual lung damage.

Inability to sustain spontaneous ventilation related to pulmonary edema and fibrosis. Based on this nursing diagnosis, you'll establish these patient outcomes. The patient will:
• recover from lung tissue damage
• resume spontaneous ventilation with treatment
• have ABG values that return to normal and remain normal.

Nursing interventions

• Maintain a patent airway by suctioning. Use sterile, nontraumatic technique. Ensure adequate humidification to help liquefy tenacious secretions.
• If the patient is on mechanical ventilation, drain any condensation from the tubing promptly to ensure maximum oxygen delivery.
• Provide alternative means of communication for the patient on mechanical ventilation.
• Be prepared to administer CPAP to the patient with severe hypoxemia.
• To maintain PEEP, suction only as needed. High-frequency jet ventilation may also be required.
• Give sedatives, as ordered, to reduce restlessness. Administer sedatives and analgesics at regular intervals if the patient is receiving neuromuscular blocking agents.
• If the patient has a pulmonary artery catheter in place, change dressings according to hospital guidelines, using strict aseptic technique.
• Reposition the patient often.
• Note and record any changes in respiratory status, temperature, or hypotension that may indicate a deteriorating condition. Notify the doctor.
• Record caloric intake. Administer tube feedings and parenteral nutrition as ordered. To promote health and prevent fatigue, arrange for alternate periods of rest and activity.
• Maintain joint mobility by performing passive range-of-motion exercises. If possible, help the patient perform active exercises.
• Provide meticulous skin care. To prevent skin breakdown, reposition the endotracheal tube from side to side every 24 hours.
• Provide emotional support. Answer the patient's and family's questions as fully as possible to allay their fears and concerns.

Monitoring

• Frequently assess the patient's respiratory status. Be alert for inspiratory retractions. Note respiratory rate, rhythm, and depth. Watch for dyspnea and accessory muscle use. Listen for adventitious or diminished breath sounds. Check for clear, frothy sputum (indicating pulmonary edema).
• Monitor the patient's level of consciousness, noting confusion or mental sluggishness.
• Be alert for signs of treatment-induced complications, including arrhythmias, DIC, GI bleeding, infection, malnutrition, paralytic ileus, pneumothorax, pulmonary fibrosis, renal failure, thrombocytopenia, and tracheal stenosis.
• Closely monitor the patient's heart rate and blood pressure. Watch for arrhythmias that may result from hypoxemia, acid-base disturbances, or electrolyte imbalance.
• With pulmonary artery catheterization, know the desired PCWP level; check readings as indicated, and watch for decreasing mixed venous oxygen saturation.
• Frequently evaluate the patient's serum electrolyte levels. Measure intake and output. Weigh the patient daily.
• Check ventilator settings frequently. Monitor ABG levels; document and report changes in arterial oxygen saturation as well as metabolic and respiratory acidosis and Pa_{O_2} changes.

• Monitor and record the patient's response to medication.
• Because PEEP may lower cardiac output, check for hypotension, tachycardia, and decreased urine output.
• Evaluate the patient's nutritional intake.
• If the patient has injuries that affect the lungs, watch for adverse respiratory changes, especially in the first few days after the injury, when his condition may appear to be improving.

Patient teaching

• Explain the disorder to the patient and his family. Tell them what signs and symptoms may occur, and review the treatment that may be required.
• Orient the patient and his family to the unit and hospital surroundings. Provide them with simple explanations and demonstrations of treatments.
• Tell the recuperating patient that recovery will take some time and that he'll feel weak for a while. Urge him to share his concerns with the staff.

Allergic purpuras

A nonthrombocytopenic purpura, allergic purpura is an acute or chronic vascular inflammation that affects the skin, joints, and GI and genitourinary (GU) tracts in association with allergy symptoms. When allergic purpura primarily affects the GI tract, with accompanying joint pain, it is called Henoch-Schönlein syndrome or anaphylactoid purpura. However, the term allergic purpura applies to purpura associated with many other conditions, such as erythema nodosum. An acute attack of allergic purpura can last for several weeks.

Fully developed allergic purpura is persistent and debilitating. This disorder affects males more commonly than females and is most prevalent in children ages 3 to 7. The prognosis is more favorable for children than for adults. The course of Henoch-Schönlein syndrome is usually benign and self-limiting, lasting 1 to 6 weeks if renal involvement is not severe.

Causes

The most common identifiable cause of allergic purpura is probably an autoimmune reaction directed against vascular walls and triggered by a bacterial infection (particularly a streptococcal infection, such as scarlet fever). Typically, upper respiratory tract infection occurs 1 to 3 weeks before the onset of signs and symptoms. Other possible causes include allergic reactions to some drugs and vaccines; allergic reactions to insect bites; and allergic reactions to some foods (such as wheat, eggs, milk, and chocolate).

Complications

Renal disease (renal failure and acute glomerulonephritis) can be fatal. Hypertension and resulting blood loss from renal damage can further complicate the patient's condition.

Assessment

An accurate patient allergy history may yield information that helps ensure a positive outcome. The patient history may include pain and bleeding due to bleeding from the mucosal surfaces of the ureters, bladder, and urethra. In 25% to 50% of patients, allergic purpura is associated with GU symptoms. Other patient complaints include moderate, transient headaches; fever; anorexia; edema of the hands, feet, or scalp; and skin lesions, accompanied by pruritus, paresthesia and, occasionally, angioneurotic edema.

The patient with Henoch-Schönlein purpura may report a hypersensitivity to aspirin and food and drug additives. Typically, the patient complains of transient or severe colic, tenesmus, constipation, vomiting, and edema. He also may report hematuria and joint pain, mostly affecting the knees and ankles. Other symptoms include bleeding or hemorrhage of the mucous membranes of the bowel, resulting in GI bleeding, occult blood in the stool and, possibly, intussusception. Such GI abnormalities may precede overt, cutaneous signs of purpura.

Inspection findings in allergic purpuras include characteristic skin lesions. Purple, macular, ecchymotic, and of varying sizes, these lesions result from vascular leakage into the skin and mucous membranes. The lesions usually appear in symmetrical patterns on the arms and legs. In children, skin lesions are generally urticarial; they expand and become hemorrhagic.

In Henoch-Schönlein purpura, inspection and palpation may disclose localized areas of edema, especially on the dorsal surfaces of the hands.

Diagnostic tests

No laboratory test clearly identifies allergic purpura (although white blood cell count and erythrocyte sedimentation rate are elevated). Diagnosis necessitates careful clinical observation, often during the second or third attack. The following laboratory test results may aid diagnosis:

- guaiac-positive stools
- hematuria identified on urinalysis
- elevated blood urea nitrogen and creatinine levels and proteinuria, indicating glomerular involvement
- normal coagulation and platelet function (with the exception of a positive tourniquet test).

Small-bowel X-rays may reveal areas of transient edema. Diagnosis must rule out other forms of nonthrombocytopenic purpura.

Treatment

In allergic purpura, treatment is usually based on symptoms; for example, severe allergic purpura may require corticosteroids to relieve edema and analgesics to alleviate joint and abdominal pain. Some patients with chronic renal disease may benefit from immunosuppression with azathioprine or corticosteroids, along with identification of the provocative allergen.

Key nursing diagnoses and patient outcomes

Body image disturbance related to skin lesions. Based on this nursing diagnosis, you'll establish these patient outcomes. The patient will:

- communicate feelings about change in body image from the appearance of skin lesions
- express positive feelings about himself
- demonstrate two new coping behaviors.

Altered renal or GI tissue perfusion related to vascular inflammation in the GU or GI tracts. Based on this nursing diagnosis, you'll establish these patient outcomes. The patient will:

- exhibit a return to normal GU or GI function or both, as evidenced by guaiac-negative stools, normal urinalysis, and alleviation of GU and GI signs and symptoms
- take precautions to prevent future infections and allergic reactions, including testing to identify the provocative allergen, if necessary.

Pain related to vascular inflammation. Based on this nursing diagnosis, you'll establish these patient outcomes. The patient will:

- identify factors that intensify pain and modify his behavior accordingly
- express a feeling of comfort and relief from pain after administration of an analgesic
- become pain free.

Nursing interventions

- If the patient experiences pain, provide analgesics as needed.
- To prevent muscle atrophy in the bedridden patient, perform passive or active range-of-motion exercises.
- Provide emotional support and reassurance, especially if the patient is temporarily disfigured by florid skin lesions.

• Administer fluids if required to maintain fluid level. Encourage fluid intake as appropriate.
• If the patient is receiving immunosuppressant therapy, provide an environment free from the risk of secondary infection.

Monitoring
• Monitor skin lesions and level of pain.
• Watch carefully for complications, including GI and GU tract bleeding, edema, nausea, vomiting, headache, hypertension (with nephritis), abdominal rigidity and tenderness, and absence of stool (with intussusception).
• If corticosteroid therapy is added, watch for signs of Cushing's syndrome and labile emotional involvement.

Patient teaching
• Teach the patient about the disease, its symptoms, and treatment.
• Explain the need to protect against infection. Advise the patient to wash his hands frequently to avoid infecting his skin lesions. Teach him to protect edematous areas because the skin over these areas breaks down easily.
• After the acute stage, direct the patient to report immediately any recurrence of symptoms (most common about 6 weeks after initial onset). Tell him to return for follow-up urinalysis as scheduled.
• Encourage maintenance of an elimination diet to help identify specific allergenic foods so that these foods can be eliminated from the patient's diet.

Alzheimer's disease

This progressive degenerative disorder of the cerebral cortex (especially the frontal lobe) accounts for more than half of all cases of dementia. An estimated 5% of people over age 65 have a severe form of this disease, and 12% suffer from mild to moderate dementia. Because this is a primary progressive dementia, the prognosis for a patient with this disease is poor.

Typically, patients die of debilitating brain disease 2 to 15 years after the onset of symptoms. The average duration of the illness before death is 8 years.

Causes
The cause of Alzheimer's disease is unknown. Nevertheless, several factors are thought to be closely connected to this disease. These include neurochemical factors, such as deficiencies of the neurotransmitters acetylcholine, somatostatin, substance P, and norepinephrine; environmental factors, such as intake of aluminum and manganese; viral factors, such as slow-growing central nervous system viruses; trauma; and genetic factors.

Researchers believe that up to 70% of Alzheimer's disease cases stem from a genetic abnormality. Recently, they located the abnormality on chromosome 21. They've also isolated a genetic substance (amyloid) that causes brain damage typical of Alzheimer's disease. The brain tissue of patients with this dementia has three distinguishing features: neurofibrillary tangles, neuritic plaques, and granulovascular degeneration.

Complications
In this disorder, complications include injury from the patient's own violent behavior or from wandering or unsupervised activity; pneumonia and other infections, especially if the patient doesn't receive enough exercise; malnutrition and dehydration, especially if the patient refuses or forgets to eat; and aspiration.

Assessment
As you assess this patient, keep in mind that the onset of this disorder is insidious; initial changes are almost imperceptible but gradually progress to serious problems. The patient history is almost always obtained from a family member or caregiver.

Teaching families about Alzheimer's disease

Counsel family members to expect progressive deterioration in the patient with Alzheimer's disease. To help them plan future patient care, discuss the stages of this relentless disease.

Bear in mind that family members may refuse to believe that the disease is advancing. So be sensitive to their concerns and, if necessary, review the information again when they're more receptive.

Forgetfulness

The patient becomes forgetful, especially of recent events. He frequently loses everyday objects, such as keys. Aware of his loss of function, he may compensate by relinquishing tasks that might reveal his forgetfulness. Because his behavior isn't disruptive and may be attributed to stress, fatigue, or normal aging, he usually doesn't consult a doctor at this stage.

Confusion

The patient has increasing difficulty with activities that require planning, decision making, and judgment, such as managing personal finances, driving a car, and performing his job. However, he does retain everyday skills, such as personal grooming. Social withdrawal occurs when the patient feels overwhelmed by a changing environment and his inability to cope with multiple stimuli. Travel is difficult and tiring. As he becomes aware of his progressive loss of function, he may become severely depressed.

Safety becomes a concern when the patient forgets to turn off appliances or to recognize unsafe situations, such as boiling water. At this point, the family may need to consider day care or a supervised residential facility.

Decline in activities of daily living

The patient at this stage loses his ability to perform daily activities, such as eating or washing, without direct supervision. Weight loss may occur. He withdraws from the family and increasingly depends on the primary caregiver. Communication becomes difficult as his understanding of written and spoken language declines. Agitation, wandering, pacing, and nighttime awakening are linked to his inability to cope with a multisensory environment. He may mistake his mirror image for a real person (pseudohallucination). Caregivers must be constantly vigilant, which may lead to physical and emotional exhaustion. They may also be angry and feel a sense of loss.

Total deterioration

In the final stage of Alzheimer's disease, the patient no longer recognizes himself, his body parts, or other family members. He becomes bedridden, and his activity consists of small, purposeless movements. Verbal communication stops, although he may scream spontaneously. Complications of immobility may include pressure ulcers, urinary tract infections, pneumonia, and contractures.

Typically, the patient history shows initial onset of very small changes, such as forgetfulness and subtle memory loss without loss of social skills and behavior patterns. It also reveals that over time the patient began experiencing recent-memory loss and had difficulty learning and remembering new information. The history also may reveal a general deterioration in personal hygiene and appearance and an inability to concentrate. (See *Teaching families about Alzheimer's disease.*)

Depending on the severity of the disease, the patient history may reveal that the patient experiences several of the following problems: difficulty with abstract thinking and activities that require judgment; progressive difficulty in communicating; a severe deterioration of memory, language, and motor function that in the more severe cases finally results in coordination loss and an inability to speak or write; repetitive actions; restlessness; negative personality changes, such as irritability, depression, paranoia, hostility, and combativeness; nocturnal awakenings; and disorientation.

The person giving the history may explain that the patient is suspicious and fearful of imaginary people and situations, misperceives his environment, misidentifies objects and people, and complains of stolen or misplaced objects.

He also may report that the patient seems overdependent on caregivers and has difficulty using correct words and may often substitute meaningless words. He may report that conversations with the patient drift off into nonsensical phrases. The patient's emotions may be described as labile. Also, the patient may laugh or cry inappropriately and have mood swings, sudden angry outbursts, and sleep disturbances.

Neurologic examination confirms many of the problems revealed during the history. In addition, it often reveals an impaired sense of smell (usually an early symptom), impaired stereognosis (inability to recognize and understand the form and nature of objects by touching them), gait disorders, tremors, and loss of recent memory. The patient with Alzheimer's disease also has a positive snout reflex. To check for this reflex, stroke or tap his lips or the area just under his nose. If he has a positive reflex, you'll observe him grimacing or puckering his lips.

If the patient is in the final stages, he typically has urinary or fecal incontinence and may twitch and have seizures.

Diagnostic tests

Alzheimer's disease is diagnosed by exclusion. Various tests, such as those described below, are performed to rule out other disorders. However, the diagnosis can't be confirmed until death, when pathologic findings come to light at autopsy.

- *Positron emission tomography* measures the metabolic activity of the cerebral cortex and may help confirm early diagnosis.
- *Computed tomography scan* in some patients shows progressive brain atrophy in excess of that which occurs in normal aging.
- *Magnetic resonance imaging* may permit evaluation of the condition of the brain and rule out intracranial lesions as the source of dementia.
- *EEG* may allow evaluation of the brain's electrical activity and may show slowing of the brain waves. It also helps identify tumors, abscesses, and other intracranial lesions that might cause the patient's symptoms.
- *Cerebrospinal fluid analysis* may help determine if the patient's signs and symptoms stem from a chronic neurologic infection.
- *Cerebral blood flow studies* may detect abnormalities in blood flow to the brain.

Treatment

No cure or definitive treatment exists for Alzheimer's disease. Therapy consists of cerebral vasodilators, such as ergoloid mesylates, isoxsuprine, and cyclandelate to enhance the brain's circulation; hyperbaric oxygen to increase oxygenation to the brain; psychostimulators, such as methylphenidate, to enhance the patient's mood; and antidepressants if depression seems to exacerbate the patient's dementia.

Most other drug therapies being tried are experimental. These include choline salts, lecithin, physostigmine, tacrine, enkephalins, and naloxone, which may slow the disease process.

Another approach to treatment includes avoiding use of antacids, aluminum cooking utensils, and aluminum-containing deodorants to help decrease aluminum intake, which is thought to be one of the environmental factors that may cause this disorder.

Key nursing diagnoses and patient outcomes

Altered nutrition: Less than body requirements, related to patient's forgetfulness. Based on this nursing diagnosis, you'll establish these patient outcomes. The patient will:
- eat meals with supervision to ensure adequate intake
- consume a well-balanced diet provided by the caregiver
- maintain his weight.

Altered thought processes related to progressive deterioration of the cerebral cortex. Based on this nursing diagnosis, you'll establish these patient outcomes. The family or caregiver will:
- provide a simple, daily routine for the patient to perform activities of daily living
- avoid or minimize change in the patient's environment
- demonstrate appropriate interventions, reorientation techniques, and coping skills.

Risk for trauma related to negative personality changes and confusion. Based on this nursing diagnosis, you'll establish these patient outcomes. The patient will:
- remain safe and protected from injury
- perform activities of daily living under supervision.

The family or caregiver will:
- seek assistance with care and consult appropriate resources, as needed, including arrangements for care in a health care facility.

Nursing interventions

- Establish an effective communication system with the patient and his family to help them adjust to the patient's altered cognitive abilities.
- Provide emotional support to the patient and his family. Encourage them to talk about their concerns. Listen to them, and answer their questions honestly.
- Because the patient may misperceive his environment, use a soft tone and a slow, calm manner when speaking to him. Allow him sufficient time to answer because his thought processes are slow, impairing his ability to communicate verbally.
- Administer ordered medications, and note their effects. If the patient has trouble swallowing, crush tablets and open capsules and mix them with a semisoft food. Always check with the pharmacist before crushing tablets or opening capsules because some drugs shouldn't be altered.
- Protect the patient from injury by providing a safe, structured environment. Provide rest periods between activities because these patients tire easily.
- Encourage the patient to exercise as ordered to help maintain mobility.
- Encourage patient independence, and allow ample time for the patient to perform tasks.
- Encourage sufficient fluid intake and adequate nutrition. Provide assistance with menu selection, and allow the patient to feed himself as much as he can. Provide a well-balanced diet with adequate fiber. Avoid stimulants, such as coffee, tea, cola, and chocolate. Give the patient semisolid foods if he has dysphagia. Insert and care for a nasogastric tube or a gastrostomy tube for feeding, as ordered.
- Because the patient may be disoriented or neuromuscular functioning may be impaired, take the patient to the bathroom at least every 2 hours and make sure he knows the location of the bathroom.
- Assist the patient with hygiene and dressing as necessary. Many patients with Alzheimer's disease are incapable of performing these tasks.

Monitoring

- Monitor the patient's neurologic function, including his emotional and mental states and motor capabilities, for changes indicating further deterioration.
- Frequently check the patient's vital signs. Watch for signs and symptoms of pneu-

monia and other infections, such as fever, chills, malaise, sputum production, or dyspnea.

• Monitor the patient's fluid and food intake to detect imbalances.
• Inspect the patient's skin for evidence of trauma, such as bruises or skin breakdown.
• Evaluate the family's or caregiver's ability to manage the patient if he is living at home.

Patient teaching

• Teach the patient's family about the disease. Explain that the cause of Alzheimer's disease is unknown. Review the signs and symptoms of the disease with them. Be sure to explain that Alzheimer's disease progresses but at an unpredictable rate and that the patient will eventually suffer complete memory loss and total physical deterioration.
• Review the diagnostic tests that will be performed and the treatment the patient will require.
• Advise the family to provide the patient with exercise. Suggest physical activities, such as walking or light housework, that occupy and satisfy the patient.
• Stress the importance of diet. Instruct the family to limit the number of foods on the patient's plate so he won't have to make decisions. If the patient has coordination problems, tell the family to cut up his food and to provide finger foods, such as fruit and sandwiches. Suggest using plates with rim guards, built-up utensils, and cups with lids and spouts.
• Encourage the family to allow the patient as much independence as possible while ensuring his and others' safety. Tell them to create a routine for all the patient's activities, which will avoid confusion. If the patient becomes belligerent, advise the family to remain calm and to try distracting him.
• Refer the family to support groups, such as the Alzheimer's Association. Set up an appointment with the social service department, which will help the family assess its needs.

Amputation

Performed to preserve function in a remaining part or, at times, to prevent death, amputation is a radical treatment for severe trauma, gangrene, cancer, vascular disease, congenital deformity, or thermal injury. It can take one of two basic forms. In a closed, or flap, amputation – the most commonly performed type – the surgeon uses skin flaps to cover the bone stump. In an open, or guillotine, amputation (a rarely performed emergency operation), he cuts the tissue and bone flush, leaving the wound open. A second operation completes repair and stump formation. Amputation may be performed at a number of sites, depending on the nature and extent of injury. (See *Common levels of amputation,* page 38.)

Procedure

The patient receives a general anesthetic (or perhaps a local anesthetic for a finger or toe amputation). In the closed technique, the surgeon incises the tissue to the bone, leaving sufficient skin to cover the stump end. He usually controls bleeding above the level of amputation by tying off the bleeding vessels with suture ties. He then saws the bone (or resects a joint), files the bone ends smooth and rounded, and removes the periosteum up about ¼" (0.6 cm) from the bone end. After ligating all vessels and dividing the nerves, he sutures opposing muscles over the bone end and to the periosteum to provide better muscle control and circulation. Next, he sutures the skin flaps closed. Placement of an incisional drain and a soft dressing completes the procedure.

In a below-the-knee amputation, the surgeon may order a rigid dressing applied over the stump in the operating

Common levels of amputation

Amputation may be performed at a wide range of sites. Review this list for common types and levels of amputation.

- *Partial foot:* removal of one or more toes and part of the foot
- *Total foot:* removal of the foot below the ankle joint
- *Ankle (Syme's amputation):* removal of the foot at the ankle joint
- *Below-the-knee:* removal of the leg 5" to 7" (12.7 to 17.8 cm) below the knee
- *Knee disarticulation:* removal of the patella, with the quadriceps brought over the end of the femur, or fixation of the patella to a cut surface between the condyles (known as the Gritti-Stokes operation)
- *Above-the-knee:* removal of the leg from 3" (7.6 cm) above the knee
- *Hip disarticulation:* removal of both the leg and hip or the leg and pelvis
- *Hemipelvectomy:* removal of a leg and half of the pelvis
- *Fingers:* removal of one or more fingers at the hinge or condyloid joints
- *Wrist disarticulation:* removal of the hand at the wrist
- *Below-the-elbow:* removal of the lower arm about 7" (17.8 cm) below the elbow
- *Elbow disarticulation:* removal of the lower arm at the elbow
- *Above-the-elbow:* removal of the arm from 3" (7.6 cm) above the elbow

room. This enables immediate postoperative fitting of a prosthesis and helps prevent contractures.

In an emergency, or guillotine, amputation, the surgeon makes a perpendicular incision through the bone and all tissue. He leaves the wound open, applying a large bulky dressing.

Complications

Amputation can cause several complications, including infection at the stump site, contractures in the remaining limb part (if exercise of the limb part is delayed), skin breakdown from improper care of the stump or an ill-fitting prosthetic device, and phantom pain. Phantom pain is a sensation of pain, itching, or numbness in the area of amputation, even though the limb or digit has been removed. It commonly develops after a major amputation and can occur as late as 2 to 3 months afterward. Because amputation of a body part can be emotionally devastating to the patient, he may develop depression, which may be severe enough to interfere with self-care and require psychiatric therapy.

Key nursing diagnoses and patient outcomes

Body image disturbance related to loss of limb or digit. Based on this nursing diagnosis, you'll establish these patient outcomes. The patient will:

- express feelings about the effect of amputation on his body image
- participate in a rehabilitation program to help adapt to the change in his body image and function
- accept his altered body image.

Risk for infection related to improper stump care. Based on this nursing diagnosis, you'll establish these patient outcomes. The patient will:

- not exhibit signs of infection (blistering, redness, or pain), abrasions, or delayed tissue and skin healing at stump site
- demonstrate correct stump hygiene and take preventive measures to avoid or minimize skin breakdown at the stump site
- apply and use his prosthesis correctly.

Pain related to surgery and phantom pain. Based on this nursing diagnosis, you'll establish these patient outcomes. The patient will:

• achieve pain relief with analgesics
• perform activities to help minimize pain, such as early ambulation and, when in bed, keeping his stump elevated on a pillow for 24 to 48 hours after surgery
• express understanding of phantom pain and be able to distinguish it from incisional pain
• experience complete disappearance of phantom pain.

Nursing interventions

When caring for an amputation patient, your major roles include preparing the patient for surgery and providing care and instruction after the amputation.

Before surgery

• If time permits, review the doctor's explanation of the scheduled amputation, answering any questions the patient may have.
• Remember that the patient faces not only the loss of a body part, with an attendant change in body image, but also the threat of loss of mobility and independence. Keep in mind, too, that loss of a limb or digit can be emotionally devastating to the patient; be sure to provide emotional support.
• If possible, arrange for the patient to meet with a well-adjusted amputee, who can provide additional reassurance and encouragement.
• Discuss postoperative care and rehabilitation measures. Demonstrate appropriate exercises to strengthen the remaining portion of the limb and maintain mobility. Such exercises may include active hip extension and abduction, and adduction for an above-the-knee amputation. Follow the doctor's or physical therapist's directions in explaining such exercises.
• The patient may be fitted with a prosthesis while hospitalized, but most often he will require more time to heal and so will be discharged before being fitted. Explain to him that the duration between amputation and fitting of the prosthesis varies, depending on wound healing, muscle tone, and overall stump condition. Stress that good stump care can speed this process and help ensure a better fit for the prosthesis. If possible, show him the types of prostheses available for his type of amputation and explain how they work.
• Point out the possibility of phantom limb sensation. Explain that the patient may "feel" sensations of pain, itching, or numbness in the area of amputation, even though the limb or digit has been removed. Reassure him that these sensations, although inexplicable, are common and should eventually disappear.
• As ordered, administer broad-spectrum antibiotics to minimize the risk of infection.

After surgery

• After the patient returns from surgery, monitor his vital signs every hour for the first 4 hours, every 2 hours for the next 4 hours, and then every 4 hours until stable. Be alert, particularly for bleeding through the dressing. Notify the doctor if any bleeding occurs.
• If ordered, elevate the stump on a pillow or other support for 24 to 48 hours; be aware, however, that this could lead to contractures. Check dressings frequently and change them as necessary. Assess drain patency, and note the amount and character of drainage.
• Assess for pain, and provide analgesics and other pain control measures, as needed. Because movement may be painful and interfere with therapy, give analgesics about 30 minutes before scheduled exercises or ambulation. Distinguish stump pain from phantom limb sensation; severe, unremitting stump pain may indicate infection or other complications.
• Keep the stump properly wrapped with elastic compression bandages. A properly applied bandage is essential to stump care; it supports soft tissue, controls edema and pain, and shrinks and molds the stump into a cone-shaped form to allow a good fit

for the prosthesis. Rewrap the stump at least twice a day to maintain tightness. As an alternative to bandages, the doctor may order that the patient wear a stump shrinker – a custom-fitted elastic stocking that fits snugly over the stump.

• If a rigid plaster dressing has been applied, care for it as you would a plaster cast for a fracture or severe sprain. Keep it from getting wet, and observe its margin for skin irritation and excessive or malodorous drainage, which may indicate infection. As the stump shrinks, the plaster dressing may loosen or fall off. If this occurs, notify the doctor and wrap the stump in an elastic compression bandage until he can replace the dressing.

• Emphasize the need for proper body alignment and regular physical therapy to condition the stump and prevent contractures and deformity. Encourage frequent ambulation, if possible, and a program of active or passive range-of-motion exercises, as ordered.

• If the patient is bedridden, encourage him to turn from side to side and to assume an alternate position – usually on his stomach – from time to time throughout the day. Frequent position changes will stretch the hip flexor muscles and prevent contractures.

• If the patient has had a leg amputation, instruct him not to prop his stump on a pillow, to avoid hip flexion contracture.

• If the patient has had a below-the-knee amputation, tell him to keep the knee extended to prevent hamstring contracture.

• Instruct the patient with a partial arm amputation to keep his elbow extended and shoulder abducted.

• If possible, give the patient information about available prostheses. Keep in mind his age and physical condition as well as the complexity and cost of the device. Generally, a child needs a relatively simple, inexpensive device that can be maintained easily and replaced at a reasonable cost when he outgrows it. An elderly patient may require a prosthesis that provides extra stability even if it means sacrificing some flexibility.

• Throughout recovery and rehabilitation, encourage the patient to adopt a positive outlook toward resuming an independent life-style. Emphasize that the prosthesis should allow him to lead a full and active life with few restrictions on activity. If he seems overly despondent or depressed, consider referring him to psychological counseling or social services.

Home care instructions

• Instruct the patient to examine his stump daily, using a hand-held mirror to visualize the entire area. Tell him to watch for and report swelling, redness, or excessive drainage as well as increased pain. Also instruct him to note and report any skin changes on the stump, including rashes, blisters, or abrasions.

• Explain that good stump hygiene will prevent irritation, skin breakdown, and infection. Tell the patient to wash the stump daily with mild soap and water and then rinse and gently dry it. Suggest that he wash the stump at night and bandage it when dry; advise against bandaging a wet stump because this may lead to skin maceration or infection. Also advise against applying body oil or lotion to the stump because this can interfere with proper fit of the prosthesis.

• Teach the patient how to apply a stump dressing. Instruct him to change dressings frequently, as necessary, and to maintain sterile technique. Explain that as the wound heals, he'll need to change the dressing less often.

• As appropriate, show the patient how to properly wrap his stump with elastic bandages or how to slip on a stump shrinker. If he's using bandages, show him how to apply them with even, moderate pressure, avoiding overtightness that could impair circulation. Suggest that he apply the bandages when he awakens in the morning and rewrap the stump at least twice a day to maintain proper compression. If he's using a shrinker, suggest that he have two available: one to wear while the other is being washed. Explain that he'll need to use elastic bandages or a stump shrinker at all times (except when bathing or exercising) until postoperative edema completely subsides and the prosthesis is properly fitted. Even after adjustment to the prosthesis, he may need to continue nighttime bandaging for many years.

• Instruct the patient to apply a clean stump sock before attaching his prosthesis. Advise him never to wear a stump sock that has any tears, holes, mends, or seams; these could cause skin irritation. Explain that as the stump shrinks over time, he may need to apply two stump socks to ensure a snug fit of the prosthesis. Tell him to notify the doctor if he needs more than two socks for proper fit or if his prosthesis feels loose for any other reason.

• Review proper care of the prosthesis. Instruct the patient never to immerse it in water, which could weaken its leather joints or hinges. Tell him to clean the device with soap and water each night before bedtime and to let it dry overnight.

• If appropriate, refer the patient to a local support group.

Amyloidosis

A rare, chronic disease, amyloidosis results in the accumulation of an abnormal fibrillar scleroprotein (amyloid), which infiltrates body organs and soft tissues. The forms of amyloidosis may differ clinically and biochemically.

A primary disease, amyloidosis may also be familial, especially in persons of Portuguese ancestry. Amyloidosis is frequently associated with carpal tunnel syndrome. It may occur in conjunction with multiple myeloma, or it may be associated with chronic infections, tuberculosis, osteomyelitis, long-term hemodialysis, or chronic inflammatory conditions such as rheumatoid arthritis. It may also accompany aging or Alzheimer's disease. Localized amyloidosis affects isolated organs with no evidence of systemic involvement.

Although the prognosis varies with the disease type, site, and extent of involvement, amyloidosis sometimes results in permanent – even life-threatening – organ damage. The average survival rate for a patient with generalized amyloidosis is about 1 to 4 years, although some patients live 10 years or more.

Causes

The precise etiology of amyloidosis is unknown. Multiple immunobiological factors are thought to contribute to this disorder.

Complications

Renal failure is the most common cause of death associated with amyloidosis; arrhythmias resulting in sudden death also are common. Other life-threatening complications of amyloidosis include GI hemorrhage, respiratory failure, intractable heart failure, and superimposed infections.

Assessment

Depending on which body site is involved, amyloidosis may cause dysfunction of the heart, respiratory tract, kidneys, GI tract, skin, peripheral nerves, joints, and liver.

The patient may have a history of an associated disease or condition. He may list decreased sensations of pain and temperature; difficulty talking, swallowing, and eating due to macroglossia; and an inability to sweat. He may also have dyspnea, a cough, light-headedness with position changes, palpitations, and increased clotting time. With GI involvement, he may report abdominal pain, constipation, diarrhea, or GI bleeding. With joint involvement, he may complain of morning stiffness and fatigue.

Inspection may reveal dyspnea with respiratory involvement and enlargement of the tongue with hindered enunciation. The patient may appear malnourished due to chronic malabsorption. With skin involvement, characteristic lesions appear as slightly raised papules or plaques found mainly in the axillary, inguinal, or anal regions or on the face, neck, ear, or tongue. With proteinuria, edema may be evident.

Palpation may reveal abdominal tenderness and an enlarged liver. The tongue may feel stiff and firm. You may be able to palpate small joint nodules.

On auscultation, you may discover distant heart sounds, crackles, or murmurs due to amyloid deposits in the subendocardium, endocardium, and myocardium, resulting in congestive heart failure (CHF) and valvular abnormalities. With GI involvement, bowel sounds may be decreased.

Neurologic testing may detect decreased muscle strength and, with peripheral nervous system involvement, decreased temperature and pain sensation.

Diagnostic tests

Definitive diagnosis requires histologic examination of a tissue biopsy specimen using a polarizing or electron microscope. After appropriate tissue staining, this technique identifies amyloid deposits. Rectal mucosa biopsy and abdominal fat pad aspiration are the best screening tests because they're less hazardous than kidney or liver biopsy. Other biopsy sites include the gingiva and skin.

Other tests depend on the site of involvement; for example, electrocardiography may show low voltage and conduction or rhythm abnormalities resembling those of myocardial infarction. Echocardiography (M-mode and two-dimensional) may detect myocardial infiltration; however, only biopsy is definitive for cardiac amyloidosis. Liver function studies are usually normal except for slightly elevated serum alkaline phosphatase levels.

Treatment

No specific treatment currently exists for amyloidosis. Management is mainly supportive and conservative. It may include drugs, such as colchicine, melphalan, and prednisone, which may decrease amyloid deposits. However, the use of melphalan and prednisone is controversial; one view holds that immunosuppressants may increase amyloid deposits. Also, melphalan therapy produces bone marrow depression.

Transplantation may be useful for amyloidosis-induced renal failure. Patients with cardiac amyloidosis require conservative treatment to prevent dangerous arrhythmias. Malnutrition caused by malabsorption in end-stage GI involvement may require total parenteral nutrition. Vitamin K for coagulopathy, analgesics for musculoskeletal pain, and tracheotomy for macroglossia may also be required.

Key nursing diagnoses and patient outcomes

Altered nutrition: Less than body requirements, related to difficulty eating caused by tongue involvement in amyloidosis. Based on this nursing diagnosis, you'll establish these patient outcomes. The patient will:

- communicate understanding of special dietary needs and plan an appropriate diet
- consume adequate calories daily
- maintain his weight.

Fluid volume excess related to compromised renal regulatory mechanisms. Based on this nursing diagnosis, you'll establish these patient outcomes. The patient will:

- maintain fluid intake equal to urine output
- communicate understanding of limiting fluids and sodium intake
- not exhibit signs of fluid overload (elevated blood pressure, CHF, and edema).

Impaired verbal communication related to tongue involvement. Based on this nursing diagnosis, you'll establish these patient outcomes. The patient will:

- communicate needs and desires without undue frustration
- use alternative means of communication when necessary
- use appropriate resources to maximize communication skills.

Nursing interventions

- Maintain the patient's nutrition and fluid balance; give analgesics to relieve pain; control constipation or diarrhea.
- Provide good mouth care for the patient with tongue involvement. If needed, refer him for speech therapy, provide an alternate method of communication, and alert the staff to his communication problem.
- When tongue involvement is present, provide gentle and adequate suctioning as indicated to prevent respiratory compromise. Keep a tracheostomy tray at the patient's bedside.
- When long-term bed rest is necessary, properly position the patient and turn him often to prevent pressure ulcers. Perform range-of-motion exercises to prevent contractures.
- Provide supportive measures, such as assistance with general hygiene and comfort, when skin lesions are present.
- Provide a safe environment to prevent injury. Be sure to test heating pads and bath water for the patient with sensory impairment.
- Provide psychological support. Exercise patience and understanding to help the patient cope with this chronic illness. Encourage the patient to use available support systems.

Monitoring

- Assess the patient's airway patency if his tongue is involved.
- Closely observe the patient for signs and symptoms of CHF (jugular vein distention, peripheral edema, crackles, dyspnea, and oliguria) and other complications associated with amyloidosis.
- Monitor electrolyte levels and coagulation studies.

Patient teaching

- Instruct the patient to move slowly when changing positions from lying or sitting to standing.
- Make sure the patient understands his medication regimen, including the names of prescribed drugs, their actions, dosages, and adverse effects.
- Teach the patient to recognize the signs and symptoms of CHF and renal failure. Tell him when to notify the doctor.

Amyotrophic lateral sclerosis

Also known as Lou Gehrig's disease (after a well-known baseball player who died of it in 1941), this disease is the most common motor neuron disease of muscular atrophy. Amyotrophic lateral sclerosis (ALS) is a chronic, progressive, and debilitating disease that is invariably fatal. It's characterized by progressive degeneration of the anterior horn cells of the spinal cord and cranial nerves and of the motor nuclei in the cerebral cortex and corticospinal tracts.

Generally, ALS affects people ages 40 to 70. Most patients with ALS succumb within 3 to 5 years, but some may live as long as 15 years. Death usually results from a complication, such as aspiration pneumonia or respiratory failure.

Reportedly, more than 30,000 Americans have ALS; about 5,000 more are newly diagnosed each year. ALS is about three times more common in men than in women.

Causes

The exact cause of ALS is unknown, but about 10% of ALS patients inherit the disease as an autosomal dominant trait. ALS may also be caused by a virus that creates metabolic disturbances in motor neurons or by immune complexes, such as those formed in autoimmune disorders.

Precipitating factors that can cause acute deterioration include severe stress, such as myocardial infarction, traumatic injury, viral infections, and physical exhaustion.

Complications

Common complications of ALS include respiratory tract infections such as pneumonia, respiratory failure, and aspiration; complications of physical immobility include pressure ulcers and contractures.

Assessment

Signs and symptoms of ALS depend on the location of the affected motor neurons and the severity of the disease. Keep in mind that muscle weakness, atrophy, and fasciculations are the principal symptoms of the disorder; that the disease may begin in any muscle group; and that eventually, all muscle groups become involved. Unlike other degenerative disorders, such as Alzheimer's disease, ALS doesn't affect mental function.

The patient's history may reveal other family members with ALS if the problem was inherited. In the early disease stages, the patient may report asymmetrical weakness first noticed in one limb. He also usually reports fatigue and easy cramping in the affected muscles. Inspection may reveal fasciculations in the affected muscles if these muscles are not concealed by adipose tissue and muscle atrophy. Fasciculations and atrophy are most obvious in the feet and hands.

As the disease progresses, the patient may report progressive weakness in muscles of the arms, legs, and trunk. Inspection reveals atrophy and fasciculations. Neurologic examination often reveals brisk and overactive stretch reflexes. Muscle strength tests confirm the reported muscle weakness.

When the disease progresses to involve the brain stem and the cranial nerves, the patient has difficulty talking, chewing, swallowing and, ultimately, breathing. In these patients, auscultation may reveal decreased breath sounds.

In some patients (about 25%), muscle weakness begins in the musculature supplied by the cranial nerves. When this occurs, initial patient history reveals difficulty talking, swallowing, and breathing. Occasionally, the patient may report choking. Inspection may reveal some shortness of breath and, occasionally, drooling.

Diagnostic tests

Although no diagnostic tests are specific to this disease, the following tests may aid in its diagnosis:

- *Electromyography* may show abnormalities of electrical activity of involved muscles.
- *Muscle biopsy* may disclose atrophic fibers interspersed among normal fibers.
- *Nerve conduction studies* are usually normal.
- *Cerebrospinal fluid analysis* reveals increased protein content in one-third of patients.
- *Computed tomography scan* and *EEG* may help rule out other disorders, including multiple sclerosis, spinal cord neoplasms, myasthenia gravis, and progressive muscular dystrophy.

Treatment

ALS has no cure. Treatment, which is supportive and based on the patient's symptoms, may include diazepam for spasticity and quinine for relief of painful muscle cramps that occur in some patients. I.V. or intrathecal administration of thyrotropin-releasing hormone temporarily improves motor function in some patients but has no long-term benefits. Riluzole (Rilutek) has been approved for use with ALS because it can increase the time the patient is able to remain ventilator free. Rehabilitative measures can help patients function effectively for a longer period, and mechanical ventilation can lengthen survival.

Key nursing diagnoses and patient outcomes

Anticipatory grieving related to the progression and ultimately fatal outcome of ALS. Based on this nursing diagnosis, you'll establish these patient outcomes. The patient will:

- express his feelings about the changes in his life resulting from ALS and future losses he will need to face
- accept feelings and behavior caused by these changes in his life
- use appropriate coping mechanisms to deal with his grief.

Impaired home maintenance management related to fatigue and loss of muscle strength to perform activities of daily living. Based on this nursing diagnosis, you'll establish these patient outcomes. The patient will:

- express his need to make home adjustments to perform activities of daily living
- identify and contact individuals or organizations to provide home assistance.

Impaired physical mobility related to progressive deterioration of the nervous system. Based on this nursing diagnosis, you'll establish these patient outcomes. The patient will:

- attain the highest degree of mobility possible, such as ambulating with assistive devices
- show no evidence of complications related to impairment of physical mobility, such as contractures or skin breakdown.

The patient or caregiver will:

- carry out the mobility regimen consistently.

Nursing interventions

- Provide emotional and psychological support to the patient and his family. Stay with the patient during periods of severe stress and anxiety. Keep in mind that because mental status remains intact while progressive physical degeneration takes place, the patient acutely perceives every change in his condition.
- Implement a rehabilitation program to help the patient maintain his independence as long as possible.
- Have the patient perform active exercises and range-of-motion exercises on unaffected muscles to help strengthen them. Stretching exercises are also helpful.
- Depending on the patient's muscular capacity, assist with bathing, personal hygiene, and transfers from wheelchair to bed. Help establish a regular bowel and bladder elimination routine.
- To prevent skin breakdown, provide good skin care when the patient's mobility decreases. Turn him often, keep his skin clean and dry, and use pressure-reducing devices, such as an alternating air mattress.
- Help the patient obtain equipment, such as a walker or a wheelchair, when this becomes necessary.
- If the patient can't talk, provide an alternate means of communication, such as message boards, eye blinks for yes and no, or a computer.
- Administer ordered medications as necessary to relieve the patient's symptoms. Crush tablets and mix them with semisolid food for the patient who has dysphagia.
- Have the patient who has breathing difficulty perform deep-breathing and coughing exercises. Suctioning, chest physiotherapy, and incentive spirometry can also prove helpful.
- If the patient chooses to use mechanical ventilation to assist his breathing, provide necessary care.
- If the patient has trouble swallowing, give him soft, semisolid foods and position him upright during meals. Have suctioning equipment available to prevent aspiration. Use a soft cervical collar to help the patient hold his head upright if he has difficulty doing so. Gastrostomy and nasogastric tube feedings may be necessary if he can no longer swallow.

Monitoring

• Evaluate the patient's neuromuscular function regularly to assess progression of deterioration.
• Frequently assess the patient's respiratory status to detect breathing difficulty.
• Carefully assess the patient with respiratory involvement for infection because respiratory complications may be fatal.
• Monitor the patient's nutritional intake for evidence of malnourishment.
• Inspect the patient's skin regularly for evidence of breakdown.

Patient teaching

• Teach the patient and his family about ALS and expected signs and symptoms. Be sure they understand that this is a progressive, incurable disease. However, explain to the patient that treatments can make him more comfortable and help him stay independent as long as possible.
• Teach the patient who has difficulty chewing to cut his food into smaller pieces or to use a blender or food processor to mince food. Suggest adding baby cereal to minced foods to help thicken them.
• Caution the patient against eating foods that stick in the mouth, such as peanut butter and chocolate. If the patient has drooling problems, suggest that he avoid foods such as grapefruit and fluids such as milk; these increase salivation.
• Teach the family how to administer gastrostomy feedings if these become necessary.
• To help the patient handle increased accumulation of secretions and dysphagia, teach him to suction himself. He should have a suction machine handy at home to reduce fear of choking.
• As the patient's condition deteriorates, teach the family how to perform comfort measures and help the patient through this difficult period.
• Refer the patient and family to the social service department. If appropriate, arrange for a home health care nurse to oversee the patient's status to provide support and to continue teaching the family about the illness.
• Prepare the patient and his family for his eventual death, and assist them in the grieving process. Patients with ALS may benefit from a hospice program or the local chapter of an ALS support group such as the Amyotrophic Lateral Sclerosis Association.

Anaphylaxis

A dramatic, acute atopic reaction, anaphylaxis is marked by the sudden onset of rapidly progressive urticaria and respiratory distress. A severe reaction may initiate vascular collapse, leading to systemic shock and possibly death.

Causes

Anaphylactic reactions result from systemic exposure to sensitizing drugs or other specific antigens. Such substances may be serums (usually horse serum), vaccines, allergen extracts (such as pollen), enzymes (L-asparaginase), hormones, penicillin and other antibiotics, sulfonamides, local anesthetics, salicylates, polysaccharides (such as iron dextran), diagnostic chemicals (sodium dehydrocholate, radiographic contrast media), foods (legumes, nuts, berries, seafood, egg albumin) and sulfite-containing food additives, insect venom (honeybees, wasps, hornets, yellow jackets, fire ants, and certain spiders) and, rarely, a ruptured hydatid cyst.

The most common anaphylaxis-causing antigen is penicillin. This drug induces a reaction in 1 to 4 of every 10,000 patients treated with it. Penicillin is most likely to induce anaphylaxis after parenteral administration or prolonged therapy.

After initial exposure to an antigen, the immune system responds by producing specific immunoglobulin (Ig) antibodies in the lymph nodes. Helper T cells enhance the process. These antibodies (IgE) then bind to membrane receptors located on mast cells (found throughout connective tissue) and basophils.

Once the body reencounters the antigen, the IgE antibodies, or cross-linked IgE receptors, recognize the antigen as foreign. This activates a series of cellular reactions that, if left unchecked, will lead to rapid vascular collapse and, ultimately, hemorrhage, disseminated intravascular coagulation, and cardiopulmonary arrest.

Complications

Untreated anaphylaxis causes respiratory obstruction, systemic vascular collapse, and death minutes to hours after the first symptoms (although a delayed or persistent reaction may occur for as long as 24 hours).

Assessment

The patient, a relative, or another responsible person will report the patient's exposure to an antigen. Immediately after exposure, the patient may complain of a feeling of impending doom or fright, weakness, sweating, sneezing, dyspnea, nasal pruritus, and urticaria. He may impress you as extremely anxious. Keep in mind that the sooner signs and symptoms begin after exposure to the antigen, the more severe the anaphylaxis.

On inspection, the patient's skin may display well-circumscribed, discrete cutaneous wheals with erythematous, raised, serpiginous borders and blanched centers. They may coalesce to form giant hives.

Angioedema may cause the patient to complain of a "lump" in his throat, or you may hear hoarseness or stridor. Wheezing, dyspnea, and complaints of chest tightness suggest bronchial obstruction. These are early signs of impending, potentially fatal respiratory failure.

Other effects may follow rapidly. The patient may report GI and genitourinary effects, including severe stomach cramps, nausea, diarrhea, and urinary urgency and incontinence. Neurologic effects include dizziness, drowsiness, headache, restlessness, and seizures. Cardiovascular effects include hypotension, shock, and cardiac arrhythmias, which may precipitate vascular collapse if untreated.

NURSING ALERT

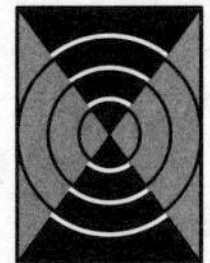

Aminophylline precaution

Be aware that rapid infusion of aminophylline may cause or aggravate severe hypotension in a patient experiencing an allergic reaction. If aminophylline must be used, administer the drug under the direct supervision of a doctor and monitor the patient's blood pressure continuously. Have emergency equipment close by.

Diagnostic tests

No tests are required to identify anaphylaxis. The patient's history and signs and symptoms establish the diagnosis. If signs and symptoms occur without a known allergic stimulus, other possible causes of shock, such as acute myocardial infarction, status asthmaticus, or congestive heart failure, must be ruled out.

Skin testing may help to identify a specific allergen. However, because skin tests can cause serious reactions, a scratch test should be done first in high-risk situations.

Treatment

Always an emergency, anaphylaxis requires an *immediate* injection of epinephrine 1:1,000 aqueous solution, 0.1 to 0.5 ml for mild signs and symptoms. If signs and symptoms are severe, repeat the dose every 5 to 20 minutes, as directed.

In the early stages of anaphylaxis, when the patient remains conscious and normotensive, give epinephrine I.M. or subcuta-

HEALTH PROMOTION POINTERS

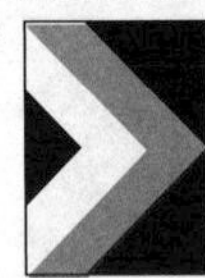

Preventing anaphylaxis

Experiencing an anaphylactic reaction can be extremely upsetting to the patient. To ease his anxiety and help prevent a future episode, instruct the patient to avoid exposure to known allergens, such as foods, drugs, and insects.

- Tell the patient not to consume the offending item in any combination or form; caution him to read food labels before purchasing and to check with restaurant personnel about the contents of menu items before ordering.
- Advise the patient to avoid insect stings by not wearing scented colognes or deodorants and by staying away from open fields and wooded areas during the insect season.
- Recommend that he carry an anaphylaxis kit whenever he's outdoors; ensure that he knows how and when to use it.
- Tell the patient to always wear medical identification naming his allergies.

neously. Speed it into circulation by massaging the injection site. In severe reactions, when the patient is unconscious and hypotensive, give the drug I.V., as ordered.

Establish and maintain a patent airway. Watch for early signs of laryngeal edema (stridor, hoarseness, and dyspnea), which may require endotracheal tube insertion or a tracheotomy and oxygen therapy.

If cardiac arrest occurs, begin cardiopulmonary resuscitation. Assist with ventilation, closed-chest cardiac massage, and sodium bicarbonate administration as ordered.

Watch for hypotension and shock. As ordered, maintain circulatory volume with volume expanders (plasma, plasma expanders, 0.9% sodium chloride solution, and albumin) as needed. As ordered, administer I.V. vasopressors, norepinephrine, and dopamine to stabilize blood pressure. Monitor blood pressure, central venous pressure, and urine output.

Key nursing diagnoses and patient outcomes

Anxiety related to the rapid deterioration in body function and a feeling of impending doom. Based on this nursing diagnosis, you'll establish these patient outcomes. The patient will:

- express feelings of anxiety
- show fewer physical symptoms of anxiety following reassurance and support from medical staff and treatment of anaphylaxis.

Decreased cardiac output related to shock, hypotension, and vascular collapse. Based on this nursing diagnosis, you'll establish these patient outcomes. The patient will:

- attain hemodynamic stability, evidenced by normal vital signs and relief of anaphylactic signs and symptoms
- not exhibit cardiac arrhythmias
- recover normal cardiac output.

Risk for suffocation related to swelling and edema in respiratory tract caused by anaphylaxis. Based on this nursing diagnosis, you'll establish these patient outcomes. The patient will:

- maintain adequate ventilation
- experience relief of respiratory symptoms, indicating that respiratory tissues have returned to normal
- identify (or try to) the offending allergen that precipitated anaphylaxis and take steps to prevent future anaphylactic episodes.

Nursing interventions

- Provide supplemental oxygen, and observe. If hypoxia continues, prepare to help insert an artificial airway.
- Insert a peripheral I.V. line for giving emergency drugs and volume expanders.
- After the initial emergency, administer other ordered medications: subcutaneous epinephrine, longer-acting epinephrine, cor-

ticosteroids, and diphenhydramine I.V. for urticaria; aminophylline I.V. for bronchospasm. (See *Aminophylline precaution.*)

- Continually reassure the patient, and explain all tests and treatments to reduce fear and anxiety. If necessary, reorient the patient to the situation and surroundings.
- If the patient undergoes skin or scratch testing, keep emergency resuscitation equipment nearby during and after the test.
- If the patient must receive a drug to which he's allergic, prevent a severe reaction by making sure he receives careful desensitization with gradually increasing doses of the antigen or with advance administration of corticosteroids. A person with a history of allergies should receive a drug with high anaphylactic potential only after cautious pretesting for sensitivity. Be sure you have resuscitation equipment and epinephrine on hand. When a patient takes a drug with high anaphylactic potential (particularly parenteral drugs), make sure he receives close medical observation.

Monitoring

- Continously assess the patient's response to treatment. Monitor his vital signs and cardiopulmonary and neurologic function. Look for complications associated with anaphylaxis, such as vascular collapse and acute respiratory insufficiency or obstruction.
- Closely observe a patient with known allergies for anaphylaxis when giving a drug with high anaphylactic potential.
- Watch for indications of serious allergic response in patients undergoing skin or scratch tests or diagnostic procedures that use radiographic contrast media, such as excretory urography, cardiac catheterization, and angiography. Notify the doctor immediately if you detect allergic signs and symptoms followed by itchy, red skin; wheals; and swelling.

Patient teaching

Help the patient avoid another allergic reaction. (See *Preventing anaphylaxis.*)

Angioplasty, percutaneous transluminal coronary

Used to treat coronary artery disease, percutaneous transluminal coronary angioplasty (PTCA) offers some patients a nonsurgical alternative to coronary artery bypass surgery. In PTCA, a tiny balloon catheter is used to dilate a coronary artery that's been narrowed by atherosclerotic plaque.

With PTCA, hospitalization usually lasts 1 to 2 days, compared with a typical 5- to 7-day stay for coronary artery bypass. The patient is usually ambulatory within a day after PTCA and can often return to work within a few weeks. Another advantage of PTCA is that it's much less costly than coronary artery bypass.

However, PTCA is an option for only a select group of patients. Usually it's indicated for patients who have myocardial ischemia documented by an electrocardiogram (ECG) or thallium scan and a lesion in the proximal portion of a single coronary artery. Recently, however, patients with multivessel disease, totally occluded coronary arteries, or acute myocardial infarction have undergone successful PTCA. In addition, patients who have had previous coronary artery bypass surgery, postthrombolytic therapy with high-grade stenosis, or who are at high risk for complications associated with coronary artery bypass surgery may be candidates for PTCA. However, patients undergoing PTCA must also be acceptable candidates for coronary artery bypass surgery in case PTCA is not successful and emergency coronary artery bypass surgery becomes necessary. Emergency coronary artery bypass surgery occurs in about 6% of PTCA patients.

PTCA is most successful when lesions are noncalcified, concentric, discrete, and smoothly tapered. Patients with a history of less than 1 year of disabling angina are preferred because their lesions tend to be softer and more compressive.

Procedure

Although PTCA is performed in the cardiac catheterization laboratory, a surgical team must stand by during the procedure in case emergency coronary artery bypass is required. Coronary arteriography is usually performed to compare the size and exact location of the lesion to previous films. As a precautionary measure, temporary pacemaker wires are inserted in case transient heart block occurs during the procedure.

After preparing and anesthetizing the catheter insertion site, the surgeon inserts a guide wire into the femoral artery by a percutaneous approach (other sites, such as the brachial artery with a cutdown approach, may be used instead). The surgeon threads the catheter into the coronary artery with the help of fluoroscopy and confirms the presence of the lesion by angiography.

Next, the surgeon introduces a small double-lumen balloon-tipped catheter through the guide wire, positions it, and repeatedly inflates the balloon with a solution of 0.9% sodium chloride and contrast medium for about 15 to 30 seconds to a pressure of 6 atmospheres. The duration of inflation and the amount of pressure used may vary, depending on the severity of the patient's symptoms and myocardial ischemia. The expanding balloon compresses the atherosclerotic plaque against the arterial wall, expanding the arterial lumen.

Quantitative measurements of the procedure's success are derived from pressure gradient measurements across the stenotic area of the artery. The balloon can be inflated repeatedly until the residual gradient decreases to about 20% or until the pressure gradient is less than 16 mm Hg. The surgeon then performs a repeat angiogram.

After completing the procedure, the surgeon leaves the catheter in place to provide access in case coronary artery occlusion develops. Afterward, the patient is returned to the intensive care unit or postanesthesia room for monitoring.

Complications

Although PTCA avoids many surgical risks, it can cause serious complications. The most dangerous, arterial dissection during dilatation, can lead to coronary artery rupture, cardiac tamponade, myocardial ischemia or infarction, or death. Another life-threatening complication is abrupt reclosure of the coronary artery. (See *Responding to abrupt reclosure of the coronary artery.*)

Other complications include myocardial infarction, closure of a side branch of a coronary artery, coronary artery spasm, decreased coronary artery blood flow, allergic reactions to contrast medium, and arrhythmias during catheter manipulation. Infrequently, thrombi may embolize, causing a cerebrovascular accident.

Key nursing diagnoses and patient outcomes

Anxiety related to seriousness of the procedure and potential complications. Based on this nursing diagnosis, you'll establish these patient outcomes. The patient will:
- express feelings of anxiety
- use support systems to assist with coping
- demonstrate diminished physical symptoms of anxiety.

Fluid volume deficit related to bleeding at the catheterization site. Based on this nursing diagnosis, you'll establish these patient outcomes. The patient will:
- maintain adequate fluid volume
- demonstrate minimal bleeding at the catheterization site
- not exhibit signs and symptoms of dehydration, such as dry mucous membranes, excessive thirst, or decreased urine output.

Pain related to potential for abrupt reclosure of the coronary artery. Based on

LIFE-THREATENING COMPLICATIONS

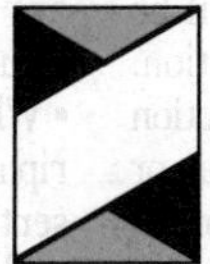

Responding to abrupt reclosure of the coronary artery

About 4% of patients undergoing PTCA will experience abrupt reclosure of the coronary artery, a life-threatening complication, within a few hours after the procedure. Risk factors for abrupt reclosure include:

- coronary artery stenosis length greater than twice the lumen diameter
- stenosis at a blood vessel bend of 45 degrees or more
- stenosis at a branching point
- stenosis-associated thrombus or filling defect
- other stenoses in the vessel undergoing dilatation
- multivessel disease.

In about 50% of patients, the blood vessels that close can be reopened by repeating the procedure; the remaining patients will require emergency coronary artery bypass surgery. Abrupt closure is precipitated by local vasospasm, extensive dissection, or thrombus formation.

Signs and symptoms

Chest pain is a cardinal symptom of abrupt coronary artery closure. You'll also note signs and symptoms of myocardial infarction, such as diaphoresis, tachycardia, and anxiety. An ECG will reveal changes in ST and T waves indicative of myocardial injury.

Emergency interventions

- Notify the doctor immediately.
- Prepare the patient for repeat PTCA and possibly coronary artery bypass surgery.
- Monitor vital signs closely.
- Watch the patient for signs of left ventricular failure, such as hypotension, decreased peripheral perfusion, distended neck veins, edema, and crackles.
- Anticipate the possibility that a fibrinogen-sparing thrombolytic agent may be ordered.

this nursing diagnosis, you'll establish these patient outcomes. The patient will:

- not develop sudden angina-like pain
- not show changes on his ECG indicative of myocardial ischemia
- not exhibit signs and symptoms of abrupt reclosure, such as diaphoresis, tachycardia, chest pain, and anxiety.

Nursing interventions

When PTCA is indicated, your major goals are to prepare the patient for the procedure, monitor his condition afterward, and provide home care instructions.

Before the procedure

- Prepare the patient for PTCA by reinforcing the doctor's explanation of the procedure, including its risks and alternatives. Tell him that a catheter will be inserted into an artery in the groin area and that he may feel pressure as the catheter moves along the vessel. Also explain that he'll be awake during the procedure and may be asked to take deep breaths to allow visualization of the radiopaque balloon catheter. He may also have to answer questions about how he's feeling and will have to notify the cardiologist if he experiences any angina. Advise him that the entire procedure lasts from 1 to 4 hours and that he'll lie flat on a hard table during that time.

• Explain that a contrast medium will be injected to outline the lesion's location. Warn the patient that during the injection he may feel a hot, flushing sensation or transient nausea. Check his history for allergies; if he's had allergic reactions to shellfish, iodine, or contrast medium, notify the doctor.
• Tell the patient that an I.V. line will be inserted. Explain that the groin area of both legs will be shaved and cleaned with an antiseptic and that he'll experience a brief stinging sensation when a local anesthetic is injected.
• Restrict the patient's food and fluid intake for at least 6 hours before the procedure or as ordered. Ensure that coagulation studies, complete blood count, serum electrolyte studies, and blood typing and crossmatching have been performed. Also, palpate the bilateral distal pulses (usually the dorsalis pedis or posterior tibial pulses) and mark them with an indelible marker to help you locate them later.
• Take the patient's vital signs and assess the color, temperature, and sensation in his extremities to serve as a baseline for posttreatment assessment. Before the patient goes to the catheterization laboratory, sedate him as ordered and put a 5-lb (2.2-kg) sandbag on the bed to be used later for applying direct pressure on the arterial puncture site.

After the procedure

• When the patient returns from the cardiac catheterization laboratory, he'll be receiving I.V. heparin and nitroglycerin. He'll require continuous arterial and ECG monitoring.
• To prevent excessive hip flexion and migration of the catheter, keep the patient's leg straight and elevate the head of the bed no more than 15 degrees; at mealtimes, elevate the head of the bed 15 to 30 degrees.
• Monitor vital signs every 15 mintues for the first hour after the procedure, then every 30 minutes for 2 hours, and then hourly for the next 5 hours. If vital signs are unstable, notify the doctor and continue to check them every 5 minutes.
• When you take vital signs, assess the peripheral pulses distal to the catheter insertion site and the color, temperature, and capillary refill time of the extremity. If pulses are difficult to palpate because of the size of the arterial catheter, use a Doppler stethoscope to hear them. Notify the doctor if pulses are absent.
• Assess the catheter insertion site for hematoma formation, ecchymosis, or hemorrhage. If an expanding ecchymotic area appears, mark the area to determine the rapidity of expansion and obtain a blood sample for a hemoglobin and hematocrit analysis, as ordered. If bleeding occurs, apply direct pressure and notify the doctor.
• Monitor cardiac rate and rhythm continuously, and notify the doctor of any changes or if the patient reports chest pain; it may signal vasospasm or coronary occlusion.
• Give I.V. fluids at a rate of at least 100 ml/hour to promote excretion of the contrast medium, but be sure to assess the patient for signs of fluid overload (distended neck veins, atrial and ventricular gallops, dyspnea, pulmonary congestion, tachycardia, hypertension, and hypoxemia).
• The arterial catheter will be removed about 18 hours after the procedure. Afterward, apply direct pressure over the insertion site for at least 30 minutes. Then apply a pressure dressing, and assess the patient's vital signs according to the same schedule you used when he first returned to the unit.

Home care instructions

• Instruct the patient to call his doctor if he experiences any bleeding or bruising at the arterial puncture site.
• Explain the necessity of taking all prescribed medications, and ensure that the patient understands their intended effects.

- Tell the patient that he can resume normal activity. Most patients experience an increased exercise tolerance.
- Instruct the patient to return for a stress thallium imaging test and follow-up angiography, as recommended by his doctor.

Ankylosing spondylitis

Also called rheumatoid spondylitis or Marie-Strümpell disease, ankylosing spondylitis primarily affects the sacroiliac, the axial spine, and the adjacent ligamentous or tendinous attachments to the bone.

Typically beginning in adults before age 40, this inflammatory disease progressively restricts spinal movement. It begins in the sacroiliac and gradually progresses to the lumbar, thoracic, and cervical spine. Bone and cartilage deterioration leads to fibrous tissue formation and eventual fusion of the spine or the peripheral joints. Symptoms progress unpredictably into remission, exacerbation, or arrest at any stage.

Ankylosing spondylitis usually occurs as a primary disorder, but it also may occur secondary to various GI, genitourinary (GU), and cutaneous disorders. For example, with GI disease, ankylosing spondylitis may occur in association with ulcerative colitis, regional enteritis, Whipple's disease, gram-negative dysentery, and yersiniosis. With GU disease, it's associated with chlamydial or mycoplasmic infections, and with cutaneous disease, it's associated with psoriasis, acne conglobata, and hidradenitis suppurativa.

In primary disease, sacroiliitis is usually bilateral and symmetrical; in secondary disease, it's usually unilateral and asymmetrical. The patient may also have extra-articular disease, such as acute anterior iritis (in about 25% of patients), proximal root aortitis and heart block, and apical pulmonary fibrosis. Rarely, extra-articular disease appears as caudal adhesive leptomeningitis and immunoglobulin A (IgA) nephropathy.

Ankylosing spondylitis affects men three to four times more often than women. Progressive disease is well recognized in men but often overlooked or missed in women, who tend to have more peripheral joint involvement.

Causes

Studies suggest a familial tendency for ankylosing spondylitis; however, the exact cause of the disease is unknown. In more than 90% of the patients with this disease, circulating immune complexes and human leukocyte-histocompatibility antigen (HLA-B27) suggest immune system activity.

Complications

Rarely, disease progression can impose severe physical restrictions on activities of daily living and occupational functions. Atlantoaxial subluxation is a rare complication of primary ankylosing spondylitis.

Assessment

Varying assessment findings depend on the disease stage. The patient may first complain of intermittent low back pain that's most severe in the morning or after inactivity and is relieved by exercise. He may also report mild fatigue, fever, anorexia, and weight loss. If he has symmetrical or asymmetrical peripheral arthritis, he may describe pain in his shoulders, hips, knees, and ankles.

The patient may also complain of pain over the symphysis pubis, which may lead to ankylosing spondylitis being mistaken for pelvic inflammatory disease.

Observe the patient's movements. Note stiffness or limited motion of the lumbar spine; pain and limited expansion of the chest, resulting from costovertebral and sternomanubrial joint involvement; and limited range of motion, resulting from hip deformity.

Diagnosing primary ankylosing spondylitis

The following are the diagnostic criteria for primary ankylosing spondylitis. For a reliable diagnosis, the patient must meet the following:
- criterion 7 and any one of criteria 1 through 5 *or*
- any five of criteria 1 through 6 if he doesn't have criterion 7.

Seven criteria

1. Axial skeleton stiffness of at least 3 months' duration relieved by exercise
2. Lumbar pain that persists at rest
3. Thoracic cage pain of at least 3 months' duration that persists at rest
4. Past or current iritis
5. Decreased lumbar range of motion
6. Decreased chest expansion (age-related)
7. Bilateral, symmetrical sacroiliitis demonstrated by radiographic studies

Inspect the spine. In advanced disease, you'll see kyphosis (caused by chronic stooping to relieve discomfort). Inspect the eyes for redness and inflammation resulting from iritis.

Palpate the affected joints. In particular, note any warmth, swelling, or tenderness.

Auscultate the heart and listen for an aortic murmur caused by regurgitation and cardiomegaly. Also auscultate the lungs. When present, upper lobe pulmonary fibrosis, which mimics tuberculosis, may reduce vital capacity to 70% or less of predicted volume.

Diagnostic tests

Diagnosis of primary ankylosing spondylitis requires meeting established criteria. (See *Diagnosing primary ankylosing spondylitis.*) Laboratory tests never confirm the diagnosis; however, the following findings may support the diagnosis:
- *Serum findings* include HLA-B27 in about 95% of patients with primary ankylosing spondylitis and up to 80% of patients with secondary disease. The absence of rheumatoid factor helps to rule out rheumatoid arthritis, which produces similar symptoms.
- *Erythrocyte sedimentation rate* and *alkaline phosphatase* and *creatine phosphokinase levels* may be slightly elevated in active disease.
- *Serum IgA levels* may be elevated.
- *X-ray studies* define characteristic changes in ankylosing spondylitis. However, these changes may not appear for up to 3 years after the disease's onset. They include bilateral sacroiliac involvement (the hallmark of the disease); blurring of the joints' bony margins in early disease; patchy sclerosis with superficial bony erosions; eventual squaring of vertebral bodies; and "bamboo spine" with complete ankylosis.

Treatment

Because no treatment reliably stops disease progression, management aims to delay further deformity by good posture, stretching and deep-breathing exercises and, if appropriate, braces and lightweight supports. Heat, ice, and nerve stimulation measures may relieve symptoms in some patients. Nonsteroidal anti-inflammatory drugs, such as aspirin, indomethacin, and sulindac, control pain and inflammation.

Severe hip involvement, which affects about 15% of patients, usually necessitates hip replacement surgery. Severe spinal involvement may require a spinal wedge osteotomy to separate and reposition the vertebrae. Usually, this surgery is reserved for selected patients because of possible spinal cord damage and a lengthy convalescence.

Key nursing diagnoses and patient outcomes

Activity intolerance related to fatigue and pain. Based on this nursing diagnosis,

you'll establish these patient outcomes. The patient will:
• maintain muscle strength and joint range of motion
• perform self-care activities to tolerance level
• adopt life-style changes that minimize pain and fatigue while increasing activity level.

Impaired physical mobility related to spinal or hip joint deformities. Based on this nursing diagnosis, you'll establish these patient outcomes. The patient will:
• attain the greatest degree of mobility possible within disease limitations
• begin to accept limitations imposed by deformity and life-style changes
• not show evidence of contractures, venous stasis, thrombus formation, skin breakdown, hypostatic pneumonia, or other complications of impaired mobility.

Pain related to effects of ankylosing spondylitis on the spinal column, joints, or both. Based on this nursing diagnosis, you'll establish these patient outcomes. The patient will:
• follow a pain management program that includes an activity and rest schedule, exercise program, and medication regimen that's not pain contingent
• obtain pain relief from analgesics
• avoid activities that cause pain.

Nursing interventions

• Keep in mind the patient's limited range of motion when planning self-care tasks and activities.
• Offer support and reassurance.
• Give analgesics as ordered.
• Apply heat locally and massage as indicated. Assess mobility and comfort levels frequently.
• Have the patient perform active range-of-motion exercises to prevent restricted, painful movement.
• Pace periods of exercise and rest to help the patient achieve comfortable energy levels and oxygenation of lungs.
• If treatment includes surgery, ensure proper body alignment and positioning.
• Because ankylosing spondylitis is a chronic, progressively crippling condition, you'll need to involve other caregivers, such as a social worker, a visiting nurse, and a dietitian.

Monitoring

• Regularly evaluate the patient's degree of mobility to detect deterioration.
• Monitor the patient's cardiopulmonary status to detect changes that may indicate cardiomegaly or pulmonary fibrosis.

Patient teaching

• To minimize deformities, advise the patient to avoid any physical activity that places stress on the back, such as lifting heavy objects.
• Teach the patient to stand upright; to sit upright in a high, straight-backed chair; and to avoid leaning over a desk.
• Instruct him to sleep in a prone position on a hard mattress and to avoid using pillows under the neck or knees.
• Advise the patient to avoid prolonged walking, standing, sitting, or driving; to perform regular stretching and deep-breathing exercises; and to swim regularly, if possible.
• Instruct the patient to have his height measured every 3 to 4 months to detect kyphosis.
• Suggest that he seek vocational counseling if work requires standing or prolonged sitting at a desk.
• Tell the patient to contact the local arthritis agency or the Ankylosing Spondylitis Association for additional information and support.

Anorectal abscess and fistula

A localized infection, anorectal abscess appears as a collection of pus due to inflammation of the soft tissue. As the abscess produces more pus, a fistula may form, creating an abnormal opening in the anal skin.

A fistula usually forms in the soft tissue beneath the muscle fibers of the sphincters (especially the external sphincter), extending into the perianal skin. The internal (primary) opening of the abscess or fistula is usually near the anal glands and crypts; the external (secondary) opening, in the perianal skin. In severe cases, this opening may communicate with the rectum.

Causes

The inflammatory process that leads to abscess may begin with an abrasion or tear in the lining of the anal canal, rectum, or perianal skin and subsequent infection with *Escherichia coli,* staphylococci, or streptococci. Such trauma may result from abrasive contact with certain objects, such as enema tips, ingested eggshells, fishbones, or very hard stools. An abscess may also develop after infection of submucosal hematomas, sclerosed hemorrhoids, or anal fissures.

Other causes include obstruction of glands in the anal area, extension of cryptitis, infection in the apocrine glands, or folliculitis in the perianal region. Certain systemic illnesses also may lead to abscess formation, including ulcerative colitis and Crohn's disease.

Complications

Anorectal abscess may lead to anorectal fistula. Either disorder can cause perineal cellulitis, scar tissue formation, and anal stricture. Rarely, peritonitis develops from internal abscess rupture.

Assessment

Signs and symptoms depend on the severity of the infection and whether or not the abscess is a chronic condition. Assessment findings also vary according to the type of abscess.

Usually, the first symptom the patient reports is rectal pain, which he usually describes as throbbing. Occasionally, diarrhea precedes the onset of rectal pain. The patient may also state that he can't sit comfortably because of the development of a hard, painful lump on one side. With a perianal abscess, the patient may report that sitting or coughing increases his pain. A submucosal or high intermuscular abscess may cause a dull, aching pain in the rectum, whereas a pelvirectal abscess typically causes no pain.

If the anorectal abscess is a chronic condition, the patient may report discharge or bleeding and anal pruritus, although an ischiorectal abscess may not produce drainage and a pelvirectal abscess won't show any local anal or external rectal signs. If he also has an anal fistula, anal pruritus and purulent discharge are commonly reported.

Depending on the infection's severity, the patient may also complain of fever, chills, nausea, vomiting, and malaise.

Inspection may reveal an erythematous lump or swelling in the anal area. If the patient has a fistula, its external opening may be visible as a pink or red elevated discharging sinus or ulcer on the skin near the anus. Palpation usually reveals tenderness over the reddened or swollen area.

Expect assessment findings to vary when you perform a digital examination, depending on the type of anorectal abscess present. A perianal abscess usually reveals no abnormalities. If the patient has an ischiorectal abscess, you'll detect a tender induration bulging into the anal canal. With a submucosal or high intermuscular abscess, you'll feel a smooth swelling of the upper part of the anal canal or lower rectum. If he has a pelvirectal abscess, the examination will reveal a tender mass high in the pelvis, perhaps extending into one of the ischiorectal fossae. If a fistula is present, you may detect a palpable, indurated tract and a depression or ulcer in the midline anteriorly or at the dentate line posteriorly.

Diagnostic tests

Sigmoidoscopy, barium enema, and colonoscopy may be performed to rule out other conditions.

Treatment

Anorectal abscesses require surgical incision and drainage, usually under caudal anesthesia. Fistulas require fistulotomy – removal of the fistula and associated granulation tissue – under caudal anesthesia. If the fistula tract is epithelialized, treatment requires fistulectomy – removal of the fistulous tract – followed by insertion of drains, which remain in place for 48 hours. Fistulas that result from an intestinal disorder, such as Crohn's disease, are usually treated conservatively because surgery is often not successful.

Key nursing diagnoses and patient outcomes

Risk for infection related to normal intestinal flora containing bacteria causing a secondary infection. Based on this nursing diagnosis, you'll establish these patient outcomes. The patient will:

- remain free of a secondary infection
- demonstrate appropriate personal hygiene and take precautions to prevent an additional infection.

Impaired tissue integrity related to abscess and fistula formation caused by the anorectal infection. Based on this nursing diagnosis, you'll establish these patient outcomes. The patient will:

- exhibit complete healing of the infected area after surgery
- identify factors that increase the risk of anorectal abscess and fistula formation
- communicate understanding of preventive measures for anorectal abscess and fistula formation, such as maintaining perianal cleanliness and avoiding constipation.

Pain related to swelling and inflamed anal tissue caused by the anorectal abscess. Based on this nursing diagnosis, you'll establish these patient outcomes. The patient will:

- obtain pain relief from analgesics
- employ additional pain control measures, such as use of ice, sitz baths, or witch hazel compresses
- become pain free with appropriate therapy.

Nursing interventions

- Before surgery, apply ice and witch hazel soaks and provide sitz baths to help ease the patient's discomfort.
- After surgery, provide adequate medication for pain relief as ordered.
- Dispose of soiled dressings properly.
- Note the time of the first postoperative bowel movement. Anticipating pain, the patient may suppress the urge to defecate; the resulting constipation would increase pressure at the wound site. Such a patient benefits from a stool-softening laxative, such as psyllium, given as soon after surgery as tolerated.

Monitoring

- Examine the wound frequently to assess proper healing. Healing should be complete within 4 to 5 weeks for perianal fistulas and 12 to 16 weeks for deeper wounds.
- Monitor the patient for signs of infection after surgery, such as fever, purulent drainage from the incision, redness, and swelling.

Patient teaching

- Explain the disorder to the patient. If diagnostic tests are scheduled, review their purpose and required preparation and aftercare.

• Emphasize that complete recovery takes time. Offer encouragement.
• Teach the patient that a diet high in fiber and fluids promotes regular bowel movements, which helps to prevent irritation of an existing abscess. Explain that straining during a bowel movement can increase abscess discomfort.
• Stress the importance of perianal cleanliness at all times, especially after bowel movements or any contact with a foreign body. Tell the patient that good hygiene helps prevent infection.
• Provide appropriate preoperative teaching if surgery will be performed. Be sure the patient understands the procedure and its possible complications.
• After surgery, reinforce the importance of diet and perianal cleanliness. Teach the patient about prescribed medications, such as analgesics or stool softeners. Also show him how to perform sitz baths if these are ordered to promote comfort.

Aortic insufficiency

In this disorder (also called aortic regurgitation), blood flows back into the left ventricle during diastole. The ventricle becomes overloaded, dilated, and eventually hypertrophies. The excess fluid volume also overloads the left atrium and eventually the pulmonary system.

Aortic insufficiency by itself occurs most commonly among males. When associated with mitral valve disease, however, it's more common among females. This disorder also may be associated with Marfan syndrome, ankylosing spondylitis, syphilis, essential hypertension, and a ventricular septal defect, even after surgical closure.

Causes

Aortic insufficiency results from rheumatic fever, syphilis, hypertension, endocarditis, or trauma. In some patients, it may be idiopathic.

Complications

Left ventricular failure usually occurs. The patient may develop fatal pulmonary edema if a fever, infection, or cardiac arrhythmia develops. The patient also risks myocardial ischemia because left ventricular dilation and elevated left ventricular systolic pressure alter myocardial oxygen requirements.

Assessment

In chronic severe aortic insufficiency, the patient may complain that he has an uncomfortable awareness of his heartbeat, especially when lying down. He may report palpitations along with a pounding head.

Dyspnea may occur with exertion, and the patient may experience paroxysmal nocturnal dyspnea with diaphoresis, orthopnea, and cough. He may become fatigued and syncopal with exertion or emotion. He may also have a history of anginal chest pain unrelieved by sublingual nitroglycerin.

On inspection, you may note that each heartbeat seems to jar the patient's entire body and that his head bobs with each systole. Inspection of arterial pulsations shows a rapidly rising pulse that collapses suddenly as arterial pressure falls late in systole. This is called a water-hammer pulse.

The patient's nail beds may appear to be pulsating. If you apply pressure at the nail tip, the root will alternately flush and pale (called Quincke's sign). Inspection of the chest may reveal a visible apical impulse. In left ventricular failure, the patient may have ankle edema and ascites.

In palpating the peripheral pulses, you may note rapidly rising and collapsing pulses (pulsus biferiens). If the patient has cardiac arrhythmias, pulses may be irregular. You'll be able to feel the apical impulse. (The apex will be displaced laterally and inferiorly.) A diastolic thrill probably will be palpable along the left sternal border, and you may be able to feel a prominent systolic thrill in the jugular notch and along the carotid arteries.

Auscultation may reveal an S_3, occasionally an S_4, and a loud systolic ejection sound. A high-pitched, blowing, decrescendo diastolic murmur is best heard at the left sternal border, third intercostal space. Use the diaphragm of the stethoscope to hear it, and have the patient sit up, lean forward, and hold his breath in forced expiration.

You also may hear a midsystolic ejection murmur at the base of the heart. It may be a grade 5 or 6 and typically is higher pitched, shorter, and less rasping than the murmur heard in aortic stenosis. Another murmur that may occur is a soft, low-pitched, rumbling, middiastolic or presystolic bruit (Austin Flint murmur). This murmur is best heard at the base of the heart.

Place the stethoscope lightly over the femoral artery, and you'll notice a booming, pistol-shot sound and a to-and-fro murmur (Duroziez's sign). Arterial pulse pressure is widened. Auscultating blood pressure may be difficult because you can auscultate the patient's pulse without inflating the cuff. To determine systolic pressure, note when Korotkoff sounds begin to muffle.

Diagnostic tests

- *Cardiac catheterization* shows reduction in arterial diastolic pressures, aortic insufficiency, other valvular abnormalities, and increased left ventricular end-diastolic pressure.
- *Chest X-rays* display left ventricular enlargement and pulmonary vein congestion.
- *Echocardiography* reveals left ventricular enlargement, dilation of the aortic annulus and left atrium, and thickening of the aortic valve. It also shows a rapid, high-frequency fluttering of the anterior mitral leaflet that results from the impact of aortic regurgitation.
- *Electrocardiography (ECG)* shows sinus tachycardia, left ventricular hypertrophy, and left atrial hypertrophy in severe disease. ST-segment depressions and T-wave inversions appear in leads I, aV_L, V_5, and V_6 and indicate left ventricular strain.

Treatment

Valve replacement is the treatment of choice and should be performed before significant ventricular dysfunction occurs. This may not be possible, however, because signs and symptoms seldom occur until after myocardial dysfunction develops.

Digitalis glycosides, a low-sodium diet, diuretics, vasodilators, and especially angiotensin-converting enzyme inhibitors are used to treat left ventricular failure. In acute episodes, supplemental oxygen may be necessary.

Key nursing diagnoses and patient outcomes

Altered cardiopulmonary tissue perfusion related to left ventricular dilation and elevated left ventricular systolic pressure. Based on this nursing diagnosis, you'll establish these patient outcomes. The patient will:

- state relief of symptoms
- identify activities that cause chest pain and avoid or seek assistance with the activity
- not show ischemic changes on his ECG.

Decreased cardiac output related to aortic regurgitation caused by damage to the aortic valve. Based on this nursing diagnosis, you'll establish these patient outcomes. The patient will:

- exhibit a pulse rate and blood pressure that remain within set limits and be free of arrhythmias
- describe signs and symptoms of decreased cardiac output, such as dizziness, syncope, clammy skin, fatigue, and dyspnea

• communicate the importance of seeking medical attention if signs and symptoms occur
• express the importance of complying with his ordered diet, medication schedule, and activity level.

Fatigue related to decreased tissue oxygenation with exertion caused by aortic insufficiency. Based on this nursing diagnosis, you'll establish these patient outcomes. The patient will:
• be able to explain the relationship of fatigue to the disease process and his activity level
• identify measures to prevent or modify fatigue
• incorporate measures to modify fatigue into his daily routine.

Nursing interventions

• If the patient needs bed rest, stress its importance. Assist with bathing if necessary. Provide a bedside commode because using a commode puts less stress on the heart than using a bedpan. Offer diversional activities that are physically undemanding.
• Alternate periods of activity and rest to prevent extreme fatigue and dyspnea.
• To reduce anxiety, allow the patient to express his concerns about the effects of activity restrictions on his responsibilities and routines. Reassure him that the restrictions are temporary.
• To improve venous return, keep the patient's legs elevated while he sits in a chair; advise him not to cross his legs.
• Place the patient in an upright position to relieve dyspnea if necessary, and administer oxygen to prevent tissue hypoxia.
• Keep the patient on a low-sodium diet. Consult a dietitian to ensure that the patient receives foods that he likes while adhering to the diet restrictions.
• If the patient is schedule for valve-replacement surgery, explain the procedure and prepare him as necessary.

Monitoring

• Observe the patient for signs of cardiac arrhythmias, which can increase the risk of pulmonary edema, as well as fever and infection.
• Assess the patient's vital signs, weight, and intake and output for changes that suggest fluid overload.
• Regularly evaluate the patient's activity tolerance and degree of fatigue.
• Monitor the patient for chest pain, which may indicate cardiac ischemia.
• Evaluate the patient's cardiopulmonary function. Notify the doctor if sudden or significant changes occur.
• Watch closely for complications and adverse reactions to drug therapy.

Patient teaching

• Advise the patient to plan for periodic rest in his daily routine to prevent undue fatigue.
• Teach the patient about diet restrictions, medications, symptoms that should be reported, and the importance of consistent follow-up care.
• Tell the patient to elevate his legs whenever he sits.

Aortic stenosis

In this disorder, the opening of the aortic valve becomes narrowed and the left ventricle exerts increased pressure to drive blood through the opening. The added work load increases the demand for oxygen, while diminished cardiac output reduces coronary artery perfusion, causes ischemia of the left ventricle, and leads to heart failure.

Signs and symptoms of aortic stenosis may not appear until the patient reaches ages 50 to 70, even though the lesion has been present since childhood. Incidence increases with age. Aortic stenosis is the most significant valvular lesion seen among elderly people. About 80% of patients with aortic stenosis are male.

Causes

Aortic stenosis may result from congenital aortic bicuspid valve (associated with coarctation of the aorta), congenital stenosis of pulmonary valve cusps, rheumatic fever or, in elderly patients, atherosclerosis.

Complications

Aortic stenosis leads to left ventricular failure, usually after age 70. It typically occurs within 4 years after the onset of signs and symptoms and is fatal in up to two-thirds of patients.

Sudden death, possibly caused by an arrhythmia, occurs in up to 20% of patients, usually around age 60.

Assessment

Even with severe aortic stenosis (narrowing to about one-third of the normal opening), the patient may be asymptomatic. Eventually, the patient will complain of dyspnea on exertion, fatigue, exertional syncope, angina, and palpitations. If left ventricular failure develops, the patient may complain of orthopnea and paroxysmal nocturnal dyspnea.

Inspection may reveal peripheral edema if the patient has left ventricular failure.

Palpation may detect diminished carotid pulses and pulsus alternans. If the patient has left ventricular failure, the apex of the heart may be displaced inferiorly and laterally. If the patient has pulmonary hypertension, you may be able to palpate a systolic thrill at the base of the heart, at the jugular notch, and along the carotid arteries. Occasionally, it may be palpable only during expiration and when the patient leans forward.

Auscultation may uncover an early systolic ejection murmur in children and adolescents who have noncalcified valves. The murmur begins shortly after S_1 and increases in intensity to reach a peak toward the middle of the ejection period. It diminishes just before the aortic valve closes.

The murmur is low-pitched, rough, and rasping and is loudest at the base in the second intercostal space. In stenosis, the murmur is at least grade 3 or 4. It disappears when the valve calcifies. A split S_2 develops as aortic stenosis becomes more severe. An S_4 reflects left ventricular hypertrophy and may be heard at the apex in many patients with severe aortic stenosis.

Diagnostic tests

- *Cardiac catheterization* reveals the pressure gradient across the valve (indicating the obstruction's severity), increased left ventricular end-diastolic pressures (indicating left ventricular function), and the location of the left ventricular outflow obstruction.
- *Chest X-rays* show valvular calcification; left ventricular enlargement; pulmonary vein congestion; and, in later stages, left atrial, pulmonary artery, right atrial, and right ventricular enlargement.
- *Echocardiography* demonstrates a thickened aortic valve and left ventricular wall and, possibly, coexistent mitral valve stenosis.
- *Electrocardiography (ECG)* reveals left ventricular hypertrophy. In advanced stages, the patient will exhibit ST-segment depression and T-wave inversion in standard leads I and aV_L and in the left precordial leads. Up to 10% of patients have atrioventricular and intraventricular conduction defects.

Treatment

Digitalis glycosides, a low-sodium diet, diuretics and, in acute cases, oxygen are used to treat heart failure. Nitroglycerin helps relieve angina.

In children who don't have calcified valves, simple commissurotomy under direct visualization is usually effective. Adults with calcified valves will need valve replacement once they become symptomatic or are at risk for developing left ventricular failure.

Percutaneous balloon aortic valvuloplasty is useful in children and young adults who have congenital aortic stenosis and in elderly patients with severe calcifications. This procedure may improve left ventricular function so that the patient can tolerate valve replacement surgery.

Key nursing diagnoses and patient outcomes

Altered cardiopulmonary tissue perfusion related to decreased coronary artery perfusion and increased demand for oxygen. Based on this nursing diagnosis, you'll establish these patient outcomes. The patient will:

- state relief of symptoms
- identify activities that cause chest pain and avoid or seek assistance with the activities
- not show ischemic changes on ECG.

Decreased cardiac output related to narrowed opening of aortic valve. Based on this nursing diagnosis, you'll establish these patient outcomes. The patient will:

- exhibit a pulse rate and blood pressure within set limits and be free of arrhythmias
- describe signs and symptoms of decreased cardiac output, such as dizziness, syncope, clammy skin, fatigue, and dyspnea
- communicate the importance of seeking medical attention if any signs and symptoms occur
- express the importance of following the prescribed diet, taking medications as ordered, and adhering to activity guidelines.

Fluid volume excess related to left ventricular failure. Based on this nursing diagnosis, you'll establish these patient outcomes. The patient will:

- express comfort in his ability to breathe
- not display signs and symptoms of fluid overload, such as shortness of breath, distended neck veins, edema, sudden unexplained weight gain, and crackles on lung auscultation
- demonstrate skill and willingness to adhere to the prescribed therapy, such as maintaining a sodium-restricted diet and measuring intake and output.

Nursing interventions

- If the patient needs bed rest, stress its importance. Assist him with bathing if necessary. Provide a bedside commode because using a commode puts less stress on the heart than using a bedpan. Offer diversional activities that are physically undemanding.
- Alternate periods of activity and rest to prevent extreme fatigue and dyspnea.
- To reduce anxiety, allow the patient to express his concerns about the effects of activity restrictions on his responsibilities and routines. Reassure him that the restrictions are temporary.
- Keep the patient's legs elevated while he sits in a chair to improve venous return to the heart.
- If necessary, place the patient in an upright position to relieve dyspnea. Administer oxygen as needed to prevent tissue hypoxia.
- Keep the patient on a low-sodium diet. Consult with a dietitian to ensure that the patient receives foods that he likes while adhering to the diet restrictions.
- Allow the patient to express his fears and concerns about the disorder, its impact on his life, and any impending surgery. Reassure him as needed.
- After cardiac catheterization, apply firm pressure to the catheter insertion site, usually in the groin. If the site bleeds, remove the pressure dressing, apply firm pressure, and contact the doctor.
- Notify the doctor of any changes in peripheral pulses distal to the insertion site, changes in cardiac rhythm and vital signs, and complaints of chest pain.

Monitoring

- After a patient has had a cardiac catheterization, monitor the insertion site every 15 minutes for at least 6 hours for signs of bleeding. Monitor the patient for chest pain, and assess his vital signs, heart rhythm, and peripheral pulses distal to the insertion site.

• Monitor the patient's vital signs, weight, and intake and output for signs of fluid overload.
• Evaluate the patient's activity tolerance and degree of fatigue.
• Monitor the patient for chest pain that may indicate cardiac ischemia; evaluate his ECG for ischemic changes.
• Regularly assess the patient's cardiopulmonary function. Notify the doctor if sudden or significant changes occur.
• Observe the patient for complications and adverse reactions to drug therapy.

Patient teaching

• Advise the patient to plan for periodic rest in his daily routine to prevent undue fatigue.
• Teach the patient about diet restrictions, medications, symptoms that should be reported, and the importance of consistent follow-up care.
• Tell the patient to elevate his legs whenever he sits.

Aplastic or hypoplastic anemias

Potentially fatal, aplastic or hypoplastic anemias result from injury to or destruction of stem cells in bone marrow or the bone marrow matrix, causing pancytopenia (anemia, leukopenia, thrombocytopenia) and bone marrow hypoplasia.

Although often used interchangeably with other terms for bone marrow failure, aplastic anemias correctly refer to pancytopenia resulting from the decreased functional capacity of a hypoplastic, fatty bone marrow. These disorders usually produce fatal bleeding or infection, particularly when they're idiopathic or stem from chloramphenicol use or infectious hepatitis. Mortality for aplastic anemias with severe pancytopenia is 80% to 90%.

Causes

Aplastic anemias usually develop when damaged or destroyed stem cells inhibit red blood cell (RBC) production. Less commonly, they develop when damaged bone marrow microvasculature creates an unfavorable environment for cell growth and maturation. About half of such anemias result from drugs (such as chloramphenicol or hair color dye), toxic agents (such as benzene), or radiation. The rest may result from immunologic factors (suspected but unconfirmed), severe disease (especially hepatitis), or preleukemic and neoplastic infiltration of bone marrow.

Idiopathic anemias may be congenital. Two such forms of aplastic anemia have been identified: congenital hypoplastic anemia (anemia of Blackfan and Diamond) develops between ages 2 and 3 months; Fanconi's syndrome, between birth and age 10. In the absence of a consistent familial or genetic history of aplastic anemia, researchers suspect that these congenital abnormalities result from an induced change during fetal development.

Complications

Life-threatening hemorrhage from the mucous membranes is the most common complication of aplastic or hypoplastic anemias. Immunosuppression can lead to secondary opportunistic infections.

Assessment

The patient's history may not help establish the disease onset because the symptoms often develop insidiously. The patient may report signs and symptoms of anemia (progressive weakness and fatigue, shortness of breath, and headache) or signs of thrombocytopenia (easy bruising and bleeding, especially from the mucous membranes [nose, gums, rectum, vagina]).

CHECKLIST

Key blood test values in aplastic or hypoplastic anemias

Characteristic blood test results are key indices of aplastic or hypoplastic anemias. Values include:

- ☐ RBC count of 1 million/mm³ or less, usually with normochromic and normocytic cells (although macrocytosis [larger-than-normal erythrocytes] and anisocytosis [excessive variation in erythrocyte size] may exist); very low absolute reticulocyte count (less than 0.5% of the total RBC count).
- ☐ Serum iron levels above 150 mcg/dl (unless bleeding occurs), but normal or slightly reduced total iron-binding capacity (below 300 mcg/dl for men and below 350 mcg/dl for women); hemosiderin is present, and tissue iron storage is visible microscopically.
- ☐ Platelet count below 130,000/mm³ and abnormal coagulation tests, reflecting decreased platelet count, such as an activated partial thromboplastin time that's greater than 36 seconds; prothrombin consumption time that's greater than 20 seconds; and a prothrombin time that is greater than 11.8 seconds in males and greater than 11.3 seconds in females.
- ☐ Neutrophil count below 47.6% (relative value) and 1,950 to 8,400/µl (absolute value).

Inspection may reveal pallor if the patient is anemic, and ecchymosis, petechiae, or retinal bleeding if thrombocytopenia is present. You may note weakness and alterations in the level of consciousness if bleeding into the central nervous system has occurred.

Auscultation may reveal bibasilar crackles, tachycardia, and a gallop murmur if severe anemia results in congestive heart failure.

The patient may also have signs and symptoms of an opportunistic infection (most commonly, a bacterial infection). Fever, oral and rectal ulcers, and sore throat may indicate the presence of an infection without characteristic inflammation.

Diagnostic tests

Confirmation of aplastic anemia requires a series of laboratory tests. (See *Key blood test values in aplastic or hypoplastic anemias.*)

Bone marrow biopsies performed at several sites may yield a dry tap or show severely hypocellular or aplastic marrow, with a varying amount of fat, fibrous tissue, or gelatinous replacement; absence of tagged iron (because the iron is deposited in the liver rather than in bone marrow) and megakaryocytes; and depression of erythroid elements.

Differential diagnosis must rule out paroxysmal nocturnal hemoglobinuria and other diseases in which pancytopenia is common.

Treatment

Effective treatment must eliminate any identifiable cause and provide vigorous supportive measures, such as packed RBC, platelet, and experimental histocompatibility antigen (HLA)-matched leukocyte transfusions. Even after elimination of the cause, recovery can take months. Bone marrow transplantation is the treatment of choice for anemia due to severe aplasia and for patients who need constant RBC transfusions.

The patient with low leukocyte counts is at risk for infection. Prevention of infection may range from frequent hand washing to filtered airflow or protective environment. The infection itself may require specific antibiotics; however, these aren't given prophylactically because they tend to encourage resistant strains of organisms. Patients with low hemoglobin counts may need respiratory support with oxygen in addition to blood transfusions.

Other appropriate forms of treatment include corticosteroids to stimulate erythroid production (successful in children, unsuccessful in adults); marrow-stimulating agents, such as androgens (which are controversial); antilymphocyte globulin (experimental); and immunosuppressant agents (if the patient doesn't respond to other therapy).

A new group of agents called colony-stimulating factors encourage the growth of specific cellular components and show some promise in trials of patients who have received chemotherapy or radiation therapy. These agents include granulocyte colony-stimulating factor, granulocyte-macrophage colony-stimulating factor, and erythropoietic stimulating factor.

Key nursing diagnoses and patient outcomes

Altered protection related to decreased platelet count. Based on this nursing diagnosis, you'll establish these patient outcomes. The patient will:

- not exhibit signs of bleeding, such as hematuria, melena, or petechiae
- recover a normal platelet count that remains normal
- state precautions to prevent or minimize bleeding.

Fatigue related to decreased tissue oxygenation resulting from decreased RBCs. Based on this nursing diagnosis, you'll establish these patient outcomes. The patient will:

- recover a normal RBC count
- perform activities of daily living without limitations
- state precautions to prevent or minimize fatigue.

Risk for infection related to decreased white blood cells (WBCs). Based on this nursing diagnosis, you'll establish these patient outcomes. The patient will:

- not exhibit signs and symptoms of infection, such as fever, chills, malaise, dysuria, or cough
- recover a normal WBC count and cultures that will remain normal
- state precautions to prevent or minimize infection.

Nursing interventions

- Focus your efforts on helping to prevent or manage hemorrhage, infection, adverse effects of drug therapy, and blood transfusion reaction.
- If the patient's platelet count is less than $20,000/mm^3$, prevent hemorrhage by avoiding I.M. injections, suggesting the use of an electric razor and a soft toothbrush, humidifying oxygen to prevent drying of mucous membranes (dry mucosa may bleed), and promoting regular bowel movements through the use of a stool softener and a diet to prevent constipation (which can cause rectal mucosal bleeding). Also, apply pressure to venipuncture sites until bleeding stops.
- Help prevent infection by washing your hands thoroughly before entering the patient's room, by making sure the patient is receiving a nutritious diet (high in vitamins and proteins) to improve his resistance, and by encouraging meticulous mouth and perianal care.
- If the patient has a low hemoglobin level, which causes fatigue, schedule frequent rest periods. Administer oxygen therapy as needed.
- Ensure a comfortable environmental temperature for a patient experiencing hypothermia.

Monitoring

- Check the patient's complete blood count with differential regularly. Report sudden or significant changes to the doctor.
- Detect bleeding promptly by checking for blood in the patient's urine and stool and assessing the skin for petechiae.

• Watch for signs and symptoms of infection, such as fever, chills, malaise, oral or rectal ulcerations, dysuria, or cough. Also monitor results of throat, urine, nasal, stool, and blood cultures, checking to be sure they are done regularly and correctly to detect infection.
• Regularly evaluate the patient's degree of fatigue and activity intolerance.
• If blood transfusions are necessary, assess for a transfusion reaction by checking the patient's temperature and watching for the development of other signs and symptoms, such as rash, urticaria, pruritus, back pain, restlessness, and shaking chills.
• To prevent aplastic anemia, monitor blood studies carefully in the patient receiving anemia-inducing drugs.

Patient teaching

• Teach the patient to avoid contact with potential sources of infection, such as crowds, soil, and standing water that can harbor organisms.
• Reassure and support the patient and his family by explaining the disease and its treatment, particularly if the patient has recurring acute episodes. Explain the purpose of all prescribed drugs, and discuss possible adverse reactions, including which ones he should report promptly.
• Tell the patient who doesn't require hospitalization that he can continue his normal life-style, with appropriate restrictions (such as regular rest periods), until remission occurs.
• Support efforts to educate the public about the hazards of toxic agents. Tell parents to keep toxic agents out of their children's reach. Encourage people who work with radiation to wear protective clothing and a radiation-detecting badge and to observe plant safety precautions. Those who work with benzene (solvent) should know that 10 parts per million is the highest safe environmental level and that a delayed reaction to benzene may develop.
• Refer the patient to the Aplastic Anemia Foundation of America for additional information and assistance.

Appendectomy

With rare exceptions, the only effective treatment for acute appendicitis is appendectomy, the surgical removal of an inflamed vermiform appendix. Commonly performed in an emergency, this surgery aims to prevent imminent rupture or perforation of the appendix. When completed before these complications can occur, appendectomy is generally effective and uneventful. If the appendix ruptures or perforates before surgery, its infected contents spill into the peritoneal cavity, possibly causing peritonitis – the most common and deadly complication of appendicitis, with a mortality of 10%.

Procedure

With the patient under general anesthesia, the surgeon makes an incision in the right lower abdominal quadrant (using either a muscle-splitting, or "gridiron," incision or a McBurney's point incision) to expose the appendix (called "open appendectomy"). He ligates the base of the appendix and places a purse-string suture in the cecum. Then he removes any excess fluid or tissue debris from the abdominal cavity and closes the incision. The use of laparoscopy for diagnosis and removal of the appendix is becoming a safe and common approach even in acute cases.

If perforation occurs, the surgeon may drain the abdominal cavity by inserting one or more Penrose drains or abdominal sump tubes (or both) before closing the incision, or he may leave the incision open. The open incisional wound then heals by secondary intention through granulation and epithelialization.

Complications

An appendectomy usually causes few complications postoperatively if the appendix is removed before inflammation has progressed to the point of perforation. Although uncommon, infection at the surgical site or a paralytic ileus may occur. If the appendix has ruptured before surgery, requiring drainage postoperatively, complications are more likely. These include local or general peritonitis, paralytic ileus, intestinal obstruction, and secondary abscesses in the pelvis or liver or under the diaphragm.

Key nursing diagnoses and patient outcomes

Risk for infection related to potential for peritonitis or formation of secondary abscesses following an appendectomy performed for a ruptured appendix. Based on this nursing diagnosis, you'll establish these patient outcomes. The patient will:

- exhibit a temperature and white blood cell count that will stay within normal range
- have an incision that will appear clean, pink, and free of purulent drainage
- show no other signs of infection.

Pain related to surgical incision or infectious process postoperatively or both. Based on this nursing diagnosis, you'll establish these patient outcomes. The patient will:

- report a decrease in incisional pain in 24 hours and eventually become pain free
- obtain pain relief from analgesics
- adhere to postoperative activity guidelines.

Risk for fluid volume deficit related to temporary cessation of oral intake caused by appendectomy. Based on this nursing diagnosis, you'll establish these patient outcomes. The patient will:

- maintain normal fluid volume, as evidenced by stable vital signs
- maintain a urine output of 30 ml or more every hour
- not exhibit signs and symptoms of dehydration, such as dry mucous membranes, poor skin turgor, thirst, and decreased urine output.

Nursing interventions

When preparing for or managing a patient with an open appendectomy, expect to implement the following interventions.

Before surgery

- Typically, you'll have little time to prepare the patient for appendectomy. Begin by reassuring him that the surgery will relieve his pain and won't interfere with normal GI functioning.
- Briefly explain the surgery, and answer any questions the patient and his family might have. Explain that before surgery he'll receive prophylactic antibiotics to prevent infection and I.V. fluids to maintain blood pressure during surgery. He may have a nasogastric (NG) tube inserted to decompress the stomach and reduce postoperative nausea and vomiting, and he'll be given a sedative and general anesthetic. Tell him that he'll awaken from the general anesthetic with a dressing over the surgical site and possibly several drains in the incision; the drains will remain in place for 3 to 5 days.
- Assure the patient that recovery is usually rapid; if no complications occur, he should be walking and gradually resuming oral feeding the day after surgery. He can expect to be discharged after 3 days and return to his normal activity level in 2 to 4 weeks.
- While awaiting surgery, place the patient in Fowler's position to reduce pain. Avoid giving analgesics, which can mask the pain that heralds rupture. Also, never apply heat to the abdomen or give cathartics or enemas; these measures could trigger rupture.
- Ensure that the patient or a responsible family member has signed a consent form.

After surgery

• After the patient awakens from the anesthetic, place him in Fowler's position to decrease the risk of any contaminated peritoneal fluid infecting the upper abdomen. Monitor his vital signs and record intake and output for 2 days after surgery. Auscultate the abdomen for bowel sounds, indicating the return of peristalsis.
• Regularly check the dressing for drainage, and change it as necessary. If abdominal drains are in place, check and record the amount and nature of drainage and maintain drain patency. Also check drainage from the NG tube, and suction as necessary.
• Encourage ambulation within 12 hours after surgery, if possible. Assist the patient as necessary. Also encourage coughing, deep breathing, and frequent position changes to prevent pulmonary complications. On the day after surgery, remove the NG tube and gradually resume oral foods and fluids, as ordered.
• Throughout the recovery period, assess the patient closely for signs of peritonitis. Watch for and report continuing pain and fever, excessive wound drainage, hypotension, tachycardia, pallor, weakness, and other signs of infection and fluid and electrolyte loss. If peritonitis develops, expect to assist with emergency treatment, including GI intubation, parenteral fluid and electrolyte replacement, and antibiotic therapy.
• After a laparoscopic appendectomy, assess the three to four small abdominal incisions and dressings. Prepare to ambulate the patient within 6 hours. Anticipate discharge in 1 to 2 days.

Home care instructions

• Instruct the patient to watch for and immediately report fever, chills, diaphoresis, nausea, vomiting, and abdominal pain.
• Teach the patient about wound care as necessary.
• After a laparoscopic appendectomy, instruct the patient to resume normal activities in about 8 to 10 days.
• Encourage the patient to keep his scheduled follow-up appointments to monitor healing and detect any complications.

Appendicitis

The most common disease requiring major surgery, appendicitis is an inflammation of the vermiform appendix, a small, fingerlike projection attached to the cecum just below the ileocecal valve. Although the appendix has no known function, it does regularly fill and empty itself of food. Appendicitis occurs when the appendix becomes inflamed from ulceration of the mucosa or obstruction of the lumen.

Appendicitis may occur at any age and affects both sexes equally; however, between puberty and age 25, it's more prevalent in males. Since the advent of antibiotics, the incidence and mortality of appendicitis have declined. If untreated, this disease is invariably fatal.

Causes

Appendicitis probably results from an obstruction of the appendiceal lumen, caused by a fecal mass, stricture, barium ingestion, or viral infection. This obstruction sets off an inflammatory process that can lead to infection, thrombosis, necrosis, and perforation.

Complications

The most common and perilous complication of appendicitis occurs when the appendix ruptures or perforates. When this happens, the infected contents spill into the abdominal cavity, causing peritonitis. Other complications include appendiceal abscess and pyelophlebitis.

Assessment

During the initial phase of appendicitis, the patient typically complains of abdominal pain. Pain may be generalized but, within a few hours, becomes localized in the right lower abdomen (McBurney's point). He may also report anorexia, nausea, and one or two episodes of vomiting. Later signs and symptoms include malaise, constipation, or diarrhea (rare). He may have a low-grade fever.

Inspection typically shows a patient who walks bent over to reduce right lower quadrant pain. When sleeping or lying supine, he may keep his right knee bent up to decrease pain.

Auscultation usually reveals normal bowel sounds. Initially, palpation and percussion disclose no localized abdominal findings except for diffuse tenderness in the midepigastrium and around the umbilicus. Later, palpation may disclose tenderness in the right lower abdominal quadrant that worsens when the patient is asked to cough or upon gentle percussion. Rebound tenderness and spasm of the abdominal muscles are also usually present.

If the appendix is positioned retrocecally or in the pelvis, abdominal tenderness may be completely absent; instead, rectal or pelvic examination reveals tenderness in the flank.

Keep in mind that abdominal rigidity and tenderness worsen as the condition progresses. Sudden cessation of abdominal pain signals perforation or infarction.

Diagnostic tests

A finding of a moderately elevated white blood cell (WBC) count, with increased numbers of immature cells, supports the diagnosis. The use of an enema containing a radiographic contrast agent (a diatrizoate meglumine and diatrizoate sodium solution) may aid the diagnosis. The radiologist attempts to fill the appendix with the contrast agent; failure of the organ to fill indicates appendicitis.

Diagnosis must rule out illnesses with similar symptoms: bladder infection, diverticulitis, gastritis, ovarian cyst, pancreatitis, renal colic, and uterine disease.

Treatment

Appendectomy is the only effective treatment. If peritonitis develops, treatment involves GI intubation, parenteral replacement of fluids and electrolytes, and administration of antibiotics.

Key nursing diagnoses and patient outcomes

Risk for fluid volume deficit related to nausea and vomiting caused by appendicitis. Based on this nursing diagnosis, you'll establish these patient outcomes. The patient will:

• maintain normal fluid volume as evidenced by normal blood pressure and urine output and absence of dehydration
• experience decreased nausea and vomiting
• recover normal GI function.

Risk for infection related to potential for ruptured or perforated appendix. Based on this nursing diagnosis, you'll establish these patient outcomes. The patient will:

• not exhibit signs and symptoms of peritonitis, including sudden cessation of abdominal pain followed by pain recurrence that intensifies and becomes constant; other signs and symptoms are fever, tachycardia, hypotension, abdominal distention, increased nausea or vomiting, and inability to pass feces or flatus
• exhibit a WBC count and temperature that will return to normal and remain normal
• state the importance of notifying a health professional immediately if pain suddenly ceases before surgery.

Pain related to inflammation of the vermiform appendix. Based on this nursing diagnosis, you'll establish these patient outcomes. The patient will:

• express understanding of why pain medication is withheld until diagnosis is confirmed
• obtain pain relief after analgesic administration
• become pain free.

Nursing interventions

- Make sure the patient with suspected or known appendicitis receives nothing by mouth until surgery is performed. Administer I.V. fluids to prevent dehydration. Never administer cathartics or enemas because they may rupture the appendix.
- Don't administer analgesics until the diagnosis is confirmed because they mask symptoms. Once the diagnosis is confirmed, analgesics may be given.
- Place the patient in Fowler's position to reduce pain. Never apply heat to the right lower abdomen; this may cause the appendix to rupture.
- Once the diagnosis is confirmed, prepare the patient for surgery.
- If peritonitis occurs, nasogastric drainage may be necessary to decompress the stomach and reduce nausea and vomiting. If so, record drainage and provide proper mouth and nose care. Expect to administer antibiotic therapy.

Monitoring

- Monitor the patient's vital signs. Also assess intake and output for signs of dehydration, such as hypotension or fluid imbalance.
- Evaluate the severity and location of abdominal pain. Notify the doctor immediately if pain suddenly ceases.
- Observe the patient for complications, such as peritonitis, appendiceal abscess, and pyelophlebitis.

Patient teaching

- Teach the patient what happens in appendicitis.
- Explain why analgesic administration may be delayed, and reassure the patient that an analgesic will be administered as soon as possible.
- Tell the patient that assuming a Fowler's position may help relieve his pain.
- Emphasize the importance of notifying a health care professional if pain is suddenly relieved without medical or surgical treatment.
- Help the patient understand the required surgery and its possible complications.

Arrhythmias

Arrhythmias result from abnormal electrical conduction or automaticity that changes heart rate and rhythm. They vary in severity, from those that are mild, asymptomatic, and require no treatment (such as sinus arrhythmia, in which heart rate increases and decreases with respiration) to catastrophic ventricular fibrillation, which requires immediate intervention.

Arrhythmias are classified according to their origin as ventricular, atrial (supraventricular), or junctional. Their effect on cardiac output and blood pressure, partially influenced by the site of origin, determines their clinical significance.

Causes

Arrhythmias may be congenital or may result from myocardial ischemia or infarction, organic heart disease, drug toxicity, or degeneration of conductive tissue necessary to maintain normal heart rhythm (sick sinus syndrome).

Complications

In a patient with a normal heart, arrhythmias typically produce few symptoms. But even in a normal heart, persistently rapid or highly irregular rhythms can strain the myocardium and impair cardiac output.

Assessment

Depending on the arrhythmia, the patient may exhibit symptoms ranging from pallor, cold and clammy extremities, reduced urine output, palpitations, and weakness to chest pains, dizziness and, if cerebral circulation is severely impaired, syncope.

Diagnostic tests

Electrocardiography (ECG) allows detection and identification of arrhythmias. (See *Types of cardiac arrhythmias,* pages 72 to 78.)

Treatment

Effective treatment aims to return pacer function to the sinus node, increase or decrease ventricular rate to normal, regain atrioventricular synchrony, and maintain normal sinus rhythm. Such treatment corrects abnormal rhythms through therapy with antiarrhythmic drugs; electrical conversion with precordial shock (defibrillation and cardioversion); physical maneuvers, such as carotid massage and Valsalva's maneuver; temporary or permanent placement of a pacemaker to maintain heart rate; and surgical removal or cryotherapy of an irritable ectopic focus to prevent recurring arrhythmias.

Arrhythmias may respond to treatment of the underlying disorder, such as correction of hypoxia. However, arrhythmias associated with heart disease may require continuing and complex treatment.

Key nursing diagnoses and patient outcomes

Altered cerebral tissue perfusion related to decreased cardiac output from an arrhythmia. Based on this nursing diagnosis, you'll establish these patient outcomes. The patient will:

- not develop complications caused by altered cerebral tissue perfusion, such as stroke or seizures
- maintain adequate cerebral perfusion, as evidenced by being oriented to time, person, and place
- maintain hemodynamic stability.

Anxiety related to potential for arrhythmia to become life-threatening. Based on this nursing diagnosis, you'll establish these patient outcomes. The patient will:

- express feelings of anxiety
- use support systems to assist with coping
- experience diminished physical symptoms of anxiety.

Decreased cardiac output related to decreased left ventricular filling time caused by the arrhythmia. Based on this nursing diagnosis, you'll establish these patient outcomes. The patient will:

- not exhibit signs of decreased cardiac output, such as hypotension and altered tissue perfusion
- recover a normal cardiac rhythm that will remain normal
- communicate understanding of medical therapy to treat and prevent arrhythmias.

Nursing interventions

- Document any arrhythmias in a monitored patient.
- Notify the doctor if a change in pulse pattern or rate occurs in an unmonitored patient or if a monitored patient exhibits an arrhythmia.
- As ordered, obtain an ECG tracing in an unmonitored patient to confirm and identify the type of arrhythmia present.
- Be prepared to initiate cardiopulmonary resuscitation, if indicated, when a life-threatening arrhythmia occurs.
- Administer medications, as ordered, and prepare to assist with medical procedures, if indicated (for example, cardioversion).
- If you suspect drug toxicity, report it to the doctor immediately and withhold the next dose.
- To prevent arrhythmias postoperatively, provide adequate oxygen and reduce heart work load while carefully maintaining metabolic, neurologic, respiratory, and hemodynamic status.
- To avoid temporary pacemaker malfunction, install a fresh battery before each insertion. Carefully secure the external catheter wires and the pacemaker box.

Monitoring

- Assess an unmonitored patient for rhythm disturbances. If the patient's pulse rate is abnormally rapid, slow, or irregular, watch for

(Text continues on page 78.)

Types of cardiac arrhythmias

This chart reviews several common cardiac arrhythmias and outlines their characteristics, causes, and treatments. For comparison, here's a normal cardiac rhythm strip and its characteristics.

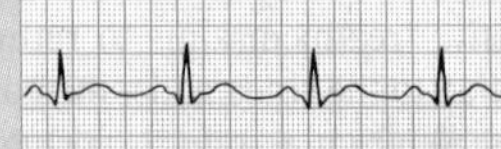

- Ventricular and atrial rates 60 to 100 beats/minute
- Regular and uniform QRS complexes and P waves
- PR interval of 0.12 to 0.2 second
- QRS duration < 0.12 second
- Identical atrial and ventricular rates, with constant PR interval.

Arrhythmia and features	Causes	Treatment
Sinus arrhythmia 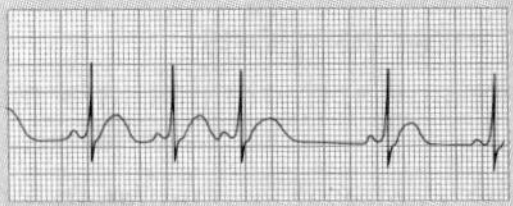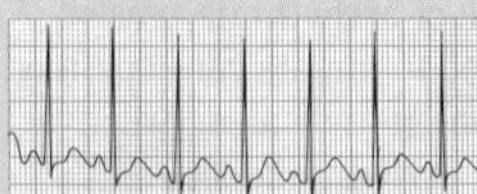 • Irregular atrial and ventricular rhythms • Normal P wave preceding each QRS complex	• A normal variation of normal sinus rhythm in athletes, children, and elderly people • Also seen in digitalis toxicity and inferior wall myocardial infarction (MI)	• Atropine, if rate decreases below 40 beats/minute
Sinus tachycardia • Atrial and ventricular rates regular • Rate > 100 beats/minute; rarely, > 160 beats/minute • Normal P wave preceding each QRS complex	• Normal physiologic response to fever, exercise, anxiety, pain, dehydration; may also accompany shock, left ventricular failure, cardiac tamponade, hyperthyroidism, anemia, hypovolemia, pulmonary embolism, anterior wall MI • May also occur with atropine, epinephrine, isoproterenol, quinidine, caffeine, alcohol, and nicotine use	• Correction of underlying cause
Sinus bradycardia 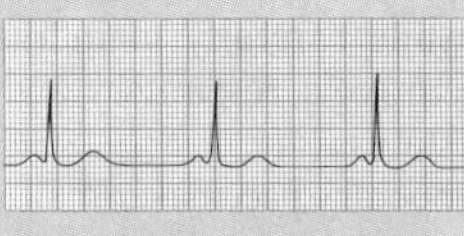 • Regular atrial and ventricular rates • Rate < 60 beats/minute • Normal P wave preceding each QRS complex	• Normal in well-conditioned heart, such as in an athlete • Increased intracranial pressure; increased vagal tone due to bowel straining, vomiting, intubation, mechanical ventilation; sick sinus syndrome; hypothyroidism; inferior wall MI • May also occur with anticholinesterase, beta blockers, digitalis glycosides, and morphine use	• For low cardiac output, dizziness, weakness, altered level of consciousness, or low blood pressure: 0.5 mg atropine every 5 minutes to total of 2 mg • Temporary pacemaker or isoproterenol, if atropine fails; may need permanent pacemaker

Types of cardiac arrhythmias *(continued)*

Arrhythmia and features	Causes	Treatment
Sinoatrial arrest or block (sinus arrest) 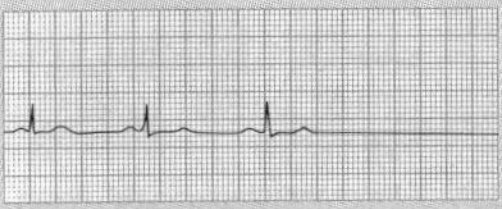 • Atrial and ventricular rhythms normal except for missing complex • Normal P wave preceding each QRS complex • Pause not equal to a multiple of the previous sinus rhythm	• Acute infection • Coronary artery disease, degenerative heart disease, acute inferior wall MI • Vagal stimulation, Valsalva's maneuver, carotid sinus massage • Digitalis, quinidine, or salicylate toxicity • Pesticide poisoning • Pharyngeal irritation caused by endotracheal intubation • Sick sinus syndrome	• Treat symptoms with atropine 0.5 mg I.V. • Temporary or permanent pacemaker for repeated episodes
Wandering atrial pacemaker 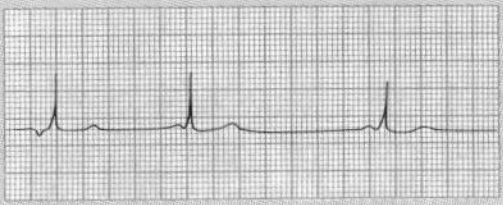 • Atrial and ventricular rates vary slightly • Irregular PR interval • P waves irregular with changing configuration, indicating they're not all from sinoatrial (SA) node or single atrial focus; may appear after the QRS complex • QRS complexes uniform in shape but irregular in rhythm	• Rheumatic carditis as a result of inflammation involving the SA node • Digitalis toxicity • Sick sinus syndrome	• No treatment if asymptomatic • Treatment of underlying cause if symptomatic
Premature atrial contraction (PAC) 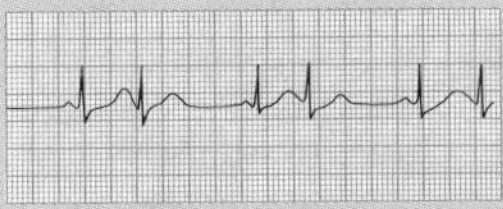 • Premature, abnormal-looking P waves, differing in configuration from normal P waves • QRS complexes after P waves, except in very early or blocked PACs • P wave often buried in the preceding T wave or identified in the preceding T wave	• Coronary or valvular heart disease, atrial ischemia, coronary atherosclerosis, heart failure, acute respiratory failure, chronic obstructive pulmonary disease (COPD), electrolyte imbalance, and hypoxia • Digitalis toxicity and aminophylline, adrenergics, or caffeine use • Anxiety	• If occurring more than six times per minute or increasing in frequency, digitalis glycosides, quinidine, verapamil, or propranolol; after revascularization surgery, propranolol • Treatment of underlying cause

(continued)

Types of cardiac arrhythmias *(continued)*

Arrhythmia and features	Causes	Treatment
Paroxysmal atrial tachycardia (paroxysmal supraventricular tachycardia) 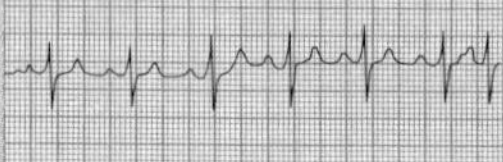 • Atrial and ventricular rates regular • Heart rate > 160 beats/minute; rarely exceeds 250 beats/minute • P waves regular but aberrant; difficult to differentiate from preceding T wave; precede QRS complexes • Sudden onset and termination of arrhythmia	• Intrinsic abnormality of atrioventricular (AV) conduction system • Physical or psychological stress, hypoxia, hypokalemia, cardiomyopathy, congenital heart disease, MI, valvular disease, Wolff-Parkinson-White syndrome, cor pulmonale, hyperthyroidism, systemic hypertension • Digitalis toxicity; caffeine, marijuana, central nervous system stimulant use	• Vagal stimulation, Valsalva's maneuver, carotid sinus massage • Adenosine by rapid I.V. bolus injection to rapidly convert arrhythmia • Propranolol, quinidine, verapamil, edrophonium to alter AV node conduction and maintain normal rhythm • Elective cardioversion, if patient is symptomatic and unresponsive to drugs
Atrial flutter 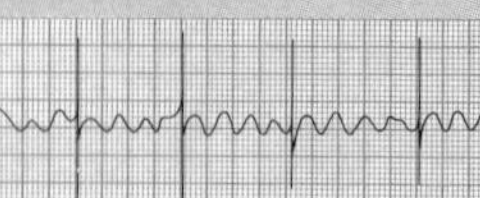 • Atrial rhythm regular; 250 to 400 beats/minute • Ventricular rate variable, depending on degree of AV block, usually 60 to 100 beats/minute • Sawtooth P-wave configuration possible (F waves) • QRS complexes uniform in shape but often irregular in rate	• Heart failure, tricuspid or mitral valve disease, pulmonary embolism, cor pulmonale, inferior wall MI, carditis • Digitalis toxicity	• Digitalis glycosides (unless arrhythmia is due to digitalis toxicity), verapamil, propranolol, or quinidine • May require synchronized cardioversion or atrial pacemaker
Atrial fibrillation 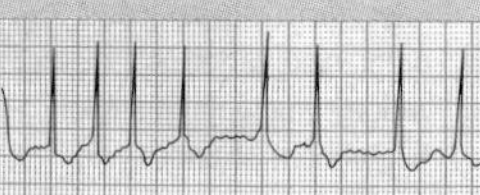 • Atrial rhythm grossly irregular; rate > 400 beats/minute • Ventricular rate grossly irregular • QRS complexes of uniform configuration and duration • PR interval indiscernible • No P waves, or erratic, irregular, baseline fibrillatory P waves	• Heart failure, COPD, thyrotoxicosis, constrictive pericarditis, ischemic heart disease, sepsis, pulmonary embolus, rheumatic heart disease, hypertension, mitral stenosis, digitalis toxicity (rarely), atrial irritation, complication of coronary bypass or valve replacement surgery • Nifedipine and digitalis glycoside use	• Digitalis glycosides (unless the cause) and quinidine to slow ventricular rate and quinidine to convert rhythm to normal sinus rhythm • May require elective cardioversion for rapid ventricular rate • Treatment of underlying cause

Types of cardiac arrhythmias *(continued)*

Arrhythmia and features	Causes	Treatment
Junctional rhythm 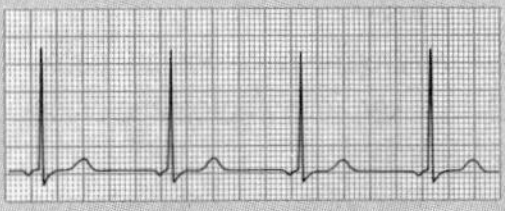 • Atrial and ventricular rates regular • Atrial rate 40 to 60 beats/minute • Ventricular rate 40 to 60 beats/minute (60 to 100 beats/minute is accelerated junctional rhythm) • P waves before, hidden in, or after QRS complex; inverted, if visible • PR interval (when present) < 0.12 second • QRS complex configuration and duration normal, except in aberrant conduction	• Inferior wall MI or ischemia, hypoxia, vagal stimulation, sick sinus syndrome • Acute rheumatic fever • Valve surgery • Digitalis toxicity	• Atropine for symptomatic slow rate • Pacemaker insertion, if refractory to drugs • Discontinuation of digitalis glycosides, if appropriate
Premature junctional contractions (junctional premature beats) 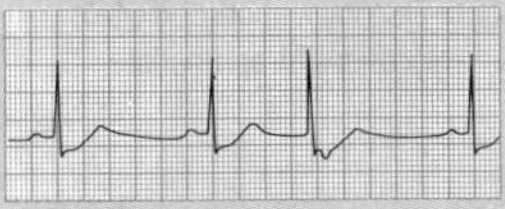 • Atrial and ventricular rhythms irregular • P waves inverted; may precede, be hidden within, or follow QRS complex • PR interval < 0.12 second, if P wave precedes QRS complex • QRS complex configuration and duration normal	• MI or ischemia • Digitalis toxicity and excessive caffeine or amphetamine use	• Correction of underlying cause • Quinidine, atropine, or disopyramide, as ordered • Discontinuation of digitalis glycosides, if appropriate • May require pacemaker
First-degree AV block 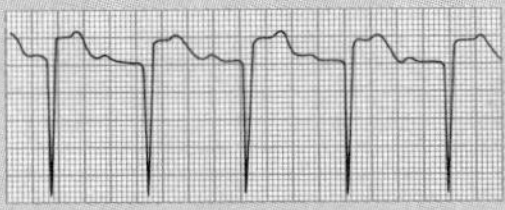 • Atrial and ventricular rhythms regular • PR interval > 0.20 second • P wave preceding each QRS complex; QRS complex normal	• May be seen in a healthy person • Inferior wall myocardial ischemia or infarction, hypothyroidism, hypokalemia, hyperkalemia • Digitalis toxicity; quinidine, procainamide, or propranolol use	• Cautious use of digitalis glycosides • Correction of underlying cause • Atropine may be used if PR interval exceeds 0.26 second or bradycardia develops

(continued)

Types of cardiac arrhythmias *(continued)*

Arrhythmia and features	Causes	Treatment
Second-degree AV block Mobitz I (Wenckebach) • Atrial rhythm regular • Ventricular rhythm irregular • Atrial rate exceeds ventricular rate • PR interval progressively, but only slightly, longer with each cycle until QRS complex disappears (dropped beat); PR interval shorter after dropped beat	• Inferior wall MI, cardiac surgery, acute rheumatic fever, and vagal stimulation • Digitalis toxicity; propranolol, quinidine, or procainamide use	• Treatment of underlying cause • Atropine or temporary pacemaker, for symptomatic bradycardia • Discontinuation of digitalis glycosides, if appropriate
Second-degree AV block Mobitz II 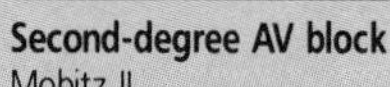 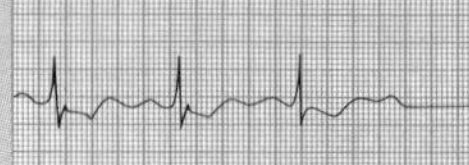 • Atrial rate regular • Ventricular rhythm regular or irregular, with varying degree of block • P-P interval constant • QRS complexes periodically absent	• Severe coronary artery disease, anterior MI, acute myocarditis • Digitalis toxicity	• Isoproterenol for symptomatic bradycardia • Temporary or permanent pacemaker • Discontinuation of digitalis glycosides, if appropriate
Third-degree AV block (complete heart block) 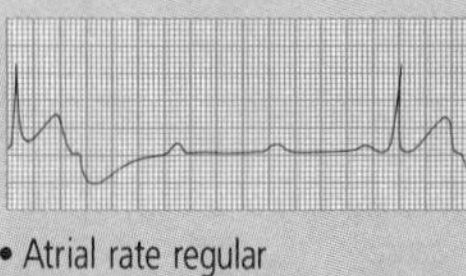 • Atrial rate regular • Ventricular rate slow and regular • No relation between P waves and QRS complexes • No constant PR interval • QRS interval normal (nodal pacemaker) or wide and bizarre (ventricular pacemaker)	• Inferior or anterior wall MI, congenital abnormality, rheumatic fever, hypoxia, postoperative complications of mitral valve replacement, Lev's disease (fibrosis and calcification that spreads from cardiac structures to the conductive tissue), and Lenegre's disease (conductive tissue fibrosis) • Digitalis toxicity	• Atropine or isoproterenol for symptomatic bradycardia • Temporary or permanent pacemaker

Types of cardiac arrhythmias *(continued)*

Arrhythmia and features	Causes	Treatment
Junctional tachycardia 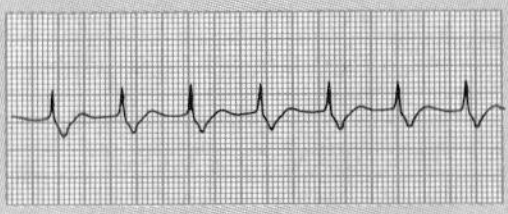 • Atrial rate > 100 beats/minute; however, P wave may be absent, be hidden in QRS complex, or precede T wave • Ventricular rate > 100 beats/minute • P wave inverted • QRS complex configuration and duration normal • Onset of rhythm often sudden, occurring in bursts	• Myocarditis, cardiomyopathy, inferior wall MI or ischemia, acute rheumatic fever, valve replacement surgery • Digitalis toxicity	• Temporary atrial pacemaker to override the rhythm • Carotid sinus massage, elective cardioversion • Propranolol, verapamil, or edrophonium • Discontinuation of digitalis glycosides, if appropriate
Premature ventricular contraction (PVC) 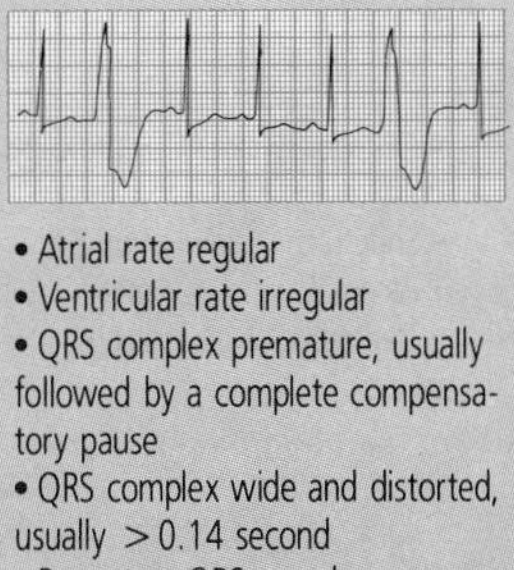 • Atrial rate regular • Ventricular rate irregular • QRS complex premature, usually followed by a complete compensatory pause • QRS complex wide and distorted, usually > 0.14 second • Premature QRS complexes occurring singly, in pairs, or in threes; alternating with normal beats; focus from one or more sites • Most ominous when clustered, multifocal, with R wave on T pattern	• Heart failure; old or acute myocardial ischemia, infarction, or contusion; myocardial irritation by ventricular catheter, such as a pacemaker; hypercapnia; hypokalemia; hypocalcemia • Drug toxicity (digitalis glycosides, aminophylline, tricyclic antidepressants, beta-adrenergics [isoproterenol or dopamine]) • Caffeine, tobacco, or alcohol use • Psychological stress; anxiety; pain; exercise	• Lidocaine I.V. bolus and drip infusion or procainamide or quinidine • Treatment of underlying cause • Discontinuation of drug causing toxicity • Potassium chloride I.V. if induced by hypokalemia

(continued)

Types of cardiac arrhythmias *(continued)*

Arrhythmia and features	Causes	Treatment
Ventricular tachycardia 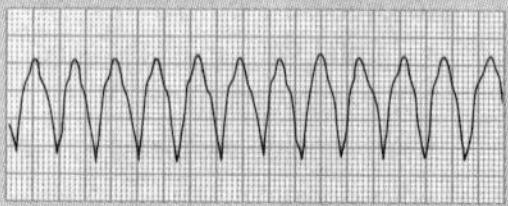 • Ventricular rate 140 to 220 beats/minute, regular or irregular • QRS complexes wide, bizarre, and independent of P waves • P waves not discernible • May start and stop suddenly	• Myocardial ischemia, infarction, or aneurysm; coronary artery disease; rheumatic heart disease; mitral valve prolapse; heart failure; cardiomyopathy; ventricular catheters; hypokalemia; hypercalcemia; pulmonary embolism • Digitalis, procainamide, epinephrine, or quinidine toxicity • Anxiety	• Lidocaine, procainamide, or bretylium I.V. • Cardiopulmonary resuscitation (CPR) if pulses are absent, following advanced cardiac life support (ACLS) protocol • Synchronous cardioversion
Ventricular fibrillation 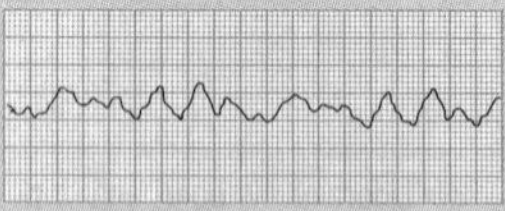 • Ventricular rhythm rapid and chaotic • QRS complexes wide and irregular; no visible P waves	• Myocardial ischemia or infarction, untreated ventricular tachycardia, R-on-T phenomenon, hypokalemia, alkalosis, hyperkalemia, hypercalcemia, electric shock, hypothermia • Digitalis, epinephrine, or quinidine toxicity	• Defibrillation • Epinephrine and lidocaine, procainamide, or bretylium I.V. • CPR • Treatment of underlying cause
Ventricular standstill (asystole) 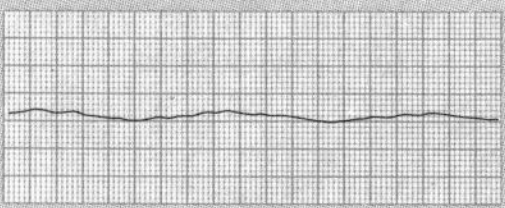 • No atrial or ventricular rate or rhythm • No discernible P waves, QRS complexes, or T waves	• Myocardial ischemia or infarction, aortic valve disease, heart failure, hypoxemia, hypokalemia, severe acidosis, electric shock, ventricular arrhythmias, atrioventricular block, pulmonary embolism, heart rupture, cardiac tamponade, hyperkalemia, electromechanical dissociation • Cocaine overdose	• CPR, following ACLS protocol • Endotracheal intubation • Pacemaker • Treatment of underlying cause

signs of hypoperfusion, such as hypotension and diminished urine output.
• Evaluate the monitored patient's ECG regularly for arrhythmia.
• Monitor for predisposing factors, such as fluid and electrolyte imbalance, and signs of drug toxicity, especially with digoxin.
• If an arrhythmia occurs, carefully monitor the patient's cardiac, electrolyte, and overall clinical status to determine the effect on cardiac output.
• When life-threatening arrhythmias develop, rapidly assess the patient's level of consciousness and pulse and respiratory rates. Monitor his ECG continuously.
• After pacemaker insertion, monitor the patient's pulse rate regularly and watch for signs of pacemaker failure and decreased cardiac output. Watch closely for prema-

ture contractions, a sign of myocardial irritation, and check threshold daily.

Patient teaching

- Explain to the patient the importance of taking all ordered medications at the proper time intervals. Teach him how to take his pulse and recognize an irregular rhythm, and instruct him to report alterations from his baseline to the doctor.
- If the patient has a permanent pacemaker, warn him about environmental and electrical hazards, as indicated by the pacemaker manufacturer. Although hazards may not present a problem, in doubtful situations a 24-hour ambulatory ECG (Holter monitoring) may be helpful. Tell the patient to report any light-headedness or syncope. Stress the importance of scheduling and keeping appointments for regular checkups.

Arterial occlusive disease

An obstruction or narrowing of the lumen of the aorta and its major branches, arterial occlusive disease interrupts blood flow, usually to the legs and feet. This disorder may affect the carotid, vertebral, innominate, subclavian, mesenteric, and celiac arteries.

Arterial occlusive disease is more common in males than in females. The prognosis depends on the location of the occlusion, the development of collateral circulation to counteract reduced blood flow and, in acute disease, the time elapsed between the development of the occlusion and its removal.

Causes

The most common cause of acute arterial occlusion is obstruction of a major artery by a clot. The occlusive mechanism may be endogenous, resulting from emboli formation, thrombosis, or plaques, or exogenous, resulting from trauma or fracture. Chronic arterial occlusive disease is a common complication of atherosclerosis.

Predisposing factors include smoking; aging; conditions such as hypertension, hyperlipidemia, and diabetes mellitus; and family history of vascular disorders, myocardial infarction, or cerebrovascular accident.

Complications

Occlusions may be acute or chronic and often cause severe ischemia, skin ulceration, and gangrene.

Assessment

Assessment findings depend on the vessel involved. (See *Detecting arterial occlusive disease,* page 80.)

Acute arterial occlusion occurs suddenly, often without warning. However, peripheral occlusion can often be recognized by the five *Ps:*

- *Pain,* the most common symptom, occurs suddenly and is localized to the affected arm or leg.
- *Pallor* results from vasoconstriction distal to the occlusion.
- *Pulselessness* occurs distal to the occlusion.
- *Paralysis and paresthesia* occur in the affected arm or leg from disturbed nerve endings or skeletal muscles.

A sixth *P,* known as *poikilothermy,* refers to temperature changes that occur distal to the occlusion, making the skin feel cool.

Diagnostic tests

- *Arteriography* demonstrates the type, location, and degree of obstruction and the establishment of collateral circulation. It is particularly useful in chronic disease or for evaluating candidates for reconstructive surgery.
- *Ultrasonography* and *plethysmography* are noninvasive tests that, in acute disease, show decreased blood flow distal to the occlusion.

Detecting arterial occlusive disease

A patient with arterial occlusive disease may have a variety of signs and symptoms, depending on which portion of the vasculature is affected by the disorder.

Site of occlusion	Signs and symptoms
Internal and external carotid arteries	Transient ischemic attacks (TIAs) due to reduced cerebral circulation produce unilateral sensory or motor dysfunction (transient monocular blindness, hemiparesis), possible aphasia or dysarthria, confusion, decreased mentation, and headache. These recurrent clinical features usually last for 5 to 10 minutes but may persist for up to 24 hours and may herald a cerebrovascular accident. Absent or decreased pulsation with an auscultatory bruit over the affected vessels.
Vertebral and basilar arteries	TIAs of brain stem and cerebellum produce binocular visual disturbances, vertigo, dysarthria, and falling down without loss of consciousness. Less common than carotid TIA.
Innominate (brachiocephalic) artery	Signs and symptoms of vertebrobasilar occlusion. Indications of ischemia (claudication) of right arm; possible bruit over right side of neck.
Subclavian artery	Subclavian steal syndrome characterized by the backflow of blood from the brain through the vertebral artery on the same side as the occlusion, into the subclavian artery distal to the occlusion; clinical effects of vertebrobasilar occlusion and exercise-induced arm claudication. Possible gangrene, usually limited to the digits.
Mesenteric artery	Bowel ischemia, infarct necrosis, and gangrene; sudden, acute abdominal pain; nausea and vomiting; diarrhea; leukocytosis; shock due to intraluminal fluid and plasma loss.
Aortic bifurcation (saddle block occlusion, a medical emergency associated with cardiac embolization)	Sensory and motor deficits (muscle weakness, numbness, paresthesia, paralysis) and ischemia (sudden pain; cold, pale legs with decreased or absent peripheral pulses) in legs.
Iliac artery (Leriche's syndrome)	Intermittent claudication of lower back, buttocks, and thighs, relieved by rest; absent or reduced femoral or distal pulses; shiny, scaly skin, subcutaneous tissue loss, and no body hair on affected limb; nail deformities; increased capillary refill time; blanching of feet on elevation; possible bruit over femoral arteries; impotence in males.
Femoral and popliteal arteries (associated with aneurysm formation)	Intermittent claudication of the calves on exertion; ischemic pain in feet; pretrophic pain (heralds necrosis and ulceration); leg pallor and coolness; shiny, scaly skin, subcutaneous tissue loss, and no body hair on affected limb; nail deformities; increased capillary refill time; blanching of feet on elevation; gangrene; no palpable pulses distal to occlusion. Auscultation over affected area may reveal a bruit.

• *Doppler ultrasonography* typically reveals a relatively low-pitched sound and a monophasic waveform.
• *Segmental limb pressures* and *pulse volume measurements* help evaluate the location and extent of the occlusion.
• *Ophthalmodynamometry* helps determine the degree of obstruction in the internal carotid artery by comparing ophthalmic artery pressure with brachial artery pressure on the affected side. More than a 20% difference between pressures suggests arterial insufficiency.
• *EEG* and a *computed tomography scan* may be necessary to rule out brain lesions.

Treatment

In mild chronic disease, treatment usually consists of supportive measures: elimination of smoking, hypertension control, walking exercise, and foot and leg care. In carotid artery occlusion, antiplatelet therapy may begin with dipyridamole and aspirin. For those patients with intermittent claudication caused by chronic arterial occlusive disease, pentoxifylline may improve blood flow through the capillaries. This drug is particularly useful for poor surgical candidates.

Thrombolytics, such as urokinase, streptokinase, and alteplase, can dissolve clots and relieve the obstruction caused by a thrombus.

Acute arterial occlusive disease usually requires surgery, such as the following:
• *Embolectomy.* A balloon-tipped Fogarty catheter is used to remove thrombotic material from the artery. Embolectomy is used mainly for mesenteric, femoral, or popliteal artery occlusion.
• *Thromboendarterectomy.* This involves the opening of the artery and removal of the obstructing thrombus and the medial layer of the arterial wall. Plaque deposits will remain intact. Thromboendarterectomy is usually performed after angiography and is often used in conjunction with autogenous vein or Dacron bypass surgery (femoropopliteal or aortofemoral).
• *Percutaneous transluminal coronary angioplasty (PTCA).* Using fluoroscopy and a special balloon catheter, PTCA dilates the stenosis or occluded artery to a predetermined diameter without overdistending it.
• *Laser surgery.* An excimer or a hot-tip laser obliterates the clot and plaque by vaporizing it.
• *Patch grafting.* This involves removal of the thrombosed arterial segment and replacement with an autogenous vein or Dacron graft.
• *Bypass graft.* Blood flow is diverted through an anastomosed autogenous or woven Dacron graft to bypass the thrombosed arterial segment.
• *Lumbar sympathectomy.* Depending on the condition of the sympathetic nervous system, this procedure may be an adjunct to reconstructive surgery.

Amputation may be necessary if arterial reconstructive surgery fails or if gangrene, uncontrollable infection, or intractable pain develops.

Other therapy includes heparin to prevent emboli (for embolic occlusion) and bowel resection after restoration of blood flow (for mesenteric artery occlusion).

Key nursing diagnoses and patient outcomes

Activity intolerance related to exercise-induced pain and ischemia in the lower extremities. Based on this nursing diagnosis, you'll establish these patient outcomes. The patient will:
• maintain muscle strength and joint range of motion
• perform self-care activities to tolerance level
• seek assistance when performing an activity, as needed, to prevent injury or trauma to tissue.

Altered peripheral or cerebral tissue perfusion related to reduced blood flow. Based on this nursing diagnosis, you'll establish these patient outcomes. The patient will:
• demonstrate adequate tissue perfusion, as evidenced by the presence of peripheral

pulses, normal skin temperature and color in the extremities, absence of pain, and being oriented to time, person, and place
• communicate understanding of precautions to avoid or minimize tissue damage
• adhere to the prescribed treatment regimen and eliminate risk factors from his life-style.

Pain related to peripheral ischemia in the lower extremities. Based on this nursing diagnosis, you'll establish these patient outcomes. The patient will:
• attain pain relief with analgesics
• identify factors that cause pain and make changes in life-style to avoid precipitating factors
• become pain free.

Nursing interventions

• Prevent trauma to the affected extremity. Use minimal-pressure mattresses, heel protectors, a foot cradle, or a footboard to reduce pressure that could lead to skin breakdown. Keep the arm or leg warm, but never use heating pads. If the patient is wearing socks, remove them frequently to check the skin.
• Avoid using restrictive clothing, such as antiembolism stockings.
• Administer analgesics, as ordered, to relieve pain.
• Allow the patient to express fears and concerns, and help him identify and use effective coping strategies.
• If the patient has experienced an embolus occlusion, expect to administer heparin or thrombolytics by continuous I.V. drip, as ordered. Use an infusion monitor or pump to ensure the proper flow rate.
• During an acute episode, wrap the patient's affected foot in soft cotton batting and reposition it frequently to prevent pressure on any one area until surgery is performed. Strictly avoid elevating or applying heat to the affected leg.
• Prepare the patient experiencing an acute episode for surgery. Explain the surgical procedure to the patient and family. Answer any questions to reduce anxiety.

Monitoring

• Regularly assess the patient's circulatory status by checking for the most distal pulses and inspecting his skin color and temperature for evidence of aortic, iliac, femoral or popliteal artery involvement. Compare findings to earlier assessments and observations.
• Evaluate the patient's neurologic status regularly for evidence of carotid, innominate, vertebral, or subclavian artery involvement. Watch for changes in level of consciousness, pupil size, and muscle strength.
• Monitor the patient for severe abdominal pain and change in bowel function by performing abdominal assessment for evidence of mesenteric artery involvement. Increasing abdominal distention and tenderness may indicate extension of bowel ischemia with resulting gangrene, or it may indicate peritonitis.
• Check the patient for signs of fluid and electrolyte imbalance. Monitor his intake and output for signs of renal failure (urine output of less than 30 ml/hour) in an acute arterial occlusive episode involving the mesenteric artery or aorta.

Patient teaching

• When preparing the patient for discharge, instruct him to watch for signs of recurrence (pain, pallor, numbness, paralysis, absence of pulse) that can result from graft occlusion or occlusion at another site. Caution against wearing constrictive clothing, crossing his legs, or wearing garters. Tell him to avoid "bumping" injuries to affected limbs.
• Warn the patient to avoid all tobacco products.
• Tell the patient to avoid temperature extremes. If he must go outside in the cold, remind him to dress warmly and take special care to keep his feet warm.
• Instruct the patient to wash his feet daily and inspect them for signs of injury or infection. Remind him to report any abnormalities to the doctor.

• Advise the patient to wear sturdy, properly fitting shoes. Refer him to a podiatrist for any foot problems.

Arthrocentesis

Commonly used as an adjunctive treatment for orthopedic disorders such as joint trauma or septic arthritis, arthrocentesis involves insertion of a needle into the joint space to aspirate excessive synovial fluid or blood or to instill corticosteroids or other anti-inflammatory drugs. It also may be performed to obtain a specimen for diagnostic testing.

Most commonly performed on the knee, arthrocentesis also may be done on the elbow, shoulder, or other joints. It's often combined with two related procedures: arthroscopy, which allows endoscopic visualization of the joint, and arthrography, an X-ray showing joint tissue and structure.

Procedure

After cleaning and sterilizing the area, the doctor injects or sprays a local anesthetic at the site. He then inserts the appropriate needle and aspirates at least 10 to 15 ml of synovial fluid from the joint. To aid aspiration, he may wrap an elastic bandage around the joint above and below the puncture site; this compresses the fluid into the site and ensures maximum aspiration.

If the doctor will be injecting medication into the joint space, he leaves the needle in the joint, detaches the fluid-filled syringe, attaches a drug-filled syringe, and injects the medication. After withdrawing the needle, he applies direct pressure over the puncture site for 2 minutes, then applies a sterile pressure dressing to control bleeding. If an excessive amount of fluid has been aspirated from the knee, an elastic bandage may be applied to improve joint stability and inhibit further fluid accumulation by compressing the joint space.

Complications

Arthrocentesis is performed under strict aseptic technique to avoid infecting the joint or contaminating the specimen. Other possible complications include intra-articular or soft-tissue hemorrhage, tendon rupture, and temporary nerve palsy.

Key nursing diagnoses and patient outcomes

Anxiety related to lack of knowledge about arthrocentesis. Based on this nursing diagnosis, you'll establish these patient outcomes. The patient will:
• express his feelings of anxiety and concerns about arthrocentesis
• state understanding of arthrocentesis and have all questions addressed before the procedure
• demonstrate reduced anxiety by remaining calm and cooperating with the doctor, as evidenced by keeping his joint in position and motionless during the procedure.

Risk for infection related to foreign object introduced into sterile joint cavity. Based on this nursing diagnosis, you'll establish these patient outcomes. The patient will:
• not exhibit signs and symptoms of infection, such as fever, increased pain, or redness and swelling at injection site.

Pain related to needle insertion into joint space and increased postprocedure activity. Based on this nursing diagnosis, you'll establish these patient outcomes. The patient will:
• experience minimal discomfort during arthrocentesis
• gradually resume normal activities to prevent overuse of affected joint.

Nursing interventions

As you prepare or manage a patient undergoing arthrocentesis, expect to implement the following interventions.

Before the procedure

• Review the procedure with the patient, reinforcing and clarifying the doctor's explanation as necessary. Explain that the patient must keep his joint in position and motionless throughout the procedure to aid the doctor and minimize the risk of complications. Point out that although he'll receive a local anesthetic, he may feel some pain as the needle is introduced into the joint space. Reassure him that this pain should resolve quickly and that he should be able to resume his normal activities soon after the procedure.

• If the patient is undergoing arthrocentesis to withdraw a synovial fluid sample for glucose analysis, restrict foods or fluids for the ordered time before the procedure.

• Make sure the patient or a responsible family member has signed a consent form. Check the patient's history for hypersensitivity to iodine compounds (such as povidone-iodine), procaine, lidocaine, or other local anesthetics. Administer a sedative, as ordered.

• Assemble the necessary equipment, including a corticosteroid suspension if necessary.

After the procedure

• Monitor the puncture site for excessive bleeding, and take steps to control it if necessary. Elevate the affected limb, and apply ice or cold packs to the joint for 24 to 36 hours to decrease pain and swelling.

• Assess for signs of infection, such as fever or increased joint pain. Report such signs promptly, and prepare to initiate antibiotic therapy as ordered. To minimize the risk of infection, handle all dressings and linens carefully and keep the puncture site clean.

Home care instructions

• Advise the patient that he can resume normal activities soon after the procedure. However, warn him to avoid overusing the affected joint for several days to prevent increased pain, swelling, and stiffness.

• Instruct the patient to immediately report increased pain, redness, swelling, or fever; explain that these signs may indicate infection, which requires prompt medical attention.

• Remind him to keep follow-up medical appointments so that the doctor can evaluate the effectiveness of treatment.

Asbestosis

This disorder is characterized by diffuse interstitial pulmonary fibrosis, resulting from prolonged exposure to airborne asbestos particles. Asbestosis may develop many years (about 15 to 20) after regular exposure to asbestos ceases. Asbestos exposure also causes pleural plaques and mesotheliomas of the pleura and the peritoneum. A potent co-carcinogen, asbestos heightens a cigarette smoker's risk for lung cancer. In fact, an asbestos worker who smokes is 90 times more likely to develop lung cancer than a smoker who never worked with asbestos.

Asbestos-related diseases may also develop in family members of asbestos workers from exposure to stray fibers shaken off the workers' clothing at home. Furthermore, asbestosis may develop in the general public from exposure to fibrous asbestos dust in public buildings, such as schools and factories, or waste piles from a nearby asbestos plant.

Causes

A form of pneumoconiosis, asbestosis follows prolonged inhalation of respirable asbestos fibers (about 50 microns long and 0.5 micron wide). The inhaled fibers travel down the airway and penetrate respiratory bronchioles and alveolar walls. They become encased in a brown, iron-rich, proteinlike sheath (ferruginous bodies or asbestosis bodies) in sputum or lung tissue. Interstitial fibrosis may develop in lower lung zones, causing pathologic changes in lung parenchyma and pleurae. Raised hyaline plaques may form in the parietal pleura and the diaphragm and in pleura adjacent to the pericardium.

Complications

Asbestosis may progress to pulmonary fibrosis with respiratory failure and cardiovascular complications, including pulmonary hypertension and cor pulmonale.

Assessment

The patient typically relates a history of occupational, family, or neighborhood exposure to asbestos fibers. The average exposure time is about 10 years. He may report exertional dyspnea. With extensive fibrosis, he may report dyspnea even at rest. In advanced disease, the patient may complain of a dry cough (may be productive in smokers), chest pain (often pleuritic), and recurrent respiratory tract infections.

Inspection findings may include tachypnea and clubbing of the fingers. With auscultation, you may hear characteristic dry crackles in the lung bases.

Diagnostic tests

- *Chest X-rays* may show fine, irregular, and linear diffuse infiltrates. If the patient has extensive fibrosis, X-rays may disclose lungs with a honeycomb or ground-glass appearance. Films may also show pleural thickening and pleural calcification, bilateral obliteration of costophrenic angles and, in later disease stages, an enlarged heart with a classic "shaggy" border.
- *Pulmonary function tests* may identify decreased vital capacity, forced vital capacity (FVC), and total lung capacity; decreased or normal forced expiratory volume in 1 second (FEV_1); normal ratio of FEV_1 to FVC; and reduced diffusing capacity for carbon monoxide when fibrosis destroys alveolar walls and thickens the alveolocapillary membrane.
- *Arterial blood gas (ABG) analysis* may reveal decreased partial pressure of oxygen in arterial blood and decreased partial pressure of carbon dioxide in arterial blood from hyperventilation.

Treatment

Chest physiotherapy techniques, such as controlled coughing and postural drainage with chest percussion and vibration, may be implemented to relieve respiratory signs and symptoms and, in advanced disease, manage hypoxia and cor pulmonale.

Aerosol therapy, inhaled mucolytics, and increased fluid intake (at least 3 liters daily) may also help relieve respiratory symptoms. Hypoxia requires oxygen administration by cannula or mask (1 to 2 liters/minute) or by mechanical ventilation if the patient's arterial oxygen level can't be maintained above 40 mm Hg.

Diuretic agents, digitalis preparations, and salt restriction may be necessary for patients with cor pulmonale. Respiratory tract infections require prompt antibiotic therapy.

Key nursing diagnoses and patient outcomes

Altered nutrition: Less than body requirements, related to fatigue caused by impaired gas exchange. Based on this nursing diagnosis, you'll establish these patient outcomes. The patient will:

- maintain adequate nutrition, as evidenced by eating a well-balanced diet
- maintain his weight within the normal range for his sex, height, and age
- plan rest periods before each meal.

Fatigue related to impaired gas exchange. Based on this nursing diagnosis, you'll establish these patient outcomes. The patient will:

- identify activities that cause fatigue
- incorporate measures as part of daily activities to modify fatigue
- exhibit reduced fatigue.

Impaired gas exchange related to asbestosis-induced pulmonary tissue changes. Based on this nursing diagnosis, you'll establish these patient outcomes. The patient will:

- maintain adequate ventilation, as evidenced by normal ABG values and decreased dyspnea

• use correct bronchial hygiene
• comply with ordered medical therapy.

Nursing interventions

• Provide supportive care, and help the patient adjust to life-style changes necessitated by chronic illness.
• Perform chest physiotherapy, including postural drainage and chest percussion and vibration for involved lobes, several times daily.
• Weigh the patient three times weekly.
• Provide high-calorie, high-protein foods. Offer small, frequent meals to conserve the patient's energy and prevent fatigue.
• Make sure the patient receives adequate fluids to loosen secretions.
• Schedule respiratory therapy at least 1 hour before or after meals. Provide mouth care after inhalational bronchodilator therapy.
• Encourage daily activity, and provide diversions as appropriate. Help conserve the patient's energy and prevent fatigue by alternating rest and activity.
• Administer medication, as ordered, and note the patient's response.

Monitoring

• Monitor for changes in baseline respiratory function. Also watch for changes in sputum quality and quantity, restlessness, increased tachypnea, and changes in breath sounds. Report these immediately.
• Be alert for complications, such as pulmonary hypertension and cor pulmonale.

Patient teaching

• Advise the patient to avoid crowds and people with known infections and to obtain influenza and pneumococcus immunizations.
• If the patient receives home oxygen therapy, explain why he needs it and show him how to operate the equipment.
• If the patient has a transtracheal catheter, teach him how to care for it. Review precautions for catheter use, and urge him to schedule appointments for follow-up care.
• Teach the patient and his family how to perform chest physiotherapy.
• Review the patient's medication regimen with him.
• Encourage the patient to follow a high-calorie, high-protein diet to meet increased energy requirements. Also, tell him to drink plenty of fluids to prevent dehydration and to help loosen secretions.
• If the patient smokes, encourage him to stop. Provide him with information or counseling, as appropriate.
• Inform the public, as appropriate, about the health hazard from asbestos exposure and ways to prevent asbestosis.

Asthma

A chronic reactive airway disorder, asthma involves episodic, reversible airway obstruction resulting from bronchospasms, increased mucus secretions, and mucosal edema. Signs and symptoms range from mild wheezing and dyspnea to life-threatening respiratory failure. Signs and symptoms of bronchial airway obstruction may or may not persist between acute episodes.

Although this common respiratory condition can strike at any age, about half of all patients with asthma are under age 10. In this age-group, asthma affects twice as many boys as girls. About one-third of patients experience asthma's onset between ages 10 and 30; in this group, incidence is the same in both sexes. Hereditary factors are also important: about one-third of all patients with asthma share the disease with at least one immediate family member.

Asthma may result from sensitivity to specific external allergens (extrinsic) or from internal, nonallergenic factors (intrinsic). Allergens that cause extrinsic asthma (atopic asthma) include pollen, animal dander, house dust or mold, kapok or feather pillows, food additives containing sulfites, and any other sensitizing substance. Extrinsic asthma begins in childhood and is commonly accompanied by other manifestations of atopy (Type I, immunoglobulin E- [IgE] mediated allergy), such as eczema and allergic rhinitis.

In intrinsic asthma (nonatopic asthma), no extrinsic substance can be identified. Most episodes are preceded by a severe respiratory tract infection (especially in adults). Irritants, emotional stress, fatigue, endocrine changes, temperature and humidity variations, and exposure to noxious fumes may aggravate intrinsic asthma attacks. In many asthmatics, especially children, intrinsic and extrinsic asthma coexist.

Causes

In asthma, the tracheal and bronchial linings overreact to various stimuli, causing episodic smooth-muscle spasms that severely constrict the airways. Mucosal edema and thickened secretions further block the airways.

IgE antibodies, attached to histamine-containing mast cells and receptors on cell membranes, initiate intrinsic asthma attacks. When exposed to an antigen, such as pollen, the IgE antibody combines with the antigen. On subsequent exposure to the antigen, mast cells degranulate and release mediators.

These mediators cause the bronchoconstriction and edema of an asthma attack. As a result, expiratory airflow decreases, trapping gas in the airways and causing alveolar hyperinflation. Atelectasis may develop in some lung regions. The increased airway resistance initiates labored breathing.

Several factors may contribute to bronchoconstriction. These include hereditary predisposition; sensitivity to allergens or irritants, such as pollutants; viral infections; aspirin, beta blockers, nonsteroidal anti-inflammatory drugs, and other drugs; tartrazine (a yellow food dye); psychological stress; cold air; and exercise.

Complications

Asthma can produce status asthmaticus and respiratory failure, which are life-threatening complications. (See *Responding to status asthmaticus,* page 88.)

Assessment

An asthma attack may begin dramatically, with simultaneous onset of severe, multiple symptoms, or insidiously, with gradually increasing respiratory distress. Typically, the patient reports exposure to a particular allergen followed by a sudden onset of dyspnea and wheezing, and tightness in the chest accompanied by a cough that produces thick, clear or yellow sputum.

The patient may complain of feeling suffocated. He may be visibly dyspneic and able to speak only a few words before pausing to catch his breath. You may also see him using accessory respiratory muscles to breathe. He may sweat profusely, and you may observe an increased anteroposterior thoracic diameter.

Percussion may produce hyperresonance. Palpation may reveal vocal fremitus. Auscultation may disclose tachycardia, tachypnea, mild systolic hypertension, harsh respirations with both inspiratory and expiratory wheezes, prolonged expiratory phase of respiration, and diminished breath sounds.

Cyanosis, confusion, and lethargy indicate the onset of life-threatening status asthmaticus and respiratory failure.

Diagnostic tests

• *Pulmonary function studies* reveal signs of airway obstructive disease (decreased flow rates and forced expiratory volume in 1 second [FEV_1]), low-normal or decreased vital capacity, and increased total lung and residual capacities. Despite abnormal findings during asthmatic episodes, pulmonary function may be normal between attacks.

Typically, the patient has decreased partial pressure of oxygen in arterial blood ($Pa{O_2}$) and partial pressure of carbon

LIFE-THREATENING COMPLICATIONS

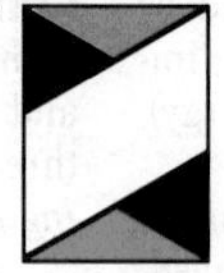

Responding to status asthmaticus

When your patient has an acute asthma attack, be alert for the signs and symptoms of status asthmaticus, such as cyanosis, confusion, and lethargy.

The flowchart at right shows the path of untreated status asthmaticus. This complication begins with impaired gas exchange and may lead to respiratory failure and eventually to death. If you detect this complication in your asthma patient, you'll need to intervene immediately.

Emergency interventions

- Notify the doctor immediately.
- Observe the patient closely for respiratory arrest. Monitor his respiratory rate continuously and other vital signs every 5 minutes. Never leave the patient alone.
- Make sure the patient receives oxygen and bronchodilator and nebulizer therapies, as ordered.
- Have emergency equipment brought to the bedside, and prepare to assist with intubation and mechanical ventilation if the patient's $Pa{CO_2}$ rises or if respiratory arrest occurs.
- Assist with drawing arterial blood samples for immediate blood gas analysis.
- Administer corticosteroids, epinephrine, sympathomimetic aerosol agents, and I.V. aminophylline, as ordered.
- Prepare to transfer the patient to the intensive care unit.

Obstructed airways impede gas exchange and increase airway resistance. The patient labors to breathe.

↓

Initially, the patient's struggle to breathe causes hyperventilation, which lowers $Pa{CO_2}$. Respiratory alkalosis and hypoxemia develop.

↓

As breathing and hypoxia tire the patient, his respiratory rate drops to normal.

↓

Later, the $Pa{CO_2}$ level rises, exceeding the baseline level, which is usually low in an asthmatic patient.

↓

The patient hypoventilates from exhaustion.

↓

Respiratory acidosis begins as $Pa{O_2}$ drops and the $Pa{CO_2}$ level continues to rise.

↓

Without treatment, the patient experiences acute respiratory failure.

dioxide in arterial blood ($Paco_2$). However, in severe asthma, $Paco_2$ may be normal or increased, indicating severe bronchial obstruction. In fact, FEV_1 will probably be less than 25% of the predicted value. Initiating treatment tends to improve the airflow. However, even when the asthma attack appears controlled, the spirometric values (FEV_1 and forced expiratory flow) remain abnormal (between 25% and 75% of vital capacity), necessitating frequent arterial blood gas (ABG) analyses or pulse oximetry measurements. Residual volume remains abnormal for the longest period—up to 3 weeks after the attack.

- *Serum IgE levels* may rise from an allergic reaction.
- *Complete blood count with differential* reveals increased eosinophil count.
- *Chest X-rays* can diagnose or monitor the progress of asthma. X-rays may show possible hyperinflation with areas of focal atelectasis.
- *ABG analysis* can detect hypoxemia and guide treatment.
- *Skin testing* may identify specific allergens. Test results are read in 1 to 2 days to detect an early reaction and then again after 4 to 5 days to reveal a late reaction.
- *Bronchial challenge testing* evaluates the clinical significance of allergens identified by skin testing.

Treatment

The best treatment for asthma is prevention by identifying and avoiding precipitating factors, such as environmental allergens or irritants. Usually, such stimuli can't be removed entirely. Desensitization to specific antigens may be more helpful in children than in adults with bronchial asthma.

Drug therapy usually includes bronchodilators and is most effective when begun soon after the onset of signs and symptoms. Drugs used include rapid-acting epinephrine, terbutaline, aminophylline, theophylline and theophylline-containing oral preparations, oral sympathomimetics, corticosteroids, and aerosolized sympathomimetics, such as metaproterenol and albuterol. (See *Taking precautions in asthma*.) ABG measurements help determine the severity of an asthma attack and the patient's response to treatment.

NURSING ALERT

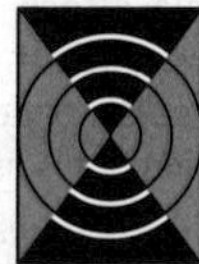

Taking precautions in asthma

When caring for a patient with asthma, keep in mind the following precautions:

- Elderly patients with hepatic or cardiac insufficiency or those taking erythromycin are predisposed to aminophylline toxicity.
- Young patients and those who smoke or take barbiturates have increased aminophylline metabolism and therefore require a larger dose of aminophylline.
- Because of their respiratory depressant effect, sedatives and narcotics are not recommended.

Low-flow oxygen may be required, as may antibiotics if infection is evident. Fluid replacement may also be necessary.

Status asthmaticus must be treated promptly to prevent progression to fatal respiratory failure. The patient with increasingly severe asthma that doesn't respond to drug therapy is usually admitted to the intensive care unit for treatment with corticosteroids, epinephrine, sympathomimetic aerosol sprays, and I.V. aminophylline. He'll need frequent ABG analysis and pulse oximetry to assess respiratory status, particularly after ventilator therapy or a change in oxygen concentration. The patient may require endotracheal intubation and mechanical ventilation if his $Paco_2$ rises.

Key nursing diagnoses and patient outcomes

Impaired gas exchange related to bronchoconstriction and mucosal edema caused by

an acute asthma attack. Based on this nursing diagnosis, you'll establish these patient outcomes. The patient will:
• exhibit resolution of his asthmatic attack
• regain normal gas exchange, as evidenced by normal ABG values and normal assessment findings of respiratory function
• recover from an acute asthma attack with no residual lung damage.

Ineffective airway clearance related to increased thick mucus secretions and fatigue. Based on this nursing diagnosis, you'll establish these patient outcomes. The patient will:
• cough and deep-breathe adequately to expectorate secretions
• demonstrate skill in conserving energy while attempting to clear airway
• maintain a patent airway.

Ineffective breathing pattern related to labored breathing. Based on this nursing diagnosis, you'll establish these patient outcomes. The patient will:
• achieve maximum lung expansion with adequate ventilation
• recover normal respiratory rate and pattern that will remain normal
• experience diminished dyspnea.

Nursing interventions

• Maintain respiratory function and relieve bronchoconstriction while allowing mucus plug expulsion.
• Control exercise-induced asthma by having the patient sit down, rest, and use diaphragmatic and pursed-lip breathing until shortness of breath subsides.
• Supervise the patient's drug regimen. Make sure he knows how to use a metered-dose inhaler properly. The addition of spacer devices may help optimize drug delivery.
• If the patient develops cushingoid adverse reactions from long-term corticosteroid therapy, expect to minimize these reactions with alternate-day dosage or use of orally inhalable corticosteroids, such as beclomethasone, flunisolide, and triamcinolone acetonide. In addition, ipratropium may be used.
• In an acute attack, find out if the patient has a nebulizer and if he has used it. The patient with asthma should have access to an albuterol or metaproterenol inhaler at all times. Instruct him to take no more than two to three puffs every 4 hours. If he needs the nebulizer before 4 hours pass, however, allow him to use it and call the doctor for further instruction. (Excessive nebulizer use can progressively weaken the patient's response and mask underlying inflammation. Extended overuse can even lead to cardiac arrest and death, although this is rare.)
• Reassure the patient during an asthma attack and stay with him. Place him in semi-Fowler's position, and encourage diaphragmatic breathing. Assist him to relax as much as possible.
• As ordered, administer humidified oxygen by nasal cannula at 2 liters/minute to ease breathing and to increase arterial oxygen saturation during an acute asthma attack. Later, adjust oxygen according to the patient's vital functions and ABG measurements.
• Administer drugs and I.V. fluids as ordered. Continue epinephrine or a sympathomimetic for a patient experiencing an acute attack. Administer aminophylline I.V. as a loading dose. Follow with I.V. drip administration, as ordered. When possible, use an I.V. infusion pump. Simultaneously, give a loading dose of corticosteroidal medication I.V. or I.M., as ordered.
• Combat dehydration with I.V. fluids until the patient can tolerate oral fluids, which will help loosen secretions.
• Encourage the patient to express his fears and concerns about his illness. Answer his questions honestly. Encourage him to identify and comply with care measures and activities that promote relaxation.

Monitoring

• Assess the patient's respiratory status for evidence of deterioration.

HEALTH PROMOTION POINTERS

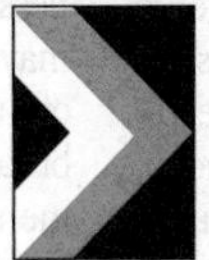

Reducing triggers

Educating the patient to reduce triggers, especially in the environment, is crucial for patients with asthma. Instruct the patient to:
- identify and avoid any foods that may trigger an attack
- wear a mask if cold weather precipitates bronchospasm
- stay indoors when the outside air quality is poor
- avoid contact with people who have respiratory infections
- use environmental control measures, such as enclosing bed items in dustproof covers; using only synthetic blankets; removing carpeting and using only synthetic, easily washable throw rugs and curtains; avoiding use of scents (perfumes and hair spray); avoiding dusty or musty places (basements, storerooms); frequent, often daily, wet dusting of rooms; avoiding exposure to smoke and cooking odors; and using air filtration devices and dehumidifiers as appropriate.

- Monitor the patient's compliance with drug therapy.
- During an acute asthma attack, watch the patient for signs of complications.
- Monitor plasma drug levels of theophylline because oral absorption may vary.
- With long-term corticosteroid therapy, watch for cushingoid adverse reactions.

Patient teaching

- Teach the patient and his family about diaphragmatic and pursed-lip breathing. Advise him to perform relaxation exercises.
- Teach the patient how to use an oral inhaler or a turbo-inhaler. Tell him about possible adverse reactions associated with his medications, and instruct him to notify the doctor if these symptoms occur.

To prevent recurring attacks:
- Show the patient how to breathe deeply. Instruct him to cough up secretions accumulated overnight and to allow time for medications to work.
- Urge the patient to drink plenty of fluids (at least six 8-oz glasses daily) to help loosen secretions and maintain hydration.
- Advise the patient to eat a well-balanced diet to prevent respiratory infection and fatigue. Teach him to avoid substances that trigger an attack. (See *Reducing triggers.*)

Atelectasis

Alveolar clusters (lobules) or lung segments that expand incompletely may produce a partial or complete lung collapse. Known as atelectasis, this phenomenon effectively removes certain regions of the lung from gas exchange. This allows unoxygenated blood to pass unchanged through these regions and produces hypoxia.

Atelectasis may be chronic or acute. The prognosis depends on prompt removal of any airway obstruction, relief of hypoxia, and reexpansion of the collapsed lung.

Causes

Atelectasis can result from bronchial occlusion by mucus plugs, bronchiectasis, or cystic fibrosis. Mucus plugs may also affect lung expansion in patients who smoke heavily. It may also result from occlusion caused by foreign bodies, bronchogenic cancer, and inflammatory lung disease.

Other causes include idiopathic respiratory distress syndrome of the newborn, oxygen toxicity, and pulmonary edema.

External compression, which inhibits full lung expansion, or any condition that makes deep breathing painful may also cause atelectasis. Such compression or pain may result from upper abdominal surgical incisions, rib fractures, pleuritic chest pain, and obesity (which elevates the diaphragm and reduces tidal volume).

What's more, lung collapse or reduced expansion may accompany prolonged immobility (which promotes ventilation of one lung area over another) or mechanical ventilation (which supplies constant small tidal volumes without intermittent deep breaths). Central nervous system depression (resulting from drug overdose, for example) eliminates periodic sighing and predisposes the patient to progressive atelectasis.

Complications

Atelectasis may cause hypoxemia and acute respiratory failure. Additionally, static secretions from atelectasis may lead to pneumonia.

Assessment

Clinical effects vary with the causes of lung collapse, the degree of hypoxia, and the underlying disease. If atelectasis affects a small lung area, the patient's symptoms may be minimal and transient. However, with massive collapse, the patient may report severe symptoms – for example, dyspnea and pleuritic chest pain.

Inspection may disclose decreased chest wall movement, cyanosis, diaphoresis, substernal or intercostal retractions, and anxiety.

Palpation may detect decreased fremitus and mediastinal shift to the affected side. Percussion may disclose dullness or flatness over lung fields. Auscultation findings may include crackles during the last part of inspiration and decreased (or absent) breath sounds with major lung involvement. Auscultation may also disclose tachycardia.

Diagnostic tests

- *Chest X-rays* are the primary diagnostic tool, although extensive areas of "microatelectasis" may exist without abnormalities appearing on the films. In widespread atelectasis, X-ray findings define characteristic horizontal lines in the lower lung zones. With segmental or lobar collapse, the films reveal characteristic dense shadows (commonly associated with hyperinflation of neighboring lung zones).
- *Bronchoscopy* may rule out an obstructing neoplasm or a foreign body if the cause of atelectasis can't be determined.
- *Arterial blood gas (ABG) analysis* may detect respiratory acidosis and hypoxemia resulting from atelectasis.
- *Pulse oximetry* may show deteriorating arterial oxygen saturation levels.

Treatment

Incentive spirometry, chest percussion, postural drainage, and frequent coughing and deep-breathing exercises may improve oxygenation in the patient with atelectasis. If these measures fail, bronchoscopy may help remove secretions. Humidity and bronchodilator medications can improve mucociliary clearance and dilate airways. These drugs may be administered by nebulizer or by a face mask device that establishes continuous positive airway pressure. Alternatively, intermittent positive-pressure breathing therapy may be ordered.

If the patient has atelectasis secondary to an obstructing neoplasm, he may need surgery or radiation therapy. To minimize the risk for atelectasis after thoracic and abdominal surgery, the patient requires analgesics to facilitate deep breathing.

Key nursing diagnoses and patient outcomes

Impaired gas exchange related to decreased availability of lung tissue for gas exchange. Based on this nursing diagnosis, you'll establish these patient outcomes. The patient will:
- not exhibit signs of hypoxia, such as change in level of consciousness, restlessness, or dyspnea
- maintain normal ABG values and pulse oximetry readings.

Ineffective breathing pattern related to decreased chest wall movement. Based on this nursing diagnosis, you'll establish these patient outcomes. The patient will:
- recover a normal respiratory rate and pattern
- achieve maximum lung expansion with adequate ventilation.

Risk for infection related to retained pulmonary secretions. Based on this nursing diagnosis, you'll establish these patient outcomes. The patient will:
- maintain a normal temperature and white blood cell count
- perform bronchial hygienic measures correctly and as ordered
- not exhibit other signs and symptoms of pulmonary infection.

Nursing interventions

- Encourage the patient recovering from surgery (or other patients at high risk for atelectasis) to perform coughing and deep-breathing exercises every 1 to 2 hours. To minimize pain during these exercises, hold a pillow tightly over the patient's incisional area. Teach the patient how to do this for himself.
- Help the patient use an incentive spirometer to encourage deep breathing.
- *Gently* reposition the patient often, and help him walk as soon as possible. Administer adequate analgesics to control pain.
- If the patient is receiving mechanical ventilation, maintain tidal volume at 10 to 15 cc/kg of the patient's body weight to ensure adequate lung expansion. Use the sigh mechanism on the ventilator, if appropriate, to intermittently increase tidal volume at the rate of 3 to 4 sighs/hour.
- Humidify inspired air, and encourage adequate fluid intake to mobilize secretions. Use postural drainage and chest percussion to remove secretions.
- Provide suctioning as needed for patients who are intubated or unable to clear their own secretions. Administer sedatives with care because these medications depress respirations and the cough reflex. They also suppress sighs. Keep in mind that the patient will cooperate minimally with treatment (or not at all) if he has pain.
- Offer ample reassurance and emotional support because the patient's limited breathing capacity may frighten him.

Monitoring

- Assess breath sounds and respiratory status frequently. Report any changes immediately.
- Evaluate the patient's ability to perform bronchial hygiene.
- Monitor pulse oximetry readings and ABG values for evidence of hypoxia.
- Observe the patient for pain if appropriate.

Patient teaching

- Teach the patient how to use the spirometer. Urge him to use it every 1 to 2 hours.
- Show the patient and his family how to perform postural drainage and percussion. Instruct the patient to maintain each position for 10 minutes and then perform chest percussion. Let him know when to cough. Also, teach coughing and deep-breathing techniques to promote ventilation and mobilize secretions.
- Encourage the patient to stop smoking or to lose weight, or to do both, if needed. Refer him to appropriate educational resources and support groups for help.
- Demonstrate comfort measures to promote relaxation and conserve energy. Advise the patient and his family to alternate periods of rest and activity to promote energy and prevent fatigue.

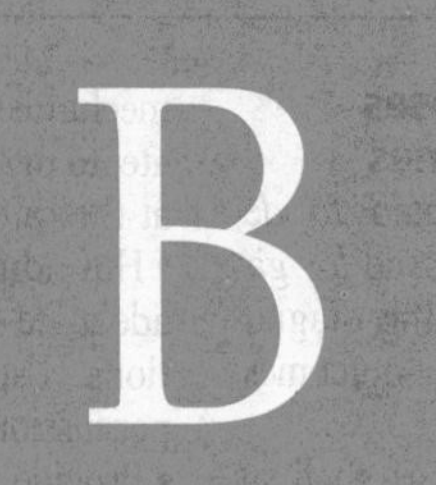

Basal cell epithelioma

This slow-growing, destructive skin tumor usually occurs in people over age 40. Basal cell epithelioma is most prevalent in blond, fair-skinned men, and it's the most common malignant tumor that affects whites. The two major types of basal cell epithelioma are noduloulcerative and superficial.

Causes

Prolonged sun exposure is the most common cause of basal cell epithelioma – 90% of tumors occur on sun-exposed areas of the body – but arsenic ingestion, radiation exposure, burns, immunosuppression and, rarely, vaccinations are other possible causes.

Although the pathogenesis is uncertain, some experts hypothesize that basal cell epithelioma originates when undifferentiated basal cells become cancerous instead of differentiating into sweat glands, sebum, and hair.

Complications

Disease progression can lead to disfiguring lesions of the eyes, nose, and cheeks.

Assessment

The patient history may reveal that the patient became aware of an odd-looking skin lesion, which prompted him to seek medical examination. The history may also disclose prolonged exposure to the sun sometime in the patient's life or other risk factors for this disease.

Inspection of the face, particularly the forehead, eyelid margins, and nasolabial folds, may reveal lesions characterized as small, smooth, pinkish, and translucent papules (early-stage noduloulcerative). Telangiectatic vessels cross the surface, and the lesions may be pigmented. As the lesions enlarge, their centers become depressed and their borders become firm and elevated. These ulcerated tumors are called rodent ulcers.

Inspection of the chest and back may disclose multiple oval or irregularly shaped, lightly pigmented plaques. These may have sharply defined, slightly elevated, threadlike borders (superficial basal cell epitheliomas).

Inspection of the head and neck may show waxy, sclerotic, yellow to white plaques without distinct borders. These plaques may resemble small patches of scleroderma and may suggest sclerosing basal cell epitheliomas (morphea-like epitheliomas).

Diagnostic tests

All types of basal cell epitheliomas are diagnosed by clinical appearance. Incisional or excisional biopsy and histologic study may help to determine the tumor type and histologic subtype.

Treatment

Depending on the size, location, and depth of the lesion, treatment may include curet-

tage and electrodesiccation, chemotherapy, surgical excision, irradiation, or chemosurgery.
• *Curettage and electrodesiccation* offer good cosmetic results for small lesions.
• *Topical fluorouracil* is often used for superficial lesions. This medication produces marked local irritation or inflammation in the involved tissue but no systemic effects.
• Microscopically controlled *surgical excision* carefully removes recurrent lesions until a tumor-free plane is achieved. After removal of large lesions, skin grafting may be required.
• *Irradiation* is used if the tumor location requires it. It's also preferred for elderly or debilitated patients who might not tolerate surgery.
• *Chemosurgery* may be necessary for persistent or recurrent lesions. It consists of periodic applications of a fixative paste (such as zinc chloride) and subsequent removal of fixed pathologic tissue. Treatment continues until tumor removal is complete.
• *Cryotherapy,* using liquid nitrogen, freezes the cells and kills them.

Key nursing diagnoses and patient outcomes

Body image disturbance related to facial disfigurement caused by lesions. Based on this nursing diagnosis, you'll establish these patient outcomes. The patient will:
• acknowledge changes in body image
• participate in decisions about care that will minimize or prevent recurrence of facial lesions
• develop and express positive feelings about himself.

Fear related to the diagnosis of cancer. Based on this nursing diagnosis, you'll establish these patient outcomes. The patient will:
• identify fears related to the diagnosis
• use available support systems to help cope with fear
• express reduced fear and manifest no physical signs or symptoms of fear.

Impaired skin integrity related to ulceration caused by basal cell epithelioma or skin irritation from therapy. Based on this nursing diagnosis, you'll establish these patient outcomes. The patient will:
• communicate and demonstrate preventive skin care measures
• exhibit a positive response to therapy and no recurrence of basal cell epithelioma
• not develop skin breakdown from therapy.

Nursing interventions

• Listen to the patient's fears and concerns. Offer reassurance when appropriate. Remain with the patient during periods of severe stress and anxiety. Provide positive reinforcement for the patient's efforts to adapt.
• Arrange for the patient to interact with others who have a similar problem.
• Assess the patient's readiness for decision making; then involve him and his family in decisions related to his care whenever possible.
• Provide reassurance and comfort measures when appropriate.

Monitoring

• Watch for complications of treatment, including local skin irritation from topically applied chemotherapeutic agents and infection.
• If applicable, watch for radiation's adverse effects, such as nausea, vomiting, hair loss, malaise, and diarrhea.

Patient teaching

• Instruct the patient to eat frequent, small, high-protein meals. Advise him to include eggnogs, blenderized foods, and liquid protein supplements if the lesion has invaded the oral cavity and is causing eating difficulty.
• To prevent disease recurrence, tell the patient to avoid excessive sun exposure and to use a strong sunscreen to protect his skin from damage by ultraviolet rays.

• Advise the patient to relieve local inflammation from topical fluorouracil with cool compresses or with corticosteroid ointment.
• Instruct the patient with noduloulcerative basal cell epithelioma to wash his face gently when ulcerations and crusting occur; scrubbing too vigorously may cause bleeding.
• As appropriate, direct the patient and his family to hospital and community support services – for example, social workers, psychologists, and cancer support groups.

Benign prostatic hyperplasia

Most men over age 50 have some prostatic enlargement or benign prostatic hyperplasia (BPH). BPH becomes symptomatic when the prostate gland enlarges sufficiently to compress the urethra and cause some overt urinary obstruction. As the prostate enlarges, it may extend toward the bladder and obstruct urine outflow by compressing or distorting the prostatic urethra. BPH also may cause a weakening of the detrusor musculature that retains urine when the rest of the bladder empties. Depending on the size of the enlarged prostate, the age and health of the patient, and the extent of the obstruction, BPH may be treated surgically or symptomatically.

Causes

The cause of BPH is unknown. It is known that circulating male hormones or androgens, specifically testosterone, and aging are necessary for BPH to develop.

Complications

Because BPH causes urinary obstruction, a patient may have one or more of the following complications:
• urinary retention or incomplete bladder emptying, leading to urinary tract infection (UTI) or calculi
• bladder wall trabeculation
• detrusor muscle hypertrophy
• bladder diverticuli and saccules
• urethral stenosis
• hydronephrosis
• overflow incontinence
• acute or chronic renal failure
• acute postobstructive diuresis.

Assessment

Clinical features of BPH depend on the extent of prostatic enlargement and the lobes affected. Characteristically, the patient complains of obstructive voiding symptoms: decreased urine stream caliber and force, an interrupted stream, urinary hesitancy, and difficulty starting urination, which results in straining and a feeling of incomplete voiding.

As the obstruction increases, the patient may report irritative voiding symptoms; frequent urination with nocturia, dribbling, urine retention, incontinence and, possibly, hematuria.

Physical examination may reveal a visible midline mass above the symphysis pubis, which represents an incompletely emptied bladder. The distended bladder can be palpated. Rectal examination discloses an enlarged prostate.

Diagnostic tests

The following tests help to confirm this diagnosis:
• *Excretory urography* may indicate urinary tract obstruction, hydronephrosis, calculi or tumors, and filling and emptying defects in the bladder.
• *Elevated blood urea nitrogen* and *serum creatinine levels* suggest impaired renal function.
• *Urinalysis* and *urine culture* show hematuria, pyuria and, when the bacterial count exceeds 100,000/mm^3, UTI.
• *Prostate-specific antigen (PSA)* levels are routinely drawn on men with prostatic symptoms to rule out prostate cancer.

When symptoms are severe, cystourethroscopy is the definitive diagnostic measure and helps to determine the best surgical procedure. It can show prostate enlargement, bladder wall changes, calculi, and a raised bladder.

Treatment

Medications can be effective in relieving symptoms of urethral obstruction caused by BPH. Alpha blockers, such as terazosin and doxazosin, relax the bladder neck and prostatic urethra. These drugs are also used for hypertension; adverse effects include hypotension, dizziness, headaches, and nasal congestion. Finasteride blocks the conversion of testosterone to dihydrotestosterone within the prostate, preventing the continued growth of BPH. It causes few adverse effects but must be taken for 6 to 12 months before the patient notices an improvement in symptoms.

Surgery is the only effective therapy for relief of acute urine retention, hydronephrosis, severe hematuria, and recurrent UTI and for palliative relief of intolerable symptoms. Continuous drainage with an indwelling urinary catheter alleviates urine retention in high-risk patients. A transurethral resection may be performed if the prostate weighs under 2 oz (56.7 g). Weight is approximated by digital examination. (See the entry "Prostatectomy.")

Other procedures involve open surgical removal of the prostate (prostatectomy). One of the following operations may be appropriate:

- *Suprapubic (transvesical) prostatectomy* is the most common and is especially useful when prostatic enlargement remains within the bladder area.
- *Perineal prostatectomy* usually is performed for a large gland in an older patient. The operation commonly results in impotence and incontinence.
- *Retropubic (extravesical) prostatectomy* allows direct visualization; potency and continence usually are maintained in about 50% of patients.

Key nursing diagnoses and patient outcomes

Altered urinary elimination related to obstruction of the urethra. Based on this nursing diagnosis, you'll establish these patient outcomes. The patient will:

- be able to empty the bladder effectively
- identify signs and symptoms of urine retention and seek medical attention.

The patient and family or caretaker will:

- demonstrate skill in managing urine elimination problem.

Risk for infection related to potential for urine retention. Based on this nursing diagnosis, you'll establish these patient outcomes. The patient will:

- have urine that will remain clear yellow, odorless, with no sediment, and free of bacteria
- not experience signs and symptoms of UTI.

Urge incontinence related to obstruction of the urethra. Based on this nursing diagnosis, you'll establish these patient outcomes. The patient will:

- regain continence
- not experience complications of urinary incontinence, such as skin breakdown
- seek medical or surgical treatment.

Nursing interventions

- Prepare the patient for diagnostic tests and surgery, as appropriate.
- Obtain a urine culture if UTI is suspected. Administer antibiotics, as ordered, for UTI, urethral procedures that involve instruments, and cystoscopy.
- If urine retention occurs, insert an indwelling urinary catheter (difficult in a patient with BPH). If the catheter can't be passed transurethrally, assist with suprapubic cystostomy (under local anesthesia).
- Avoid giving a patient with BPH decongestants, tranquilizers, alcohol, antidepressants, or anticholinergics because these drugs can worsen obstruction.

Monitoring

- Monitor and record the patient's vital signs, intake and output, and daily weight. Watch closely for signs of postobstructive diuresis (such as increased urine output and hypotension), which may lead to serious dehydration, lowered blood volume, shock, electrolyte losses, and anuria.
- Observe the patient for signs and symptoms of UTI, such as dysuria or changes in urine appearance.

Patient teaching

- If an indwelling urinary catheter has been used to maintain urine flow until surgery can be done, the patient may experience urinary frequency, dribbling and, occasionally, hematuria after the catheter has been removed. Reassure him and his family that he'll gradually regain urinary control.
- Teach the patient to recognize the signs of UTI. Urge him to immediately report these signs to the doctor because infection can worsen obstruction.
- Instruct the patient to follow the prescribed oral antibiotic regimen, and tell him the indications for using gentle laxatives.
- Urge the patient to seek medical care immediately if he can't void, if he passes bloody urine, or if he develops a fever.
- Advise the patient that it may take several months of medical therapy before symptoms improve; emphasize the importance of regular follow-up.

Bladder cancer

Benign or malignant tumors may develop on the bladder wall surface or grow within the wall itself and quickly invade underlying muscles. About 90% of bladder cancers are transitional cell carcinomas, arising from the transitional epithelium of mucous membranes. They may result from malignant transformation of benign papillomas. Less common bladder tumors include adenocarcinomas and squamous cell carcinomas.

Bladder tumors are most prevalent in people over age 50, are more common in men than in women, and occur more often in densely populated industrial areas. Bladder cancer is the fourth most common cause of cancer deaths in men over age 75.

Despite treatment, the patient with superficial disease has up to an 80% chance for recurrence. Only about 10% of superficial bladder cancers develop into invasive disease; in invasive disease, however, the patient's chances for metastasis increase up to 90%. With treatment, about 50% of patients with invasive cancer experience complete remission; 20% have partial remission.

Causes

Certain substances, such as 2-naphthylamine, tobacco, and nitrates, may predispose a person to transitional cell tumors. This places certain industrial workers (including rubber workers, weavers, aniline dye workers, hairdressers, petroleum workers, spray painters, and leather finishers) at high risk for developing these tumors. The latency period between exposure to the carcinogen and development of signs and symptoms of a tumor is about 18 years.

Squamous cell carcinoma of the bladder is common in geographic areas where schistosomiasis is endemic, such as Egypt. What's more, it's also associated with chronic bladder irritation and infection in people with renal calculi, indwelling urinary catheters, chemical cystitis that's caused by cyclophosphamide, and pelvic irradiation.

Complications

If bladder cancer progresses, complications include bone metastases and problems resulting from tumor invasion of contiguous viscera.

Assessment

The patient typically reports gross, painless, intermittent hematuria (often with clots). He may complain of suprapubic pain after voiding (which suggests invasive lesions). Other signs and symptoms include bladder irritability, urinary frequency, nocturia, and dribbling. If the patient reports flank pain, he may have an obstructed ureter.

Diagnostic tests

• To confirm a bladder cancer diagnosis, the patient typically undergoes *cystoscopy* and *biopsy.* If the test results show cancer cells, further studies will determine the cancer stage and treatment. (See *Comparing staging systems for bladder cancer,* page 100.)

Cystoscopy should be performed when hematuria first appears. If the patient receives an anesthetic during the procedure, he also may undergo a bimanual examination to detect whether the bladder is fixed to the pelvic wall.

• *Excretory urography* can identify a large, early-stage tumor or an infiltrating tumor; delineate functional problems in the upper urinary tract; assess hydronephrosis; and detect rigid deformity of the bladder wall.

• *Urinalysis* can detect blood and malignant cells in the urine.

• *Retrograde cystography* can evaluate bladder structure and integrity. The test results can also help confirm a bladder cancer diagnosis.

• *Bone scan* can detect metastases.

• *Computed tomography scan* or *magnetic resonance imaging* can define the thickness of the involved bladder wall and disclose enlarged retroperitoneal lymph nodes.

• *Ultrasonography* can detect metastases in tissues beyond the bladder and can also distinguish a bladder cyst from a bladder tumor.

• *Laboratory tests,* such as a complete blood count and chemistry profile, may be ordered to evaluate conditions such as anemia, which are associated with bladder cancer.

Treatment

The cancer's stage and the patient's lifestyle, other health problems, and mental outlook will influence selection of therapy. Surgery, chemotherapy, and radiation therapy may be used.

Superficial bladder tumors are typically removed cystoscopically by *transurethral resection* and electrically by *fulguration.* This approach usually is effective treatment if the tumor hasn't invaded the muscle. Additional tumors may also develop, however, and fulguration may then have to be repeated every 3 months for years. Once the tumors penetrate the muscle layer or recur frequently, cystoscopy with fulguration is no longer an appropriate treatment choice.

Intravesical chemotherapy is used for treating superficial tumors (especially tumors in several sites) and for preventing recurrence of tumors. This approach directly washes the bladder with drugs that fight the cancer. Commonly used antitumor agents include thiotepa, doxorubicin, and mitomycin.

Intravesical administration of the live, attenuated *bacille Calmette-Guérin vaccine* has been effective in the treatment of superficial bladder cancers, particularly primary and relapsed carcinoma in situ.

Tumors too large to be treated by cystoscopy require *segmental bladder resection.* This surgical approach removes a full-thickness section of the bladder and is practical only if the tumor isn't located near the bladder neck or ureteral orifices. Bladder instillations of thiotepa after transurethral resection also may be useful therapy.

Comparing staging systems for bladder cancer

Staging helps determine the most appropriate treatment for bladder cancer. One of two staging systems may be used: the tumor, node, metastasis (TNM) system or the Jewett-Strong-Marshall (JSM) system.

Both systems distinguish superficial bladder cancers from invasive bladder cancers, which penetrate bladder muscle and may spread to other sites. In the chart below, a dash indicates that a grade can't be determined.

TNM system	Stage	JSM system
Superficial tumor		
TX	Primary tumor can't be assessed	–
T0	No tumor	0
Tis	Carcinoma in situ	0
Ta	Noninvasive papillary tumor	0
Invasive tumor		
T1	Tumor invades subepithelial connective tissue	–
T2	Tumor invades superficial muscle (inner half)	B1
T3a	Tumor invades deep muscle	B2
T3b	Tumor invades perivesical fat	C
T4	Tumor invades prostate, uterus, vagina, pelvic wall, or abdominal wall	D1
NX	Regional lymph nodes can't be assessed	–
N0	No evidence of lymph node involvement	–
N1	Metastasis in a single lymph node, 2 cm or less in greatest dimension	D1
N2	Metastasis in a single lymph node, between 2 and 5 cm in greatest dimension, or metastases to several lymph nodes, none greater than 5 cm in greatest dimension	–
N3	Metastasis in a lymph node more than 5 cm in greatest dimension	–
MX	Distant metastasis can't be assessed	–
M0	No evidence of distant metastasis	–
M	Distant metastasis	D2

For patients with infiltrating bladder tumors, the treatment of choice is *radical cystectomy.*

Treatment for patients with advanced bladder cancer includes cystectomy to remove the tumor, radiation therapy, and combination systemic chemotherapy with cisplatin, the most active agent. Other agents include methotrexate, vinblastine, and doxorubicin. In some instances, this combined treatment successfully arrests the disease.

Key nursing diagnoses and patient outcomes

Altered urinary elimination related to changes in bladder function. Based on this nursing diagnosis, you'll establish these patient outcomes. The patient will:
- maintain adequate urine elimination through natural or artifical means
- recognize and report changes in urine elimination pattern to the doctor
- adhere to the prescribed treatment plan used to eradicate cancer cells in the bladder.

Fear related to potential radical changes in body image and possibly death from bladder cancer. Based on this nursing diagnosis, you'll establish these patient outcomes. The patient will:
- express his fears
- seek help in coping with fears from support groups, family, and friends
- express reduced fear and demonstrate no physical signs of fear.

Pain related to urinary tract infection or cancer cell invasion to surrounding tissues. Based on this nursing diagnosis, you'll establish these patient outcomes. The patient will:
- seek medical care for pain relief
- express feelings of relief and comfort after analgesic administration or other therapy to treat complication responsible for the pain
- become pain free.

Nursing interventions

- Listen to the patient's fears and concerns. Stay with him during episodes of severe stress and anxiety, and provide psychological support, as needed. As appropriate, encourage the patient to express feelings and concerns about the extent of the cancer, the surgical procedure, an altered body image (especially if he undergoes urinary diversion surgery), and sexual dysfunction.
- To relieve discomfort, administer ordered analgesics for pain as necessary. Implement comfort measures and provide distractions that will enable the patient to relax.
- As appropriate, implement measures to prevent or alleviate complications of treatment.

Monitoring

- Monitor the patient's intake and output. Question him regularly about changes in his urine elimination pattern to detect changes in his condition.
- Observe the patient's urine for signs of hematuria (reddish tint to gross bloodiness) or infection (cloudy, foul smelling, with sediment present).
- Monitor the patient's laboratory tests, such as changes in white blood cell differential, indicating possible bone marrow suppression from chemotherapy.
- If the patient is being given intravesical chemotherapy, watch closely for myelosuppression, chemical cystitis, and skin rash.
- If the patient is receiving chemotherapy, watch for complications from the particular drug regimen.

Patient teaching

- Inform the patient what to expect from the diagnostic tests. For example, make sure he understands that anesthesia may be given to him before undergoing cystoscopy. After the test results are known, explain their implications to the patient and his family.
- Instruct the patient and family about the types of treatment that are being planned for him.
- Teach the patient and family to recognize and manage adverse effects of chemotherapy.
- Teach the patient and family how to care for urinary diversions, if performed; arrange for home care follow up if necessary.
- Stress the importance of notifying the doctor if the patient develops signs and

symptoms of urinary tract infection or other sudden changes in his condition.
• Refer the patient to the American Cancer Society as appropriate.

Bone marrow transplantation

The treatment of choice for aplastic anemia and severe combined immunodeficiency diseases, bone marrow transplantation involves the infusion of fresh or stored bone marrow into a recipient. The procedure may also be used to treat acute leukemia, chronic leukemia, lymphoma, multiple myeloma, and certain solid tumors.

The bone marrow used in the transplantation may be obtained by autologous, syngeneic, or allogeneic means. In an *autologous* donation, the bone marrow is harvested from the patient before he receives chemotherapy or radiation therapy, or while he's in remission, and then frozen for later use.

In a *syngeneic* donation, bone marrow is taken from the patient's identical twin. Obviously, syngeneic donations are rare. But, when possible, they are the ideal type. That's because an identical twin has healthy bone marrow that is histologically identical to the patient's own tissue.

The most common type of transplant involves an *allogeneic* donation. For this procedure, bone marrow is obtained from a histocompatible individual. This is usually a sibling, although it's possible for an unrelated donor to meet the requirements. Because the donor's and patient's tissue don't match perfectly, the patient must receive medications to suppress his immune system. Even then, the procedure isn't always successful.

A new method, *peripheral stem cell* transplantation, involves the collection of peripheral stem cells, usually after the patient has been treated with chemotherapy or growth factors to increase the number of circulating stem cells. The cells are stored and later reinfused into the patient after high-dose chemotherapy and, possibly, radiotherapy.

Procedure

If the patient will be receiving his own bone marrow, the donation will have been made 2 weeks earlier and frozen. For a syngeneic or allogeneic transplant, doctors will obtain the donor bone marrow in the operating room the same day as the transplant. (See *Teaching about marrow donation.*)

The transplantation procedure itself will occur at the patient's bedside. Just before the procedure, administer an antihistamine or analgesic, as ordered, to minimize adverse reactions. In the case of an allogeneic or syngeneic donation, someone will bring the bone marrow to the patient's room as soon as it's obtained. For an autologous donation, the marrow will be allowed to thaw. Then, as soon as the marrow has been made available or has thawed, the doctor will infuse it into the patient through a central venous catheter.

The rate of infusion varies, depending on the volume of marrow being infused. Once infused, the marrow cells will migrate to the patient's marrow cavity, where they'll begin to proliferate. This process, called engraftment, takes from 10 days to 4 weeks.

Complications

During infusion, potential complications include volume overload, anaphylaxis, and pulmonary fat emboli. After infusion, the patient may develop an infection or abnormal bleeding. If the bone marrow was obtained from an allogeneic donor, the patient may develop graft-versus-host disease (GVHD). This serious complication can occur anywhere from a few days to years after transplantation.

Key nursing diagnoses and patient outcomes

Risk for injury related to GVHD as a result of bone marrow transplantation. Based on this nursing diagnosis, you'll establish these patient outcomes. The patient will:
• identify the early signs and symptoms of GVHD and express the importance of seeking immediate medical attention if any should occur
• not experience permanent damage to any body organ or system as a result of GVHD.

Risk for infection related to immunosuppression caused by chemotherapy and radiation used to prepare the patient for bone marrow transplantation. Based on this nursing diagnosis, you'll establish these patient outcomes. The patient will:
• not exhibit any signs and symptoms of infection, and his temperature will remain normal
• regain, and then maintain, a normal white blood cell count
• remain free of infection.

Altered protection related to potential for bleeding caused by immunosuppression as a result of chemotherapy and radiation used to prepare patient for bone marrow transplantation. Based on this nursing diagnosis, you'll establish these patient outcomes. The patient will:
• not exhibit any signs of bleeding
• regain and then maintain a normal platelet count.

Nursing interventions

When caring for a patient receiving bone marrow transplantation, your responsibilities will focus on educating the patient and on protecting him from potential complications.

Before the procedure

• Reinforce the doctor's explanation of bone marrow transplantation. Give the patient and his family time to discuss the procedure fully to be sure they understand its risks and benefits. Make sure they know that, if the transplant fails, the patient may die. Then ensure that the patient or a responsible family member has signed a consent form.
• Inform the patient that, because his white blood cells will be depleted, he'll be at high risk for infection immediately after the procedure and may remain in reverse isolation for several weeks. Explain that

Teaching about marrow donation

When a patient is scheduled for a syngeneic or allogeneic bone marrow transplant, you'll need to prepare the donor for the procedure. To begin, make sure the donor understands the risks of the procurement procedure. Give him an opportunity to ask questions and express his concerns or fears.

Tell him that he'll be taken to the operating room for the procedure and that, once there, the doctor will insert a needle in his iliac crest and aspirate bone marrow. The procedure will require multiple aspirations. Reassure the donor that he'll receive either a general or epidural anesthetic and that he won't feel any pain during the procedure.

Inform the donor that the doctor will aspirate between 500 and 1,000 ml of bone marrow and that the procedure will take 1½ to 2 hours. Explain that, once the marrow is obtained, it will be filtered to remove bone and fat particles and then mixed with an anticoagulant. It will then be placed in a blood administration bag and taken to the patient's room for immediate infusion.

Tell the donor that, after the procedure, he'll be taken to the recovery room. Let him know that the sites where the doctor removed the marrow will be covered with pressure dressings. Warn him that he'll probably feel pain when he wakes up, but reassure him that the nurse will give him medication to relieve it.

contact with his family will be limited during this time.

• Prepare the patient for the pretransplant regimen. Explain that he will receive chemotherapy or radiation therapy (or both) to kill any residual cancer cells.

• During this pretransplant regimen, expect to see adverse reactions, such as bone marrow suppression, diarrhea, fever, cystitis, nausea, vomiting, and mucositis. Administer prophylactic antiemetics, as ordered. Monitor intake and output and administer fluids to prevent fluid and electrolyte imbalances and cystitis.

• Before the procedure begins, make sure that diphenhydramine and epinephrine are readily available to manage transfusion reactions. Start an I.V. line for hydration and record vital signs. Obtain an administration set (without a filter, which can trap the marrow cells) for the bone marrow infusion.

During the procedure

• Once the transfusion has begun, take the patient's vital signs at least every 15 minutes for 1 hour, every 30 minutes for the next 2 hours, and then every hour for another 4 hours. The patient's vital signs will help you promptly recognize such reactions as fever, dyspnea, and hypotension.

• Monitor the patient for other reactions, such as bronchospasm, urticaria, erythema, chest pain, and back pain. Administer ordered medications to relieve these symptoms.

After the procedure

• Continue to monitor the patient's vital signs closely, and assess the patient every 4 hours for any signs of infection, such as fever or chills. Because the patient is already pancytopenic from the pretransplant regimen, he's at risk for hemorrhage as well as infection. Maintain strict asepsis when caring for him, and take measures to protect him from injury. The doctor may also order blood or platelet transfusions (or both), and the patient may be placed in a room with laminar flow to further reduce the possibility of infection.

• Draw blood for laboratory analysis, as ordered, and monitor the patient's hematologic status. Notify the doctor immediately of any changes.

• On the seventh day after the transplant, begin to watch for symptoms of GVHD, such as dermatitis, hepatitis, hemolytic anemia, and thrombocytopenia.

Home care instructions

• Tell the patient and family about infection control measures and bleeding precautions.

• Teach the patient and his family how to care for the central venous catheter.

• Instruct the patient and his family about his medication regimen, including how to administer his medications.

• Tell the patient and his family about potential complications and what signs and symptoms to be alert for. Stress the importance of contacting the doctor *immediately* if any should occur.

• Make sure the patient and his family have emergency telephone numbers, such as those for the doctor managing his post-transplant follow-up care, the health care facility where the bone marrow transplant was performed, and ambulance services.

• Stress the need to keep follow-up medical appointments so that the doctor can monitor his progress and detect complications.

• If the patient is a child, explain to the parents that his growth may be impaired by bone marrow transplantation. Tell them to monitor their child's growth; if it lags, he may need hormonal therapy.

Bone tumors, primary malignant

Sarcomas of the bone, primary malignant bone tumors are rare, constituting less than 0.5% of all malignant tumors. Most bone tumors result from metastasis from another malignant tumor.

Primary bone tumors occur more commonly in males than in females and especially in children and adolescents, although some types occur in people ages 35 to 60.

Causes

Although the cause of primary malignant bone tumors remains unknown, some researchers hypothesize that they arise in centers of rapid skeletal growth because children and young adults with these tumors seem to be much taller than average. Other theories point to heredity factors, trauma, and excessive radiotherapy as causes.

Prior exposure to carcinogens, an underlying condition such as Paget's disease, or radiation exposure has been linked with the development of osteogenic sarcomas, chondrosarcomas, and fibrosarcomas.

Primary malignant bone tumors may originate in osseous or nonosseous tissue. (See *Types of primary malignant bone tumors,* page 106.) Osseous tumors arise from the bony structure itself as well as from cartilage, fibrous tissue, and bone marrow. They include osteogenic sarcoma (the most common), parosteal osteogenic sarcoma, chondrosarcoma (malignant cartilage tumor), and malignant giant cell tumor. Together, these make up 60% of all malignant bone tumors.

Nonosseous tumors arise from hematopoietic, vascular, and neural tissues. These include Ewing's sarcoma, fibrosarcoma, and chordoma. Osteogenic and Ewing's sarcomas are the most common bone tumors of children.

Complications

A life-threatening complication, hypercalcemia commonly occurs from excessive calcium release associated with tumor destruction of bone. When the calcium reaches a level that exceeds the renal and GI capacity to excrete it, the calcium blood level rises above normal.

Assessment

The patient may complain of bone pain and describe it as a dull ache. The pain is usually localized, although it may be referred from the hip or spine. The patient may describe the pain as more intense at night and note that movement doesn't aggravate the pain.

Inspection may reveal weakness in the affected limb; you may also note that the patient walks with a limp. In late stages, the patient may appear cachectic, with fever and impaired mobility.

Palpation may disclose a mass or tumor, possibly accompanied by swelling. You may also find a pathologic fracture.

Diagnostic tests

A biopsy (by incision or aspiration) confirms primary malignant bone tumors. Bone X-rays and radioisotope bone and computed tomography scans delineate the tumor size. A patient with sarcoma also usually has elevated serum alkaline phosphatase levels.

Treatment

The focus of treatment is preserving the limb as well as controlling the cancer. Surgical resection of the tumor (often with preoperative radiation and postoperative chemotherapy) saves many limbs from amputation. Some hospitals may perform both preoperative and postoperative radiation therapy and chemotherapy or various other combinations.

Sometimes treatment calls for radical surgery, such as hemipelvectomy. When any type of surgical amputation is indicated, a 3″ to 4″ (8- to 10-cm) margin of healthy tissue should be left.

Intensive chemotherapy combines cyclophosphamide, vincristine, doxorubicin, and dacarbazine. Adjuvant therapies include immunotherapy with interferon and

Types of primary malignant bone tumors

Type	Clinical features	Treatment
Osseous origin		
Osteogenic sarcoma	• Osteoid tumor present in specimen • Arises from bone-forming osteoblast and bone-digesting osteoclast • Occurs most commonly in femur but also in tibia and humerus; occasionally, in fibula, ileum, vertebra, or mandible • Usually occurs in men ages 10 to 30	• Surgery (tumor resection, high thigh amputation, hemipelvectomy) • Radiation therapy • Chemotherapy • Combination of above
Parosteal osteogenic sarcoma	• Develops on surface of bone instead of interior; progresses slowly • Occurs most commonly in distal femur; occurs in tibia, humerus, and ulna also • Usually develops in women ages 30 to 40	• Surgery (tumor resection, possible amputation, hemipelvectomy) • Chemotherapy • Combination of above
Chondrosarcoma	• Develops from cartilage • Doesn't cause pain; grows slowly; locally recurrent and invasive • Occurs most commonly in pelvis, proximal femur, ribs, and shoulder girdle • Usually develops in men ages 30 to 50	• Hemipelvectomy, surgical resection (ribs) • Radiation therapy (palliative) • Chemotherapy
Malignant giant cell tumor	• Arises from benign giant cell tumor • Most common in long bones, especially in knee • Usually develops in women ages 18 to 50	• Curettage • Total excision • Radiation therapy
Nonosseous origin		
Ewing's sarcoma	• Originates in bone marrow and invades shafts of long and flat bones • Usually affects legs, most commonly femur, innominate bones, ribs, tibia, humerus, vertebra, and fibula; may spread to lungs • Causes increasingly severe and persistent pain • Usually develops in men ages 10 to 20	• High-voltage radiation therapy (tumor is very radiosensitive) • Chemotherapy to slow growth • Amputation (only if no evidence of metastases)
Fibrosarcoma	• Occurs relatively rarely; originates in fibrous tissue of bone; invades long or flat bones (femur, tibia, mandible); also involves periosteum and overlying muscle • Usually develops in men ages 30 to 40	• Amputation • Radiation therapy • Chemotherapy • Bone grafts (with low-grade fibrosarcoma)
Chordoma	• Derived from embryonic remnants of notochord; progresses slowly • Occurs at end of vertebral column and in spheno-occipital, sacrococcygeal, and vertebral areas; causes constipation and visual problems • Usually develops in men ages 50 to 60	• Surgical resection (often resulting in neural defects) • Radiation therapy (palliative, or when surgery isn't applicable, as in occipital area)

hyperthermia, which is still under investigation.

Key nursing diagnoses and patient outcomes

Body image disturbance related to amputation of a limb. Based on this nursing diagnosis, you'll establish these patient outcomes. The patient will:
- express feelings about amputation's effects on his body image
- participate in a rehabilitation program to learn how to adapt to change in body image and function
- accept change in body image.

Impaired physical mobility related to the presence of a primary malignant bone tumor affecting the function of the extremity. Based on this nursing diagnosis, you'll establish these patient outcomes. The patient will:
- maintain physical strength and joint mobility in the affected limb
- not develop complications related to physical immobility, such as skin breakdown or contractures
- regain mobility of the affected limb through treatment or the use of a prosthesis.

Pain related to malignant bone tumor. Based on this nursing diagnosis, you'll establish these patient outcomes. The patient will:
- obtain pain relief after analgesic administration
- avoid activities that increase pain or seek assistance to minimize pain
- become pain free with treatment.

Nursing interventions

- Administer analgesics as necessary. Make sure the patient has received his analgesic before morning care or any activity that may increase pain. If necessary, brace him with pillows, keeping the affected part at rest.
- Provide foods high in protein, vitamins, and folic acid. Administer laxatives if necessary. Encourage fluids to prevent dehydration, and record intake and output.
- Because the patient may have thrombocytopenia, make sure he uses a soft toothbrush and an electric razor to avoid bleeding. Don't give I.M. injections or take rectal temperatures. Be careful not to bump the patient's arms or legs; low platelet count causes bruising.
- During radiation therapy or chemotherapy, take measures to reduce adverse reactions, such as providing the patient with plenty of fluids to drink and saline mouthwash for gargling.
- Prepare the patient for amputation, if indicated. Throughout treatment, be sensitive to the enormous emotional strain of amputation. Encourage communication, and help the patient set realistic goals.
- Listen to the patient's fears and concerns, and offer reassurance when appropriate. Stay with the patient during periods of severe stress and anxiety.

Monitoring

- Regularly monitor the patient's degree of pain and the effectiveness of analgesics and other pain relief measures, such as positioning or guided imagery.
- Evaluate the patient's coping ability and emotional state for signs of severe anxiety, depression, or inability to cope.
- During radiation therapy, monitor the patient for such adverse reactions as nausea, vomiting, and dry skin with excoriation.
- During chemotherapy, watch for such complications as infection and for expected adverse reactions, including nausea, vomiting, mouth ulcers, and alopecia.

Patient teaching

- Help the patient and his family understand the disease. Reinforce the doctor's explanations, and provide information that will help the patient and his family make informed decisions about treatment.
- Prepare the patient for the effects of surgery, if indicated.

• Stress the importance of getting plenty of rest and sleep to promote recovery, but encourage some physical exercise.
• Emphasize the importance of sound nutrition. Ask the dietitian to provide instruction for the patient and his family.
• Teach the patient and his family about the complications associated with prescribed treatments. Teach them measures to alleviate or minimize these adverse reactions.
• As appropriate, refer the patient and his family to the social service department, home health care agencies, and support groups such as the American Cancer Society.
• Try to help the patient develop a positive attitude toward recovery, and urge him to resume an independent life-style. If the patient is elderly, refer him to community health services as necessary.

Botulism

This life-threatening paralytic illness results from an exotoxin produced by the gram-positive, anaerobic bacillus *Clostridium botulinum.* It occurs as botulism food poisoning or wound botulism.

Botulism occurs worldwide and affects adults more often than children. The incidence of botulism in the United States had been declining, but the current trend toward home canning has resulted in an upswing in recent years.

The mortality rate is about 25%, with death most often caused by respiratory failure during the first week of illness. Onset within 24 hours of ingestion signals critical and potentially fatal illness.

Causes

Botulism usually results from eating improperly preserved foods, such as home-canned fruits and vegetables, sausages, and smoked or preserved fish or meat. Rarely, it results from wound infection with *C. botulinum.*

Complications

Botulism can result in respiratory failure and paralytic ileus.

Assessment

The patient may report having eaten home-canned food 12 to 36 hours before the onset of symptoms.

The patient may complain of vertigo, dry mouth, sore throat, weakness, nausea, vomiting, constipation, and diarrhea. Concurrently or up to 3 days later, he may report diplopia, blurred vision, dysarthria, and dysphagia from cranial nerve impairment. Later, he may experience dyspnea from muscle weakness or paralysis. His body temperature will remain normal.

The patient may appear alert and oriented on inspection. Ocular signs may include ptosis and dilated, nonreactive pupils. Oral mucous membranes commonly appear dry, red, and crusted.

Palpation may reveal abdominal distention with absent bowel sounds.

Further assessment may disclose descending weakness or paralysis of muscles in the extremities or trunk – the major physical finding in botulism. The patient's deep tendon reflexes may be intact, diminished, or absent. He won't have pathologic reflexes or sensory impairment.

Diagnostic tests

Identification of the exotoxin in the patient's serum, stool, or gastric contents or in the suspected food confirms the diagnosis. An electromyogram showing diminished muscle action potential after a single supramaximal nerve stimulus also is diagnostic.

Diagnosis must rule out conditions often confused with botulism, such as Guillain-Barré syndrome, myasthenia gravis, cerebrovascular accident, staphylococcal food poisoning, tick paralysis, chemical intoxication, carbon monoxide poisoning, fish poisoning, trichinosis, and diphtheria.

Treatment

For adults, treatment consists of I.V. or I.M. administration of botulinum antitoxin (available through the Centers for Disease Control and Prevention).

Early elective tracheotomy and ventilatory assistance can be lifesaving in respiratory failure. The patient will need nasogastric suctioning and total parenteral nutrition (TPN) if he develops significant paralytic ileus.

Key nursing diagnoses and patient outcomes

Altered nutrition: Less than body requirements, related to adverse GI symptoms and inability to swallow. Based on this nursing diagnosis, you'll establish these patient outcomes. The patient will:

- consume enough calories daily to prevent weight loss
- consume a balanced diet naturally or artificially to prevent nutritional deficits
- not exhibit signs and symptoms of malnutrition.

Impaired physical mobility related to progressive weakness and paralysis of muscles. Based on this nursing diagnosis, you'll establish these patient outcomes. The patient will:

- regain muscle use and strength
- show no evidence of complications, such as contractures, venous stasis, thrombus formation, or skin breakdown.

Ineffective breathing pattern related to decreased respiratory muscle function. Based on this nursing diagnosis, you'll establish these patient outcomes. The patient will:

- maintain adequate ventilation
- maintain normal arterial blood gases (ABGs)
- recover an effective breathing pattern that will remain effective.

Nursing interventions

- If you suspect the patient ate contaminated food, obtain a careful history of his food intake for the past several days. Determine if other family members exhibit similar symptoms and have eaten the same food.
- If the patient ate the food within several hours, induce vomiting, begin gastric lavage, and give a high enema to purge any unabsorbed toxin from the bowel. Family members or friends who have eaten the same food also should receive this treatment.
- If clinical signs of botulism appear, have the patient admitted to the intensive care unit (isolation isn't required).
- Before giving the antitoxin, obtain an accurate patient history of allergies, especially to horses, and perform a skin test. Then administer botulinum antitoxin, as ordered, to neutralize any circulating toxin. Keep epinephrine 1:1,000 (for subcutaneous administration) and emergency airway equipment available.
- If the patient has difficulty swallowing, initiate nasogastric tube feedings or TPN, as ordered. Suction the patient as needed.
- Administer I.V. fluids, as ordered.
- Turn the patient often, and encourage deep-breathing exercises. Position him in proper alignment, and assist with range-of-motion exercises.
- If the patient has difficulty speaking, try to anticipate his needs. Assure him that this symptom will pass, and establish an alternative method of communication.
- Because botulism sometimes is fatal, keep the patient and family informed about the course of the disease.
- Immediately report all cases of botulism to local public health authorities.

Monitoring

- Monitor cardiac and respiratory function carefully. Assess vital capacity frequently; report reduced vital capacity, reduced inspiratory effort, or respiratory distress.

• If the patient is on mechanical ventilation, monitor his ABGs to detect signs of hyperventilation or hypoventilation.
• Observe the patient carefully for abnormal neurologic signs.
• Closely assess and record the patient's neurologic function, including bilateral motor status (reflexes and ability to move his arms and legs). Check the patient's cough and gag reflexes.
• Monitor intake and output.
• After administering botulinum antitoxin, watch for anaphylaxis or other hypersensitivity reactions as well as serum sickness.

Patient teaching

• If ingestion of contaminated food is suspected but the patient returns home before neurologic symptoms occur, advise him and his family to watch for such signs as weakness, blurred vision, and slurred speech. Tell them to return the patient to the hospital immediately if such signs appear.
• To help prevent botulism in the future, encourage the patient and his family to use proper techniques in processing and preserving foods. Warn them to avoid even *tasting* food from a bulging can or one with a peculiar odor and to sterilize by boiling any utensil that contacts suspected food. Explain that eating even a small amount of food contaminated with botulism toxin can prove fatal.

Bowel resection with anastomosis

Surgical resection of diseased intestinal tissue and anastomosis of the remaining segments helps treat localized obstructive disorders, including diverticulosis (with an area of acute diverticulitis or abscess formation), intestinal polyps, adhesions that cause bowel dysfunction, and malignant or benign intestinal lesions. It's the preferred surgical technique for localized bowel cancer but not for wide-spread carcinoma, which usually requires massive resection with creation of a temporary or permanent colostomy or an ileostomy. (See the entry "Bowel resection with ostomy.")

Procedure

After the patient has received a general anesthetic, the surgeon makes the abdominal incision. The incision site varies, depending on the pathology's location. The surgeon limits the resection to the diseased area and a wide margin of surrounding normal tissue. After excising the diseased colonic tissue, the surgeon then anastomoses the remaining bowel segments to restore patency. End-to-end anastomosis provides the most physiologically sound junction and is the quickest to perform, but it requires that the approximated bowel segments be large enough to prevent postoperative obstruction at the anastomosis site. Side-to-side anastomosis minimizes the danger of obstruction, but this lengthy procedure may be contraindicated in an emergency. After the anastomosis is complete, the surgeon closes the incision and applies a sterile dressing.

Complications

Several complications can occur in a patient who has had a bowel resection with anastomosis. These include bleeding or leakage from the anastomosis site, peritonitis and resultant sepsis, postresection obstruction, and problems common to all patients undergoing abdominal surgery, such as wound infection and atelectasis.

Key nursing diagnoses and patient outcomes

Risk for infection related to anastomotic leak or spillage (or both) of intestinal contents into the abdominal cavity during surgery. Based on this nursing diagnosis, you'll establish these patient outcomes. The patient will:

• maintain a temperature and white blood cell count within normal limits
• have an incision that's clean and free of inflammation and purulent drainage
• not experience signs and symptoms of peritonitis, such as abdominal distention or increased abdominal pain.

Ineffective breathing pattern related to guarded respirations secondary to the abdominal incision. Based on this nursing diagnosis, you'll establish these patient outcomes. The patient will:
• maintain adequate ventilation, as exhibited by normal respiratory rate and rhythm and normal arterial blood gas values postoperatively
• demonstrate proper breathing techniques, such as splinting the incision and using incentive spirometry postoperatively
• change position and cough and deep-breathe every 2 to 4 hours postoperatively.

Nursing interventions

In caring for a patient undergoing bowel resection with anastomosis, your major roles include surgical preparation and postoperative care tailored to his condition.

Before surgery

• Explain that the surgery will remove a diseased portion of the patient's bowel and will connect the remaining healthy segments. Keep in mind that the patient and his family will probably have many questions about the surgery and its effect on the patient's life-style. Take the time to listen to their concerns and to answer their questions.
• Discuss anticipated postoperative care measures. Tell the patient that he'll awaken from surgery with a nasogastric (NG) tube in place to drain air and fluid from the intestinal tract and prevent distention. Explain that when peristalsis returns, usually within 2 to 3 days, the tube will be removed. Tell him to anticipate ambulation on the first day after surgery to promote return of peristalsis. Also prepare him for the presence of an I.V. line, which will provide fluid replacement, and abdominal drains.
• To reduce the risk of postoperative atelectasis and pneumonia, teach the patient how to cough and deep-breathe properly and emphasize the need to do so regularly throughout the recovery period. Demonstrate incisional splinting to protect the sutures and reduce discomfort.
• Before surgery, as ordered, administer antibiotics to reduce intestinal flora and laxatives or enemas to remove fecal contents.
• Ensure that the patient or a responsible family member has signed a consent form.

After surgery

• For the first few days after surgery, carefully monitor intake and output and weigh the patient daily. Maintain fluid and electrolyte balance through I.V. replacement therapy, and check the patient regularly for signs of dehydration, such as decreased urine output and poor skin turgor.
• Keep the NG tube patent. Warn the patient that, if the tube becomes dislodged, he should never attempt to reposition it himself; doing so could damage the anastomosis.
• To detect possible complications, carefully monitor the patient's vital signs and closely assess his overall condition. Remember that anastomotic leakage may produce only vague symptoms at first; watch for low-grade fever, malaise, slight leukocytosis, and abdominal distention and tenderness. Also be alert for more extensive hemorrhage from acute leakage; watch for signs of hypovolemic shock (precipitous drop in blood pressure and pulse rate, respiratory difficulty, decreased level of consciousness) and bloody stool or wound drainage.
• Observe the patient for signs of peritonitis or sepsis, caused by leakage of bowel contents into the abdominal cavity. Remember that a patient receiving antibiotics or total parenteral nutrition is at increased

risk for sepsis. Sepsis also may result from "wicking" of colonic bacteria up the NG tube to the oral cavity; to prevent this problem, provide frequent mouth and tube care.

• Provide meticulous wound care, changing dressings often. Check dressings and drainage sites frequently for signs of infection (purulent drainage, foul odor) or fecal drainage. Also watch for sudden fever, especially when accompanied by abdominal pain and tenderness.

• Regularly assess the patient for signs of postresection obstruction. Examine the abdomen for distention and rigidity, auscultate for bowel sounds, and note passage of any flatus or feces.

• Once the patient regains peristalsis and bowel function, take steps to prevent constipation and straining during defecation, both of which can damage the anastomosis. Encourage him to drink plenty of fluids, and administer a stool softener or other laxatives, as ordered. Note and record the frequency and amount of all bowel movements as well as characteristics of the stool.

• Encourage regular coughing and deep breathing to prevent atelectasis; remind him to splint the incision site as necessary.

Home care instructions

• Instruct the patient to record the frequency and character of bowel movements and to notify the doctor of any changes in his normal pattern. Warn against using laxatives without consulting his doctor.

• Caution the patient to avoid abdominal straining and heavy lifting until the sutures are completely healed and the doctor grants permission to do so.

• Instruct the patient to maintain the prescribed semibland diet until his bowel has healed completely (usually 4 to 8 weeks after surgery). In particular, urge him to avoid carbonated beverages and gas-producing foods.

• Because extensive bowel resection may interfere with the patient's ability to absorb nutrients from food, emphasize the importance of taking prescribed vitamin supplements.

Bowel resection with ostomy

A bowel resection with ostomy involves the excision of diseased bowel and the creation of a stoma on the outer abdominal wall to allow elimination of feces. This surgery is performed for such intestinal maladies as inflammatory bowel disease, familial adenomatous polyposis, diverticulitis, and especially advanced colorectal cancer if conservative surgery and other treatments aren't successful or if the patient develops acute complications, such as obstruction, abscess, or fistula.

Depending on the nature and location of the problem, the surgeon will perform one of several types of procedures. For instance, some obstructions of the ascending, transverse, descending, or sigmoid colon require a colostomy with removal of the affected bowel segments. Cancer of the rectum often mandates abdominal perineal resection, which involves wide resection of the rectum, surrounding tissues, and lymph nodes, with formation of a permanent colostomy. Perforated sigmoid diverticulitis, Hirschsprung's disease, rectovaginal fistula, and penetrating trauma often call for temporary colostomy to interrupt the intestinal flow and allow healing of inflamed or injured bowel segments.

A small bowel obstruction, on the other hand, may require resection and formation of an ileostomy from the proximal ileum. Severe, widespread colonic obstruction may require total or near total removal of the colon and rectum and creation of an ileostomy. A permanent ileostomy requires that the patient wear a drainage appliance or pouch over the stoma to contain the constant fecal drainage.

Instead of a conventional stoma, patients with ulcerative colitis or familial adenomatous polyposis may be candidates for either of two surgical advances: the creation of an ileoanal reservoir or a Kock ileostomy. Both are continent diversions in which the patient retains stool until draining it. Both techniques eliminate the need to wear an external pouch or drainage bag.

Procedure

After the patient receives an anesthetic, the surgeon makes an incision in the abdominal wall. The location depends on the area of the bowel to be resected and the type of ostomy required. After excising the diseased bowel segment and, in the case of colon cancer, several more inches of bowel beyond the margins of the tumor, the surgeon creates the stoma used to drain fecal content. (See *Types of intestinal stomas,* page 114.)

For an abdominoperineal resection, the surgeon makes a low abdominal incision and divides the sigmoid colon. He brings the proximal end of the colon out through another, smaller abdominal incision to create an end stoma, which results in a permanent colostomy. He then makes a wide perineal incision and resects the anus, rectum, and distal portion of the sigmoid colon. He closes the abdominal wound and places one or more abdominal drains; he usually leaves the perineal wound open but may pack it with gauze or close it and place several Penrose drains.

For an ileostomy, the surgeon resects all or part of the colon and rectum (proctocolectomy). He creates a permanent ileostomy by bringing the end of the ileum out through a small abdominal incision, typically located in the right lower quadrant between the anterosuperior iliac spine and the umbilicus, and fashions a stoma.

For an ileoanal reservoir, the surgeon performs a colectomy and creates a loop or end stoma for a temporary ileostomy. He then strips the rectal mucosa to prevent recurrence of the disease, forms an internal pouch with a portion of the ileum, and performs a pouch-anal anastomosis. The temporary ileostomy is required to allow adequate healing of the internal pouch and all anastomosis sites and to allow for an increase in the capacity of the internal reservoir through fluid instillations postoperatively. It is closed after 3 or 4 months.

For a Kock ileostomy, the surgeon first performs a proctocolectomy, in which he removes the colon, the rectum, and the anus and closes the anus. He then constructs a reservoir from a loop of the terminal ileum that is folded and sutured together and then cut. A portion of the ileum is intussuscepted to form a nipple valve, and the upper part of the sutured and cut ileum is pulled down and sutured to form a pouch. The nipple valve, which shuts tight against pressure from a filled pouch, is used to create a stoma by pulling it through the abdominal wall and suturing it flush with the skin.

Both standard colostomy and end ileostomy have been created through a laparoscopic approach.

Complications

Common complications of ostomies include hemorrhage, sepsis, ileus, and fluid and electrolyte imbalance from excessive drainage through the stoma. Skin excoriation may occur around the stoma from contact with acidic digestive enzymes in the drainage, and irritation may occur from pressure of the ostomy pouch.

Complications associated with the ileoanal reservoir include sepsis and pelvic abscess. The Kock ileostomy may result in an incompetent nipple valve, leading to leakage or difficulties with intubating the valve.

Ostomates commonly exhibit some degree of emotional and psychological prob-

Types of intestinal stomas

The surgeon may construct a stoma from the large intestine in one of three ways: end, loop, or double barrel.

End stoma

To form an end stoma, the surgeon pulls a section of the intestine through the outer abdominal wall, everts the section, and sutures it to the skin. An ostomy with an end stoma can be either temporary or permanent.

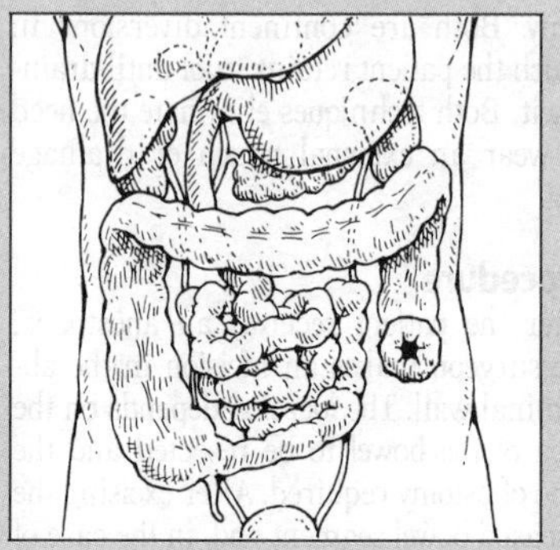

Loop stoma

To create a loop stoma, the surgeon brings a loop of intestine out through an abdominal incision to the abdominal surface and supports it with a rod or bridge (usually removed 5 to 7 days after surgery). He then opens the anterior wall of the bowel loop with a small incision to provide fecal diversion. The result is one stoma with a proximal, functioning limb and a distal, nonfunctioning limb. The surgeon then closes the wound around the exposed intestinal loop.

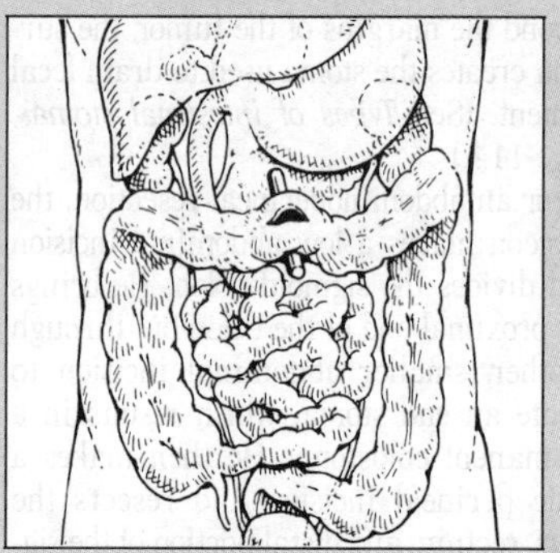

Double-barrel stoma

To create a double-barrel stoma, the surgeon divides the intestine and brings both the proximal and distal ends through the abdominal incision to the abdominal surface. He makes a small incision in the proximal stoma for fecal drainage. The distal stoma, also referred to as a mucous fistula, leads to the inactive intestine and is left intact.

Later, when the intestinal injury has healed or the inflammation has subsided, the colostomy is reversed and the divided ends of the intestine are anastomosed to restore intestinal integrity.

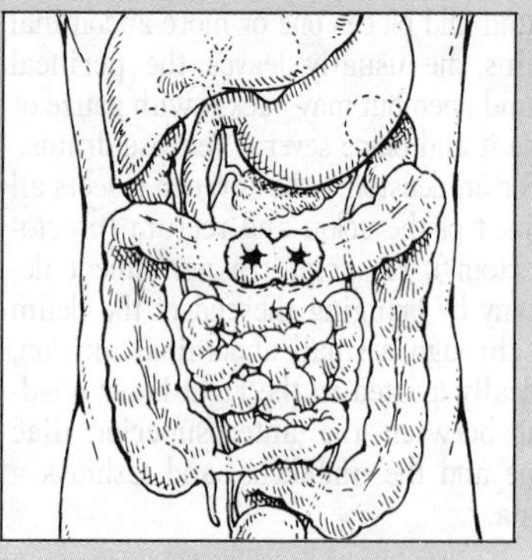

lems, such as depression and anxiety, related to altered body image and worries about life-style changes associated with the stoma and ostomy pouch.

Key nursing diagnoses and patient outcomes

Impaired skin integrity related to skin contact with acidic digestive enzymes at the stoma site. Based on this nursing diagnosis, you'll establish these patient outcomes. The patient will:

- demonstrate skill and diligence in performing ostomy care
- remain free of skin breakdown at the stoma site.

Risk for fluid volume deficit related to loss of fluids and electrolytes from ostomy drainage. Based on this nursing diagnosis, you'll establish these patient outcomes. The patient will:

- not experience signs of dehydration, such as decreased urine output, poor skin turgor, and dry mucous membranes
- not develop excessive drainage from the ostomy
- maintain normal fluid and electrolyte balance with adequate oral intake of fluids and electrolytes.

Nursing interventions

In caring for a patient undergoing a bowel resection with ostomy, you'll prepare him for surgery, monitor his progress afterward, and provide home care instructions.

Before surgery

- If emergency surgery is necessary, briefly explain that the diseased or injured bowel portion will be repaired, if possible, and isolated to allow healing. Mention that a small portion of the unaffected bowel will be brought to an opening in the skin to allow elimination.
- If immediate surgery isn't required, supplement the doctor's explanation of the surgery as necessary and answer all questions in clear, simple terms. Explain all preoperative and postoperative procedures and equipment that the patient may experience. Include family members or caregivers in your discussion, if appropriate.
- Prepare the patient for postoperative pain, and mention that analgesics will be provided.
- Describe the type of ostomy the patient will have and explain how fecal matter drains through it. Try using simple illustrations to facilitate your explanation. Discuss selection and use of ostomy appliances; if possible, show him the actual appliances. Prepare him for the foul smell and consistency of fecal drainage. This consistency varies, depending on the location of the stoma, from a constant watery stool with an ileostomy to a soft, semisolid stool with a colostomy in the descending colon.
- Inform the colostomy patient that he'll initially wear a pouch to collect fecal drainage. Point out that if the colostomy is placed in the descending or sigmoid colon, he may learn to control bowel movements by irrigating the colostomy. If he does learn bowel control, he may no longer need to use a pouch.
- Reassure the patient that once he becomes comfortable with the ostomy management routine, he should be able to resume his normal level of activity with few restrictions.
- Before surgery, arrange for a visit with an enterostomal therapist, who can provide more detailed information. The therapist can also help the patient select the best location for the stoma. If possible, arrange for the patient to meet with well-adjusted ostomy patients (from groups such as the United Ostomy Association) before undergoing surgery; these people can share their personal insights into the realities of living with and caring for a stoma.
- If chronic bowel disease has seriously compromised the patient's condition, evaluate his nutritional and fluid status for 3 to 4 days before surgery (if time per-

mits). Typically, the patient will be receiving total parenteral nutrition (TPN) to prepare him for the physiologic stress of surgery. Record the patient's fluid intake and output and weight daily, and watch for early signs of dehydration. Expect to draw periodic blood samples for hematocrit and hemoglobin determinations. Be prepared to transfuse blood, if ordered.

• If the patient is on long-term, low-dose corticosteroid therapy, continue to administer the drug to prevent rebound adrenocortical insufficiency. Explain that the drug will be withdrawn gradually after surgery. Also administer antibiotics, as ordered, to reduce intestinal flora.

• Ensure that the patient or a responsible family member has signed a consent form.

After surgery

• In the immediate postoperative period, carefully monitor the patient's intake and output. Maintain fluid and electrolyte balance, and watch for signs of dehydration: decreased urine output, poor skin turgor, and electrolyte imbalance. Provide analgesics, as ordered. Be especially alert for pain in the patient with an abdominoperineal resection because of the extent and location of the incisions.

• Note and record the color, consistency, and odor of fecal drainage from the stoma. If the patient has a double-barrel colostomy, check for mucus drainage from the inactive (distal) stoma. The nature of fecal drainage is determined by the type of ostomy surgery; generally, the more colon tissue that is preserved, the more closely drainage will resemble normal stool. For the first few days after surgery, fecal drainage probably will be mucoid (and possibly slightly blood tinged) and mostly odorless. Report excessive blood or mucus content, which could indicate hemorrhage or infection.

• Observe the patient for signs of peritonitis or sepsis, caused by leakage of bowel contents into the abdominal cavity. Remember that patients receiving antibiotics or TPN are at an increased risk for sepsis.

• Provide meticulous wound care, changing dressings often. Check dressings and drainage sites frequently for signs of infection (purulent drainage, foul odor) or fecal drainage. If the patient has had an abdominoperineal resection, irrigate the perineal area as ordered.

• Regularly check the stoma and the surrounding skin for irritation and excoriation, which may develop from contact with fecal drainage or from pressure caused by an overfilled or improperly fitted drainage pouch. Take measures to correct any such problems. Also observe the stoma's appearance. The stoma should look smooth, cherry-red, and slightly edematous; immediately report any discoloration or excessive swelling, which may indicate circulatory problems that could lead to ischemia.

• The patient with a Kock pouch will return from surgery with a catheter inserted in the stoma to drain fecal matter from the reservoir and prevent it from filling and placing pressure on the sutures. Be sure the catheter is connected to low intermittent suction or to straight drainage, as ordered. Check the patency of the catheter regularly, and irrigate it as ordered with 20 to 30 ml of 0.9% sodium chloride solution every 2 to 4 hours to prevent obstruction. If no complications develop, the color of the pouch drainage will change 2 to 4 days after surgery from blood tinged to greenish brown, indicating the return of peristalsis. When this occurs, give the patient clear liquids and gradually introduce low-residue solids. Clamp and unclamp the pouch catheter to increase its capacity as ordered by the surgeon.

• During the recovery period, don't neglect the patient's emotional needs. Encourage him to express his feelings and concerns; if he's anxious and depressed, reassure him that these common postoperative reactions should fade as he adjusts to the ostomy. Continue to arrange for visits by an enterostomal therapist, if possible.

Home care instructions

• Instruct the patient with an ileostomy to change the drainage pouch every 3 to 4 days. Also emphasize meticulous skin care around the stoma site. Discuss dietary restrictions and suggestions for preventing stoma blockage, diarrhea, flatus, and odor. Explain the need for maintaining a high fluid intake to help ensure fluid and electrolyte balance. This is especially important in times of increased fluid loss, such as during periods of hot weather or bouts of diarrhea. Warn the patient to avoid alcohol, laxatives, and diuretics, which will increase fluid loss and may contribute to an imbalance. Tell the patient to report persistent diarrhea through the stoma, which can quickly lead to fluid and electrolyte imbalance.

• Teach the patient with an ileoanal reservoir temporary ileostomy management and, after the pouch has healed and if needed, how to irrigate the pouch. Explain that after the ileostomy is reversed, perianal skin care with the use of skin sealants or moisture barriers is essential. Tell the patient that initially he will have 10 to 12 small-volume bowel movements daily but that they will decrease to approximately six a day as the diet is advanced and the reservoir expands. Inform him that some incontinence during the adaptation phase is common. Explain the signs and symptoms of inflammation of the reservoir. They include increased stool frequency, pelvic discomfort, fever, and malaise. Treatment usually involves antibiotics such as metronidazole.

• Explain to the patient with a Kock pouch that the catheter remains in place for 4 to 6 weeks after surgery. After it's removed, teach the patient how to empty the pouch by inserting a lubricated #28 French Silastic catheter through the stoma. He can empty the pouch while sitting or standing, though the latter position usually gives better results. Tell him he can also quicken drainage by contracting his abdominal muscles. Provide guidelines for draining the pouch. For example, right after surgery, the pouch usually holds 70 to 100 ml. One month later, it will hold about 200 ml. After 6 months, it will hold about 600 ml and need to be emptied three or four times a day. Be sure the patient knows to carry a catheter with him at all times. Between intubations, tell him to cover the stoma with gauze to prevent mucus from soiling his clothes. Before applying the gauze, he should wash the stomal area with warm water and dry it. Demonstrate how to irrigate the pouch. Suggest irrigation weekly or whenever undigested food obstructs drainage.

• Teach the colostomy patient how to apply, remove, and empty the pouch. If appropriate, teach the patient with a descending or sigmoid colostomy how to irrigate the ostomy with warm tap water to gain some control over elimination. Emphasize that continence can usually be achieved with dietary control and bowel retraining. Instruct him to change the appliance every 3 to 4 days and to wash the stoma site with warm water and soap without emollients to prevent skin irritation and excoriation.

• Tell the patient recovering from an abdominoperineal resection to take sitz baths to help relieve perineal discomfort. Instruct him to refrain from intercourse until the perineum heals.

• Encourage the ostomy patient to discuss his feelings about resuming sexual intercourse. Mention that the drainage pouch will not dislodge if the device is empty and fitted properly. Suggest avoiding foods and fluids for several hours before intercourse.

• Remind the patient and his family that depression commonly occurs after ostomy surgery. Advise the patient to seek counseling, however, if depression persists or becomes severe.

• Ensure visiting nurse follow-up to reinforce teaching and provide initial assistance.

Brain tumors, malignant

Slightly more common in men than in women, malignant brain tumors (gliomas and schwannomas) have an overall incidence of 5 per 100,000. They cause central nervous system (CNS) changes by invading and destroying tissues and by secondary effect – mainly compression of the brain, cranial nerves, and cerebral vessels; cerebral edema; and increased intracranial pressure (ICP).

Tumors can occur at any age. In adults, incidence is highest between ages 40 and 60, and the most common tumor types are gliomas and meningiomas. They usually occur above the covering of the cerebellum (supratentorial tumors).

Most tumors in children occur before age 1 or between ages 2 and 12. The most common are astrocytomas, medulloblastomas, ependymomas, and brain stem gliomas. Brain tumors are one of the most common causes of cancer death in children.

Causes

The cause of brain tumors is unknown.

Complications

In malignant brain tumors, life-threatening complications from increasing ICP include coma, respiratory or cardiac arrest, and brain herniation.

Assessment

The patient's history usually reveals an insidious onset of signs and symptoms. If the brain tumor has already been diagnosed, his history may also show an early misdiagnosis – a common occurrence.

Signs and symptoms result from increased ICP. Specific assessment findings vary with the type of tumor, its location, and the degree of invasion. Neurologic assessment findings often help to pinpoint the location of the tumor. (See *Brain tumors: Site-specific signs and symptoms,* page 119, and *Assessment findings in malignant brain tumors,* pages 120 and 121.)

Diagnostic tests

Skull X-rays, brain scans, computed tomography and magnetic resonance imaging scans, and cerebral angiography help locate the tumor. Biopsy of the lesion allows identification of the histologic type and grading of the tumor. Grade 1 tumors are well differentiated; grade 2, moderately well differentiated; grade 3, poorly differentiated; and grade 4, extremely poorly differentiated. The higher the grade, the poorer the prognosis.

The patient may also receive a lumbar puncture. However, if increased ICP is suspected, a lumbar puncture is not performed.

Treatment

Specific treatments vary with the tumor's histologic type, radiosensitivity, and location. Such treatments may include surgery, radiation therapy, chemotherapy, and decompression of increased ICP with diuretics, corticosteroids or, possibly, ventriculoatrial or ventriculoperitoneal shunting of the CSF. (See *Responding to brain herniation,* page 123.)

Treatment of a glioma usually consists of resection by craniotomy. Radiation therapy and chemotherapy follow resection. The combination of carmustine, lomustine, or procarbazine with radiation therapy is more effective than radiation treatment alone.

For low-grade cystic cerebellar astrocytomas, surgical resection permits long-term survival. For other astrocytomas, treatment consists of repeated surgery, radiation therapy, and shunting of fluid from obstructed CSF pathways. Radiation therapy works best in radiosensitive astrocytomas; some astrocytomas are radioresistant.

Treatment for oligodendrogliomas and ependymomas includes surgical resection and radiation therapy. Medulloblastomas

(Text continues on page 122.)

Brain tumors: Site-specific signs and symptoms

A brain tumor usually produces signs and symptoms specific to its location. Recognizing these typical effects helps identify the tumor site and guide treatment before and after surgery. It can also help you spot life-threatening complications, such as increasing ICP and imminent brain herniation. A brain tumor may cause all, some, or none of the effects listed below.

Hypothalamus
(Possible pituitary area tumor extending upward)
- Diabetes insipidus
- Temperature control loss

Frontal lobe
- Expressive or Broca's aphasia (dominant hemisphere)
- Contralateral seizures
- Contralateral motor weakness
- Personality and behavioral changes

Subfrontal lobe
Cranial nerve I (olfactory)
- Smell loss

Midbrain
Cranial nerve III (oculomotor)
- Ptosis
- Diplopia
- Dilated pupil
- Inability to gaze up, down, or inward (all ipsilateral)

Cerebellum
- Disturbed gait
- Impaired balance
- Incoordination

Pituitary (sella turcica)
- Amenorrhea
- Cushingoid signs and symptoms
- Galactorrhea
- Impotence
- Visual field deficits

Cerebellopontile angle
Cranial nerve VII (facial)
- Ipsilateral facial muscle drooping

Cranial nerve VIII (acoustic)
- Tinnitus
- Hearing loss

Occipital lobe
- Visual agnosia (inability to name objects)
- Visual field deficits

Medulla
Cranial nerve IX (glossopharyngeal)
- Difficulty swallowing

Cranial nerve X (vagus)
- Gag and cough reflex loss
- Difficulty swallowing
- Hoarseness
- Projectile vomiting

Cranial nerve XI (spinal accessory)
- Inability to shrug shoulders or turn head toward tumor side

Cranial nerve XII (hypoglossal)
- Tongue protrusion (deviating toward tumor side)
- Respiratory pattern changes

Parietal lobe
- Dyslexia (left side)
- Position sense loss
- Perceptual problems
- Contralateral sensory disturbances
- Visual field deficits

Pons
Cranial nerve V (trigeminal)
- Ipsilateral facial or forehead sensation loss
- Corneal reflex loss

Cranial nerve VI (abducens)
- Ipsilateral inability to gaze outward

Cranial nerve VII (facial)
- Ipsilateral facial muscle drooping

Temporal lobe
- Auditory hallucinations
- Impaired memory (with bilateral tumor)
- Personality changes
- Psychomotor seizures
- Visual field deficits
- Receptive or Wernicke's aphasia (dominant hemisphere)
- Dysarthria

Assessment findings in malignant brain tumors

Tumor and characteristics	Assessment findings
Astrocytoma • Second most common malignant glioma, accounting for 10% of all gliomas • Occurs at any age; incidence higher in males than in females • Occurs most often in central and subcortical white matter; may originate in any part of the CNS • Cerebellar astrocytomas usually confined to one hemisphere	*General* • Headache and mental activity changes • Decreased motor strength and coordination • Seizures and scanning speech • Altered vital signs *Localizing* • Third ventricle: changes in mental activity and level of consciousness, nausea, and pupillary dilation and sluggish light reflex; paresis or ataxia in later stages • Brain stem and pons: ipsilateral trigeminal, abducens, and facial nerve palsies in early stages; cerebellar ataxia, tremors, and other cranial nerve deficits later • Third or fourth ventricle or aqueduct of Sylvius: secondary hydrocephalus • Thalamus or hypothalamus: various endocrine, metabolic, autonomic, and behavioral changes
Ependymoma • Rare glioma; most common in children and young adults • Located most often in fourth and lateral ventricles	*General* • Increased ICP and obstructive hydrocephalus • Other assessment findings similar to those of oligodendroglioma
Glioblastoma multiforme • Most common glioma, accounting for 60% of all gliomas • Peak incidence between ages 50 and 60; more common in men • Unencapsulated, highly malignant; grows rapidly and infiltrates the brain; may be enormous before diagnosed • Occurs most often in cerebral hemispheres (frontal and temporal lobes) • Occupies more than one lobe of affected hemisphere; may spread to opposite hemisphere by corpus callosum; may metastasize into CSF, producing tumors in distant parts of the nervous system	*General* • Increased ICP (nausea, vomiting, headache, papilledema) • Mental and behavioral changes • Altered vital signs (increased systolic pressure, widened pulse pressure, respiratory changes) • Speech and sensory disturbances • In children, irritability and projectile vomiting *Localizing* • Midline: headache (bifrontal or bioccipital) that's worse in morning; intensified by coughing, straining, or sudden head movements • Temporal lobe: psychomotor seizures • Central region: focal seizures • Optic and oculomotor nerves: visual defects • Frontal lobe: abnormal reflexes and motor responses
Medulloblastoma • Rare glioma • Incidence highest in children ages 4 to 6 • Affects males more than females • Frequently metastasizes by way of CSF	*General* • Increased ICP *Localizing* • Brain stem and cerebrum: papilledema, nystagmus, hearing loss, perception of flashing lights, dizziness, ataxia, paresthesia of the face, cranial nerve palsies, hemiparesis, suboccipital tenderness; compression of supratentorial area produces other symptoms

Assessment findings in malignant brain tumors *(continued)*

Tumor and characteristics	Assessment findings
Meningioma • Most common nonmalignant brain tumor, constituting 20% of primary brain tumors • Occurs most frequently among people in their 50s; rare in children; more common in females than in males (ratio 3:2) • Arises from the meninges • Common locations include parasagital area, sphenoidal ridge, anterior part of the base of the skull, cerebellopontile angle, and spinal canal • Benign, well-circumscribed, highly vascular tumor that compresses underlying brain tissue by invading overlying skull	*General* • Headache, seizures, vomiting, and changes in mental activity. Other assessment findings similar to those of schwannomas *Localizing* • Skull changes (bony bulge) over tumor • Sphenoidal ridge, indenting optic nerve: unilateral visual changes and papilledema • Prefrontal parasagital: personality and behavioral changes • Motor cortex: contralateral motor changes • Anterior fossa compressing both optic nerves and frontal lobes: headaches and bilateral vision loss • Pressure on cranial nerves, causing varying symptoms
Oligodendroglioma • Third most common glioma, accounting for less than 5% of all gliomas • Occurs in middle adult years; more common in women than in men • Slow-growing	*General* • Mental and behavioral changes • Decreased visual acuity and other visual disturbances • Increased ICP *Localizing* • Temporal lobe: hallucinations and psychomotor seizures • Central region: seizures (one muscle group or unilateral) • Midbrain or third ventricle: pyramidal tract symptoms (dizziness, ataxia, paresthesia of the face) • Brain stem and cerebrum: nystagmus, hearing loss, dizziness, ataxia, paresthesia of the face, cranial nerve palsies, hemiparesis, suboccipital tenderness, loss of balance
Schwannoma (acoustic neurinoma, neurilemoma, cerebellopontile angle tumor) • Accounts for about 10% of all intracranial tumors • Onset of symptoms between ages 30 and 60; higher incidence in women than in men • Affects the craniospinal nerve sheath, usually cranial nerve VIII; also, V and VII, and to a lesser extent, VI and X on the same side as the tumor • Benign, but often classified as malignant because of its growth patterns; slow growing – may be present for years before symptoms occur	*General* • Unilateral hearing loss with or without tinnitus • Stiff neck and suboccipital discomfort • Secondary hydrocephalus • Ataxia and uncoordinated movements of one or both arms due to pressure on brain stem and cerebellum *Localizing* • V: early signs including facial hypoesthesia and paresthesia on the side of hearing loss; unilateral loss of corneal reflex • VI: diplopia • VII: paresis progressing to paralysis (Bell's palsy) • X: weakness of palate, tongue, and nerve muscles on same side as tumor

call for surgical resection and possibly intrathecal infusion of methotrexate or another antineoplastic drug. Meningiomas require surgical resection, including dura mater and sometimes bone.

For schwannomas, microsurgical technique allows complete resection of the tumor and preservation of facial nerves. Although schwannomas are moderately radioresistant, treatment still calls for postoperative radiation therapy.

Treatment for malignant brain tumors also includes chemotherapy with nitrosoureas, which cross the blood-brain barrier and allow other chemotherapeutics to go through as well. Intrathecal and intra-arterial administration maximizes drug action.

Palliative measures for gliomas, astrocytomas, oligodendrogliomas, and ependymomas include dexamethasone for cerebral edema and antacids and histamine receptor antagonists for stress ulcers. These tumors and schwannomas may also require anticonvulsants.

New treatments under investigation include bone marrow transplantation and hyperthermia.

Treatment of brain tumors can cause several complications. Although rare, surgery can result in immediate or delayed CNS infections, with symptoms that mimic tumor progression or recurrence. If fever or rapidly progressive neurologic symptoms develop, bacterial and fungal cultures will confirm the infection.

Early delayed radiation encephalopathy may stem from temporary demyelination. Anorexia, somnolence, lethargy, and headache occur 2 to 6 weeks after the therapy but resolve spontaneously in approximately 6 weeks.

Late delayed radiation encephalopathy stems from brain necrosis and small-vessel occlusion. Symptoms can mimic disease advancement and may include intracranial hypertension and focal neurologic dysfunction. Both are irreversible and potentially fatal complications.

Corticosteroid therapy predisposes the patient to cushingoid symptoms, GI ulceration, and steroid psychosis (if used in the long term).

Key nursing diagnoses and patient outcomes

Altered role performance related to neurologic deficits caused by a malignant brain tumor. Based on this nursing diagnosis, you'll establish these patient outcomes. The patient will:
- identify limitations imposed by changes in neurologic function
- seek assistance in performing activities related to role performance as dictated by tumor growth or adverse reactions
- continue to function in his usual role as much as possible.

Sensory/perceptual alterations (potential for all areas to be affected) related to neurologic deficits caused by a malignant brain tumor. Based on this nursing diagnosis, you'll establish these patient outcomes. The patient will:
- use adaptive equipment (glasses, hearing aid) as needed
- remain safe in his environment.

The patient or caregiver will:
- take an active role in preventing sensory deprivation and isolation.

Powerlessness related to potential for inability to control cancer growth or adverse effects of a malignant brain tumor. Based on this nursing diagnosis, you'll establish these patient outcomes. The patient will:
- express feelings of powerlessness over tumor growth and adverse reactions
- participate in planning care and managing adverse reactions
- express feeling of having regained a sense of control.

Nursing interventions

- Carefully document the occurrence, nature, and duration of seizure activity.
- Maintain a patent airway.
- Take steps to protect the patient's safety.

LIFE-THREATENING COMPLICATIONS

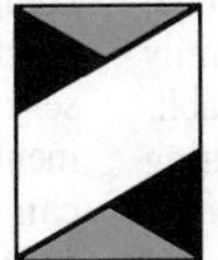

Responding to brain herniation

Brain herniation occurs when an expanding brain tumor increases ICP beyond compensatory levels. Without prompt intervention, coma, respiratory arrest, and death can result.

Two paths of herniation

Brain hernias develop through two main paths. Brain tissue can herniate through the tentorial notch or the foramen magnum (or both).

Herniation through the tentorial notch can occur as central or uncal herniation. In central herniation, the cerebral hemisphere is compressed against the incisura, causing compression of the midbrain. Uncal herniation occurs when the uncus presses upon the tentorial notch, compressing the upper brain stem and entrapping the ipsilateral third cranial nerve.

Herniation through the foramen magnum results when increased intracranial pressure compresses the cerebellum and medulla oblongata through the foramen magnum. Herniation through the foramen magnum isn't clinically distinguishable from central or uncal herniation.

Signs and symptoms

Be alert for these signs and symptoms of brain herniation in your patient:

- Rapidly deteriorating level of consciousness
- Change in pupil size (dilation in uncal herniation; pinpoint in central herniation) and reaction (rapidly becoming nonreactive)
- Rapid change in respirations, leading to respiratory arrest
- Deteriorating motor response, leading to decorticate or decerebrate posturing
- Cranial nerve dysfunction

Emergency interventions

- Notify the doctor immediately.
- Prepare for possible respiratory or cardiac arrest or both. Have emergency equipment brought to the bedside.
- Maintain a patent airway.
- Expect to administer an osmotic diuretic, such as mannitol, and corticosteroids I.V. to decrease cerebral edema.
- Prepare the patient for transfer to the intensive care unit or, if necessary, to the operating room for an emergency craniotomy.

- Administer anticonvulsant drugs, as ordered.
- Use hypothermia blankets before and after surgery to keep the patient's temperature down and minimize cerebral metabolic demands.
- As ordered, administer corticosteroids and osmotic diuretics, such as mannitol, and restrict fluid intake to reduce cerebral edema.
- Prepare the patient for surgery, as indicated.
- Before chemotherapy, give prochlorperazine or another antiemetic, as ordered, to minimize nausea and vomiting.
- Because brain tumors may cause residual neurologic deficits that handicap the patient physically or mentally, begin rehabilitation early. Consult with occupational and physical therapists to encourage independence in daily activities. As necessary, provide aids for self-care and mobilization, such as bathroom rails for wheelchair patients. If the patient is aphasic, arrange for consultation with a speech pathologist.

• Throughout therapy, provide emotional support to help the patient and his family cope with the treatment, potential disabilities, and changes in life-style resulting from his tumor.

Monitoring

• Closely observe the patient for seizure activity.
• Watch for changes in the patient's neurologic status and be alert for increased ICP.
• Evaluate respiratory changes carefully. An abnormal respiratory rate and depth may indicate rising ICP or herniation of the cerebellar tonsils from expanding infratentorial mass.
• Monitor the patient's temperature carefully. Fever commonly follows hypothalamic anoxia, but it can also indicate meningitis.
• Regularly evaluate the patient's fluid and electrolyte balance to prevent dehydration.
• Observe and report signs of stress ulcers: abdominal distention, pain, vomiting, and tarry stools. Administer antacids, as ordered.
• Monitor the patient receiving radiation therapy postoperatively for signs of infection and sinus formation. Because radiation may cause brain inflammation, also watch for signs of rising ICP.

Patient teaching

• Because some of the antineoplastic agents (carmustine, lomustine, semustine, and procarbazine, for example) used as adjuncts to radiation therapy and surgery can cause delayed bone marrow depression, tell the patient to watch for and immediately report any signs of infection or bleeding that appear within 4 weeks after the start of chemotherapy.
• As appropriate, explain adverse effects of chemotherapy and other treatments. Explain what actions the patient can take to alleviate them.
• Tell the patient and family the early signs of tumor recurrence, and encourage their compliance with the treatment regimen.
• Refer the patient to resource and support services, such as the social service department, home health care agencies, American Brain Tumor Foundation, and the American Cancer Society.

Breast cancer

The most frequent anatomic site for a cancer diagnosis in women is the breast, although lung cancer accounts for more deaths in the female population. The disease seldom occurs in men.

Breast cancer may develop any time after puberty, but most cases are diagnosed in women between ages 60 and 79. Five-year survival rates show increasing improvement because of earlier diagnosis and better treatment. Mortality rates, however, haven't changed in the past 50 years.

The most reliable breast cancer detection method is regular breast self-examination, followed by immediate professional evaluation of any abnormality noticed. Mammography is another important detection method, and it is probably responsible for an increase in the number of reported cases.

Causes

The causes of breast cancer remain elusive. Significant risk factors include a family history of breast cancer (mother, sister, grandmother, aunt) and being a woman over age 45 and premenopausal. Other probable risk factors being investigated include a long menstrual cycle, early onset of menses, or late menopause; first pregnancy after age 35; a high-fat diet; endometrial or ovarian cancer; radiation exposure; estrogen therapy; antihypertensive therapy; alcohol and tobacco use; and preexisting fibrocystic disease.

About half of all breast cancers develop in the upper outer quadrant, the section containing the most glandular tissue. The second most common cancer site is the nipple, where all the breast ducts converge. The next most common site is the upper inner quadrant, followed by the lower outer quadrant and, finally, the lower inner quadrant.

Growth rates vary. Theoretically, slow-growing breast cancer may take up to 8 years to become palpable at 3/8" (1 cm). Breast cancer spreads by way of the lymphatic system and the bloodstream through the right side of the heart to the lungs and to the other breast, chest wall, liver, bone, and brain.

The estimated breast cancer growth rate is called its doubling time, or the time it takes malignant cells to double in number. Survival time is based on tumor size and the number of involved lymph nodes.

Classified by histologic appearance and the lesion's location, breast cancer may be described as:

- *adenocarcinoma* (ductal) – arising from the epithelium
- *intraductal* – developing within the ducts (includes Paget's disease)
- *infiltrating* – occurring in the breast's parenchymal tissue
- *inflammatory (rare)* – growing rapidly and causing overlying skin to become edematous, inflamed, and indurated
- *lobular carcinoma in situ* – involving the lobes of glandular tissue
- *medullary or circumscribed* – enlarging tumor with rapid growth rate.

Coupled with a staging system, these classifications provide a clearer picture of the cancer's extent. The most common system for staging, both before and after surgery, is the tumor, node, metastasis (TNM) system. (See *Staging breast cancer,* page 126.)

Assessment

The patient most often reports that she detected a painless lump or mass in her breast or that she noticed a thickening of breast tissue. Otherwise, the disease most commonly appears on a mammogram before a lesion becomes palpable. The patient's health history may indicate several significant risk factors for breast cancer.

Inspection of the patient's breast may reveal clear, milky, or bloody nipple discharge, nipple retraction, scaly skin around the nipple, and skin changes, such as dimpling, peau d'orange, or inflammation. Arm edema, which is also identified on inspection, may indicate advanced nodal involvement.

Palpation may identify a hard lump, mass, or thickening of breast tissue. Palpation of the cervical supraclavicular and axillary nodes may also disclose lumps or enlargement.

Complications

Disease progression and metastasis of breast cancer lead to site-specific complications, including infection, decreased mobility if breast cancer metastasizes to the bone, central nervous system effects if the tumor metastasizes to the brain, and respiratory problems if the disease spreads to the lung.

Diagnostic tests

- *Mammography,* the essential test for breast cancer, can detect a tumor too small to palpate.
- *Fine-needle aspiration* and *excisional biopsy* provide cells for histologic examination to confirm the diagnosis.
- *Ultrasonography* can distinguish between a fluid-filled breast cyst and a solid mass.
- *Chest X-rays* can pinpoint metastases in the chest.
- *Scans* of the bone, brain, liver, and other organs can detect metastases to distant sites.
- *Laboratory tests,* such as alkaline phosphatase levels and liver function, can uncover distant metastases.
- *Hormonal receptor assay* can determine whether the tumor is estrogen- or progesterone-dependent. This test guides deci-

Staging breast cancer

Cancer staging helps form a prognosis and a treatment plan. For breast cancer, most clinicians use the TNM system developed by the American Joint Committee on Cancer.

Primary tumor

TX—primary tumor can't be assessed
T0—no evidence of primary tumor
Tis—carcinoma in situ: intraductal carcinoma, lobular carcinoma in situ, or Paget's disease of the nipple with no tumor
T1—tumor 2 cm or less in greatest dimension
T1a—tumor 0.5 cm or less in greatest dimension
T1b—tumor more than 0.5 cm but not more than 1 cm in greatest dimension
T1c—tumor more than 1 cm but not more than 2 cm in greatest dimension
T2—tumor more than 2 cm but not more than 5 cm in greatest dimension
T3—tumor more than 5 cm in greatest dimension
T4—tumor of any size that extends to the chest wall or skin
T4a—tumor extends to the chest wall
T4b—tumor accompanied by edema (including peau d'orange), ulcerated breast skin, or satellite skin nodules on the same breast
T4c—both T4a and T4b
T4d—inflammatory carcinoma

Regional lymph nodes

NX—regional lymph nodes can't be assessed
N0—no evidence of nodal involvement
N1—movable ipsilateral axillary nodal involvement
N2—ipsilateral axillary nodal involvement with nodes fixed to one another or to other structures
MX—distant—ipsilateral internal mammary nodal involvement

Distant metastasis

MX—distant metastasis can't be assessed
M0—no evidence of distant metastasis
M1—distant metastasis (including metastasis to ipsilateral supraclavicular nodes)

Staging categories

Breast cancer progresses from mild to severe as follows:
Stage 0—Tis, N0, M0
Stage I—T1, N0, M0
Stage IIA—T0, N1, M0; T1, N1, M0; T2, N0, M0
Stage IIB—T2, N1, M0; T3, N0, M0
Stage IIIA—T0, N2, M0; T1, N2, M0; T2, N2, M0; T3, N1 or N2, M0
Stage IIIB—T4, any N, M0; any T, N3, M0
Stage IV—any T, any N, M1

sions to use therapy that blocks the action of the estrogen hormone that supports tumor growth.

Treatment

The choice of treatment for breast cancer usually reflects the disease's stage and type, the woman's age and menopausal status, and the disfiguring effects of the surgery. Appropriate therapy may include any combination of surgery, radiation, chemotherapy, and hormonal therapy.

Surgical options include lumpectomy, partial mastectomy, total mastectomy, and modified radical mastectomy. Modified radical mastectomy has replaced radical mastectomy as the most extensively used surgical procedure for treating breast cancer.

Before or after tumor removal, primary radiation therapy may be effective for a patient who has a small tumor in early stages without distant metastases. Radiation therapy can also prevent or treat local recurrence. Furthermore, preoperative breast irradiation helps to "sterilize" the field, making the tumor more manageable surgically–especially in inflammatory breast cancer.

Various cytotoxic drug combinations may be administered either as adjuvant or primary therapy.

Chemotherapy relies on a combination of drugs, such as cyclophosphamide, fluorouracil, methotrexate, doxorubicin, vincristine, and prednisone. A typical regimen is cyclophosphamide, methotrexate, and fluorouracil; it's used for premenopausal and postmenopausal women.

Hormonal therapy blocks the uptake of estrogen and other hormones that may nourish breast cancer cells. For example, antiestrogen therapy (specifically tamoxifen, which is effective against tumors identified as estrogen-receptor-positive) is used in postmenopausal women. Alternatively, the patient may receive antiandrogen (aminoglutethimide), androgen (fluoxymesterone), estrogen (diethylstilbestrol), or progestin (megestrol) therapy.

Key nursing diagnoses and patient outcomes

Altered nutrition: Less than body requirements, related to adverse effects of radiation or chemotherapy used to treat breast cancer. Based on this nursing diagnosis, you'll establish these patient outcomes. The patient will:
- maintain her weight
- consume a well-balanced diet
- recover her appetite and GI function.

Decisional conflict related to more than one treatment option available for breast cancer. Based on this nursing diagnosis, you'll establish these patient outcomes. The patient will:
- be well informed about pros and cons of each treatment option
- seek a second opinion
- make a well-informed decision about her breast cancer treatment choice.

Fear related to potential for metastatic breast disease. Based on this nursing diagnosis, you'll establish these patient outcomes. The patient will:
- express her fears and concerns
- use available support systems and seek information about breast cancer from reputable sources to assist in coping with fear
- express less fear and show fewer physical signs and symptoms of fear.

Nursing interventions

- Always evaluate the patient's feelings about her illness, and determine her level of knowledge and expectations.
- Administer analgesics for pain, as needed.
- Perform comfort measures to promote relaxation and relieve anxiety.
- If immobility develops late in the disease, prevent complications by frequently repositioning the patient, using a convoluted foam mattress, and providing skin care (particularly over bony prominences).
- Provide measures to relieve adverse effects of treatment.

Monitoring

- Watch for treatment complications, such as nausea, vomiting, anorexia, leukopenia, thrombocytopenia, GI ulceration, and bleeding.
- Monitor the patient's weight and nutritional intake for evidence of malnutrition.
- Inspect the skin for redness, irritation, and skin breakdown if immobility occurs.
- In late disease, monitor the patient's pain level and the efficacy of administered analgesics and nonpharmacologic measures.
- Assess the patient's and family's ability to cope, especially if the cancer is terminal.

Patient teaching

- Provide clear, concise explanations of all procedures and prescribed treatments.
- Instruct the patient or caregiver how to manage adverse effects of treatment.
- Teach the patient how to examine her breasts. (See *Breast self-examination.*)

HEALTH PROMOTION POINTERS

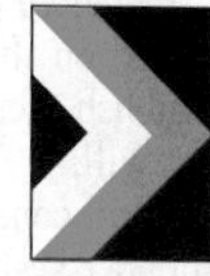

Breast self-examination

This is an inexpensive, risk-free method of detecting breast cancer. Early detection gives the patient a better chance for long-term survival.

• Teach the patient how and when to perform self-examination: every month after the menstrual period for the menstruating female and once a month at the same time each month for males and nonmenstruating females.
• Review the signs for breast cancer: lump or mass in the breast, changes in breast symmetry or size, changes in breast skin (thickening, dimpling, edema, peau d'orange appearance, or ulceration), changes in skin temperature (a hot, warm, or pink area), unusual nipple drainage or discharge, changes in the nipple (itching, burning, erosion, or retraction), and pain.
• Advise the patient to have a baseline mammogram between ages 35 and 40 and to follow up every 1 to 2 years for ages 40 to 49 and every year for age 50 and older.

• Women who have had breast cancer in one breast are at higher risk for cancer in the other breast or for recurrent cancer in the chest wall. Therefore, urge the patient to continue examining the other breast and to comply with follow-up treatment.
• Refer the patient and family to hospital and community support services.

Bronchiectasis

Marked by chronic abnormal dilation of the bronchi and destruction of the bronchial walls, bronchiectasis can occur throughout the tracheobronchial tree, or it may be confined to one segment or lobe. It's usually bilateral and involves the basilar segments of the lower lobes.

The disease has three forms: cylindrical (fusiform), varicose, and saccular (cystic). It affects people of both sexes and all ages. With antibiotics available to treat acute respiratory tract infections, the incidence of bronchiectasis has dramatically decreased over the past 20 years. Its incidence is highest among Inuit populations in the Northern Hemisphere and the Maoris of New Zealand. Bronchiectasis is irreversible.

Causes

Bronchiectasis results from conditions associated with repeated damage to bronchial walls and with abnormal mucociliary clearance, which causes a breakdown of supporting tissue adjacent to the airways. Such conditions include:
• cystic fibrosis
• immune disorders (agammaglobulinemia, for example)
• recurrent, inadequately treated bacterial respiratory tract infections (such as tuberculosis)
• complications of measles, pneumonia, pertussis, or influenza
• obstruction (by a foreign body, a tumor, or stenosis) with recurrent infection
• inhalation of corrosive gas or repeated aspiration of gastric juices
• congenital anomalies (rare), such as bronchomalacia, congenital bronchiectasis, and Kartagener's syndrome (bronchiectasis, sinusitis, and dextrocardia), and various rare disorders, such as immotile cilia syndrome.

In the patient with bronchiectasis, sputum stagnates in the dilated bronchi and leads to secondary infection, characterized by inflammation and leukocytic accumulations. Additional debris collects in and occludes the bronchi. Building pressure from the retained secretions induces mucosal injury.

Complications

Advanced bronchiectasis may produce chronic malnutrition and amyloidosis, right ventricular failure, and cor pulmonale.

Assessment

Patient complaints commonly include frequent bouts of pneumonia or a history of coughing up blood or blood-tinged sputum. The patient typically reports a chronic cough that produces copious, foul-smelling, mucopurulent secretions (up to several cups daily). He may also report dyspnea, weight loss, and malaise.

Inspection of the patient's sputum may show a cloudy top layer, a central layer of clear saliva, and a heavy, thick, purulent bottom layer. In advanced disease, the patient may have clubbed fingers and toes and cyanotic nail beds.

If the patient also has a complicating condition, such as pneumonia or atelectasis, percussion may detect dullness over lung fields. Auscultation may reveal coarse crackles during inspiration over involved lobes or segments and occasional wheezes. With complicating atelectasis or pneumonia, you may hear diminished breath sounds during auscultation.

Diagnostic tests

- *Bronchography* may be ordered for patients who are considering surgery or for those with recurrent or severe hemoptysis. In bronchography, a radiopaque contrast medium outlines the bronchial walls, allowing X-ray images to display the location and extent of disease.
- *Chest X-rays* show peribronchial thickening, atelectatic areas, and scattered cystic changes that suggest bronchiectasis.
- *Bronchoscopy* helps to identify the source of secretions or the bleeding site in hemoptysis.
- *Sputum culture* and a *Gram stain* identify predominant pathogens.
- *Complete blood count* can detect anemia and leukocytosis.
- *Pulmonary function studies* detect decreased vital capacity, expiratory flow, and hypoxemia; these tests also help evaluate disease severity, therapeutic effectiveness, and the patient's suitability for surgery.

Depending on the patient and his condition, additional tests may include urinalysis and electrocardiography. If the health care team suspects cystic fibrosis as the underlying cause of bronchiectasis, a sweat electrolyte test may be ordered.

Treatment

Antibiotic therapy (oral or I.V.) for 7 to 10 days – or until sputum production decreases – is the principal treatment. Bronchodilators and postural drainage and chest percussion help remove secretions if the patient has bronchospasm and thick, tenacious sputum. Occasionally, bronchoscopy may be used to remove secretions. Oxygen therapy may be used for hypoxia. Segmental resection or lobectomy may be recommended for severe hemoptysis.

The only cure for bronchiectasis is the surgical removal of the affected lung portion. However, the patient with bronchiectasis affecting both lungs probably won't benefit from surgery.

Key nursing diagnoses and patient outcomes

Altered nutrition: Less than body requirements, related to chronic malnutrition caused by advanced bronchiectasis. Based on this nursing diagnosis, you'll establish these patient outcomes. The patient will:

- consume enough calories to regain weight lost and to maintain a normal weight
- consume a nutritionally balanced diet daily
- take measures to minimize fatigue during the day so he will have enough strength to eat at mealtimes.

Impaired gas exchange related to damage to the bronchial walls caused by bronchiectasis. Based on this nursing diagnosis, you'll establish these patient outcomes. The patient will:

- maintain adequate gas exchange with treatment measures
- have arterial blood gas (ABG) values that reflect adequate gas exchange.

Ineffective airway clearance related to abnormal mucociliary clearance and stagnated sputum in bronchi. Based on this nursing diagnosis, you'll establish these patient outcomes. The patient will:

- perform effective bronchial hygiene skillfully and regularly
- exhibit clearing airways with therapy
- demonstrate skill in conserving energy when attempting to clear his airways.

Nursing interventions

- Provide supportive care, and help the patient adjust to the life-style changes that irreversible lung damage necessitates.
- Administer antibiotics, as ordered, and record the patient's response to this medication.
- Give oxygen as needed.
- Perform chest physiotherapy, including postural drainage and chest percussion for involved lobes, several times a day, especially in the early morning and before bedtime.
- Provide a warm, quiet, comfortable environment. Also, help the patient to alternate rest and activity periods.
- Give the patient well-balanced, high-calorie meals. Offer small, frequent meals or nutritional supplements.
- Make sure the patient receives adequate hydration to help thin secretions and promote easier removal.
- Give frequent mouth care to remove foul-smelling sputum. Provide the patient with tissues and a waxed bag in which to dispose of the contaminated tissues.
- If surgery is to be performed, prepare the patient. After surgery, give meticulous postoperative care. Also, encourage deep breathing and position changes every 2 hours and provide chest-tube care.

Monitoring

- Monitor the patient's respiratory rate and pattern regularly.
- Assess gas exchange by monitoring ABG values as ordered.
- Observe the patient's breath sounds and sputum production for changes that might indicate a respiratory infection or worsening of condition.
- Watch for developing complications, such as right ventricular failure and cor pulmonale.
- If surgery is performed, monitor the patient's vital signs, respiratory status, and incision postoperatively for signs of complications, such as wound infection or atelectasis.

Patient teaching

- Show family members how to perform postural drainage and percussion. Also, teach the patient coughing and deep-breathing techniques to promote good ventilation and assist in secretion removal. Instruct him to maintain each postural drainage position for 10 minutes. Then direct the caregiver in performing percussion and instructing the patient to cough.
- If appropriate, advise the patient to stop smoking because it stimulates secretions and irritates the airways. Refer the patient to a local smoking-cessation group.
- Instruct the patient to avoid air pollutants and people with known upper respiratory tract infections.
- Direct the patient to take medications (especially antibiotics) exactly as ordered. Make sure he knows the adverse reactions associated with his medications. Instruct him to notify the doctor if any of these reactions occur.
- Teach the patient to dispose of all secretions properly to avoid spreading the infection to others. Advise him to wash his hands thoroughly after disposing of contaminated tissues.

• Urge the patient to keep up-to-date in his immunization schedule to prevent childhood diseases.
• Encourage the patient to rest as much as possible.
• Discuss dietary measures. Encourage the patient to follow a balanced, high-protein diet. Suggest that he eat small, frequent meals. Explain that milk products may increase the viscosity of secretions.
• Encourage the patient to drink plenty of fluids to thin secretions and to aid expectoration.
• If the patient needs surgery, offer complete preoperative and postoperative instructions. Forewarn the patient if he will have an I.V. line and chest tubes. Explain the reason for these procedures.

Bronchitis, chronic

A form of chronic obstructive pulmonary disease, chronic bronchitis is marked by excessive production of tracheobronchial mucus that's sufficient to cause a cough for at least 3 months each year for 2 consecutive years. The severity of the disease is linked to the amount of cigarette smoke or other pollutants inhaled and the duration of the inhalation. A respiratory tract infection typically exacerbates the cough and related symptoms. However, few patients with chronic bronchitis develop significant airway obstruction. About 20% of men have chronic bronchitis.

Causes

Cigarette smoking is the most common cause of chronic bronchitis, although some studies suggest a genetic predisposition to the disease as well.

The disease is directly correlated to heavy pollution and is more prevalent in people exposed to organic or inorganic dusts and noxious gases. Children of parents who smoke are at higher risk for respiratory tract infections that can lead to chronic bronchitis.

Chronic bronchitis results in hypertrophy and hyperplasia of the bronchial mucous glands, increased goblet cells, ciliary damage, squamous metaplasia of the columnar epithelium, and chronic leukocytic and lymphocytic infiltration of bronchial walls. Additional effects include widespread inflammation, airway narrowing, and mucus within the airways – all producing resistance in the small airways and, in turn, a severe ventilation-perfusion imbalance.

Complications

Chronic bronchitis can lead to cor pulmonale, pulmonary hypertension, right ventricular hypertrophy, and acute respiratory failure.

Assessment

The patient's history typically reflects a longtime smoker who has frequent upper respiratory tract infections. Usually, the patient seeks treatment for a productive cough and exertional dyspnea. He may describe his cough as initially prevalent in the winter months but gradually becoming a year-round problem with increasingly severe episodes. He also typically reports progressively worsening dyspnea that takes increasingly longer to subside.

Inspection usually reveals a cough, producing copious gray, white, or yellow sputum. The patient may appear cyanotic. And he may use accessory respiratory muscles for breathing (a "blue bloater"). Vital signs usually include tachypnea; other typical findings include substantial weight gain.

Palpation may disclose pedal edema and neck vein distention. Auscultation findings include wheezing, prolonged expiratory time, and rhonchi.

Diagnostic tests

• *Chest X-rays* may show hyperinflation and increased bronchovascular markings.

• *Pulmonary function tests* demonstrate increased residual volume, decreased vital capacity and forced expiratory flow, and normal static compliance and diffusing capacity.
• *Arterial blood gas analysis* displays decreased partial pressure of oxygen in arterial blood and normal or increased partial pressure of carbon dioxide in arterial blood.
• *Sputum culture* may reveal many microorganisms and neutrophils.
• *Electrocardiography* may detect atrial arrhythmias; peaked P waves in leads II, III, and aV_F; and occasionally right ventricular hypertrophy.

Treatment

The most effective treatment is for the patient to stop smoking and to avoid air pollutants as much as possible. Antibiotics can be used to treat recurring infections. Bronchodilators may relieve bronchospasm and facilitate mucus clearance. Adequate fluid intake is essential, and chest physiotherapy may be needed to mobilize secretions. Ultrasonic or mechanical nebulizer treatments may help to loosen and mobilize secretions. Occasionally, the patient will respond to corticosteroid therapy. Diuretics may be used to treat edema, and oxygen may be necessary to treat hypoxia.

Key nursing diagnoses and patient outcomes

Altered nutrition: Less than body requirements, related to inability to eat properly because of fatigue. Based on this nursing diagnosis, you'll establish these patient outcomes. The patient will:
• consume enough calories to regain weight lost and maintain weight within normal range
• consume a well-balanced diet daily
• not develop signs of malnutrition.

Fatigue related to impaired gas exchange. Based on this nursing diagnosis, you'll establish these patient outcomes. The patient will:
• identify activities that increase fatigue
• take measures to conserve energy and prevent or minimize fatigue
• seek assistance, as needed, to perform activities of daily living.

Ineffective airway clearance related to increased tracheobronchial secretions. Based on this nursing diagnosis, you'll establish these patient outcomes. The patient will:
• perform bronchial hygiene skillfully and regularly
• maintain effective airway clearance
• have the energy to clear his airway properly.

Nursing interventions

• Answer the patient's questions, and encourage him and his family to express their concerns about the illness. Include the patient and his family in care decisions. Refer them to other support services as appropriate.
• As needed, perform chest physiotherapy, including postural drainage and chest percussion and vibration for involved lobes several times daily.
• Provide the patient with a high-calorie, protein-rich diet. Offer small, frequent meals to conserve the patient's energy and prevent fatigue.
• Make sure the patient receives adequate fluids (at least 3 liters a day) to loosen secretions.
• Schedule respiratory therapy for the patient at least 1 hour before or after meals. Provide mouth care after bronchodilator inhalation therapy.
• Encourage daily activity, and provide diversional activities as appropriate. To conserve the patient's energy and prevent fatigue, help him to alternate periods of rest and activity.
• Administer medications, as ordered, and note the patient's response to them.

Monitoring

• Assess the patient for changes in baseline respiratory function. Evaluate sputum

quality and quantity, restlessness, increased tachypnea, and altered breath sounds. Report changes immediately.
• Monitor the patient's weight by weighing him three times weekly. Assess for edema.
• Evaluate the patient's nutritional status regularly.
• Watch the patient for signs and symptoms of respiratory infection, such as fever, increased cough and sputum production, and purulent sputum.

Patient teaching

• Advise the patient to avoid crowds and people with known infections and to obtain influenza and pneumococcus immunizations.
• If the patient is receiving home oxygen therapy, explain the treatment rationale. Show him how to operate the equipment.
• Teach the patient and family how to perform postural drainage and chest percussion. Instruct the patient to maintain each position for 10 minutes before a caregiver performs percussion and the patient coughs. Also teach the patient coughing and deep-breathing techniques to promote good ventilation and to remove secretions.
• Review all medications, including dosages, adverse effects, and purposes. Teach the patient how to use an inhaler. Advise him to report any adverse reactions to the doctor immediately.
• Encourage the patient to eat high-calorie, protein-rich meals and to drink plenty of fluids to prevent dehydration and help loosen secretions.
• If the patient smokes, encourage him to stop. Provide him with smoking-cessation resources or counseling if necessary.
• Urge the patient to avoid inhaled irritants, such as automobile exhaust fumes, aerosol sprays, and industrial pollutants.
• Warn the patient that exposure to blasts of cold air may precipitate bronchospasm. Suggest that he avoid cold, windy weather or that he cover his mouth and nose with a scarf or mask if he must go outside.
• If the patient takes theophylline, warn him that cigarette or marijuana smoking significantly increases plasma clearance of theophylline. Also, patients who quit smoking should notify the doctor because they may experience the onset of adverse effects of higher blood levels of theophylline.
• If appropriate, describe the signs and symptoms of peptic ulcer disease. Instruct the patient to check his stools every day for blood and to notify the doctor if he has persistent nausea, vomiting, heartburn, indigestion, constipation, diarrhea, or bloody stools.

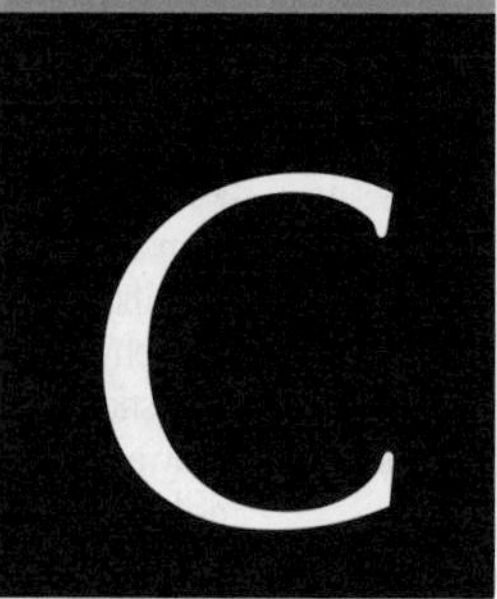

Calcium imbalance

Calcium plays an indispensable role in cell permeability, the formation of bones and teeth, blood coagulation, transmission of nerve impulses, and normal muscle contraction. Nearly all of the body's calcium is found in the bones. The remaining exists in serum in three forms: ionized or free calcium (the only active, or available, calcium), calcium bound to protein, and calcium combined with citrate or other organic ions.

Maintaining stable levels of ionized calcium in the serum is critical to neurologic function. The parathyroid glands regulate ionized calcium and determine its resorption into bone, absorption from the GI mucosa, and excretion in urine and feces.

Causes

Hypocalcemia may result from:

- inadequate intake of calcium and vitamin D, in which inadequate levels of vitamin D inhibit intestinal absorption of calcium
- hypoparathyroidism as a result of injury, disease, or surgery that reduces or eliminates secretion of parathyroid hormone (PTH), which is necessary for calcium absorption and normal serum calcium levels
- malabsorption or loss of calcium from the GI tract, caused by increased intestinal motility from severe diarrhea or laxative abuse, from inadequate levels of vitamin D or PTH, or from a reduction in gastric acidity.
- severe infections or burns, in which diseased and burned tissue traps calcium from the extracellular fluid
- alkalosis, in which calcium forms a complex with bicarbonate, causing diminished levels of ionized calcium and inducing symptoms of hypocalcemia
- pancreatic insufficiency, which may cause malabsorption of calcium and subsequent calcium loss in feces; in acute pancreatitis, hypocalcemia varies in degree with the disorder's severity and is of unknown origin
- renal failure or use of loop diuretics, resulting in excessive excretion of calcium
- hypomagnesemia, which causes decreased PTH secretion and blocks the peripheral action of that hormone
- hyperphosphatemia, which causes calcium levels to decrease as phosphorus levels rise
- extensive administration of citrated blood, which may result in citrate binding with calcium
- osteoblast metastases, which is attributed to increased calcium influx into osteoblastic lesions.

Hypercalcemia may result from:

- hyperparathyroidism, a primary cause, which increases serum calcium levels by promoting calcium absorption from the intestine, resorption from bone, and reabsorption from the kidneys
- hypervitaminosis D, which may increase absorption of calcium from the intestine
- certain cancers, such as multiple myeloma, lymphoma, squamous cell carcinoma of the lung, and breast cancer, which raise serum

calcium levels by destroying bone or by releasing PTH or a PTH-like substance, osteoclast-activating factor, prostaglandins and, perhaps, a sterol resembling vitamin D
• multiple fractures and prolonged immobilization, which release bone calcium and raise the serum calcium level.

Other causes of hypercalcemia include milk-alkali syndrome, renal failure, sarcoidosis, hyperthyroidism, adrenal insufficiency, thiazide diuretics, and excessive administration of calcium during cardiopulmonary arrest.

CHECKLIST

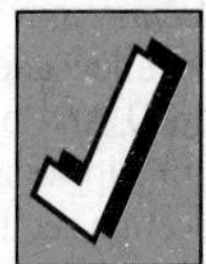

Identifying calcium imbalance

Serum calcium levels help you identify a patient's calcium imbalance. To identify *hypocalcemia,* look for:

- ☐ total serum calcium level less than 8.5 mg/dl
- ☐ ionized serum calcium level under 4.5 mg/dl.

To identify *hypercalcemia,* look for:

- ☐ total serum calcium level greater than 10.5 mg/dl
- ☐ ionized serum calcium level above 5.3 mg/dl.

Note: Because about one-half of serum calcium is bound to albumin, you must consider changes in serum protein levels when interpreting serum calcium levels.

Complications

Severe hypocalcemia can lead to laryngeal spasm, seizures and, possibly, respiratory arrest. Cardiac arrhythmias may also occur.

In hypercalcemia, serum calcium levels greater than 13.5 mg/dl may cause coma and cardiac arrest. Hypercalcemia may also lead to renal calculi.

Assessment

The history of a patient with *hypocalcemia* may disclose risk factors, such as hypothyroidism or renal failure. The patient may report digital and perioral paresthesia and muscle cramps. Inspection may reveal twitching, carpopedal spasm, tetany, and seizures. Auscultation sometimes detects cardiac arrhythmias. Also, a physical examination may uncover reliable indicators of hypocalcemia, including hyperactive reflexes, a positive Trousseau's sign, and a positive Chvostek's sign.

A patient with *hypercalcemia* may have a history of risk factors such as excessive ingestion of vitamin D or prolonged immobilization. He may complain of lethargy, weakness, anorexia, constipation, nausea, vomiting, and polyuria. Family members may report personality changes.

During assessment, the patient may appear confused or, in severe cases, comatose. Neuromuscular assessment may reveal weakness, with hyporeflexia and decreased muscle tone.

Diagnostic tests

For key diagnostic tests, see *Identifying calcium imbalance.* Supplemental tests include:

• *Sulkowitch's urine test* may reveal increased calcium precipitation in hypercalcemia.
• *Electrocardiogram (ECG)* results are significant for lengthened QT interval, prolonged ST segment, and arrhythmias in hypocalcemia. In hypercalcemia, the QT interval shortens. Ventricular arrhythmias may occur with severe hypercalcemia.

Treatment

Treatment aims to correct acute imbalance and provide follow-up maintenance therapy. It also aims to correct the underlying cause.

Mild *hypocalcemia* may require only a diet adjustment to allow adequate intake of calcium, vitamin D, and protein, possibly with oral calcium supplements.

Acute hypocalcemia requires immediate correction by I.V. administration of calcium gluconate, which is usually preferable to calcium chloride. If the hypocalcemia is related to hypomagnesemia, magnesium replacement may be necessary because the hypocalcemia often doesn't respond to calcium therapy alone.

Chronic hypocalcemia requires vitamin D supplements to facilitate GI calcium absorption. To correct mild deficiency, the amount of vitamin D found in most multivitamin preparations is adequate. For severe deficiency, vitamin D is used in four forms: ergocalciferol (vitamin D_2), cholecalciferol (vitamin D_3), calcitriol, and dihydrotachysterol, a synthetic form of vitamin D_2.

If *hypercalcemia* produces no symptoms, treatment may consist only of managing the underlying cause. If the imbalance produces symptoms, treatment primarily eliminates excess serum calcium through hydration with 0.9% sodium chloride solution, which promotes calcium excretion in urine. Loop diuretics, such as ethacrynic acid and furosemide, also promote calcium excretion. (Thiazide diuretics are contraindicated in hypercalcemia because they inhibit calcium excretion.)

Corticosteroids, such as prednisone and hydrocortisone, help treat sarcoidosis, hypervitaminosis D, and certain tumors. Plicamycin can also lower serum calcium levels and is especially effective against hypercalcemia secondary to certain tumors. Calcitonin may also be helpful in certain instances. Administration of I.V. phosphates can be hazardous to the patient and is used only when other treatments prove ineffective.

Key nursing diagnoses and patient outcomes

For *hypocalcemia:*

Altered nutrition: Less than body requirements related to inadequate intake of calcium and vitamin D in diet. Based on this nursing diagnosis, you'll establish these patient outcomes. The patient will:

- identify food sources rich in calcium and vitamin D
- consume a diet high in calcium and vitamin D
- develop a total serum calcium level within normal range.

Pain related to hypocalcemia-induced muscle cramps. Based on this nursing diagnosis, you'll establish these patient outcomes. The patient will:

- state and carry out appropriate interventions for pain relief
- experience relief of muscle cramps.

For *hypercalcemia:*

Altered urinary elimination related to hypercalcemia-induced polyuria. Based on this nursing diagnosis, you'll establish these patient outcomes. The patient will:

- have a total serum calcium level within the normal range
- maintain a normal balance between intake and output.

Impaired physical mobility related to hypercalcemia-induced muscle weakness. Based on this nursing diagnosis, you'll establish these patient outcomes. The patient will:

- show no evidence of complications related to impaired physical mobility, such as contractures, venous stasis, thrombus formation, or skin breakdown
- adhere to his treatment regimen, which will prevent or minimize further elevations in serum calcium level.

Nursing interventions

For patients with hypocalcemia:

- Using a volumetric infusion pump, administer calcium gluconate I.V. slowly, in dextrose 5% in water. Don't infuse more than 1 g/hour, except in an emergency. (See *Administering calcium gluconate safely.*)
- Give oral calcium supplements, as ordered, 1 to 1½ hours after meals. If GI up-

set occurs, administer the supplements with milk.

• Provide a quiet, safe, stress-free environment for the patient. Observe seizure precautions for patients with severe hypocalcemia.

• If the patient is symptomatic, keep a tracheotomy tray and manual resuscitation bag at the bedside in case of laryngeal spasm.

For patients with hypercalcemia:

• Increase fluid intake to dilute calcium in serum and urine and to prevent renal damage and dehydration.

• Administer loop diuretics (not thiazide diuretics), as ordered. Provide acid-ash drinks, such as cranberry juice, because calcium salts are more soluble in acid than in alkali.

• Ambulate the patient as soon as possible. Handle the patient with chronic hypercalcemia gently to prevent pathologic fractures. If the patient is bedridden, reposition him frequently and encourage range-of-motion exercises to promote circulation and prevent urinary stasis and calcium loss from bone.

• Provide a safe environment. Keep the bed's side rails raised and the bed in the lowest position with the wheels locked.

• Orient the patient to his surroundings, as needed.

Monitoring

For patients with hypocalcemia:

• Watch for the disorder in patients at risk, such as those receiving massive transfusions of citrated blood and those with chronic diarrhea, severe infections, and insufficient dietary intake of calcium and protein (especially elderly patients).

• Assess the patient's respiratory status, including rate, depth, pattern, and rhythm. Be alert for stridor, dyspnea, or crowing.

• Monitor serum calcium levels every 12 to 24 hours, and report any decrease.

• If possible, monitor the patient for ECG changes. Notify the doctor if ventricular arrhythmias or heart block develops.

NURSING ALERT

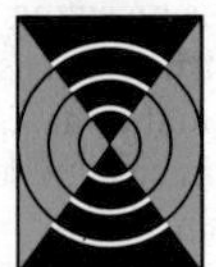

Administering calcium gluconate safely

Give I.V. calcium gluconate slowly, in dextrose 5% in water. Never use 0.9% sodium chloride because of possible renal calcium loss. What's more, never add calcium gluconate I.V. to solutions containing bicarbonate; precipitation will occur.

• When giving calcium supplements, frequently check pH level because an alkalotic state that exceeds a pH of 7.45 inhibits calcium ionization.

• Check for Trousseau's and Chvostek's signs, and report positive signs to the doctor.

• When administering calcium solutions, watch for anorexia, nausea, and vomiting – possible signs of overcorrection, resulting in hypercalcemia.

• Observe the I.V. site for signs of infiltration because calcium can cause tissue sloughing.

• If the patient is receiving calcium chloride, watch for abdominal discomfort.

• Monitor the patient closely for a possible drug interaction if he's receiving a digitalis glycoside with large doses of oral calcium supplements; watch for signs and symptoms of digitalis toxicity (anorexia, nausea, vomiting, yellow vision, and cardiac arrhythmias).

For patients with hypercalcemia:

• Frequently assess the patient's level of consciousness.

• Watch for signs of congestive heart failure in patients receiving diuresis therapy with 0.9% sodium chloride solution.

• When administering loop diuretics, monitor intake and output and strain urine for renal calculi.

• If the patient is receiving digitalis, watch for signs of toxicity, such as anorexia, nausea, vomiting, and an irregular pulse.
• Monitor serum calcium levels frequently. Report increasing levels.
• Check ECG results and vital signs frequently. Observe for arrhythmias if hypercalcemia is severe.

Patient teaching

For patients with hypocalcemia:
• To prevent hypocalcemia, be sure to advise all patients – especially elderly patients – to eat foods rich in calcium, vitamin D, and protein, such as fortified milk and cheese. Explain how important calcium is for normal bone formation and blood coagulation. Discourage chronic use of laxatives.
• If the patient requires oral calcium preparations or vitamin D supplements, make sure he understands his regimen.

For patients with hypercalcemia:
• To prevent recurrence of hypercalcemia, suggest a low-calcium diet with increased fluid intake.
• Review nonprescription medications that are high in calcium, and advise the patient to avoid these. Also caution him not to take megadoses of vitamin D.
• Stress the importance of increased fluid intake (up to 3 liters in nonrestricted patients) to minimize the possibility of renal calculi formation.

Candidiasis

Also known as candidosis and moniliasis, this usually mild, superficial fungal infection can lead to severe disseminated infections and fungemia in an immunocompromised patient. In most cases, the causative fungi infect the nails (paronychia), skin (diaper rash), or mucous membranes, especially the oropharynx (thrush), vagina (vaginitis), esophagus, and GI tract.

These fungi may enter the bloodstream and invade the kidneys, lungs, endocardium, brain, or other structures, causing serious systemic infection. Such systemic infection predominates among drug abusers and hospitalized patients (particularly diabetic and immunosuppressed patients).

The prognosis varies, depending on the patient's resistance. The incidence of candidiasis continues to rise because of increasing use of I.V. antibiotic therapy and increasing numbers of immunocompromised patients in the acute care setting.

Causes

Most cases of candidiasis result from infection with *Candida albicans* or *C. tropicalis,* although eight other potentially disease-causing strains exist among the more than 150 species of *Candida.* One of the normal flora of the GI tract, mouth, vagina, and skin, *C. albicans* causes infection when some change in the body permits its sudden proliferation. The changes may be triggered by rising blood glucose levels from diabetes mellitus; lowered resistance from such diseases as cancer; immunosuppressant drug therapy; radiation; aging; or irritation from dentures.

The infecting organism may enter the body because of I.V. or urinary catheterization, drug abuse, total parenteral nutrition, or surgery. The most common precipitator is the use of broad-spectrum antibiotics, such as tetracycline. These agents decrease the number of normal bacterial flora and permit the number of fungi, including candidal organisms, to increase.

A mother with vaginitis can transmit the organism (as oral thrush) to the neonate during vaginal delivery.

Complications

The most common complications include *Candida* dissemination with organ failure of the kidneys, brain, GI tract, eyes, lungs, and heart.

Assessment

The patient's history may reveal an underlying illness, such as cancer, diabetes, or human immunodeficiency virus infection; a recent course of antibiotic or antineoplastic therapy; or drug abuse.

Depending on the infection site, superficial infection may cause the following signs and symptoms:

• Skin – scaly, erythematous, papular rash, possibly covered with exudate and erupting in breast folds, between fingers, and at the axillae, groin, and umbilicus (in diaper rash, papules appear at the edges of the rash)
• Nails – red, swollen, darkened nail beds; occasionally, purulent discharge; sometimes the nail separates from the nail bed.
• Esophageal mucosa – occasionally, scales in the mouth and throat
• Vaginal mucosa – white or yellow discharge, with local excoriation; white or gray raised patches on vaginal walls, with local inflammation
• Oropharyngeal mucosa – cream-colored or bluish white lacelike patches of exudate on the tongue, mouth, or pharynx that reveal bloody engorgement when scraped; pain and a burning sensation in the mouth and throat may occur.

If the patient has systemic disease, he also may report myalgia, arthralgia, chills with a high and spiking fever, prostration, and rash. Other specific complaints vary, depending on the infection site:

• Lungs – hemoptysis, cough; coarse breath sounds in the lung fields infected by *Candida*
• Kidneys – flank pain, dysuria, hematuria, cloudy urine with casts
• Brain – headache, nuchal rigidity, seizures, focal neurologic deficits
• Eyes – blurred vision, orbital or periorbital pain, exudate, floating scotomata, and lesions with a white, cotton-ball appearance seen during ophthalmoscopy
• Endocardium – chest pain and arrhythmias; auscultation may reveal a systolic or diastolic murmur with endocarditis.

Diagnostic tests

Detection of candidal organisms by a Gram stain of skin or vaginal scrapings, pus, or sputum or of skin scrapings prepared in potassium hydroxide solution confirms the diagnosis.

Tests for systemic infection include blood and tissue cultures.

Treatment

Initial treatment aims to improve the underlying condition that predisposes the patient to candidiasis. For example, measures may be taken to control diabetes or, if possible, to discontinue antibiotic therapy or catheterization.

For superficial candidiasis, the doctor may prescribe an antifungal medication, such as nystatin. Amphotericin B and gentian violet are effective for candidiasis of the skin and nails. Rarely used because it stains the skin purple, gentian violet is effective for paronychial candidiasis, thrush, and vaginitis. Clotrimazole, fluconazole, and miconazole are effective in mucous membrane and vaginal candidiasis. And ketoconazole or fluconazole is the primary choice for chronic candidiasis of the mucous membranes.

Treatment for systemic infection consists mainly of I.V. amphotericin B, but flucytosine or miconazole may be added.

Key nursing diagnoses and patient outcomes

Altered oral mucous membrane related to the presence of exudative patches in the oral cavity. Based on this nursing diagnosis, you'll establish these patient outcomes. The patient will:

• demonstrate appropriate oral hygiene practices
• experience increased comfort
• recover normal mucous membranes that appear pink and moist upon inspection.

Impaired skin integrity related to skin rash and possible exudate. Based on this nursing diagnosis, you'll establish these patient outcomes. The patient will:

NURSING ALERT

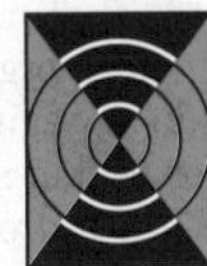

Oral anesthetic precaution

When using a topical anesthetic to relieve pain caused by oral candidiasis, use the smallest amount necessary. Using an excessive amount may suppress the the patient's gag reflex and lead to aspiration.

- demonstrate appropriate skin care practices
- avoid complications, such as abscesses or sepsis
- regain normal skin appearance, as exhibited by the disappearance of rash and exudate and the absence of breaks in the skin.

Altered sexuality patterns related to vaginal infection. Based on this nursing diagnosis, you'll establish these patient outcomes. The patient will:

- comply with the prescribed medication regimen
- express an understanding that sexual activity may resume after the infection resolves
- resume normal sexual activity.

Nursing interventions

- Observe standard precautions.
- Provide a nonirritating mouthwash to loosen tenacious secretions and a soft toothbrush to avoid irritation.
- Relieve mouth discomfort with a topical anesthetic, such as lidocaine or benzocaine, at least 1 hour before meals. (See *Oral anesthetic precaution.*)
- Apply cornstarch, nystatin powder, or dry padding in intertriginous areas of obese patients to prevent irritation and candidal growth.
- Record dates of I.V. catheter insertion and replace the catheter according to your hospital's policy, to prevent phlebitis.
- Provide appropriate supportive care for patients with systemic infections. If the patient is receiving amphotericin B for systemic candidiasis, premedicate him with aspirin, antihistamines, or antiemetics, as ordered, to help reduce adverse reactions.
- Prepare to give a blood transfusion if ordered and if the patient has a low platelet count. Low platelet count may be related to underlying disease or treatment with amphotericin B.

Monitoring

- Frequently check the vital signs of a patient with a systemic infection.
- Check high-risk patients daily, especially those receiving antibiotics. Watch for patchy areas, irritation, sore throat, oral and gingival bleeding, and other signs of superinfection. If you note a vaginal discharge, document the color and amount.
- Carefully monitor intake and output and potassium levels while the patient is receiving medication.
- If the patient has renal involvement, carefully monitor blood urea nitrogen, serum creatinine, and urine blood and protein levels.
- Assess the patient with candidiasis for underlying systemic causes, such as diabetes mellitus. If the patient is receiving amphotericin B for systemic candidiasis, he may have severe chills, fever, anorexia, nausea, vomiting, hypokalemia, and renal impairment.

Patient teaching

- Demonstrate comprehensive oral hygiene practices, and have the patient perform a return demonstration. Recommend that the patient use alkaline mouth care products because increased acidity promotes candidal growth.
- Tell the patient who's using nystatin solution to swish it around in his mouth for several minutes before swallowing. Be

sure he knows not to scrape the lesions but to coat them with the medication.

• Suggest a soft diet for the patient with severe dysphagia. Advise the patient with mild dysphagia to chew food thoroughly.

• Encourage a woman in her third trimester of pregnancy to be examined for vaginitis to protect her infant from thrush infection at birth.

• Direct the patient with dyspareunia to take intravaginal medication as prescribed. Listen to her concerns and reassure her that sexual impairment should resolve when her infection subsides. Tell her that her sexual partner usually won't need concomitant treatment.

Cardiac tamponade

A rapid rise in intrapericardial pressure impairs diastolic filling of the heart in cardiac tamponade. The rise in pressure usually results from blood or fluid accumulation in the pericardial sac. If fluid accumulates rapidly, as little as 250 ml can create an emergency situation. Slow accumulation and rise in pressure, as in pericardial effusion associated with cancer, may not produce immediate signs and symptoms because the fibrous wall of the pericardial sac can gradually stretch to accommodate as much as 1 to 2 liters of fluid.

Causes

Cardiac tamponade may be idiopathic (Dressler's syndrome) or may result from:

• effusion (in cancer, bacterial infections, tuberculosis and, rarely, acute rheumatic fever)

• hemorrhage from trauma (such as gunshot or stab wounds of the chest, perforation by catheter during cardiac or central venous catheterization, or after cardiac surgery)

• hemorrhage from nontraumatic causes (such as rupture of the heart or great vessels or anticoagulant therapy in a patient with pericarditis)

• viral, postirradiation, or idiopathic pericarditis

• acute myocardial infarction

• chronic renal failure during dialysis

• drug reaction (procainamide, hydralazine, minoxidil, isoniazid, penicillin, methysergide, and daunorubicin)

• connective tissue disorders (such as rheumatoid arthritis, systemic lupus erythematosus, rheumatic fever, vasculitis, and scleroderma).

Complications

Pressure resulting from fluid accumulation in the pericardium decreases ventricular filling and cardiac output, resulting in cardiogenic shock and death if untreated.

Assessment

The patient's history may show a disorder that can cause cardiac tamponade. He may report acute pain and dyspnea, which forces him to sit upright and lean forward to ease breathing and lessen the pain. He may be orthopneic, diaphoretic, anxious, restless, and pale or cyanotic. You may note neck vein distention produced by increased venous pressure, although this may not be present if the patient is hypovolemic.

Palpation of the peripheral pulses may disclose rapid, weak pulses. Palpation of the upper quadrant may reveal hepatomegaly.

Percussion may detect a widening area of flatness across the anterior chest wall, indicating a large effusion. Hepatomegaly may also be noted.

Auscultation of the blood pressure may demonstrate a decreased arterial blood pressure, pulsus paradoxus (an abnormal inspiratory drop in systemic blood pressure greater than 15 mm Hg), and narrow pulse pressure.

Heart sounds may be muffled. A quiet heart with faint sounds usually accompanies only severe tamponade and occurs within minutes of the tamponade, as happens with cardiac rupture or trauma. The lungs are clear.

Diagnostic tests

The following test results are characteristic:

- *Chest X-rays* show a slightly widened mediastinum and enlargement of the cardiac silhouette.
- *Electrocardiography (ECG)* is useful to rule out other cardiac disorders. The QRS amplitude may be reduced, and electrical alternans of the P wave, QRS complex, and T wave may be present. Generalized ST-segment elevation is noted in all leads.
- *Pulmonary artery pressure monitoring* detects increased right atrial pressure, right ventricular diastolic pressure, and central venous pressure.
- *Echocardiography* records pericardial effusion with signs of right ventricular and atrial compression.

Treatment

The goal of treatment is to relieve intrapericardial pressure and cardiac compression by removing accumulated blood or fluid. Pericardiocentesis (needle aspiration of the pericardial cavity) or surgical creation of an opening dramatically improves systemic arterial pressure and cardiac output with aspiration of as little as 25 ml of fluid. A drain may be inserted into the pericardial sac to drain the effusion. This may be left in until the effusion process stops or the corrective action (pericardial window) is performed. In the case of infection, antibiotics can be instilled through the drain, clamped, and later drained off.

In the hypotensive patient, trial volume loading with I.V. 0.9% sodium chloride solution with albumin and perhaps an inotropic drug, such as dopamine, is necessary to maintain cardiac output.

Depending on the cause of tamponade, additional treatment may include:

- in traumatic injury, blood transfusion or a thoracotomy to drain reaccumulating fluid or to repair bleeding sites
- in heparin-induced tamponade, the heparin antagonist protamine
- in warfarin-induced tamponade, vitamin K.

Key nursing diagnoses and patient outcomes

Altered tissue perfusion (cerebral, renal, cardiopulmonary) related to decreased cardiac output caused by cardiac tamponade. Based on this nursing diagnosis, you'll establish these patient outcomes. The patient will:

- regain and maintain normal tissue perfusion
- remain alert and oriented to time, person, and place
- maintain normal renal function as exhibited by a urine output of at least 30 ml/hour
- not experience any cardiac arrhythmias.

Decreased cardiac output related to impaired diastolic filling of the heart caused by increased intrapericardial pressure. Based on this nursing diagnosis, you'll establish these patient outcomes. The patient will:

- exhibit a normal pulse and blood pressure
- maintain adequate cardiac output.

Ineffective breathing pattern related to chest pain caused by cardiac tamponade. Based on this nursing diagnosis, you'll establish these patient outcomes. The patient will:

- demonstrate a respiratory rate that fluctuates no more than 5 breaths/minute from the baseline
- maintain arterial blood gas values within the normal range
- be able to breathe easily.

Nursing interventions

- If the patient isn't in the intensive care unit already, transfer him there immediately.

• Infuse I.V. solutions and inotropic drugs such as dopamine, as ordered, to maintain the patient's blood pressure.
• Administer oxygen therapy as needed.
• Prepare the patient for pericardiocentesis, a thoracotomy, or central venous pressure (CVP) line insertion, as indicated.
• Provide supportive care as indicated by the patient's condition and the underlying cause of the tamponade.
• Reassure the patient to reduce anxiety.

Monitoring

• Check for signs of increasing tamponade, increasing dyspnea, and arrhythmias.
• Watch for a decrease in CVP and a concomitant rise in blood pressure following treatment, which indicate relief of cardiac compression.
• Monitor the patient's respiratory status for signs of respiratory distress, such as severe tachypnea or changes in the patient's level of consciousness.

Patient teaching

• If the patient is not acutely ill, briefly teach him about his condition and explain why it is occurring. Tell him how the condition will be treated, and explain each new procedure before beginning.
• Stress the importance of alerting the nurse if symptoms worsen.

Cardiogenic shock

Sometimes called pump failure, cardiogenic shock is a condition of diminished cardiac output that severely impairs tissue perfusion. Cardiogenic shock occurs as a serious complication in nearly 15% of all patients who are hospitalized with acute myocardial infarction (MI). It typically affects patients whose area of infarction involves 40% or more of left ventricular muscle mass; in such patients, mortality may exceed 85%. Most patients with cardiogenic shock die within 24 hours of onset. The prognosis for those who survive is poor.

Causes

Cardiogenic shock can result from any condition that causes significant left ventricular dysfunction with reduced cardiac output, such as MI (most common), myocardial ischemia, papillary muscle dysfunction, and end-stage cardiomyopathy.

Other causes include myocarditis and depression of myocardial contractility after cardiac arrest and prolonged cardiac surgery. Mechanical abnormalities of the ventricle, such as acute mitral or aortic insufficiency or an acutely acquired ventricular septal defect or ventricular aneurysm, may also result in cardiogenic shock.

Regardless of the cause, left ventricular dysfunction initiates a series of compensatory mechanisms that attempt to increase cardiac output and, in turn, maintain vital organ function. As cardiac output falls, aortic and carotid baroreceptors activate sympathetic nervous responses. These compensatory responses increase heart rate, left ventricular filling pressure, and peripheral resistance to flow in order to enhance venous return to the heart. The action initially stabilizes the patient but later causes deterioration with rising oxygen demands on the already compromised myocardium. These events constitute a vicious circle of low cardiac output, sympathetic compensation, myocardial ischemia, and even lower cardiac output.

Complications

Death usually ensues because the vital organs can't overcome the deleterious effects of extended hypoperfusion.

Assessment

Typically, the patient's history includes a disorder (such as MI or cardiomyopathy) that severely decreases left ventricular function. Patients with underlying cardiac disease may complain of anginal pain because of decreased myocardial perfusion and oxygenation. Urine output is usually less than 20 ml/hour.

Inspection usually reveals pale skin, decreased sensorium, and rapid, shallow respirations. Palpation of peripheral pulses may detect a rapid, thready pulse. The skin feels cold and clammy.

Auscultation of blood pressure usually discloses a mean arterial pressure of less than 60 mm Hg and a narrowing pulse pressure. In a patient with chronic hypotension, the mean pressure may fall below 50 mm Hg before he exhibits any signs of shock. Auscultation of the heart detects gallop rhythm, faint heart sounds and, possibly (if shock results from rupture of the ventricular septum or papillary muscles), a holosystolic murmur.

Although many of these clinical features also occur in heart failure and other shock syndromes, they are usually more profound in cardiogenic shock. Patients with pericardial tamponade may have distant heart sounds.

Diagnostic tests

- *Pulmonary artery pressure monitoring* reveals increased pulmonary artery pressure (PAP) and pulmonary capillary wedge pressure (PCWP), reflecting a rise in left ventricular end-diastolic pressure (preload) and heightened resistance to left ventricular emptying (afterload) caused by ineffective pumping and increased peripheral vascular resistance. Thermodilution catheterization reveals a reduced cardiac index.
- *Invasive arterial pressure monitoring* shows systolic arterial pressure less than 80 mm Hg caused by impaired ventricular ejection.
- *Arterial blood gas analysis* may show metabolic and respiratory acidosis and hypoxia.
- *Electrocardiography (ECG)* demonstrates possible evidence of acute MI, ischemia, or ventricular aneurysm.
- *Serum enzyme measurements* display elevated levels of creatine kinase (CK), lactate dehydrogenase (LDH), aspartate aminotransferase (formerly SGOT), and alanine aminotransferase (formerly SGPT), which indicate MI or ischemia and suggest heart failure or shock. CK-MB (an isoenzyme of CK that occurs in cardiac tissue) and LDH isoenzyme levels may confirm acute MI.
- *Cardiac catheterization* and *echocardiography* reveal other conditions that can lead to pump dysfunction and failure, such as cardiac tamponade, papillary muscle infarct or rupture, ventricular septal rupture, pulmonary emboli, venous pooling (associated with venodilators and continuous or intermittent positive-pressure breathing), and hypovolemia.

Treatment

Treatment aims to enhance cardiovascular status by increasing cardiac output, improving myocardial perfusion, and decreasing cardiac work load with combinations of cardiovascular drugs and mechanical-assist techniques.

I.V. drugs may include dopamine, a vasopressor that increases cardiac output, blood pressure, and renal blood flow; amrinone or dobutamine, inotropic agents that increase myocardial contractility; and norepinephrine, when a more potent vasoconstrictor is necessary. Nitroprusside, a vasodilator, may be used with a vasopressor to further improve cardiac output by decreasing peripheral vascular resistance (afterload) and reducing left ventricular end-diastolic pressure (preload). However, the patient's blood pressure must be adequate to support nitroprusside therapy and must be monitored closely.

Treatment may also include the intra-aortic balloon pump (IABP), a mechanical-assist device that attempts to improve coronary artery perfusion and decrease cardiac work load. The inflatable balloon pump is inserted through the femoral artery into the descending thoracic aorta. The balloon inflates during diastole to increase coronary artery perfusion pressure and deflates before systole (before the aortic valve opens) to reduce resistance to ejection (afterload) and therefore lessen cardiac work load. Improved ventricular ejection, which significantly improves cardiac output, and a subsequent vasodilation in the peripheral vessels lead to lower preload volume.

When drug therapy and IABP insertion fail, a ventricular-assist pump (an experimental device) may be used.

Key nursing diagnoses and patient outcomes

Altered cardiopulmonary tissue perfusion related to decreased cardiac output caused by left ventricular dysfunction. Based on this nursing diagnosis, you'll establish these patient outcomes. The patient will:
- not exhibit cardiac arrhythmias
- remain free of chest pain
- exhibit arterial blood gas values within the normal range.

Decreased cardiac output related to left ventricular dysfunction caused by myocardial injury. Based on this nursing diagnosis, you'll establish these patient outcomes. The patient will:
- have a heart rate and blood pressure within the normal range
- regain and maintain a normal cardiac output.

Fear related to threat of death caused by cardiogenic shock. Based on this nursing diagnosis, you'll establish these patient outcomes. The patient will:
- identify and verbalize his fears
- use support systems to diminish his fears
- exhibit fewer physical symptoms of fear.

NURSING ALERT

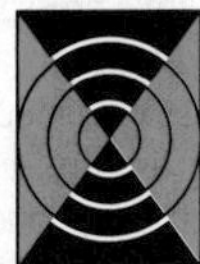

I.V. infusion precaution in abdominal trauma

Don't start an I.V. infusion in the legs of a patient who is in shock and who has sustained abdominal trauma. The infused fluid may escape into the abdomen through a ruptured blood vessel.

Nursing interventions

- In the intensive care unit (ICU), start I.V. infusions of 0.9% sodium chloride or lactated Ringer's solution, using a large-bore (14G to 18G) catheter, which allows easier administration of later blood transfusions. (See *I.V. infusion precaution in abdominal trauma.*)
- Administer oxygen by face mask or artificial airway to ensure adequate oxygenation of tissues. Adjust the oxygen flow rate to a higher or lower level, as blood gas measurements indicate. Many patients will need 100% oxygen, and some will require 5 to 15 cm H_2O of positive end-expiratory or continuous positive airway pressure ventilation.
- Administer an osmotic diuretic, such as mannitol, if ordered to increase renal blood flow and urine output.
- When a patient is on the IABP, move him as little as possible. Never flex the patient's "ballooned" leg at the hip because this may displace or fracture the catheter. Never place the patient in a sitting position for any reason (including chest X-rays) while the balloon is inflated; the balloon will tear through the aorta and result in immediate death.
- If the patient becomes hemodynamically stable, gradually reduce the frequency of balloon inflation to wean him from the IABP.
- To ease emotional stress, plan your care to allow frequent rest periods and provide as much privacy as possible. Allow family members to visit and comfort the patient as much as possible.
- Allow the family to express their anger, anxiety, and fear.

Monitoring

- Monitor and record blood pressure, pulse, respiratory rate, and peripheral pulses every 1 to 5 minutes until the patient stabilizes.

Record hemodynamic pressure readings every 15 minutes. Monitor cardiac rhythm continuously. Systolic blood pressure less than 80 mm Hg usually results in inadequate coronary artery blood flow, cardiac ischemia, arrhythmias, and further complications of low cardiac output. When blood pressure drops below 80 mm Hg, increase the oxygen flow rate and notify the doctor immediately.

A progressive drop in blood pressure accompanied by a thready pulse generally signals inadequate cardiac output from reduced intravascular volume. Notify the doctor, and increase the I.V. infusion rate.

• Using a pulmonary artery catheter, closely monitor PAP, PCWP and, if equipment is available, cardiac output. A high PCWP indicates heart failure, increased systemic vascular resistance, decreased cardiac output, and decreased cardiac index and should be reported immediately.

• Insert an indwelling urinary catheter if necessary to measure hourly urine output. If output is less than 30 ml/hour in adults, increase the fluid infusion rate but watch for signs of fluid overload, such as an increase in PCWP. Notify the doctor if urine output doesn't improve.

• Determine how much fluid to give by checking blood pressure, urine output, central venous pressure (CVP), or PCWP. (To increase accuracy, measure CVP at the level of the right atrium, using the same reference point on the chest each time.) Whenever the fluid infusion rate is increased, watch for signs of fluid overload, such as an increase in PCWP.

• Monitor arterial blood gas values, complete blood count, and electrolyte levels.

• During therapy, assess skin color and temperature and note any changes. Cold, clammy skin may be a sign of continuing peripheral vascular constriction, indicating progressive shock.

• During use of the IABP, assess pedal pulses and skin temperature and color to ensure adequate peripheral circulation. Check the dressing over the insertion site frequently for bleeding, and change it according to hospital protocol. Also check the site for hematoma or signs of infection, and culture any drainage.

• When weaning the patient from the IABP, watch for ECG changes, chest pain, and other signs of recurring cardiac ischemia as well as for shock.

Patient teaching

• Because the patient and his family may be anxious about the ICU and about the IABP and other devices, offer explanations and reassurance.

• Prepare the patient and his family for a probable fatal outcome, and help them find effective coping strategies.

Carpal tunnel release

If rest, splinting, and corticosteroid injections fail to relieve carpal tunnel syndrome, surgery may be necessary to decompress the median nerve. Surgery almost always relieves pain and restores function in the wrist and hand.

Procedure

The surgeon can choose from several approaches to carpal tunnel release. However, the selected technique must involve complete transection of the transverse carpal tunnel ligament to ensure adequate median nerve decompression.

In one of the more popular techniques, the surgeon makes an incision around the thenar eminence to expose the flexor retinaculum, which he then transects to relieve pressure on the median nerve. Depending on the extent of nerve compression, he also may perform neurolysis to free flattened nerve fibers. Neurolysis involves stretching the nerve, which relieves tension and loosens surrounding adhesions.

Complications

Although carpal tunnel release is relatively simple and generally risk free, certain complications may arise. These include hematoma formation, infection, painful scar formation, and tenosynovitis.

Key nursing diagnoses and patient outcomes

Altered peripheral tissue perfusion related to postoperative swelling and potential hematoma. Based on this nursing diagnosis, you'll establish these patient outcomes. The patient will:
- not develop a hematoma postoperatively
- maintain normal neurovascular function
- experience minimal swelling.

Pain related to high risk for developing tenosynovitis. Based on this nursing diagnosis, you'll establish these patient outcomes. The patient will:
- not experience signs of tenosynovitis, such as excessive tenderness, pain, or a crackling sound with motion of the affected wrist
- become pain free.

Risk for infection related to surgical incision of wrist. Based on this nursing diagnosis, you'll establish these patient outcomes. The patient will:
- exhibit and maintain a serum white blood cell count and temperature within the normal range
- have an incision that will remain pink and dry and heal normally
- not develop an infection.

Nursing interventions

When caring for a patient undergoing a carpal tunnel release, your primary responsibilities will include instructing the patient and monitoring for postoperative complications.

Before surgery

- Reinforce the purpose of the planned surgery. Tell the patient that the procedure should relieve the pain in his wrist and help him regain full use of his hand. Outline the steps of surgery, tailoring your explanation to the particular procedure the doctor has chosen as well as to the patient's level of understanding.
- Explain to the patient that before surgery, the affected arm will be shaved and cleaned and he'll be given a local anesthetic. Reassure him that although he may feel some pressure, the anesthetic will ensure a pain-free operation.
- Discuss postoperative care measures. Point out that he'll have a dressing wrapped around his hand and lower arm, which usually will remain in place for 1 to 2 days after surgery. Explain that he may experience pain once the anesthetic wears off but that analgesics will be available.
- Teach him the rehabilitative exercises that he'll be asked to do during the recovery period: gentle range-of-motion exercises with the wrist and fingers to prevent muscle atrophy. Demonstrate these exercises, and have him perform a return demonstration. Note, however, that severe pain may prevent him from doing so.

After surgery

- After the patient returns from surgery, monitor his vital signs and carefully assess circulation and sensory and motor function in the affected arm and hand. Keep the hand elevated to reduce swelling and discomfort.
- Check the dressing often for unusual drainage or bleeding, which may indicate infection. Assess for pain and provide analgesics as needed. Report severe, persistent pain or tenderness, which may point to tenosynovitis or hematoma formation.
- Encourage the patient to perform his wrist and finger exercises daily to improve circulation and enhance muscle tone. If these exercises are painful, have him perform them with his wrist and hand immersed in warm water. (Have him wear a surgical glove if his dressing is still in place.)
- Assess the need for home care and follow-up with activities of daily living, especially if the patient lives alone.

Home care instructions

- Instruct the patient to keep the incision site clean and dry. Tell him to cover it with a surgical or rubber glove when immersing it in water for exercises or when taking a bath or shower.
- Teach the patient how to change the dressing. Instruct him to do so once a day until healing is complete.
- Tell the patient to notify the doctor if redness, swelling, pain, or excessive drainage persists at the operative site.
- Encourage the patient to continue daily wrist and finger exercises. However, warn him against overusing the affected wrist or against lifting any object heavier than a thin magazine.
- If the patient's carpal tunnel syndrome is job related, suggest that he seek occupational counseling to help him find more suitable employment.

Carpal tunnel syndrome

The most common nerve entrapment syndrome, carpal tunnel syndrome results from compression of the median nerve in the wrist where it passes through the carpal tunnel. (See *Locating the carpal tunnel.*)

The median nerve controls motions in the forearm, wrist, and hand, such as turning the wrist toward the body, flexing the index and middle fingers, and many thumb movements. It also supplies sensation to the index, middle, and ring fingers. Compression of this nerve causes loss of movement and sensation in the wrist, hand, and fingers. Carpal tunnel syndrome usually occurs in women between ages 30 and 60 and may pose a serious occupational health problem. It may also occur in people who move their wrists continuously – for example, butchers, computer operators, and concert pianists. Any strenuous use of the hands – sustained grasping, twisting, or flexing – aggravates the condition.

Causes

The exact cause of carpal tunnel syndrome is unknown. However, the syndrome may result from amyloidosis or from an edema-producing condition such as diabetes, rheumatoid arthritis, pregnancy, premenstrual fluid retention, renal failure, and heart failure.

Repetitive wrist motions involving excessive flexion or extension also cause the carpal tunnel structures (tendons, for example) to swell and press the median nerve against the transverse carpal ligament. Dislocation or an acute sprain may damage the median nerve. Some experts think that a vitamin B_6 deficiency contributes to carpal tunnel syndrome.

Complications

Continued use of the affected wrist may increase tendon inflammation, compression, and neural ischemia. Wrist function will decrease. Untreated carpal tunnel syndrome can produce permanent nerve damage with loss of movement and sensation.

Assessment

The history may disclose that the patient's occupation or hobby requires strenuous or repetitive use of the hands. It may reveal a hormonal condition, wrist injury, rheumatoid arthritis, or other condition that causes swelling in carpal tunnel structures.

The patient may complain of weakness, pain, burning, numbness, or tingling in one or both hands. Paresthesia may affect the thumb, forefinger, middle finger, and half of the ring finger. She may report that the paresthesia worsens at night and in the morning (because of vasodilation and venous stasis). She may also report that the pain spreads to the forearm and, in severe cases, as far as the shoulder. She can usually relieve the pain by shaking her hands vigorously or dangling her arms at her sides. Inspection and palpation may show that the patient can't make a fist; her fin-

Locating the carpal tunnel

The carpal tunnel lies between the longitudinal tendons of the hand-flexing forearm muscles (not shown) and the transverse carpal ligament. Note the median nerve and flexor tendons passing through the tunnel on their way from the forearm to the hand.

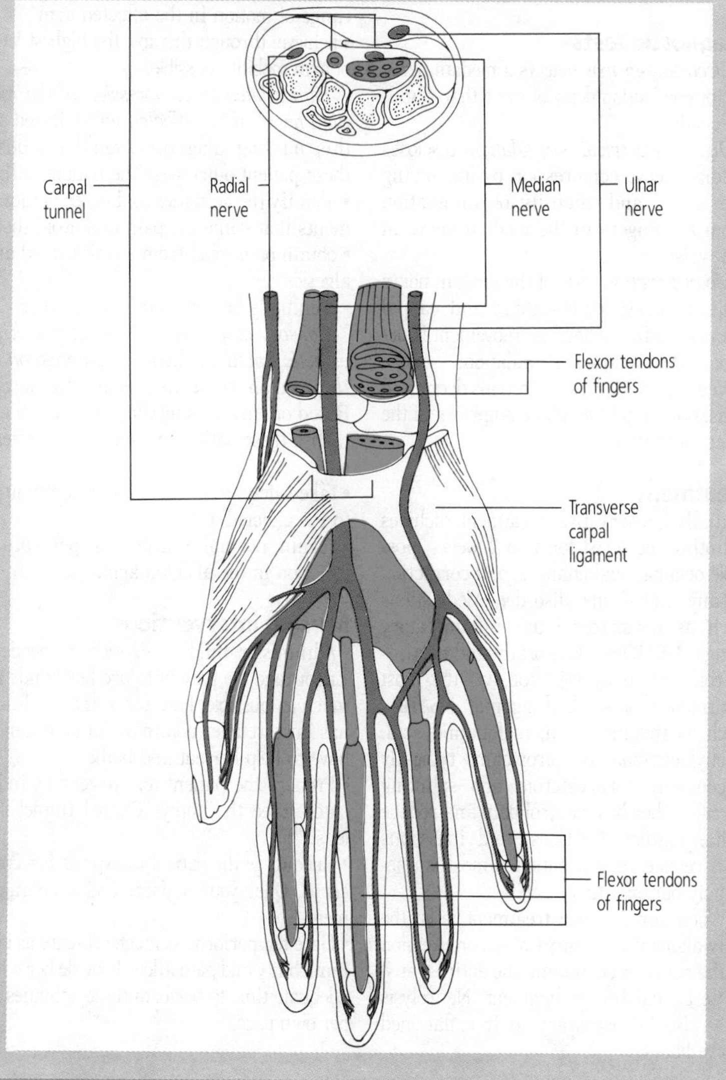

gernails may be atrophied, with surrounding dry, shiny skin. Light percussion of the transverse carpal ligament over the median nerve causes pain, burning, numbness, or tingling in the hand and fingers (Tinel's sign). Flexion of the wrist for about 30 seconds causes pain or numbness in the hand or fingers (Phalen's sign).

Diagnostic tests

- *Electromyography* detects a median nerve motor conduction delay of more than 5 milliseconds.
- *Digital electrical stimulation* discloses median nerve compression by measuring the length and intensity of stimulation from the fingers to the median nerve in the wrist.
- *Motor function tests* of the median nerve indicate nerve compression and carpal tunnel syndrome because movement is delayed after electrical stimulation.
- *Neuromuscular testing* reveals decreased sensation to light touch or pinpricks in the affected fingers.

Treatment

Initially conservative, treatment includes splinting the wrist for 1 to 2 weeks, possible occupational changes, and correction of any underlying disorder. Medications such as nonsteroidal anti-inflammatory drugs (NSAIDs) taken orally and corticosteroids given by injection are the most commonly prescribed agents. NSAIDs, such as indomethacin, mefenamic acid, phenylbutazone, or piroxicam, typically accompany corticosteroid and splinting therapy. They help control pain and reduce inflammation. Corticosteroid injections will reduce inflammation almost immediately but only temporarily.

When conservative treatment fails, the only alternative is surgical decompression of the nerve by sectioning the entire transverse carpal tunnel ligament. Neurolysis may also be necessary to free flattened nerve fibers.

Key nursing diagnoses and patient outcomes

Impaired physical mobility related to weakness or pain caused by entrapment of the median nerve in the wrist. Based on this nursing diagnosis, you'll establish these patient outcomes. The patient will:

- maintain normal muscle strength and range of motion in the affected arm
- achieve, through therapy, the highest level of arm mobility possible.

Pain related to compression of the median nerve in the affected wrist. Based on this nursing diagnosis, you'll establish these patient outcomes. The patient will:

- identify the activities and types of movements that stimulate pain and avoid them
- obtain pain relief from administered analgesics
- eventually become totally pain free.

Sensory or perceptual alterations (kinesthetic, tactile) related to compression of the median nerve in the affected wrist. Based on this nursing diagnosis, you'll establish these patient outcomes. The patient will:

- take safety precautions to prevent injury to the affected arm
- regain normal sensory or perceptual function in the affected arm.

Nursing interventions

- Administer mild analgesics as needed. Encourage the patient to use her hands as much as possible; however, if the condition has impaired her dominant hand, you may have to help her eat and bathe.
- Prepare the patient for surgery as indicated. (See the entry "Carpal tunnel release.")
- Encourage the patient to express her concerns. Offer your support and encouragement.
- Have her perform as much self-care as her immobility and pain allow. Provide her with adequate time to perform these activities at her own pace.

Monitoring

• Monitor the effectiveness of analgesics and other forms of therapy used to relieve the patient's discomfort.

• Regularly assess the patient's degree of physical immobility. Notify the patient's doctor if impairment worsens.

Patient teaching

• Teach the patient how to apply a splint. Advise her not to make it too tight. Show her how to remove the splint to perform gentle range-of-motion exercises (which should be done daily).

• Advise the patient who is about to be discharged to occasionally exercise her hands in warm water. If she's using a sling, tell her to remove it several times a day to exercise her elbow and shoulder.

• Suggest occupational counseling for the patient who has to change jobs because of carpal tunnel syndrome.

• Review the prescribed medication regimen. Emphasize that drug therapy may require 2 to 4 weeks before maximum effect is achieved. If the regimen includes indomethacin, mefenamic acid, phenylbutazone, or piroxicam, advise taking the drug with foods or antacids to avoid stomach upset. List possible adverse reactions. Tell the patient which adverse reactions require immediate medical attention.

• If the patient is pregnant, advise her to avoid NSAIDs because their effects on the fetus aren't known.

Cataract

A common cause of gradual vision loss, a cataract is an opacity of the lens or the lens capsule of the eye. Light shining through the cornea is blocked by the clouded lens. This, in turn, blurs the image cast onto the retina. As a result, the brain interprets a hazy image.

Cataracts commonly affect both eyes, but each cataract progresses independently. Exceptions are traumatic cataracts, which are usually unilateral, and congenital cataracts, which may remain stationary. Cataracts are most prevalent in persons over age 70. Surgery restores vision in about 95% of patients.

Causes

Cataracts are classified by their causes:

• *Senile cataracts* develop in elderly people, probably because of chemical changes in lens proteins.

• *Congenital cataracts* occur in neonates from inborn errors of metabolism or from maternal rubella infection during the first trimester of pregnancy. These cataracts may also result from a congenital anomaly or from genetic causes. Transmission is usually autosomal dominant; however, recessive cataracts may be sex linked.

• *Traumatic cataracts* develop after a foreign body injures the lens with sufficient force to allow aqueous or vitreous humor to enter the lens capsule.

• *Complicated cataracts* occur secondary to uveitis, glaucoma, retinitis pigmentosa, or retinal detachment. They can also occur with systemic disease, such as diabetes, hypoparathyroidism, or atopic dermatitis, or from ionizing radiation or infrared rays.

• *Toxic cataracts* result from drug or chemical toxicity with ergot, dinitrophenol, naphthalene, and phenothiazines.

Complications

Without surgery, a cataract eventually leads to complete vision loss.

Assessment

Typically, the patient complains of painless, gradual vision loss. He may also report a blinding glare from headlights when he drives at night, poor reading vision, and an annoying glare and poor vision in bright sunlight. If he has a central opacity, the patient may report seeing better in dim light than in bright light. That's because this cataract is nuclear, and as the pupil dilates, the patient can see around the opacity.

Inspection with a penlight may reveal a milky white pupil and, with an advanced cataract, a grayish white area behind the pupil.

Diagnostic tests

• *Indirect ophthalmoscopy* reveals a dark area in the normally homogeneous red reflex.
• *Slit-lamp examination* confirms the diagnosis of a lens opacity.
• *Visual acuity testing* confirms the degree of vision loss.

Treatment

Surgical lens extraction and implantation of an intraocular lens to correct the visual deficit is the treatment for a cataract. (See the entry "Cataract removal.")

Key nursing diagnoses and patient outcomes

Fear related to complete loss of vision caused by untreated cataracts. Based on this nursing diagnosis, you'll establish these patient outcomes. The patient will:
• identify and verbalize his fears
• request information about cataracts to diminish his fears
• state that his fears have been reduced.

Risk for injury related to decrease in vision caused by the cataract. Based on this nursing diagnosis, you'll establish these patient outcomes. The patient will:
• take precautions to protect himself from injury
• not sustain an injury.

Sensory or perceptual alterations (visual) related to diminishing ability to see properly as a result of the cataract. Based on this nursing diagnosis, you'll establish these patient outcomes. The patient will:
• discuss how his visual loss affects his life-style and institute measures to compensate
• resume a functional life-style
• regain lost vision.

Nursing interventions

• Prepare the patient, as appropriate, for cataract surgery.
• Provide a safe environment. For example, keep bed side rails raised and assist the patient with activities as needed.
• Allow the patient to express his fears and anxieties about his visual loss.

Monitoring

• Check the patient's vision regularly.

Patient teaching

• Explain how and why cataracts form.
• Stress the importance of regular ophthalmic examinations to monitor the degree of visual impairment and to determine when surgery can be performed. Encourage the patient to have the cataract removed.
• Caution the patient to take safety precautions until the cataract can be removed, including avoidance of night driving.

Cataract removal

Lens opacities, called cataracts, can be removed by one of two techniques. In the first technique, intracapsular cataract extraction (ICCE), the entire lens is removed, most commonly with a cryoprobe.

In the other technique, extracapsular cataract extraction (ECCE), the patient's anterior capsule, cortex, and nucleus are removed, leaving the posterior capsule intact. This technique may be carried out using manual extraction, irrigation and aspiration, or phacoemulsification. ECCE represents the primary treatment for congenital and traumatic cataracts. It's characteristically used to treat children and young adults because the posterior capsule adheres to the vitreous until about age 20. By leaving the posterior capsule undisturbed, ECCE avoids disruption and loss of vitreous.

Immediately after removal of the natural lens, many patients receive an intraocular lens implant. An implant is especially well suited for elderly patients who are unable to use eyeglasses or contact lenses (because of arthritis or tremors, for example).

Procedure

The patient may receive a local or general anesthetic.

For a review of cataract removal procedures, see *Comparing methods of cataract removal,* page 154. After cataract removal, the surgeon may insert a lens implant. After enlarging the incision, he'll implant the lens into the capsular sac. If he implants the lens without sutures, he'll administer miotic agents, such as pilocarpine, to prevent the iris from dilating too widely and causing the lens to slip.

In both ICCE and ECCE, the surgeon may also perform a peripheral iridectomy to reduce intraocular pressure and may briefly instill alpha-chymotrypsin, a proteolytic enzyme, in the anterior chamber to dissolve resistant zonular fibers. After the procedure, the surgeon may administer miotics to constrict the pupil. Then he'll close the sutures, instill antibiotic drops or ointment, and patch and shield the eye.

Complications

Cataract removal can cause numerous complications. Fortunately, most can be corrected. Complications include pupillary block, corneal decompensation, vitreous loss, hemorrhage, cystoid macular edema, lens dislocation, secondary membrane opacification, and retinal detachment.

Key nursing diagnoses and patient outcomes

Pain related to elevated intraocular pressure postoperatively. Based on this nursing diagnosis, you'll establish these patient outcomes. The patient will:

- exhibit an intraocular pressure within normal limits postoperatively
- remain free from severe pain.

Impaired home maintenance management related to visual disturbances following cataract removal. Based on this nursing diagnosis, you'll establish these patient outcomes. The patient will:

- be able to care for himself at home following cataract removal
- identify resources to help with self-care if necessary.

Sensory or perceptual alterations (visual) related to potential complications caused by cataract removal. Based on this nursing diagnosis, you'll establish these patient outcomes. The patient will:

- remain free from eye complications following cataract removal
- demonstrate improved or normal visual acuity postoperatively.

Nursing interventions

When caring for a patient undergoing a cataract removal, your main duties will involve instructing the patient and taking measures to prevent postoperative complications.

Before surgery

- Explain the planned surgical technique to the patient. Tell him that he'll receive mydriatics and cycloplegics to dilate the eye and facilitate cataract removal, that he'll receive osmotics and antibiotics to reduce the risk of infection, and that he may receive a sedative to help him relax.
- Inform the patient that after surgery he'll have to wear an eye patch temporarily to prevent traumatic injury and infection. Instruct him to call for help when getting out of bed, and tell him that he should sleep on the unaffected side to reduce ocular pressure. Explain to the patient that he'll temporarily experience loss of depth perception and decreased peripheral vision on the operative side.
- If ordered, perform an antiseptic facial scrub to reduce the risk of infection. Ensure that the patient has signed a consent form.

Comparing methods of cataract removal

Cataracts can be removed by intracapsular or extracapsular techniques.

Intracapsular cataract extraction

In this technique, the surgeon makes a partial incision at the superior limbus arc. He then removes the lens using specially designed forceps or a cryoprobe, which freezes and adheres to the lens to facilitate its removal.

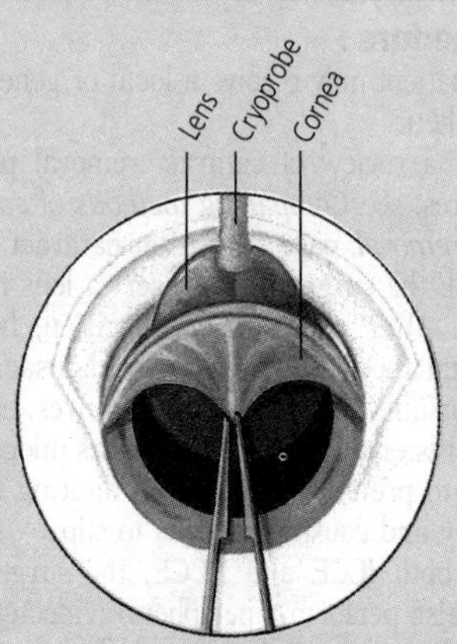

Extracapsular cataract extraction

In this technique, the surgeon may use irrigation and aspiration or phacoemulsification. In the former approach, the surgeon makes an incision at the limbus, opens the anterior lens capsule with a cystotome, and exerts pressure from below to express the lens. He then irrigates and suctions the remaining lens cortex.

In phacoemulsification, he uses an ultrasonic probe to break the lens into minute particles, which are aspirated by the probe.

Irrigation and aspiration

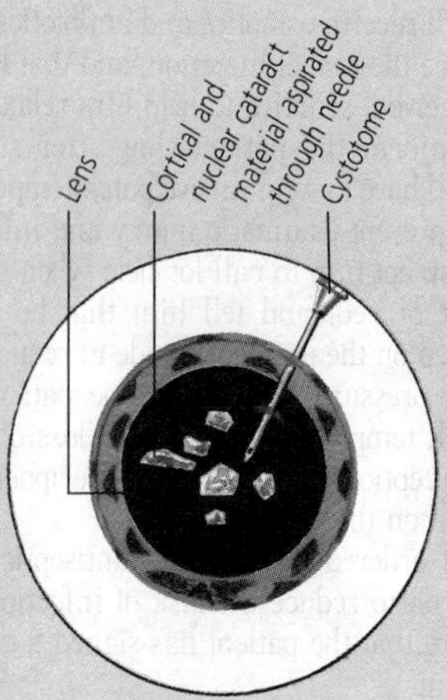

Phacoemulsification

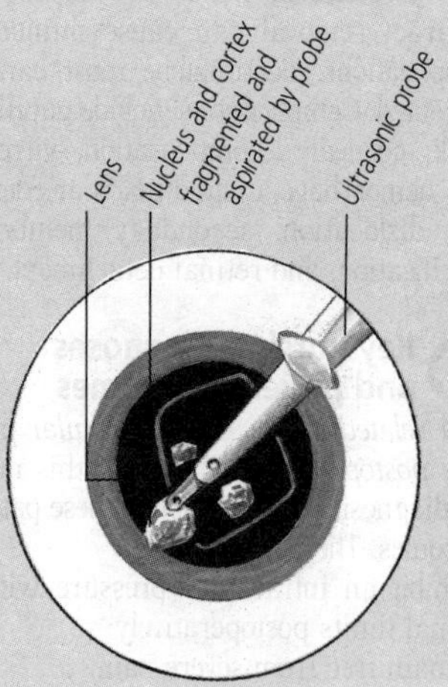

After surgery

- After the patient returns to his room, notify the doctor if severe pain, bleeding, increased drainage, or fever occurs. Also report any increased intraocular pressure.
- Because of the change in the patient's depth perception, keep the side rails of his bed raised, assist him with ambulation, and observe other safety precautions.
- Maintain the eye patch, and have the patient wear an eye shield, especially when sleeping. Tell him to continue wearing the shield during sleep for several weeks, as ordered.

Home care instructions

- Warn the patient to immediately contact the doctor if sudden eye pain, red or watery eyes, photophobia, or sudden visual changes occur.
- Instruct the patient to avoid activities that raise intraocular pressure, including heavy lifting, bending, straining during defecation, or vigorous coughing and sneezing. Tell him not to exercise strenuously for 6 to 10 weeks.
- Explain that follow-up appointments are necessary to monitor the results of the surgery and to detect any complications.
- Teach the patient or a family member how to instill eyedrops and ointments and how to change the eye patch.
- Suggest that the patient wear dark glasses to relieve the glare that he might experience.
- If the patient will be wearing eyeglasses, explain that changes in his vision can present safety hazards. To compensate for loss of depth perception, show him how to use up-and-down head movements to judge distances. To overcome the loss of peripheral vision on the operative side, teach him to turn his head fully in that direction to view objects to his side.
- If the patient will be wearing contact lenses, teach him how to insert, remove, and care for his lenses or have him arrange to visit a doctor routinely for removal, cleaning, and reinsertion of extended-wear lenses.

Cerebral aneurysm

This localized dilation of a cerebral artery results from a weakness in the arterial wall. Its most common form is the saccular (berry) aneurysm, a saclike outpouching in a cerebral artery. (See *Comparing aneurysm types,* page 156.) Cerebral aneurysms commonly rupture, causing subarachnoid hemorrhage. Sometimes bleeding also spills into the brain tissue and subsequently forms a clot. This may result in potentially fatal increased intracranial pressure (ICP) and brain tissue damage.

Most cerebral aneurysms occur at bifurcations of major arteries in the circle of Willis and its branches. An aneurysm can produce neurologic symptoms by exerting pressure on the surrounding structures, such as the cranial nerves.

Cerebral aneurysms are much more common in adults than in children. Incidence is slightly higher in women than in men, especially women in their late 40s or early to middle 50s, but cerebral aneurysm may occur at any age. In about 20% of patients, multiple aneurysms occur.

The prognosis is usually guarded but depends on the patient's age and neurologic condition, the presence of other diseases, and the extent and location of the aneurysm. About half the patients who suffer subarachnoid hemorrhages die immediately. With new and better treatment, the prognosis is improving.

Causes

Cerebral aneurysm results from a congenital defect of the vessel wall, head trauma, hypertensive vascular disease, advanced age, infection, or atherosclerosis, which can weaken the vessel wall.

Complications

Potentially fatal complications after rupture of an aneurysm include subarachnoid hemorrhage and brain tissue infarction.

Comparing aneurysm types

Review the following to familiarize yourself with the various types of aneurysms.

Saccular (berry) aneurysm
- Most common type
- Secondary to congenital weakness of media
- Usually occurs at major vessel bifurcations
- Occurs at the circle of Willis
- Has a neck or stem
- Has a sac that may be partly filled with a blood clot

Fusiform (spindle-shaped) aneurysm
- Occurs with atherosclerotic disease
- Characterized by irregular vessel dilation
- Develops on internal carotid or basilar arteries
- Rarely ruptures
- Produces brain and cranial nerve compression or CSF obstruction

Mycotic aneurysm
- Rare
- Associated with septic emboli that occur secondary to bacterial endocarditis
- Develops when emboli lodge in the arterial lumen, causing arteritis; the arterial wall weakens and dilates

Dissecting aneurysm
- Caused by arteriosclerosis, head injury, syphilis, or trauma during angiography
- Develops when blood is forced between layers of arterial walls, stripping intima from the underlying muscle layer

Traumatic aneurysm
- Develops in the carotid system
- Associated with fractures and intimal damage
- May thrombose spontaneously

Giant aneurysm
- Similiar to saccular, but larger—1⅛" (3 cm) or more in diameter
- Behaves like a space-occupying lesion, producing cerebral tissue compression and cranial nerve damage
- Associated with hypertension

Charcot-Bouchard aneurysm
- Microscopic
- Associated with hypertension
- Involves basal ganglia or brain stem

Cerebral vasospasm, probably the most common cause of death after rupture, occurs in about 40% of all patients after subarachnoid hemorrhage occurs.

Other possible complications of a cerebral aneurysm include rebleeding, which usually occurs within the first 24 to 48 hours after rupture, 7 to 10 days after the initial rupture, or anytime within the first 6 months; meningeal irritation from blood in the subarachnoid space; and hydrocephalus, which can occur weeks or even months after rupture if blood obstructs the fourth ventricle.

Assessment

Most cerebral aneurysms produce no symptoms until rupture occurs. A history may have to be obtained from a family member if the patient is unconscious or severely neurologically impaired.

Usually, the patient's history reveals the onset of an unusually severe headache that is accompanied by nausea, vomiting and, commonly, loss of consciousness. The patient or family member may report that rupture of the aneurysm was preceded by a period of activity, such as exercise, labor and delivery, or sexual intercourse. The patient also may have a history of hypertension, infection, or head injury.

Occasionally, rupture of a cerebral aneurysm occurs as a slow leak, causing premonitory symptoms that last for several days, such as headache, stiff back and legs, and intermittent nausea. (See *Early symptoms of cerebral aneurysm.*)

Other findings vary with the location of the aneurysm and the extent and severity of hemorrhage. Bleeding causes meningeal irritation, which can result in nuchal rigidity, back and leg pain, fever, restlessness, irritability, occasional seizures, and blurred vision. If the aneurysm is adjacent to the oculomotor nerve, ptosis and vision disturbances (diplopia and vision loss) may occur. If the bleeding extends into the brain tissue, hemiparesis, unilateral sensory deficits, dysphagia, visual defects, and altered consciousness may occur.

To describe the status of patients with ruptured cerebral aneurysm, the following grading system has been developed:

- *Grade I (minimal bleeding)*–patient is alert, with no neurologic deficit; he may have a slight headache and nuchal rigidity.
- *Grade II (mild bleeding)*–patient is alert with a mild to severe headache, nuchal rigidity and, possibly, third nerve palsy.
- *Grade III (moderate bleeding)*–patient is confused or drowsy, with nuchal rigidity and, possibly, a mild focal deficit.
- *Grade IV (severe bleeding)*–patient is stuporous, with nuchal rigidity and, possibly, mild to severe hemiparesis.
- *Grade V (moribund [often fatal])*–if nonfatal, patient is in deep coma or decerebrate.

Age greater than 70 or the presence of other systemic diseases increases the grade by one.

NURSING ALERT

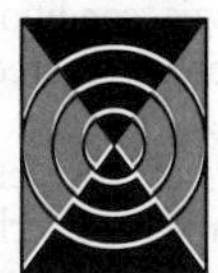

Early symptoms of cerebral aneurysm

Although cerebral aneurysms usually rupture without warning, they sometimes leak blood for up to several days, causing premonitory symptoms of impending rupture.

If your patient reports nuchal rigidity, stiff back and legs, and intermittent nausea, notify the doctor immediately. "Warning leaks" can occur a few hours to a few days before severe bleeding, which causes cerebral damage, coma, and death.

Diagnostic tests

The following tests help establish a diagnosis, which, unfortunately, usually follows aneurysmal rupture:

- *Angiography* confirms the location of a cerebral aneurysm.
- *Lumbar puncture* can detect blood in the cerebrospinal fluid (CSF), but this procedure is contraindicated if the patient shows signs of increased ICP.
- *EEG* commonly shows flattened or depressed T waves.
- *Computed tomography scan* locates the clot and identifies hydrocephalus, areas of infarction, and extent of blood spillage within the cisterns around the brain.
- *Magnetic resonance imaging* may help locate the aneurysm and the bleeding.

Treatment

Initial emergency treatment includes oxygenation and ventilation. To reduce the risk of rebleeding, the doctor may then attempt to repair the aneurysm. Usually, surgical repair is done by clipping, ligating, or wrapping the aneurysm neck with muscle. The timing of surgery is controversial; many patients with grade III or higher with anterior circulation aneurysms go to surgery within 1 to 3 days.

After surgical repair, the patient's condition depends on the extent of damage from the initial bleed and the degree of successful treatment of the resulting complications. Surgery can't improve the patient's neurologic condition unless it removes a hematoma or reduces the compression effect.

When surgical correction poses too much risk (in very elderly patients and those with heart, lung, or other serious diseases), when the aneurysm is in a particularly dangerous location, or when vasospasm necessitates a delay in surgery, the patient may receive conservative treatment. This includes:
• bed rest in a quiet, darkened room, with the head of the bed flat or raised less than 30 degrees; if immediate surgery isn't possible, such bed rest may continue for 4 to 6 weeks
• avoidance of caffeine, other stimulants, and aspirin
• codeine or another analgesic, as needed
• hydralazine or another antihypertensive agent, if the patient is hypertensive
• a vasoconstrictor to maintain blood pressure at the optimum level (20 to 40 mm Hg above normal), if necessary
• corticosteroids to reduce cerebral edema and meningeal irritation
• phenobarbital or another sedative to keep the patient relaxed.

Key nursing diagnoses and patient outcomes

Altered thought processes related to neurologic impairment caused by a ruptured cerebral aneurysm. Based on this nursing diagnosis, you'll establish these patient outcomes. The patient will:
• remain free from injury
• exhibit normal thought processes
• be oriented to time, person, and place.

Altered cerebral tissue perfusion related to inadequate oxygenation of cerebral tissue caused by bleeding from a ruptured cerebral aneurysm. Based on this nursing diagnosis, you'll establish these patient outcomes. The patient will:
• regain adequate cerebral tissue perfusion as exhibited by being oriented to time, person, and place
• demonstrate normal neurologic function.

Risk for injury related to increased ICP caused by a ruptured cerebral aneurysm. Based on this nursing diagnosis, you'll establish these patient outcomes. The patient will:
• have a normal ICP
• experience no signs of permanent neurologic injury, such as paralysis, speech impairment, or memory loss
• remain free from injury.

Nursing interventions

• Establish and maintain a patent airway as needed.
• Administer supplemental oxygen.
• Position the patient to promote pulmonary drainage and prevent upper airway obstruction.
• Following hospital policy, suction secretions from the airway as necessary to prevent hypoxia and vasodilation from carbon dioxide accumulation. Suction for fewer than 20 seconds to avoid increased ICP.
• Monitor pulse oximetry levels and arterial blood gas levels, as ordered. Use these levels as a guide to determine appropriate needs for supplemental oxygen.
• Prepare the patient for an emergency craniotomy, if indicated. (See the entry "Craniotomy.")
• If surgery can't be performed immediately, institute aneurysm precautions to minimize the risk of rebleeding and to avoid increasing the patient's ICP. Limit the patient's visitors, restrict his fluid intake, and tell the patient to avoid performing Valsalva's maneuver.
• Administer hydralazine or another antihypertensive agent, as ordered.
• Turn the patient often. Encourage deep breathing and leg movement. Assist with active range-of-motion exercises; if the patient is paralyzed, perform passive range-of-motion exercises.

• Apply elastic stockings or compression boots to the patient's legs to reduce the risk of deep vein thrombosis.
• Provide frequent nose and mouth care.
• Give fluids, as ordered, and monitor I.V. infusions to avoid overhydration, which may increase ICP.
• If the patient has facial weakness, assist him during meals; assess his gag reflex, and place the food in the unaffected side of his mouth.
• If the patient can't swallow, insert a nasogastric tube, as ordered, and give all tube feedings slowly.
• Institute measures to prevent skin breakdown; secure nasogastric tube by taping the tube so it doesn't press against the nostril.
• If the patient can eat, provide a high-bulk diet (bran, salads, and fruit) to prevent straining during defecation, which can increase ICP.
• Obtain an order for a stool softener, such as dioctyl sodium sulfosuccinate, or a mild laxative, and administer as ordered. Don't force fluids.
• Implement a bowel elimination program based on previous habits. If the patient is receiving steroids, check the stool for blood.
• If the patient has third or facial nerve palsy, administer artificial tears to the affected eye, and tape the eye shut at night to prevent corneal damage.
• Raise the bed's side rails to protect the patient from injury. If possible, avoid using restraints because these can cause agitation and raise ICP.
• Provide emotional support to the patient and his family. To minimize stress, encourage the patient to use relaxation techniques. Encourage him to express his concerns if he's able.

Monitoring
• Monitor the patient for signs of increasing ICP, such as restlessness, weakness, or a changed speech pattern.
• Watch for decreased level of consciousness (LOC), unilaterally enlarged pupil, onset or worsening of hemiparesis or motor deficit, increased blood pressure, decreased heart rate, worsened or sudden headache, renewed or persistent vomiting, and renewed or worsened nuchal rigidity. These signs and symptoms may be indicative of an enlarging aneurysm, rebleeding, an intracranial clot, vasospasm, or another complication; report them immediately.
• Carefully monitor the patient's blood pressure. Report any significant changes, particularly a rise in systolic pressure.
• Frequently check the patient's arterial blood gas values, intake and output, and vital signs.
• Avoid taking the patient's temperature rectally because this could stimulate the vagus nerve and lead to cardiac arrest.

Patient teaching
• Teach the patient, if possible, and his family about his condition. Encourage family members to adopt a realistic attitude, but don't discourage hope. Answer questions honestly.
• Explain all tests, neurologic examinations, treatments, and procedures to the patient even if he's unconscious.
• Warn the patient who will be treated conservatively to avoid all unnecessary physical activity.
• If surgery will be performed, provide preoperative teaching if the patient's condition permits. Be sure the patient, if possible, and the family understand the surgery and its possible complications. Reinforce the doctor's explanations as necessary.
• Before discharge, make a referral to a home health care nurse or a rehabilitation center when necessary.
• Teach family members to recognize and immediately report signs of rebleeding, such as headache, nausea, vomiting, and changes in LOC.

Cerebrovascular accident

Also known as stroke, cerebrovascular accident (CVA) is a sudden impairment of cerebral circulation in one or more of the blood vessels supplying the brain. CVA interrupts or diminishes oxygen supply and commonly causes serious damage or necrosis in brain tissues. The sooner circulation returns to normal after CVA, the better the chances for complete recovery. However, about half of those who survive CVA remain permanently disabled and experience a recurrence within weeks, months, or years.

CVA is the third most common cause of death in the United States today and the most common cause of neurologic disability. It strikes 500,000 persons each year; half of them die as a result. Although it mostly affects older adults, it can strike people of any age and occurs most commonly in men, especially blacks.

CVAs are classified according to their course of progression. The least severe is the transient ischemic attack (TIA), which results from a temporary interruption of blood flow, most often in the carotid and vertebrobasilar arteries. A progressive stroke, or stroke-in-evolution (thrombus-in-evolution), begins with slight neurologic deficit and worsens in a day or two. In a completed stroke, neurologic deficits are maximal at onset.

Causes

Major causes of CVA include cerebral thrombosis, embolism, and hemorrhage.

Thrombosis is the most common cause of CVA in middle-aged and elderly people. CVA results from obstruction of a blood vessel. Typically, the main site of the obstruction is the extracerebral vessels, but sometimes it's intracerebral.

Embolism, the second most common cause of CVA, can occur at any age, especially among patients with a history of rheumatic heart disease, endocarditis, posttraumatic valvular disease, myocardial fibrillation and other cardiac arrhythmias, or after open-heart surgery. It usually develops rapidly – in 10 to 20 seconds – and without warning. Most often the left middle cerebral artery is the embolus site.

Hemorrhage, the third most common cause of CVA, may also occur suddenly at any age. Such hemorrhage results from chronic hypertension or aneurysms, which cause sudden rupture of a cerebral artery.

Factors that increase the risk of CVA include a history of TIAs, atherosclerosis, hypertension, arrhythmias, electrocardiogram changes, rheumatic heart disease, diabetes mellitus, gout, postural hypotension, cardiac enlargement, high serum triglyceride levels, lack of exercise, use of oral contraceptives, smoking, and a family history of cerebrovascular disease.

Complications

Among the many possible complications of CVA are unstable blood pressure from loss of vasomotor control; fluid imbalances; malnutrition; sensory impairment, including vision problems; and infection, such as encephalitis, brain abscess, and pneumonia. Altered level of consciousness (LOC), aspiration, contractures, and pulmonary emboli also may occur.

Assessment

Clinical features of CVA vary with the artery affected (and, consequently, the portion of the brain it supplies), the severity of the damage, and the extent of collateral circulation that develops to help the brain compensate for decreased blood supply.

When assessing a patient who may have experienced a CVA, remember this: If the CVA occurs in the left hemisphere, it produces signs and symptoms on the right side; if it occurs in the right hemisphere, signs and symptoms appear on the left side. However, a CVA that causes cranial nerve damage produces signs of cranial nerve dysfunction on the same side as the hemorrhage or infarct.

The patient's history, obtained from a family member or friend if necessary, may uncover one or more risk factors for CVA. The history may also reveal either a sudden onset of hemiparesis or hemiplegia or a gradual onset of dizziness, mental disturbances, or seizures. The patient or a family member may also report that the patient lost consciousness or suddenly developed aphasia. Speaking with the patient during history taking may reveal communication problems, such as dysarthria, dysphasia or aphasia, and apraxia.

Neurologic examination identifies most of the physical findings associated with CVA. These may include unconsciousness or changes in LOC, such as a decreased attention span, difficulties with comprehension, forgetfulness, and a lack of motivation. If conscious, the patient may exhibit anxiety along with communication and mobility difficulties. Inspection may reveal related urinary incontinence.

Motor function and muscle strength tests often show a loss of voluntary muscle control and hemiparesis or hemiplegia on one side of the body. In the initial phase, flaccid paralysis with decreased deep tendon reflexes may occur. These reflexes return to normal after the initial phase, along with an increase in muscle tone and, in some cases, muscle spasticity on the affected side.

Vision testing often reveals hemianopia on the affected side of the body and, in patients with left-sided hemiplegia, problems with visual-spatial relations.

Sensory assessment may reveal sensory losses, ranging from slight impairment of touch to the inability to perceive the position and motion of body parts. The patient also may have difficulty interpreting visual, tactile, and auditory stimuli. (See *Reviewing neurologic deficits in CVA,* page 162.)

Diagnostic tests

- *Cerebral angiography* details disruption or displacement of the cerebral circulation by occlusion or hemorrhage. It's the test of choice for examination of the entire cerebral artery.
- *Digital subtraction angiography* evaluates the patency of the cerebral vessels and identifies their position in the head and neck. It also detects and evaluates lesions and vascular abnormalities.
- *Computed tomography (CT) scan* detects structural abnormalities, edema, and lesions, such as nonhemorrhagic infarction and aneurysms. Thus, it differentiates CVA from imitative disorders, such as primary metastatic tumor and subdural, intracerebral, or epidural hematoma. Patients who experience a TIA usually have a CT scan done within 72 hours of the onset of symptoms.
- *Positron emission tomography* provides data on cerebral metabolism and cerebral blood flow changes, especially in ischemic stroke.
- *Single-photon emission tomography* identifies cerebral blood flow and helps diagnose cerebral infarction.
- *Magnetic resonance imaging (MRI)* allows evaluation of the lesion's location and size without exposing the patient to radiation. MRI doesn't distinguish hemorrhage, tumor, and infarction as well as CT scanning does, but it is superior in imaging the cerebellum and the brain stem.
- *Transcranial Doppler studies* examine the size of intracranial vessels using blood flow velocity.
- *Cerebral blood flow studies* measure blood flow to the brain and help detect abnormalities.
- *Ophthalmoscopy* may show signs of hypertension and atherosclerotic changes in retinal arteries.
- *EEG* may detect reduced electrical activity in an area of cortical infarction. This test proves especially useful when CT scan results are inconclusive. It can also differentiate seizure activity from CVA.
- *Neuropsychological tests* evaluate simple to complex mental and verbal abilities and may include a personality inventory.

Reviewing neurologic deficits in CVA

CVA can leave one patient with mild hand weakness and another with complete unilateral paralysis. In both patients, the functional loss reflects damage to the brain area normally perfused by the occluded or ruptured artery. But the damage doesn't stop there. The resulting hypoxia and ischemia produce edema that affects distal parts of the brain, causing further neurologic deficits.

Most CVAs occur in the anterior cerebral circulation and cause symptoms related to damage in the middle cerebral artery, internal carotid artery, or anterior cerebral artery. CVAs can also occur in the posterior circulation. These originate in the vertebral arteries and result in signs and symptoms caused by damage to the vertebral or basilar artery and posterior cerebral artery, resulting in higher mortality. Described below are the signs and symptoms that accompany CVA at the following sites.

Middle cerebral artery

The patient may experience aphasia, dysphasia, reading difficulty (dyslexia), writing inability (dysgraphia), visual field cuts, and hemiparesis on the affected side (more severe in the face and arm than in the leg).

Internal carotid artery

The patient may complain of headaches. Expect to find weakness, paralysis, numbness, sensory changes, and visual disturbances such as blurring on the affected side. You may also detect altered LOC, bruits over the carotid artery, aphasia, dysphasia, and ptosis.

Anterior cerebral artery

You may note confusion, weakness, and numbness (especially of the arm) on the affected side; paralysis of the contralateral foot and leg with accompanying footdrop; incontinence; loss of coordination; impaired motor and sensory functions; and personality changes (flat affect, distractibility).

Vertebral or basilar artery

The patient may complain of numbness around the lips and mouth and dizziness. You may note weakness on the affected side; visual deficits, such as color blindness, lack of depth perception, and diplopia; poor coordination; dysphagia; slurred speech; amnesia; and ataxia.

Posterior cerebral artery

The patient may experience visual field cuts, sensory impairment, dyslexia, coma, and cortical blindness from ischemia in the occipital area. Usually, paralysis is absent.

Appropriate baseline laboratory studies include urinalysis, coagulation studies, complete blood count, serum osmolality, and tests for electrolyte, glucose, triglyceride, creatinine, and blood urea nitrogen levels.

Treatment

Medical management of CVA commonly includes physical rehabilitation, dietary and drug regimens to help decrease risk factors, possibly surgery, and care measures to help the patient adapt to specific deficits, such as speech impairment and paralysis.

Depending on the CVA's cause and extent, the patient may undergo a craniotomy to remove a hematoma, endarterectomy to remove atherosclerotic plaques from the inner arterial wall, or extracranial-intracranial bypass to circumvent an artery that's blocked by occlusion or stenosis. Ventricular shunts may be necessary to drain cerebrospinal fluid.

Medications useful in CVA include:
• anticonvulsants, such as phenytoin or phenobarbital, to treat or prevent seizures
• stool softeners, such as dioctyl sodium sulfosuccinate, to avoid straining
• corticosteroids, such as dexamethasone, to minimize associated cerebral edema
• analgesics, such as codeine, to relieve headache that may follow hemorrhagic CVA; usually, aspirin is contraindicated in hemorrhagic CVA because it increases bleeding tendencies, but it may be useful in preventing TIAs
• anticoagulants, such as heparin, coumadin, or aspirin, if the CVA is related to thrombus or embolus.

Key nursing diagnoses and patient outcomes

Impaired home maintenance management related to permanent neurologic deficits caused by CVA. Based on this nursing diagnosis, you'll establish these patient outcomes. The patient will:
• identify changes needed to promote maximum health and safety at home
• seek help from resources and support systems to achieve adequate home maintenance
• remain living successfully at home.

Impaired verbal communication related to neurologic damage to speech center in brain caused by CVA. Based on this nursing diagnosis, you'll establish these patient outcomes. The patient will:
• use adaptive equipment or speech therapy to improve his ability to communicate
• communicate his needs, thoughts, and feelings without frustration.

Self-esteem disturbance related to sudden devastating change in body function caused by CVA. Based on this nursing diagnosis, you'll establish these patient outcomes. The patient will:
• verbalize his feelings about his self-esteem
• engage in activities that help him achieve higher physical and emotional wellness
• express a positive self-image.

Nursing interventions

• During the acute phase, maintain a patent airway and oxygenation. Loosen constricting clothes. Watch for ballooning of the cheek on the affected side with respiration. If the patient is unconscious, position him on his side to allow secretions to drain and prevent aspiration; if necessary, suction the secretions. Insert an artificial airway, and start mechanical ventilation or supplemental oxygen if necessary.
• Maintain fluid and electrolyte balance. If the patient can take liquids orally, offer them as often as fluid limitations permit. Administer I.V. fluids, as ordered; never give too much too fast because this can increase ICP.
• Offer the urinal or bedpan every 2 hours. If the patient is incontinent, he may need an indwelling urinary catheter, but this should be avoided if possible because of the risk of infection.
• Ensure adequate nutrition. Check for gag reflex before offering small oral feedings of semisolid foods. Place the food tray within the patient's visual field. Have the patient sit upright and tilt his head slightly forward when eating. If the patient has dysphagia or one-sided facial weakness, give him semisoft foods and tell him to chew on the unaffected side of his mouth. If oral feedings aren't possible, insert a nasogastric tube for tube feedings, as ordered.
• Manage GI problems. Prevent the patient from straining during defecation because this increases ICP. Modify the patient's diet; administer stool softeners, as ordered; and give laxatives, if necessary. If the patient vomits (usually during the first few days), keep him positioned on his side to prevent aspiration.

• Provide careful mouth care. Clean and irrigate the patient's mouth to remove food particles. Care for his dentures as needed.
• Provide meticulous eye care. Remove secretions with a cotton ball and 0.9% sodium chloride solution. Instill eyedrops, as ordered. Patch the patient's affected eye if he can't close his eyelid.
• Position the patient, and align his extremities correctly. Use high-topped sneakers to prevent footdrop and contracture and a convoluted foam, flotation, or pulsating mattress to prevent pressure ulcers. To decrease the possibility of pneumonia, turn the patient at least every 2 hours. Elevate the affected hand to control dependent edema, and place it in a functional position.
• Assist the patient with exercise. Perform range-of-motion (ROM) exercises for both the affected and unaffected sides. Teach and encourage the patient to use his unaffected side to exercise his affected side.
• Give medications, as ordered, and watch for and report adverse reactions.
• Establish and maintain communication with the patient. If he's aphasic, set up a simple method of communicating basic needs. Then remember to phrase your questions so he'll be able to answer using this system. Repeat yourself quietly and calmly (remember, he isn't deaf) and use gestures if necessary to help him understand. Even the unresponsive patient can hear, so don't say anything in his presence you wouldn't want him to hear and remember.
• Provide psychological support, and establish rapport with the patient. Set realistic short-term goals. Spend time with him, involve his family in his care when possible, and explain his deficits and strengths. Remember that building rapport may be difficult because of the mood changes that may result from brain damage or as a reaction to being dependent.
• Protect the patient from injury. For example, keep the bed's side rails up at all times; pad the rails if the patient tends to bang them with his feet or arms.
• Prepare patient for surgery, if indicated. (See the entry "Craniotomy.")

Monitoring

• During the acute phase, monitor blood pressure, LOC, pupillary changes, motor function (voluntary and involuntary movements), sensory function, speech, skin color, temperature, signs of increased ICP, and nuchal rigidity or flaccidity. Remember, if CVA is impending, blood pressure rises suddenly, pulse rate is rapid and bounding, and the patient may complain of headache. Record observations, and report any significant changes to the doctor.
• Monitor the patient's respiratory status closely for evidence of respiratory depression, aspiration, or infection. Also watch for signs of pulmonary emboli, such as chest pains, shortness of breath, dusky color, tachycardia, fever, and changed sensorium. If the patient is unresponsive, monitor his arterial blood gas levels often and alert the doctor to increased partial pressure of carbon dioxide or decreased partial pressure of oxygen.
• Monitor the patient's fluid and electrolyte status as well as nutritional intake for evidence of dehydration, electrolyte imbalance, or malnutrition.
• Assess the patient regularly for evidence of complications such as skin breakdown, contractures, or infection.
• Monitor the patient's progress in his rehabilitation program, if appropriate.

Patient teaching

• Teach the patient and his family about the disorder. Explain the diagnostic tests, treatments, and rehabilitation the patient will undergo.
• If surgery is scheduled, provide preoperative teaching. Be sure the patient and family understand the surgery and its possible effects.
• If necessary, teach the patient to comb his hair, dress, and wash. With the aid of

a physical and an occupational therapist, obtain appliances, such as hand bars by the toilet and ramps, as needed. If speech therapy is indicated, encourage the patient to begin as soon as possible. To reinforce teaching, involve the patient's family in all aspects of rehabilitation. With their cooperation and support, devise a realistic discharge plan, and let them help decide when the patient can return home.

• Explain the need to follow the ordered exercise program. Then teach the patient how to perform ROM exercises for the arm or leg affected by the CVA or teach a family member how to perform passive ROM exercises. Reinforce the importance of wearing slings, splints, or other ordered devices to prevent complications.

• If a special diet, such as a weight-reduction diet for an obese patient, is prescribed, have the dietitian teach the patient about the diet. Reinforce the dietitian's explanation as necessary.

• Explain the need to report any signs of an impending CVA, such as severe headache, drowsiness, confusion, extremity weakness, and dizziness. Emphasize the importance of regular follow-up visits.

• Teach the patient and, if necessary, a family member about the schedule, dosage, actions, and adverse effects of prescribed medications including antiplatelet drugs, such as aspirin and dipyridamole, and vasodilators, such as isoxsuprine. Make sure the patient taking aspirin realizes that he cannot substitute acetaminophen for aspirin.

• Teach the patient and his family about the need for safety measures. For example, recommend installing grab bars near the toilet and bathtub, removing throw rugs, and securing carpets to the floor.

• To decrease the possibility of another CVA, teach the patient and family about the need to correct risk factors. For example, if the patient smokes, refer him to a stop-smoking program. Teach the patient about the importance of maintaining an ideal weight and the need to control diseases such as diabetes or hypertension. Advise all patients (especially those at high risk) about the importance of following a low-cholesterol, low-salt diet; increasing activity; avoiding prolonged bed rest; and minimizing stress.

• Encourage the patient and family to contact a local support group and to obtain additional information from the National Institute of Neurological and Communicative Disorders and Stroke. Refer the patient to local home health care agencies as necessary.

Cervical cancer

The third most common cancer of the female reproductive system, cervical cancer is classified as either preinvasive or invasive.

Preinvasive cancer ranges from minimal cervical dysplasia, in which the lower third of the epithelium contains abnormal cells, to carcinoma in situ, in which the full thickness of epithelium contains abnormally proliferating cells (also known as cervical intraepithelial neoplasia). Preinvasive cancer is curable in 75% to 90% of patients with early detection and proper treatment. If untreated, it may progress to invasive cervical cancer, depending on the form.

In invasive disease, cancer cells penetrate the basement membrane and can spread directly to contiguous pelvic structures or disseminate to distant sites via lymphatic routes. Invasive cancer of the uterine cervix accounts for 4,900 deaths annually in the United States. In 95% of cases, the histologic type is squamous cell carcinoma, which varies from well-differentiated cells to highly anaplastic spindle cells. Only 5% of cases are adenocarcinomas. Invasive cancer typically occurs between ages 30 and 50; rarely, under age 20. Women age 65 or older account for 24% of new cases and 40% of deaths.

Causes

Although the cause is unknown, several predisposing factors have been associated with cervical cancer: frequent intercourse at a young age (under 16), multiple sexual partners, multiple pregnancies, and human papillomavirus (HPV), or other bacterial or viral venereal infections.

Other risk factors include low socioeconomic status, smoking, exposure to diethylstilbestrol, vitamin A and C deficiency and, possibly, use of oral contraceptives.

Complications

Disease progression can cause flank pain from sciatic nerve or pelvic wall invasion and hematuria and renal failure associated with bladder involvement.

Assessment

Preinvasive cancer produces no symptoms or other clinical changes. In early invasive cervical cancer, the patient's history will include abnormal vaginal bleeding, such as a persistent vaginal discharge that may be yellowish, blood-tinged, and foul-smelling; postcoital pain and bleeding; and bleeding between menstrual periods or unusually heavy menstrual periods. The patient's history may suggest one or more of the predisposing factors for this disease.

If the cancer has advanced into the pelvic wall, the patient may report gradually increasing flank pain, which can indicate sciatic nerve involvement. Leakage of urine may point to metastasis into the bladder with formation of a fistula. Leakage of feces may indicate metastasis to the rectum with fistula development.

Inspection may disclose vaginal discharge or leakage of urine or feces.

Diagnostic tests

- *Papanicolaou (Pap) test* identifies abnormal cells, and *colposcopy* determines the source of the abnormal cells seen on the Pap test.
- *Cone biopsy* is performed if endocervical curettage is positive.

Additional studies, such as lymphangiography, cystography, and major organ and bone scans, can detect metastasis. (See *Staging cervical cancer.*)

Treatment

Accurate clinical staging will determine the type of treatment. Preinvasive lesions may be treated with total excisional biopsy, loop electrosurgical excision procedure, cryosurgery, laser destruction, conization (followed by frequent Pap test follow-ups) or, rarely, hysterectomy. Therapy for invasive squamous cell carcinoma may include radical hysterectomy and radiation therapy (internal, external, or both). Rarely, pelvic exenteration may be performed for recurrent cervical cancer.

Key nursing diagnoses and patient outcomes

Fear related to potential for cervical cancer to become invasive. Based on this nursing diagnosis, you'll establish these patient outcomes. The patient will:
- identify and verbalize her fears
- use at least one fear-reducing coping mechanism daily, such as asking questions about treatment progress.
- state that her fears have diminished; she will also not experience any physical signs or symptoms of fear.

Impaired tissue integrity related to changes in cervical tissue caused by cervical cancer. Based on this nursing diagnosis, you'll establish these patient outcomes. The patient will:
- understand the treatment regimen and verbalize the need for adequate fluid and nutritional intake to promote tissue healing
- experience a cessation of vaginal discharge
- exhibit, upon physical examination, healing cervical tissue.

Pain related to invasive cervical cancer. Based on this nursing diagnosis, you'll establish these patient outcomes. The patient will:

Staging cervical cancer

Treatment decisions depend on accurate staging. The International Federation of Gynecology and Obstetrics defines cervical cancer stages as follows:

Stage 0
Carcinoma in situ, intraepithelial carcinoma

Stage I
Cancer confined to the cervix (extension to the corpus should be disregarded)

Stage IA
Preclinical malignant lesions of the cervix (diagnosed only microscopically)

Stage IA1
Minimal microscopically evident stromal invasion

Stage IA2
Lesions detected microscopically, measuring 5 mm or less from the base of the epithelium, either surface or glandular, from which it originates; lesion width shouldn't exceed 7 mm

Stage IB
Lesions measuring more than 5 mm deep and 7 mm wide, whether seen clinically or not (preformed space involvement shouldn't alter the staging but should be recorded for future treatment decisions)

Stage II
Extension beyond the cervix but not to the pelvic wall; the cancer involves the vagina but hasn't spread to the lower third

Stage IIA
No obvious parametrial involvement

Stage IIB
Obvious parametrial involvement

Stage III
Extension to the pelvic wall; on rectal examination, no cancer-free space exists between the tumor and the pelvic wall; the tumor involves the lower third of the vagina; this includes all cases with hydronephrosis or nonfunctioning kidney

Stage IIIA
No extension to the pelvic wall

Stage IIIB
Extension to the pelvic wall and hydronephrosis, nonfunctioning kidney, or both

Stage IV
Extension beyond the true pelvis or involvement of the bladder or the rectal mucosa

Stage IVA
Spread to adjacent organs

Stage IVB
Spread to distant organs

• obtain pain relief through administered analgesics
• become free from pain through therapy.

Nursing interventions

• Listen to the patient's fears and concerns, and offer reassurance when appropriate. Encourage her to use relaxation techniques to promote comfort during the diagnostic procedures.
• If you assist with a biopsy, drape and prepare the patient as for a routine Pap test and pelvic examination. Have a container of formaldehyde ready to preserve

the specimen during transfer to the pathology laboratory. Assist the doctor as needed, and provide support for the patient throughout the procedure.

- If you assist with laser therapy, drape and prepare the patient as for a routine Pap test and pelvic examination. Assist the doctor as necessary, and provide support for the patient throughout the procedure.
- Prepare the patient for surgery, if indicated. (See the entries "Cryosurgery" or "Hysterectomy," as appropriate.)
- Prepare the patient for internal radiation therapy, if indicated. (See the entry "Radiation, internal.")
- Institute measures to prevent or alleviate complications, as indicated.

Monitoring

- Monitor the patient's response to therapy through frequent Pap tests and cone biopsies, as ordered.
- Watch for complications related to therapy by listening to and observing the patient, monitoring laboratory studies, and obtaining frequent vital signs.

Patient teaching

- Explain to the patient who's having a biopsy performed that she may feel pressure, minor abdominal cramps, or a pinch from the punch forceps. Reassure her that the pain will be minimal because the cervix has few nerve endings.
- Explain any surgical or therapeutic procedure to the patient, including what to expect both before and after the procedure.
- After excisional biopsy or laser therapy, tell the patient to expect a discharge or spotting for about 1 week. Advise her not to douche, use tampons, or engage in sexual intercourse during this time. Caution her to report signs of infection. Stress the need for a follow-up Pap test and a pelvic examination in 3 to 4 months and periodically thereafter.
- Review the possible complications of the type of therapy ordered. Remind the patient to watch for and report uncomfortable adverse reactions.
- Reassure the patient that this disease and its treatment shouldn't radically alter her life-style or prohibit sexual intimacy.
- Explain the importance of complying with follow-up visits to the gynecologist and oncologist. Stress the value of follow-up visits in detecting disease progression or recurrence.

Chancroid

A sexually transmitted disease, chancroid (or soft chancre) is characterized by painful genital ulcers and inguinal adenitis.

Chancroid occurs worldwide but is particularly common in tropical countries. The infection is on the rise in the United States and is associated with increased risk for human immunodeficiency virus (HIV) infection. It affects males more often than females.

The incubation period varies but typically ranges from 5 to 7 days. Chancroidal lesions may heal spontaneously and usually respond well to treatment when no secondary infections are present.

Causes

Chancroid results from *Haemophilus ducreyi,* a short, nonmotile, gram-negative bacillus. Poor personal hygiene may predispose men – especially those who are uncircumcised – to this disease.

Complications

Phimosis and urethral fistulas may occur in men.

Assessment

The patient may report unprotected sexual contact with an infected person or with unknown or multiple partners. He may complain of pain associated with ulcers and lymphadenopathy. He also may experience headaches and malaise (in 50% of patients).

An inspection of the genital area initially reveals single or multiple papules surrounded by erythema. These rapidly become pustular and then ulcerate. The ulcers are nonindurated with ragged edges, have a base of granulation tissue, and bleed easily. They range from 1 to 2 mm in diameter.

You may observe the ulcers on the prepuce, frenulum, coronal sulcus, shaft, or glans penis in a male patient. In a female patient, you may note ulcers on the labia, fourchette, vestibule, clitoris, cervix, or anus, although many women are asymptomatic. Rarely, you'll observe lesions on the tongue, lip, or breast.

When you inspect the inguinal area within 2 to 3 weeks of onset, you're likely to observe unilateral lymphadenopathy with overlying erythema. If the patient hasn't received treatment, you may observe suppuration with bubo formation. Rupture of the abscess may follow.

On palpation, you may note tender, fluctuant inguinal nodes.

Diagnostic tests

Blood agar cultures provide a reliable diagnosis 75% of the time. Gram stains of ulcer exudate or bubo aspirate are 50% reliable. Biopsy confirms the diagnosis but is used only in resistant cases or when cancer is suspected.

Dark-field examination and serologic testing rule out other sexually transmitted diseases (genital herpes, syphilis, lymphogranuloma venereum) that cause similar ulcers.

Treatment

The first choice for treatment is 500 mg of oral erythromycin four times a day for 7 days or 250 mg of ceftriaxone given I.M. in a single dose.

Alternatively, the patient can receive 500 mg of oral ciprofloxacin twice a day for 3 days. In areas where resistance to trimethoprim is uncommon, the patient can receive co-trimoxazole (160 mg trimethoprim and 800 mg sulfamethoxazole) twice a day for 7 days.

Aspiration of fluid-filled nodes and careful personal hygiene help prevent the infection from spreading.

Key nursing diagnoses and patient outcomes

Altered sexuality patterns related to need for abstinence during therapy. Based on this nursing diagnosis, you'll establish these patient outcomes. The patient will:
- express an understanding of the need to refrain from sexual intercourse during therapy
- not resume usual patterns of sexual intercourse until healing has occurred; at that time, he'll take measures to prevent reinfection, such as using a condom during sexual intercourse.

Impaired skin integrity related to genital or inguinal ulcers caused by chancroid. Based on this nursing diagnosis, you'll establish these patient outcomes. The patient will:
- verbalize how and why the ulcers occurred
- adhere to the treatment regimen and demonstrate his ability to perform routine skin care
- experience a resolution of the infection, as exhibited by healed ulcers and the return of normal skin integrity.

Pain related to ulcers caused by chancroid. Based on this nursing diagnosis, you'll establish these patient outcomes. The patient will:
- obtain pain relief from administered analgesics
- become free from pain through therapy.

Nursing interventions

- Use standard precautions whenever you may come into contact with genital secretions – for instance, when collecting specimens and performing a physical examination.

- Administer anti-infective medications and, possibly, analgesics, as ordered. Make sure the patient isn't allergic to the medication before giving the first dose.
- Provide topical care by washing the affected area with soap and water, followed by a bactericidal agent. Don't allow the area to remain moist; this can enhance the growth of the organism.
- Report all cases of chancroid to the local board of health if required in your state.
- Examine the patient's sexual contacts, and refer them for treatment, even if they're asymptomatic.

Monitoring

- Monitor the effectiveness of analgesic administration by asking patient to rate his pain before and after receiving the drug.
- Inspect the ulcers for signs of healing as well as signs of localized infection (such as drainage or increased redness, swelling, or discomfort).

Patient teaching

- Instruct the patient to take his anti-infective medication for the period prescribed.
- Teach the patient not to apply creams, lotions, or oils on or near his genitalia or on other lesion sites. Doing so may enhance the spread of the disease.
- Advise the patient to abstain from sexual contact until follow-up evaluation shows that healing is complete (usually about 2 weeks after treatment begins).
- Instruct the patient to wash his genitalia three times daily with soap and water. If he's uncircumcised, tell him to retract the foreskin to thoroughly clean the glans penis.
- Counsel the patient about HIV infection. Also, recommend HIV testing because of the heightened risk chancroid causes.
- Inform the patient that condoms may provide protection from future infection.

Chemotherapy

Chemotherapy is the use of one or more drugs to destroy cancer cells or suppress their growth. A single drug typically gives a limited response, but if two or more drugs are used, long remissions or cures may occur. Unfortunately, remissions and cures aren't always possible. That's because many cancers become resistant to chemotherapeutic drugs. Also, the toxic effects of some drugs may prevent dosages high enough to effectively destroy the cancer cells. (See *How chemotherapeutic drugs disrupt the cell cycle.*)

Because many types of cancer exist, various types and combinations of chemotherapeutic drugs must be used. Classified according to mechanism of action, these drugs include alkylating agents, antimetabolites, antibiotic antineoplastic agents, and hormonal antineoplastic agents.

Alkylating agents can inhibit cell division at any point in the cell cycle, but they're particularly effective in the late G_1 and S phases. Examples of alkylating agents include busulfan, carmustine (BCNU), cisplatin, ifosfamide, and mechlorethamine. Given alone or with other drugs, they help treat chronic and acute leukemias, non-Hodgkin's lymphomas, multiple myeloma, melanoma, sarcoma, and cancers of the breast, ovaries, uterus, lung, brain, testes, bladder, prostate, and stomach.

Antimetabolites structurally resemble natural metabolites. As a result, they can become involved in processes associated with the natural metabolites – that is, the synthesis of nucleic acids and proteins. However, the antimetabolites differ sufficiently from the natural metabolites to interfere with this synthesis. Because the antimetabolites are cell-cycle specific and primarily affect cells that actively synthesize deoxyribonucleic acid (DNA), they are referred to as S-phase specific. Examples of antimetabolites include mercaptopurine and thioguanine, which inhibit purine

How chemotherapeutic drugs disrupt the cell cycle

Chemotherapeutic drugs may be either cell-cycle specific or cell-cycle nonspecific. Cell-cycle-specific drugs, such as methotrexate, act at one or more cell-cycle phases. Cell-cycle-nonspecific drugs, such as busulfan, can act on both replicating and resting cells.

Note: The drugs listed in this diagram are only examples of cell-cycle-specific agents.

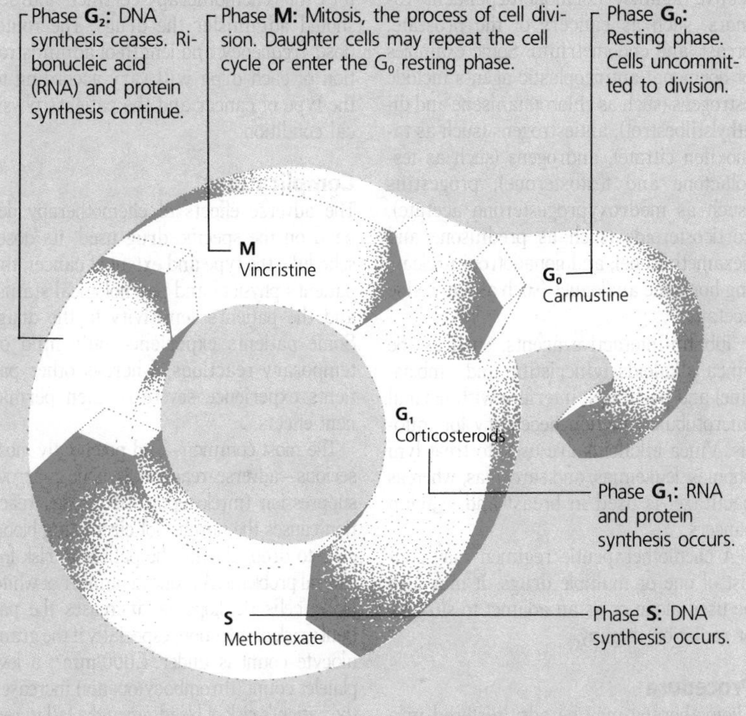

synthesis; cytarabine, floxuridine, and fluorouracil, which inhibit pyrimidine synthesis; and methotrexate, which prevents reduction of folic acid to dihydrofolate reductase. Cancers that respond to the action of antimetabolites include acute leukemia, breast cancer, adenocarcinomas of the GI tract, non-Hodgkin's lymphomas, and squamous cell carcinomas of the head, neck, and cervix.

Antibiotic antineoplastic agents achieve their effects by binding with DNA. These drugs inhibit the cellular processes of normal and malignant cells and are cell-cycle nonspecific, except for bleomycin, which causes its major effects in the G_2 phase of the cell cycle. Examples of antibiotic antineoplastics include bleomycin, dactinomycin, doxorubicin, and mitomycin, which are used mainly to treat carcinomas, sarcomas, and lymphomas; daunorubicin, which is used in acute nonlymphoblastic leukemia; and mitoxantrone, which is used to treat acute nonlymphocytic leukemia and breast cancer.

Hormonal antineoplastic agents inhibit cancer growth in specific tissues without directly causing toxicity. Although the mechanisms of action are not completely understood, hormonal therapies prove effective against hormone-dependent tumors, such as cancers of the prostate, breast, and endometrium. Some examples of hormonal antineoplastic agents include estrogens (such as chlorotrianisene and diethylstilbestrol), antiestrogens (such as tamoxifen citrate), androgens (such as testolactone and testosterone), progestins (such as medroxyprogesterone acetate), corticosteroids (such as prednisone and dexamethasone), and gonadotropin-releasing hormone analogues (such as leuprolide acetate).

Tubulin-interactive agents, such as the vinca alkaloids (vincristine and vinblastine) and paclitaxel, interfere with normal microtubule function necessary for mitosis. Vinca alkaloids are used to treat lym phomas, leukemias, and sarcomas, whereas paclitaxel is used in breast and ovarian cancers.

A chemotherapeutic regimen may consist of one or multiple drugs. It may also be used alone or as an adjunct to surgery or radiation therapy.

Procedure

Chemotherapy may be administered in a hospital, ambulatory care setting, or in the patient's home. The drugs are typically given intermittently to allow healthy tissues time to recover and to minimize adverse reactions. Chemotherapy may be given by any one of a number of routes, including I.M., I.V., S.C., intra-arterially, orally, topically, intracavitarily, intravesically, and intrathecally.

Of these routes, the I.V. route is the most common for administering chemotherapeutic drugs because whether given through a peripheral or central line, it delivers the drug directly to the body's tissues. On occasion, a patient may require continuous chemotherapy, in which case an ambulatory infusion pump may be used.

Only trained personnel, using a laminar airflow hood, should reconstitute chemotherapeutic drugs. Furthermore, only doctors or chemotherapy-certified nurses should administer the drugs. The route, dose, frequency, and length of administration of each drug will vary according to the type of cancer and the patient's physical condition.

Complications

The adverse effects of chemotherapy depend on the specific drug used, its dose, schedule, the type and extent of cancer, the patient's physical and psychological status, and the patient's sensitivity to the drug. Some patients experience only mild or temporary reactions, whereas other patients experience severe or even permanent effects.

The most common—and potentially most serious—adverse reaction is bone marrow suppression (myelosuppression). This reaction causes the number of circulating blood cells to drop, placing the patient at risk for several problems. A reduced number of white blood cells (leukopenia) increases the patient's risk of infection, especially if the granulocyte count is under 1,000/mm^3; a low platelet count (thrombocytopenia) increases the patient's risk of bleeding; and a fall in red blood cells can lead to anemia.

Other common adverse reactions include nausea and vomiting (which can lead to fluid and electrolyte imbalances), stomatitis, and alopecia. Also, because some chemotherapeutic agents are vesicants, significant tissue damage may occur if the drug leaks outside the vein.

Some patients may also experience psychological complications, such as depression and altered body image, resulting both from the disease process and the treatment regimen.

Key nursing diagnoses and patient outcomes

Altered nutrition: Less than body requirements related to adverse GI reactions caused by chemotherapy. Based on this nursing diagnosis, you'll establish these patient outcomes. The patient will:
- regain lost weight and maintain weight within a normal range
- obtain relief from adverse GI reactions through the administration of antiemetics and topical oral anesthetics; this will allow the patient to consume a well-balanced, high-protein diet and to drink at least 2 liters of fluid daily
- remain free from protein calorie malnutrition.

Fatigue related to adverse reactions caused by chemotherapy. Based on this nursing diagnosis, you'll establish these patient outcomes. The patient will:
- pace activities to avoid exacerbating fatigue
- obtain adequate sleep
- perform low-intensity exercise when energy level is good, and rest or nap when energy level is low
- maintain adequate nutrition and hydration.

Risk for infection related to myelosuppression caused by chemotherapy. Based on this nursing diagnosis, you'll establish these patient outcomes. The patient will:
- verbalize an understanding of precautions used to prevent or minimize infection and then demonstrate those precautions
- not develop an infection
- regain a normal white blood cell count after chemotherapy is completed.

Nursing interventions

When caring for a patient receiving chemotherapy, your responsibilities range from instructing and supporting the patient to observing for adverse reactions that may occur.

Before therapy

- Determine the educational needs of the patient and family, and provide patient teaching as indicated. Answer all questions, and provide explanations if the patient appears confused about his disease process or treatment regimen.
- Teach the patient the potential adverse effects of chemotherapy, and explain the interventions that can be used to treat those effects.
- Provide emotional support to the patient and his family.
- Ensure that the patient has signed an informed consent document.
- Gather the patient's past medical and drug history, and perform a complete physical assessment. Pay attention to the patient's laboratory test results (particularly the complete blood count), nutritional status, rehabilitation needs, and self-care ability.
- Develop a plan of care for managing the patient's symptoms, identifying both long-term and short-term needs.
- Instruct the patient to tell his doctor or nurse immediately if he experiences any adverse reactions during therapy, such as burning or irritation at the treatment site, nausea, or vomiting. (See *Managing common adverse effects of chemotherapy,* pages 174 and 175.)
- Examine the patient's veins, starting with the hands and proceeding to the forearm, to identify a viable route of drug administration. If you'll be administering a vesicant agent, avoid sites in the wrist or dorsum of the hand.
- Don't use an existing I.V. line to administer chemotherapy. Instead, perform a new venipuncture proximal to the old site. Then test vein patency by infusing 10 to 20 ml of 0.9% sodium chloride solution. Never test vein patency by infusing the chemotherapeutic drug.
- Administer any premedications, such as antiemetics, as ordered to minimize adverse effects.

(Text continues on page 176.)

Managing common adverse effects of chemotherapy

Adverse effect	Nursing actions	Home care instructions
Bone marrow depression (leukopenia, thrombocytopenia, anemia)	• Establish baseline white blood cell (WBC) and platelet counts, hemoglobin levels, and hematocrit before therapy begins. Monitor studies during therapy. • If WBC count drops suddenly or falls below 2,000/mm³, stop the drug and notify the doctor. Initiate reverse isolation if absolute granulocyte count falls below 1,000/mm³. Report a platelet count below 100,000/mm³. If necessary, assist with transfusion. • Monitor temperature orally every 4 hours, and regularly inspect the skin and body orifices for signs of infection. Observe for petechiae, easy bruising, and bleeding. Check for hematuria, and monitor the patient's blood pressure. Be alert for signs of anemia. • Limit S.C. and I.M. injections. If these are necessary, apply pressure for 3 to 5 minutes after injection to prevent leakage or hematoma. Report unusual bleeding after injection. • Take precautions to prevent bleeding. Use extra care with razors, nail trimmers, dental floss, toothbrushes, and other sharp or abrasive objects. • Give vitamin and iron supplements, as ordered. Provide a diet high in iron.	• Instruct the patient to immediately report fever, chills, sore throat, lethargy, unusual fatigue, or pallor. • Warn him to avoid exposure to persons with infections during chemotherapy and for several months after it. • Explain that the patient and his family shouldn't receive immunizations during or shortly after chemotherapy since an exaggerated reaction may occur. • Tell the patient to avoid activities that could cause traumatic injury and bleeding. Advise him to report any episodes of bleeding or bruising to the doctor. • Tell him to eat high-iron foods, such as liver and spinach. • Stress the importance of follow-up blood studies after completion of treatment.
Anorexia	• Assess the patient's nutritional status before and during chemotherapy. Weigh him weekly or as ordered. • Explain the need for adequate nutrition despite the loss of appetite.	• Encourage the patient's family to supply favorite foods to help him maintain adequate nutrition. • Suggest that the patient eat small, frequent meals.
Nausea and vomiting	• Before chemotherapy begins, administer antiemetics, as ordered, to reduce the severity of these reactions. • Monitor and record the frequency, character, and amount of vomitus. • Monitor serum electrolyte levels, and provide total parenteral nutrition if necessary.	• Teach the patient and his family how to insert antiemetic suppositories. • Tell the patient to take the drug on an empty stomach, with meals, or at bedtime. GI upset indicates that the drug is working. Instruct him to report any vomiting to the doctor. • Tell him to follow a high-protein diet.

Managing common adverse effects of chemotherapy *(continued)*

Adverse effect	Nursing actions	Home care instructions
Diarrhea and abdominal cramps	• Assess the frequency, color, consistency, and amount of diarrhea. Give antidiarrheals, as ordered. • Assess the severity of cramps, and observe for signs of dehydration and acidosis, which may indicate electrolyte imbalance. • Encourage fluids and, if ordered, give I.V. fluids and potassium supplements. • Provide good skin care, especially to the perianal area.	• Teach the patient how to use antidiarrheals, and instruct him to report diarrhea to the doctor. • Encourage him to maintain adequate fluid intake and to follow a bland, low-fiber diet. • Explain that good perianal hygiene can help prevent skin breakdown and infection.
Stomatitis	• Before drug administration, observe for dry mouth, erythema, and white patchy areas on the oral mucosa. Be alert for bleeding gums or complaints of a burning sensation when drinking acidic liquids. • Emphasize the principles of good mouth care with the patient and his family. • Provide mouth care every 4 to 6 hours with 0.9% sodium chloride solution or half-strength hydrogen peroxide. Coat the oral mucosa with milk of magnesia. Avoid lemon-glycerin swabs because they tend to reduce saliva and change mouth pH. • To make eating more comfortable, apply a topical viscous anesthetic, such as lidocaine, before meals. Administer special mouthwashes, as ordered. • Consult the dietitian to provide bland foods at medium temperatures. • Treat cracked or burning lips with petroleum jelly.	• Teach the patient good mouth care. Instruct him to rinse his mouth with 1 tsp of salt dissolved in 8 oz (236 ml) of warm water or hydrogen peroxide diluted to half strength with water. • Advise him to avoid acidic, spicy, or extremely hot or cold foods. • Instruct the patient to report stomatitis to the doctor, who may order a change in medication.
Alopecia	• Reassure the patient that alopecia is usually temporary. • Inform him that he may experience discomfort before hair loss starts.	• Suggest to the patient that he have his hair cut short to make thinning hair less noticeable. • Advise washing his hair with a mild shampoo and avoiding frequent brushing or combing. • Suggest wearing a hat, scarf, toupee, or wig.

During therapy

- Provide a relaxed environment.
- To protect your skin from contact with the chemotherapeutic drug, wear latex gloves, a nonpermeable gown, and protective eyewear whenever preparing or administering chemotherapeutic agents.
- Nonvesicant agents are typically administered by I.V. push or admixed in a bag of I.V. fluid. Vesicant agents are given I.V. push through the side port of a rapidly infusing I.V. line.
- Monitor the patient closely for signs of a hypersensitivity reaction or extravasation. Check the I.V. catheter for a blood return after injecting each 5 ml of medication or according to your hospital's policy. Keep emergency medications on hand to treat hypersensitivity reactions or extravasations.
- If you suspect an extravasation, stop the infusion immediately. Leave the needle in place, and notify the patient's doctor. Be familiar with your hospital's policy for treating drug extravasations.
- Infuse 20 ml of 0.9% sodium chloride solution between each chemotherapeutic medication and before discontinuing the I.V. line.

After therapy

- Dispose of used needles and syringes carefully. Leave the needles intact and place them in a leakproof, puncture-resistant container for incineration. Dispose of I.V. bags, bottles, gloves, and tubing in a covered trash container. Remove all chemotherapy trash for incineration.
- Wash your hands thoroughly after giving any chemotherapeutic drug, even though you've used gloves.
- Observe the patient for adverse reactions and be prepared to provide appropriate nursing care.
- For 48 hours after drug administration, wear latex gloves when handling items contaminated with the patient's excreta.

Home care instructions

- Teach the patient and his family how to manage the adverse effects of chemotherapy at home.
- Inform the patient and family that the blood count nadir will usually occur 12 to 24 days after the last dose of chemotherapy. Caution them that myelosuppression will be the most severe at this time and that they'll need to take precautions against bleeding and infection. Tell the patient to notify his doctor at once if he develops unusual bleeding or any signs or symptoms of infection.
- Make sure the patient has correct phone numbers for his doctor, his nurse, or other resource personnel so that he can report adverse reactions promptly.
- Make appointments for follow-up laboratory studies and doctor visits, as indicated.
- Help the patient plan for his home needs. Evaluate whether the patient's home environment is safe and whether he'll have any rehabilitation needs. Refer the patient to a home health care agency if indicated.
- Provide the patient and his family with a list of local resources, such as the American Cancer Society.

Chest drainage

Insertion of a tube into the pleural space helps treat pneumothorax, hemothorax, empyema, pleural effusion, or chylothorax. It is also routinely inserted at the completion of a thoracotomy. The tube allows drainage of blood, fluid, pus, or air from the pleural space. In pneumothorax, it restores negative pressure to the pleural space by means of an underwater-seal drainage system. The water in the system prevents air from being sucked back into the pleural space during inspiration. (If the leak is through the bronchi and cannot be sealed, suction applied to the underwater-seal system removes air from the pleural space faster than it can collect.) As negative pleural pressure is restored, the lung can reinflate.

Procedure

Position the patient on his unaffected side. After the doctor injects the local anesthetic at the insertion site, help the patient hold still while the doctor makes a small incision and tunnels the tube through the tissue into the pleural space. Usually, the doctor places the tube anteriorly near the second or third intercostal space if he wants to remove air; laterally and slightly posteriorly at about the eighth intercostal space if he wants to remove fluid. He may place tubes at both locations if he wishes to remove both air and fluid.

As soon as the doctor inserts the tube into the pleural space, connect the external end of the tube to the underwater-seal drainage system. The doctor stabilizes the proximal end by suturing the tube into place. Apply petroleum gauze and a dry sterile dressing. As ordered, tape the tube to the patient's chest wall distal to the insertion site to help prevent accidental dislodgment. Tape all tube connections and regulate suction, as ordered.

Complications

Complications include lung puncture, bleeding, or additional hemothorax at the insertion site. Chest tube obstruction or blockage of the air vent in the underwater-seal drainage system may cause tension pneumothorax, a life-threatening complication. (See *Combating tension pneumothorax,* page 178.)

Key nursing diagnoses and patient outcomes

Ineffective breathing pattern related to thoracic pain and decreased lung expansion. Based on this nursing diagnosis, you'll establish these patient outcomes. The patient will:
- exhibit increased lung expansion
- display easy, unlabored respirations at a rate of 12 to 28 breaths/minute.

Impaired physical mobility related to thoracic pain and discomfort. Based on this nursing diagnosis, you'll establish these patient outcomes. The patient will:
- maintain full range of motion in his affected arm and shoulder
- resume physical mobility after analgesic administration.

Fear related to pain and chest tube procedure. Based on this nursing diagnosis, you'll establish these patient outcomes. The patient will:
- express his fears and concerns
- verbalize an understanding of why the chest tube is necessary
- demonstrate no physical signs of fear related to the chest tube and chest drainage.

Nursing interventions

When caring for a patient with chest tubes, much of your care will center on monitoring for, and preventing, complications.

Before the procedure

- If time permits, explain the procedure to the patient. Tell him the chest tube will help him breathe more easily. Take his vital signs to serve as a baseline and be sure that a signed consent form is obtained. Then administer a sedative, as ordered.
- Collect necessary equipment, including a thoracotomy tray and an underwater-seal drainage system. Prepare lidocaine for local anesthesia, as directed. While the doctor cleans the insertion site with povidone-iodine solution, set up the underwater-seal drainage system according to the manufacturer's instructions and place it at bedside, below the patient's chest level. Stabilize the unit to avoid knocking it over.

After the procedure

- Once the patient's chest tube is stabilized, have him take several deep breaths to inflate his lungs fully and to help push pleural air out through the tube. Take his vital signs immediately after tube insertion and then every 15 minutes or as or-

LIFE-THREATENING COMPLICATIONS

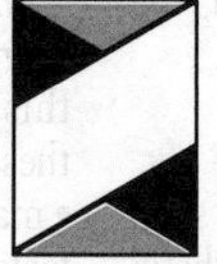

Combating tension pneumothorax

Tension pneumothorax is a life-threatening complication that may be fatal if not treated promptly. Air becomes entrapped within the pleural space, which can result from either dislodgment or obstruction of the chest tube. Either way, increasing positive pressure within the patient's chest cavity compresses the affected lung and the mediastinum, shifting them toward the opposite lung. The result is markedly impaired venous return and cardiac output, leading to cardiac arrest.

Recognizing the signs and symptoms

Suspect tension pneumothorax if the patient develops these signs and symptoms: cyanosis, air hunger, agitation, hypotension, tachycardia, and profuse diaphoresis.

As part of your assessment, palpate the patient's face, neck, and chest wall for subcutaneous emphysema. Also check to see if the patient's trachea has deviated from its normal midline position; this is a telltale sign of tension pneumothorax. Auscultate his lungs for decreased or absent breath sounds on the affected side, and percuss the chest for hyperresonance.

Emergency interventions

If you suspect a tension penumothorax, take these steps:

- Notify the patient's doctor immediately.
- Be prepared to assist with reinsertion of the chest tube or insertion of a large-bore needle to relieve air pressure in the thorax.
- Inspect the chest drainage unit for kinks in the tubing. Correct any mechanical problems immediately.
- Expect to administer a high concentration of oxygen to treat hypoxia.
- Continue to monitor vital signs and vital functions.

dered until the patient's condition is stabilized.

- Change the dressing over the chest tube site daily. At the same time, clean the site and remove any drainage.
- Prepare the patient for a chest X-ray to verify tube placement and to assess the outcome of treatment. As ordered, arrange for daily X-rays to monitor his progress.
- Palpate the patient's chest above the tube for subcutaneous emphysema, and notify the doctor of any increase.
- Routinely assess the function of the patient's chest tube. Describe and record the amount of drainage on the intake and output sheet. Once most of the air has been removed, the drainage system should bubble only during forced expiration unless the patient has a bronchopleural fistula. However, constant bubbling in the system when suction is attached may indicate a loose connection or that the tube has advanced slightly out of the patient's chest. Promptly correct any loose connections to prevent complications.
- If the chest tube becomes dislodged, cover the opening immediately with petroleum gauze and apply pressure to prevent negative inspiratory pressure from sucking air into the patient's chest. Call the doctor, and have an assistant obtain the equipment necessary for tube reinsertion while you continue to keep the opening closed. Reassure the patient and monitor him closely for signs of tension pneumothorax.

• The doctor will remove the patient's chest tube when the lung has fully reexpanded. As soon as the tube is removed, apply an airtight, sterile petroleum dressing.

Home care instructions

• Typically, the patient will be discharged with a chest tube only if it's being used to drain a loculated empyema, since this doesn't require an underwater-seal drainage system. Teach this patient how to care for his tube, dispose of drainage and soiled dressings properly, and perform wound care and dressing changes.

• Teach the patient with a recently removed chest tube how to clean the wound site and change dressings. Tell him to report any signs of infection.

Chlamydial infections

Urethritis in men, cervicitis in women, and – much less commonly in the United States – lymphogranuloma venereum in both sexes all result from chlamydial infections. And all are linked to one organism: *Chlamydia trachomatis.* These infections are the most common sexually transmitted diseases in the United States, afflicting an estimated 4 million Americans each year.

Children born of infected mothers may contract associated otitis media, pneumonia, and trachoma inclusion conjunctivitis during passage through the birth canal. Although trachoma inclusion conjunctivitis seldom occurs in the United States, it's a leading cause of blindness in Third World countries.

Causes

Transmission of *C. trachomatis,* an intracellular obligate bacterium, primarily follows vaginal or rectal intercourse or oral-genital contact with an infected person. Because signs and symptoms of chlamydial infections commonly appear late in the course of the disease, sexual transmission of the organism usually occurs unknowingly.

Complications

Left untreated, chlamydial infections can lead to acute epididymitis, salpingitis, pelvic inflammatory disease (PID) and, eventually, sterility. In pregnant women, chlamydial infections are associated with spontaneous abortion, premature rupture of membranes, premature delivery, and neonatal death, although a direct link with *C. trachomatis* hasn't been established.

Complications of lymphogranuloma venereum include urethral and rectal strictures, perirectal abscesses, and rectovesical-rectovaginal and ischiorectal fistulas. Elephantiasis with enlargement of the penis or vulva occasionally occurs.

Assessment

The patient may have a history of unprotected sexual contact with an infected person, an unknown partner, or multiple sex partners. He also may have another sexually transmitted disease or have had one in the past.

Symptoms vary with the specific type of chlamydial infection; many patients have no symptoms. If the patient has cervicitis, she may complain of pelvic pain and dyspareunia. If PID develops, she may report severe abdominal pain, nausea, vomiting, fever, chills, breakthrough bleeding, and bleeding after intercourse. A woman with urethral syndrome may experience dysuria and urinary frequency.

A male patient with urethritis may complain of dysuria, urinary frequency, and pruritus. If epididymitis develops, he may complain of severe scrotal pain. Prostatitis may cause lower back pain, urinary frequency, dysuria, nocturia, and painful ejaculation.

If the infection involves the rectum, the patient may complain of diarrhea, tenesmus, and pruritus.

A patient with lymphogranuloma venereum may have such systemic signs and symptoms as myalgia, headache, weight loss, backache, fever, and chills.

Inspection by speculum of the patient with cervicitis may reveal cervical erosion and mucopurulent discharge. Inspection of a male patient with urethritis may disclose urethral discharge, which may be copious and purulent, and meatal erythema. If he develops epididymitis, you'll note scrotal swelling and urethral discharge.

In a patient with proctitis, you may note mucopurulent discharge and diffuse or discrete ulceration in the rectosigmoid colon. Inspection of a patient with lymphogranuloma venereum may reveal a primary lesion – a painless vesicle or nonindurated ulcer. Such an ulcer usually is 2 to 3 mm in diameter and occurs on the glans or shaft of the penis; on the labia, vagina, or cervix; or in the rectum. It commonly goes unnoticed.

If a female patient with cervicitis develops PID, palpation reveals tenderness over the lower quadrant, abdominal distention and, sometimes, rigidity.

Palpation of a patient with lymphogranuloma venereum may reveal enlarged inguinal lymph nodes, especially in a male patient. These nodes may become fluctuant, tender masses. Regional nodes draining the initial lesion may enlarge and appear as a series of bilateral buboes. Untreated buboes may rupture and form sinus tracts that discharge a thick, yellow, granular secretion. The patient eventually may develop a scar or an indurated inguinal mass.

Diagnostic tests

Laboratory tests provide definitive diagnosis of chlamydial infection. A swab culture from the infection site (urethra, cervix, or rectum) usually establishes urethritis, cervicitis, salpingitis, endometritis, and proctitis. Culture of aspirated blood, pus, or cerebrospinal fluid establishes epididymitis, prostatitis, and lymphogranuloma venereum.

If the infection site is accessible, the doctor may first attempt direct visualization of cell scrapings or exudate with Giemsa stain or fluorescein-conjugated monoclonal antibodies. However, tissue cell cultures are more sensitive and specific.

Serologic studies to determine previous exposure to *C. trachomatis* include complement fixation tests and immunofluorescence microscopy. The enzyme-linked immunosorbent assay detects the *C. trachomatis* antibody as effectively as the immunofluorescence microscopy test and is useful as a screening test.

Treatment

The recommended first-line treatment for chlamydial infection may consist of either 100 mg of doxycycline four times a day for 7 to 21 days or 500 mg of erythromycin four times a day for 7 days. Alternatively, the patient can receive 300 mg of ofloxacin every 12 hours for 7 days.

A patient with lymphogranuloma venereum needs extended treatment. A pregnant woman with a chlamydial infection should receive erythromycin stearate.

Key nursing diagnoses and patient outcomes

Altered urinary elimination related to urethritis caused by a chlamydial infection. Based on this nursing diagnosis, you'll establish these patient outcomes. The patient will:

- not develop any complications associated with urethritis
- reestablish a normal urinary elimination pattern.

Knowledge deficit related to transmission of chlamydial infections. Based on this nursing diagnosis, you'll establish these patient outcomes. The patient will:

- express an interest in learning about chlamydial infections
- request information about chlamydial infections

• verbalize an understanding of chlamydial infections, their treatment, and measures to take to prevent reinfection.

Pain related to infectious process caused by chlamydial infection. Based on this nursing diagnosis, you'll establish these patient outcomes. The patient will:
• experience relief from pain following administration of analgesics
• become pain free with treatment.

Nursing interventions
• Use standard precautions when examining the patient, giving patient care, and handling contaminated material. Double-bag all soiled dressings and contaminated instruments.
• Examine and test the patient's sexual contacts for chlamydial infection.
• Check the newborn infant of an infected mother for signs of infection. Take specimens for culture from the infant's eyes, nasopharynx, and rectum. Positive rectal cultures will peak by 5 to 6 weeks postpartum.
• If required in your state, report all cases of chlamydial infection to local public health authorities for follow-up on sexual contacts. (The doctor or laboratory personnel may have done this already.)

Monitoring
• Monitor the patient for complications.
• Monitor the patient's compliance with treatment, and evaluate the effectiveness of treatment.

Patient teaching
• Teach the patient the dosage requirements of his prescribed medication. Stress the importance of taking all of his medication, even after symptoms subside.
• Teach the patient to follow proper hygiene measures.
• To prevent eye contamination, tell the patient to avoid touching any discharge and to wash his hands before touching his eyes.
• To prevent reinfection during treatment, recommend that the patient either abstain from intercourse or use condoms.
• Urge the patient to inform sexual partners of his infection so that they can seek treatment also. Explain that they should receive treatment regardless of their test results.
• Suggest that the patient and his sexual partners receive testing for the human immunodeficiency virus.
• Tell the patient to return for follow-up testing.

Chloride imbalance

Hypochloremia and hyperchloremia are chloride imbalances. A deficient serum level of the anion chloride results in hypochloremia; an excessive serum chloride level causes hyperchloremia. A predominantly extracellular anion, chloride accounts for two-thirds of all serum anions.

Secreted by the stomach mucosa as hydrochloric acid, chloride provides an acid medium conducive to digestion and activation of enzymes. It also participates in maintaining acid-base and body water balances, influences the osmolality or tonicity of extracellular fluid (ECF), plays a role in oxygen and carbon dioxide exchange in red blood cells, and helps activate salivary amylase (which, in turn, activates the digestive process).

Causes
Hypochloremia may result from:
• decreased chloride intake or absorption, as in low dietary sodium intake, sodium deficiency, potassium deficiency, or metabolic alkalosis; prolonged use of mercurial diuretics; or administration of I.V. dextrose without electrolytes
• excessive chloride loss, resulting from prolonged diarrhea or diaphoresis; or loss of hydrochloric acid in gastric secretions

CHECKLIST

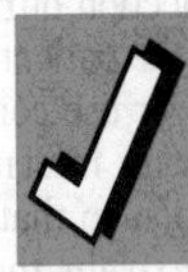

Identifying chloride imbalance

Serum chloride values are key to discerning a chloride imbalance. Use the following guidelines to determine whether your patient has a chloride imbalance:

- Hypochloremia: confirmed by a serum chloride level under 95 mEq/liter. Supportive values with metabolic alkalosis include a serum pH over 7.45 and serum carbon dioxide levels greater than 32 mEq/liter.
- Hyperchloremia: confirmed by a serum chloride level greater than 106 mEq/liter. With metabolic acidosis, serum pH is under 7.35 and serum carbon dioxide levels are less than 22 mEq/liter.

due to vomiting, gastric suctioning, or gastric surgery.

Hyperchloremia may result from:

- excessive chloride intake or absorption – as in hyperingestion of ammonium chloride or ureterointestinal anastomosis – allowing reabsorption of chloride by the bowel
- hemoconcentration, caused by dehydration
- compensatory mechanisms for other metabolic abnormalities, as in metabolic acidosis, brain stem injury causing neurogenic hyperventilation, and hyperparathyroidism.

Complications

Hypochloremia may result in depressed respirations, leading to respiratory arrest. Hyperchloremia may cause coma.

Assessment

The patient's history may reveal risk factors for hypochloremia or hyperchloremia.

When hypochloremia is associated with hyponatremia, physical assessment may detect characteristic muscle weakness and twitching because renal chloride loss always accompanies sodium loss and sodium reabsorption is not possible without chloride.

However, if chloride depletion results from metabolic alkalosis secondary to loss of gastric secretions, chloride is lost independently of sodium. Inspection may note tetany and shallow, depressed breathing. Neuromuscular assessment may find muscle hypertonicity.

Because of the natural affinity of sodium and chloride ions, hyperchloremia usually produces clinical effects associated with hypernatremia and resulting ECF volume excess. On inspection, you may note agitation, pitting edema, and dyspnea. Vital signs may reflect tachycardia and hypertension.

When hyperchloremia is associated with metabolic acidosis (due to base bicarbonate excretion by the kidneys), inspection may reveal deep, rapid breathing. Neurologic assessment may reveal weakness, diminished cognitive ability and, ultimately, coma.

Diagnostic tests

See *Identifying chloride imbalance.*

Treatment

For hypochloremia, treatment aims to correct the condition that causes excessive chloride loss and to give an oral replacement, such as salty broth.

When oral therapy isn't possible or when emergency measures are necessary, treatment may include I.V. administration of 0.9% sodium chloride solution (if hypovolemia is present) or chloride-containing drugs, such as ammonium chloride, to increase serum chloride levels and potassium chloride for metabolic alkalosis.

For severe hyperchloremic acidosis, treatment consists of sodium bicarbonate I.V. to raise serum bicarbonate levels and permit renal excretion of the chloride anion because bicarbonate and chloride compete for combination with sodium. For mild hyperchloremia, lactated Ringer's solution is administered; it converts to bicarbonate in the liver, thus increasing base bicarbonate to correct acidosis.

In either kind of chloride imbalance, treatment must correct the underlying disorder.

Key nursing diagnoses and patient outcomes

For hypochloremia:

Risk for injury related to inability of body to maintain homeostasis without adequate chloride ions. Based on this nursing diagnosis, you'll establish these patient outcomes. The patient will:

- not become injured if muscle weakness occurs
- recover and maintain a normal serum chloride level.

Ineffective breathing pattern related to weakness of respiratory muscles caused by hypochloremia. Based on this nursing diagnosis, you'll establish these patient outcomes. The patient will:

- maintain adequate ventilation, as evidenced by normal arterial blood gas levels and an absence of signs and symptoms of hypoxia
- recover and maintain a normal breathing pattern.

For hyperchloremia:

Altered thought processes related to adverse neurologic effects of hyperchloremia on cognitive function. Based on this nursing diagnosis, you'll establish these patient outcomes. The patient will:

- remain free from injury
- recover and maintain a normal serum chloride level
- become oriented to time, person, and place.

Fluid volume excess related to simultaneous increase in sodium caused by natural affinity of sodium for chloride. Based on this nursing diagnosis, you'll establish these patient outcomes. The patient will:

- tolerate restricted intake of fluids, sodium, and chloride without physical or emotional discomfort
- recover a normal fluid balance, as exhibited by the absence of edema, balanced intake and output records, and normal serum sodium and chloride levels.

Nursing interventions

When managing a patient with a chloride imbalance, your interventions will vary, depending upon whether the patient has hypochloremia or hyperchloremia.

For hypochloremia:

- Provide foods high in chloride, such as salty broth.
- Implement measures to correct the underlying cause of the imbalance, as indicated.
- Administer oral or I.V. chloride supplements, as ordered, if deficiency is severe, oral intake is restricted, or dietary adjustment is not effective.
- If the patient has muscle weakness, initiate measures to prevent injury. Assist the patient with ambulation. Keep personal articles within easy reach.

For hyperchloremia:

- Insert an I.V. line, and administer lactated Ringer's solution or sodium bicarbonate, as ordered.
- If the patient shows altered thought processes due to hyperchloremic acidosis, provide a safe environment.

Monitoring

For hypochloremia:

- Monitor serum chloride levels frequently, particularly during I.V. therapy.
- Watch for signs of hyperchloremia, which would indicate overcorrection, or continued hypochloremia, which would indicate insufficient correction. Be alert for respiratory difficulty.

• To detect hypochloremia, monitor laboratory results (serum electrolyte levels and arterial blood gas values) and fluid intake and output of patients who are vulnerable to chloride imbalance, particularly those recovering from gastric surgery. Record and report excessive or continuous loss of gastric secretions. Also report prolonged infusion of dextrose in water without 0.9% sodium chloride solution.

For hyperchloremia:

• Check serum electrolyte levels every 3 to 6 hours. If the patient is receiving high doses of sodium bicarbonate, watch for signs of overcorrection (metabolic alkalosis, respiratory depression) or lingering signs of hyperchloremia, which indicate inadequate treatment.

• If sodium excess is also present, assess for signs of fluid overload.

• If the patient shows altered thought processes, assess his neurologic status frequently for signs of deterioration.

• Assess respiratory function. Rapid, deep respirations, a compensatory mechanism, may accompany hyperchloremic acidosis.

• To detect hyperchloremia, check laboratory results for elevated serum chloride or potassium imbalance if the patient is receiving I.V. solutions containing sodium chloride, and monitor fluid intake and output. Also, watch for signs of metabolic acidosis. When administering I.V. fluids containing lactated Ringer's solution, monitor the flow rate according to the patient's age, physical condition, and bicarbonate level. Report any irregularities promptly.

Patient teaching

• Explain all tests and procedures to the patient and his family.

• Discuss food sources of sodium, potassium, and chloride with the patient experiencing hypochloremia.

Cholecystectomy

When drug therapy, dietary changes, and supportive treatments fail to control gallbladder or biliary duct disease, the patient's gallbladder may need to be removed. Known as a cholecystectomy, this procedure helps restore biliary flow from the liver to the small intestine. The procedure may be performed either as abdominal surgery, which uses one large abdominal incision, or as a laparoscopic procedure, which uses several small abdominal incisions.

After gallbladder resection, choledochoduodenostomy (anastomosis of the common bile duct to the duodenum) or choledochojejunostomy (anastomosis of the common bile duct to the jejunum) may be necessary to restore biliary flow.

Procedure

Both abdominal and laparoscopic cholecystectomies are performed under general anesthesia. An abdominal cholecystectomy begins with a right subcostal or paramedial incision. The surgeon then surveys the abdomen and uses laparotomy packs to isolate the gallbladder from the surrounding organs. After identifying biliary tract structures, he may use cholangiography or ultrasonography to help identify gallstones. Using a choledoscope, he directly visualizes the bile ducts and inserts a Fogarty balloon-tipped catheter to clear the ducts of stones.

The surgeon ligates and divides the cystic duct and artery and removes the entire gallbladder. Typically, he performs a choledochotomy: the insertion of a T tube into the common bile duct to decompress the biliary tree and prevent bile peritonitis during healing. He may also insert a Penrose drain into the ducts. After completion of the surgery and, if necessary, implantation of the T tube, the surgeon removes blood and debris from the abdomen, closes the incision, and applies a dressing.

For a laparoscopic cholecystectomy, the surgeon begins by making a small incision just above the umbilicus and injecting either carbon dioxide or nitrous oxide into the abdominal cavity. This inflates the abdomen and lifts the abdominal wall away from the abdominal organs, allowing the surgeon to identify the gallbladder readily. He then connects a trocar to an insufflator and inserts it through the incision. Next, he passes a thin, flexible optical instrument, called a laparoscope, through the trocar. The laparoscope allows the surgeon to view the intra-abdominal contents.

At this time, the patient is placed in Trendelenburg's position. This causes the small intestines to fall out of the pelvis, making room for the initial needle and trocar insertion. Then, while looking through the laparoscope, the surgeon makes three incisions in the patient's right upper quadrant: one 2″ (5 cm) below the xiphoid process in the midline; one 1″ (2 cm) below the right costal margin in the midclavicular line; and one in the anterior axillary line at the level of the umbilicus.

While continuing to look through the laparoscope, the surgeon passes instruments through the three incisions in the right upper quadrant. He uses these to clamp and then tie off the cystic duct and to excise the gallbladder. The gallbladder is then removed through the umbilical opening. After this, the surgeon sutures all four incisions and places a dressing over each one.

Complications

Although relatively rare, complications from cholecystectomy can be grave. Peritonitis, for instance, may occur from obstructed biliary drainage and resultant leakage of bile into the peritoneum. Postcholecystectomy syndrome, marked by fever, jaundice, and pain, may occur. As in all abdominal surgeries, postoperative atelectasis may result from hampered respiratory excursion if an abdominal surgical approach was used. If a laparoscopic approach was used, bile duct or small bowel injury may occur during introduction of the trocar.

Other complications include superficial wound infection, prolonged ileus, urine retention, and retained gallstones.

Key nursing diagnoses and patient outcomes

Ineffective breathing patterns related to guarded respirations caused by one or more incisions in the right upper quadrant of the abdomen. Based on this nursing diagnosis, you'll establish these patient outcomes. The patient will:
- not exhibit any signs of hypoxia, such as restlessness, shortness of breath, and confusion
- regain and maintain a normal breathing pattern.

Risk for infection related to potential for leakage of biliary drainage into the abdominal cavity. Based on this nursing diagnosis, you'll establish these patient outcomes. The patient will:
- have a normal temperature, white blood cell count, and liver function studies; these values will remain normal
- exhibit an incision that is clean and free of inflammation and purulent drainage
- not experience any signs and symptoms of peritonitis, such as abdominal distention or increased abdominal pain.

Pain related to one or more surgical incisions. Based on this nursing diagnosis, you'll establish these patient outcomes. The patient will:
- verbalize a decrease in pain within 24 hours
- express relief from pain after analgesic administration
- become pain free after healing is complete.

Nursing interventions

With a cholecystectomy patient, your major roles include instruction and care tailored to the patient's condition.

Before surgery

- Explain the planned surgery to the patient using clear, simple terms and diagrams. Reassure him that the surgery will relieve his symptoms. Also reassure him that his recovery should be rapid and uneventful and that he should be allowed to resume his full range of activities within 4 to 6 weeks.
- If the patient is scheduled for an abdominal surgical approach, warn the patient that, after surgery, he'll have a nasogastric tube (NG) in place for 1 to 2 days and an abdominal drain at the incision site for 3 to 5 days. If appropriate, tell him that a T tube will be inserted in the common bile duct during surgery to drain excess bile and allow removal of retained stones. Explain that the T tube may remain in place for up to 2 weeks, depending on the surgery, and that he may be discharged with it still in place.
- If the patient is scheduled for a laparoscopic approach, tell the patient that an indwelling urinary catheter will be inserted into his bladder and an NG tube into his stomach after general anesthesia has been administered. Reassure him that these tubes will be removed in the postanesthesia room following the procedure. Explain that he will have three small incisions in the right upper quadrant of his abdomen and one small incision in his umbilicus. Each of these incisions will be covered with a small sterile dressing postoperatively. Also inform him that he may be discharged the day of surgery or the day after.
- Teach the patient how to perform coughing and deep-breathing exercises to prevent postoperative atelectasis, which can lead to pneumonia. Tell him that an analgesic can be administered before these exercises to relieve discomfort.
- Monitor and, if necessary, help stabilize the patient's nutritional status and fluid balance. Such measures may include administering vitamin K, blood transfusions, or glucose and protein supplements. Twenty-four hours before surgery, administer only clear liquids. Then, after midnight the night before surgery or as ordered, withhold all food and fluid.
- Administer preoperative medications and assist with insertion of an NG tube.
- Ensure that the patient or a responsible family member has signed a consent form.

After surgery

- When the patient returns from surgery, place him in low Fowler's position. As ordered, attach the NG tube to low intermittent suction. Monitor the amount and characteristics of drainage from the NG tube as well as from any abdominal drains. Check dressings frequently and change as necessary.
- If the patient has a T tube in place, frequently assess the position and patency of the tube and drainage bag. The drainage bag should be level with his abdomen to prevent excessive drainage. Also note the amount and characteristics of drainage; bloody or blood-tinged bile normally occurs for only the first few hours after surgery. Provide meticulous skin care around the tube insertion site to prevent irritation.
- After a few days, expect to remove the NG tube, if present, and begin to introduce foods: first liquids, then gradually soft solids. As ordered, clamp the T tube for an hour before and an hour after each meal to allow bile to travel to the intestine to aid digestion. If the patient has had a laparoscopic cholecystectomy, expect him to begin clear liquids when fully recovered from general anesthesia and to resume his normal diet the day of or the day after surgery.
- Be alert for signs of postcholecystectomy syndrome (such as fever, abdominal pain, and jaundice) and other complications involving obstructed bile drainage. For several days after surgery, monitor vital signs and record intake and output every 8 hours. If any complications occur, report them to the doctor and collect urine and stool samples for laboratory analysis of bile content.

• Assist the patient with ambulation on the first postoperative day, unless contraindicated. Have him cough, deep-breathe, and perform incentive spirometry every 4 hours; as ordered, provide analgesics to ease discomfort during these exercises. Assess his respiratory status every 2 hours to detect hypoventilation and signs of atelectasis.

Home care instructions

• If the patient is being discharged with a T tube in place, show him how to care for it, stressing the need for meticulous tube care.
• Tell the patient to immediately report any signs of biliary obstruction: fever, jaundice, pruritus, pain, dark urine, and clay-colored stools.
• Tell the patient that, although there are typically no dietary restrictions, he may wish to avoid excessive fat intake for 4 to 6 weeks.

Cholelithiasis, cholecystitis, and related disorders

The leading biliary tract disease, cholelithiasis is the formation of stones or calculi (gallstones) in the gallbladder. The prognosis is usually good with treatment unless infection occurs. In that case, the prognosis depends on the infection's severity and its response to antibiotics.

The formation of gallstones can give rise to a number of related disorders.

In cholecystitis, the gallbladder becomes acutely or chronically inflamed, usually because a gallstone becomes lodged in the cystic duct, causing painful gallbladder distention. The acute form is most common during middle age; the chronic form, among elderly persons. The prognosis is good with treatment.

In choledocholithiasis, gallstones pass out of the gallbladder and lodge in the common bile duct, causing partial or complete biliary obstruction. The prognosis is good unless infection occurs.

In cholangitis, the bile duct becomes infected; this disorder is commonly associated with choledocholithiasis and may follow percutaneous transhepatic cholangiography. Nonsuppurative cholangitis usually responds rapidly to antibiotic treatment. Suppurative cholangitis has a poor prognosis unless surgery to correct the obstruction and drain the infected bile is performed promptly.

In gallstone ileus, a gallstone obstructs the small bowel. Typically, the gallstone travels through a fistula between the gallbladder and small bowel and lodges at the ileocecal valve. This condition is most common in elderly persons. The prognosis is good with surgery.

Generally, gallbladder and duct diseases occur during middle age. Between ages 20 and 50, they're six times more common in women, but the incidence in men and women equalizes after age 50. The incidence rises with each succeeding decade.

Causes

These related disorders all stem from a common cause: formation of calculi. Although the exact cause of gallstone formation is unknown, abnormal metabolism of cholesterol and bile salts clearly plays an important role.

A number of risk factors have been identified that predispose a person to calculi formation. These include:
• a high-calorie, high-cholesterol diet, associated with obesity
• elevated estrogen levels from oral contraceptive use, postmenopausal hormone-replacement therapy, or pregnancy
• the use of clofibrate
• diabetes mellitus, ileal disease, hemolytic disorders, hepatic disease, or pancreatitis.

The disorder that develops depends on where in the gallbladder or biliary tract the calculi collect. For example, cholelithiasis results when gallstones form and

Where calculi collect

Possible locations for calculi include these sites.

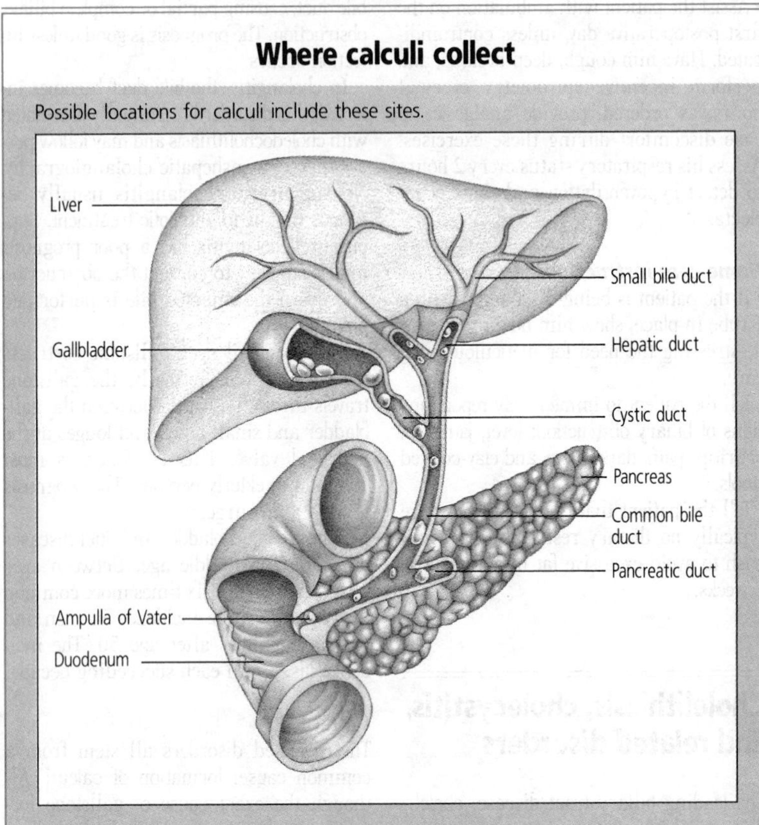

remain in the gallbladder. Cholecystitis, choledocholithiasis, cholangitis, and gallstone ileus usually develop after a gallstone lodges in a duct or in the small bowel, causing an obstruction. (See *Where calculi collect.*)

Acute cholecystitis also may result from conditions that alter the gallbladder's ability to fill or empty. These conditions include trauma, reduced blood supply to the gallbladder, prolonged immobility, chronic dieting, adhesions, prolonged anesthesia, and narcotic abuse.

Complications

Each of these disorders produces its own set of complications.

Cholelithiasis may lead to any of the disorders associated with gallstone formation: cholangitis, cholecystitis, choledolithiasis, and gallstone ileus.

Cholecystitis can progress to gallbladder complications, such as empyema, hydrops or mucocele, or gangrene. Gangrene may lead to perforation, resulting in peritonitis, fistula formation, pancreatitis, and porcelain gallbladder. Other complications include chronic cholecystitis and cholangitis.

Choledocholithiasis may lead to cholangitis, obstructive jaundice, pancreatitis, and secondary biliary cirrhosis.

Cholangitis may progress to septic shock and death, especially in the suppurative form.

Gallstone ileus may cause bowel obstruction, which can lead to intestinal perforation, peritonitis, septicemia, secondary infection, and septic shock.

Assessment

Although gallbladder disease may produce no symptoms (even when X-rays reveal gallstones), acute cholelithiasis, acute cholecystitis, and choledocholithiasis produce symptoms of a classic gallbladder attack.

In a gallbladder attack, the patient typically complains of sudden onset of severe steady or aching pain in the midepigastric region or the right upper abdominal quadrant. He may describe this pain as radiating to his back, between the shoulder blades, over the right shoulder blade, or just to the shoulder area. This type of pain is known as biliary colic and is the most characteristic symptom of gallbladder disease. It's often severe enough to send him to the emergency department.

Often, the patient reports that the attack followed eating a fatty meal or a large meal after fasting for an extended time. The attack may have occurred in the middle of the night, suddenly awakening him. He may also report nausea, vomiting, and chills; a low-grade fever may be assessed.

The patient may report a history of milder GI symptoms that preceded the acute attack. He may have experienced these symptoms for some time before seeking treatment. Such symptoms may include indigestion, vague abdominal discomfort, belching, and flatulence after eating meals or snacks rich in fats.

During an acute attack, inspection confirms that the patient is in severe pain and reveals pallor, diaphoresis, and exhaustion. If he has chronic cholecystitis, inspection of the skin, sclerae, and oral mucous membranes may confirm jaundice; inspection of urine and stool specimens may reveal dark-colored urine and clay-colored stools.

Tachycardia may be noted on palpation. Light palpation of the abdomen may disclose tenderness over the gallbladder, which increases on inspiration. If a calculus-filled gallbladder without ductal obstruction is palpated, a painless, sausagelike mass can be felt. Auscultation may reveal hypoactive bowel sounds if the patient has acute cholecystitis.

If the patient has cholangitis, he may report a history of choledocholithiasis and classic symptoms of biliary colic. On inspection, jaundice and pain may be evident. He may also have a spiking fever with chills.

In gallstone ileus, the patient may complain of colicky pain, which may persist for several days, sometimes with nausea and vomiting. You may note abdominal distension on inspection. Auscultation may reveal absent bowel sounds if the patient has a complete bowel obstruction.

Diagnostic tests

Ultrasonography and X-rays detect gallstones. Specific procedures include the following:

- *Plain abdominal X-rays* identify gallstones if they contain enough calcium to be radiopaque. X-rays are also helpful in identifying porcelain gallbladder, limy bile, and gallstone ileus.
- *Ultrasonography of the gallbladder* confirms cholelithiasis in most patients and distinguishes between obstructive and nonobstructive jaundice; calculi as small as 2 mm can be detected.
- *Oral cholecystography* confirms the presence of gallstones, although this test is gradually being replaced by ultrasonography.
- *Technetium-labeled iminodiacetic acid scan of the gallbladder* indicates cystic duct obstruction and acute or chronic cholecystitis if the gallbladder can't be seen.

• *Percutaneous transhepatic cholangiography,* imaging performed under fluoroscopic control, supports the diagnosis of obstructive jaundice and visualizes calculi in the ducts.
• *Blood studies* may reveal elevated levels of serum alkaline phosphatase, lactate dehydrogenase, aspartate aminotransferase (formerly SGOT), and total bilirubin. The white blood cell count is slightly elevated during a cholecystitis attack.

Treatment

Surgery, usually elective, remains the most common treatment for gallbladder and duct disease. Surgery is usually recommended if the patient has symptoms frequent enough to interfere with his regular routine; if he has any complications of gallstones; or if he has had a previous attack of cholecystitis.

Procedures may include cholecystectomy; cholecystectomy with operative cholangiography; choledochostomy; exploration of the common bile duct or, possibly, laparoscopic cholecystectomy.

If the patient's gallstones are radiolucent and consist totally or in part of cholesterol, he may be a candidate for gallstone dissolution therapy. In this treatment, oral chenodeoxycholic acid or ursodiol are used to partially or completely dissolve gallstones. However, this treatment has several limitations, including the need for prolonged treatment, the fact that it dissolves only small calculi, the high incidence of adverse reactions, and the frequency of calculus reformation after treatment ends.

Other, more direct, methods may be used to remove the gallstones. One of these is insertion of a percutaneous transhepatic biliary catheter under fluoroscopic guidance, which permits visualization of the calculi and their removal using a basket-shaped tool called a Dormia basket. Another calculus-removal technique is endoscopic retrograde cholangiopancreatography (ERCP). In this procedure, the calculi are removed with a balloon or basketlike tool passed through an endoscope. Both of these techniques permit decompression of the biliary tree, allowing bile to flow.

Another technique, lithotripsy, breaks up gallstones using ultrasonic waves. It has been used successfully in some patients with radiolucent calculi. (See the entry "Lithotripsy.")

If the patient is asymptomatic or has recovered from a first attack of biliary colic, noninvasive treatment may be attempted. This treatment includes a low-fat diet with replacement of the fat-soluble vitamins A, D, E, and K and administration of bile salts to facilitate digestion and vitamin absorption.

During an acute attack, medications include narcotics for pain relief; antispasmodics and anticholinergics to relax smooth muscles and decrease ductal tone and spasm; and antiemetics to reduce nausea and vomiting. A nasogastric tube may also be inserted and connected to intermittent low-pressure suction to relieve vomiting.

In patients with severe acute cholecystitis, I.V. fluids and I.V. antibiotic therapy are often given before surgery. Cholestyramine may be given if the patient has obstructive jaundice with severe itching from accumulation of bile salts in the skin.

The patient with nonsuppurative cholangitis usually responds quickly to antibiotic therapy. Suppurative cholangitis requires antibiotic therapy, prompt surgical correction of the obstruction, and drainage of the infected bile.

Key nursing diagnoses and patient outcomes

Risk for fluid volume deficit related to nausea and vomiting caused by cholecystitis. Based on this nursing diagnosis, you'll establish these patient outcomes. The patient will:
• maintain an adequate fluid balance as exhibited by equal intake (I.V. if necessary) and output and normal blood pressure
• not exhibit signs and symptoms of dehydration

• experience a cessation of nausea and vomiting.

Risk for infection related to biliary obstruction caused by one or more gallstones lodging in a duct or the small intestine. Based on this nursing diagnosis, you'll establish these patient outcomes. The patient will:

• maintain a normal temperature and white blood cell count
• not exhibit other signs and symptoms of infection, such as chills or acute abdominal pain.

Pain related to inflammation of the gallbladder caused by a gallstone becoming lodged in the cystic duct. Based on this nursing diagnosis, you'll establish these patient outcomes. The patient will:

• express relief from pain following analgesic administration
• become pain free following removal of lodged gallstone.

Nursing interventions

• If the patient will be managed without invasive procedures, provide a low-fat diet and smaller, more frequent meals to help prevent attacks of biliary colic. Replace vitamins A, D, E, and K, and administer bile salts, as ordered.
• As ordered, administer narcotic and anticholinergic medications to relieve pain and antiemetics to relieve nausea and vomiting.
• If the patient develops nausea or vomits, stay with him and withhold food and fluids.
• If the patient has cholangitis, administer antibiotics, as ordered.
• After percutaneous transhepatic biliary catheterization or ERCP to remove gallstones, the patient should receive nothing by mouth until his gag reflex returns.
• Prepare the patient for surgery, if indicated. (See the entry "Cholecystectomy.")

Monitoring

• Evaluate the effectiveness of medication, and watch for possible adverse reactions.
• If the patient vomits or has nausea, assess his vital signs and monitor his intake and output for signs of a fluid deficit.
• If the patient has cholangitis, monitor his vital signs closely. Watch for signs of severe toxicity, including confusion, septicemia, and septic shock.
• If the patient has had a percutaneous transhepatic biliary catheterization or ERCP, monitor his intake and output, keeping in mind that urine retention can be a problem. Observe the patient for complications, including cholangitis and pancreatitis.

Patient teaching

• Teach the patient about the disease and the reasons for his symptoms.
• Explain scheduled diagnostic tests, reviewing pretest instructions and necessary aftercare.
• If a low-fat diet is prescribed, suggest ways to implement it. If necessary, ask the dietitian to reinforce your instructions. Be sure the patient understands how dietary changes help to prevent biliary colic.
• Review the proper use of prescribed medications, explaining their desired effects. Point out possible adverse reactions, especially those that warrant a call to the doctor.
• Reinforce the doctor's explanation of the ordered treatment, such as surgery, ERCP, or lithotripsy. Be sure the patient fully understands the possible complications, if any, associated with the treatments.

Chronic fatigue and immune dysfunction syndrome

Also called chronic fatigue syndrome, chronic Epstein-Barr virus, myalgic encephalomyelitis, and yuppie flu, this syndrome is characterized by incapacitating fatigue. The patient's symptoms may wax and wane, but they are often severely debilitating and may last for months or years.

Although most prevalent among professionals in their 20s and 30s, the syndrome affects people of all ages, occupations, and income levels. The diagnosis is more common in women than in men or children, especially women under age 45. Sporadic incidence as well as epidemic clusters have been observed.

Causes

The precise cause of chronic fatigue syndrome isn't known. Although the syndrome originally was attributed to the Epstein-Barr virus, that hypothesis has since been rejected on the basis of serologic and epidemiologic observation.

Several other causative viruses have been proposed and investigated, including cytomegalovirus, herpes simplex virus types 1 and 2, human herpesvirus 6, Inoue-Melnick virus, human adenovirus 2, enteroviruses, measles virus, and a retrovirus that resembles human T-cell lymphotropic virus type II. The onset in some patients suggests a viral cause, but whether the syndrome results from a new or a reactivated infection isn't known.

Another theory holds that some symptoms may result from an overactive immune system. In addition, genetic predisposition, age, hormonal balance, neuropsychiatric factors, sex, previous illness, environment, and stress appear to have a role in the syndrome.

Complications

Chronic fatigue syndrome causes few complications. Its debilitating nature, however, greatly influences the patient's sense of well-being.

Assessment

The patient characteristically complains of prolonged, overwhelming fatigue, along with other signs and symptoms, including sore throat, myalgia, and cognitive dysfunction. The Centers for Disease Control and Prevention uses a working case definition to group symptoms and severity. (See *Diagnostic criteria in chronic fatigue syndrome.*) When assessing the patient, keep in mind that this definition was developed for research purposes, not clinical use. Use the definition as a guide, not as the basis for determining the patient's need for care.

Diagnostic tests

No definitive test exists for this disorder. Diagnostic testing should include studies to rule out other illnesses, such as Epstein-Barr virus, leukemia, and lymphoma.

Some patients with chronic fatigue syndrome have reduced natural killer cell cytotoxicity, abnormal CD4+:CD8 T-cell ratio, decreases in immunoglobulin subclasses, mild lymphocytosis, circulating immune complexes, and increased levels of antimicrosomal antibodies. But because these findings vary from patient to patient, they're of uncertain clinical significance.

A psychiatric screening may aid diagnosis because many patients have an underlying psychiatric disorder. Also, they commonly experience depression and anxiety after the syndrome's onset.

Treatment

Polyribonucleotide, an investigational antiviral agent and immunomodulator, is in clinical trials as a treatment for this disease.

Acyclovir, I.V. immune globulin, and I.M. magnesium sulfate also have been studied, but acyclovir has been found no better than a placebo. The role of immune globulin remains unclear after two clinical trials that yielded contradictory results. I.M. magnesium sulfate can improve the patient's energy and emotional state and relieve pain.

Treatment focuses on supportive care. The patient with myalgia or arthralgia can benefit from nonsteroidal anti-inflammatory drugs. A patient who sleeps excessively can receive an antidepressant such as fluoxetine. A patient who has trouble

Diagnostic criteria in chronic fatigue syndrome

The Centers for Disease Control and Prevention uses two major and several minor criteria for diagnosing chronic fatigue and immune dysfunction syndrome. Keep in mind that they were developed for research purposes, not clinical use.

Major criteria

The patient has persistent or relapsing debilitating fatigue or must tire easily, with no previous history of similar symptoms. The fatigue doesn't resolve with bed rest and is severe enough that the patient can maintain an average level of activity of less than 50% of normal for at least 6 months.

A thorough evaluation that includes a patient history, a physical examination, and appropriate laboratory findings has ruled out other clinical conditions that produce similar symptoms.

Minor criteria

In addition to the criteria above, the patient must exhibit at least eight of the following symptoms, or six symptoms plus at least two signs. He must have first experienced these at the same time or after the onset of fatigue, and they must have persisted or recurred for at least 6 months. The signs must be documented by a doctor on at least two occasions, at least 1 month apart.

Symptoms

- Reported mild fever (oral temperature of 99.5° to 101.5° F [37.5° to 38.6°C]), as measured by the patient or chills
- Sore throat
- Painful anterior or posterior cervical or axillary lymph nodes
- Unexplained generalized muscle weakness
- Muscle discomfort or myalgia
- Generalized fatigue that persists for 24 hours or longer after levels of exercise that the patient could have tolerated easily when healthy
- Migratory arthralgia without joint swelling or redness
- One or more neuropsychiatric complaints (photophobia, transient visual scotomata, forgetfulness, excessive irritability, confusion, difficulty thinking, inability to concentrate, depression)
- Sleep disturbance (hypersomnia or insomnia)
- Description of the main symptom complex as first developing over a few hours to a few days (considered equivalent to the symptoms above in meeting the requirements of the case definition)

Signs

- Low-grade fever: an oral temperature of 99.5° to 101.5° F (37.5° to 38.6° C) or rectal temperature of 100° to 103.8° F (37.8° to 39.9° C)
- Nonexudative pharyngitis
- Palpable or tender anterior or posterior cervical or axillary lymph nodes 3/4" (2 cm) in diameter

sleeping or who experiences pain may benefit from amitriptyline.

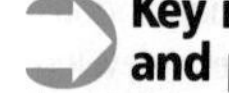

Key nursing diagnoses and patient outcomes

Activity intolerance related to fatigue caused by chronic fatigue and immune dysfunction syndrome. Based on this nursing diagnosis, you'll establish these patient outcomes. The patient will:

- maintain normal muscle mass, strength, and joint range of motion
- express a willingness to maximize his activity level
- perform self-care activities as tolerated.

Fatigue related to the cause of chronic fatigue and immune dysfunction syndrome. Based on this nursing diagnosis, you'll establish these patient outcomes. The patient will:
• identify activities that increase fatigue and avoid or change those activities
• incorporate measures to modify fatigue, such as a regular exercise program
• reattain his normal energy level.

Self-esteem disturbance related to debilitating nature of chronic fatigue and immune dysfunction syndrome. Based on this nursing diagnosis, you'll establish these patient outcomes. The patient will:
• verbalize his feelings related to his self-esteem
• take steps to achieve a higher level of physical and emotional wellness
• describe at least two positive personal qualities.

Nursing interventions

• Give the patient emotional support through the often long period of diagnostic testing and the protracted, often debilitating course of illness.
• Refer the patient for counseling as needed and to a local support group, if available. Make sure that the group advocates helping the patient lead as normal a life as possible. If necessary, refer him to a mental health center or a career counselor.

Monitoring

• Monitor the patient's activity level, and assess his degree of fatigue when performing activities of daily living.
• Monitor the patient's emotional response to his illness, and evaluate his ability to cope.

Patient teaching

• Suggest that the patient decrease activities when his fatigue is greatest. But advise him to avoid bed rest, which has no proven therapeutic value. A graded exercise program, although often difficult for the patient to accept, may help him feel better. Stress the importance of starting with a short exercise period and slowly increasing exercise time.
• If the patient needs medication, explain the medication regimen. If the doctor prescribes an antidepressant, explain how the medication can help relieve other signs and symptoms, such as sleep pattern disturbances and appetite changes.
• Help the patient return to a normal lifestyle. Begin by helping him plan a gradual return to work.

Cirrhosis

A chronic hepatic disease, cirrhosis is characterized by diffuse destruction and fibrotic regeneration of hepatic cells. As necrotic tissue yields to fibrosis, this disease alters liver structure and normal vasculature, impairs blood and lymph flow, and ultimately causes hepatic insufficiency.

Cirrhosis is the ninth most common cause of death in the United States and, among patients ages 35 to 55, the fourth leading cause of death. The disease, which can occur at any age, occurs in four main types: Laënnec's, postnecrotic, biliary, and cardiac. Laënnec's cirrhosis, the most common type, is most prevalent among malnourished alcoholic men; it accounts for more than half of all cirrhosis cases in the United States. Postnecrotic cirrhosis is more common in women than in men and is the most common type worldwide.

Causes

The factors that lead to the development of cirrhosis are not clearly defined. A genetic factor appears to be important, with familial tendencies to develop cirrhosis or possess a sensitivity to alcohol in some individuals. However, many alcoholics don't develop cirrhosis, whereas others develop the disease even though their nutritional status is adequate.

Cirrhosis has a diverse etiology, reflecting the varied clinical types:

- Laënnec's cirrhosis (alcoholic, nutritional, or portal cirrhosis) stems from chronic alcoholism and malnutrition.
- Postnecrotic cirrhosis usually results as a complication of viral hepatitis. This type also may occur after exposure to liver toxins, such as arsenic, carbon tetrachloride, or phosphorus.
- Biliary cirrhosis results from prolonged biliary tract obstruction or inflammation.
- Cardiac cirrhosis is associated with protracted venous congestion in the liver caused by right ventricular failure.
- In addition, some patients develop idiopathic cirrhosis.

Complications

Depending on the amount of liver damage, cirrhosis can lead to such complications as portal hypertension, bleeding esophageal varices, hepatic encephalopathy, hepatorenal syndrome, and death. (See *What happens in portal hypertension,* pages 196 and 197.)

Assessment

Signs and symptoms are similar for all types, regardless of the cause. However, clinical manifestations vary depending on when in the course of the disease the patient seeks treatment.

In the early stage, the patient may experience only vague signs and symptoms, but typically he complains of abdominal pain, diarrhea, fatigue, nausea, and vomiting. Later, as the disease progresses, he may complain of chronic dyspepsia, constipation, pruritus, and weight loss. He may report a tendency for easy bleeding, such as frequent nosebleeds, easy bruising, or bleeding gums.

During history taking, you may uncover alcoholism or other diseases or conditions, such as acute viral hepatitis, biliary tract disorders, congestive heart failure, recent blood transfusions, or viral infections.

In a head-to-toe approach, inspection reveals these common signs: telangiectasis on the cheeks; spider angiomas on the face, neck, arms, and trunk; gynecomastia; umbilical hernia; distended abdominal blood vessels; ascites; testicular atrophy; palmar erythema; clubbed fingers; thigh and leg edema; ecchymosis; and jaundice.

In the early phase of the disease, palpation finds the liver to be large and firm with a sharp edge. Later, scar tissue causes the liver to decrease in size; at this point, if the liver is palpable, its edge is nodular. Palpation also reveals an enlarged spleen.

Diagnostic tests

A thorough workup consisting of laboratory and other diagnostic tests is required to confirm the diagnosis, establish the type of cirrhosis, and pinpoint complications.

- *Liver biopsy.* The definitive test for cirrhosis, biopsy detects hepatic tissue destruction and fibrosis.
- *Abdominal X-rays.* Films show liver size and reveal cysts or gas within the biliary tract or liver, liver calcification, and massive ascites.
- *Computed tomography and liver scans.* These studies determine liver size, identify liver masses, and visualize hepatic blood flow and obstruction.
- *Esophagogastroduodenoscopy.* This study reveals bleeding esophageal varices, stomach irritation or ulceration, or duodenal bleeding and irritation.
- *Blood studies.* Liver enzymes (alanine aminotransferase [formerly SGPT], aspartate aminotransferase [formerly SGOT]), total serum bilirubin, and indirect bilirubin levels are elevated. Total serum albumin and protein levels decrease; prothrombin time is prolonged. Hemoglobin, hematocrit, and serum electrolyte levels decrease. Vitamins A, C, and K are deficient.
- *Urine and stool studies.* Urine levels of bilirubin and urobilinogen increase; fecal urobilinogen levels fall.

LIFE-THREATENING COMPLICATIONS

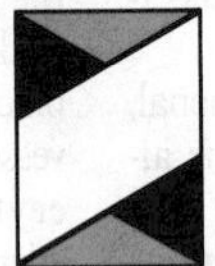

What happens in portal hypertension

Portal hypertension — elevated pressure in the portal vein — occurs when blood flow meets increased resistance from fibrotic tissue that has developed as a result of diffuse destruction of hepatic cells. The disorder, a common result of cirrhosis, may also stem from mechanical obstruction and occlusion of the hepatic veins (Budd-Chiari syndrome).

As pressure in the portal vein rises, blood backs up into the spleen and flows through collateral channels to the venous system, bypassing the liver. Consequently, portal hypertension produces dilated tortuous collateral veins in the submucosa of the lower esophagus known as esophageal varices.

Bleeding esophageal varices

In many patients, the first sign of portal hypertension is bleeding from esophageal varices. Esophageal varices commonly cause massive hematemesis that can quickly result in hemorrhage and hypovolemic shock. If bleeding is not stopped, the patient will die.

Emergency interventions

If you suspect bleeding esophageal varices in a patient, follow these steps:

- While you stay with the patient, send someone to notify the patient's doctor.
- Monitor the patient's vital signs continuously for signs of hypovolemic shock.
- Prepare to administer vasopressin, 0.2 to 0.4 units/minute I.V., to reduce portal venous pressure.
- Institute measures to alleviate hypovolemic shock, such as infusing blood or a crystalloid or colloid volume expander, as indicated.
- Assist with gastric intubation and esophageal balloon tamponade.
- Transfer the patient to the intensive care unit.
- If the patient continues to bleed or rebleeds, prepare to assist with sclerotherapy.
- If the patient still continues to bleed, prepare to send him to the operating room for a portal-systemic shunt insertion.

Treatment

Therapy aims to remove or alleviate the underlying cause of cirrhosis, prevent further liver damage, and prevent or treat complications. Vitamins and nutritional supplements promote healing of damaged hepatic cells and improve the patient's nutritional status. Sodium consumption is usually restricted to 500 mg/day and liquid intake is limited to 1,500 ml/day to help manage ascites and edema.

Drug therapy requires special caution because the cirrhotic liver can't detoxify harmful substances efficiently. Antacids may be prescribed to reduce gastric distress and decrease the potential for GI bleeding. Potassium-sparing diuretics, such as furosemide, may be used to reduce ascites and edema. However, diuretics require careful monitoring because fluid and electrolyte imbalance may precipitate hepatic encephalopathy. Vasopressin may be indicated for esophageal varices. Alcohol is prohibited, and sedatives should be avoided.

In patients with ascites, paracentesis may be used as a palliative treatment to relieve abdominal pressure. However, surgical intervention may be required to divert ascites into venous circulation; if so, a

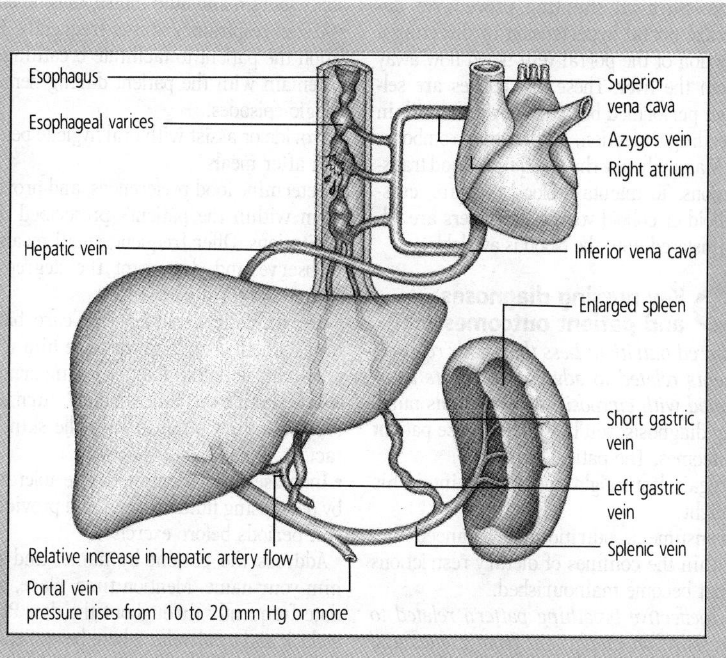

peritoneovenous shunt is used. Shunt insertion results in weight loss, decreased abdominal girth, increased sodium excretion from the kidneys, and improved urine output.

To control bleeding from esophageal varices or other GI hemorrhage, nonsurgical measures are attempted first. These include gastric intubation and esophageal balloon tamponade. In gastric intubation, a tube is inserted and the stomach is lavaged until the contents are clear. If the bleeding is assessed as a gastric ulcer, antacids and histamine antagonists are administered.

In esophageal balloon tamponade, bleeding vessels are compressed to stanch blood loss from esophageal varices. Several forms of balloon tamponade are available, including the Sengstaken-Blakemore method, the esophagogastric tube method, and the Minnesota tube method.

Sclerotherapy is performed if the patient continues to experience repeated hemorrhagic episodes despite conservative treatment. A sclerosing agent is injected into the oozing vessels. This agent traumatizes epithelial tissue, which causes thrombosis and leads to sclerosis. If bleeding from the varices doesn't stop within 2 to 5 minutes, a second injection is given below the bleeding site. Sclerotherapy also may be performed prophylactically on nonbleeding varices.

As a last resort, portal-systemic shunts may be used for patients with bleeding esophageal varices and portal hypertension. Surgical shunting procedures decrease portal hypertension by diverting a portion of the portal vein blood flow away from the liver. These procedures are seldom performed because they can result in bleeding, infection, and shunt thrombosis.

Massive hemorrhage requires blood transfusions. To maintain blood pressure, crystalloid or colloid volume expanders are administered until the blood is available.

Key nursing diagnoses and patient outcomes

Altered nutrition: Less than body requirements related to adverse GI effects associated with cirrhosis. Based on this nursing diagnosis, you'll establish these patient outcomes. The patient will:
- regain lost weight and then maintain his weight
- consume a nutritionally balanced diet within the confines of dietary restrictions
- not become malnourished.

Ineffective breathing pattern related to pressure on diaphragm from ascites and changes in liver function. Based on this nursing diagnosis, you'll establish these patient outcomes. The patient will:
- be free of respiratory distress
- not exhibit dyspnea or hypoxia (cyanosis, restlessness).

Risk for injury related to potential for bleeding esophageal varices caused by increased portal hypertension. Based on this nursing diagnosis, you'll establish these patient outcomes. The patient will:
- not develop bleeding esophageal varices
- adhere to the treatment regimen to prevent further liver damage and complications such as esophageal varices.

- adhere to the treatment regimen to prevent further liver damage and complications such as esophageal varices.

Nursing interventions

- Administer diuretics, potassium, and protein or vitamin supplements, as ordered. Restrict sodium and fluid intake, as ordered.
- Assess respiratory status frequently. Position the patient to facilitate breathing.
- Remain with the patient during hemorrhagic episodes.
- Provide or assist with oral hygiene before and after meals.
- Determine food preferences, and provide them within the patient's prescribed diet limitations. Offer frequent, small meals.
- Observe and document the degree of sclerae and skin jaundice.
- Give the patient frequent skin care, bathe him without soap, and massage him with emollient lotions. Keep his fingernails short. Handle the patient gently; turn and reposition him often to keep the skin intact.
- Increase the patient's exercise tolerance by decreasing fluid volumes and providing rest periods before exercise.
- Address the patient by name, and tell him your name. Mention time, place, and date frequently throughout the day. Place a clock and a calendar where he can easily see them.
- Use appropriate safety measures to protect the patient from injury. Avoid physical restraints if possible.
- Allow the patient to express his feelings about having cirrhosis. Offer psychological support and encouragement when appropriate. Offer him and his family a realistic evaluation of his present health status, and communicate hope for the immediate future.
- Prepare the patient for necessary medical procedures (such as paracentesis, gastric intubation, esophageal ballon tamponade, sclerotherapy, or portal-systemic shunt insertion), and assist with the procedures as needed.

Monitoring

- Monitor vital signs, intake and output, and electrolyte levels to determine fluid volume status.
- To assess fluid retention, measure and record abdominal girth every shift. Weigh the patient daily, and document his weight.
- Observe for bleeding gums, ecchymoses, epistaxis, and petechiae.
- Inspect stools for amount, color, and consistency. Test stools and vomitus for occult blood.
- Watch for signs of anxiety, epigastric fullness, restlessness, and weakness.
- Observe closely for signs of behavioral or personality changes. Report increasing stupor, lethargy, hallucinations, or neuromuscular dysfunction. Arouse the patient periodically to determine level of consciousness. Watch for asterixis, a sign of developing encephalopathy.

Patient teaching

- To minimize the risk of bleeding, warn the patient against taking nonsteroidal anti-inflammatory drugs. Suggest using an electric razor and a soft toothbrush.
- Explain the importance of avoiding activities that increase intra-abdominal pressure, such as heavy lifting, vigorous coughing, and straining to have a bowel movement.
- Advise the patient that rest and good nutrition conserve energy and decrease metabolic demands on the liver. Urge him to eat frequent, small meals. Teach him to alternate periods of rest and activity to reduce oxygen demand and prevent fatigue.
- Tell the patient how he can conserve energy while performing activities of daily living. For example, suggest that he sit on a bench while bathing or dressing.
- Stress the need to avoid infections and abstain from alcohol. Refer the patient to Alcoholics Anonymous if appropriate.

Coal worker's pneumoconiosis

Also known as black lung, coal miner's disease, miner's asthma, anthracosis, and anthracosilicosis, coal worker's pneumoconiosis is a progressive nodular pulmonary disease. The disease occurs in two forms: simple and complicated. With the simple form, the patient has characteristically limited lung capacity. In this patient, complicated coal worker's pneumoconiosis (also known as progressive massive fibrosis) may develop. In the complicated form, fibrous tissue masses form in the lungs.

A person's risk for coal worker's pneumoconiosis depends on various factors, including how long he has been exposed to coal dust (usually 15 or more years), the intensity of his exposure (dust count and size of inhaled particles), his proximity to the mine site, the silica content of the coal (anthracite has the highest silica content), and his susceptibility. The highest incidence of this disease is among anthracite miners in the eastern United States.

Causes

Inhalation and prolonged retention of respirable coal dust particles (less than 5 microns wide) cause coal worker's pneumoconiosis. In the simple form, macules (coal dust–laden macrophages) form around terminal and respiratory bronchioles and are surrounded by a halo of dilated alveoli. At the same time, supporting tissues atrophy and harden, causing permanent small-airway dilation (focal emphysema). Simple coal worker's pneumoconiosis may progress to the complicated form – most likely if the disease begins after a relatively short exposure.

Complicated coal worker's pneumoconiosis may involve one or both lungs. Fibrous tissue masses enlarge and coalesce, grossly distorting pulmonary structures as the disease progressively destroys vessels, alveoli, and airways.

Complications

Pulmonary hypertension, cor pulmonale, and pulmonary tuberculosis can complicate coal worker's pneumoconiosis. In cigarette smokers, chronic bronchitis and emphysema can also complicate the disease.

Assessment

Whether the patient has simple or complicated coal worker's pneumoconiosis, the patient history will disclose exposure to coal dust. In the simple form, the patient is typically asymptomatic, especially if he's a nonsmoker.

If the patient has complicated coal worker's pneumoconiosis, the patient history may reveal exertional dyspnea and a cough. This patient may state that he occasionally coughs up inky-black sputum (from avascular necrosis and cavitation).

Additionally, the patient may report a productive cough with milky, gray, clear, or coal-flecked sputum or yellow, green, or thick sputum with recurrent bronchial and pulmonary infections.

Inspection may reveal a barrel chest. Percussion may uncover hyperresonant lungs with areas of dullness. On auscultation, you'll hear diminished breath sounds, crackles, rhonchi, and wheezes.

Diagnostic tests

• *Chest X-rays* in simple coal worker's pneumoconiosis show small opacities (less than 10 mm in diameter). These opacities may inhabit all lung zones but appear more prominent in the upper lung zones. In complicated coal worker's pneumoconiosis, X-rays may show one or more large opacities (3⁄8″ to 2″ [1 to 5 cm] in diameter). Some may exhibit cavitation.

• *Pulmonary function studies* indicate a vital capacity that's normal in simple coal worker's pneumoconiosis but decreased in the complicated form; decreased forced expiratory volume in 1 second (FEV_1) in the complicated form; and a normal ratio of FEV_1 to forced vital capacity.

The ratio of residual volume to total lung capacity is normal in the simple form but decreased in the complicated form. Diffusing capacity for carbon monoxide – significantly below normal in the complicated form – reflects alveolar septal destruction and pulmonary capillary obliteration.

• *Arterial blood gas analysis* typically shows normal partial pressure of oxygen (Pao_2) in simple coal worker's pneumoconiosis but decreased Pao_2 in complicated disease. Partial pressure of carbon dioxide ($Paco_2$) is normal in the simple form (possibly decreasing in hyperventilation) but may increase if the patient is hypoxic and has severely impaired alveolar ventilation.

Treatment

Appropriate treatment aims to relieve respiratory symptoms, manage hypoxia and cor pulmonale, and avoid respiratory tract irritants and infections. Treatment also includes observation for developing tuberculosis.

Respiratory signs and symptoms may be relieved by bronchodilator therapy with theophylline or aminophylline (if bronchospasm is reversible), oral or inhaled beta-adrenergics (such as metaproterenol), corticosteroids (such as oral prednisone or aerosolized beclomethasone), or inhalable cromolyn sodium. Chest physiotherapy may be used to mobilize and remove secretions.

Other measures include increased fluid intake (at least 3 qt [3 liters] daily) and respiratory therapy with aerosolized preparations, inhaled mucolytics, and intermittent positive-pressure breathing or incentive spirometry. Diuretic agents, digitalis glycosides, and sodium restriction may be ordered to treat cor pulmonale.

In serious illness, oxygen may be administered by cannula or mask (usually 1 to 2 liters/minute) if the patient has chronic hypoxia or by mechanical ventilation if Pao_2 falls below 40 mm Hg.

Respiratory tract infections require prompt administration of antibiotics.

Key nursing diagnoses and patient outcomes

Fatigue related to hypoxia caused by impaired gas exchange as a result of coal worker's pneumoconiosis. Based on this nursing diagnosis, you'll establish these patient outcomes. The patient will:
• identify activities that cause or increase fatigue
• modify daily routine to allow for rest periods
• perform self-care without fatigue.

Impaired gas exchange related to fibrotic lung tissue masses caused by coal worker's pneumoconiosis. Based on this nursing diagnosis, you'll establish these patient outcomes. The patient will:
• maintain normal arterial blood gas values
• not have any signs of hypoxia, such as irritability, restlessness, change in skin color, change in level of consciousness, or shortness of breath while at rest.

Knowledge deficit related to complex treatment regimen required to manage coal worker's pneumoconiosis. Based on this nursing diagnosis, you'll establish these patient outcomes. The patient will:
• express an interest in learning how to manage coal worker's pneumoconiosis
• learn how to perform measures used to manage coal worker's pneumoconiosis
• verbalize an understanding of, and demonstrate the skill needed to perform, necessary respiratory care measures.

Nursing interventions

• Help the patient adjust to life-style changes necessitated by chronic illness. Answer his questions, and encourage him to express his concerns. Include the patient and his family in care-related decisions.
• Provide the patient with high-calorie, high-protein foods, and offer small, frequent meals to conserve his energy and prevent fatigue.
• Make sure the patient receives adequate fluids to loosen secretions.
• Perform chest physiotherapy, including postural drainage and chest percussion and vibration, several times daily.
• Schedule respiratory therapy at least 1 hour before or after meals. Provide mouth care after inhalation therapy.
• If the patient requires incentive spirometry, assist him to a comfortable sitting or semi-Fowler's position to promote optimal lung expansion.
• Encourage daily activity. Provide diversional activities as appropriate. To conserve the patient's energy and prevent fatigue, alternate periods of rest and activity.
• Administer medications, as ordered. Record the patient's response to drug therapies.

Monitoring

• Assess for changes in baseline respiratory function. Be alert for changes in sputum quality and quantity. Watch for restlessness, increased tachypnea, and changes in breath sounds. Report these changes immediately.
• Watch for complications such as pulmonary hypertension, cor pulmonale, and tuberculosis.

Patient teaching

• Advise the patient to avoid crowds and people with known infections and to obtain influenza and pneumococcus immunizations.
• If the patient receives home oxygen therapy, explain its purpose. Teach him how to use the equipment.
• Teach the patient and his family how to perform chest physiotherapy with postural drainage and chest percussion. Advise the patient to maintain each position for about 10 minutes and then to perform percussion and coughing exercises. Also teach him coughing and deep-breathing tech-

niques to promote good ventilation and to remove secretions.

- Show the patient how to use an incentive spirometer properly, and tell him why he needs it.
- Explain the patient's medication regimen to him and his family. Discuss the dosages, adverse effects, and purposes of prescribed drugs.
- Encourage the patient to follow a high-calorie, high-protein diet and to drink plenty of fluids to prevent dehydration and help loosen secretions.
- If the patient smokes, urge him to stop. Provide him with further information, or refer him for counseling.
- As appropriate, provide information about coal worker's pneumoconiosis, including prevention. Educate workers and employers concerning the importance of wearing effective respirators in the workplace.

Colorectal cancer

The second most common visceral neoplasm in the United States and Europe, colorectal cancer is equally distributed between men and women. It occurs more frequently in those over age 40.

Malignant tumors of the colon or rectum are almost always adenocarcinomas. About half of these are sessile lesions of the rectosigmoid area; the rest, polypoid lesions.

Colorectal cancer progresses slowly, remaining localized for a long time. Unless the tumor has metastasized, the 5-year survival rate is relatively high: about 80% for rectal cancer and more than 85% for colon cancer. If left untreated, the disease is invariably fatal.

Causes

Although the exact cause of colorectal cancer is unknown, studies show a greater incidence in areas of higher economic development, suggesting a relation to diet (excess animal fat, particularly beef, and low fiber).

Other risk factors for colorectal cancer include diseases of the digestive tract, a history of ulcerative colitis (in which case cancer usually starts in 11 to 17 years), familial polyposis (cancer almost always develops by age 50), and a family history of the disease (first-degree relatives).

Complications

As the tumor grows and encroaches on the abdominal organs, abdominal distention and intestinal obstruction occur. Anemia may develop if rectal bleeding isn't treated.

Assessment

Signs and symptoms depend on the tumor's location. If it develops on the colon's right side, the patient probably won't have signs and symptoms in the early stages because the stool is still in liquid form in that part of the colon. He may have a history of black, tarry stools, however, and report anemia, abdominal aching, pressure, and dull cramps. As the disease progresses, he may complain of weakness, diarrhea, constipation, anorexia, weight loss, and vomiting.

A tumor on the left side of the colon causes symptoms of obstruction even in the early disease stages because stools are more completely formed when they reach this part of the colon. The patient may report rectal bleeding (often ascribed to hemorrhoids), intermittent abdominal fullness or cramping, and rectal pressure.

As the disease progresses, constipation, diarrhea, or ribbon- or pencil-shaped stools may develop. The patient may note that the passage of flatus or stool relieves his pain. He may also report obvious bleeding during defecation, dark or bright red blood in the feces, and mucus in or on the stools.

A patient with a rectal tumor may report a change in bowel habits, often beginning with an urgent need to defecate on arising ("morning diarrhea") or constipation alternating with diarrhea. He also may notice blood or mucus in the stools and complain of a sense of incomplete evacuation. Late in the disease, he may complain of pain that begins as a feeling of rectal fullness and progresses to a dull, sometimes constant ache confined to the rectum or sacral region.

Inspection of the abdomen may reveal distention or visible masses. Abdominal veins may appear enlarged and visible from portal obstruction. The inguinal and supraclavicular nodes may also appear enlarged. You may note abnormal bowel sounds on abdominal auscultation. Palpation may reveal abdominal masses. Right-side tumors usually feel bulky; tumors of the transverse portion are more easily detected.

Diagnostic tests

Several tests support a diagnosis of colorectal cancer:

- *Digital rectal examination* can detect almost 15% of colorectal cancers. Specifically, it can detect suspicious rectal and perianal lesions.
- *Fecal occult blood test* can detect blood in stools, a warning sign of rectal cancer.
- *Proctoscopy* or *sigmoidoscopy* permits visualization of the lower GI tract. It can detect up to 66% of colorectal cancers.
- *Colonoscopy* permits visual inspection and photography of the colon up to the ileocecal valve and provides access for polypectomies and biopsies of suspected lesions.
- *Excretory urography* verifies bilateral renal function and allows inspection for displacement of the kidneys, ureters, or bladder by a tumor pressing against these structures.
- *Barium enema studies,* using a dual contrast of barium and air, allow the location of lesions that aren't detectable manually or visually. Barium examination shouldn't precede colonoscopy or excretory urography because barium sulfate interferes with these tests.
- *Computed tomography scan* allows better visualization if a barium enema yields inconclusive results or if metastasis to the pelvic lymph nodes is suspected.
- *Carcinoembryonic antigen,* although not specific or sensitive enough for early diagnosis of colorectal cancer, permits patient monitoring before and after treatment to detect metastasis or recurrence.

Treatment

The most effective treatment for colorectal cancer is surgery to remove the malignant tumor and adjacent tissues, along with any lymph nodes that may contain cancer cells. After surgery, treatment continues with chemotherapy, radiation therapy, or both. (See *Staging colorectal cancer,* page 204.)

The type of surgery depends on tumor location:

- *Cecum and ascending colon.* Tumors in these areas call for right hemicolectomy (for advanced disease). Surgery may include resection of the terminal segment of the ileum, cecum, ascending colon, and right half of the transverse colon with corresponding mesentery.
- *Proximal and middle transverse colon.* Surgery consists of right colectomy that includes the transverse colon and mesentery corresponding to midcolic vessels or segmental resection of the transverse colon and associated midcolic vessels.
- *Sigmoid colon.* Surgery usually is limited to the sigmoid colon and mesentery.
- *Upper rectum.* A tumor in this area usually requires anterior or low anterior resection. A newer method, using a stapler, allows for much lower resections than previously possible.
- *Lower rectum.* Abdominoperineal resection and permanent sigmoid colostomy are required.

If metastasis has occurred, or if the patient has residual disease or a recurrent inoperable tumor, he needs chemotherapy. Drugs used in such treatment commonly include fluorouracil combined with lev-

Staging colorectal cancer

Named for pathologist Cuthbert Dukes, the Dukes cancer classification assigns tumors to four stages. These stages (with substages) reflect the extent of bowel mucosa and bowel wall infiltration, lymph node involvement, and metastasis. Use this summary to clarify your patient's cancer stage and prognosis.

Stage A

Malignant cells are confined to the bowel mucosa, and the lymph nodes contain no cancer cells. Treated promptly, about 80% of these patients remain disease-free 5 years later.

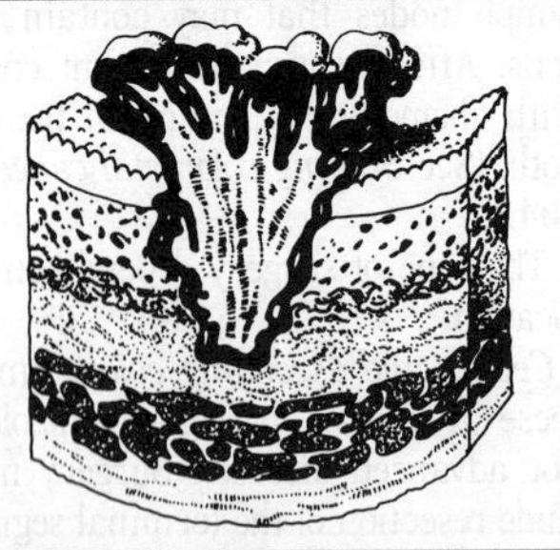

Stage B

Malignant cells extend through the bowel mucosa but remain within the bowel wall. The lymph nodes are normal. In substage B_2, all bowel wall layers and immediately adjacent structures contain malignant cells, but the lymph nodes remain normal. About 50% of patients with substage B_2 survive for 5 or more years.

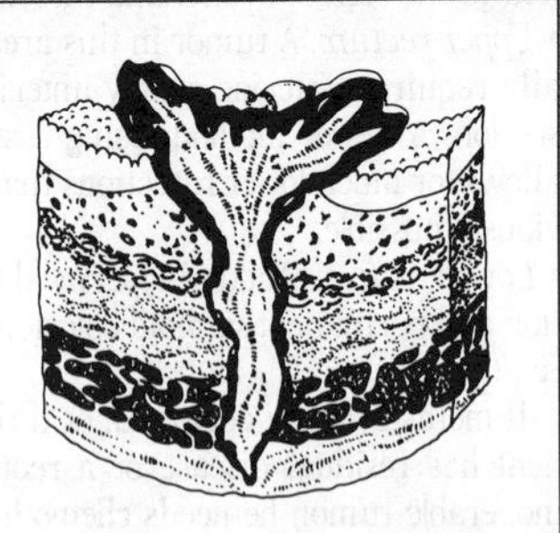

Stage C

Malignant cells extend into the bowel wall and the lymph nodes. In substage C_2, malignant cells extend through the entire thickness of the bowel wall. The lymph nodes also contain malignant cells. The 5-year survival rate for patients with stage C disease reaches about 25%.

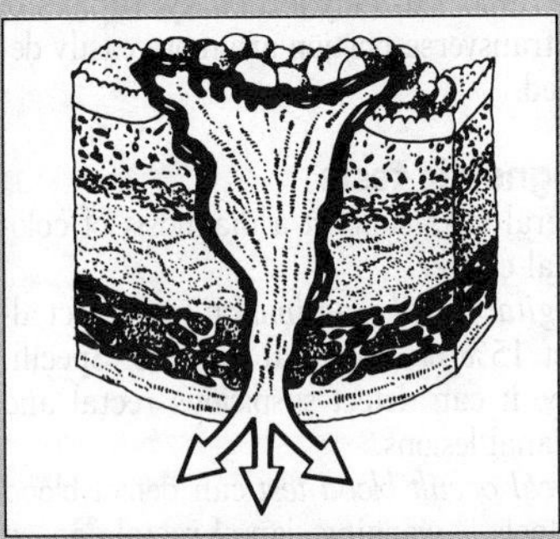

Stage D

Metastasized to distant organs by way of the lymph nodes and mesenteric vessels, malignant cells typically lodge in the lungs and liver. Only 5% of patients with stage D cancer survive 5 or more years.

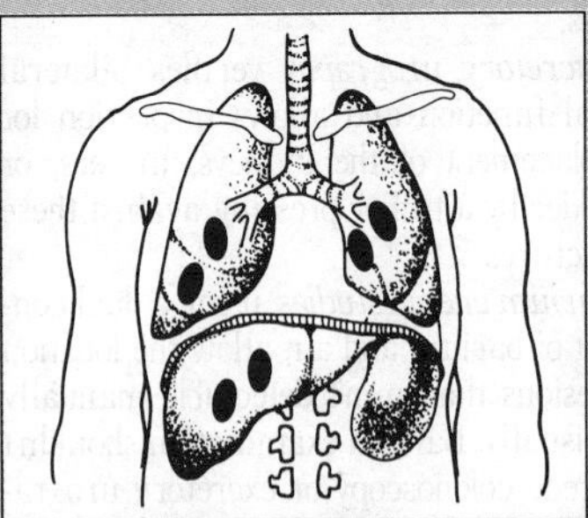

amisole or leucovorin. Researchers are evaluating the effectiveness of fluorouracil with recombinant interferon alfa-2a.

Radiation therapy, used before or after surgery, induces tumor regression.

Key nursing diagnoses and patient outcomes

Constipation related to presence of a cancerous tumor in the colon or rectal area. Based on this nursing diagnosis, you'll establish these patient outcomes. The patient will:

- relieve constipation with changes in lifestyle (such as a high-fiber diet, exercise, and adequate fluid intake) or medication until treatment is complete
- regain normal bowel pattern with treatment.

Diarrhea related to presence of a cancerous tumor in the colon or rectal area. Based on this nursing diagnosis, you'll establish these patient outcomes. The patient will:

- control diarrhea with medication until treatment can be completed
- not exhibit any sign of fluid and electrolyte imbalance
- develop a normal elimination pattern with treatment, either naturally or through an ostomy.

Fear related to potential for colorectal cancer to recur or metastasize. Based on this nursing diagnosis, you'll establish these patient outcomes. The patient will:

- express his fears about being diagnosed with colorectal cancer
- use situational support systems to diminish his fears
- use at least one fear-reducing behavior, such as asking questions about treatment progress or making decisions about care, each day
- manifest no physical signs or symptoms of fear

Nursing interventions

- Prepare the patient for surgery, as indicated. (See the entries "Bowel resection with anastomosis" and "Bowel resection with ostomy.")
- Provide comfort measures and reassurance for patients undergoing radiation therapy.
- Prepare the patient for the adverse effects of chemotherapy, and take steps to minimize these effects. For example, offer the patient a 0.9% sodium chloride mouthwash to help deter mouth ulcers.
- To help prevent infection, use strict aseptic technique when caring for I.V. catheters. Change I.V. tubing and sites as directed by hospital policy. Have the patient wash his hands before and after meals and after going to the bathroom.
- Listen to the patient's fears and concerns, and stay with him during periods of severe stress and anxiety.
- Encourage the patient to identify actions and care measures that will promote his comfort and relaxation. Try to perform these measures, and encourage the patient and his family to do so, too.
- Whenever possible, include the patient and his family in care decisions.

Monitoring

- Monitor the patient's bowel patterns.
- Monitor the patient's diet modifications, and assess the adequacy of his nutritional intake.
- If the patient is receiving radiation therapy, watch for adverse reactions, such as nausea, vomiting, hair loss, and malaise. Likewise, if the patient is receiving chemotherapy, be prepared for common adverse reactions while watching for complications such as infection.

Patient teaching

- Throughout therapy, answer the patient's questions and tell him what to expect from surgery and other therapy.
- Explain to the patient's family that their positive reactions will foster the patient's adjustment.
- Direct the patient to follow a high-fiber diet.

HEALTH PROMOTION POINTERS

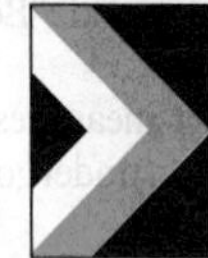

Reducing the risk of colorectal cancer

Screening and early detection are key to reducing the risk of colorectal cancer.
• Instruct the patient and family about the following guidelines from the American Cancer Society: annual digital rectal examination from age 40, periodic sigmoidoscopy and colonoscopy, and annual stool for occult blood beginning at age 50.
• Teach the patient about high-fiber diets—fiber appears to provide protection by increasing stool bulk, shortening intestinal transit time, and altering the flora of the colon.

• Advise the patient about foods to eat and those to avoid.
• Caution him to take laxatives or antidiarrheal medications only as prescribed by his doctor.
• Stress the need for regular check-ups due to an increased risk for developing another primary cancer. The patient should have annual screening and follow-up testing.
• Explain radiation therapy or chemotherapy, as appropriate. Be sure he understands the adverse reactions that usually occur and the measures he can take to decrease their severity or prevent their occurrence.
• Inform the patient about screening and early detection. (See *Reducing the risk of colorectal cancer.*)
• Refer the patient to a home health care agency that can check on his physical care at home.

Common variable immunodeficiency

This immunodeficiency disorder is marked by gradual deterioration of humoral (B-cell) immunity, resulting in increased risk of infection. (Symptoms often occur after infancy and childhood; the disorder manifests itself between ages 25 and 40.) It affects both sexes equally and normal life span, pregnancy, and offspring aren't affected.

Common variable immunodeficiency (also known as acquired agammaglobulinemia or common variable agammaglobulinemia) may be associated with autoimmune diseases and cancer.

Causes

The cause is unknown. Most patients have a normal circulating B-cell count but defective synthesis or release of immunoglobulins. Many also exhibit progressive deterioration of cell-mediated (T-cell) immunity. Although unproven, a genetic influence occurs in siblings. Family members are at higher risk of hypogammaglobulinemia, selective IgA deficiency, and autoimmune disease.

Complications

Complications include a spruelike syndrome with diarrhea, malabsorption, steatorrhea, and a protein-losing enteropathy. *Giardia lamblia* GI infection and upper and lower respiratory tract infections also occur.

Assessment

Review the patient's history. Investigate disorders, such as pyogenic bacterial infections, which are characteristic of common variable immunodeficiency. Be alert also for a history of chronic rather than acute infections. Recurrent sinopulmonary infections, chronic bacterial conjunctivitis, atrophic gastritis with pernicious anemia, and malabsorption (often associated with infestation by *G. lamblia*) are usually the first clues to common variable immunodeficiency. Also, suspect the disorder in an adult patient with unexplained bronchiectasis. Other initial signs and symptoms include fever, weight loss, and a palpable spleen and lymph nodes.

Diagnostic tests

Characteristic diagnostic markers in this disorder are decreased serum IgM, IgA, and IgG levels detected by immunoelectrophoresis and a normal circulating B-cell count. Plasma cells seldom appear in the lymph nodes, bone marrow, and spleen but may be found in intestinal lamina propria. Rheumatoid factor and positive Coombs' test findings may be present. Antigenic stimulation confirms an inability to produce specific antibodies; cell-mediated immunity may be intact or delayed.

X-rays usually show signs of chronic lung disease or sinusitis. Regular X-ray and pulmonary function studies monitor infection in the lungs.

Treatment

Care and treatment measures for patients with common variable immunodeficiency include weekly or monthly injections of immune globulin to help maintain the immune response. Antibiotics are preferred for combating infection.

Key nursing diagnoses and patient outcomes

Altered nutrition: Less than body requirements related to spruelike syndrome caused by common variable immunodeficiency. Based on this nursing diagnosis, you'll establish these patient outcomes. The patient will:

- regain lost weight and then maintain his weight within the normal range
- consume a nutritionally balanced diet
- not develop malnutrition.

Fluid volume deficit related to GI infection or spruelike syndrome caused by common variable immunodeficiency. Based on this nursing diagnosis, you'll establish these patient outcomes. The patient will:

- identify signs and symptoms of fluid volume deficit (such as dry mucous membranes, concentrated urine, decreased urine output, and thirst) and report them if they occur
- regain and then maintain a normal fluid balance.

Risk for infection related to increased incidence of respiratory and GI infections caused by common variable immunodeficiency. Based on this nursing diagnosis, you'll establish these patient outcomes. The patient will:

- identify signs and symptoms of a GI or respiratory infection
- identify the factors that can cause GI or respiratory infections and verbalize an understanding of the measures needed to prevent them from occurring
- not develop a GI or respiratory infection.

Nursing interventions

- Because immune globulin administration causes significant pain, administer injections deep into a large muscle mass, such as the gluteal or thigh muscle. Massage well. If the dose is more than 1.5 ml, divide it. Then, inject the divided doses into more than one site. For frequent injections, rotate the injection sites. Because immune globulin is composed primarily of IgG, the patient may also need fresh-frozen plasma infusions to provide IgA and IgM.
- As ordered, administer antibiotics and chest physiotherapy, including additional hydration and mucolytics, to forestall or treat infection.
- Institute diet therapy, as recommended, to counteract the depleting effects of malabsorption syndrome and anemias. Be sure to involve the dietitian and doctor in devising an optimal nutrition plan.

Monitoring

- Monitor the patient's nutritional intake, weight, and bowel patterns. Watch for signs of malnutrition.
- Monitor the patient's complete blood count with differential regularly, as or-

dered, to detect evidence of anemia or infection.

- Observe the patient for signs and symptoms of a GI infection (such as nausea, vomiting, diarrhea, and abdominal pain) or a respiratory infection (such as productive cough, fever, and shortness of breath).

Patient teaching

- To help avoid severe infection, teach the patient and his family how to recognize its early signs and symptoms. Warn him to avoid crowds and people who have active infections.
- Stress the importance of good nutrition and regular follow-up care. A cooked-food diet (one that contains no raw foods) may help reduce bacteria in foods and beverages.
- Explain to the patient that secondary conditions may coexist with the immunodeficiency. Advise him that these may require additional or specialized treatment.

Complement deficiencies

Complement is a series of circulating enzymatic serum proteins with nine functional components, labeled C1 through C9. Complement deficiency or dysfunction may increase susceptibility to infection and seems to be related to certain autoimmune disorders.

Theoretically, any complement component may be deficient or dysfunctional, and many such disorders are under investigation. However, primary complement deficiencies are rare. The most common include C2, C6, and C8 deficiencies and C5 familial dysfunction. (See *Major disorders associated with complement deficiencies.*) More common secondary complement abnormalities have been confirmed in patients with lupus erythematosus, in some with dermatomyositis, in one with scleroderma (and in his family), and in a few patients with gonococcal and meningococcal infections.

The prognosis varies with the abnormality and the severity of associated diseases.

Causes

Primary complement deficiencies are inherited as autosomal recessive traits, except for deficiency of C1 esterase inhibitor, which is autosomal dominant. Secondary deficiencies may follow complement-fixing (complement-consuming) immunologic reactions, such as drug-induced serum sickness, acute streptococcal glomerulonephritis, and acute active systemic lupus erythematosus.

Normally, IgG or IgM reacts with antigens as part of an immune response, activating C1, which then combines with C4, initiating the classical complement pathway, or cascade. (An alternative complement pathway involves the direct activation of C3 by the serum protein properdin, bypassing the initial components [C1, C4, and C2] of the classical pathway.) Complement then combines with the antigen-antibody complex and undergoes a sequence of complicated reactions that amplify the immune response against the antigen. This complex process is called complement fixation. Any deficiency in complement interferes with this system.

Complications

C1 esterase inhibitor deficiency may lead to severe or even fatal swelling of the larynx.

Assessment

Signs and symptoms vary with the specific deficiency.

A patient with C2 or C3 deficiency or C5 familial dysfunction is likely to have signs and symptoms of a bacterial infection, which may involve several body systems simultaneously. Your assessment may also show signs of such collagen vascular diseases as lupus erythematosus and chronic

Major disorders associated with complement deficiencies

A deficiency of a specific complement may be linked to a particular disorder. Study the following list to help you better understand this link.

Deficiency	Associated clinical conditions
C1q	Glomerulonephritis, systemic lupus erythematosus (SLE)
C1r	SLE-like syndrome
C2	SLE, discoid lupus erythematosus, juvenile rheumatoid arthritis, glomerulonephritis
C3	Recurrent pyogenic infections, glomerulonephritis
C4	SLE-like syndrome
C5	Recurrent disseminated neisserial infections, SLE
C6	Recurrent disseminated neisserial infections
C7	Recurrent disseminated neisserial infections, Raynaud's phenomenon
C8	Recurrent disseminated neisserial infections
C9	None identified
Properdin	Recurrent pyogenic infections, fulminant meningococcemia
C1 esterase inhibitor	Hereditary angioedema, increased incidence of several autoimmune diseases

renal failure in a patient with C2 deficiency. And, in a patient with a C1 esterase inhibitor deficiency, you may observe periodic swelling in the face, hands, abdomen, or throat that may lead to airway obstruction.

Diagnostic tests

Diagnosis of a complement deficiency is difficult and requires careful interpretation of both clinical features and laboratory results. Various complement deficiencies cause a low total serum complement level. Specific assays may help confirm deficiency of specific complement components. For example, immunofluorescence of glomerular tissues in glomerulonephritis that reveals complement components and IgG strongly suggests complement deficiency.

Treatment

Although primary complement deficiencies have no known cure, the associated infections, collagen vascular disease, and renal disease require prompt treatment. Transfusion of fresh-frozen plasma replaces complement components, but this treatment is controversial because it doesn't cure complement deficiencies and provides only transient beneficial effects. Although helpful, bone marrow transplantation can cause potentially fatal graft-versus-host disease. Anabolic steroids and antifibrinolytic agents reduce acute swelling in patients with C1 esterase inhibitor deficiency.

Key nursing diagnoses and patient outcomes

Altered protection related to complement deficiencies. Based on this nursing diag-

nosis, you'll establish these patient outcomes. The patient will:
• identify the risks associated with his complement deficiency
• verbalize an understanding of how to protect himself by maintaining a balanced diet, conserving his energy, and obtaining adequate rest.

Risk for infection related to a complement deficiency. Based on this nursing diagnosis, you'll establish these patient outcomes. The patient will:
• take precautions to prevent infections
• remain free from infection.

Risk for suffocation related to potential for swelling of the larynx caused by a C1 esterase inhibitor deficiency. Based on this nursing diagnosis, you'll establish these patient outcomes. The patient will:
• identify the early signs of laryngeal swelling (such as a feeling of fullness in the throat and difficulty swallowing or talking) and verbalize the importance of seeking immediate medical attention if these signs occur
• maintain a patent airway at all times.

Nursing interventions

• Administer medications, as ordered. These include antibiotics, transfusions of fresh-frozen plasma and, for C1 esterase inhibitor deficiencies, anabolic steroids and antifibrinolytic agents.
• To maintain adequate ventilation, provide chest physiotherapy as needed to the patient with a respiratory tract infection.
• Prepare the patient for bone marrow transplantation, if indicated. (See the entry "Bone marrow transplantation.")
• When caring for a patient with C1 esterase inhibitor deficiency, be prepared for emergency management of laryngeal edema that may result from angioedema. Keep airway equipment on hand.
• Provide support to the patient or his family, if he's a child. Help them identify and use effective coping strategies. Refer them to a counselor, if needed.

Monitoring

• Closely monitor the intake and output, serum electrolyte levels, and acid-base balance of a patient with renal infection. Also, watch for signs of renal failure.
• Closely monitor the patient with C1 esterase inhibitor deficiency for laryngeal edema and respiratory distress.
• Monitor the patient for signs and symptoms of an infection, such as fever, chills, productive cough, nausea, vomiting, and diarrhea.

Patient teaching

• Teach the patient or his family the importance of avoiding infection, how to recognize its early signs and symptoms, and the need for prompt treatment if it occurs.

Conization

The definitive treatment for microinvasive cervical cancer, cervical conization involves the removal of a cone-shaped portion of the cervix. The procedure may also be used to diagnose cervical disorders such as an abnormal Papanicolaou smear, in which case it may be called a cone biopsy. Conization has largely been replaced by colposcopy for diagnostic purposes.

Procedure

After the patient has received a general or local anesthetic, the surgeon uses a cold scalpel (cold knife) or laser to cut a circular incision around the external os of the cervix. He then removes a cone-shaped piece of tissue, takes biopsies at the apex, and sutures the cervix. He may conclude by performing a dilatation and curettage.

Complications

Short-term complications include uterine perforation, heavy bleeding, and infection. Long-term complications include cervical stenosis, infertility, decreased cervical mucus, and premature labor due to cervical incompetence in future pregnancies.

Key nursing diagnoses and patient outcomes

Fear related to potential for future complications, such as infertility or premature labor, caused by cervical conization. Based on this nursing diagnosis, you'll establish these patient outcomes. The patient will:
- express her fears about the effect of conization on future fertility and pregnancy
- use available support systems to help her cope with her fears
- use at least one effective fear-reducing behavior when feeling fearful.

Risk for infection related to invasive procedure. Based on this nursing diagnosis, you'll establish these patient outcomes. The patient will:
- identify the signs and symptoms of infection and verbalize an understanding of the importance of reporting them if they occur
- remain free of purulent, malodorous vaginal drainage.

Impaired tissue integrity of the cervix related to surgical trauma caused by conization. Based on this nursing diagnosis, you'll establish these patient outcomes. The patient will:
- remain free from discomfort
- experience a normal healing process, without complications such as infection or stenosis.

Nursing interventions

When caring for a patient scheduled for a cervical conization, expect to implement the following interventions.

Before surgery

- Review the procedure with the patient, and answer her questions. Provide emotional support.
- Tell her what to expect after surgery. Inform her that she'll have some vaginal drainage for which she'll receive a perineal pad. Warn her that she may experience abdominal cramping along with some pelvic and low back pain after the procedure. Reassure her that these symptoms are normal and that they will soon disappear.
- Ensure that preliminary studies have been completed, including a medical history, physical examination, Papanicolaou (Pap) test, urinalysis, and hematocrit and hemoglobin measurements. Notify the doctor of any abnormalities.
- Be sure the patient has followed preoperative directions for fasting and used an enema to empty her colon before admission. Remind her that she'll be groggy after the procedure and won't be able to drive if general anesthesia is used. Make sure she has arranged transportation.
- Ask the patient to void before you administer any preoperative medications. Start I.V. fluids, as ordered.
- Make sure that the patient has signed a consent form.

After surgery

- After surgery, administer analgesics, as ordered. Expect the patient to have moderate cramping and pelvic and low back pain, but be sure to report any continuous, sharp abdominal pain that doesn't respond to analgesics.
- Monitor the patient's vital signs and vaginal drainage. Report profuse or purulent drainage to the doctor.
- Administer fluids, as tolerated, and allow food if the patient requests it. Keep the bed's side rails raised, and, if appropriate, help the patient walk to the bathroom until the effects of general anesthesia have worn off.

Home care instructions

- Instruct the patient to report any signs of infection. Tell her to use analgesics to control pain but to report any unrelenting sharp pain.
- Inform her that spotting and discharge may last a week or longer and that her periods may be heavier than normal for the first two or three menstrual cycles after

the procedure. Tell her to report any bright red blood.
• Instruct her to schedule an appointment with her doctor for follow-up care.

Corneal transplant

In a corneal transplant, or keratoplasty, healthy corneal tissue from a human donor replaces a damaged part of the cornea. Corneal transplants help restore corneal clarity lost through injury, inflammation, ulceration, or chemical burns. They may also correct corneal dystrophies, such as keratoconus, the abnormal thinning and bulging of the central portion of the cornea.

A corneal transplant can take one of two forms: a full-thickness penetrating keratoplasty, involving excision and replacement of the entire cornea, or a lamellar keratoplasty, which removes and replaces a superficial layer of corneal tissue. The full-thickness procedure, the more common of the two, produces a high degree of clarity and restores vision in 95% of patients.

A lamellar transplant is used if damage is limited to the anterior stroma or if the patient is uncooperative and may be expected to exert pressure on the eye after surgery. The degree of clarity produced by a lamellar transplant rarely matches that of a full-thickness graft. As a treatment for dystrophies, its success depends on the type and extent of the abnormality.

Because the cornea is avascular and doesn't recover as rapidly as other parts of the body, healing may take up to a year. Usually, sutures remain in place and vision isn't completely functional until healing is complete.

Procedure

In a full-thickness keratoplasty, the surgeon cuts a "button" from the donor cornea and a button from the host cornea, sized to remove the abnormality. Next, he anchors the donor button in place with extremely fine sutures. To end the procedure, he patches the eye and tapes a shield in place over it.

In a lamellar, or partial-thickness, keratoplasty, the surgeon excises a shallower layer of corneal tissue in both the donor and host corneas. He then peels away the excised layers of tissue and sutures the donor graft in place. As in the full-thickness procedure, he patches the eye and applies a rigid shield.

Complications

Graft rejection occurs in about 15% of patients; it may happen at any time during the patient's life. Uncommon complications include wound leakage, loosening of the sutures, dehiscence, and infection.

Key nursing diagnoses and patient outcomes

Anxiety related to potential for graft rejection following a corneal transplant. Based on this nursing diagnosis, you'll establish these patient outcomes. The patient will:
• verbalize his feelings of anxiety
• develop effective coping behaviors
• maintain autonomy and independence, without being handicapped by fears or phobic behavior.

Risk for infection related to surgical procedure and use of ophthalmic corticosteroid medication that may mask infection. Based on this nursing diagnosis, you'll establish these patient outcomes. The patient will:
• not exhibit inflammation or drainage in his operative eye
• not develop an infection in his operative eye.

Sensory or perceptual alterations (visual) related to photophobia in the operative eye caused by corneal transplant. Based on this nursing diagnosis, you'll establish these patient outcomes. The patient will:
• express an understanding of the need to wear dark glasses whenever he's exposed to bright light

• report a gradual reduction in photophobia
• report a cessation of photophobia after healing is complete.

Nursing interventions

With a corneal transplant patient, your major roles include watching for complications and instructing the patient how to care for his eye.

Before surgery

• Explain the transplant procedure to the patient, and answer any questions he may have. Advise him that healing will be slow and that his vision may not be completely restored until the sutures are removed, which may be in about a year.
• Tell the patient that most corneal transplants are performed under local anesthesia and that he can expect momentary burning during injection of the anesthetic. Explain to him that the procedure will last for about an hour and that he must remain still until it has been completed.
• Tell the patient that analgesics will be available after surgery since he may experience a dull aching. Inform him that a bandage and protective shield will be placed over the eye.
• As ordered, administer a sedative or an osmotic agent to reduce intraocular pressure. Ensure that the patient has signed a consent form.

After surgery

• After the patient recovers from the anesthetic, assess for and immediately report sudden, sharp, or excessive pain; bloody, purulent, or clear viscous drainage; or fever. As ordered, instill corticosteroid eyedrops or topical antibiotics to prevent inflammation and graft rejection.
• Instruct the patient to lie on his back or on his unaffected side, with the bed flat or slightly elevated, as ordered. Also have him avoid rapid head movements, hard coughing or sneezing, bending over, and other activities that could increase intraocular pressure; likewise, he shouldn't squint or rub his eyes.
• Remind the patient to ask for help in standing or walking until he adjusts to changes in his vision. And make sure that all his personal items are within his field of vision.

Home care instructions

• Teach the patient and his family to recognize the signs of graft rejection (inflammation, cloudiness, drainage, and pain at the graft site.) Instruct them to immediately notify the doctor if any of these signs occur. Emphasize that rejection can occur many years after surgery; stress the need for assessing the graft *daily* for the rest of the patient's life. Also remind the patient to keep regular appointments with his doctor.
• Tell the patient to avoid activities that increase intraocular pressure, including extreme exertion; sudden, jerky movements; lifting or pushing heavy objects; or straining during defecation.
• Explain that photophobia, a common adverse reaction, gradually decreases as healing progresses. Suggest wearing dark glasses in bright light.
• Teach the patient how to correctly instill prescribed eyedrops.
• Remind the patient to wear an eye shield when sleeping.

Coronary artery bypass grafting

Coronary artery bypass grafting (CABG) circumvents an occluded coronary artery with an autogenous graft (usually a segment of the saphenous vein from the leg or internal mammarian artery), thereby restoring blood flow to the myocardium.

Performed to prevent a myocardial infarction (MI) in a patient with acute or chronic myocardial ischemia, CABG is one of the most commonly performed surgeries today in the United States. The need for CABG is determined from the results of cardiac catherization and patient symptomology. Prime candidates for CABG include patients who have any of the following: medically uncontrolled angina interfering with the patient's life-style; left main coronary artery stenosis; severe proximal left anterior descending coronary artery stenosis; three-vessel disease with proximal stenoses or left ventricular dysfunction; and three-vessel disease with normal left ventricular function at rest but with inducible ischemia and poor exercise capacity.

If successful, CABG can relieve anginal pain, improve cardiac function, and possibly enhance the patient's quality of life. CABG techniques vary according to the patient's condition and the number of arteries being bypassed.

Procedure

After the patient has received general anesthesia, surgery begins with graft harvesting; the surgeon makes a series of incisions in the patient's thigh or calf and removes a saphenous vein segment for grafting. Most surgeons prefer using a segment of the internal mammarian artery because this provides an artery doing the job of an artery.

Once the grafts are obtained, the surgeon performs a medial sternotomy and exposes the heart. He then initiates cardiopulmonary bypass. (See *Understanding cardiopulmonary bypass.*) To reduce myocardial oxygen demands during surgery and to protect the heart, he induces cardiac hypothermia and standstill by injecting a cold cardioplegic solution (potassium-enriched saline solution) into the aortic root.

After the patient is fully prepared, the surgeon sutures one end of the venous graft to the ascending aorta and the other end to a patent coronary artery distal to the occlusion. He sutures the graft in a reversed position to promote proper blood flow. He repeats this procedure for each artery he bypasses.

Once the grafts are in place, he flushes the cardioplegic solution from the heart and discontinues cardiopulmonary bypass. He then implants epicardial pacing electrodes, inserts a chest tube, closes the incision, and applies a sterile dressing.

Complications

CABG can cause many postoperative complications, including arrhythmias, hypertension or hypotension, cardiac tamponade, thromboembolism, hemorrhage, postpericardiotomy syndrome, and MI. Noncardiac complications include cerebral vascular accident, postoperative depression or emotional instability, pulmonary embolism, decreased renal function, and infection. Also, problems such as graft rupture or closure or the development of atherosclerosis in other coronary arteries may need repeat surgery.

Key nursing diagnoses and patient outcomes

Decreased cardiac output related to hypothermia, recovery from general anesthesia, and complications such as arrhythmias, fluid and electrolyte imbalances, and pericardial tamponade. Based on this nursing diagnosis, you'll establish these patient outcomes. The patient will:

- maintain an adequate cardiac output, as evidenced by a normal blood pressure and pulse rate
- maintain adequate tissue perfusion as evidenced by a urine output of at least 30 ml/hour and by being oriented to time, person, and place
- not develop complications, such as arrhythmias, fluid and electrolyte imbalances, or pericardial tamponade, which could alter his cardiac output.

Risk for injury related to fluid and electrolyte imbalances caused by the use of cardiopulmonary bypass during CABG. Based on this nursing diagnosis, you'll es-

Understanding cardiopulmonary bypass

Open-heart surgery often involves a technique known as cardiopulmonary bypass to divert blood from the heart and lungs to an extracorporeal circuit with a minimum of hemolysis and trauma. As shown in this simplified diagram, the cardiopulmonary bypass (or "heart-lung") machine uses a mechanical pump to provide ventricular pumping action, an oxygenator to perform gas exchange, and a heat exchanger to cool the blood and lower the metabolic rate during surgery.

To perform this procedure, the surgeon inserts catheters into the right atrium or the inferior or superior vena cava for blood removal and into the ascending aorta for blood return. Then, after heparinizing the patient and priming the pump with fluid to replace diverted venous blood, the surgeon switches on the machine. The pump draws blood from the vena cava catheters into the machine, where it passes through a filter, oxygenator, heat exchanger, and another filter and bubble trap before being returned to arterial circulation. During cardiopulmonary bypass, an anesthesiologist or perfusionist maintains mean arterial pressure by adjusting the rate of perfusion or by infusing fluids or vasopressor drugs.

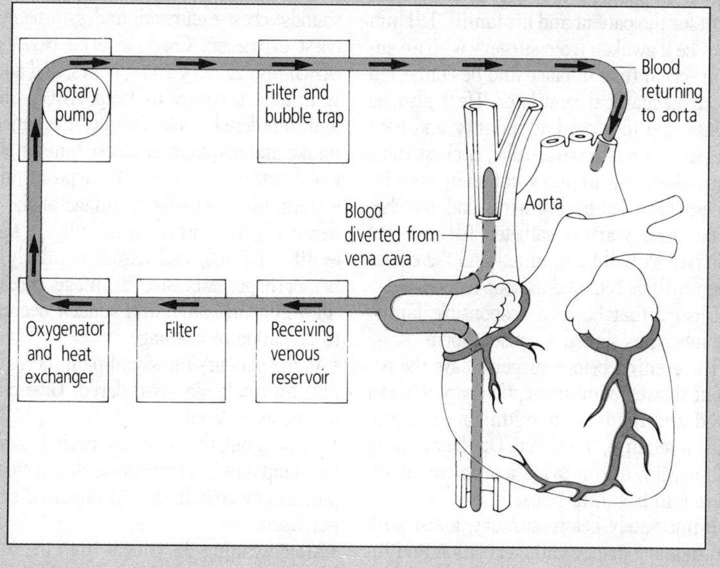

tablish these patient outcomes. The patient will:

- not become injured because of a fluid or electrolyte imbalance
- regain and maintain normal fluid balance postoperatively, as evidenced by a balanced fluid intake and output
- exhibit and maintain serum electrolyte levels within normal limits.

Hypothermia related to cooling procedures used during CABG. Based on this nursing diagnosis, you'll establish these patient outcomes. The patient will:

• regain and then maintain a normal temperature
• not shiver (which increases heart rate, blood pressure, and myocardial oxygen requirement) during the postoperative rewarming process.

Nursing interventions

When caring for a CABG patient, your major roles include patient instruction and caring for the patient's changing cardiovascular needs.

Before surgery

• Begin by reinforcing the doctor's explanation of the surgery. Next, explain the complex equipment and procedures used in the intensive care unit or postanesthesia room. If possible, arrange a tour of the unit for the patient and his family. Tell him that he'll awaken from surgery with an endotracheal tube in place and be connected to a mechanical ventilator. He'll also be connected to a cardiac monitor and have in place a nasogastric tube, a chest tube, an indwelling urinary catheter, arterial lines, epicardial pacing wires and, possibly, a pulmonary artery catheter. Tell him that discomfort will be minimal and the equipment will be removed as soon as possible.
• Ensure that he or a responsible family member has signed a consent form.
• The evening before surgery, have the patient shower with antiseptic soap. Restrict food and fluids after midnight, and provide a sedative, if ordered. On the morning of surgery, also provide a sedative, as ordered, to help him relax.
• Immediately before surgery, assist with pulmonary artery catheterization and insertion of arterial lines. Then begin cardiac monitoring.

After surgery

• Following CABG, look for signs of hemodynamic compromise, such as severe hypotension, decreased cardiac output, and shock. Check and record vital signs every 5 to 15 minutes until the patient's condition stabilizes. Monitor the electrocardiogram for disturbances in heart rate and rhythm. If you detect serious abnormalities, notify the doctor and be prepared to assist with epicardial pacing or, if necessary, cardioversion or defibrillation.
• To ensure adequate myocardial perfusion, keep arterial pressure within the limits set by the doctor. Usually, mean arterial pressure below 70 mm Hg results in inadequate tissue perfusion; pressure above 110 mm Hg can cause hemorrhage and graft rupture. Monitor pulmonary artery, central venous, and left atrial pressures, as ordered.
• Frequently evaluate the patient's peripheral pulses, capillary refill time, and skin temperature and color, and auscultate for heart sounds; report any abnormalities. Also evaluate tissue oxygenation by assessing breath sounds, chest excursion, and symmetry of chest expansion. Check arterial blood gas (ABG) results every 2 to 4 hours, and adjust ventilator settings to keep ABG values within ordered limits. Monitor the patient's intake and output, and assess him for electrolyte imbalance, especially hypokalemia.
• Maintain chest tube drainage at the ordered negative pressure (usually -10 to -40 cm H_2O), and assess regularly for hemorrhage, excessive drainage (greater than 200 ml/hour), and sudden decrease or cessation of drainage.
• As the patient's incisional pain increases, give an analgesic, as ordered. Give other drugs, as ordered.
• Throughout the recovery period, assess for symptoms of cerebrovascular accident, pulmonary embolism, and impaired renal perfusion.
• After weaning the patient from the ventilator and removing the endotracheal tube, promote chest physiotherapy. Start him on incentive spirometry, and encourage him to cough, turn frequently, and deep-breathe. Assist him with range-of-motion exercises, as ordered, to enhance peripheral circulation and prevent thrombus formation.
• Monitor the elderly patient closely for complications. (See *After a CABG*.)

EXPERT GERIATRIC CARE

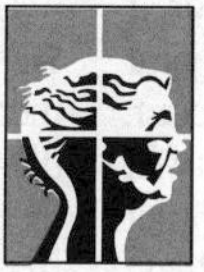

After a CABG

Elderly patients are at high risk for developing complications after a CABG because they have a smaller margin of physiologic reserve and a decreased ability to compensate or adapt to change. Infection, hemorrhage, blood pressure changes, and fluid and electrolyte imbalances are more problematic in the elderly. Inelasticity of blood vessels, poor nutritional status, increased risk for infection, and decreased cardiac, respiratory, and renal reserves can cause complications to occur more often. Watch for the following complications when caring for an elderly patient after a CABG.

Respiratory complications

Because of age-related changes in the respiratory system, coupled with the stresses of surgery and interventions to sustain ventilation, perfusion, and gas exchange, the elderly patient has a higher risk of developing postoperative respiratory complications such as pneumonia.

Delayed wound healing

Because of the slowed rated of skin cell turnover, wound healing may be delayed, thus, the patient is at greater risk for wound infection. Surgery can diminish the patient's reserves, and the vascular changes associated with normal aging can impair the blood flow necessary for proper wound healing.

Cardiovascular complications

Changes in the heart muscle and blood vessels predispose the elderly patient to cardiac complications. Symptoms of a myocardial infarction (MI) may be subtle; dyspnea, rather than chest pain, is the most common sign. Because the elderly patient has less lean body mass, which influences the creatine kinase and creatinine clearance levels, laboratory results after an MI can also be confusing. Arrhythmias are especially serious due to the patient's reduced tolerance of decreased cardiac output.

Gastrointestinal complications

Slowing of the intestinal transit time, a normal age-related change, can result in constipation and, possibly, intestinal obstruction.

Neurologic complications

New or overwhelming surroundings, such as a cardiac intensive care unit, can have a strong impact on the elderly patient's ability to determine what's going on, thus leading to confusion. He may also be somewhat reluctant to complain of pain.

Age-related changes can also affect medication pharmacodynamics and pharmacokinetics, placing the elderly patient at higher risk of adverse reactions.

Home care instructions

- Instruct the patient to watch for and notify the doctor of any signs of infection (fever, sore throat, or redness, swelling, or drainage from the leg or chest incisions) or possible arterial reocclusion (angina, dizziness, dyspnea, rapid or irregular pulse, or prolonged recovery time from exercise).
- Explain that postpericardiotomy syndrome often develops after open-heart sur-

gery. Tell the patient to call his doctor if such symptoms as fever, muscle and joint pain, weakness, or chest discomfort occur.
- Prepare the patient for the possibility of postoperative depression, which may not develop until weeks after discharge. Reassure him that this depression is normal and should pass quickly.
- Make sure the patient understands the dose, frequency of administration, and possible adverse effects of all prescribed medications.
- Encourage the patient to follow his prescribed diet, especially noting any sodium and cholesterol restrictions. Explain that this diet can help reduce the risk of recurrent arterial occlusion.
- Instruct him to maintain a balance between activity and rest. Tell him to try to sleep at least 8 hours a night, to schedule a short rest period for each afternoon, and to rest frequently when engaging in tiring physical activity. As appropriate, tell him he can climb stairs, engage in sexual activity, take baths and showers, and do light chores. Tell him to avoid lifting heavy objects (greater than 20 lb [9 kg]), driving a car, or doing strenuous work (such as lawn mowing or vacuuming) until his doctor grants permission. If the doctor has prescribed an exercise program, encourage the patient to follow it.
- Refer the patient to a local chapter of the Mended Hearts Club and the American Heart Association for information and support.

Coronary artery disease

The dominant effect of coronary artery disease is the loss of oxygen and nutrients to myocardial tissue because of diminished coronary blood flow. Fatty fibrous plaques, calcium-plaque deposits, or combinations of both narrow the lumens of coronary arteries, reducing the volume of blood that can flow through them.

This disease is nearly epidemic in the Western world. Coronary artery disease is more prevalent in men, whites, and middle-aged and elderly people than in women or in people of other races and ages. More than 50% of men age 60 or older show signs of coronary artery disease on autopsy.

Causes

Atherosclerosis, the most common cause of coronary artery disease, has been linked to many risk factors. Some risk factors, such as the following, can't be controlled:
- *Age.* Atherosclerosis usually occurs after age 40.
- *Sex.* Men are eight times more susceptible than premenopausal women.
- *Heredity.* A positive family history of coronary artery disease increases the risk.
- *Race.* White men are more susceptible than nonwhite men; nonwhite women are more susceptible than white women.

However, the patient can modify other risk factors, such as the following, with good medical care and appropriate lifestyle changes:
- *Blood pressure.* Systolic blood pressure that is greater than 160 mm Hg or diastolic blood pressure that is greater than 95 mm Hg increases the risk.
- *Serum cholesterol levels.* Increased low-density lipoprotein and decreased high-density lipoprotein levels substantially heighten the risk.
- *Smoking.* Cigarette smokers are twice as likely to have a myocardial infarction and four times as likely to experience sudden death. The risk dramatically drops within 1 year after smoking ceases.
- *Obesity.* Added weight augments the risk for diabetes mellitus, hypertension, and elevated serum cholesterol levels.
- *Physical activity.* Regular exercise reduces the risk.
- *Stress.* Added stress or type A personality increases the risk.
- *Diabetes mellitus.* This disorder raises the risk, especially in women.

Understanding coronary artery spasm

In coronary artery spasm, a spontaneous, sustained contraction of one or more coronary arteries causes ischemia and dysfunction of the heart muscle. This disorder may also cause Prinzmetal's angina and even myocardial infarction in patients with unoccluded coronary arteries.

Causes

The direct cause of coronary artery spasm is unknown, but possible contributing factors include:

- altered influx of calcium across the cell membrane
- intimal hemorrhage into the medial layer of the blood vessel
- hyperventilation
- elevated catecholamine levels
- fatty buildup in the lumen.

Signs and symptoms

The major symptom of coronary artery spasm is angina. But unlike classic angina, this pain commonly occurs spontaneously and may be unrelated to physical exertion or emotional stress; it may, however, follow cocaine use. It is usually more severe than classic angina, lasts longer, and may be cyclic—recurring every day at the same time. Ischemic episodes may cause arrhythmias, altered heart rate, lower blood pressure and, occasionally, fainting caused by decreased cardiac output. Spasm in the left coronary artery may result in mitral valve prolapse, producing a loud systolic murmur and, possibly, pulmonary edema, with dyspnea, crackles, and hemoptysis. Myocardial infarction and sudden death may occur.

Treatment

After diagnosis by coronary angiography and 12-lead ECG, the patient may receive calcium channel blockers (verapamil, nifedipine, or diltiazem) to reduce coronary artery spasm and to decrease vascular resistance, and nitrates (nitroglycerin or isosorbide dinitrate) to relieve chest pain. During cardiac catheterization, the patient with clean arteries may receive ergotamine to induce the spasm and aid in the diagnosis.

Nursing interventions

When caring for a patient with coronary artery spasm, explain all necessary procedures and teach him how to take his medications safely. For calcium antagonist therapy, monitor the patient's blood pressure, pulse rate, and cardiac rhythm strips to detect arrhythmias.

For nifedipine and verapamil therapy, monitor digoxin levels and check for signs of digitalis toxicity. Because nifedipine may cause peripheral and periorbital edema, watch for fluid retention.

Because coronary artery spasm is sometimes associated with atherosclerotic disease, advise the patient to stop smoking, avoid overeating, use alcohol sparingly, and maintain a balance between exercise and rest.

- *Other modifiable factors.* Increased levels of serum fibrinogen and uric acid, elevated hematocrit, reduced vital capacity, high resting heart rate, thyrotoxicosis, and use of oral contraceptives heighten the risk.

Uncommon causes of reduced coronary artery blood flow include dissecting aneurysms, infectious vasculitis, syphilis, and congenital defects in the coronary vascular system. Coronary artery spasms may also impede blood flow. (See *Understanding coronary artery spasm.*)

Complications

When a coronary artery goes into spasm or is occluded by plaques, blood flow to the myocardium supplied by that vessel decreases, causing angina pectoris. Failure to remedy the occlusion causes ischemia and, eventually, myocardial tissue infarction.

Assessment

The classic symptom of coronary artery disease is angina, the direct result of inadequate flow of oxygen to the myocardium. The patient usually describes it as a burning, squeezing, or crushing tightness in the substernal or precordial chest that may radiate to the left arm, neck, jaw, or shoulder blade. Typically, the patient clenches his fist over his chest or rubs his left arm when describing the pain. Nausea, vomiting, fainting, sweating, and cool extremities may accompany the tightness.

Angina commonly occurs after physical exertion but may also follow emotional excitement, exposure to cold, or a large meal. Angina can also develop during sleep and may awaken the patient.

The patient's history will suggest any pattern to the type and onset of pain. If the pain is predictable and relieved by rest or nitrates, it's called stable angina. If it increases in frequency and duration and is more easily induced, it's referred to as unstable or unpredictable angina. Unstable angina generally indicates extensive or worsening disease and, untreated, may progress to myocardial infarction. An effort-induced pain that occurs with increasing frequency and with decreasing provocation is referred to as crescendo angina. If severe pain occurs at rest without provocation, it's called variant or Prinzmetal's angina.

Inspection may reveal evidence of atherosclerotic disease, such as xanthelasma and xanthoma. Ophthalmoscopic inspection may show increased light reflexes and arteriovenous nicking, suggesting hypertension, an important risk factor for coronary artery disease.

Palpation can uncover thickened or absent peripheral arteries, signs of cardiac enlargement, and abnormal contraction of the cardiac impulse, such as left ventricular akinesia or dyskinesia.

Auscultation may detect bruits, an S_3, an S_4, or a late systolic murmur (if mitral insufficiency is present).

Diagnostic tests

Diagnostic measures include the following:

- *Electrocardiography (ECG)* during angina shows ischemia, as demonstrated by T-wave inversion or ST-segment depression and, possibly, arrhythmias, such as premature ventricular contractions. ECG results may or may not be normal during pain-free periods. Arrhythmias may occur without infarction, secondary to ischemia.
- *Treadmill* or *bicycle exercise test* may provoke chest pain and ECG signs of myocardial ischemia in response to physical exertion. Monitoring of electrical rhythm may demonstrate T-wave inversion or ST-segment depression in the ischemic areas.
- *Coronary angiography* reveals coronary artery stenosis or obstruction, collateral circulation, and the arteries' condition beyond the narrowing.
- *Myocardial perfusion imaging* with thallium-201 during treadmill exercise detects ischemic areas of the myocardium, visualized as "cold spots."

Treatment

The goal of treatment in patients with angina is to reduce myocardial oxygen demand or increase the oxygen supply and reduce pain. Activity restrictions may be required to prevent onset of pain. Rather than eliminating activities, performing them more slowly often averts pain. Stress-reduction techniques are also essential, especially if known stressors precipitate pain.

Drug therapy consists primarily of nitrates, such as nitroglycerin, isosorbide dinitrate, or beta-adrenergic blockers.

Obstructive lesions may need atherectomy or coronary artery bypass graft surgery, using vein or arterial grafts. Percutaneous transluminal coronary angioplasty (PTCA) may be performed during cardiac catheterization to compress fatty deposits and relieve occlusion. (See the entries "Angioplasty, percutaneous transluminal coronary" and "Coronary artery bypass grafting.")

Laser angioplasty corrects occlusion by vaporizing fatty deposits with the excimer or hot-tip laser device.

Rotational ablation (or rotational atherectomy) removes atheromatous plaque with a high-speed, rotating burr covered with diamond crystals.

Because coronary artery disease is so widespread, prevention is important. Dietary restrictions aimed at reducing intake of calories (in obesity) and of salt, fats, and cholesterol minimize the risk, especially when supplemented with regular exercise. Abstention from smoking and reduction of stress are also essential.

Other preventive actions include control of hypertension (with diuretics or beta blockers), control of elevated serum cholesterol or triglyceride levels (with antilipemics, such as clofibrate), and measures to minimize platelet aggregation and the danger of blood clots (with aspirin, for example).

Key nursing diagnoses and patient outcomes

Altered cardiopulmonary tissue perfusion related to reduced blood flow to the myocardium caused by coronary artery spasm or occlusion. Based on this nursing diagnosis, you'll establish these patient outcomes. The patient will:

- maintain adequate myocardial tissue perfusion, as exhibited by a normal heart rate and rhythm and the absence of ischemic ECG changes
- verbalize an understanding of the prescribed medical regimen and relate the importance of seeking follow-up care for the rest of his life.

Pain related to inadequate oxygen flow to the myocardium as a result of reduced myocardial blood flow. Based on this nursing diagnosis, you'll establish these patient outcomes. The patient will:

- experience a reduction in the severity and frequency of anginal pain episodes by complying with medical or surgical therapy
- identify the factors that trigger anginal pain
- verbalize an understanding of what he needs to do when anginal pain occurs.

Activity intolerance related to an imbalance between myocardial oxygen supply and demand. Based on this nursing diagnosis, you'll establish these patient outcomes. The patient will:

- identify the activities he needs to avoid and the activities for which he must obtain assistance
- conserve energy while performing his daily activities
- participate in a medically supervised exercise program that will help him develop collateral myocardial circulation and increase his activity tolerance level.

Nursing interventions

- Keep nitroglycerin available for immediate use. Instruct the patient to call immediately whenever he feels chest, arm, or neck pain and before taking nitroglycerin.
- After a cardiac catheterization, review the expected course of treatment with the patient and his family. Also, to counter the diuretic effect of the dye, increase the I.V. flow rate and make sure the patient drinks plenty of fluids. Add potassium to the I.V. fluid, as ordered.
- Prepare the patient for PTCA or bypass surgery, as indicated.

Monitoring

- During anginal episodes, monitor blood pressure and heart rate. Take a 12-lead ECG during anginal episodes before administering nitroglycerin or other nitrates. Record duration of pain, amount of medication required to relieve it, and accompanying symptoms.
- Ask the patient to grade the severity of his pain on a scale of 1 to 10. This allows him to give his individual assessment of

HEALTH PROMOTION POINTERS

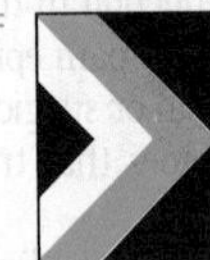

Reducing the risk of coronary artery disease

To reduce the patient's risk for coronary artery disease, certain risk factors can be altered. Teach the patient about:

- stress reduction techniques
- diets low in fat and cholesterol
- exercise and weight reduction programs
- smoking cessation
- caffeine intake reduction
- alcohol limitations or restrictions
- medical follow-up for such disorders as diabetes and hypertension.

pain as well as of the effectiveness of pain-relieving medications.

- Following cardiac catheterization, monitor the patient's catheter site for bleeding, evaluate his distal pulses, and periodically check his serum potassium level.
- After rotational ablation, monitor the patient for chest pain, hypotension, coronary artery spasm, and bleeding from the catheter site. Provide heparin and antibiotics for 24 to 48 hours, as ordered.

Patient teaching

- Explain cardiac catheterization to the patient. Make sure he understands its purpose and risks and possible indications for other interventional therapies (such as PTCA, bypass surgery, or atherectomy).
- If the patient is scheduled for surgery, explain the procedure and events.
- Help the patient more effectively cope with stress and identify activities that precipitate pain.
- Stress the need to follow the prescribed drug regimen.
- Explain that recurrent angina symptoms after PTCA or rotational ablation may signal recurring obstruction.
- Encourage the patient to maintain the prescribed low-sodium diet and if the patient is also obese, start a low-calorie diet.
- Encourage regular, moderate exercise. Refer the patient to a cardiac rehabilitation center or cardiovascular fitness program.
- Discuss issues surrounding sexual activity and possible modifications. Review the patient's medications – impotency occurs commonly with many cardiac medications.
- If necessary, refer the patient to a program to stop smoking. (See *Reducing the risk of coronary artery disease.*)

Cor pulmonale

Also called right ventricular hypertrophy, cor pulmonale occurs at the end stage of various chronic disorders that affect lung function or structure (except those stemming from congenital heart disease or diseases that affect the left side of the heart).

Cor pulmonale follows some disorders of the lungs, pulmonary vessels, chest wall, or respiratory control center. Because cor pulmonale often occurs late in chronic obstructive pulmonary disease (COPD) and other irreversible diseases, its prognosis is poor.

The disorder accounts for about 25% of all types of heart failure, and it's most common in patients who smoke and who have COPD.

Causes

In cor pulmonale, pulmonary hypertension increases the heart's work load. To compensate, the right ventricle hypertrophies to force blood through the lungs. However, the compensatory mechanism begins to fail, and larger amounts of blood remain in the right ventricle at the end of diastole. This causes ventricular dilation. In response to hypoxia, the bone marrow produces more red blood cells, resulting in polycythemia. Then, the blood's viscosity increases, further aggravating pulmonary hypertension, increasing the right ventricle's work load, and causing heart failure.

Cor pulmonale may result from:

- disorders that affect pulmonary parenchyma (such as pulmonary fibrosis, pneumoconiosis, cystic fibrosis, periarteritis nodosa, and tuberculosis)
- pulmonary diseases that affect the airways (such as COPD and bronchial asthma)
- vascular diseases (such as vasculitis, pulmonary emboli, or external vascular obstruction resulting from a tumor or an aneurysm)
- chest wall abnormalities, including thoracic deformities (such as kyphoscoliosis and pectus excavatum)
- other external factors, including obesity, living at a high altitude, and neuromuscular disorders (such as muscular dystrophy and poliomyelitis).

Complications

Cor pulmonale eventually may lead to biventricular failure. Depending on the severity of cor pulmonale, hepatomegaly, edema, ascites, and pleural effusions may develop. Because of polycythemia, the risk of thromboembolism also increases.

Assessment

As long as the heart can compensate for the increased pulmonary vascular resistance, your patient will report signs and symptoms associated with the underlying disorder, occurring mostly in the respiratory system. The patient is most likely to complain of a chronic productive cough, exertional dyspnea, wheezing respirations, fatigue, and weakness.

Cor pulmonale progresses with dyspnea (even at rest) that worsens on exertion, tachypnea, orthopnea, edema, weakness, and right upper quadrant discomfort. Chest examination typically discloses characteristics of the underlying lung disease.

On inspection, you may find such signs of cor pulmonale (and right ventricular failure) as dependent edema and distended neck veins. Drowsiness and alterations in consciousness may also occur.

Palpation may disclose tachycardia and a weak pulse (from decreased cardiac output); an enlarged and tender liver; hepatojugular reflux; and a prominent parasternal or epigastric cardiac impulse.

Chest auscultation yields various findings, depending on the cause of cor pulmonale. If the patient also has COPD, auscultation may detect crackles, rhonchi, and diminished breath sounds. With disease secondary to upper airway obstruction or damage to the respiratory control center, auscultation findings may be normal except for a right ventricular lift, a gallop rhythm, and a loud pulmonic component of S_2.

If the patient has tricuspid insufficiency, you'll hear a pansystolic murmur at the lower left sternal border. The murmur's intensity increases when the patient inhales, distinguishing it from a murmur caused by mitral valve disease. Also, you may hear a right ventricular early murmur that increases on inspiration and can be heard at the left sternal border or over the epigastrium. You may also auscultate a systolic pulmonary ejection sound.

Diagnostic tests

- *Pulmonary artery catheterization* shows increased right ventricular and pulmonary artery pressures, resulting from increased pulmonary vascular resistance. Both right ventricular systolic and pulmonary artery systolic pressures will be over 30 mm Hg. Pulmonary artery diastolic pressure will be above 15 mm Hg.
- *Echocardiography* or *angiography* demonstrates right ventricular enlargement.
- *Chest X-rays* reveal large central pulmonary arteries and right ventricular enlargement.
- *Arterial blood gas (ABG) analysis* detects decreased partial pressure of oxygen (Pao_2) – usually less than 70 mm Hg and never more than 90 mm Hg.

NURSING ALERT

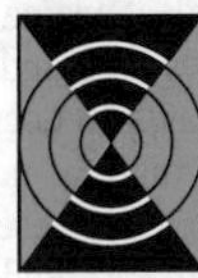

Oxygen administration precautions

If your patient with cor pulmonale needs oxygen, double-check his condition. If he also has underlying COPD, don't administer high concentrations of oxygen. This could precipitate respiratory depression.

• *Electrocardiography (ECG)* discloses arrhythmias, such as premature atrial and ventricular contractions and atrial fibrillation during severe hypoxia. The ECG may also show right bundle-branch block, right axis deviation, prominent P waves and inverted T wave in right precordial leads, and right ventricular hypertrophy.
• *Pulmonary function tests* provide values consistent with underlying pulmonary disease.
• *Hematocrit* is typically over 50%.
• *Serum hepatic enzyme levels* show an elevated serum level of aspartate aminotransferase (formerly SGOT) with hepatic congestion and decreased liver function.
• *Serum bilirubin level* may be elevated if liver dysfunction and hepatomegaly are present.

Treatment

Therapy for the patient with cor pulmonale aims to reduce hypoxemia, increase exercise tolerance and, when possible, correct the underlying condition.

Besides bed rest, treatment may include digitalis glycosides, such as digoxin, and antibiotics for an underlying respiratory tract infection. (Usually, sputum culture and sensitivity tests determine which antibiotic the patient receives.) To treat primary pulmonary hypertension, the patient may receive a potent pulmonary artery vasodilator, such as diazoxide, nitroprusside, or hydralazine.

The patient may need oxygen administered by mask or cannula in concentrations ranging from 24% to 40%, depending on PaO_2 values. In acute disease, therapy may also include mechanical ventilation. (See *Oxygen administration precautions.*)

The patient may benefit from a low-sodium diet, restricted fluid intake and, possibly, a diuretic (furosemide, for example) to reduce edema.

Occasionally, the patient with cor pulmonale may require phlebotomy to decrease red blood cell mass. Anticoagulation with small doses of heparin can decrease the risk for thromboembolism.

Depending on the underlying cause, some treatment variations may be indicated. For example, the patient may need a tracheotomy if he has an upper airway obstruction. He may require corticosteroids if he has vasculitis or an autoimmune disorder.

Key nursing diagnoses and patient outcomes

Activity intolerance related to hypoxemia caused by cor pulmonale. Based on this nursing diagnosis, you'll establish these patient outcomes. The patient will:
• identify controllable factors and activities that cause fatigue and dyspnea
• demonstrate methods of conserving energy while carrying out daily activities
• seek assistance as needed to perform activities of daily living.

Fluid volume excess related to right ventricular failure caused by cor pulmonale. Based on this nursing diagnosis, you'll establish these patient outcomes. The patient will:
• tolerate restricted fluid and sodium intake without physical or emotional discomfort
• maintain normal fluid balance, as exhibited by no weight gain, intake and output balance, and the absence of edema.

Risk for injury related to potential for polycythemia-induced thromboembolism. Based on this nursing diagnosis, you'll establish these patient outcomes. The patient will:

- use measures to prevent emboli formation, such as performing passive exercises, wearing antiembolism stockings, and changing his position regularly
- comply with anticoagulation therapy or scheduled phlebotomy, as ordered
- not develop a thromboembolism.

Nursing interventions

- Listen to the patient's fears and concerns about his illness. Remain with him when he feels severe stress and anxiety. Encourage him to identify actions and care measures that promote comfort and relaxation. Include him in care-related decisions whenever possible.
- Plan a nutritious diet carefully with the patient and the staff dietitian. Because the patient may tire easily, provide small, frequent feedings rather than three heavy meals. Avoid scheduling respiratory treatments immediately before meals.
- Prevent fluid retention by limiting the patient's fluid intake to 1,000 to 2,000 ml daily and by providing a low-sodium diet. Clarify the need for restricting fluids, especially if the patient has underlying COPD. (Most patients with COPD are encouraged to drink up to 10 glasses of water daily.)
- Reposition the bedridden patient often to prevent atelectasis.
- Provide meticulous respiratory care, including oxygen therapy and, for COPD patients, pursed-lip breathing exercises. Encourage the patient to rinse his mouth after respiratory therapies.
- Pace patient care activities to avoid patient fatigue.

Monitoring

- Monitor serum potassium levels closely if the patient takes a diuretic. Low serum potassium levels can potentiate the risk for arrhythmias associated with digitalis glycoside therapy.
- Be alert for complaints that signal digitalis toxicity, such as anorexia, nausea, vomiting, and seeing a yellow halo around an object. Monitor for cardiac arrhythmias.
- Periodically, measure ABG levels and watch for such signs of respiratory failure as change in pulse rate; deep, labored respirations; and increased fatigue produced by exertion.

Patient teaching

- Before the patient's discharge, make sure he understands the importance of maintaining a low-sodium diet, weighing himself daily, and immediately reporting edema. Teach him to detect edema by pressing the skin over his shins with one finger, holding it for 1 to 2 seconds, and then checking for a finger impression. He should report a weight gain of 2 to 3 lb (0.9 to 1.4 kg) over 1 to 2 days to his doctor or nurse at once.
- Instruct the patient to schedule frequent rest periods and to perform his breathing exercises regularly.
- Because pulmonary infection usually exacerbates cor pulmonale (and COPD), advise the patient to watch for and immediately report early signs of infection, such as increased sputum production, change in sputum color, increased coughing or wheezing, chest pain, fever, and tightness in the chest. Tell the patient to avoid crowds and people known to have infections, especially during the flu season.
- Warn the patient to avoid using nonprescription medications, such as sedatives, that may depress ventilatory drive. Teach him to check his radial pulse before taking digoxin or any digitalis glycoside. Instruct the patient to notify the doctor if he detects a pulse rate change.
- Urge the patient to discuss influenza and pneumonia immunizations with the doctor. Assist him to obtain the vaccines, if appropriate.

• Instruct the patient to add potassium-rich foods to his daily diet if he takes a potassium-wasting diuretic.
• If the patient needs suctioning or supplemental oxygen therapy at home, refer him to a social service agency that can help him obtain the equipment and care. As needed, arrange for follow-up examinations.
• If appropriate, discuss smoking cessation programs with the patient. Encourage him to quit smoking.

Craniotomy

This procedure involves creation of a surgical incision into the skull, thereby exposing the brain for treatment. These treatments may include ventricular shunting, excision of a tumor or abscess, hematoma aspiration, and aneurysm clipping.

Procedure

The surgical approach to a supratentorial craniotomy can be frontal, parietal, temporal, occipital, or a combination of these areas. If structures below the tentorium are involved, the surgical approach to an infratentorial craniotomy utilizes an incision slightly above the neck in the back of the skull. In the operating room just before surgery, the anesthetist will start a peripheral I.V. line, a central venous pressure (CVP) line, and an arterial line. The CVP line provides access to remove air should an air embolus occur—a particular risk when posterior fossa surgery is performed in the sitting position.

After the patient receives a general anesthetic, the surgeon marks an incision line and cuts through the scalp to the cranium, forming a scalp flap that he folds to one side. He then bores four or five holes through the skull in the corners of the cranial incision and cuts out a bone flap. After pulling aside or removing the bone flap, he incises and retracts the dura, exposing the brain. (See *Craniotomy: A window to the brain.*)

The surgeon then proceeds with the surgery. Afterward, he reverses the incision procedure and covers the site with a sterile dressing.

Complications

Craniotomy has many potential complications, including infection, vasospasm, hemorrhage, air embolism, respiratory compromise, increased intracranial pressure (ICP), diabetes insipidus, syndrome of inappropriate secretion of diuretic hormone, seizures, and cranial nerve damage; the degree of risk depends largely on the patient's condition and the surgery's complexity.

Key nursing diagnoses and patient outcomes

Altered cerebral tissue perfusion related to the surgical procedure performed during a craniotomy. Based on this nursing diagnosis, you'll establish these patient outcomes. The patient will:
• exhibit a postoperative mental status equal to or better than his preoperative status
• not demonstrate a new neurologic deficit postoperatively.

Risk for injury related to potential for increased ICP following a craniotomy. Based on this nursing diagnosis, you'll establish these patient outcomes. The patient will:
• exhibit an intracranial pressure within normal limits of 0 to 10 mm Hg
• not demonstrate such signs of increased intracranial pressure as worsening mental status or pupillary changes, or such focal signs as increasing weakness in an extremity.

Fear related to potential for permanent physical or psychological impairment as a result of the surgical procedure performed during a craniotomy. Based on this nursing diagnosis, you'll establish these patient outcomes. The patient will:
• be able to identify and verbalize his fears

Craniotomy: A window to the brain

To perform a craniotomy, the surgeon incises the skin, clamps the aponeurotic layer, and retracts the skin flap. He then incises and retracts the muscle layer and scrapes the periosteum off the skull.

Next, using an air-driven or electric drill, he drills a series of burr holes in the corners of the skull incision. During drilling, warm saline solution is dripped into the burr holes and the holes are suctioned to remove bone dust. Once drilling is complete, the surgeon uses a dural elevator to separate the dura from the bone around the margin of each burr hole. He then saws between the burr holes to create a bone flap. He either leaves this flap attached to the muscle and retracts it or detaches the flap completely and removes it. In either case, the flap is wrapped to keep it moist and protected.

Finally, the surgeon incises and retracts the dura, exposing the brain.

Initial incision

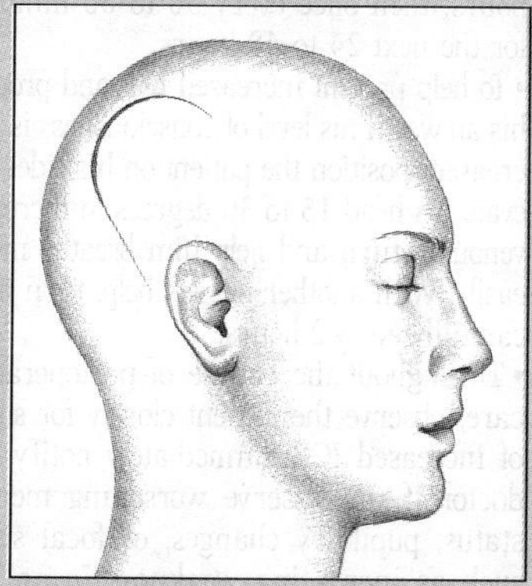

Retraction of skin flap

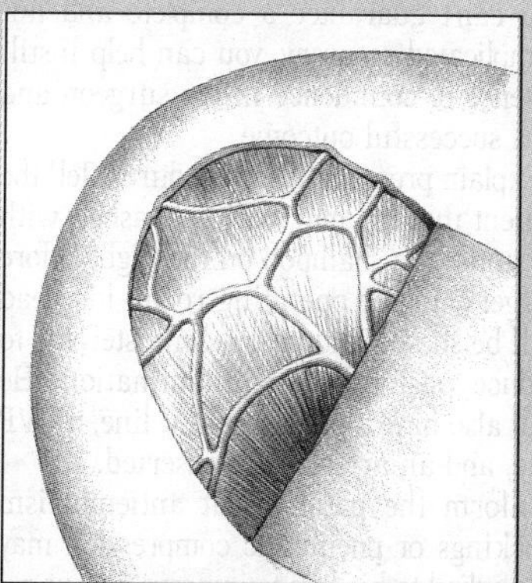

Burr holes drilled

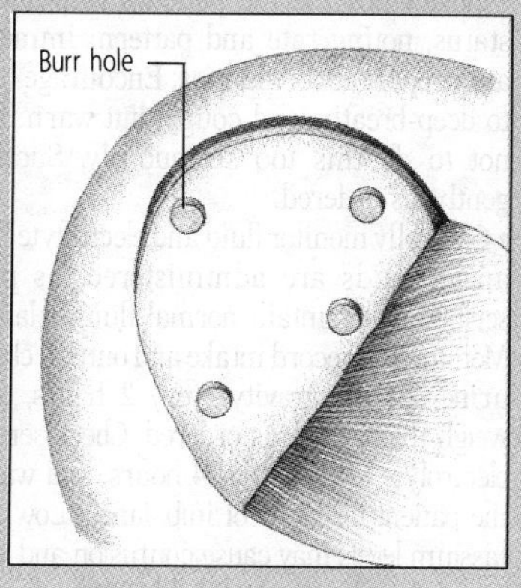

Brain exposed

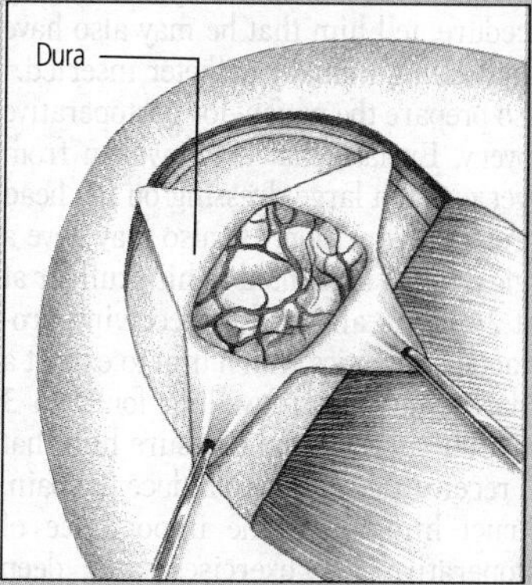

• request assistance from support systems to diminish his fears
• use at least one effective fear-reducing behavior each day preoperatively and postoperatively.

Nursing interventions

When preparing for or managing a patient with a craniotomy, expect to implement the following interventions.

Before surgery

• Help the patient and family cope with the surgery by clarifying the doctor's explanation and by encouraging them to ask questions. When answering their questions, be informative and honest. While you can't guarantee a complete and uncomplicated recovery, you can help instill a sense of confidence in the surgeon and in a successful outcome.
• Explain preoperative procedures. Tell the patient that his hair will be washed with an antiseptic shampoo on the night before surgery. In the operating room, his head will be shaved and he'll receive steroids to reduce postoperative inflammation. He will also have a peripheral I.V. line, a CVP line, and an arterial line inserted.
• Inform the patient that antiembolism stockings or pneumatic compression may be applied to his legs to improve venous return and reduce the risk of thrombophlebitis. And because craniotomy is a lengthy procedure, tell him that he may also have an indwelling urinary catheter inserted.
• Also prepare the patient for postoperative recovery. Explain that he'll awaken from surgery with a large dressing on his head to protect the incision. He also may have a surgical drain implanted in his skull for at least 24 hours and will be receiving prophylactic antibiotics. Warn him to expect a headache and facial swelling for 2 to 3 days after surgery, and reassure him that he'll receive medication to reduce the pain. Instruct him about the importance of postoperative leg exercises and deep breathing. Explain that, if all goes well, he should be ambulatory within 2 to 3 days after surgery. The doctor will usually remove the sutures within 7 to 10 days.
• Before surgery, perform a complete neurologic assessment. Carefully record your assessment data to use as a baseline for postoperative evaluation.
• Because the patient will go to the intensive care unit after surgery, arrange a preoperative visit for him and his family. Explain the equipment, and introduce them to the staff.

After surgery

• After surgery, carefully monitor the patient's vital signs and neurologic status. Check him every 15 minutes for the first 4 hours, then once every 30 to 60 minutes for the next 24 to 48 hours.
• To help prevent increased ICP and protect his airway if his level of consciousness is decreased, position the patient on his side. Elevate his head 15 to 30 degrees to increase venous return and help him breathe more easily. With another nurse's help, turn him carefully every 2 hours.
• Throughout the course of postoperative care, observe the patient closely for signs of increased ICP. Immediately notify the doctor if you observe worsening mental status, pupillary changes, or focal signs such as increasing weakness in an extremity.
• Closely observe the patient's respiratory status, noting rate and pattern. Immediately report abnormalities. Encourage him to deep-breathe and cough, but warn him not to do this too strenuously. Suction gently, as ordered.
• Carefully monitor fluid and electrolyte balance. Fluids are administered, as prescribed, to maintain normal fluid balance. Monitor and record intake and output, check urine specific gravity every 2 hours, and weigh the patient, as ordered. Check serum electrolyte levels every 24 hours, and watch the patient for signs of imbalance. Low potassium levels may cause confusion and stupor; reduced sodium and chloride levels may

produce weakness, lethargy, and even coma. Because fluid and electrolyte imbalance can precipitate seizures, report any of these signs immediately.

• Provide good wound care. Make sure the dressing stays dry and in place and that it's not too tight. Dressing tightness is usually related to soft-tissue swelling. If the patient has a closed drainage system, periodically check drain patency and note and document the amount and characteristics of any discharge. Notify the doctor of excessive bloody drainage, possibly indicating cerebral hemorrhage, or of clear or yellow drainage, which may indicate a cerebrospinal fluid leak. Also monitor the patient for signs of wound infection, such as fever and purulent drainage.

• Finally, provide supportive care. Ensure a quiet, calm environment to minimize anxiety and agitation and help lower ICP. Administer anticonvulsants, as ordered, and maintain seizure precautions. Provide other ordered medications, such as steroids to prevent or reduce cerebral edema, stool softeners to prevent increased ICP from straining during defecation, and analgesics to relieve pain.

Home care instructions

• Before discharge, teach the patient proper wound care techniques. Tell him to keep the suture line dry and to regularly clean the incision with hydrogen peroxide and saline solution. Instruct him to evaluate the incision regularly for redness, warmth, or tenderness and to report any of these findings to the doctor.

• If the patient is self-conscious about his appearance, suggest that he wear a wig, hat, or scarf until his hair grows back. As his hair begins to grow back, tell him to apply a lanolin-based lotion to keep his scalp supple and decrease itching. Remind him not to apply lotion to the suture line.

• Remind the patient to continue taking prescribed anticonvulsant medications to minimize the risk for seizures. Depending on the type of surgery performed, he may need to continue anticonvulsant therapy for up to 12 months after surgery. Also remind him to report any adverse drug effects, such as excessive drowsiness or confusion.

Crohn's disease

A type of inflammatory bowel disease, Crohn's disease can affect any part of the GI tract but usually involves the terminal ileum and upper colon. The disease extends through all layers of the intestinal wall and may involve regional lymph nodes and the mesentery.

Crohn's disease is most prevalent in adults ages 20 to 40. It is two to three times more common in Jews and least common in Blacks. The disease is not considered a predisposing factor for colon or rectal cancer.

Crohn's disease has a varied nomenclature. When it affects only the small bowel, it is also known as regional enteritis. If the disorder also involves the colon or only affects the colon, it is known as Crohn's disease of the colon. (Crohn's disease of the colon also has been termed granulomatous colitis—an inaccurate term because not all patients develop granulomas.)

Causes

Although researchers are still probing the etiology of Crohn's disease, possible causes include allergies and other immune disorders, lymphatic obstruction, and infection (although no infecting organism has been isolated). Genetic factors may also play a role: Crohn's disease sometimes occurs in monozygotic twins, and up to 5% of patients with the disease have one or more affected relatives. However, no simple pattern of inheritance has been identified.

Inflammation spreads slowly and progressively, beginning with lymphadenia and obstructive lymphedema in the submucosa, where Peyer's patches develop in the intestinal mucosa. Lymphatic obstruction causes edema, with mucosal ulceration and development of fissures, abscesses and, sometimes, granulomas. The mucosa may acquire a characteristic "cobblestone" look.

As the disease progresses, fibrosis occurs, thickening the bowel wall and narrowing the lumen. Serositis (serosal inflammation) also develops, causing inflamed bowel loops to adhere to other diseased or normal loops. This may result in bowel shortening. Because inflammation usually occurs segmentally, the bowel may become a patchwork of healthy and diseased segments. Eventually, the diseased parts of the bowel become thicker, more narrow, and shorter.

Complications

Anal fistula, resulting from severe diarrhea and enzymatic corrosion of the perineal area, is the most common complication. A perineal abscess may also develop during the active inflammatory state. Fistulas may develop to the bladder or vagina or even to the skin in an old scar area. Other complications include intestinal obstruction, nutritional deficiencies (caused by malabsorption and maldigestion) and, rarely, peritonitis.

Assessment

Generally, the patient reports signs and symptoms of gradual onset, marked by periods of remission and exacerbation. Because signs and symptoms may be intermittent, he may have postponed seeking medical attention for some time.

The patient typically complains of fatigue, fever, abdominal pain, diarrhea (usually without obvious bleeding) and, occasionally, weight loss. Questioning may reveal that his diarrhea worsens after emotional upset or after ingestion of poorly tolerated foods, such as milk, fatty foods, and spices.

The patient with regional enteritis, often a young adult, may report similar signs and symptoms as well as anorexia, nausea, and vomiting. Typically, this patient describes his abdominal pain as steady, colicky, or cramping. It usually occurs in the right lower abdominal quadrant.

On inspection, the patient's stool may appear soft or semiliquid, without gross blood (a distinguishing clinical feature from the bloody diarrhea seen in ulcerative colitis). Palpation may reveal tenderness in the right lower abdominal quadrant; it may also disclose an abdominal mass, indicating adherent loops of bowel.

Diagnostic tests

- *Laboratory analysis* to detect occult blood in stools is usually positive.
- *Small-bowel X-rays* may show irregular mucosa, ulceration, and stiffening.
- *Barium enema* that reveals the string sign (segments of stricture separated by normal bowel) supports the diagnosis. This test may also show fissures and narrowing of the lumen.
- *Sigmoidoscopy* and *colonoscopy* may show patchy areas of inflammation, thus helping to rule out ulcerative colitis. These studies may also reveal the characteristic coarse irregularity (cobblestone appearance) of the mucosal surface. When the colon is involved, discrete ulcerations may be evident.
- *Biopsy,* performed during sigmoidoscopy or colonoscopy, reveals granulomas in up to half of all specimens.
- *Laboratory test findings* indicate increased white blood cell count and erythrocyte sedimentation rate. Other findings include hypokalemia, hypocalcemia, hypomagnesemia, and decreased hemoglobin levels.

Treatment

Effective management of Crohn's disease requires drug therapy and significant life-style changes, including physical rest and dietary restrictions. In debilitated patients, treatment includes total parenteral nutrition to maintain nutrition while resting the bowel.

Drug therapy, designed to combat inflammation and relieve symptoms, may include:

- corticosteroids, such as prednisone, to reduce signs and symptoms of diarrhea,

pain, and bleeding by decreasing inflammation
- immunosuppressant agents, such as azathioprine, to suppress the body's response to antigens
- sulfasalazine to reduce inflammation
- metronidazole to treat perianal complications
- antidiarrheals, such as diphenoxylate and atropine, to combat diarrhea (contraindicated in patients with significant bowel obstruction)
- narcotics to control pain and diarrhea.

Life-style changes, such as stress reduction and reduced physical activity, help to rest the bowel, giving it time to heal. Also essential are dietary changes that decrease bowel activity while still providing adequate calories and nutrition. Dietary modifications include elimination of high-fiber foods (no fruits or vegetables) and foods that irritate the mucosa (such as dairy products, and spicy and fatty foods). Foods that stimulate excessive intestinal activity (such as carbonated or caffeinated beverages) also should be avoided. Vitamins may be prescribed to compensate for the bowel's inability to absorb them.

If complications develop, surgery may be required. Indications for surgery include bowel perforation, massive hemorrhage, fistulas, or acute intestinal obstruction. Colectomy with ileostomy is often necessary in patients with extensive disease of the large intestine and rectum.

Key nursing diagnoses and patient outcomes

Altered nutrition: Less than body requirements related to malabsorption and diarrhea caused by Crohn's disease. Based on this nursing diagnosis, you'll establish these patient outcomes. The patient will:
- regain lost weight and then maintain his weight
- eat a well-balanced diet while obeying dietary restrictions and taking ordered nutritional supplements.
- not become malnourished.

Diarrhea related to bowel changes as a result of Crohn's disease. Based on this nursing diagnosis, you'll establish these patient outcomes. The patient will:
- not develop a fluid and electrolyte disturbance because of diarrhea
- obtain relief from diarrhea by making appropriate changes in his diet and lifestyle and by taking prescribed antidiarrheal agents
- experience a cessation of diarrhea after treatment.

Pain related to inflammation of the bowel caused by Crohn's disease. Based on this nursing diagnosis, you'll establish these patient outcomes. The patient will:
- avoid stressful situations and foods that contribute to bowel inflammation
- experience a relief of pain after analgesic administration
- become pain free with treatment.

Nursing interventions

- Provide emotional support to the patient and his family. Listen to the patient's concerns, and help him cope.
- Schedule patient care to include rest periods throughout the day.
- Provide the patient with a diet that is high in protein, calories, and vitamins. Also try providing frequent, small meals throughout the day rather than three large meals.
- If patient is receiving parenteral nutrition, provide meticulous site care.
- Give iron supplements and blood transfusions, as ordered.
- Administer medications, as ordered.
- Provide good patient hygiene and meticulous oral care if the patient is restricted to nothing by mouth. After each bowel movement, provide careful skin care. Always keep a clean, covered bedpan within the patient's reach. Ventilate the room to eliminate odors.
- Prepare the patient for surgery, if indicated. (See the entries "Bowel resection with anastomosis" and "Bowel resection with ostomy.")

Monitoring

- Record fluid intake and output (including the amount of stools), and weigh the patient daily. Watch for dehydration, and maintain fluid and electrolyte balance. Be alert for signs of intestinal bleeding (bloody stools); check stools for occult blood.
- If the patient is receiving total parenteral nutrition, monitor his condition closely.
- If the patient is receiving steroids, watch for adverse reactions, such as GI bleeding. Remember that steroids can mask signs of infection.
- Monitor hemoglobin and hematocrit levels.
- Evaluate the effectiveness of medication administration, and watch for adverse reactions.
- Monitor the patient for complications. Watch for fever and pain on urination, which may signal bladder fistula. Abdominal pain, fever, and a hard, distended abdomen may indicate intestinal obstruction.

Patient teaching

- Teach the patient about the disease, its symptoms, and its complications. Explain ordered diagnostic tests; make sure he's aware of all pretest dietary restrictions or other pretest guidelines. Answer his questions.
- Emphasize the importance of adequate rest. Explain that limiting physical activity helps to reduce intestinal motility and promote healing.
- Encourage the patient to identify and reduce sources of stress in his life. If stress clearly aggravates his disease, teach him stress-management techniques or refer him for counseling.
- Be sure the patient understands prescribed dietary changes. Emphasize the need for a restricted diet, which may be trying, especially for a young patient. Refer him to a dietitian for further instruction, if necessary.
- Give the patient a list of foods to avoid, including milk products, spicy or fried high-residue foods, raw vegetables and fruits, and whole-grain cereals. Advise him to avoid carbonated, caffeinated, or alcoholic beverages (because they increase intestinal activity) and extremely hot or cold foods or fluids (because they increase flatus). Remind him to take supplemental vitamins, if prescribed.
- Teach the patient about prescribed medications, their desired effects, and possible adverse reactions. Urge him to call his doctor if adverse reactions occur.
- If the patient smokes, encourage him to quit and assist him in joining a smoking-cessation program. Point out that smoking can aggravate his disease by altering bowel motility.
- Instruct the patient to notify his doctor if he experiences signs and symptoms of complications, such as fever, fatigue, weakness, a rapid heart rate, abdominal cramping or pain, vomiting, or acute diarrhea.
- If the patient is scheduled for surgery, provide preoperative teaching. Reinforce the doctor's explanation of the surgery, and mention possible complications.

Cryosurgery

Often performed in the doctor's office, cryosurgery refers to the destruction of tissue by the application of extreme cold. The procedure is used to treat dermatologic conditions such as actinic and seborrheic keratoses, leukoplakia, molluscum contagiosum, condyloma acuminatum, verrucae, and sometimes early basal cell epitheliomas and squamous cell carcinomas. It's also used to treat gynecologic conditions such as cervicitis, chronic cervical erosion, cervical polyps, and condyloma accuminata as well as ophthalmic conditions such as cataracts and retinal tears or holes.

Cryosurgery's success depends on the type of lesion, the extent and depth of the freeze, and the duration between freezing and thawing. A slow thaw destroys lesions most effectively.

Liquid nitrogen and nitrous oxide (N_2O) are the most commonly used cryogens. Carbon dioxide and freon are less frequently used. At −320° F (−196° C), liquid nitrogen is by far the most powerful cryogen. It's especially useful for treating cancers, which resist cold well because of their vascularity. N_2O is often favored for less extensive procedures, since the surgeon can more easily control its effects.

Procedure

The procedure varies with the area being treated. For dermatologic cryosurgery, the surgeon may give a local anesthetic depending on the type and extensiveness of the lesion. He'll then determine the correct temperature and depth for freezing. For superficial lesions, he can often determine this simply by palpating and observing the lesion. For skin cancers, however, he'll use thermocouple needles and a tissue temperature monitor (pyrometer) to be sure that tissue at the deepest part of the lesion has been adequately frozen.

If the surgeon is using thermocouple needles, assist him as he inserts and secures them into the base of the tumor. (See *Positioning thermocouple needles,* page 234.) Next, clean the operative site with povidone-iodine solution. The surgeon will then use either a cotton-tipped applicator that has been dipped into liquid nitrogen or the complex cryosurgical unit to freeze the lesion. He may refreeze a tumor several times to ensure its destruction; for each cycle, monitor and record the number of seconds that elapse until the tissue reaches −4° F (−20° C) and the number of seconds that it takes the tissue to thaw. After cryosurgery, leave the area uncovered.

For gynecologic cryosurgery, the patient will come to the doctor's office one week after a menstrual cycle. Anesthesia is usually not given. Place the patient in the lithotomy position. The doctor will then insert a speculum into the vagina. After locating and inspecting the cervix, he'll slide the cryoprobe through the speculum and place it against the cervix. This will freeze the tissue, which will later become necrotic and slough off. After the procedure, tell the patient to expect a heavy, watery discharge for the next several weeks. Warn her that the discharge will be heavy enough to require that she wear a peripad.

For ophthalmic cryosurgery, the doctor will first instill mydriatic and anesthetic eyedrops into the affected eye. Then, once the patient's eye dilates and becomes numb, he'll position the cryoprobe. Typically, he'll place the cryoprobe on the conjunctiva, directly over the anterior retinal break. However, if he'll be treating the posterior retinal area, he'll first cut an opening in the conjunctiva and rotate the eye to expose a large portion of the sclera. After the procedure, apply a patch to the affected eye. (See the entry "Cataract removal.")

Complications

Complications, when they occur, are usually minor. They include hypopigmentation (from destruction of melanocytes) and secondary infection. Rarely, the procedure may damage blood vessels, nerves, and tear ducts. Following gynecologic cryosurgery, cervical stenosis may result if too large an area of the cervix is frozen at one time.

Key nursing diagnoses and patient outcomes

Risk for infection related to change in tissue integrity caused by cryosurgery. Based on this nursing diagnosis, you'll establish these patient outcomes. The patient will:
- maintain a normal temperature and white blood cell count
- not have a purulent drainage from the treated area
- remain free from infection.

Pain related to tissue sensitivity to extreme cold as a result of cryosurgery. Based on this nursing diagnosis, you'll establish these patient outcomes. The patient will:
- express a relief of pain after analgesic administration

Positioning thermocouple needles

During cryosurgery, you may be responsible for positioning thermocouple needles and then operating them according to the surgeon's direction. These needles measure the temperature of the tissue at its tip and help the doctor gauge the depth of freezing—a vitally important factor when destroying cancerous lesions. The needle may be placed in any of several positions.

Precise temperature measurement can be difficult because a variation of only 1 mm in the needle's position can translate into a difference of 50° to 59° F (10° to 15° C). For that reason, you'll usually place two or more needles in different areas to increase the accuracy of the reading.

In this illustration, the needle is shown inserted at an angle so that its tip rests about 5 mm below the base of the tumor to give a direct reading of tissue temperature. In this position, the temperature reading may be affected by chilling of the shaft within the frozen tissue, but the error isn't likely to be significant.

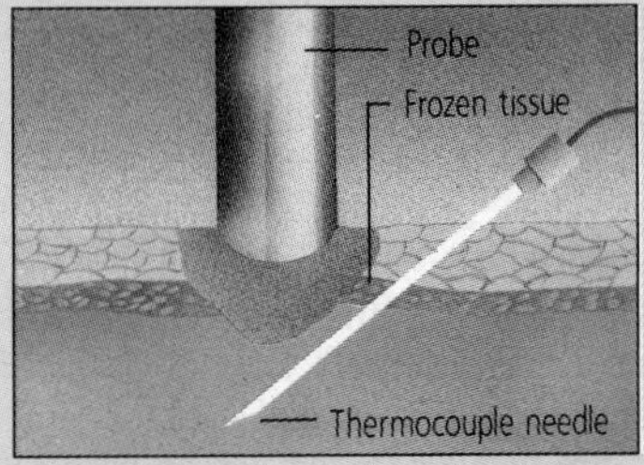

Here the probe is placed about 5 mm to one side of the frozen tissue at a depth of about 3 mm. In this position, it will register the same temperature as the probe above because both probe tips are about the same distance from the frozen tissue.

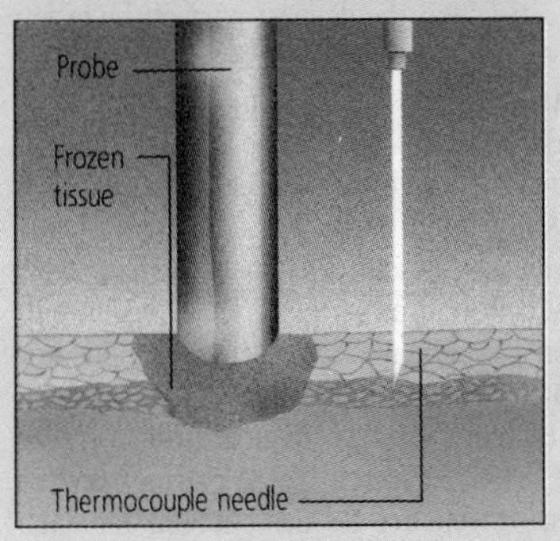

- take precautions to prevent bumping or injuring the treated area
- become pain free after healing is complete.

Body image disturbance related to transient skin changes caused by dermatologic cryosurgery. Based on this nursing diagnosis, you'll establish these patient outcomes. The patient will:

- verbalize his feelings about transient changes in body image
- not cover the treated area with anything other than a loose dressing when outdoors
- express positive feelings about his body image.

Nursing interventions

When caring for a patient undergoing cryosurgery, your primary responsibilities will include instructing the patient and preparing for and assisting with the procedure.

Before surgery

• Ask the patient if he has any known allergies or hypersensitivities, especially to lidocaine, iodine, or cold.

• Most patients will be unfamiliar with cryosurgery, so briefly explain the procedure and its intended purpose. Outline the basic steps of the procedure to the patient.

• Tell the patient that he'll initially feel cold, followed by burning, during the procedure. Caution him to remain as still as possible to prevent inadvertent freezing of unaffected tissue.

• Inform the patient having gynecologic cryosurgery that she may experience headache, dizziness, flushing, or cramping during the procedure. Reassure her that these adverse reactions are transient.

• After providing the patient with this overview, gather the necessary equipment. If you'll be using thermocouple needles and a pyrometer, obtain them as well; make sure they're sterile and in proper working order. You may also need tape to secure the needles to the base of the lesion, and you'll need a watch or clock with a second hand to time the thaw and freeze cycles accurately. Obtain the local anesthetic, alcohol swabs, and gauze.

• Some surgeons use gentian violet or a surgical marker to delineate the margins of the lesion. If necessary, obtain the appropriate marker.

• Check to be sure the patient or a responsible family member has signed a consent form.

• Position the patient comfortably and as required by the particular site being treated. If necessary, shield his eyes or ears to prevent damage.

After surgery

• After dermatologic cryosurgery, clean the area gently with a cotton-tipped applicator soaked in hydrogen peroxide. Because cryosurgery doesn't cause bleeding, you needn't apply a bandage. In fact, occlusive dressings are contraindicated.

• After gynecologic cryosurgery, monitor the type and amount of vaginal drainage.

• After ophthalmic cryosurgery, remove the eye patch when the anesthesia has worn off.

• If necessary, apply an ice bag to relieve swelling and give analgesics to relieve pain, as ordered. Cryosurgery may cause considerable pain, especially if it was performed on or near the lips, eyes, eyelids, tongue, or plantar surfaces of the feet. Generalized headache may persist for more than an hour after freezing of a scalp tumor.

Home care instructions

• Tell the patient to expect pain, but tell him he may take the prescribed analgesic as needed.

• Tell the dermatologic patient to expect pain, redness, and swelling and that a blister will form within 6 hours of treatment. Ordinarily, it will flatten within a few days and slough off in 2 to 3 weeks. Serous exudation may follow during the 1st week, accompanied by the development of a crust or eschar.

• Warn the dermatologic patient that the blister may be large and may bleed. Warn him not to touch it, to promote healing and prevent infection. Tell him that if the blister becomes uncomfortable or interferes with daily activities, he should call the doctor, who can decompress it with a sterile blade or pin.

• Tell the dermatologic patient to clean the area gently with soap and water, alcohol, or a cotton-tipped applicator soaked in hydrogen peroxide, as ordered. To prevent hypopigmentation, instruct him to cover the wound with a loose dressing when he's outdoors. After the wound heals, he should apply a sunscreen over the area.

• Tell the gynecologic patient that she will have a watery vaginal discharge for several weeks. Warn her not to use tampons and to avoid sexual intercourse while the discharge is present because the cervix is very fragile during this time.

• Emphasize the importance of calling the doctor immediately if the dermatologic patient experiences extreme pain, a widening area of erythema, oozing (of other than serous material), or fever; if the gynecologic patient experiences a vaginal discharge other than a watery appearance and fever; and if the ophthalmic patient experiences sudden changes in vision or an increase in eye pain.
• If the patient had a cancerous lesion destroyed, urge him to have regular checkups since cancers may recur.

Cryptosporidiosis

This intestinal infection typically results in acute, self-limited diarrhea. However, in immunocompromised patients, cryptosporidiosis causes chronic, severe, and life-threatening symptoms.

The disease is prevalent in immunocompromised patients, such as malnourished children, patients with hypogammaglobulinemia, and those who receive immunosuppressants for cancer therapy or organ transplantation. It's especially prevalent in patients with acquired immunodeficiency syndrome (AIDS), in whom the incidence can be as high as 30%.

Cryptosporidiosis occurs worldwide. In addition to immunocompromised patients, children, foreign travelers, and medical personnel caring for patients with the disease are at particular risk. Incidence in children with gastroenteritis in Western countries ranges from 1% to 4%; in developing countries, up to 11% of children with gastroenteritis have cryptosporidiosis.

Cryptosporidiosis is increasingly recognized as a major cause of diarrhea in the United States. An outbreak in Milwaukee in 1993, caused by contamination of the public water supply, resulted in an estimated 400,000 cases. Other outbreaks have been traced to contaminated swimming pools and fresh-pressed apple cider.

Causes

Cryptosporidiosis is caused by the protozoan *Cryptosporidium*. These small spherules inhabit the microvillus border of the intestinal epithelium. There, the protozoa shed infected oocysts into the intestinal lumen, where they pass into the feces.

These oocysts are particularly hardy, resisting destruction by routine water chlorination. This increases the risk for infection spreading through contact with contaminated water. The disease can also be transmitted by means of contaminated food and person-to-person contact.

Complications

Complications can be particularly severe in immunocompromised patients. In these patients, profuse, watery diarrhea can lead to severe fluid and electrolyte depletion and malnutrition. Rectal excoriation and breakdown can also result.

If the biliary tract becomes affected, papillary stenosis, sclerosing cholangitis, or cholecystitis can occur.

Assessment

Although asymptomatic infections can occur in both normal and immunocompromised patients, the typical patient with cryptosporidiosis develops symptoms after an incubation period of about 7 days. (The incubation period may be less in an immunocompromised patient.) The patient initially complains of watery, nonbloody diarrhea. Other signs include abdominal pain, anorexia, nausea, fever, and weight loss. In the 10% of patients who develop biliary tract involvement, right upper abdominal pain may be severe. Signs and symptoms usually subside within 2 weeks but may recur sporadically for months to years.

The history of an immunocompromised patient typically reveals a more gradual onset of symptoms. Such a patient may also develop more severe diarrhea with daily fluid losses as high as 20 liters.

For all patients, auscultation of the abdomen may reveal hyperactive bowel sounds. Palpation may reveal abdominal tenderness.

Diagnostic tests

Cryptosporidiosis often goes undetected as the cause of profuse diarrhea because the acid-fast stain needed to detect the organism isn't routinely used. However, the acid-fast stain as well as microscopic examination of stool samples reveals the presence of oocysts. If too few oocysts are excreted to be seen readily under microscopic examination, Sheather's cover-slip flotation method can make detection easier by concentrating the oocysts.

The infecting organisms can also be detected by light and electron microscopy at the apical surfaces of intestinal epithelium obtained through biopsies of the small bowel. Although serologic tests exist, their value in diagnosing acute or chronic infections in immunocompromised patients hasn't been determined. With biliary tract involvement, studies may reveal an elevated alkaline phosphatase level, gallbladder wall thickening, and dilated bile ducts.

Treatment

Although no treatment currently exists that can eradicate the infecting organism, several medications, such as zidovudine, spiramycin, diclazuril, and azithromycin, are being investigated to control the disease in patients with AIDS.

Treatment consists of supportive measures, including fluid replacement (to prevent dehydration) and administration of analgesics (to relieve pain) and antidiarrheal and antiperistaltic agents (to control diarrhea). Occasionally, a patient – especially one who is immunocompromised – may require I.V. hyperalimentation therapy to maintain adequate nutrition.

Key nursing diagnoses and patient outcomes

Diarrhea related to intestinal infection. Based on this nursing diagnosis, you'll establish these patient outcomes. The patient will:
• remain free of problems associated with diarrhea, such as malnutrition, fluid and electrolyte imbalance, and skin breakdown
• regain normal bowel elimination pattern
• demonstrate appropriate personal hygiene, including proper handwashing to prevent transmission.

Risk for fluid volume deficit related to fluid loss from diarrhea. Based on this nursing diagnosis, you'll establish these patient outcomes. The patient will:
• remain free of signs and symptoms of fluid volume deficit
• maintain adequate intake and output.

Risk for impaired skin integrity related to anal irritation from diarrhea. Based on this nursing diagnosis, you'll establish these patient outcomes. The patient will:
• demonstrate measures to adequately clean and dry anal area after each bowel movement
• remain free of irritation and excoriation
• maintain intact skin.

Nursing interventions

• Institute standard precautions.
• Administer analgesics, antidiarrheal and antiperistaltic agents, and antibiotics, as ordered. Watch the patient for signs of adverse reactions as well as therapeutic effects.
• Apply perirectal protective cream to prevent excoriation and skin breakdown.
• Encourage small, frequent meals to help prevent nausea.

Monitoring

• Closely monitor the patient's fluid and electrolyte balance.
• Encourage an adequate intake of fluids, especially those rich in electrolytes.
• Monitor the patient's fluid intake and output, and weigh him daily to evaluate the need for fluid replacement. Watch him closely for signs of dehydration, and provide fluid replacement as ordered.
• If the patient is receiving I.V. nutritional therapy, monitor him carefully. Provide

meticulous skin care to maintain skin integrity at the I.V. site.

Patient teaching

• Teach the patient about his medications. Make sure he understands how to take the drugs and which adverse reactions to watch for. Stress the importance of calling his doctor immediately if he develops an adverse reaction.

• Teach the patient and his family to recognize the signs and symptoms of dehydration, including weight loss, poor skin turgor, oliguria, irritability, and dry flushed skin. Tell them to report such findings to the doctor.

• Teach the patient and his family about good personal hygiene, especially proper hand-washing technique. Explain to them how to safely handle potentially infectious material, such as soiled bed sheets.

• Advise the patient's family members and close contacts to have their stools tested.

Cushing's syndrome

Chronic glucocorticoid excess leads to development of symptoms and physical features known as Cushing's syndrome. The most common cause is iatrogenic, resulting from chronic glucocorticoid therapy. Spontaneous Cushing's syndrome is caused by abnormalities of the pituitary or adrenal or because of adrenocorticotropic hormone (ACTH) secretion by nonpituitary tumors. Cushing's disease is defined as the specific type of Cushing's syndrome caused by excessive pituitary ACTH secretion from a pituitary tumor.

Causes

In about 70% of patients, Cushing's syndrome results from excess production of ACTH and consequent hyperplasia of the adrenal cortex. ACTH overproduction may stem from pituitary hypersecretion (Cushing's disease), an ACTH-producing tumor in another organ (particularly bronchogenic or pancreatic carcinoma), or administration of synthetic glucocorticoids or ACTH. In the remaining 30% of patients, Cushing's syndrome results from a cortisol-secreting adrenal tumor, which is usually benign.

Complications

The stimulating and catabolic effects of cortisol produce the complications of Cushing's syndrome. Increased calcium resorption from bone may lead to osteoporosis and pathologic fractures. Peptic ulcer may result from increased gastric secretions, pepsin production, and decreased gastric mucus. Increased hepatic gluconeogenesis and insulin resistance can cause impaired glucose tolerance. Overt diabetes mellitus occurs in fewer than 20% of patients.

Frequent infections or slow wound healing due to decreased lymphocyte production and suppressed antibody formation may occur. Suppressed inflammatory response may mask even a severe infection.

Hypertension due to sodium and water retention is common and may lead to ischemic heart disease and congestive heart failure. Menstrual disturbances and sexual dysfunction also occur. Decreased ability to handle stress may result in psychiatric problems, ranging from mood swings to frank psychosis.

Assessment

The patient may report using synthetic steroids. She may complain of fatigue, muscle weakness, sleep disturbances, water retention, amenorrhea, decreased libido, irritability, and emotional lability. Additionally, she may list signs and symptoms similar to those of hypoglycemia. Inspection may reveal a spectrum of characteristic signs and symptoms, including thin hair, a moon-shaped face from fluid retention, hirsutism, acne, a buffalo-humplike back, and thin extremities from muscle wasting. Other observable features are petechiae, ecchymoses, and purplish striae; delayed wound healing; and swollen ankles. Auscultation typically reveals hypertension.

Diagnostic tests

Diagnosis of Cushing's syndrome depends on a demonstrated increase in cortisol production and the failure to suppress endogenous cortisol secretion after administration of dexamethasone. Initial screening may consist of a 24-hour urine test to determine free cortisol excretion rate in addition to the tests described below. Failure to suppress plasma and urine cortisol levels confirms the diagnosis of Cushing's syndrome.

A high-dose dexamethasone suppression test can determine if Cushing's syndrome results from pituitary dysfunction (Cushing's disease). In this diagnostic test, dexamethasone suppresses plasma cortisol levels, and urine 17-hydroxycorticosteroid (17-OHCS) and 17-ketosteroid levels fall to 50% or less of basal levels. Failure to suppress these levels indicates that the syndrome results from an adrenal tumor or a nonendocrine, corticotropin-secreting tumor. This test can produce false-positive results.

In a stimulation test, administration of metyrapone, which blocks cortisol production by the adrenal glands, tests the ability of the pituitary gland and the hypothalamus to detect and correct low levels of plasma cortisol by increasing corticotropin production. The patient with Cushing's disease reacts to this stimulus by secreting an excess of plasma corticotropin as measured by levels of urine 17-OHCS. If the patient has an adrenal or a nonendocrine corticotropin-secreting tumor, the pituitary gland – which is suppressed by the high cortisol levels – cannot respond normally, so steroid levels remain stable or fall.

Radiologic evaluation for Cushing's syndrome seeks to locate the causative tumor in the pituitary gland or the adrenals. Tests include ultrasonography, a computed tomography scan, and magnetic resonance imaging enhanced with gadolinium.

Treatment

Management to restore hormone balance and reverse Cushing's syndrome may necessitate radiation, drug therapy, or surgery.

Pituitary-dependent Cushing's syndrome with adrenal hyperplasia may require bilateral adrenalectomy, hypophysectomy, or pituitary irradiation. Nonendocrine corticotropin-producing tumors require excision of the tumor, followed by drug therapy with mitotane, metyrapone, or aminoglutethimide. Aminoglutethimide and cyproheptadine decrease cortisol levels and have been beneficial for many cushingoid patients. Aminoglutethimide alone, or in combination with metyrapone, may also be useful in metastatic adrenal carcinoma.

Before surgery, the patient with cushingoid symptoms requires management to control hypertension, edema, diabetes, and cardiovascular manifestations and to prevent infection. Glucocorticoid administration the morning of surgery can help prevent acute adrenal insufficiency during surgery. Cortisol therapy is essential during and after surgery to help the patient tolerate the physiologic stress imposed by removal of the pituitary or adrenal glands. If normal cortisol production resumes, steroid therapy may gradually be tapered and eventually discontinued. However, bilateral adrenalectomy or total hypophysectomy mandates lifelong steroid replacement therapy to correct hormonal deficiencies.

Key nursing diagnoses and patient outcomes

Body image disturbance related to changes caused by Cushing's syndrome. Based on this nursing diagnosis, you'll establish these patient outcomes. The patient will:

- verbalize her feelings about her changed body image
- express positive feelings about herself.

Risk for infection related to suppressed inflammatory response caused by excessive corticosteroid production. Based on this nursing diagnosis, you'll establish these patient outcomes. The patient will:

- maintain a normal temperature and white blood cell count and differential
- remain free from infection
- take precautions to avoid, or decrease her risk for, infection.

Risk for injury related to the stimulating and catabolic adverse effects of excessive corticosteroid production on body tissue. Based on this nursing diagnosis, you'll establish these patient outcomes. The patient will:

- identify the early signs and symptoms of complications associated with Cushing's syndrome and state the importance of seeking medical attention if they occur
- express an understanding of measures to prevent complications, such as obtaining adequate rest, eating a well-balanced diet, complying with the treatment regimen, and taking precautions against infection
- remain free from injury.

Nursing interventions

- Consult a dietitian to plan a diet high in protein and potassium but low in calories, carbohydrates, and sodium.
- Use protective measures to reduce the risk for infection. If necessary, provide a private room and institute reverse isolation precautions. Use meticulous handwashing technique.
- Schedule activities around the patient's rest periods to avoid fatigue. Gradually increase activity as tolerated.
- Institute safety precautions to minimize the risk for injury from falls. Help the patient walk to avoid bumps and bruises.
- Help the bedridden patient turn and reposition herself every 2 hours. Use extreme caution while moving the patient to minimize skin trauma and bone stress. Provide frequent skin care, especially over bony prominences. Provide support with pillows and a convoluted foam mattress.
- Encourage the patient to verbalize her feelings about body image changes and sexual dysfunction. Offer emotional support and a positive, realistic assessment of her condition. Help her to develop coping strategies. Include the family (or significant other) as a support system, and help them to develop positive coping mechanisms to deal with the patient. Refer her to a mental health professional for additional counseling, if necessary.
- Prepare the patient for surgery, as indicated. (See the entries "Adrenalectomy" and "Hypophysectomy," as appropriate.)

Monitoring

- Monitor the patient's vital signs, intake and output, weight, and daily serum electrolyte levels.
- Monitor the patient's nutritional intake, and assess her for nutritional imbalances.
- Assess the patient for signs and symptoms of diabetes mellitus, such as polyuria, polyphagia, polydipsia, fatigue, weight loss, and an elevated serum glucose level.
- Inspect regularly for skin breakdown.
- Watch the patient for other complications of Cushing's syndrome, such as a peptic ulcer, osteoporosis, fluid and electrolyte imbalances, psychiatric disorders, and infection.

Patient teaching

- Encourage the patient to wear a medical identification bracelet and carry her medication with her at all times.
- Teach the patient and family (or significant other) protective measures to decrease stress and infections. For example, she should get adequate rest and avoid fatigue, eat a balanced diet, and avoid people with infections. Also teach her relaxation and stress-reduction techniques.
- Stress the importance of lifelong follow-up care.

Cystectomy

Partial or total removal of the urinary bladder and surrounding structures may be necessary to treat advanced bladder cancer or, rarely, other bladder disorders such as interstitial cystitis. Cystectomy may be partial, simple, or radical. (See *Types of cystectomy.*)

Procedure

In a partial cystectomy, the surgeon makes a midline incision from the umbilicus to the symphysis pubis. He then opens the bladder and removes the tumor along with a small portion of healthy tissue. To complete the procedure, he closes the wound, leaving a Penrose drain and suprapubic catheter in place.

In a simple cystectomy, the surgeon first makes a midline abdominal incision. He then removes the entire bladder, leaving only a portion of the urethra.

In a radical cystectomy, the surgeon also removes, in addition to the bladder, the seminal vesicles and prostate in male patients and the uterus, ovaries, fallopian tubes, and anterior vagina in female patients. Depending on the extent of the cancer, the surgeon may also remove the urethra and surrounding lymph nodes.

To complete either a simple or radical cystectomy, the surgeon provides for urinary diversion by attaching the ureters to an external collection device, such as a cutaneous ureterostomy, ileal conduit, or continent urinary neobladder.

Complications

Immediately after surgery, potential complications include bleeding, hypotension, and nerve injury (such as to the genitofemoral or peroneal nerve). Later complications include anuria, stoma stenosis, urinary tract infection, pouch leakage, electrolyte imbalance, stenosis of the ureteroileal junction, and vascular compromise. Radical and simple cystectomy may also cause psychological problems relating to changes in the patient's body image and loss of sexual or reproductive function.

Key nursing diagnoses and patient outcomes

Altered urinary elimination related to removal of bladder. Based on this nursing diagnosis, you'll establish these patient outcomes. The patient will:

- be able to eliminate urine through either a stoma or by self-catheterization
- not develop complications caused by urinary diversion
- demonstrate ability to manage the altered route of urinary elimination.

Risk for infection related to manipulation of bowel and instrumentation in the abdominal cavity. Based on this nursing diagnosis, you'll establish these patient outcomes. The patient will:

- maintain a normal temperature and white blood cell count and differential
- display a clean, pink incision and conduit site that are free from purulent drainage
- remain free of all signs and symptoms of infection.

Types of cystectomy

In cystectomy, the surgery may be partial, simple, or radical.

Partial cystectomy involves resection of a portion of the bladder wall. Commonly preserving bladder function, this surgery is most often indicated for a single, easily accessible bladder tumor.

Simple or total cystectomy, which involves resection of the entire bladder, is indicated for benign conditions limited to the bladder. It may also be performed as a palliative measure, such as to stop bleeding, when the cancer isn't curable.

Radical cystectomy is generally indicated for muscle-invasive primary bladder carcinoma. Besides removing the bladder, this procedure entails removing several surrounding structures. Because this surgery is so extensive, it typically produces impotence in men and sterility in women.

Whenever the entire bladder is removed, the patient will require a permanent urinary diversion, such as an ileal conduit or continent urinary pouch.

Pain related to extensive abdominal surgery needed to perform a cystectomy. Based on this nursing diagnosis, you'll establish these patient outcomes. The patient will:
- verbalize a relief of pain after administration of an analgesic
- use diversional activities, such as position change or distraction, to help minimize pain
- become pain free after healing is complete.

Nursing interventions

When caring for a cystectomy patient, you'll typically focus on instructing the patient and monitoring for complications.

Before surgery

- Review the surgery with the patient and his family, if appropriate. Pay special attention to the patient's emotional state since he will probably be anxious. Help allay his fears by listening to his concerns and answering his questions. If the patient is undergoing simple or radical cystectomy, he will also be concerned about the effects of a urinary diversion on his life-style. Reassure him that such diversion need not interfere with his normal activities, and arrange for a visit by an enterostomal therapist, who can provide additional information.
- If the patient is scheduled for radical cystectomy, you will need to address concerns about the inevitable loss of sexual or reproductive function.
- Explain to the patient that he will awaken in an intensive care unit (ICU) after a radical cystectomy. He will return to his own hospital room following a partial cystectomy unless complications occur in the perioperative period. Mention that he will have a nasogastric (NG) tube, a central venous catheter, and an indwelling urinary catheter in place and a drain at the surgical site. Tell him that he will not be able to eat or drink until the return of bowel function and that he will be given I.V. fluids during this period. After that, he can resume oral fluids and eventually progress to solids. If possible, arrange for the patient and his family to visit the ICU before surgery to familiarize themselves with the unit and meet the staff.
- Perform a standard bowel preparation as ordered. Antibiotics administered orally (such as neomycin) or parenterally (such as cefazolin) are used prophylactically to reduce colonic microbial flora. To further clean the bowel, high colonic enemas (administered until they run clear) or oral polyethylene glycol–electrolyte solution (PEG-ES), a nonabsorbable osmotic agent, are given. Large amounts of PEG-ES (4 liters) are administered over 3 to 4 hours; diarrhea begins within 1 hour.

After surgery

- Monitor the amount and character of urine drainage every hour. Report output of less than 30 ml/hour, which may indicate retention. (Other signs of retention include bladder distention and spasms in a partial cystectomy.) If output is low, check the patency of the indwelling urinary catheter or stoma, as appropriate, and irrigate as ordered.
- Monitor vital signs closely. Watch especially for signs of hypovolemic shock: increased pulse and respiratory rate, hypotension, diaphoresis, and pallor. (Be especially alert for hemorrhage if the doctor has ordered anticoagulant therapy to reduce the risk of pulmonary embolism.) Periodically, inspect the stoma (if present) and incision site for bleeding and observe urine drainage for frank hematuria and clots. Slight hematuria normally occurs for several days after surgery but should clear thereafter. Test all drainage from the NG tube, abdominal drains, indwelling urinary catheter, and urine collection appliance for blood, and notify the doctor of positive findings.
- Observe the wound site and all drainage for signs of infection. Change abdominal dressings frequently, using sterile technique.

- Periodically ask the patient about incisional pain and, if he has had a partial cystectomy, about bladder spasms as well. Provide analgesics as ordered. You may also be asked to administer an antispasmodic such as oxybutynin.
- To prevent pulmonary complications associated with prolonged immobility, encourage frequent position changes, coughing, deep breathing and, if possible, early ambulation. Assess respiratory status regularly.
- Provide care for the type of urinary diversion present.
- Continue to offer the patient emotional support throughout the recovery period to help him accept changes in body image and, if appropriate, sexual function. If possible, refer the patient and his family for psychological and sexual counseling to further aid this adjustment.

Home care instructions

- Explain to the patient that incisional pain and fatigue will probably last for several weeks after discharge. Tell him to notify the doctor if these effects persist or worsen.
- Instruct the patient to watch for and report any signs of urinary tract infection (fever, chills, flank pain, and decreased urine volume) or wound infection (redness, swelling, and purulent drainage at the incision site). Also, tell him to report persistent hematuria.
- Make sure the patient or a family member understands how to care for his type of urinary diversion and where to obtain needed supplies. If needed, arrange for visits by a home care nurse who can reinforce urinary diversion care measures and provide emotional support. You may also want to refer the patient to a support group, such as a local chapter of the United Ostomy Association, if a stoma is present.
- Stress the importance of follow-up examinations to evaluate healing and recurrence of cancer.

Cystic fibrosis

A chronic, progressive, inherited disease, cystic fibrosis affects the exocrine (mucus-secreting) glands. The disease is transmitted as an autosomal recessive trait and is the most common fatal genetic disease of white children. When both parents are carriers of the recessive gene, they have a 25% chance of transmitting the disease with each pregnancy. (See *How the cystic fibrosis gene is transmitted,* page 244.)

Cystic fibrosis increases the viscosity of bronchial, pancreatic, and other mucus gland secretions, obstructing glandular ducts. The accumulation of thick, tenacious secretions in the bronchioles and alveoli causes respiratory changes, eventually leading to severe atelectasis and emphysema.

The disease also causes characteristic GI effects in the intestines, pancreas, and liver. Obstruction of the pancreatic ducts results in a deficiency of trypsin, amylase, and lipase, which prevents the conversion and absorption of fat and protein in the intestinal tract. This interferes with the digestion of food and the absorption of fat-soluble vitamins (A, D, E, and K). In the pancreas, fibrotic tissue, multiple cysts, thick mucus, and fat replace the acini (small, saclike swellings normally found in this gland), producing signs of pancreatic insufficiency (insufficient insulin production, abnormal glucose tolerance, and glycosuria).

The incidence of cystic fibrosis is highest in people of northern European ancestry (about 1 in 2,000 live births). The disease is less common in Blacks (1 in 17,000 live births), Native Americans, and Asians. It occurs with equal frequency in both sexes.

Cystic fibrosis is incurable. But as medical research seeks to find better treatment, life expectancy has greatly increased. One-half of all patients with cystic fibrosis today are over age 28. Many survive to age 40, and a few have survived to age 50 or older.

How the cystic fibrosis gene is transmitted

Parents of a child with cystic fibrosis will be concerned about how the causative gene is transmitted and what their chances are of having another child with cystic fibrosis. Tell them that cystic fibrosis results from an autosomal recessive gene.

Explain to the parents that genes are either dominant or recessive. The weaker recessive genes manifest themselves only when paired with another recessive gene. At conception, an embryo normally receives two genes—one from each parent. If both parents carry the recessive gene for cystic fibrosis, each offspring has a 25% chance of having the disease. Explain that special laboratories offer prenatal testing for parents of children with cystic fibrosis. Mention that about 75% of cystic fibrosis patients have the cystic fibrosis gene. Researchers are still exploring gene mutations in the remaining 25%. Advise parents to seek up-to-date information from a genetic counselor.

As shown below, *C* represents the dominant gene, and *c* represents the recessive gene. The unaffected noncarrier—*CC*—has inherited the dominant gene from each parent and won't have cystic fibrosis. *Cc* and *cC* are unaffected carriers; each child has inherited one dominant gene and one recessive gene for cystic fibrosis. Because both genes must be recessive for cystic fibrosis to develop, these children won't have the disease, but they can pass the recessive gene to their offspring.

The affected person—*cc*—has inherited the recessive gene from both parents and has cystic fibrosis. He will pass the recessive cystic fibrosis gene on, if he has offspring.

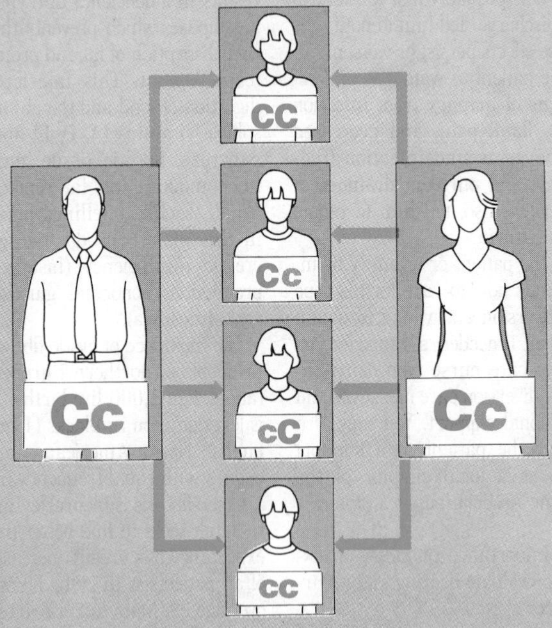

Causes

Cystic fibrosis is inherited as an autosomal recessive trait. The responsible gene is on chromosome 7. Researchers have found that most cases of cystic fibrosis arise from a mutation in this gene that causes it to encode a single amino acid, resulting in an abnormal protein that adversely affects membrane transport.

The defective protein resembles other transmembrane transport proteins. However, it lacks a phenylalanine that appears in proteins produced by normal genes. Researchers speculate that this abnormal protein may interfere with chloride transport by preventing adenosine triphosphate from binding to the protein or by interfering with activation by protein kinases. This leads to dehydration and mucosal thickening in the respiratory and intestinal tracts and may explain the characteristic elevated sweat chloride levels that occur in cystic fibrosis.

However, this abnormal protein is only the major defect in the cystic fibrosis gene. Other gene mutations remain to be found.

Complications

Cystic fibrosis can cause bronchiectasis, pneumonia, atelectasis, hemoptysis, dehydration, distal intestinal obstructive syndrome, malnutrition, gastroesophageal reflux, nasal polyps, rectal prolapse, and cor pulmonale. Other inevitable complications include hepatic disease, diabetes, pneumothorax, arthritis, pancreatitis, and cholecystitis.

A deficiency of fat-soluble vitamins can lead to clotting problems, retarded bone growth, and delayed sexual development. Males may experience azoospermia; females may experience secondary amenorrhea.

Hypochloremia and hyponatremia from increased sodium and chloride concentrations in sweat can induce cardiac arrhythmias and potentially fatal shock, especially in hot weather, when sweating is profuse.

Biliary obstruction and fibrosis may prolong neonatal jaundice. In some patients, cirrhosis and portal hypertension may lead to esophageal varices, episodes of hematemesis and, occasionally, hepatomegaly.

Assessment

A neonate with cystic fibrosis shows meconium ileus – a failure to excrete meconium, the dark green mucilaginous material found in the intestine at birth. Your assessment of such an infant may reveal signs of intestinal obstruction, such as abdominal distention, vomiting, constipation, and dehydration.

Other signs, which may be apparent soon after birth or years later, include major aberrations in sweat gland and GI functions (sweat gland dysfunction ranks as the most consistent abnormality). The patient may also complain of frequent upper respiratory tract infections, dyspnea, paroxysmal cough, frequent bouts of pneumonia, and other types of severe respiratory dysfunction.

A young child typically has a history of poor weight gain and poor growth, despite a healthy appetite. The parents may describe the child's stools as frequent, bulky, foul-smelling, and pale.

Inspection of the child may reveal a barrel chest, cyanosis, and clubbing of the fingers and toes. He may cough up tenacious, yellow-green sputum. Palpation may show a distended abdomen. On auscultation, you may hear wheezy respirations and crackles.

Diagnostic tests

- A *sweat test* confirms cystic fibrosis. It shows elevated electrolyte (sodium and chloride) concentrations in sweat in a patient with pulmonary disease or pancreatic insufficiency. The sweat test (stimulation of sweat glands, collection of specimens, and laboratory analysis) shows that the volume of sweat is normal but that it has an increased weight because of concentrated chloride and sodium. (Sweat normally has a sodium concentration of less than 40 mEq/liter; in cystic fibrosis, this rises to more than 60 mEq/liter.)

The sodium and chloride concentrations of sweat normally rise with age, but any value greater than 50 mEq/liter, even in adults, strongly suggests cystic fibrosis and calls for repeated testing.

- *Deoxyribonucleic acid (DNA) testing* can locate the presence of the Delta 508 deletion and help to confirm the diagnosis. Most cystic fibrosis patients have this deletion, although the disease can also cause more than 100 other mutations. In some families, DNA analysis may allow prenatal diagnosing, which can identify about 70% of white carriers.
- *Chest X-rays* help diagnose a respiratory obstruction and monitor its progress.
- *Pulmonary function tests* evaluate lung function.
- *Arterial blood gas analysis* helps determine pulmonary status.
- *Sputum culture* allows the detection of concurrent infectious diseases.
- *Examination of duodenal contents* for pancreatic enzymes and *stools* for trypsin can confirm pancreatic insufficiency; trypsin is absent in more than 80% of children with cystic fibrosis.

Treatment

Because cystic fibrosis has no cure, treatment aims to help the patient lead as normal a life as possible. The specific treatments depend on the organ systems involved.

To combat electrolyte loss through sweat, the patient should generously salt his food and, during hot weather, take salt supplements.

To offset pancreatic enzyme deficiencies, the patient can take oral pancreatic enzymes with meals and snacks. Such supplements improve absorption and digestion and help satisfy hunger on a reasonable calorie intake. The patient should also follow a diet that's low in fat and high in protein and calories and that includes supplements of vitamins A, D, E, and K.

To manage pulmonary dysfunction, the patient should undergo physical therapy, nebulization to loosen secretions followed by postural drainage, and breathing exercises several times daily to help remove secretions from the lungs. He shouldn't receive antihistamines, which have a drying effect on mucous membranes and make expectoration of mucus difficult or impossible.

A patient with pulmonary infection needs intermittent nebulization and postural drainage to relieve obstruction and loosen and remove mucopurulent secretions. In acute cases, he also needs aggressive treatment with broad-spectrum antibiotics and oxygen therapy as needed.

To prevent the recurrence of respiratory tract infections, which are more likely in hot, dry air, the patient can use an air conditioner and a humidifier.

In advanced stages of cystic fibrosis, the patient may require heart-lung transplantation.

Since the discovery of the basic genetic defect of cystic fibrosis, new treatments have been explored in some centers. Experimental treatments include drugs, such as DNase and amiloride, and gene therapy. Researchers have targeted the lungs for gene therapy because the most serious pathology occurs there. They hope to insert corrected genetic material into lung stem cells, which produce new lung cells. Lung stem cells might be reached through an aerosolized delivery system currently under study.

Key nursing diagnoses and patient outcomes

Altered nutrition: Less than body requirements related to adverse effects in the intestines, pancreas, and liver caused by cystic fibrosis. Based on this nursing diagnosis, you'll establish these patient outcomes. The patient will:

- express an understanding of dietary restrictions and demonstrate skill in choosing the correct foods

• take salt and pancreatic enzyme supplements correctly
• not develop malnutrition.

Ineffective airway clearance related to the viscosity of respiratory sections caused by cystic fibrosis. Based on this nursing diagnosis, you'll establish these patient outcomes. The patient will:
• express an understanding of his need to remain hydrated, perform bronchial hygiene measures, and take medications as ordered
• along with his caregiver, demonstrate skill in performing bronchial hygiene measures, including chest physiotherapy
• keep a patent airway and maintain arterial blood gases at baseline levels.

Ineffective individual coping related to chronic nature of disease, complex treatment regimen, and loss of normal life span as a result of having cystic fibrosis. Based on this nursing diagnosis, you'll establish these patient outcomes. The patient will:
• verbalize an understanding of the relationship between his emotional state and his behavior
• identify effective and ineffective coping techniques
• use available support systems, such as family, friends, and a psychotherapist, to develop and maintain effective coping skills.

Nursing interventions

• Give medications, as ordered. Administer pancreatic enzymes with meals and snacks.
• Perform chest physiotherapy, including postural drainage and chest percussion designed for all lobes, several times a day, as ordered.
• Administer oxygen therapy, as ordered. Check arterial oxygen saturation levels using pulse oximetry.
• Provide a well-balanced, high-calorie, high-protein diet for the patient. Include plenty of fats, which, though difficult for the patient to digest, are nutritionally necessary. Give him enzyme capsules to help combat most of the effects of fat malabsorption. Include vitamin A, D, E, and K supplements if laboratory analysis indicates any deficiencies.
• Make sure the patient receives plenty of liquids to prevent dehydration, especially in warm weather.
• Provide exercise and activity periods for the patient to promote health. Encourage him to perform breathing exercises to help improve his ventilation.
• Provide the young child with play periods, and enlist the help of the physical therapy department. Some pediatric hospitals have play therapists, who provide essential playtime for young patients.
• Provide emotional support to the parents of children with cystic fibrosis. Because it's an inherited disease, the parents may feel enormous guilt. Encourage them to discuss their fears and concerns, and answer their questions as honestly as possible.
• Be flexible with care and visiting hours during hospitalization to allow the child to continue school and friendships.
• Include the family in all phases of the child's care. If the child is an adolescent, he may want to perform much of his own treatment protocol. Encourage him to do so.

Monitoring

• Monitor the patient's nutritional intake, and assess him regularly for nutritional imbalances.
• Monitor the patient's respiratory status, including the quality of sputum production, to determine the effectiveness of respiratory care measures. Also evaluate the patient regularly for signs of a respiratory infection.
• Monitor the patient's and his family's ability to cope with the patient's illness.

Patient teaching

• Inform the patient and his family about the disease, and thoroughly explain all treatment measures. Make sure they know about tests that can determine if family members carry the cystic fibrosis gene.

• Teach the patient and his family breathing exercises and postural drainage techniques, and advise them to perform these several times daily. Stress the importance of following the regimen.
• Teach the patient and his family about all the medications the patient may be receiving. Explain possible adverse reactions, and urge them to notify the doctor if these reactions occur.
• Instruct the patient and his family about aerosol therapy, including intermittent nebulizer treatments before postural drainage. Tell them that these treatments help to loosen secretions and dilate bronchi.
• Stress the importance of supplemental pancreatic enzyme therapy in combating malabsorption. Tell the patient and the family that the patient should take the supplements with both snacks and meals.
• Emphasize the importance of a well-balanced, high-calorie, high-protein diet. Also, encourage the patient to eat salty foods to compensate for sodium chloride lost in sweat and to drink plenty of fluids to prevent dehydration.
• If the doctor prescribes aerobic exercises, teach these to the patient and review their importance in respiratory muscle and cardiopulmonary function and in improved activity tolerance.
• Discuss the importance of lifelong follow-up care. Stress the need to keep all regular appointments.
• Teach the patient and his family the signs of infection or sudden change in the patient's condition that they should report to the doctor. These include increased cough, decreased appetite, sputum that thickens or contains blood, shortness of breath, and chest pain.
• Help the patient and his family cope with the realization that cystic fibrosis can shorten the patient's life. Encourage the whole family to use the resources available in their cystic fibrosis center, and help them to find appropriate support groups.
• Advise the parents of a child with the disease not to be overly protective. Help them instead to explore ways to enhance the patient's quality of life and to foster responsibility and independence in their child from an early age. Stress the importance of good communication so that the patient may express his fears and concerns.
• If the patient is at the end stage of the disease, help him and his family deal with his approaching death.
• Refer the patient and his family to the Cystic Fibrosis Foundation for further information.

Cytomegalovirus infection

Also called generalized salivary gland disease and cytomegalic inclusion disease, cytomegalovirus (CMV) occurs worldwide. A herpesvirus, the disease is transmitted by human contact.

About four out of five persons over age 35 have been infected with CMV, usually during childhood or early adulthood. In most, the disease is so mild that it's overlooked. However, CMV can be devastating to a fetus or to an immunosuppressed patient.

Causes

The infection results from the cytomegalovirus, an ether-sensitive, deoxyribonucleic acid virus belonging to the herpes family. CMV has been found in the saliva, urine, semen, breast milk, feces, blood, and vaginal and cervical secretions of infected people.

Transmission occurs through direct contact with secretions and excretions, through blood transfusions, through the placenta, and through transplanted organs (patients who receive organs from a CMV-seropositive donor run a 90% chance of contracting the infection). CMV in cervical secretions can infect a sexual partner or an infant during passage through the birth canal. CMV is reaching epidemic proportions in female prostitutes and sexually active homosexual men as CMV antibody titers in these groups approach 100%.

The disease probably spreads through the body in lymphocytes or mononuclear cells to the lungs, liver, GI tract, eyes, and central nervous system, where it often produces inflammatory reactions.

Complications

Immunosuppressed patients, such as those with acquired immunodeficiency syndrome, may develop opportunistic infections, such as pneumonia, hepatitis, ulceration of the GI tract, retinitis, and encephalopathy.

Assessment

The adult patient's history may reveal an immunosuppressive condition. He may complain of mild, nonspecific clinical symptoms, such as fatigue, myalgia, and headache, or he may have no symptoms.

Other immunosuppressed patients may suffer extensive organ involvement. For example, a patient with CMV pneumonia may complain of a nonproductive cough and dyspnea with hypoxia. A patient with CMV colitis may report explosive watery diarrhea. A patient with CMV ulcerative disease may have GI bleeding. And a patient with CMV retinitis may complain of blurred vision and scotoma, which can progress to blindness in one or both eyes.

Fever is common. In an immunocompetent patient with CMV mononucleosis, 3 or more weeks of irregular high fever may be the only symptom.

Inspection findings vary in immunosuppressed patients. With respiratory involvement, you may note tachypnea, shortness of breath, cyanosis, and coughing but seldom sputum production. With liver involvement, you may note jaundice and spider angiomas.

Palpation in all CMV patients may reveal splenomegaly and hepatomegaly.

Diagnostic tests

Isolating the virus or demonstrating rising serologic titers allows diagnosis of CMV. Complement fixation studies, hemagglutination inhibition antibody tests and, in congenital infections, indirect immunofluorescent tests for CMV immunoglobulin M antibody may be performed. Chest X-ray typically shows bilateral, diffuse, white infiltrates.

The perfection of the CMV early antigen test has led to improved diagnosis and early treatment.

Treatment

Although antiviral therapy for herpesviruses has had encouraging results, CMV is more difficult to prevent and treat than other herpesviruses. Ganciclovir and, less frequently, acyclovir prove helpful for certain patients, although relapse may occur. One experimental drug, foscarnet, looks promising.

Key nursing diagnoses and patient outcomes

Fatigue related to prolonged infectious process because of difficuty in treating CMV infection. Based on this nursing diagnosis, you'll establish these patient outcomes. The patient will:

- identify activities that increase fatigue
- schedule adequate rest periods throughout the day and seek assistance with activities that increase fatigue
- experience a decrease in fatigue and regain his normal level of energy when treatment is completed.

Risk for infection related to susceptibility to opportunistic infections as the CMV infection spreads throughout the body. Based on this nursing diagnosis, you'll establish these patient outcomes. The patient will:

- take precautionary measures (such as obtaining adequate rest, eating a well-balanced diet, and remaining well hydrated) to prevent opportunistic infections
- not develop an opportunistic infection.

Hyperthermia related to inflammatory process of a CMV infection. Based on this

nursing diagnosis, you'll establish these patient outcomes. The patient will:
• exhibit a decrease in temperature after the administration of antipyretic medications
• not experience complications related to hyperthermia, such as dehydration or seizures
• regain and maintain a normal temperature.

Nursing interventions

• Institute standard precautions before coming into contact with the patient's blood or other body fluids. Secretion precautions are especially important for infants known to be shedding CMV.
• Administer medications to treat symptoms, as needed.
• Offer nutritionally adequate meals. If the patient has diarrhea, increase fluids to replace those lost.
• Provide emotional support and counseling to the parents of a child with severe CMV infection. Help them find support systems, and coordinate referrals to other health care professionals.
• For the patient with impaired vision, provide a safe environment and encourage optimal independence. Make referrals to community resources as needed.
• For the patient with respiratory involvement, administer oxygen and assist with ventilation, as needed. Position the patient in a semi-Fowler's or sitting position to facilitate ventilation.

Monitoring

• Monitor the patient's vital signs, especially his temperature and intake and output.
• Monitor the patient for signs and symptoms of opportunistic infections.
• If the patient has splenomegaly, monitor him for signs of rupture and protect him from excess activity and injury.
• If the patient has respiratory involvement, monitor his respiratory status closely.
• If the patient has diarrhea, monitor the number and characteristics of stools passed. Also observe for signs and symptoms of fluid and electrolyte imbalance.

Patient teaching

• Advise female health care workers trying to become pregnant to have CMV titers drawn to identify their risk of contracting the infection. A study done by the Centers for Disease Control and Prevention showed that 50% of pregnant women exposed to CMV also had fetal exposure, with 20% of the fetuses contracting the infection.
• Urge the patient to wash his hands thoroughly to help prevent contagion.
• Warn an immunosuppressed or pregnant patient to avoid contact with any person who has confirmed or suspected CMV infection.
• Tell an immunosuppressed patient who is CMV-seronegative to carry this information with him and to relay it to any caregiver. This way, he won't be given CMV-positive blood.

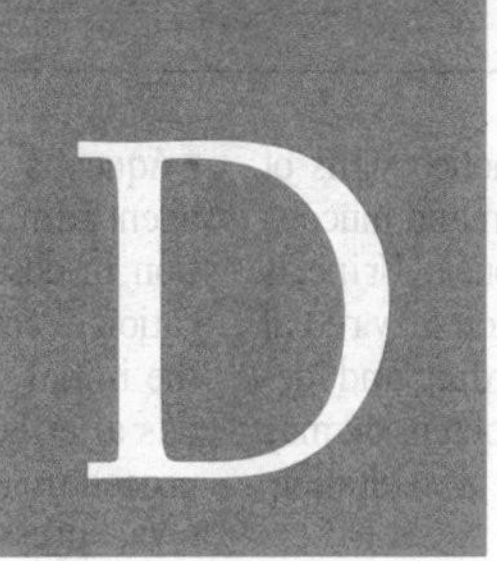

Diabetes insipidus

A deficiency of vasopressin (also called antidiuretic hormone) causes this metabolic disorder characterized by excessive fluid intake and hypotonic polyuria. The disorder may start in childhood or early adulthood (the median age of onset is 21) and occurs more commonly in men than in women.

In uncomplicated diabetes insipidus, with adequate water replacement, the prognosis is good, and patients usually lead normal lives. However, in patients with an underlying disorder, such as cancer, the prognosis varies.

Causes

The most common cause is failure of vasopressin secretion in response to normal physiologic stimuli (pituitary or neurogenic diabetes insipidus). A less common cause is failure of the kidneys to respond to vasopressin (congenital nephrogenic diabetes insipidus).

Two types of pituitary diabetes insipidus exist: primary and secondary. The primary form affects about 50% of patients. Familial or idiopathic in origin, this form may occur in neonates as a result of congenital malformation of the central nervous system (CNS), infection, trauma, or tumor.

Secondary pituitary diabetes insipidus results from intracranial neoplastic or metastatic lesions, hypophysectomy or other types of neurosurgery, a skull fracture, or head trauma – which damages the neurohypophyseal structures. This disease can also result from infection, granulomatous disease, and vascular lesions.

A transient form of diabetes insipidus also occurs during pregnancy, usually after the fifth or sixth month of gestation. The condition usually reverses spontaneously after delivery.

Complications

Untreated diabetes insipidus can produce hypovolemia, hyperosmolality, circulatory collapse, unconsciousness, and CNS damage. These complications are most likely to occur if the patient has an impaired (or no) thirst mechanism.

A prolonged increase in urine flow may produce chronic complications, such as bladder distention, enlarged calyces, hydroureter, and hydronephrosis. Complications may result from underlying conditions, such as metastatic brain lesions, head trauma, and infections.

Assessment

The patient's history shows an abrupt onset of extreme polyuria (usually 4 to 16 liters/day of dilute urine, but sometimes as much as 30 liters/day), extreme thirst, and consumption of extraordinary volumes of fluid. The patient may report weight loss, dizziness, weakness, constipation, slight to moderate nocturia and, in severe cases, fatigue from inadequate rest caused by frequent voiding and excessive thirst.

On inspection, you may notice signs of dehydration, such as dry skin and mucous membranes, fever, and dyspnea. Urine is pale and voluminous. Palpation may reveal poor skin turgor, tachycardia, and decreased muscle strength. Hypotension may be present on blood pressure auscultation.

Diagnostic tests

To distinguish diabetes insipidus from other types of polyuria, the doctor may order the following tests:

- *Urinalysis* reveals almost colorless urine of low osmolality (50 to 200 mOsm/kg of water, less than that of plasma) and of low specific gravity (less than 1.005).
- *Dehydration test* is a simple, reliable way to diagnose diabetes insipidus and differentiate vasopressin deficiency from other forms of polyuria. It compares urine osmolality after dehydration with urine osmolality after vasopressin administration. In diabetes insipidus, the rise in urine osmolality after vasopressin administration exceeds 9%. Patients with pituitary diabetes insipidus respond to exogenous vasopressin with decreased urine output and increased urine specific gravity. Those with nephrogenic diabetes insipidus show no response to vasopressin.
- *Plasma and urinary vasopressin evaluations* are too expensive and time-consuming to use regularly but are occasionally necessary if osmolality measures are inconclusive.

In critically ill patients, diagnosis may be based on the following laboratory values only:

- urine osmolality – below 200 mOsm/kg
- urine specific gravity – below 1.005
- serum osmolality – above 300 mOsm/kg
- serum sodium – above 147 mEq/liter.

Treatment

Until the cause of diabetes insipidus is identified and eliminated, administration of vasopressin or a vasopressin stimulant can control fluid balance and prevent dehydration:

- Aqueous vasopressin is a replacement agent administered by subcutaneous injection in doses of 5 to 10 units with a duration of action of 3 to 6 hours. It's used in the initial management of diabetes insipidus after head trauma or a neurosurgical procedure.
- Vasopressin tannate (in oil), an I.M. preparation in a 1.5 to 5 unit/ml suspension, is given in doses of 0.3 to 1 ml, as required. Duration is 24 to 72 hours.
- Desmopressin acetate, a synthetic vasopressin analogue, exerts prolonged antidiuretic activity and has no pressor effects. It's given intranasally in doses of 0.1 to 0.4 ml or subcutaneously in doses of 2 to 4 mcg. Duration of action is 12 to 24 hours, making it the drug of choice.
- Lypressin is a synthetic vasopressin replacement given as a short-acting nasal spray. It has significant disadvantages: variable absorption rate, nasal congestion and irritation, ulcerated nasal passages (with repeated use), substernal chest tightness, coughing, and dyspnea (after accidental inhalation of large doses).
- Chlorpropamide, an oral antidiabetic agent used in patients who have residual release of vasopressin, stimulates or potentiates the action of submaximal amounts of vasopressin on the renal tubules and reduces polyuria. It may be given with clofibrate.

Key nursing diagnoses and patient outcomes

Altered urinary elimination related to polyuria. Based on this nursing diagnosis, you'll establish these patient outcomes. The patient will:

- express an understanding of how the prescribed medication can control polyuria
- recover and maintain normal urine output volume with drug therapy.

Fluid volume deficit related to polyuria. Based on this nursing diagnosis, you'll establish these patient outcomes. The patient will:

• recover and maintain normal fluid volume as evidenced by equal intake and output
• exhibit normal serum osmolality and sodium levels
• not have complications related to fluid volume deficit.

Knowledge deficit related to diabetes insipidus and the prescribed treatment. Based on this nursing diagnosis, you'll establish these patient outcomes. The patient and caregiver will:
• express a desire to learn about his condition and therapy
• communicate an understanding of how his prescribed treatment can control the symptoms of diabetes insipidus
• correctly administer vasopressin nasally or subcutaneously.

Nursing interventions

• Institute safety precautions if the patient complains of dizziness or weakness.
• Make sure the patient has easy access to the bathroom or bedpan, and answer his call signals promptly.
• Give vasopressin cautiously to a patient with coronary artery disease because the drug may cause vasoconstriction.
• If the patient is taking chlorpropamide, provide adequate caloric intake, and keep orange juice or another carbohydrate handy to treat hypoglycemic episodes.
• Provide meticulous skin and mouth care. Use a soft toothbrush and mild mouthwash to avoid trauma to the oral mucosa, and apply petroleum jelly, as needed, to cracked or sore lips. Use alcohol-free skin care products and apply emollient lotion after baths.
• Urge the patient to verbalize his feelings. Offer encouragement and a realistic assessment of his situation. Identify his strengths for use in developing coping strategies. Refer him to a mental health professional for counseling, if necessary.

Monitoring

• Keep accurate records of hourly fluid intake and urine output, vital signs, and daily weight.
• Monitor urine specific gravity and serum electrolyte and blood urea nitrogen levels.
• During dehydration testing, watch for signs of hypovolemic shock. Monitor blood pressure, pulse rate, body weight, and changes in mental or neurologic status.
• Monitor patients taking chlorpropamide for signs of hypoglycemia. Watch for decreasing urine output and increasing urine specific gravity between doses. Check laboratory values for hyponatremia and hypoglycemia.
• If the patient is receiving vasopressin for coronary artery disease, monitor for electrocardiogram changes and exacerbation of angina.
• Monitor serum osmolality and sodium levels with drug therapy.

Patient teaching

• Encourage the patient to maintain adequate fluid intake during the day to prevent severe dehydration, but to limit fluids in the evening to prevent nocturia.
• Instruct the patient and his family to identify and report signs of severe dehydration and impending hypovolemia.
• Tell the patient to record his weight daily, and teach him and his family how to monitor intake and output and how to use a hydrometer to measure urine specific gravity.
• Inform the patient and his family about long-term hormone replacement therapy. Inform them that the medication must be taken as prescribed and must not be discontinued abruptly without the doctor's advice. Teach them how to give subcutaneous or I.M. injections and how to use nasal applicators. Discuss the drug's adverse effects and when to report them.
• Advise the patient to wear a medical identification bracelet and to carry his medication with him at all times.

Diabetes mellitus

A chronic disease of absolute or relative insulin deficiency or resistance, diabetes mellitus is characterized by disturbances in carbohydrate, protein, and fat metabolism. Insulin transports glucose into the cells for use as energy and storage as glycogen. It also stimulates protein synthesis and free fatty acid storage in the adipose tissues. Insulin deficiency compromises the body tissues' access to essential nutrients for fuel and storage.

The disorder occurs in two primary forms: Type I, insulin-dependent diabetes mellitus, and the more prevalent Type II, non-insulin-dependent diabetes mellitus. Several secondary forms also exist, resulting from conditions such as pancreatic disease, pregnancy, hormonal or genetic syndromes, or ingestion of certain drugs, chemicals, or toxins.

Diabetes mellitus is thought to affect about 3.1% of the U.S. population (7.8 million diagnosed cases). About half of those affected are undiagnosed. Incidence is equal in males and females and rises with age.

Causes

Type I diabetes results from destruction of the beta cells in the pancreas. By the time the disorder becomes apparent, about 80% of the beta cells have been destroyed. This destruction almost certainly results from an autoimmune process, although details are obscure. The genes that predispose a person to Type I diabetes are found in the HLA region of chromosome 6, which contains genes that control immune response. Patients with autoantibodies to islet cell antigens, insulin, or glutamic acid decarboxylase are most likely to develop Type I diabetes. Although viruses have been suggested to cause Type I diabetes, their mechanism of action has not been proven. Further studies of risk factors and their interactions are needed to provide details about the cause and management of Type I diabetes.

In insulitis, the islets are infiltrated with activated T lymphocytes, and the beta cells are mistaken as foreign by the immune system. Cytotoxic antibodies develop and act in concert with cell-mediated immune mechanisms to destroy the beta cells.

Type II diabetes may arise from abnormal insulin secretion and resistance to insulin action in target tissues. This may be caused by primary islet cell abnormality. Acquired insulin resistance, usually obesity-related, may be required for hyperglycemia to develop.

The causes of secondary diabetes vary. Physiologic or emotional stress may induce prolonged elevation of stress hormone levels (cortisol, epinephrine, glucagon, and growth hormone), which subsequently elevates blood glucose and places increased demands on the pancreas. Pregnancy causes weight gain and increased estrogen and placental hormone levels. Certain medications, including thiazide diuretics, adrenal corticosteroids, and oral contraceptives, antagonize the effects of insulin.

Complications

Two acute metabolic complications of diabetes are diabetic ketoacidosis (DKA) and hyperosmolar hyperglycemic nonketotic syndrome (HHNS). These life-threatening conditions require immediate medical intervention. (See *Distinguishing between DKA and HHNS,* pages 256 and 257, for more detailed information.)

Patients with diabetes mellitus also have a higher risk for various systemic chronic illnesses. The most common chronic complications include cardiovascular and peripheral vascular disease, retinopathy, nephropathy, diabetic dermopathy, and peripheral and autonomic neuropathy.

Peripheral neuropathy usually affects the hands and feet and may cause numbness or pain. Autonomic neuropathy manifests itself in several ways, including gastroparesis (leading to delayed gastric emptying and a feeling of nausea and fullness after meals), nocturnal diarrhea, impotence, and postural hypotension.

Hyperglycemia impairs the patient's resistance to infection because the glucose content of the epidermis and urine encourages bacterial growth. The patient is, therefore, susceptible to skin and urinary tract infections and vaginitis.

Assessment

The patient with Type I diabetes usually reports rapidly developing symptoms. With Type II diabetes, the patient's symptoms are usually vague and long-standing and develop gradually. Patients with Type II diabetes generally report a family history of diabetes mellitus, gestational diabetes or the delivery of a baby weighing more than 9 lb (4 kg), severe viral infection, autoimmune dysfunction, other endocrine disease, recent stress or trauma, or use of drugs that increase blood glucose levels.

Patients with both types of diabetes may report symptoms related to hyperglycemia, such as polyuria, polydipsia, polyphagia, weight loss, and fatigue. Or they may complain of weakness; vision changes; frequent skin infections; dry, itchy skin; sexual problems; and vaginal discomfort – all symptoms of complications.

Inspection may show retinopathy or cataract formation. Skin changes – especially on the legs and feet – represent impaired peripheral circulation. Muscle wasting and loss of subcutaneous fat may be evident in Type I diabetes; Type II is characterized by thin, muscular limbs and fat deposits around the face, neck, and abdomen.

Palpation may detect poor skin turgor and dry mucous membranes related to dehydration. Decreased peripheral pulses, cool skin temperature, and decreased reflexes may also be palpable. Auscultation may reveal orthostatic hypotension. Patients with DKA may have a characteristic "fruity" breath odor because of increased acetone production.

CHECKLIST

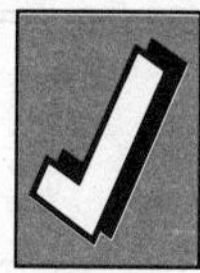

Key abnormal test values in diabetes mellitus

In nonpregnant adults, one of the following findings confirms a diagnosis of diabetes mellitus:

- ☐ symptoms of uncontrolled diabetes (for example, polyuria, polydipsia, ketonuria, and rapid weight loss) and a glucose level of 200 mg/dl or higher in a random sample of blood.
- ☐ a fasting plasma glucose level of 140 mg/dl or higher on at least two occasions.
- ☐ an oral glucose tolerance test result showing the glucose level above 200 mg/dl at 2 hours and on at least one other occasion during the test (despite normal results during the fasting phase of the test).

Diagnostic tests

For critical test values, see *Key abnormal test values in diabetes mellitus.* An ophthalmologic examination may show diabetic retinopathy. Other tests include urinalysis for acetone and blood testing for glycosylated hemoglobin (hemoglobin A), which reflects recent glucose control.

Treatment

Effective treatment of diabetes normalizes the blood glucose level and decreases complications. In Type I diabetes, goals are achieved with insulin replacement, diet, and exercise. Current forms of insulin replacement therapy include single-dose, mixed-dose, split-mixed-dose, and multiple-dose regimens. The multiple-dose regimens may be implemented with an insulin pump.

(Text continues on page 258.)

NURSING PRIORITY

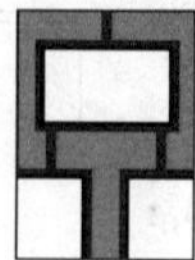

Distinguishing between DKA and HHNS

DKA and HHNS are two acute complications of diabetes. Use the flowchart below to help distinguish between these two complications when assessing your patient.

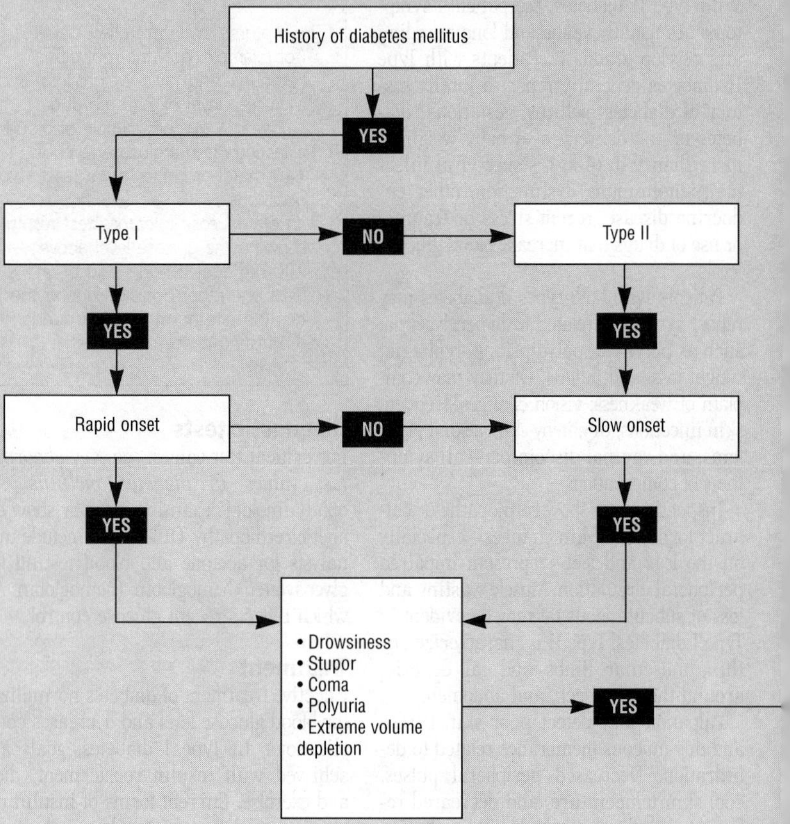

History of diabetes mellitus

YES

Type I

NO

Type II

YES

YES

Rapid onset

NO

Slow onset

YES

YES

- Drowsiness
- Stupor
- Coma
- Polyuria
- Extreme volume depletion

YES

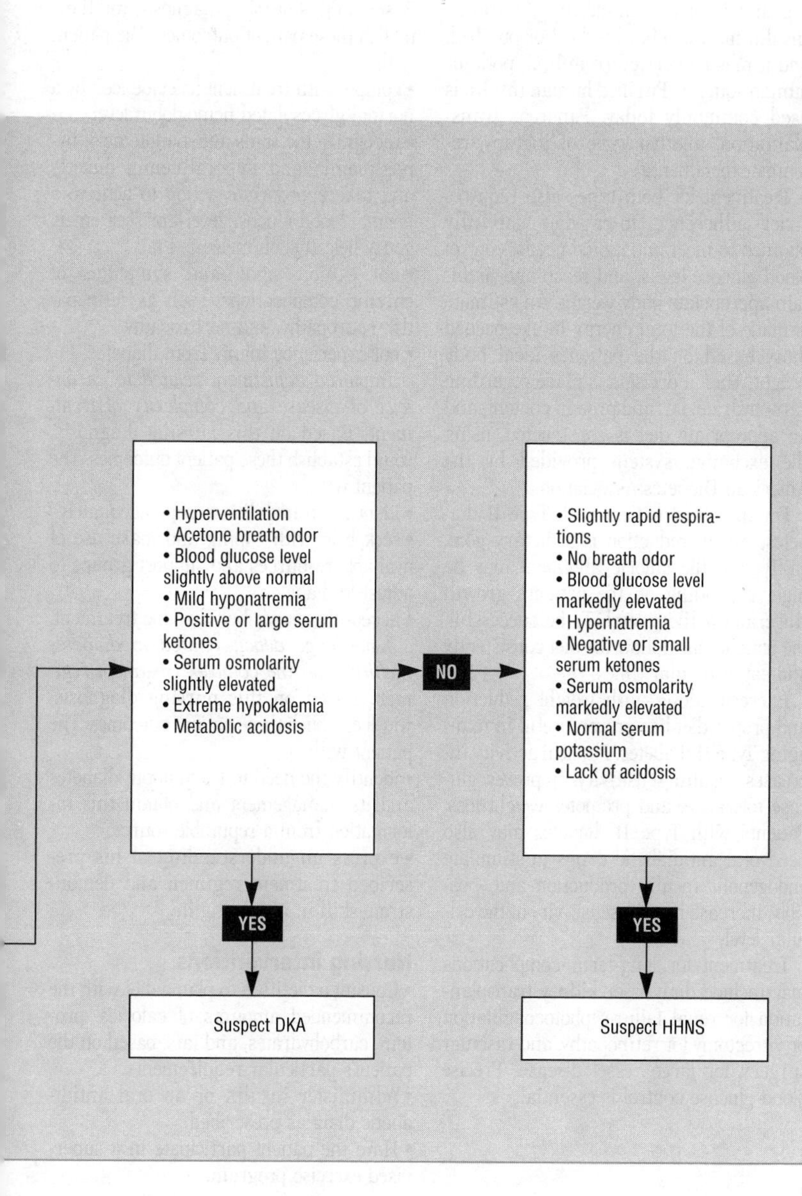

• Hyperventilation
• Acetone breath odor
• Blood glucose level slightly above normal
• Mild hyponatremia
• Positive or large serum ketones
• Serum osmolarity slightly elevated
• Extreme hypokalemia
• Metabolic acidosis
NO
• Slightly rapid respirations
• No breath odor
• Blood glucose level markedly elevated
• Hypernatremia
• Negative or small serum ketones
• Serum osmolarity markedly elevated
• Normal serum potassium
• Lack of acidosis
YES
Suspect DKA
YES
Suspect HHNS

Insulin may be rapid-acting (regular), intermediate-acting (NPH), long-acting (ultralente), or a combination of rapid-acting and intermediate-acting (Mixtard). Insulin may also be standard or purified, and it may be derived from beef, pork, or human sources. Purified human insulin is used commonly today. Pancreas transplantation, another type of therapy, remains experimental.

Treatment for both types also requires strict adherence to a diet carefully planned to meet nutritional needs, control blood glucose levels, and reach and maintain appropriate body weight. An estimate is made of the total energy intake needed daily based on the patient's ideal body weight. Then a decision is made regarding carbohydrate, fat, and protein content, and an appropriate diet is constructed, using the exchange system provided by the American Diabetes Association.

For the obese patient with Type II diabetes, weight reduction is a dietary goal. In Type I, the calorie allotment may be high, depending on the patient's growth stage and activity level. To be successful, the patient must follow the diet consistently and eat at regular times.

Exercise along with weight reduction and proper diet has proven useful in managing Type II diabetes. Physical activity increases insulin sensitivity, improves glucose tolerance, and promotes weight loss. Patients with Type II diabetes may also need oral antidiabetic drugs to stimulate endogenous insulin production and, possibly, increase insulin sensitivity at the cellular level.

Treatment for long-term complications may include dialysis or kidney transplantation for renal failure, photocoagulation or vitrectomy for retinopathy, and vascular surgery for large vessel disease. Precise blood glucose control is essential.

Key nursing diagnoses and patient outcomes

Risk for injury related to complications. Based on this nursing diagnosis, you'll establish these patient outcomes. The patient will:

- comply with treatment as evidenced by a normal glycosylated hemoglobin level
- recognize the signs and symptoms of hypoglycemia and hyperglycemia quickly and take appropriate action to achieve a normal blood glucose level – or seek emergency help if such measures fail
- not exhibit signs and symptoms of chronic complications, such as retinopathy, neuropathy, and nephropathy
- not experience injury from diabetes.

Impaired adjustment related to chronicity of disease and complexity of treatment. Based on this nursing diagnosis, you'll establish these patient outcomes. The patient will:

- identify an inability to cope adequately
- seek help with coping and make use of available resources and support groups to adjust to diabetes
- accept the prescribed diabetic treatment.

Knowledge deficit related to diabetes mellitus and the complex treatment regimen. Based on this nursing diagnosis, you'll establish these patient outcomes. The patient will:

- identify the need to learn about diabetes and its management and obtain this information from a reputable source
- express an understanding of his prescribed treatment regimen and demonstrate skill in managing it.

Nursing interventions

- Consult a dietitian to plan a diet with the recommended amounts of calories, protein, carbohydrates, and fats, based on the patient's particular requirements.
- Administer insulin or an oral antidiabetic drug as prescribed.
- Have the patient participate in a supervised exercise program.

• Treat hypoglycemic reactions promptly by giving carbohydrates in the form of fruit juice, hard candy, honey or, if the patient is unconscious, glucagon or I.V. dextrose. Treat hyperglycemic crises with I.V. fluids, insulin and, possibly, potassium replacement, as ordered.
• Provide meticulous skin care, especially to the feet and legs. Treat all injuries, cuts, and blisters promptly. Avoid constricting hose, slippers, or bed linens. Refer the patient to a podiatrist.
• Encourage the patient to verbalize his feelings about diabetes and its effects on life-style and life expectancy.
• Assist the patient to develop coping strategies. Refer him and his family to a counselor or support group.

Monitoring

• Keep accurate records of vital signs, weight, fluid intake, urine output, and caloric intake. Monitor serum glucose and urine acetone levels.
• Monitor for acute complications of diabetic therapy, especially hypoglycemia. Also be alert for signs of ketoacidosis (acetone breath, dehydration, weak and rapid pulse, and Kussmaul's respirations) and HHNS (polyuria, thirst, neurologic abnormalities, and stupor).
• Monitor diabetic effects on the cardiovascular, peripheral vascular, and nervous systems.
• Observe for signs of urinary tract and vaginal infections, and monitor the patient's urine for protein, an early sign of nephropathy.
• Look for signs and symptoms of diabetic neuropathy (numbness or pain in the hands and feet, footdrop, and neurogenic bladder).
• Monitor the patient's compliance with his prescribed diabetic regimen.

Patient teaching

• Stress the importance of strictly complying with the prescribed therapy. Discuss diet, medications, exercise, monitoring techniques, hygiene, and how to prevent and recognize hypoglycemia and hyperglycemia. (See *The elderly and diabetes mellitus*.)
• Emphasize how blood glucose control affects long-term health.
• Teach the patient how to care for his feet: He should wash them daily, carefully dry between his toes, and inspect for corns, calluses, redness, swelling, bruises, and breaks in the skin. He should report any skin changes to the doctor. Advise him to wear comfortable, nonconstricting shoes and never to walk barefoot.
• Recommend regular ophthalmologic examinations.
• Describe the signs and symptoms of diabetic neuropathy, and emphasize the need for safety precautions because decreased sensation can mask injuries.
• Teach the patient how to manage his diabetes when he has a minor illness, such as a cold, flu, or upset stomach.
• Teach the patient and family how to monitor the patient's diet and use food exchange lists.

EXPERT GERIATRIC CARE

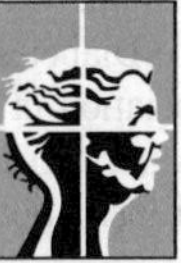

The elderly and diabetes mellitus

Teach the elderly patient how to care for his diabetes mellitus by:
• assessing him for sensory deficits, such as decreased visual acuity, hearing, and fine touch, which can impact on his learning and ability to independently manage the disease
• providing appropriate audiovisual materials, such as large-print pamphlets, slow-paced videotapes, and slide presentations
• suggesting modifications for insulin aids, such as an insulin pen or syringe magnifier to help draw up the insulin.

• Encourage the patient and family to contact the Juvenile Diabetes Foundation, the American Association of Diabetes Educators, and the American Diabetes Association for more information.

Dilatation and curettage or evacuation

Two of the most commonly performed gynecologic procedures, dilatation and curettage (D&C) and dilatation and evacuation (D&E) involve cervical expansion (dilatation) to allow access to the endocervix and uterus. In a D&C, a curette is used to scrape endometrial tissue; in a D&E, suction is applied to extract the uterine contents.

A D&C provides treatment for an incomplete abortion, controls abnormal uterine bleeding, and can secure an endometrial or endocervical tissue sample for cytologic study. A D&E can also be used for an incomplete or a therapeutic abortion, usually up to 12 weeks of gestation but occasionally as late as 16 weeks.

Procedure

After receiving a local or general anesthetic, the patient is placed in the dorsal lithotomy position. The doctor performs a preliminary bimanual pelvic examination. Then he exposes the cervix and checks the depth and direction of the uterine cavity. (In a D&E, this confirms gestational size.) He then dilates the cervical canal.

In a D&C, the doctor next explores the uterine cavity, removing any polyps. If he suspects cervical or uterine cancer, he obtains specimens for biopsy from the endocervical canal. Then he performs standard curettage to remove the superficial layer of the endometrium, taking tissue specimens from the four quadrants of the cervix. If he performs a D&C to treat an incomplete abortion, he also removes the remaining products of conception.

In a D&E, the doctor uses a suction curette to extract the contents of the uterus. He then explores the uterine cavity to ensure complete removal of the products of conception.

Complications

Potential complications include uterine perforation, hemorrhage, and infection. If cervical trauma occurs during these procedures, subsequent pregnancies may be affected. In fact, such trauma can lead to spontaneous abortion, cervical incompetence, or premature birth.

Key nursing diagnoses and patient outcomes

Anticipatory grieving related to loss of fetus. Based on this nursing diagnosis, you'll establish these patient outcomes. The patient will:

• express feelings related to loss of a fetus
• use support systems to help with coping.

Risk for cervical trauma. Based on this nursing diagnosis, you'll establish these patient outcomes. The patient will:

• not experience cervical trauma during the procedure
• not develop problems in future pregnancies associated with cervical trauma.

Nursing interventions

For the patient having a D&C or D&E, your major roles include instruction, postsurgical care, and emotional support.

Before surgery

• Review the procedure with the patient and answer her questions. Tell her that she may have some uterine cramping during the procedure and that she'll have some vaginal drainage and a perineal pad in place afterward. Explain that temporary abdominal cramping and pelvic and low back pain normally occur after the procedure.

• Ensure that preliminary studies have been completed, including a history, physical examination, urinalysis, Papanicolaou test, and hematocrit and hemoglobin measurements. Alert the doctor to any abnormalities.
• Be sure that the patient has followed preoperative directions for fasting and used an enema to empty her colon before admission. Remind her that she'll be groggy after the procedure and won't be able to drive. Make sure that she has arranged transportation.
• Ask the patient to void before you administer any preoperative medications, such as meperidine or diazepam. Start I.V. fluids, as ordered (either dextrose 5% in water or 0.9% sodium chloride solution), to facilitate administration of the anesthetic. For D&C or D&E, the patient may receive a general anesthetic, a regional paracervical block, or a local anesthetic.
• Offer emotional support and allow the patient to verbalize her feelings.
• Make sure that the patient has given informed consent for the procedure.

After surgery
• Administer analgesics, as ordered. Expect the patient to have moderate cramping and pelvic and low back pain, but report any continuous, sharp abdominal pain that doesn't respond to analgesics. This may indicate perforation of the uterus.
• Monitor the patient for hemorrhage and signs of infection, such as purulent, foul-smelling vaginal drainage. Also check the color and volume of urine; hematuria indicates infection. Report any of these signs immediately.
• Administer fluids, as tolerated, and allow food if the patient requests it. Keep the bed's side rails raised. Help the patient walk to the bathroom, if appropriate.

Home care instructions
• Instruct the patient to report any signs of infection. Tell her to use analgesics to control pain but to report any unrelenting sharp pain.
• Inform her that spotting and discharge may last 1 week or longer, but she should report any bright red blood.
• Instruct her to schedule an appointment with the doctor for a routine checkup.
• Tell her to resume activity as tolerated, but to follow her doctor's instructions for vigorous exercise and sexual intercourse. They're usually discouraged until after the follow-up visit.
• Advise her to seek birth control counseling, if needed, and refer her to an appropriate center. Also advise her to seek psychological counseling, if indicated.

Diphtheria

Acute, highly contagious, and toxin-mediated, diphtheria usually infects the respiratory tract, primarily involving the tonsils, nasopharynx, and larynx. Cutaneous, stool, and wound diphtheria are the most common types in the United States, often resulting from nontoxigenic strains. The GI and urinary tracts, conjunctivae, and ears seldom are involved.

Thanks to effective immunization, diphtheria has become rare in many parts of the world, including the United States. Since 1972, however, the incidence of cutaneous diphtheria has increased, especially in the Pacific Northwest and the Southwest. It's particularly likely to strike in areas where crowding and poor hygienic conditions prevail. Most victims are children under age 15. Mortality from diphtheria can be as high as 10%.

Causes
Diphtheria is caused by *Corynebacterium diphtheriae,* a gram-positive rod. Transmission usually occurs through intimate contact or by airborne respiratory droplets from apparently healthy carriers or convalescing patients. Many more people

LIFE-THREATENING COMPLICATIONS

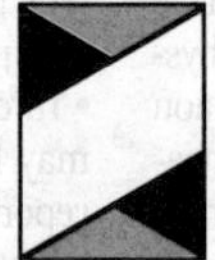

Anticipating diphtheria hazards

When caring for a patient with diphtheria, be alert for these potentially life-threatening hazards.

- *Anaphylaxis* after administering antitoxin, antibiotics, or both. Monitor for signs and symptoms, and keep epinephrine 1:1,000 and resuscitative equipment handy.
- *Thrombophlebitis* after giving erythromycin.
- *Airway obstruction,* which could require a tracheotomy.
- *Shock,* which can develop suddenly as a result of systemic vascular collapse, airway obstruction, or anaphylaxis.
- *Myocarditis,* which causes a sudden decrease in pulse rate, an irregular heartbeat, and pallor.
- *Heart murmurs and ECG changes,* especially ventricular fibrillation. Because ventricular fibrillation is a common cause of sudden death in diphtheria patients, be prepared to intervene immediately.

carry this disease than contract active infection.

Diphtheria is more prevalent during the colder months because of closer person-to-person contact indoors, but it can be contracted at any time of the year.

Complications

The extensive pseudomembrane formation and swelling that occur during the first few days of the disease may cause respiratory obstruction in addition to other life-threatening complications (see *Anticipating diphtheria hazards*). The disease may also be complicated by polyneuritis (primarily affecting motor fibers but possibly also sensory neurons), encephalitis, cerebral infarction, bacteremia, renal failure, pulmonary emboli, and bronchopneumonia caused by *C. diphtheriae* or other superinfecting organisms. Serum sickness may result from antitoxin therapy.

Assessment

The patient's history may reflect inadequate immunization and an exposure period of less than 1 week. The patient may complain of a sore throat (the most common complaint in adults) and dysphagia; a child is more likely to complain of nausea and vomiting. The patient also may complain of chills, a rasping cough, and hoarseness and may have a temperature of 100° to 102° F (37.8° to 38.9° C).

Inspection may reveal a characteristic thick, patchy, grayish green membrane over the mucous membranes of the pharynx, larynx, tonsils, soft palate, and nose.

If the patient develops respiratory obstruction, inspection will reveal stridor, suprasternal and substernal retraction and, possibly, cyanosis, restlessness, and tachypnea. In cutaneous diphtheria, you'll note skin lesions that resemble impetigo.

During palpation, you may feel enlarged cervical lymph nodes. If the patient has an obstructed airway, auscultation may disclose diminished breath sounds.

Your assessment may reveal palatal and pharyngeal paralysis, ocular or ciliary paralysis, progressive muscle weakness, and paresthesia in neurologic involvement. You may observe signs of peripheral neuritis 2 to 3 months after the onset of illness.

Diagnostic tests
When cultures of throat organisms or of specimens taken from suspicious lesions identify *C. diphtheriae,* the diphtheria diagnosis is confirmed. Electrocardiogram (ECG) abnormalities may indicate myocardium involvement.

Treatment
Initial therapy is based on clinical findings and begins even before culture results confirm the diagnosis. Standard treatment includes diphtheria antitoxin administered by I.M. or I.V. infusion. Antibiotics, such as penicillins and erythromycin, eliminate organisms from the upper respiratory tract and elsewhere so that the patient doesn't remain a carrier. Other measures prevent complications (for example, airway maintenance to prevent possible suffocation).

Key nursing diagnoses and patient outcomes
Risk for suffocation related to airway obstruction from pseudomembrane formation and infected, swollen throat structures. Based on this nursing diagnosis, you'll establish these patient outcomes. The patient will:
- receive immediate emergency help for signs of respiratory obstruction, such as stridor, cyanosis, restlessness, or hypoxia
- continue to have an open airway.

Ineffective airway clearance related to pseudomembrane formation and swollen throat structures. Based on this nursing diagnosis, you'll establish these patient outcomes. The patient will:
- cough effectively and expectorate sputum
- have normal arterial blood gas levels and clear breath sounds
- experience adequate ventilation.

Impaired skin integrity related to lesions caused by cutaneous diphtheria. Based on this nursing diagnosis, you'll establish these patient outcomes. The patient will:
- show skill in caring for skin lesions
- not develop complications from skin lesions, such as skin breakdown or secondary infection
- regain skin integrity when the infection is eradicated.

Nursing interventions
- Obtain culture specimens, as ordered.
- Administer humidified oxygen, as ordered, and elevate the head of the bed to prevent pressure on the diaphragm and compromised breathing.
- Administer drugs, as ordered. Before giving diphtheria antitoxin, which is made from horse serum, review eye and skin test results identifying the patient's sensitivity level. *Note:* Although time-consuming and hazardous, desensitization should be attempted if test results indicate sensitivity to diphtheria antitoxin–the only specific treatment available. If test results are normal, antitoxin is usually administered before laboratory confirmation of the diagnosis because mortality increases when drug administration is delayed.
- Offer frequent, small feedings of liquids and soft foods to the patient with mild to moderate dysphagia. Give parenteral fluids, as ordered, to a patient who can't swallow. Suction, as needed, to prevent aspiration.
- Maintain strict infection and isolation precautions until two consecutive nasopharyngeal culture results are negative for *C. diphtheriae*–at least 1 week after drug therapy stops.
- Report all cases of diphtheria to local public health authorities; follow up on others who have been exposed to the patient, if appropriate.
- If the patient sustains paralysis, assist him to begin a rehabilitation program to restore optimal functioning.

Monitoring
- Watch for anaphylaxis after giving antitoxin or antibiotics, such as penicillin.

• Watch for thrombophlebitis in patients who receive erythromycin therapy.
• Assess respiratory effort and status. Report stridor, cyanosis, and alterations in consciousness and oxygen saturation.
• Inspect the skin regularly in patients with cutaneous diphtheria.
• Monitor neuromuscular function for weakness, paralysis, or sensory changes. Notify the doctor of these changes.

Patient teaching

• Teach the patient the proper technique for disposing of nasopharyngeal secretions.
• Explain the need for follow-up testing. Prepare the patient to expect a prolonged convalescence.
• Inform the patient's family about diphtheria. Explain that treating exposed people with antitoxin remains controversial. If family members haven't been immunized, suggest that they arrange to receive diphtheria toxoid (which is usually given as combined diphtheria and tetanus toxoids or as a combination including pertussis vaccine for children under age 6).
• Stress the need for childhood immunizations to all parents.

Disseminated intravascular coagulation

Also known as consumption coagulopathy and defibrination syndrome, disseminated intravascular coagulation (DIC) complicates conditions that accelerate clotting, causing small-blood-vessel occlusion, organ necrosis, depletion of circulating clotting factors and platelets, and activation of the fibrinolytic system. This, in turn, can provoke severe hemorrhage.

Clotting in the microcirculation usually affects the kidneys and extremities but may occur in the brain, lungs, pituitary and adrenal glands, and GI mucosa. Other conditions, such as vitamin K deficiency, hepatic disease, and anticoagulant therapy, may cause a similar hemorrhage.

Although usually acute, DIC may be chronic in cancer patients. The prognosis depends on early detection and treatment, the severity of the hemorrhage, and treatment of the underlying condition.

Causes

DIC may result from:
• infection – gram-negative or gram-positive septicemia; viral, fungal, or rickettsial infection; protozoal infection
• obstetric complications – abruptio placentae, amniotic fluid embolism, retained dead fetus, eclampsia, septic abortion, postpartum hemorrhage
• neoplastic disease – acute leukemia, metastatic carcinoma, lymphomas
• disorders that produce necrosis – extensive burns and trauma, brain tissue destruction, transplant rejection, hepatic necrosis, anorexia nervosa
• other disorders and conditions – heatstroke, shock, poisonous snakebite, cirrhosis, fat embolism, incompatible blood transfusion, drug reactions, cardiac arrest, surgery necessitating cardiopulmonary bypass, giant hemangioma, severe venous thrombosis, purpura fulminans, adrenal disease, adult respiratory distress syndrome, diabetic ketoacidosis, pulmonary embolism, and sickle cell anemia.

Why such conditions and disorders lead to DIC is unclear. Regardless of how DIC begins, the typical accelerated clotting results in generalized activation of prothrombin and a consequent excess of thrombin. Excess thrombin converts fibrinogen to fibrin, producing fibrin clots in the microcirculation. This process consumes exorbitant amounts of coagulation factors (especially platelets, factor V, prothrombin, fibrinogen, and factor VIII), causing thrombocytopenia, deficiencies in factors V and VIII, hypoprothrombinemia, and hypofibrinogenemia.

Circulating thrombin activates the fibrinolytic system, which lyses fibrin clots into fibrinogen degradation products (FDPs). The hemorrhage that occurs may be due largely to the anticoagulant activity of FDPs, as well as to depletion of plasma coagulation factors.

Complications

DIC may be complicated by renal failure, hepatic damage, cerebrovascular accident, ischemic bowel, or respiratory distress. Hypoxia and anoxia can occur and can lead to severe striated muscle pain. Shock and coma can also result. After fibrinolysis, severe to fatal hemorrhaging of vital organs can occur without warning.

Assessment

The most significant clinical feature of DIC is abnormal bleeding *without* a history of a hemorrhagic disorder. Signs and symptoms are related to bleeding and thrombosis. Bleeding problems are usually more common than thrombotic problems unless coagulation occurs to a greater extent than fibrinolysis.

The patient history may include one of the causes of DIC. And although bleeding may occur from any site, the patient may report signs of bleeding into the skin, such as cutaneous oozing, petechiae, ecchymoses, and hematomas. If the patient is receiving treatment for another disorder when this problem occurs, he may also have bleeding from surgical or invasive procedure sites, such as incisions or venipuncture sites.

Other reported signs and symptoms may include nausea; vomiting; severe muscle, back, and abdominal pain; chest pain; hemoptysis; epistaxis; seizures; and oliguria.

Inspection may reveal petechiae and other signs of bleeding into the skin, acrocyanosis, and dyspnea. On palpation, you may detect reduced peripheral pulses. Auscultation may disclose decreased blood pressure, and neurologic assessment may reveal mental status changes, including confusion.

Diagnostic tests

Abnormal bleeding in the absence of a known hematologic disorder suggests DIC. The following initial laboratory findings reflect coagulation deficiencies:

- decreased platelet count – less than 100,000/mm^3
- reduced fibrinogen levels – less than 150 mg/dl
- prolonged prothrombin time – more than 15 seconds
- prolonged partial thromboplastin time – more than 60 to 80 seconds
- increased FDPs – often greater than 45 mcg/ml, or positive at less than 1:100 dilution
- positive D-dimer test (specific fibrinogen test for DIC) – positive at less than 1:8 dilution.

Other supportive data include prolonged thrombin time, positive fibrin monomers, diminished levels of factors V and VIII, fragmentation of red blood cells (RBCs), and decreased hemoglobin levels (less than 10 g/dl). Final confirmation of the diagnosis may be difficult because many of these test results also occur in other disorders (primary fibrinolysis, for example). However, the FDP and D-dimer tests are considered specific and diagnostic of DIC.

Treatment

Successful management of DIC requires prompt recognition and adequate treatment of the underlying disorder. Treatment may be supportive (when the underlying disorder is self-limiting, for example) or highly specific. If the patient isn't actively bleeding, supportive care alone may reverse DIC. Active bleeding may require administration of blood, fresh-frozen plasma, platelets, or packed RBCs to support hemostasis.

Heparin therapy is controversial. It may be used early in the disease to prevent microclotting but may be considered a last resort in the patient who is actively bleeding. If thrombosis occurs, heparin therapy is usually mandatory. In most cases, it's administered in combination with transfusion therapy.

Key nursing diagnoses and patient outcomes

Altered peripheral tissue perfusion related to small vessel occlusion. Based on this nursing diagnosis, you'll establish these patient outcomes. The patient will:
- demonstrate continuing-to-strong peripheral pulses
- not show changes in skin color and temperature in the extremities
- maintain tissue perfusion and cellular oxygenation in extremities.

Risk for fluid volume deficit related to blood loss. Based on this nursing diagnosis, you'll establish these patient outcomes. The patient will:
- not show signs of fluid volume deficit
- maintain adequate fluid volume as evidenced by equal intake and output volumes and stable vital signs.

Fatigue related to decreased hemoglobin because of bleeding. Based on this nursing diagnosis, you'll establish these patient outcomes. The patient will:
- rest frequently to combat fatigue
- seek help when performing activities of daily living to conserve energy
- recover his normal energy level when DIC resolves.

Nursing interventions

- Administer prescribed analgesics for pain as necessary.
- Reposition the patient every 2 hours, and provide meticulous skin care to prevent skin breakdown.
- Administer oxygen therapy as ordered.
- To prevent clots from dislodging and causing fresh bleeding, don't vigorously rub these areas when washing. Use a 1:1 solution of hydrogen peroxide and water to help remove crusted blood.
- If bleeding occurs, use pressure, cold compresses, and topical hemostatic agents to control it; effective agents may include an absorbable gelatin sponge, a microfibrillar collagen hemostat, or thrombin.
- After giving an injection or removing an I.V. catheter or needle, apply pressure to the injection site for at least 10 minutes. Alert other staff members to the patient's tendency to hemorrhage. Limit venipunctures whenever possible.
- Protect the patient from injury. Enforce complete bed rest during bleeding episodes. If the patient is very agitated, pad the bed rails.
- Perform bladder irrigations as ordered for genitourinary (GU) bleeding.
- If the patient can't tolerate activity because of blood loss, provide frequent rest periods.
- Inform the family of the patient's progress. Prepare them for his appearance (I.V. lines, nasogastric tubes, bruises, dried blood). Provide emotional support and encouragement, and listen to the patient's and family's concerns. As needed, enlist the aid of a social worker, chaplain, and other members of the health care team in providing such support.

Monitoring

- Monitor intake and output hourly in acute DIC, especially when administering blood products. Watch for transfusion reactions and signs of fluid overload.
- To measure the amount of blood lost, weigh dressings and linen and record drainage.
- Weigh the patient daily, particularly in renal involvement.
- Watch for bleeding from the GI and GU tracts. If you suspect intra-abdominal bleeding, measure the patient's abdominal girth at least every 4 hours, and observe closely for signs of shock.
- Monitor the results of serial blood studies (particularly hematocrit, hemoglobin levels, and coagulation times).
- Test all stools and urine for occult blood.
- Check all venipuncture sites frequently for bleeding.

Patient teaching
Explain the disorder to the patient and his family. Focus on early recognition of signs of abnormal bleeding, prompt treatment of the underlying disorders, and prevention of further bleeding.

Diverticular disease

In this disorder, bulging pouches (diverticula) in the GI wall push the mucosal lining through the surrounding muscle. The most common site for diverticula is in the sigmoid colon, but they may develop anywhere, from the proximal end of the pharynx to the anus. Other typical sites are the duodenum, near the pancreatic border or the ampulla of Vater, and the jejunum. Diverticular disease of the stomach is rare and may be a precursor of peptic or neoplastic disease. Diverticular disease of the ileum (Meckel's diverticulum) is the most common congenital anomaly of the GI tract. (See *Meckel's diverticulum.*)

Diverticular disease has two clinical forms. In *diverticulosis,* diverticula are present but don't cause symptoms. In *diverticulitis,* a far more serious disorder, diverticula become inflamed and may cause obstruction, infection, and hemorrhage.

Most common in adults ages 45 and older, diverticular disease affects about 30% of adults over age 60. Diverticulosis is less common in nations where diets contain abundant natural bulk and fiber.

Causes

A diverticulum develops when high intraluminal pressure is exerted on weaker areas – for example, points where blood vessels enter the intestine – causing a break in the muscular continuity of the GI wall. The pressure in the intestinal lumen forces the intestine out, creating a pouch (diverticulum).

Diet, especially highly refined foods, may be a contributing factor. Lack of fiber reduces fecal residue, narrows the bowel lumen, and leads to higher intra-abdominal pressure during defecation.

Diverticulitis occurs when retained undigested food mixed with bacteria accumulates in the diverticulum, forming a hard mass (fecalith). This substance cuts off the blood supply to the diverticulum's

Meckel's diverticulum

In Meckel's diverticulum, a blind tube (such as the appendix) opens into the distal ileum near the ileocecal valve. This congenital abnormality results when the intra-abdominal portion of the yolk sac fails to close completely during fetal development. It occurs in about 2% of the population, mostly in males.

Complications

Uncomplicated Meckel's diverticulum produces no symptoms, but complications cause melena and abdominal pain, especially around the umbilicus. The lining of the diverticulum may be either gastric mucosa or pancreatic tissue. This disorder may lead to peptic ulceration, perforation, and peritonitis and may resemble acute appendicitis.

Meckel's diverticulum may also cause bowel obstruction when a fibrous band that connects the diverticulum to the abdominal wall, the mesentery, or other structures snares a loop of the intestine. This may cause intussusception into the diverticulum, or volvulus near the diverticular attachment to the back of the umbilicus or another intra-abdominal structure.

Meckel's diverticulum should be considered in patients with GI obstruction or hemorrhage, especially when routine GI X-rays are negative.

Treatment

Treatment is surgical resection of the inflamed bowel and antibiotic therapy if infection occurs.

thin walls, increasing its susceptibility to attack by colonic bacteria. Inflammation follows bacterial infection.

Complications

Diverticulitis causes most complications. In severe diverticulitis, the diverticula can rupture, producing abscesses or peritonitis. Diverticular rupture occurs in up to 20% of such patients.

Diverticulitis also may lead to intestinal obstruction, resulting from edema or spasm related to inflammation or, in chronic diverticulitis, from fibrosis and adhesions that narrow and seal the bowel lumen.

Other complications include rectal hemorrhage or portal pyemia (generalized septicemia with abscess formation) from arterial or venous erosion. Occasionally, the inflamed colon segment may produce a fistula by adhering to the bladder or other organs.

In elderly patients, a rare complication of diverticulosis (without diverticulitis) is hemorrhage from colonic diverticula, usually in the right colon. Such hemorrhage is usually mild to moderate and easily controlled. Occasionally, bleeding may be life-threatening.

Assessment

Usually, the patient with diverticulosis has no symptoms. Occasionally, he may report intermittent pain in the left lower abdominal quadrant, which may be relieved by defecation or the passage of flatus. The patient may also report alternating bouts of constipation and diarrhea. The assessment usually reveals no clinical findings. Rarely, palpation may disclose abdominal tenderness in the left lower quadrant.

The patient with diverticulitis may have a history of diverticulosis, diagnosed incidentally (possibly during radiographic studies). Investigation of dietary history commonly reveals low fiber consumption. He may report recent consumption of foods containing seeds or kernels, such as tomatoes, nuts, popcorn, or strawberries, or indigestible roughage, such as celery or corn. Seeds and undigested roughage can block the neck of a diverticulum, causing diverticulitis.

The patient with diverticulitis typically complains of moderate pain in the left lower abdominal quadrant, which he may describe as dull or steady. Straining, lifting, or coughing may aggravate the pain. Other signs and symptoms include mild nausea, gas, and intermittent bouts of constipation, sometimes accompanied by rectal bleeding. Some patients report diarrhea.

On inspection, the patient with diverticulitis may appear distressed. Palpation may confirm his reports of left lower quadrant pain. He may have a low-grade fever.

In acute diverticulitis, the patient may report muscle spasms and show signs of peritoneal irritation. Palpation may reveal guarding and rebound tenderness. Rectal examination may disclose a tender mass if the inflamed area is close to the rectum.

Diagnostic tests

- *Barium studies* confirm the diagnosis. An upper GI series confirms or rules out diverticulosis of the esophagus and upper bowel; a barium enema confirms or rules out diverticulosis of the lower bowel. Barium-filled diverticula can be single, multiple, or clustered like grapes and may have a wide or narrow mouth. Barium outlines, but doesn't fill, diverticula blocked by impacted feces. In patients with acute diverticulitis, a barium enema may rupture the bowel, so this procedure isn't done before the acute phase resolves.
- *Radiography* may reveal colonic spasm if irritable bowel syndrome accompanies diverticular disease.
- *Biopsy* rules out cancer; however, a colonoscopic biopsy isn't recommended during acute diverticular disease because of the strenuous bowel preparation it requires.

• *Blood studies* may show leukocytosis and an elevated erythrocyte sedimentation rate in diverticulitis, especially if the diverticula are infected.
• *Stool tests* detect occult blood in 20% of patients with diverticulitis.

Treatment

Patient management depends on the type of diverticular disease and the severity of symptoms. Asymptomatic diverticulosis generally requires no treatment. Intestinal diverticulosis that causes pain, mild GI distress, constipation, or difficult defecation may respond to a liquid or bland diet, stool softeners, and occasional doses of mineral oil. These measures relieve symptoms, minimize irritation, and decrease the risk of progression to diverticulitis. After pain subsides, patients also benefit from a high-residue diet and bulk medication, such as psyllium.

Treatment of mild diverticulitis without signs of perforation aims to prevent constipation and combat infection. Therapy may include bed rest, a liquid diet, stool softeners, a broad-spectrum antibiotic, meperidine to control pain and relax smooth muscle, and an antispasmodic, such as propantheline, to control muscle spasms.

For more severe diverticulitis, treatment consists of the above measures and I.V. therapy. A nasogastric (NG) tube to relieve intra-abdominal pressure is usually required.

Patients who hemorrhage need blood replacement and careful monitoring of fluid and electrolyte balance. Such bleeding usually stops spontaneously. If it continues, angiography and infusion of vasopressin into the bleeding vessel is effective. Rarely, surgery may be required.

A colon resection to remove a diseased segment of intestine may be required to treat diverticulitis that fails to respond to medical treatment or that causes severe recurrent attacks in the same area. A temporary colostomy may be created to allow the inflamed bowel to rest.

Key nursing diagnoses and patient outcomes

Constipation related to changes in the intestinal tract. Based on this nursing diagnosis, you'll establish these patient outcomes. The patient will:
• identify factors in his life-style that predispose him to constipation
• change personal habits and thereby encourage a normal elimination pattern
• regain and maintain a normal elimination pattern.

Risk for infection related to the diverticulum's susceptibility to bacterial activity. Based on this nursing diagnosis, you'll establish these patient outcomes. The patient will:
• maintain a normal temperature and white blood cell count
• not have signs and symptoms of an intestinal infection, such as abdominal distention or pain, diarrhea, or nausea and vomiting
• remain free of intestinal infection.

Pain related to inflammation. Based on this nursing diagnosis, you'll establish these patient outcomes. The patient will:
• express feelings of comfort after analgesic administration
• not have pain when diverticulitis resolves.

Nursing interventions

• Keep in mind that diverticulitis, which produces more serious symptoms and complications, usually requires more interventions than diverticulosis.
• Administer antibiotics, stool softeners, and antispasmodics, as ordered. For severe pain, administer analgesics such as meperidine, as ordered.
• Maintain bed rest for the patient with acute diverticulitis. Don't let him lift, strain, bend, cough, or perform any other actions that increase intra-abdominal pressure.
• Maintain the diet as ordered. The patient having an acute attack is usually on a liquid diet. If symptoms are severe or if he

has nausea and vomiting or abdominal distention, insert an NG tube and attach it to intermittent suction, as ordered. Make sure the patient receives nothing by mouth, and administer ordered I.V. fluids. As symptoms subside, gradually advance the diet.

• If diverticular bleeding occurs, the patient may require angiography and catheter placement for vasopressin infusion. If so, prepare him for the procedure as ordered.

• If the patient will undergo surgery, provide routine preoperative care. (See the entries "Bowel resection with anastomosis" and "Bowel resection with ostomy.") Also perform any special required procedures, such as administering antibiotics or providing a specific diet for several days preoperatively.

• If the patient expresses anxiety, provide psychological support. Listen to his concerns and offer reassurance, when appropriate.

Monitoring

• When administering medications, monitor the patient for desired effects and possible adverse reactions.

• Inspect all stools carefully for color and consistency. Note the frequency of bowel movements.

• Monitor the patient for signs and symptoms of complications. Watch for temperature elevation, increasing abdominal pain, blood in stools, and leukocytosis.

• If the patient has had angiography for catheter placement and vasopressin infusion, inspect the insertion site frequently for bleeding. Check pedal pulses often, and keep the patient from flexing his legs at the groin. Also watch for signs and symptoms of vasopressin-induced fluid retention (apprehension, abdominal cramps, seizures, oliguria, anuria) and severe hyponatremia (hypotension; rapid, thready pulse; cold, clammy skin; cyanosis).

Patient teaching

• Instruct the patient to notify the doctor if he has a temperature above 101° F (38.3° C); abdominal pain that's severe or that lasts for more than 3 days; or blood in his stools. Emphasize that these symptoms indicate complications.

• In uncomplicated diverticulosis, focus your patient teaching on bowel and dietary habits.

• Explain what diverticula are and how they form. Teach the patient about necessary diagnostic tests and prescribed treatments.

• Be sure the patient understands the desired actions and possible adverse effects of his prescribed medications.

• Review recommended dietary changes. Encourage the patient to drink 2 to 3 quarts of fluid daily. Emphasize the importance of dietary roughage and the harmful effects of constipation and straining during a bowel movement. Advise him to increase his intake of foods high in undigestible fiber, such as fresh fruits and vegetables, whole grain breads, and wheat or bran cereals. Warn that a fiber-rich diet may temporarily cause flatulence.

• Advise the patient to relieve constipation with stool softeners or bulk-forming cathartics. Instruct him to take bulk-forming cathartics with plenty of water; if swallowed dry, they may absorb enough moisture in the mouth and throat to swell and obstruct the esophagus or trachea.

• Provide preoperative teaching as appropriate. Reinforce the doctor's explanation of the surgery, and discuss possible complications.

• If a colostomy is constructed during surgery, teach the patient how to care for it. Arrange for a visit with an enterostomal therapist.

Dysfunctional uterine bleeding

Dysfunctional uterine bleeding (DUB) refers to abnormal endometrial bleeding without recognizable organic lesions. Prognosis varies with the cause. DUB is the indication for almost 25% of gynecologic surgery.

Causes

DUB usually results from an imbalance in the hormonal-endometrial relationship whereby estrogen persistently and unopposedly stimulates the endometrium. Sustained high estrogen levels result from polycystic ovary syndrome, obesity, immaturity of the hypothalamic-pituitary-ovarian mechanism (in postpubertal teenagers and perimenopausal women), and anovulation from vigorous exercise, stress, malnutrition, and certain medications.

Usually the endometrium shows no pathologic changes. But in chronic unopposed estrogen stimulation (for example from a hormone-producing ovarian tumor), the endometrium may exhibit hyperplastic or malignant changes.

Complications

Anemia is a complication of DUB. The condition may also have social consequences, affecting work or school performance.

Assessment

The patient with DUB typically reports episodes of vaginal bleeding between menses (metrorrhagia), heavy or prolonged menses (longer than 8 days [hypermenorrhea]) or a menstrual cycle fewer than 18 days (chronic polymenorrhea).

Diagnostic tests

- Initial tests are performed to rule out pregnancy, coagulation disorders, genital tract lesions, and endocrine imbalances.
- Transvaginal ultrasound is used to provide an anatomical evaluation for the etiology.
- Hysteroscopy may be used to view the endocervix and the endometrial cavity and obtain tissue specimens for biopsy.
- Dilatation and curettage (D&C) and endometrial tissue analyses confirm the diagnosis by revealing endometrial hyperplasia.
- Hematocrit and hemoglobin levels determine the need for blood or iron replacement.

Treatment

High-dose estrogen-progestin combination therapy (oral contraceptives), the primary treatment, is designed to control endometrial growth and reestablish a normal menstrual cycle. These drugs are usually administered four times daily for 5 to 7 days, even though bleeding usually stops in 12 to 24 hours. (The patient's age and the cause of bleeding help determine the drug choice and dosage.)

In patients over age 35, endometrial biopsy is necessary before the start of estrogen therapy to rule out endometrial adenocarcinoma. Progestin therapy for 10 days each month is a necessary alternative in some women, such as those susceptible to the adverse effects of estrogen (thrombophlebitis, for example).

If drug therapy fails, a D&C serves as a supplementary treatment (by removal of a large portion of the bleeding endometrium). Also, a D&C can help determine the original cause of hormonal imbalance and can aid in planning further therapy.

Regardless of the primary treatment, the patient may need iron replacement or transfusions of packed cells or whole blood because of anemia caused by recurrent bleeding.

Key nursing diagnoses and patient outcomes

Altered sexuality patterns. Based on this nursing diagnosis, you'll establish these patient outcomes. The patient will:

- express feelings about changes in sexual activity

• resume normal sexual activity when DUB subsides.

Anxiety related to DUB as a possible cancer sign. Based on this nursing diagnosis, you'll establish these patient outcomes. The patient will:
• express feelings of anxiety
• use support systems to assist with coping
• show fewer physical signs and symptoms of anxiety.

Fatigue related to DUB-induced anemia. Based on this nursing diagnosis, you'll establish these patient outcomes. The patient will:
• identify measures to prevent or modify fatigue
• recover and retain normal hemoglobin and hematocrit levels
• regain a normal energy level.

Nursing interventions

• Encourage the patient and her partner to verbalize their feelings about DUB and its effect on their relationship. Offer emotional support and reassurance.
• Help the patient identify her strengths and use them to develop coping strategies.

Monitoring

• Monitor the patient's bleeding pattern, including the duration and amount of bleeding.
• Monitor the patient's response to therapy.

Patient teaching

• Explain the normal menstrual cycle. Ask the patient to keep a menstrual calendar to assist in the diagnosis and to document the effectiveness of treatment.
• Explain the benefits of adhering to the prescribed hormonal therapy. Instruct the patient to take her medication exactly as ordered and to avoid abruptly discontinuing it.
• Explain all procedures and treatment options to the patient to allay anxiety.
• Urge the patient to schedule regular checkups to assess treatment effectiveness.

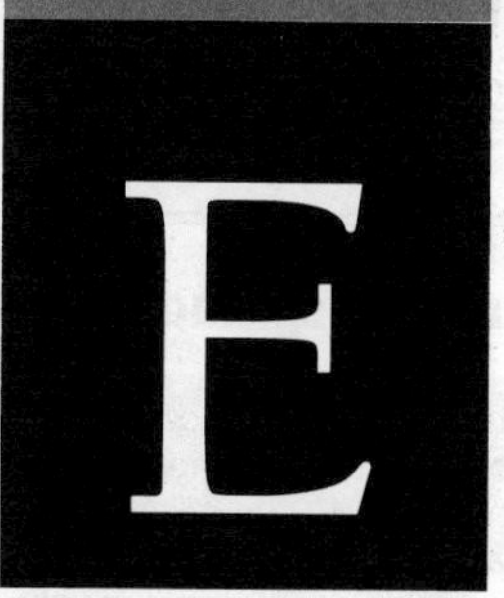

Ebola virus infection

One of the most frightening viruses to emerge from the African subcontinent, the Ebola virus first appeared in 1976. An unclassified ribonucleic acid (RNA) virus, Ebola is morphologically similar to the Marburg virus. Both viruses cause headache, malaise, myalgia, and high fever, progressing to severe diarrhea, vomiting, and internal and external hemorrhage.

The prognosis for Ebola virus infection is extremely poor, with a mortality as high as 90%. The incubation period ranges from 2 to 21 days.

Causes

Ebola virus infection is caused by an unclassified RNA virus that is passed from person to person by direct contact with infected blood, body secretions, or organs. Nosocomial and community-acquired transmission can occur. Contaminated needles can also cause the infection. Transmission through semen may occur up to 7 weeks after clinical recovery. The virus remains contagious even after the patient has died.

Complications

As the infection progresses, severe complications, including liver and kidney dysfunction, dehydration, and hemorrhage, may develop. In pregnant women, the Ebola virus leads to abortion and massive hemorrhage. Death usually results during the second week of illness from organ failure or hemorrhage.

Assessment

The patient's health history usually reveals contact with an infected person. However, no clear line of infection may be apparent at the beginning of an Ebola virus outbreak. The patient usually complains of flulike symptoms, which first appear within 3 days of infection.

As the virus spreads through the body, inspection reveals bruising as capillaries rupture and dead blood cells infiltrate the skin. A maculopapular eruption appears after the fifth day of infection. The patient may also display melena, hematemesis, epistaxis, and bleeding gums. In the final stages of the disease, the skin blisters and sloughs off, blood seeps from all body orifices, and the patient begins vomiting his liquefied internal organs.

Diagnostic tests

Specialized laboratory tests reveal specific antigens or antibodies and may show the isolated virus. As with other types of hemorrhagic fever, tests also demonstrate neutrophil leukocytosis, hypofibrinogenemia, thrombocytopenia, and microangiopathic hemolytic anemia.

Treatment

No cure exists for Ebola virus infection; treatment is providing intensive supportive care. Administration of I.V. fluids helps offset the effects of severe dehydration. The patient

Preventing the spread of Ebola virus

Practicing standard precautions generally prevents transmission of Ebola virus. However, as the patient develops diarrhea and begins vomiting and hemorrhaging, the risk of transmission is greatly increased. To prevent the spread of this deadly disease, the CDC recommends the following guidelines:

- Keep the patient in isolation throughout the course of the disease.
- If possible, place the patient in a negative-pressure room at the beginning of hospitalization to avoid the need for transfer as the disease progresses.
- Restrict nonessential staff members from entering the patient's room.
- Make sure that anyone who enters the patient's room wears gloves and a gown to prevent contact with any surface in the room that may have been soiled.
- Use barriers to prevent skin or mucous membrane exposure to blood or other body fluids, secretions, or excretions when caring for the patient.
- If you must come within 3′ (1 m) of the patient, also wear a face shield or surgical mask and goggles or eyeglasses with side shields.
- *Don't* reuse gloves or gowns unless they have been completely disinfected.
- Make sure any patient who dies of the disease is promptly buried or cremated. Precautions to prevent contact with the patient's body fluids and secretions should continue even after the patient's death.

may receive replacement of plasma heparin before the onset of clinical shock.

Key nursing diagnoses and patient outcomes

Impaired skin integrity related to severe diarrhea. Based on this nursing diagnosis, you'll establish these patient outcomes. The patient will:

- remain free of skin breakdown
- clean himself thoroughly after each loose bowel movement
- demonstrate measures to keep perianal area clean.

Risk for fluid volume deficit related to progressive viral infection. Based on this nursing diagnosis, you'll establish these patient outcomes. The patient will:

- maintain adequate fluid balance
- tolerate fluid replacement as needed
- remain free from fluid imbalance.

Risk for infection related to severe skin sloughing. Based on this nursing diagnosis, you'll establish these patient outcomes. The patient will:

- maintain skin integrity
- remain free of infection.

Fear related to severe, incurable viral infection. Based on this nursing diagnosis, you'll establish these patient outcomes. The patient will:

- verbalize concerns with caregivers and family about the disease
- demonstrate positive coping mechanisms.

Nursing interventions

- Follow the guidelines for standard precautions published by the Centers for Disease Control and Prevention (CDC). (See *Preventing the spread of Ebola virus.*)
- Watch for any changes in the patient's respiration rate and pattern.
- Closely monitor the patient's fluid and electrolyte balance; monitor intake and output.
- Check the results of complete blood count and coagulation studies for signs of blood loss and coagulopathy.

• Assess the patient daily for petechiae, ecchymoses, and oozing blood.
• Test stools, urine, and vomitus for occult blood; watch for frank bleeding.
• Protect all areas of petechiae and ecchymoses from further injury.
• Monitor the patient's family and other close contacts for fever and other signs of infection.
• Provide emotional support for the patient and family during the course of this devastating disease. Encourage the patient and family to ask questions and discuss any concerns they have about the disease and its treatment.
• Notify the local health department as appropriate.

Patient teaching

• Teach the patient's family about Ebola virus infection.
• Explain the importance of reporting any signs of bleeding.
• Explain the purpose of any diagnostic tests and procedures that the patient may undergo.

Emphysema

The most common cause of death from respiratory disease in the United States, emphysema is one of several diseases usually labeled collectively as chronic obstructive pulmonary disease (COPD).

Emphysema appears to be more prevalent in men than in women; about 65% of patients with well-defined emphysema are men; about 35% are women. Postmortem findings reveal few adult lungs without some degree of emphysema.

Causes

Emphysema may be caused by a deficiency of alpha$_1$-antitrypsin and by cigarette smoking. Recurrent inflammation associated with the release of proteolytic enzymes from lung cells causes the air spaces distal to the terminal bronchioles to enlarge abnormally and irreversibly. This leads to the destruction of alveolar walls, which results in a breakdown of elasticity.

Complications

Recurrent respiratory tract infections, cor pulmonale, and respiratory failure may complicate emphysema. Between 20% and 25% of patients with COPD develop peptic ulcer disease. Additionally, alveolar blebs and bullae may rupture, leading to spontaneous pneumothorax or pneumomediastinum.

Assessment

The patient history may disclose that the patient is a longtime smoker. The patient may report shortness of breath, a chronic cough and, possibly, anorexia with resultant weight loss and a general feeling of malaise.

Inspection may show a barrel-chested patient who breathes through pursed lips and who uses accessory muscles. You may notice peripheral cyanosis, clubbed fingers and toes, and tachypnea.

Palpation may reveal decreased tactile fremitus and decreased chest expansion. Percussion may disclose hyperresonance. On auscultation, you may hear decreased breath sounds, crackles, and wheezing during inspiration, a prolonged expiratory phase with grunting respirations, and distant heart sounds.

Diagnostic tests

• *Chest X-rays* in advanced disease may show a flattened diaphragm, reduced vascular markings at the lung periphery, overaeration of the lungs, a vertical heart, enlarged anteroposterior chest diameter, and a large retrosternal air space.
• *Pulmonary function tests* typically indicate increased residual volume and total lung capacity, reduced diffusing capacity, and increased inspiratory flow.
• *Arterial blood gas (ABG) analysis* usually shows reduced partial pressure of oxygen

in arterial blood and normal partial pressure of carbon dioxide in arterial blood until late in the disease.
• *Electrocardiography* may reveal tall, symmetrical P waves in leads II, III, and aV_F; vertical QRS axis; and signs of right ventricular hypertrophy late in the disease.
• *Red blood cell (RBC) count* usually demonstrates an increased hemoglobin level late in the disease when the patient has persistent severe hypoxia.

Treatment

Emphysema management usually includes I.V. or oral bronchodilators (such as aminophylline) and inhaled bronchodilators (such as albuterol) to promote mucociliary clearance; antibiotics to treat respiratory tract infection; and immunizations to prevent influenza and pneumococcal pneumonia. I.V. steroids (such as Solu-Medrol or Solu-Cortef) may be used to mediate any inflammatory response.

Other treatment measures include adequate hydration and (in selected patients) chest physiotherapy to help mobilize secretions.

Some patients may need oxygen therapy (at low settings) to correct hypoxia and also transtracheal catheterization to receive oxygen at home. Counseling about avoiding smoking and air pollutants is necessary.

Key nursing diagnoses and patient outcomes

Activity intolerance caused by fatigue related to chronic tissue hypoxia. Based on this nursing diagnosis, you'll establish these patient outcomes. The patient will:
• identify controllable factors that contribute to fatigue
• skillfully conserve energy while performing daily activities at a tolerable level
• seek assistance when necessary to complete an activity.

Impaired gas exchange related to lung tissue changes caused by recurrent inflammation. Based on this nursing diagnosis, you'll establish these patient outcomes. The patient will:
• have adequate ventilation
• maintain a respiratory rate at baseline level
• not exhibit signs of acute hypoxia, such as confusion, restlessness, or severe anxiety.

Ineffective airway clearance related to increased bronchial secretions caused by recurrent lung inflammation. Based on this nursing diagnosis, you'll establish these patient outcomes. The patient will:
• cough effectively
• expectorate sputum to keep the airway open
• skillfully perform bronchial hygiene to clear secretions from the airway.

Nursing interventions

• If ordered, perform chest physiotherapy, including postural drainage and chest percussion and vibration, several times daily.
• Schedule respiratory treatments at least 1 hour before or after meals. Provide the patient with mouth care after bronchodilator therapy.
• Provide a high-calorie, protein-rich diet to promote health and healing. Give small, frequent meals to conserve the patient's energy and prevent fatigue.
• Make sure the patient receives adequate fluids (at least 3 liters a day) to loosen secretions.
• Encourage daily activity, and provide diversionary activities as appropriate. To conserve energy and prevent fatigue, have the patient alternate rest and activity periods.
• Administer medications, as ordered, and record the patient's response.
• Provide supportive care, and help the patient adjust to life-style changes imposed by a chronic illness.
• Answer the patient's questions about his illness honestly. Encourage him to express his fears and concerns, and stay with him during periods of extreme stress and anxiety.
• Include the patient and his family in care-related decisions. Refer them to appropriate support services as needed.

Monitoring

• Monitor the patient's respiratory function regularly. Perform the activities needed for ABG analyses and pulmonary function studies, as ordered.
• Monitor the patient's RBC count for increases (warning signs of increasing lung and vascular congestion).
• Watch for complications, such as respiratory tract infections, cor pulmonale, spontaneous pneumothorax, respiratory failure, and peptic ulcer disease.

Patient teaching

• Advise the patient to avoid crowds and people with known infections. Also advise him to obtain influenza and pneumococcus immunizations.
• If the patient is receiving home oxygen therapy, explain treatment rationales and proper use of equipment. If the patient requires a transtracheal catheter, instruct him about catheter care, precautions, and follow-up care.
• Teach the patient and family how to perform postural drainage and chest percussion. The patient should maintain each position for about 10 minutes – during this time, a family member should perform percussion and direct the patient to cough. Also teach the patient coughing and deep-breathing techniques to promote good ventilation and mobilize secretions.
• Review the patient's medications and explain the rationale, dosage, and adverse effects related to the prescribed drug. Instruct him to report adverse reactions to the doctor immediately. Show him how to use an inhaler correctly, if appropriate.
• Encourage the patient to eat high-calorie, protein-rich foods. Urge him to drink plenty of fluids to prevent dehydration and to help loosen secretions.
• If the patient smokes, urge him to stop. Provide him with smoking cessation resources or counseling, if necessary.
• Urge the patient to avoid respiratory irritants, such as automobile exhaust fumes, aerosol sprays, and industrial pollutants.
• Warn the patient that exposure to blasts of cold air may precipitate bronchospasm. Tell him to avoid cold, windy weather and to cover his mouth and nose with a scarf or mask if he must go outside.
• If appropriate, describe signs and symptoms of peptic ulcer disease. Instruct the patient to check his stools every day for blood and to notify the doctor if he has persistent nausea, vomiting, heartburn, indigestion, constipation, diarrhea, or bloody stools.
• Inform the patient about signs and symptoms that suggest ruptured alveolar blebs and bullae. Explain the seriousness of possible spontaneous pneumothorax. Urge him to notify the doctor if he feels sudden, sharp pleuritic pain that's exacerbated by chest movement, breathing, or coughing.

Encephalitis

A severe inflammation of the brain, encephalitis is characterized by intense lymphocytic infiltration of brain tissues and the leptomeninges. This causes cerebral edema, degeneration of the brain's ganglion cells, and diffuse nerve cell destruction.

Encephalitis is usually caused by a mosquito-borne or, in some areas, a tick-borne virus. However, transmission by other means may occur through ingestion of infected goat's milk and accidental injection or inhalation of the virus. (See *Types of encephalitis,* page 278.)

Causes

Encephalitis usually results from infection with arboviruses specific to rural areas. In urban areas, encephalitis is usually caused by enteroviruses (coxsackievirus, poliovirus, and echovirus). Other causes include herpesvirus, mumps virus, adenoviruses, and demyelinating diseases af-

Types of encephalitis

Eastern (equine) encephalitis may produce permanent neurologic damage and is often fatal. It occurs in the eastern regions of North, Central, and South America. Western (equine) encephalitis occurs throughout the western hemisphere; California encephalitis, throughout the United States; St. Louis encephalitis, in Florida and in the western and southern United States; and Venezuelan encephalitis, in South America.

Between World War I and the Depression, a type of encephalitis known as lethargic encephalitis, von Economo's disease, or sleeping sickness occurred with some regularity. The causative virus was never clearly identified, and the disease is rare today. Even so, the term sleeping sickness persists and is often mistakenly used to describe other types of encephalitis as well.

ter measles, varicella, rubella, or vaccination.

Complications

Potential complications associated with viral encephalitis include bronchial pneumonia, urine retention, urinary tract infection, pressure ulcers, and coma. Seizure disorder, parkinsonism, and mental deterioration may also occur.

Assessment

Depending on the severity of the disease, all forms of viral encephalitis have similar clinical features. The severity of arbovirus encephalitis may range from subclinical to rapidly fatal necrotizing disease. Herpes encephalitis also produces signs and symptoms that vary from subclinical to acute and usually fatal fulminating disease.

If encephalitis is the primary illness, the patient may be acutely ill when he seeks treatment because the nonspecific symptoms that occur before the onset of acute neurologic symptoms aren't recognized as signs of encephalitis. Thus, patient history may include reports of systemic symptoms, such as headache, muscle stiffness, malaise, sore throat, and upper respiratory tract symptoms, that existed for several days before the onset of neurologic symptoms.

After neurologic symptoms occur, patient history may reveal the sudden onset of altered levels of consciousness, from lethargy or drowsiness to stupor. The patient or a family member may also report the occurrence of seizures, which may be the only presenting sign of encephalitis.

On neurologic examination, the patient may be confused, disoriented, or hallucinating. He may also demonstrate tremor, cranial nerve palsies, exaggerated deep tendon reflexes, absent superficial reflexes, and paresis or paralysis of the extremities. Additionally, the patient may complain of a stiff neck when the head is bent forward.

Vital signs usually reveal fever. The patient may also experience nausea and vomiting.

If the cerebral hemispheres are involved, assessment findings may include aphasia; involuntary movements identified on inspection; ataxia; sensory defects, such as disturbances of taste and smell; and poor memory retention.

Diagnostic tests

During an encephalitis epidemic, diagnosis is readily made from clinical findings and patient history. However, sporadic cases are difficult to distinguish from other febrile illnesses, such as gastroenteritis or meningitis. The following tests help establish a diagnosis:

• *Blood analysis* or, rarely, *cerebrospinal fluid (CSF) analysis* identifies the virus and confirms the diagnosis. The common viruses that also cause herpes, measles, and mumps are easier to identify than arboviruses. Arboviruses and herpesviruses

can be isolated by inoculating young mice with a specimen taken from the patient.
• *Serologic studies* in herpes encephalitis may show rising titers of complement-fixing antibodies.
• *Lumbar puncture* discloses CSF pressure elevated in all forms of encephalitis. Despite inflammation, *CSF analysis* often reveals clear fluid. White blood cell count and protein levels in CSF are slightly elevated, but the glucose level remains normal.
• *EEG* reveals abnormalities, such as generalized slowing of waveforms.
• *Computed tomography scan* may be ordered to check for temporal lobe lesions that indicate herpesvirus and to rule out cerebral hematoma.

Treatment

The antiviral agent vidarabine monohydrate is effective only against herpes encephalitis and only if it's administered before the onset of coma.

Treatment of all other forms of encephalitis is supportive. Drug therapy includes reduction of intracranial pressure (ICP) with I.V. mannitol and corticosteroids (to reduce cerebral inflammation and resulting edema); phenytoin or another anticonvulsant, usually given I.V.; sedatives for restlessness; and aspirin or acetaminophen to relieve headache and reduce fever.

Other supportive measures include adequate fluid and electrolyte intake to prevent dehydration; appropriate antibiotics for associated infections, such as pneumonia or sinusitis; maintenance of the patient's airway; administration of oxygen to maintain arterial blood gas levels; and maintenance of nutrition, especially during coma. Isolation is unnecessary.

Key nursing diagnoses and patient outcomes

Altered thought processes related to brain cell dysfunction. Based on this nursing diagnosis, you'll establish these patient outcomes. The patient will:
• remain safe from injury
• regain orientation to time, person, and place and remain oriented after the infection is eradicated.

Hyperthermia related to infection. Based on this nursing diagnosis, you'll establish these patient outcomes. The patient will:
• regain a normal temperature with antipyretic agents and maintain a normal temperature when the infection is eradicated
• not sustain brain damage because of hyperthermia.

Impaired physical mobility related to neurologic dysfunction. Based on this nursing diagnosis, you'll establish these patient outcomes. The patient will:
• not develop complications while mobility is impaired
• skillfully perform the prescribed mobility regimen to prevent complications
• regain normal physical mobility when encephalitis is eliminated.

Nursing interventions

• Maintain adequate fluid intake to prevent dehydration, but avoid fluid overload, which may increase cerebral edema.
• Maintain adequate nutrition. Give small, frequent meals, or supplement meals with nasogastric tube or parenteral feedings.
• As ordered, give vidarabine by slow I.V. infusion only.
• To prevent constipation and minimize the risk of increased ICP resulting from straining at stool, provide a mild laxative or stool softener.
• Carefully position the patient to prevent joint stiffness and neck pain, and turn him often. Assist with range-of-motion exercises.
• Provide thorough mouth care.
• Maintain a quiet environment. Darkening the room may decrease headache. If the patient naps during the day and is restless at night, plan daytime activities to minimize napping and promote nighttime sleep.

- If the patient has seizures, take precautions to protect him from injury.
- Because the illness and frequent diagnostic tests can be frightening, provide emotional support and reassurance to the patient and family.
- If the patient becomes delirious or confused, try to reorient him often. Putting a calendar or a clock in his room may help.

Monitoring

- During the acute phase of the illness, assess the patient's neurologic function often. Observe his level of consciousness and signs of increased ICP (increasing restlessness, plucking at the bedcovers, vomiting, seizures, and changes in pupil size, motor function, and vital signs). Also watch for cranial nerve involvement (ptosis, strabismus, diplopia), abnormal sleep patterns, and behavioral changes.
- Measure and record intake and output; monitor for fluid and electrolyte imbalance.
- When administering vidarabine, watch for adverse reactions, such as tremor, dizziness, hallucinations, anorexia, nausea, vomiting, diarrhea, pruritus, rash, and anemia. Also watch for adverse effects from other drugs. Check infusion sites often to prevent problems such as infiltration and phlebitis.
- Watch for complications associated with bed rest, such as skin breakdown, constipation, and muscle weakness.

Patient teaching

- Teach the patient and his family about the disease and its effects. Explain diagnostic tests and treatments. Be sure to explain procedures to the patient even if he's comatose.
- Explain that behavior changes caused by encephalitis are usually transitory, but permanent problems sometimes occur. If a neurologic deficit is severe and appears permanent, refer the patient to a rehabilitation program as soon as the acute phase passes.

Endarterectomy

Carotid endarterectomy is a surgical procedure that removes atheromatous plaque from the inner lining of the carotid arteries. This improves intracranial perfusion by increasing blood flow through the carotid arteries.

Carotid endarterectomy may help patients with reversible ischemic neurologic deficit or a completed cerebrovascular accident (CVA). Patients who experience transient ischemic attacks (TIAs), syncope, and dizziness and those who have high-grade asymptomatic or ulcerative lesions may also benefit from this procedure.

Other beneficiaries of carotid endarterectomy include patients with concurrent coronary artery disease. The procedure may relieve both conditions in one operation (in patients who are neurologically stable and otherwise good surgical risks). Because carotid lesions commonly lead to CVA in both symptomatic and asymptomatic patients, some surgeons consider this operation a prophylactic treatment for CVA. However, many intraoperative and postoperative risks are associated with the procedure, making it unsuitable for some patients (see *Risk levels in carotid endarterectomy*).

Procedure

Cervical block anesthesia and sedatives are usually used, which allow the patient to be closely monitored. Alternatively, light general anesthesia may be used during a carotid endarterectomy so that brain waves can be assessed.

An incision is made along the anterior border of the sternocleidomastoid or transversely in a skin crease in the neck. Once the incision is made, the common carotid artery, external carotid artery, and internal carotid artery (ICA) are exposed and the carotid artery is clamped to evaluate perfusion. If cerebral perfusion is inadequate, a shunt is inserted to permit blood

Risk levels in carotid endarterectomy

Is your patient a good candidate for a carotid endarterectomy? One tool for evaluating the patient's chances for a good outcome is the risk-benefit guide below.

Grade 1 patients have the least risk of surgical failure and may benefit the most from carotid endarterectomy. Grade 4 patients have the highest risk and may benefit the least.

Grade 1

Patients classified as grade 1 are under age 70. Medical risk factors, such as diabetes or hyperlipidemia, and lifestyle risk factors, such as alcohol abuse or cigarette smoking, may make patients appear older physiologically than their stated age.

Grade 1 patients have bilateral or unilateral focal carotid stenosis and no fixed neurologic deficits. They're considered neurologically stable.

Grade 2

These patients appear clinically equal to patients in grade 1. However, in grade 2, angiographic findings are more extensive; for example, coexisting stenosis of the ICA in the siphon area, extensive involvement of the vessel to be operated on, or occlusion of the opposite ICA.

Grade 3

These patients have angiographic evidence of significant lesions similar to that of patients in grade 2. However, grade 3 patients also have significant medical risk factors that will complicate surgery, such as coronary artery disease, myocardial infarction (within 6 months), blood pressure above 180/110 mm Hg, chronic obstructive pulmonary disease, severe obesity, or a physiologic age over 70.

Grade 4

Patients in this classification are neurologically unstable and represent the greatest surgical risk. Neurologic instability includes a CVA in progress, frequent uncontrolled TIAs, or multiple neurologic deficits from previous cerebral infarctions.

flow past the obstruction in the carotid artery and to ensure adequate cerebral circulation during surgery.

Once the carotid artery is stabilized, a heparin infusion is started to prevent thrombosis. The affected arteries are then incised and the plaque is dissected. Next, the artery is patched with an autogenous saphenous vein or prosthetic material and closed. If a shunt is in place, it's removed before complete closure.

Complications

The most common complication of carotid endarterectomy is blood pressure lability. Transient hypertension also occurs frequently from manipulation of the carotid body. Perioperative CVA, the most serious complication, may result from the embolization of debris during dissection.

Temporary or permanent loss of carotid body function may occur. Blood pressure and ventilation normally increase in response to hypoxia; however, with the loss of carotid body function, blood pressure and ventilation decrease in response to hypoxia. Other complications include rethrombosis, postoperative respiratory distress caused by tracheal compression from a hematoma, and wound infection at the surgical site.

An uncommon complication is a sudden increase in cerebral blood flow, which can lead to ipsilateral vascular headaches, seizures, and intracerebral hemorrhage.

Rarely, vocal cord paralysis may arise from manipulation of the vagus nerve.

Key nursing diagnoses and patient outcomes

Risk for injury related to possible complications of surgery. Based on this nursing diagnosis, you'll establish these patient outcomes. The patient will:
• not develop complications
• maintain normal vital signs or regain them quickly postoperatively
• have unchanged or improved neurologic, cardiac, and respiratory function.

Risk for suffocation related to potential tracheal compression from a hematoma at the surgical site. Based on this nursing diagnosis, you'll establish these patient outcomes. The patient will:
• maintain adequate ventilation
• not develop signs and symptoms of respiratory distress
• not complain of unusual pressure and not have excessive swelling in his neck.

Altered protection related to temporary or permanent loss of carotid body function. Based on this nursing diagnosis, you'll establish these patient outcomes. The patient will:
• be aware of the signs and symptoms of hypoxia so he'll know when to seek medical attention
• wear or carry medical identification. In an emergency, this alerts health care professionals to look for deviations in the signs of hypoxia the patient may exhibit.

Nursing interventions

When preparing the patient for carotid endarterectomy or caring for him afterward, implement these interventions.

Before surgery

• To reduce their anxiety, teach the patient and family about the procedure and answer their questions.
• Discuss the location of the lesion. Also describe the atherosclerotic process so the patient can modify risk factors after surgery.
• Explain all preoperative diagnostic tests used to evaluate carotid disease, including periorbital ultrasonography, ocular pneumoplethysmography, carotid phonoangiography, computed tomography scan, and cerebral angiography. If the patient has concurrent coronary artery disease, also explain electrocardiography (ECG), coronary angiography, and the treadmill exercise stress test.
• Give the patient and family a tour of the intensive care unit to help prepare them for the postoperative course.
• Explain postoperative care, and warn the patient and family what I.V. lines, hemodynamic measuring devices, tubes, and machinery will be connected to the patient.
• Tell the patient that he'll have some postoperative discomfort or pain but that pain medication will be available.
• Inform the patient that a nurse will check his neurologic status, including level of consciousness, orientation, extremity strength, speech, and fine hand movements, every hour after surgery. Explain that this is routine, not an indication that he isn't doing well.
• Before surgery, help the doctor insert a radial arterial catheter to monitor arterial blood gases and blood pressure.
• Ensure that a baseline EEG is done before the patient is anesthetized.

After surgery

• Monitor vital signs every 15 minutes for the first hour until the patient is stable. Lowered blood pressure and elevated heart rate and respirations could indicate cerebral ischemia.
• Perform a neurologic assessment every hour for the first 24 hours. Check extremity strength, fine hand movements, speech, level of consciousness, and orientation.
• Monitor intake and output hourly for the first 24 hours.

• Perform continuous cardiac monitoring for the first 24 hours. Take an ECG if the patient has any chest pain or arrhythmias – many patients undergoing this procedure also have coronary artery disease.

Home care instructions

• Teach the patient and family surgical wound care. Review the signs and symptoms of infection (fever, sore throat, or redness, swelling or drainage from the wound), and tell them to call the doctor immediately if these occur.
• Encourage the patient to stop smoking, reduce lipid levels, lose weight, and lower any other risk factors.
• Be sure the patient understands the dosage and possible adverse effects of all prescribed medications.
• If the patient has had a CVA and needs follow-up care, refer him and his family to a home health care agency.
• Teach the patient how to manage any neurologic, sensory, or motor deficits that occurred during surgery.
• Tell the patient to contact the doctor immediately if any new neurologic symptoms occur (reocclusion occurs in 1.5% to 23% of patients).
• Emphasize the importance of regular checkups.

Endocarditis

An infection of the endocardium, heart valves, or cardiac prosthesis, endocarditis results from bacterial or fungal invasion.

In infective endocarditis, fibrin and platelets cluster on valve tissue and engulf circulating bacteria or fungi. This produces friable verrucous vegetation. The vegetation may cover the valve surfaces, causing deformities and destruction of valvular tissue. It may also extend to the chordae tendineae, causing them to rupture and leading to valvular insufficiency.

Sometimes vegetation forms on the endocardium, usually in areas altered by rheumatic, congenital, or syphilitic heart disease. It also may form on normal surfaces. Vegetative growth on the heart valves, endocardial lining of a heart chamber, or endothelium of a blood vessel may embolize to the spleen, kidneys, central nervous system, and lungs. (See *Recognizing infarction sites in endocarditis,* page 284.)

Endocarditis can be classified as native valve endocarditis, endocarditis in I.V. drug users, and prosthetic valve endocarditis. It can be acute or subacute. Untreated, endocarditis is usually fatal. With proper treatment, however, about 70% of patients recover. The prognosis is worst when endocarditis causes severe valvular damage – leading to insufficiency and left ventricular failure – or when it involves a prosthetic valve.

Causes

Acute infective endocarditis usually results from bacteremia that follows septic thrombophlebitis, open-heart surgery involving prosthetic valves, or skin, bone, and pulmonary infections.

The most common causative organisms are group A nonhemolytic streptococci, staphylococci, and enterococci. However, almost any organism can cause endocarditis, including *Neisseria gonorrhoeae, Pseudomonas, Salmonella, Streptobacillus, Serratia marcescens,* bacteroids, *Haemophilus, Brucella, Mycobacterium, N. meningitidis, Listeria, Legionella,* diphtheroids, enteric gram-negative bacilli, spirochetes, rickettsiae, chlamydiae, and the fungi *Candida* and *Aspergillus.*

Subacute infective endocarditis typically occurs in people with acquired valvular or congenital cardiac lesions. It can also follow dental, genitourinary (GU), gynecologic, and GI procedures. The most common infecting organisms are *Streptococcus viridans,* which normally inhabits the upper respiratory tract, and *Enterococcus faecalis,* found in GI and perineal flora.

Recognizing infarction sites in endocarditis

In 12% to 35% of patients with subacute endocarditis, embolization from vegetating lesions or diseased valve tissue may produce typical characteristics of splenic, renal, cerebral, or pulmonary infarction or peripheral vascular occlusion.

- Splenic infarction causes pain in the left upper quadrant, radiating to the left shoulder, and abdominal rigidity.
- Renal infarction causes hematuria, pyuria, flank pain, and decreased urine output.
- Cerebral infarction causes hemiparesis, aphasia, and other neurologic deficits.
- Pulmonary infarction causes cough, pleuritic pain, pleural friction rub, dyspnea, and hemoptysis. These signs are most common in right-sided endocarditis, which typically occurs among I.V. drug abusers and after cardiac surgery.
- Peripheral vascular occlusion causes numbness and tingling in an arm, leg, finger, or toe or signs of impending peripheral gangrene.

Preexisting conditions, including rheumatic valvular disease, congenital heart disease, mitral valve prolapse, degenerative heart disease, calcific aortic stenosis (in elderly people), asymmetrical septal hypertrophy, Marfan syndrome, syphilitic aortic valve, I.V. drug abuse, and long-term hemodialysis with an arteriovenous shunt or fistula, can predispose a person to endocarditis. However, up to 40% of affected patients have no underlying heart disease.

Complications

Typically, the heart compensates for the malfunctioning valves for years until left ventricular failure, valve stenosis or regurgitation, or myocardial erosion sets in. Also, vegetative growth on the valves can cause embolic debris to lodge in the small vasculature of the visceral tissue.

Assessment

The patient may have a history of an underlying predisposing condition. He may complain of nonspecific symptoms, such as weakness, fatigue, weight loss, anorexia, arthralgia, night sweats, and an intermittent fever that may recur for weeks.

Inspection may reveal petechiae of the skin (especially common on the upper anterior trunk) and the buccal, pharyngeal, or conjunctival mucosa, and splinter hemorrhages under the nails. Rarely, you may see Osler's nodes (tender, raised, subcutaneous lesions on the fingers or toes), Roth's spots (hemorrhagic areas with white centers on the retina), and Janeway lesions (purplish macules on the palms or soles). Clubbing of the fingers may be present in patients with long-standing disease.

Auscultation may reveal a murmur in all patients except those with early acute endocarditis and I.V. drug users with tricuspid valve infection. The murmur is usually loud and regurgitant, which is typical of the underlying rheumatic or congenital heart disease. A murmur that changes suddenly or a new murmur that develops in the presence of fever is a classic physical sign of endocarditis.

Percussion and palpation may reveal splenomegaly in long-standing disease.

In patients who have developed left ventricular failure, your assessment may reveal dyspnea, tachycardia, bibasilar crackles, and neck vein distention.

Diagnostic tests

Three or more blood cultures during a 24- to 48-hour period identify the causative organism in up to 90% of patients. The remaining 10% may have negative blood cultures, possibly suggesting fungal or difficult-to-diagnose infections, such as *H. parainfluenzae.* Other abnormal but nonspecific laboratory results include:

- normal or elevated white blood cell count and differential
- abnormal histiocytes (macrophages)
- normocytic, normochromic anemia (in subacute infective endocarditis)
- elevated erythrocyte sedimentation rate and serum creatinine levels
- positive serum rheumatoid factor in about half of all patients with endocarditis after the disease is present for 6 weeks
- proteinuria and microscopic hematuria.

Echocardiography may identify valvular damage in up to 80% of patients with native valve disease. It also may show atrial fibrillation and other arrhythmias that accompany valvular disease.

Treatment

The goal of treatment is to eradicate all of the infecting organisms from the vegetation. Therapy should start promptly and continue over several weeks. Selection of an anti-infective drug is based on the infecting organism and sensitivity studies. If blood cultures are negative, the doctor may want to determine the *probable* infecting organism. I.V. antibiotic therapy usually lasts about 4 weeks.

Supportive treatment includes bed rest, aspirin for fever and aches, and sufficient fluid intake. Severe valvular damage, especially aortic regurgitation or infection of a cardiac prosthesis, may require corrective surgery if refractory heart failure develops or if an infected prosthetic valve must be replaced.

Key nursing diagnoses and patient outcomes

Activity intolerance related to oxygen supply deficit caused by decreased cardiac output. Based on this nursing diagnosis, you'll establish these patient outcomes. The patient will:

- sustain normal blood pressure, pulse, and respirations during limited activity
- conserve energy while performing daily activities to tolerance level
- express an understanding of the symptoms of activity intolerance occurring from a deficit in oxygen supply or use.

Decreased cardiac output related to aortic regurgitation. Based on this nursing diagnosis, you'll establish these patient outcomes. The patient will:

- maintain hemodynamic stability, evidenced by a normal blood pressure and pulse rate
- not have chest pain or arrhythmias
- maintain adequate cardiac output.

Risk for injury related to potential for embolization of other organs from vegetating lesions or diseased valve tissue. Based on this nursing diagnosis, you'll establish these patient outcomes. The patient will:

- not exhibit signs and symptoms of organ dysfunction from embolization
- maintain normal organ function in all body systems.

Nursing interventions

- Stress the importance of bed rest. Assist the patient with bathing, if necessary. Provide a bedside commode because this method puts less stress on the heart than using a bedpan. Offer diversional activities that are physically undemanding.
- Before giving antibiotics, obtain the patient's history of allergies and take blood cultures. Administer antibiotics on time to maintain consistent drug levels in the blood. Monitor therapeutic levels.
- To reduce the risk of infiltration or inflammation at the I.V. site, rotate venous access sites.
- Provide supportive care as indicated.
- To reduce anxiety, allow the patient to express his concerns about the effects of activity restrictions on his responsibilities and routines. Reassure him that the restrictions are temporary.

Monitoring

- Watch for signs of embolization (hematuria, pleuritic chest pain, left upper quadrant pain, paresis), a common occurrence

during the first 3 months of treatment. Tell the patient to watch for and report these signs, which may indicate impending peripheral vascular occlusion or splenic, renal, cerebral, or pulmonary infarction.
• Monitor the patient's renal status (including blood urea nitrogen levels, creatinine clearance levels, and urine output) to check for signs of renal emboli and drug toxicity.
• Assess cardiovascular status frequently, and watch for signs of left ventricular failure, such as dyspnea, hypotension, tachycardia, tachypnea, crackles, neck vein distention, edema, and weight gain. Check for changes in cardiac rhythm or conduction.
• Evaluate arterial blood gas values, as needed, to ensure adequate oxygenation.
• Observe for signs of infiltration or inflammation at the venipuncture site, a possible complication of long-term I.V. therapy.

Patient teaching

• Teach the patient about the anti-infectives he'll continue to take. Stress the importance of taking the medication and restricting his activities for as long as the doctor orders.
• Tell the patient to watch closely for fever, anorexia, and other signs of relapse about 2 weeks after treatment stops.
• Make sure the susceptible patient understands the need for prophylactic antibiotics before, during, and after dental work, childbirth, and GU, GI, or gynecologic procedures.
• Teach the patient how to recognize symptoms of endocarditis, and tell him to notify the doctor immediately if such symptoms occur.

Endometriosis

When endometrial tissue appears outside the lining of the uterine cavity, endometriosis results. Such ectopic tissue is generally confined to the pelvic area, most commonly around the ovaries, uterovesical peritoneum, uterosacral ligaments, and the cul-de-sac, but it can appear anywhere in the body.

This ectopic endometrial tissue responds to normal stimulation in the same way that the endometrium does. During menstruation, the ectopic tissue bleeds, which causes inflammation of the surrounding tissues. This inflammation causes fibrosis, leading to adhesions, which produce pain and infertility.

Active endometriosis usually occurs between ages 30 and 40, especially in women who postpone childbearing; it's uncommon before age 20. Severe symptoms of endometriosis may have an abrupt onset or may develop over many years. This disorder usually becomes progressively severe during the menstrual years but tends to subside after menopause.

Causes

The direct cause is unknown, but familial susceptibility or recent hysterotomy may predispose a woman to endometriosis. Although neither of these possible predisposing factors explains all the lesions in endometriosis or their location, research focuses on the following possible causes:
• *Transportation* (retrograde menstruation). During menstruation, the fallopian tubes expel endometrial fragments that implant outside the uterus.
• *Formation in situ.* Inflammation or a hormonal change triggers metaplasia.
• *Induction* (a combination of transportation and formation in situ). The endometrium chemically induces undifferentiated mesenchyma to form endometrial epithelium. (This is the most likely cause.)
• *Immune system defects.* Endometriosis may result from a specific defect in cell-mediated immunity. Researchers have documented higher titers of antibodies to endometrial antigens in patients with this disorder.

Complications

The primary complication of endometriosis is infertility. Other complications include spontaneous abortion, anemia due to excessive bleeding, and emotional problems due to infertility.

Assessment

The patient may complain of cyclic pelvic pain, infertility, and acquired dysmenorrhea. The patient typically reports pain in the lower abdomen, vagina, posterior pelvis, and back. This pain usually begins from 5 to 7 days before menses, reaches a peak, and lasts for 2 to 3 days. It differs from primary dysmenorrheal pain, which is more cramplike and concentrated in the abdominal midline. However, the severity of pain doesn't necessarily indicate the extent of the disease.

Other clinical features depend on the ectopic tissue site. The patient may report a history of infertility and profuse menses (oviducts and ovaries). She may complain of deep-thrust dyspareunia (ovaries and cul-de-sac); suprapubic pain, dysuria, and hematuria (bladder); painful defecation, rectal bleeding with menses, and pain in the coccyx or sacrum (rectovaginal septum and colon); nausea and vomiting that worsen before menses, and abdominal cramps (small bowel and appendix).

Palpation may detect multiple tender nodules on uterosacral ligaments or in the rectovaginal septum. These nodules enlarge and become more tender during menses. Palpation may also uncover ovarian enlargement in the presence of endometrial cysts on the ovaries or thickened, nodular adnexa (as in pelvic inflammatory disease).

Diagnostic tests

- *Laparoscopy* confirms the diagnosis and identifies the stage of the disease. A scoring and staging system created by the American Fertility Society quantifies endometrial implants according to size, character, and location. Stage I signifies minimal disease (1 to 5 points); Stage II, mild disease (6 to 15 points); Stage III, moderate disease (16 to 40 points); and Stage IV, severe disease (more than 40 points).
- *Barium enema* rules out bowel disease.

Treatment

The stage of the disease and the patient's age and desire to have children determine the course of treatment.

Conservative therapy for young women who want to have children includes androgens, such as danazol, which produce a temporary remission in Stages I and II. Progestins and oral contraceptives are also useful in relieving symptoms. Newer treatment involves gonadotropin-releasing analogues, which suppress estrogen production. This causes atrophic changes in the ectopic endometrial tissue, which allows healing.

Laparoscopy, used for diagnostic purposes, can also be used therapeutically to lyse adhesions, remove small implants, and cauterize implants. Laparoscopy also permits laser vaporization of implants. This surgery is usually followed with hormonal therapy to suppress the return of endometrial implants.

When the patient has ovarian masses, surgery may be needed to rule out cancer. Conservative surgery is possible, but the treatment of choice for women who don't want to bear children or for extensive disease (Stages III and IV) is a total abdominal hysterectomy with bilateral salpingo-oophorectomy.

Minor gynecologic procedures are contraindicated immediately before and during menstruation.

Key nursing diagnoses and patient outcomes

Chronic pain related to cyclic inflammation of surrounding tissue resulting in fibrosis. Based on this nursing diagnosis, you'll establish these patient outcomes. The patient will:

• express comfort after administration of analgesics
• use diversional activities to help relieve pain.

Fatigue related to anemia caused by excessive bleeding. Based on this nursing diagnosis, you'll establish these patient outcomes. The patient will:
• stagger her activities of daily living and take frequent rest periods to minimize fatigue
• seek assistance with activities that cause fatigue
• regain and maintain normal hemoglobin levels.

Ineffective individual coping related to infertility. Based on this nursing diagnosis, you'll establish these patient outcomes. The patient will:
• express an understanding of the relationship between emotional state and behavior
• identify effective and ineffective coping techniques
• use available support systems, such as family, friends, or a mental health professional, to develop and maintain effective coping skills.

Nursing interventions

• Encourage the patient and her partner to verbalize their feelings about the disorder and its effect on their relationship. Offer emotional support. Stress the need for open communication before and during intercourse to minimize discomfort and frustration.
• Help the patient develop effective coping strategies. Refer her and her partner to a mental health professional for additional counseling, if necessary. Encourage her to contact a support group, such as the Endometriosis Association.

Monitoring

• If the patient bleeds excessively with menses, monitor for signs and symptoms of anemia. Check hemoglobin levels as ordered.
• Monitor the patient's response to therapy.

Patient teaching

• Explain all procedures and treatment options. Clarify any misconceptions about the disorder, associated complications, and fertility.
• Advise adolescents to use sanitary napkins instead of tampons. This can help prevent retrograde flow in girls with a narrow vagina or small vaginal meatus.
• Because infertility is a possible complication, counsel the patient who wants children not to postpone childbearing.
• Recommend that the patient have an annual pelvic examination and a Papanicolaou test.

Epididymitis

Infection of the epididymis, the testis' cordlike excretory duct, is one of the most common infections of the male reproductive tract. It usually affects adults and is rare before puberty.

Causes

Epididymitis usually results from pyogenic organisms, such as *Escherichia coli,* chlamydia, *Neisseria gonorrhoeae,* and *Pseudomonas aeruginosa.* Infection usually results from established urinary tract infection or prostatitis extending to the epididymis through the lumen of the vas deferens. Rarely, epididymitis is secondary to a distant infection, such as pharyngitis or tuberculosis, that spreads through the lymphatic system or, less commonly, the bloodstream.

Trauma may reactivate a dormant infection or initiate a new one. In addition, epididymitis is a complication of prostatectomy and may also result from chemical irritation by extravasation of urine through the vas deferens.

Complications

Epididymitis may spread to the testis, causing orchitis. Bilateral epididymitis may cause sterility.

Assessment

The patient may complain of unilateral, dull, aching pain radiating to the spermatic cord, lower abdomen, and flank and of an extremely heavy feeling in the scrotum. He also may have erythema, a high fever, and malaise and may exhibit a characteristic waddle – an attempt to protect the groin and scrotum during walking. An acute hydrocele may occur as a reaction to the inflammatory process.

Diagnostic tests

- *Urinalysis.* Increased white blood cell (WBC) count indicates infection.
- *Urine culture and sensitivity tests.* Findings may identify the causative organism.
- *Culture of urethral discharge or prostatic secretions.* Results may identify the organism causing the infection.
- *Serum WBC count.* A count of more than 10,000/mm^3 indicates infection. If orchitis also is present, the diagnosis must be made cautiously because symptoms mimic those of testicular torsion, a condition that requires urgent surgical intervention.

Treatment

The goal of treatment is to reduce pain and swelling and combat infection. Therapy must begin immediately, particularly in a patient with bilateral epididymitis, because sterility is always a threat.

During the acute phase, treatment consists of bed rest, scrotal elevation with towel rolls or adhesive strapping, broad-spectrum antibiotics, and analgesics. An ice bag applied to the area may reduce swelling and relieve pain (heat is contraindicated because it may damage germinal cells, which are viable only at or below normal body temperature). When pain and swelling subside and permit walking, an athletic supporter may prevent pain. Corticosteroids may be prescribed to help counteract inflammation, but their use is controversial.

Prevention of constipation during treatment is important because constipation may increase pain.

Key nursing diagnoses and patient outcomes

Altered sexuality patterns related to inability to engage in sexual activity because of discomfort. Based on this nursing diagnosis, you'll establish these outcomes. The patient and his partner will:
- voice feelings about changes in their sexuality patterns
- express an understanding that these changes are temporary
- resume normal sexuality patterns when epididymitis is resolved.

Risk for injury related to potential for sterility. Based on this nursing diagnosis, you'll establish these patient outcomes. The patient will:
- express concerns and fears about possible sterility
- comply with the prescribed treatment regimen, thus reducing his risk of becoming sterile
- not become sterile because of epididymitis.

Pain related to inflamed tissue. Based on this nursing diagnosis, you'll establish these patient outcomes. The patient will:
- express feelings of comfort after analgesic administration
- use nonpharmacologic measures, such as ice and scrotal support, to help alleviate pain
- become pain free when epididymitis is resolved.

Nursing interventions

- Because the patient usually is very uncomfortable, administer analgesics as necessary. Allow him to rest in bed, legs slightly apart, with testes elevated on a towel roll. Suggest that he wear nonconstrictive, lightweight clothing until the swelling subsides. Apply ice packs as needed for comfort.

• Administer antibiotics and antipyretics, as ordered. If epididymitis is secondary to a sexually transmitted disease (STD), treat the disease with appropriate antibiotics.

• If the patient faces the possibility of sterility, suggest supportive counseling as necessary.

Monitoring

• Watch closely for signs of abscess formation (a localized, hot, red, tender area) or extension of the infection into the testes. Closely monitor temperature, and ensure adequate fluid intake.

• Monitor the patient's pain level and response to analgesics and nonpharmacologic measures for pain relief.

Patient teaching

• If the patient will be taking antibiotics after discharge, emphasize the importance of completing the prescribed regimen, even after symptoms subside.

• Suggest that the patient wear scrotal support while sitting, standing, or walking.

• If epididymitis is secondary to an STD, encourage the patient to use a condom during sexual intercourse and to notify sexual partners so that they can be adequately treated for infection.

Epilepsy

Also known as seizure disorder, epilepsy is a condition of the brain characterized by a susceptibility to recurrent seizures. Seizures are paroxysmal events associated with abnormal electrical discharges of neurons in the brain. In most patients, this condition doesn't affect intelligence. Epilepsy probably affects 0.5% to 2% of the population and usually occurs in patients under age 20. However, about 80% of patients have good seizure control with strict adherence to prescribed treatment.

Causes

About half the cases of epilepsy are idiopathic. No specific cause can be found, and the patient has no other neurologic abnormalities. Nonidiopathic epilepsy may be caused by:

• genetic abnormalities, such as tuberous sclerosis and phenylketonuria
• perinatal injuries
• metabolic abnormalities, such as hypocalcemia, hypoglycemia, and pyridoxine deficiency
• brain tumors or other space-occupying lesions
• infections, such as meningitis, encephalitis, or brain abscess
• traumatic injury, especially if the dura mater was penetrated
• ingestion of toxins, such as mercury, lead, or carbon monoxide
• cerebrovascular accident.

Researchers also have detected hereditary EEG abnormalities in some families, and certain seizure disorders appear to have a familial incidence.

Complications

Associated complications may occur during a seizure. These include anoxia from airway occlusion by the tongue or vomitus and traumatic injury. Such traumatic injury could result from a fall at the onset of a generalized tonic-clonic seizure; the rapid, jerking movements that occur during or after a generalized tonic-clonic seizure; or a fall or sudden movement sustained while the patient is confused or has an altered level of consciousness.

Assessment

Depending on the type and cause of the seizure, signs and symptoms vary. (See *Differentiating among seizure types,* pages 292 and 293.) Physical findings may be normal if the assessment is performed when the patient isn't having a seizure and the cause is idiopathic. If the seizure is associated with an underlying problem, the patient's history and physical examination should reveal signs and symptoms of that problem unless the seizure was caused by a brain tumor, which may produce no other symptoms.

In many cases, the patient's history reveals that seizure occurrence is unpredictable and unrelated to activities. Occasionally, a patient may report precipitating factors or events – for example, that the seizures always take place at a particular time, such as during sleep, or after a particular circumstance, such as lack of sleep or emotional stress. The patient may also report nonspecific changes, such as headache, mood changes, lethargy, and myoclonic jerking, occurring up to several hours before the onset of a seizure.

Patients who experience a generalized seizure may describe an aura, which represents the beginning of abnormal electrical discharges within a focal area of the brain. Typical auras may include a pungent smell, GI distress (nausea or indigestion), a rising or sinking feeling in the stomach, a dreamy feeling, an unusual taste, or a visual disturbance, such as a flashing light, that precedes seizure onset by a few seconds or minutes.

The patient may describe how the seizures affect his life-style, activities of daily living, and coping mechanisms. The patient's history may also reveal occurrence of status epilepticus. (See *Status epilepticus,* page 290.)

If you observe the patient during a seizure, be sure to note the type of seizure he's experiencing. Otherwise, details of what occurs during a seizure – obtained from a family member or friend, if necessary – may help to identify the seizure type.

Diagnostic tests

- *EEG.* Paroxysmal abnormalities may confirm the diagnosis of epilepsy by providing evidence of the continuing tendency to have seizures. A negative EEG doesn't rule out epilepsy because the paroxysmal abnormalities occur intermittently. The EEG also helps guide the prognosis and can help to classify the disorder.
- *Computed tomography scan.* This scan provides density readings of the brain and may indicate abnormalities in internal structures.
- *Magnetic resonance imaging.* This procedure helps identify the cause of the seizure because it provides clear images of the brain in regions where bone normally hampers visualization.

Other helpful tests include serum glucose and calcium studies, skull X-rays, lumbar puncture, brain scan, and cerebral angiography.

Treatment

Typically, treatment for epilepsy consists of drug therapy specific to the type of seizure. The most commonly prescribed drugs include phenytoin, carbamazepine, phenobarbital, and primidone administered individually for generalized tonic-clonic seizures and complex partial seizures. Valproic acid, clonazepam, and ethosuximide are commonly prescribed for absence seizures.

If drug therapy fails, treatment may include surgical removal of a demonstrated focal lesion to attempt to end seizures. Surgery is also performed when epilepsy results from an underlying problem, such as intracranial tumors, brain abscess or cysts, and vascular abnormalities.

Key nursing diagnoses and patient outcomes

Fear related to potential for seizures. Based on this nursing diagnosis, you'll establish these patient outcomes. The patient will:

- express feelings of fear related to seizures
- express an understanding of the importance of compliance with therapy to reduce seizure risk

Differentiating among seizure types

The hallmark of epilepsy is recurring seizures, which can be classified as partial or generalized. Some patients may be affected by more than one type.

Partial seizures

Arising from a localized area in the brain, these seizures cause specific symptoms. In some patients, partial seizure activity may spread to the entire brain, causing a generalized seizure. Partial seizures include simple partial (jacksonian motor-type and sensory-type), complex partial (psychomotor or temporal lobe), and secondarily generalized partial seizures.

Simple partial (jacksonian motor-type) seizure

This type begins as a localized motor seizure, which is characterized by a spread of abnormal activity to adjacent areas of the brain. Typically, the patient experiences a stiffening or jerking in one extremity, accompanied by a tingling sensation in the same area. For example, the seizure may start in the thumb and spread to the entire hand and arm. The patient seldom loses consciousness, although the seizure may secondarily progress to a generalized tonic-clonic seizure.

Simple partial (sensory-type) seizure

Perception is distorted in this type of seizure. Symptoms can include hallucinations, flashing lights, tingling sensations, a foul odor, vertigo, or déjà vu.

Complex partial (psychomotor or temporal lobe) seizure

Symptoms of this seizure type are variable but usually include purposeless behavior. The patient may experience an aura and exhibit overt signs, including a glassy stare, picking at his clothes, aimless wandering, lip smacking or chewing motions, and unintelligible speech. A seizure may last for a few seconds or as long as 20 minutes. Afterward, mental confusion may last for several minutes; as a result, an observer may mistakenly suspect intoxication with alcohol or drugs, or psychosis. The patient has no memory of his actions during the seizure.

Secondarily generalized partial seizure

This type of seizure can be either simple or complex and can progress to generalized seizures. An aura may precede the progression. Loss of consciousness occurs immediately or within 1 to 2 minutes of the start of the progression.

- use available support systems to assist in coping with fear.

Risk for injury related to potential for seizures. Based on this nursing diagnosis, you'll establish these patient outcomes. The patient will:

- instruct family members, friends, and co-workers on how to protect him from injury during a seizure
- not become injured during a seizure.

Social isolation related to the stigma attached to behavior exhibited during a seizure. Based on this nursing diagnosis, you'll establish these patient outcomes. The patient will:

- express his negative feelings about seizures and communicate an understanding of epilepsy
- recover from negative feelings associated with social isolation
- return to active participation in society.

Nursing interventions

- Administer anticonvulsant therapy, as prescribed. When administering phenytoin I.V., use a large vein, administer slowly (usually 50 mg/minute), and mix only with 0.9% sodium chloride solution.
- Protect the patient from injury during seizures.
- Prepare the patient for surgery, if necessary. Provide preoperative and postop-

Generalized seizures
As the term suggests, these seizures cause a generalized electrical abnormality within the brain. They include several distinct types.

Absence seizure
This type occurs most often in children, although it may affect adults as well. It usually begins with a brief change in level of consciousness, indicated by blinking or rolling of the eyes, a blank stare, and slight mouth movements. The patient retains his posture and continues preseizure activity without difficulty. Typically, a seizure lasts from 1 to 10 seconds. The impairment is so brief that the patient is sometimes unaware of it. If not properly treated, these seizures can recur as often as 100 times a day. An absence seizure may progress to a generalized tonic-clonic seizure.

Myoclonic seizure
Also called bilateral massive epileptic myoclonus, this seizure type is marked by brief, involuntary muscular jerks of the body or extremities, which may occur in a rhythmic manner, and a brief loss of consciousness.

Generalized tonic-clonic seizure
Typically, this seizure begins with a loud cry, precipitated by air rushing from the lungs through the vocal cords. The patient falls to the ground, losing consciousness. The body stiffens (tonic phase) and then alternates between episodes of muscle spasm and relaxation (clonic phase). Tongue biting, incontinence, labored breathing, apnea, and subsequent cyanosis may also occur. The seizure stops in 2 to 5 minutes, when abnormal electrical conduction of the neurons is completed. The patient then regains consciousness but is somewhat confused and may have difficulty talking. If he can talk, he may complain of drowsiness, fatigue, headache, muscle soreness, and arm or leg weakness. He may fall into a deep sleep after the seizure.

Akinetic seizure
Characterized by a general loss of postural tone and a temporary loss of consciousness, this type occurs in young children. Sometimes it's called a drop attack because it causes the child to fall.

erative care appropriate for the type of surgery he'll undergo.
• Provide emotional support. Encourage the patient and family to express their fears and concerns. Suggest counseling to help them cope.

Monitoring
• Monitor the patient continuously during seizures.
• If the patient is taking antiseizure medications, constantly monitor for toxic signs and symptoms, such as slurred speech, ataxia, lethargy, dizziness, drowsiness, nystagmus, irritability, nausea, and vomiting. Also monitor him closely when administering I.V. phenytoin.
• Monitor the patient's compliance with anticonvulsant drug therapy.
• Observe the patient's emotional response to having epilepsy.

Patient teaching
• Support the patient and family by developing an understanding of epilepsy and the myths and misconceptions surrounding it. Answer any questions the patient and family may have about the condition. Help them cope by dispelling some of the myths – for example, that epilepsy is contagious. Assure them that epilepsy is con-

LIFE-THREATENING COMPLICATIONS

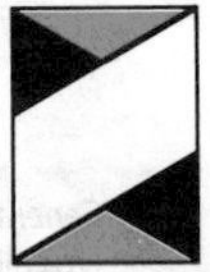

Status epilepticus

A continuous seizure state, status epilepticus can occur in all seizure types and is considered an emergency. It can result from abrupt withdrawal of antiseizure medications, hypoxic or metabolic encephalopathy, acute head trauma, or septicemia secondary to encephalitis or meningitis.

Signs and symptoms

Three types of status epilepticus exist. Patients with *generalized tonic-clonic status epilepticus,* the most life-threatening form, have continuous generalized tonic-clonic seizures with no intervening return of consciousness. Respiratory distress also occurs. In the second type, *petit mal status,* the patient may exhibit 200 to 300 "absences" per day. In the third type, partial or focal status or *epilepsia continua,* focal seizures occur continuously or regularly, and the patient usually remains conscious unless generalization occurs.

Emergency interventions

- Notify the doctor immediately but don't leave the patient unattended.
- Ensure a patent airway.
- Draw blood for glucose, electrolyte, blood urea nitrogen, arterial blood gas, and creatine phosphokinase levels to determine possible cause, and establish an I.V. line.
- Be prepared to administer I.V. medication to stop seizure activity. The most commonly used I.V. drugs are diazepam, phenytoin, and phenobarbital; dextrose 50% (when seizures are secondary to hypoglycemia); and thiamine (in the presence of chronic alcoholism or withdrawal).

trollable for most patients who follow a prescribed regimen of medication and that most patients maintain a normal life-style.

• Explain the need for compliance with the prescribed drug schedule. Assure the patient that anticonvulsants are safe when taken as ordered. Reinforce dosage instructions and find methods to help the patient remember to take medications. Stress the importance of taking the medication regularly at a scheduled time. Caution the patient to monitor the amount of medication so that he doesn't run out of it.

• Teach the patient about the medication's possible adverse effects – drowsiness, lethargy, hyperactivity, confusion, visual and sleep disturbances – all of which indicate the need for dosage adjustment. Tell him that phenytoin therapy may lead to hyperplasia of the gums, which may be relieved by conscientious oral hygiene. Instruct the patient to report adverse reactions immediately.

• Explain the importance of having anticonvulsant blood levels checked at regular intervals even if the seizures are under control.

• Instruct the patient to eat regular meals and to check with his doctor before dieting. Explain that maintaining adequate glucose levels provides the necessary energy for central nervous system neurons to work normally.

• Teach the patient the following measures to help him control and decrease the occurrence of seizures:

– Take the exact dose of medication at the times prescribed. Missing doses, doubling doses, or taking extra doses can cause a seizure.

– Eat balanced, regular meals. Low blood glucose levels (hypoglycemia) and inadequate vitamin intake can lead to seizures.

– Be alert for odors that may trigger an attack. Advise the patient and his family to inform the doctor of any strong odors they notice at the time of a seizure.

– Limit alcohol intake. In fact, the patient should check with the doctor to find out whether he should drink *any* alcoholic beverages.

– Get enough sleep. Excessive fatigue can precipitate a seizure.

– Treat a fever early during an illness. If the patient can't reduce a fever, he should notify the doctor.

– Learn to control stress. If appropriate, suggest learning relaxation techniques, such as deep-breathing exercises.

– Avoid trigger factors, for example, flashing lights, hyperventilation, loud noises, heavy musical beats, video games, and television.

• If the patient is a candidate for surgery, provide appropriate preoperative teaching. Explain the care that the patient can expect postoperatively.

• Know which social agencies in your community can help patients with epilepsy. Refer the patient to the Epilepsy Foundation of America for general information and to the state motor vehicle department for information about a driver's license.

• Teach the patient's family how to care for the patient during a seizure. This is especially important if the patient experiences generalized tonic-clonic seizures, which may necessitate first aid. Instruct the family to:

– avoid restraining the patient during a seizure

– help the patient to a lying position, loosen any tight clothing, and place something flat and soft, such as a pillow, jacket, or hand, under his head

– clear the area of hard objects

– avoid forcing anything into the patient's mouth if his teeth are clenched

– avoid using a tongue blade or spoon, which could lacerate the mouth and lips or displace teeth, precipitating respiratory distress

– protect the patient's tongue, if his mouth is open, by placing a soft object (such as folded cloth) between his teeth

– turn the patient's head to the side to provide an open airway

– reassure the patient after the seizure subsides by telling him that he's all right, orienting him to time and place, and informing him that he's had a seizure.

Escherichia coli and other Enterobacteriaceae infections

Enterobacteriaceae – a family of mostly aerobic, gram-negative bacilli – cause local and systemic infections, including an invasive diarrhea that resembles shigellosis and, more often, a noninvasive, toxin-mediated diarrhea that resembles cholera. With other bacilli of this family, *Escherichia coli* causes most nosocomial infections.

The prognosis in mild to moderate infection is good. But severe infection requires immediate fluid and electrolyte replacement to avoid fatal dehydration, especially among children, in whom the risk of death may be quite high.

The incidence of *E. coli* infection is highest among travelers returning from other countries, particularly Mexico (noninvasive), Southeast Asia (noninvasive), and South America (invasive). *E. coli* infection also causes other diseases, especially in people whose resistance is low.

Causes

Although some strains of *E. coli* exist as part of the normal GI flora, infection usually comes from nonindigenous strains. For example, noninvasive diarrhea results from two toxins produced by enterotoxigenic or enteropathogenic strains of *E. coli.* These toxins interact with intestinal juices and promote excessive loss of chloride and water. In the invasive form, *E. coli* directly invades the intestinal mucosa without producing enterotoxins, thereby causing local irritation, inflammation, and diarrhea. Normal strains can cause infection in immunocompromised patients.

Transmission can occur directly from an infected person or indirectly by ingestion of contaminated food or water or by contact with contaminated utensils. Incubation takes 12 to 72 hours.

Complications

Bacteremia, severe dehydration, life-threatening electrolyte disturbances, acidosis, and shock can result.

Assessment

Recent travel to another country, ingestion of contaminated food or water, or recent close contact with a person experiencing diarrhea may be part of the patient history.

The cardinal symptom is diarrhea. In the noninvasive form, watery diarrhea begins abruptly, along with cramping abdominal pain. In the invasive form, abdominal cramps are accompanied by diarrheal stools that may contain blood and pus. The patient may report that vomiting and anorexia precede diarrhea. He also may typically report a low-grade fever that occurs on the first and second days of infection.

With dehydration, you'll note dry skin and mucous membranes (with decreased skin turgor) and sunken eyes. Expect to see signs and symptoms of hyponatremia, hypokalemia, hypomagnesemia, and hypocalcemia from electrolyte losses caused by vomiting and diarrhea.

In dehydration, auscultation may reveal hyperactive bowel sounds and orthostatic hypotension; palpation may reveal a rapid, thready pulse.

Diagnostic tests

Because certain strains of *E. coli* normally reside in the GI tract, culturing is of little value.

A firm diagnosis requires sophisticated identification procedures, such as bioassays, which are expensive, time-consuming and, consequently, not widely available. Diagnosis must rule out salmonella infection and shigellosis, other common infections that produce similar signs and symptoms.

Treatment

Appropriate treatment consists of enteric precautions, correction of fluid and electrolyte imbalances and, in an immunocompromised patient, I.V. antibiotics based on the organism's drug sensitivity. For severe diarrhea that poses a risk of dehydration, bismuth subsalicylate or opium tincture may be ordered.

Key nursing diagnoses and patient outcomes

Diarrhea related to intestinal irritation. Based on this nursing diagnosis, you'll establish these patient outcomes. The patient will:

- not experience complications associated with diarrhea, such as fluid and electrolyte imbalances and skin breakdown
- recover and maintain a normal bowel pattern
- identify causative factors and preventive measures.

Risk for fluid volume deficit related to fluid loss from diarrhea. Based on this nursing diagnosis, you'll establish these patient outcomes. The patient will:

- not exhibit signs and symptoms of dehydration
- maintain adequate fluid balance.

Risk for impaired skin integrity related to anal irritation caused by diarrhea. Based on this nursing diagnosis, you'll es-

tablish these patient outcomes. The patient will:
• clean, dry, and lubricate the anal area after each bowel movement
• not experience skin breakdown from diarrhea.

Nursing interventions

• Institute standard precautions for all patients to prevent transmission of the organism to healthy people.
• Replace fluids and electrolytes as needed.
• Use proper hand-washing technique.
• Clean the perianal area and lubricate it after each episode of diarrhea. Provide a room deodorizer.
• Give nothing by mouth; administer antibiotics, as ordered; and maintain body warmth.
• During epidemics, screen all hospital personnel and visitors for diarrhea, and prevent people with the disorder from having direct patient contact. Report cases to local public health authorities.
• Resistant strains of *E. coli* develop in patients on antibiotic therapy. Obtain routine surveillance cultures, and evaluate culture and sensitivity results, as indicated.

Monitoring

• Keep accurate intake and output records. Measure stool volume and note the presence of blood and pus. Also monitor for decreased serum sodium and chloride levels and signs of gram-negative septic shock.
• Watch for signs of dehydration. Monitor vital signs to detect early indications of circulatory collapse.

Patient teaching

• Explain proper hand-washing technique to hospital personnel and patients and their families. Stress the importance of washing hands before eating or preparing food and after defecating, changing diapers, or having any contact with feces.
• Advise travelers to other countries to avoid unbottled water, ice, unpeeled fruit, and uncooked vegetables.
• If the patient will be cared for at home, teach him the signs of dehydration and tell him to seek prompt medical attention if these occur.

Esophageal cancer

Most common in men over age 60, esophageal cancer is nearly always fatal. The disease occurs worldwide, but incidence varies geographically. It's most commonly found in Japan, Russia, China, the Middle East, and the Transkei region of South Africa, where esophageal cancer has reached almost epidemic proportions. In the United States, more than 8,000 cases of esophageal cancer are reported annually.

Esophageal tumors are usually fungating and infiltrating. In most cases, the tumor partially constricts the lumen of the esophagus. Regional metastasis occurs early by way of submucosal lymphatics, often fatally invading adjacent vital intrathoracic organs. If the patient survives primary extension, the liver and lungs are the usual sites of distant metastases. Unusual metastasis sites include the bone, kidneys, and adrenal glands.

Most cases (98%) arise in squamous cell epithelium, although a few are adenocarcinomas and, fewer still, melanomas and sarcomas. About half the squamous cell cancers occur in the lower portion of the esophagus, 40% in the midportion, and the remaining 10% in the upper or cervical esophagus. Regardless of cell type, the prognosis for esophageal cancer is grim: 5-year survival rates are less than 5%, and most patients die within 6 months of diagnosis.

Causes

Although the cause of esophageal cancer is unknown, several predisposing factors have been identified. These include chronic irritation from heavy smoking or excessive use of alcohol; stasis-induced inflammation, as in achalasia or stricture; previous head and neck tumors; and nutritional deficiency, as in untreated sprue and Plummer-Vinson syndrome.

Complications

Direct invasion of adjoining structures may lead to severe complications, such as mediastinitis, tracheoesophageal or bronchoesophageal fistula (causing an overwhelming cough when swallowing liquids), and aortic perforation with sudden exsanguination.

Other complications include an inability to control secretions, obstruction of the esophagus, and loss of lower esophageal sphincter control, which can result in aspiration pneumonia.

Assessment

Early in the disease, the patient may report a feeling of fullness, pressure, indigestion, or substernal burning. He may also tell you he uses antacids to relieve GI upset. Later, he may complain of dysphagia and weight loss. The degree of dysphagia varies, depending on the extent of disease. At first, the dysphagia is mild, occurring only after the patient eats solid foods, especially meat. Later, the patient has difficulty swallowing coarse foods and, in some cases, liquids.

The patient may complain of hoarseness (from laryngeal nerve involvement), a chronic cough (possibly from aspiration), anorexia, vomiting, and regurgitation of food. This results from the tumor size exceeding the limits of the esophagus. He may also complain of pain on swallowing or pain that radiates to his back.

If you observe the patient in the late stages of the disease, he appears very thin, cachectic, and dehydrated.

Diagnostic tests

- *X-rays of the esophagus, with barium swallow and motility studies,* delineate structural and filling defects and reduced peristalsis.
- *Chest X-rays* or *esophagography* may reveal pneumonitis.
- *Esophagoscopy, punch and brush biopsies,* and *exfoliative cytologic tests* confirm esophageal tumors.
- *Bronchoscopy* (which is usually performed after an esophagoscopy) may reveal tumor growth in the tracheobronchial tree.
- *Endoscopic ultrasonography* of the esophagus combines endoscopy and ultrasound technology to measure the depth of penetration of the tumor.
- *Computed tomography scan* may help diagnose and monitor esophageal lesions.
- *Magnetic resonance imaging scan* permits evaluation of the esophagus and adjacent structures.
- *Liver function studies* and other laboratory tests may reveal abnormalities. If so, a *liver scan* and *mediastinal tomography scan* can help reveal the extent of the disease. (See *Staging esophageal cancer.*)

Treatment

Esophageal cancer usually is advanced when diagnosed, so surgery and other treatments can only relieve disease effects.

Palliative therapy consists of treatment to keep the esophagus open, including esophageal dilation, laser therapy, and radiation therapy. Radical surgery can excise the tumor and resect either the esophagus alone or the stomach and esophagus. Either the stomach (gastric pull-up) or a portion of the colon (colon interposition) may be used to replace the esophagus. Chemotherapy and radiation therapy can slow the growth of the tumor. Gastrostomy or jejunostomy can help provide adequate nutrition. A prosthesis can be used to seal any fistula that develops. Endoscopic laser treatment and bipolar electrocoagulation can help restore swallowing by vaporizing cancerous tissue. If the tumor is in the upper esophagus, however, the laser can't be positioned properly.

Analgesics are used for pain control.

Key nursing diagnoses and patient outcomes

Altered nutrition: Less than body requirements, related to impaired swallowing. Based on this nursing diagnosis, you'll establish these patient outcomes. The patient will:

- ingest a high-calorie, nutritionally balanced diet naturally or artificially through gastrostomy feedings or parenteral nutrition
- maintain weight
- not have signs and symptoms of malnutrition.

Risk for aspiration related to esophageal blockage. Based on this nursing diagnosis, you'll establish these patient outcomes. The patient will:

- expectorate secretions without aspiration
- consent to treatments that help prevent aspiration, such as a gastrostomy if he has trouble drinking liquids
- not develop aspiration pneumonia.

Impaired swallowing related to obstruction. Based on this nursing diagnosis, you'll establish these patient outcomes. The patient will:

- consent to treatments that improve swallowing, such as periodic dilatation of the esophagus
- not develop malnutrition, aspiration pneumonia, or other complications of impaired swallowing.

Nursing interventions

- Provide high-calorie, high-protein foods. If the patient has trouble swallowing solids, puree or liquefy his food and offer a commercially available nutritional supplement. As ordered, provide tube feedings, and prepare him for supplementary parenteral nutrition.
- To prevent food aspiration, place the patient in Fowler's position for meals and allow plenty of time to eat. If he regurgitates food after eating, provide mouth care.
- Administer ordered analgesics for pain relief as necessary. Provide comfort measures, such as repositioning, and distractions to help decrease discomfort.
- Protect the patient from infection.

Staging esophageal cancer

The prognosis and treatment of esophageal cancer depend on its type and stage. Using the TNM (tumor, node, metastasis) system, the American Joint Committee on Cancer has established the following stages for esophageal cancer.

Primary tumor

TX—primary tumor can't be assessed
T0—no evidence of primary tumor
Tis—carcinoma in situ
T1—tumor invades lamina propria or submucosa
T2—tumor invades muscularis propria
T3—tumor invades adventitia
T4—tumor invades adjacent structures

Regional lymph nodes

NX—regional lymph nodes can't be assessed
N0—no regional lymph node metastasis
N1—regional lymph node metastasis

Distant metastasis

MX—distant metastasis can't be assessed
M0—no known distant metastasis
M1—distant metastasis

Staging categories

Esophageal cancer progresses from mild to severe as follows:
Stage 0—Tis, N0, M0
Stage I—T1, N0, M0
Stage IIA—T2, N0, M0; T3, N0, M0
Stage IIB—T1, N1, M0; T2, N1, M0
Stage III—T3, N1, M0; T4, any N, M0
Stage IV—any T, any N, M1

• Prepare the patient for a gastrostomy, as indicated. When using a gastrostomy tube for nutritional support, give food slowly—by gravity—in prescribed amounts (usually 200 to 500 ml). Offer the patient something to chew before each feeding. This promotes gastric secretions and provides some semblance of normal eating.
• Prepare the patient for surgery used to treat esophageal cancer, as indicated.
• After chemotherapy, take steps to decrease adverse effects, such as providing normal saline mouthwash to help prevent mouth ulcers. Allow the patient plenty of rest, and administer medications, as ordered, to reduce adverse effects.
• Throughout therapy, answer the patient's questions, and tell him what to expect from surgery and other therapies. Listen to his fears and concerns, and stay with him during periods of severe anxiety.
• Encourage the patient to identify actions and care measures that will promote his comfort and relaxation. Try to perform these measures, and encourage the patient and his family to do so, too.
• Whenever possible, include the patient in care decisions.
• Anticipate referral to home care to assist with follow-up, teaching, patient care, and support.

Monitoring

• Monitor the patient's food and fluid intake.
• After surgery to treat esophageal cancer, monitor vital signs, fluid and electrolyte balance, and intake and output. Immediately report any unexpected changes in the patient's condition. Also monitor for complications, such as infection, fistula formation, pneumonia, empyema, and malnutrition.
• If an anastomosis to the esophagus was performed, watch for signs of an anastomotic leak.
• If the patient had a prosthetic tube inserted, monitor for signs of blockage or dislodgment. This can cause perforation of the mediastinum or precipitate tumor erosion.
• After radiation therapy, monitor the patient for complications, such as esophageal perforation, pneumonitis and fibrosis of the lungs, and myelitis of the spinal cord.
• After chemotherapy, monitor for complications, such as bone marrow suppression and GI reactions.

Patient teaching

• Explain the procedures the patient will undergo after surgery—closed chest drainage, nasogastric suctioning, and placement of gastrostomy tubes.
• If appropriate, teach the family gastrostomy tube care. This includes checking tube patency before each feeding, providing skin care around the tube, and keeping the patient upright during and after feedings.
• Stress the importance of adequate nutrition. Ask a dietitian to instruct the patient and his family. If the patient has difficulty swallowing solids, instruct him to puree or liquefy his food and to follow a high-calorie, high-protein diet to minimize weight loss. Also, recommend that he add a commercially available, high-calorie supplement to his diet.
• Encourage the patient to follow as normal a routine as possible after recovery from surgery and during radiation therapy and chemotherapy. This will help him maintain a sense of control and reduce complications associated with immobility.
• Advise the patient to rest between activities and to stop any activity that tires him or causes pain.
• Refer the patient and his family to appropriate organizations, such as the American Cancer Society.

Esophageal diverticula

Occurring as hollow outpouchings of the esophageal wall, esophageal diverticula develop in three main areas: just above the upper esophageal sphincter (Zenker's diverticulum, the most common type), near the midpoint of the esophagus (a midesophageal diverticulum), and just above the lower esophageal sphincter (an epiphrenic diverticulum, the rarest type). Diverticula may involve one or more layers of the mucosa.

Generally, esophageal diverticula occur later in life, but they can also affect infants and children. The disorder is three times more common in men than in women. Epiphrenic diverticula usually occur in middle-aged men. Zenker's diverticulum usually occurs in men over age 60.

Causes

Esophageal diverticula are due to either primary muscular abnormalities that may be congenital or to inflammatory processes adjacent to the esophagus. Zenker's diverticulum results from developmental muscle weakness of the posterior pharynx above the border of the cricopharyngeal muscle. The pressure of swallowing aggravates this weakness, as does contraction of the pharynx before relaxation of the sphincter, resulting in development of diverticula.

A midesophageal diverticulum may be a response to scarring and pulling on esophageal walls by an external inflammatory process, such as tuberculosis, or by traction from old adhesions. Another cause may be propulsion associated with esophageal motor abnormalities, such as diffuse esophageal spasm. An epiphrenic diverticulum probably results from traction and pulsation or from esophageal motor disturbances, such as diffuse esophageal spasm and achalasia.

Complications

Regurgitation of saliva or food particles may lead to aspiration, causing pulmonary complications, such as bronchitis, bronchiectasis, and lung abscess. The disorder may also lead to esophageal perforation.

Assessment

In the early stage of Zenker's diverticulum, the patient may report recent weight loss, which he may attribute to difficulty eating. The patient history may reveal dysphagia and regurgitation of saliva and food particles soon after eating. In the later stage, the esophageal opening may be almost completely blocked. The patient may describe regurgitation of food particles he consumed several days earlier. He may also hear gurgling sounds in his neck when he's swallowing liquids.

Other signs and symptoms of Zenker's diverticulum include nocturnal coughing, a bad taste in the mouth and, rarely, bleeding. Halitosis may be obvious. Inspection may reveal a swelling at the side of the neck caused by food trapped in the diverticulum.

Midesophageal and epiphrenic diverticula usually produce no symptoms in early stages. In later stages, the patient may complain of dysphagia and heartburn.

Diagnostic tests

- *Barium swallow* usually confirms the diagnosis by showing a characteristic outpouching.
- *Esophagoscopy* may rule out another lesion as the cause of the problem. However, the procedure must be performed with extreme care because it risks rupturing the diverticulum by passing the scope into it rather than into the lumen of the esophagus, a special danger with Zenker's diverticulum.

Treatment

For Zenker's diverticulum, treatment is usually palliative, including a bland diet, thorough chewing, and drinking water after eating to flush out the sac. However, severe symptoms or a large diverticulum require surgery to remove the sac or facilitate drainage. An esophagomyotomy may be necessary to prevent recurrence.

A midesophageal or an epiphrenic diverticulum typically requires no therapy because it usually produces no symptoms or complications. If symptoms occur, treatment includes antacids and an antireflux regimen. If the diverticulum becomes very large and causes symptoms, surgical removal may be indicated. Distal myotomy is usually performed if the diverticulum is associated with esophageal motor abnormalities.

If surgery is necessary, then, depending on the patient's nutritional status, treatment may also include insertion of a nasogastric tube (passed carefully to prevent perforation) and tube feedings to prepare for the stress of surgery.

Key nursing diagnoses and patient outcomes

Altered nutrition: Less than body requirements, related to dysphagia. Based on this nursing diagnosis, you'll establish these patient outcomes. The patient will:

- consume a nutritionally balanced diet in a form that he can swallow
- regain lost weight and maintain a desirable weight
- not exhibit signs and symptoms of malnutrition.

Risk for aspiration related to regurgitation of food particles and saliva. Based on this nursing diagnosis, you'll establish these patient outcomes. The patient will:

- employ measures to prevent aspiration, such as keeping his head elevated for at least 2 hours after eating and using massage or postural drainage to empty any visible outpouching in the neck before lying down
- not aspirate.

Impaired swallowing related to muscular abnormalities. Based on this nursing diagnosis, you'll establish these patient outcomes. The patient will:

- adjust food consistency to facilitate swallowing
- not develop complications of dysphagia, such as malnutrition and aspiration pneumonia.

Nursing interventions

- If the patient regurgitates food and mucus, protect him from aspiration by positioning him with his head elevated or turned to one side.
- If the patient has dysphagia, record well-tolerated foods and note circumstances that ease swallowing. If necessary, provide a "blenderized" diet, with vitamin or protein supplements.
- If the patient with a midesophageal or an epiphrenic diverticulum has discomfort, administer ordered antacids and provide antireflux care: Keep his head elevated; maintain him in an upright position for 2 hours after eating; provide small, frequent meals; control chronic coughing; and avoid constrictive clothing.
- If surgery is scheduled, perform required preoperative and postoperative care.
- Support the patient emotionally, especially if he's upset and concerned about his symptoms.

Monitoring

- Regularly assess the patient's nutritional status (weight, caloric intake, physical appearance).
- Monitor the patient's degree of discomfort and the effectiveness of treatment.
- Monitor for respiratory signs and symptoms that suggest aspiration.

Patient teaching

- Teach the patient about his disorder. Explain necessary diagnostic tests and treatments.
- Emphasize the need to chew food thoroughly to prevent food particles from becoming trapped in the diverticulum.
- Teach the patient how to perform massage or postural drainage to prevent aspiration. He should use these techniques to empty any visible outpouching in the neck before lying down.
- If surgery is necessary, provide complete preoperative teaching. Make sure the patient understands the surgical approach, its desired effects, and possible complications.

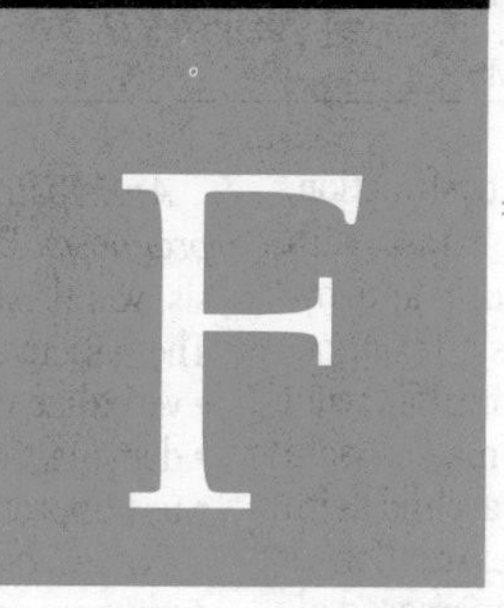

Fanconi's syndrome (de Toni-Fanconi syndrome)

Fanconi's syndrome is a renal disorder that produces malfunctions of the proximal renal tubules, leading to hyperkalemia, hypernatremia, glycosuria, phosphaturia, aminoaciduria, uricosuria, bicarbonate wasting and, eventually, retarded growth and development and rickets. Because treatment of Fanconi's syndrome is usually unsuccessful, it often leads to end-stage renal failure, and the patient may survive only a few years after its onset.

Causes

Idiopathic congenital Fanconi's syndrome is most prevalent in children and affects both sexes equally. Onset of the hereditary form usually occurs during the first 6 months of life, although another hereditary form also occurs in adults. The more serious adult form of this disease is acquired Fanconi's syndrome; it is secondary to Wilson's disease, cystinosis, galactosemia, or exposure to a toxic substance (heavy metal poisoning).

Fanconi's syndrome produces characteristic changes in the proximal renal tubules, such as shortening of the connection to glomeruli by an abnormally narrow segment (swan's neck) – a result of the atrophy of epithelial cells and loss of proximal tubular mass volume.

Assessment

Changes in the proximal renal tubules result in decreased tubular reabsorption of glucose, phosphate, amino acid, bicarbonate, potassium and, occasionally, water. An infant with Fanconi's syndrome appears normal at birth, although his birth weight may be low. At about age 6 months, the infant shows failure to thrive, weakness, dehydration (associated with polyuria, vomiting, and anorexia), constipation, acidosis, cystine crystals in the corneas and conjunctivas, and peripheral retinal pigment degeneration. Typically, the skin is yellow and has little pigmentation, even in summer. Refractory rickets or osteomalacia may be severe, and linear growth is slow. Bicarbonate loss causes acidosis; potassium loss, weakness; and water loss, dehydration. Renal calculi rarely occur.

In adults, symptoms of Fanconi's syndrome are secondary to hypophosphatemia, hypokalemia, and glycosuria. Their clinical effects include osteomalacia, muscle weakness and paralysis, and metabolic acidosis.

Diagnostic tests

Diagnosis requires evidence of excessive 24-hour urinary excretion of glucose, phosphate, amino acids, bicarbonate, and potassium (generally, serum values correspond to the decrease in these components). Other diagnostic test results include elevated phosphorus and nitrogen levels with increased renal dysfunction, and increased alkaline phosphatase with rickets. Hyperchloremic acidosis and hypokalemia support the diagnosis. (*Caution:* Glucose tolerance test is contraindicated for these patients, because it may cause a fatal shocklike reaction.) In a child with refractory rickets, growth retardation is evident; serum sample shows increased alkaline phosphatase and, with renal dysfunction, decreased calcium.

Treatment

Treatment is symptomatic, with replacement therapy appropriate to the patient's specific deficiencies. For example, a patient with rickets receives large doses of vitamin D; with acidosis and hypokalemia, supplements containing a flavored mixture of sodium and potassium citrate; and with hypocalcemia, calcium supplements (close monitoring is necessary to prevent hypercalcemia). When diminishing renal function causes hyperphosphatemia, treatment includes aluminum hydroxide antacids to bind phosphate in the intestine and prevent its absorption. Acquired Fanconi's syndrome requires treatment of the underlying cause. End-stage Fanconi's syndrome occasionally requires dialysis. Other treatment is symptomatic.

Key nursing diagnoses and patient outcomes

Risk for injury related to electrolyte disturbances. Based on this nursing diagnosis, you'll establish these patient outcomes. The patient will:
- remain free of injury
- exhibit electrolyte levels within normal limits.

Risk for fluid volume deficit related to polyuria and vomiting. Based on this nursing diagnosis, you'll establish these patient outcomes. The patient will:
- maintain adequate fluid balance
- demonstrate a reduction in polyuria and vomiting.

Anticipatory grieving related to poor prognosis. Based on this nursing diagnosis, you'll establish these patient outcomes. The patient and family will:
- verbalize concerns about the disease
- demonstrate positive coping mechanisms
- use appropriate support services.

Knowledge deficit related to the disease, treatment, and prognosis. Based on this nursing diagnosis, you'll establish these patient outcomes. The patient and family will:
- verbalize information about the disease and its treatment
- identify signs and symptoms of problems
- demonstrate understanding of medication therapy and need for follow up.

Nursing interventions

- Monitor renal function closely. Make sure 24-hour urine specimens are collected accurately.
- Watch for fluid and electrolyte imbalances, particularly hypokalemia and hyponatremia.
- Monitor the patient for signs of disturbed regulatory function characterized by anemia and hypertension; and uremic symptoms characteristic of renal failure (oliguria, anorexia, vomiting, muscle twitching, and pruritus).
- Help the patient with acquired Fanconi's syndrome or the parents of an infant with inherited Fanconi's syndrome understand the seriousness of this disease (including the possibility of dialysis) and the need to comply with drug and dietary therapy.
- If the patient has rickets, help him accept the changes in his body image.
- Because the prognosis for acquired Fanconi's syndrome is poor, the patient may be apathetic about taking medication. Encourage him to comply with therapy.
- Instruct the patient with acquired Fanconi's syndrome to follow a diet for chronic renal failure, as ordered.
- Refer patient and family to appropriate support services, as needed.

Femoral and popliteal aneurysms

Because these aneurysms occur in the two major peripheral arteries, they're also known as peripheral arterial aneurysms. They may be *fusiform* (spindle-shaped) or *saccular* (pouchlike). Fusiform types are three times more common than saccular forms. They may be singular or multiple segmental lesions, often affecting both legs, and may accompany other arterial aneurysms located in the abdominal aorta or the iliac arteries.

This condition is most common in men over age 50. Elective surgery before complications arise greatly improves the prognosis.

Causes

Femoral and popliteal aneurysms usually result from progressive atherosclerotic changes in the arterial walls (medial layer). Rarely, they result from congenital weakness in the arterial wall. They may also result from trauma (blunt or penetrating), bacterial infection, or peripheral vascular reconstructive surgery (which causes "suture line" aneurysms, also called false aneurysms, whereby a blood clot forms a second lumen).

Complications

If thrombosis, emboli, or gangrene occurs, poor tissue perfusion to areas distal to the aneurysm may require amputation.

Assessment

The patient may complain of pain in the popliteal space when a popliteal aneurysm is large enough to compress the medial popliteal nerve. Inspection may reveal edema and venous distention if the vein is compressed.

Femoral and popliteal aneurysms can produce signs and symptoms of severe ischemia in the leg or foot resulting from acute thrombosis within the aneurysmal sac, embolization of mural thrombus fragments and, rarely, rupture.

In acute aneurysmal thrombosis, the patient may complain of severe pain. Inspection may reveal distal petechial hemorrhages from aneurysmal emboli. The affected leg or foot may show loss of color. Palpation of the affected leg or foot may indicate coldness and a loss of pulse. Gangrene may develop.

Bilateral palpation that reveals a pulsating mass above or below the inguinal ligament in femoral aneurysm and behind the knee in popliteal aneurysm usually confirms the diagnosis. When thrombosis has occurred, palpation detects a firm, nonpulsating mass.

Diagnostic tests

Arteriography or ultrasonography may help resolve doubtful situations. Arteriography may also detect associated aneurysms, especially those in the abdominal aorta and the iliac arteries. Ultrasonography may also help determine the size of the femoral or popliteal artery.

Treatment

Femoral and popliteal aneurysms require surgical bypass and reconstruction of the artery, usually with an autogenous saphenous vein graft replacement. Arterial occlusion that causes severe ischemia and gangrene may require leg amputation.

Key nursing diagnoses and patient outcomes

Altered peripheral tissue perfusion related to acute thrombosis within the aneurysmal sac or embolization of mural thrombosis fragments. Based on this nursing diagnosis, you'll establish these patient outcomes. The patient will:
- maintain tissue perfusion and cellular oxygenation demonstrated by the presence of peripheral pulses in the affected extremity

• not develop complications from altered tissue perfusion, such as skin breakdown or gangrene.

Anxiety related to potential for amputation of affected extremity. Based on this nursing diagnosis, you'll establish these patient outcomes. The patient will:
• express any feelings of anxiety and concern
• use available support systems to assist with coping
• cope with anxiety by being involved in decisions about his care.

Pain related to severe ischemia of the affected extremity caused by acute aneurysmal thrombosis. Based on this nursing diagnosis, you'll establish these patient outcomes. The patient will:
• seek medical attention immediately if severe pain occurs
• become pain free when severe ischemia is relieved.

Nursing interventions

• Administer prophylactic antibiotics, antihypertensives, or anticoagulants, as ordered.
• Prepare the patient for surgery.
• Provide emotional support. Address the patient's concerns and answer his questions to help allay anxiety.

Monitoring

• Assess and record the patient's circulatory status, noting the location and quality of peripheral pulses in the patient's affected leg.
• Examine the patient's extremity for pain, pallor, pulselessness, paresthesias, and paralysis. Compare the affected extremity to the unaffected extremity. Note any differences and inform the doctor.
• Inspect the incisional area for signs of healing. Report any bleeding or drainage on dressing.
• Monitor for complications, such as skin breakdown or gangrene, in the affected leg.

Patient teaching

• Teach the patient and family what an aneurysm is and how it occurs.
• If the patient is receiving anticoagulants, suggest measures to prevent accidental bleeding, such as using an electric razor.
• Tell the patient to report immediately any signs of bleeding (bleeding gums, tarry stools, easy bruising).
• Explain the importance of follow-up blood studies to monitor anticoagulant therapy.
• Warn the patient to avoid trauma, tobacco, and aspirin.
• Provide preoperative and postoperative teaching.
• Instruct the patient to avoid prolonged sitting after surgery.
• Provide instructions about how to care for the incision site after surgery.

Fibrocystic breast changes

Also known as mammary dysplasia or chronic cystic mastitis, fibrocystic breast changes represent the most common benign breast condition. The epithelium of the breast responds to fluctuating levels of estrogen and progesterone, causing women to experience breast tenderness and fullness during the luteal phase of the menstrual cycle.

Previously, this hormonally induced, cyclic pain and lumpiness was called a disease. Today, however, many health care professionals feel this term is inaccurate because studies show that about 50% of all women ages 20 to 50 have clinical signs and nearly 90% have histologic signs of fibrocystic changes, which suggests that fibrocystic changes are a normal variation.

Fibrocystic changes respond to the changes of the menstrual cycle, and a patient may actually observe a lessening in the size of a lump when her menses begins.

Causes

Fibrocystic changes are probably caused by an imbalance of estrogen and progesterone. This imbalance distorts the normal changes of the menstrual cycle and causes an exaggerated response of breast tissue to cyclic levels of ovarian hormones.

Complications

Fibrocystic breast changes seldom cause complications, although the signs and symptoms may progress. Rarely, a patient who undergoes biopsy for a benign breast lump is found to have atypical hyperplasia. This clinical finding, combined with a family history of breast cancer, may increase the risk of breast cancer.

Assessment

The patient may report painful, multiple breast masses (cysts) that change rapidly in size. She may say that the cysts are painful and enlarge during the premenstrual period or that the pain intensifies then. This pain may be described as a localized painful area if she has a large, fluid-filled cyst. If small cyst formation occurs, the patient may have a more diffuse tenderness. She may also notice nipple discharge.

Palpation may reveal breasts that feel dense, with areas of irregularity and nodularity or lumpiness.

Diagnostic tests

- *Aspiration* is performed to determine if a cyst is fluid-filled or a solid neoplasm. The color of the aspirated fluid indicates the age of the mass. Straw-colored fluid suggests a recently formed cyst; dark green fluid, an older cyst; dark red fluid, a recent trauma.
- *Mammography* may indicate changes in the mass.
- *Ultrasonography* may help to differentiate between a solid and a fluid-filled mass.
- *Surgical excision* may be necessary if the mammogram indicates changes in the mass or if fluid can't be aspirated from the cyst.

Treatment

The most common treatment for fibrocystic change is hormone administration. Although some experts disagree, diet changes to exclude methylxanthines (particularly caffeine in coffee, tea, cola, and chocolate) and to include vitamins E, A, and B complex may make the patient more comfortable.

Daily administration of danazol, a synthetic androgen, can significantly reduce or eliminate fibrocystic breast symptoms. However, danazol can produce unpleasant adverse reactions, such as menstrual irregularities, weight gain, increased facial hair, and voice deepening.

Key nursing diagnoses and patient outcomes

Fear related to potential for breast changes to be cancerous. Based on this nursing diagnosis, you'll establish these patient outcomes. The patient will:

- verbalize her fears
- perform activities that will help reduce fear, such as monthly breast self-examinations and regular checkups
- show decreased physical symptoms of fear.

Body image disturbance related to areas of breast irregularity and lumpiness. Based on this nursing diagnosis, you'll establish these patient outcomes. The patient will:

- communicate feelings about changes in body image
- express positive feelings about herself.

Pain related to cyst formation. Based on this nursing diagnosis, you'll establish these patient outcomes. The patient will:

- take measures to reduce or relieve pain, such as applying ice packs and wearing a bra 24 hours a day
- adhere to dietary recommendations and hormonal therapy used to treat fibrocystic breast changes and thus relieve pain

• express feelings of comfort with therapy.

Nursing interventions

Provide emotional support to the patient. Encourage her to verbalize her feelings about the disorder and the changes in her body.

Monitoring

• Monitor the patient for adverse reactions to medication therapy.
• Monitor closely for breast changes.

Patient teaching

• Explain diagnostic studies and their effects and significance. Clarify any misconceptions about malignancy.
• If the patient is in pain, teach her ways to decrease discomfort, such as wearing a bra 24 hours a day, applying ice packs to the breasts, restricting sodium intake, and taking salicylates or other anti-inflammatory drugs. Advise her that the moderate to severe pain may cease spontaneously within 1 year.
• Teach other self-care activities, such as eliminating caffeine and taking vitamins, if found to be helpful.
• Encourage the patient to perform a breast self-examination every month after her menstrual cycle.
• Stress the importance of regular examinations to detect early breast changes.
• Encourage her to follow the American Cancer Society's guidelines for mammography screening:
– baseline mammography at ages 35 to 40
– repeat mammography every 2 years from ages 40 to 50
– annual mammography after age 50.

Folic acid deficiency anemia

A common, slowly progressive megaloblastic anemia, folic acid deficiency anemia is most prevalent in infants, adolescents, pregnant and breast-feeding women, alcoholics, elderly people, and patients with malignant or intestinal diseases.

Causes

Alcohol abuse suppressing the metabolic effects of folate is probably the most common cause of folic acid deficiency anemia. Additional causes include:

• poor diet (common in alcoholics, narcotic addicts, and elderly people who live alone).
• impaired absorption (due to intestinal dysfunction from such disorders as celiac disease, tropical sprue, regional jejunitis, and bowel resection).
• bacteria competing for available folic acid.
• excessive cooking of foods, which destroys the available nutrients.
• prolonged drug therapy with such drugs as anticonvulsants, estrogens, and methotrexate.
• increased folic acid requirements during pregnancy and in patients with neoplastic diseases and some skin diseases, such as exfoliative dermatitis.

Complications

Folic acid deficiency anemia produces no complications.

Assessment

The patient's history may reveal severe, progressive fatigue, the hallmark of folic acid deficiency. Associated findings include shortness of breath, palpitations, diarrhea, nausea, anorexia, headaches, forgetfulness, and irritability. The impaired oxygen-carrying capacity of the blood from lowered hemoglobin levels may produce complaints of weakness and light-headedness.

Inspection may reveal generalized pallor and jaundice. The patient may appear wasted. Cheilosis and glossitis may be present. Folic acid deficiency anemia doesn't cause neurologic impairment unless it's associated with vitamin B_{12} deficiency.

Diagnostic tests

The Schilling test and a therapeutic trial of vitamin B_{12} injections distinguish between folic acid deficiency anemia and pernicious anemia. Significant findings on blood studies include macrocytosis, decreased reticulocyte count, increased mean corpuscular volume, abnormal platelet count, and serum folate levels below 4 mg/ml.

Treatment

Medical treatment consists primarily of folic acid supplements and elimination of contributing causes. Supplements may be given orally (1 to 5 mg/day) or parenterally (to patients who are severely ill, have malabsorption, or can't take oral medication). Many patients respond favorably to a well-balanced diet. (See *Foods high in folic acid.*)

Key nursing diagnoses and patient outcomes

Altered nutrition: Less than body requirements, related to adverse GI effects. Based on this nursing diagnosis, you'll establish these patient outcomes. The patient will:

- identify foods high in folic acid
- consume a diet high in folic acid
- no longer show signs and symptoms of folic acid deficiency.

Fatigue related to folic acid deficiency. Based on this nursing diagnosis, you'll establish these patient outcomes. The patient will:

- express an understanding of the relationship between fatigue and folic acid deficiency
- employ measures to prevent or lessen fatigue
- regain his normal energy level as folic acid deficiency resolves.

Impaired physical mobility related to weakness caused by reduced hemoglobin levels. Based on this nursing diagnosis, you'll establish these patient outcomes. The patient will:

- maintain functional mobility
- not develop complications due to impaired physical mobility
- regain normal physical mobility as hemoglobin levels return to normal and folic acid deficiency resolves.

HEALTH PROMOTION POINTER

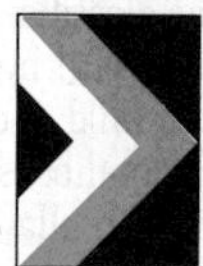

Foods high in folic acid

Folic acid (pteroylglutamic acid, folacin) is found in most body tissues, where it acts as a coenzyme in metabolic processes involving 1-carbon transfer. It's essential for formation and maturation of red blood cells and for synthesis of deoxyribonucleic acid. Although its body stores are comparatively small (about 70 mg), this vitamin is plentiful in most well-balanced diets.

However, because folic acid is water-soluble and heat-labile, it's easily destroyed by cooking. Also, about 20% of folic acid intake is excreted unabsorbed. Insufficient daily folic acid intake (less than 50 mcg/day) usually induces folic acid deficiency within 4 months. Below is a list of foods high in folic acid content; encourage your patient to consume these foods.

Food	mcg/100 g
Asparagus spears	109
Beef liver	294
Broccoli spears	54
Collards (cooked)	102
Mushrooms	24
Oatmeal	33
Peanut butter	57
Red beans	180
Wheat germ	305

Nursing interventions

- If the patient has severe anemia, plan activities, rest periods, and diagnostic tests to conserve his energy.

• If the patient has glossitis, emphasize the importance of good oral hygiene. Suggest the regular use of a mild or diluted mouthwash and a soft toothbrush. Oral anesthetics may be used to allay discomfort.
• Because a sore mouth and tongue make eating painful, ask the dietitian to give the patient only nonirritating foods. If these symptoms make talking difficult, supply a pad and pencil or some other aid to facilitate nonverbal communication; explain this problem to the family.
• To ensure accurate Schilling test results, make sure that all urine over a 24-hour period is collected and that the specimens remain uncontaminated by bacteria.
• Provide a well-balanced diet, including foods high in folate, such as dark green leafy vegetables, organ meats, eggs, milk, oranges, bananas, dry beans, and whole-grain breads. Offer between-meal snacks, and encourage the family to bring favorite foods from home.

Monitoring

• Monitor the patient's complete blood count, platelet count, and serum folate levels as ordered.
• Monitor pulse rate often. If tachycardia occurs, the patient's activities are too strenuous.
• Monitor fluid and electrolyte balance, particularly in the patient who has severe diarrhea and is receiving parenteral fluid replacement therapy.
• Advise the patient to report signs and symptoms of decreased perfusion to vital organs: dyspnea, chest pain, dizziness.

Patient teaching

• To prevent folic acid deficiency anemia, emphasize the importance of a well-balanced diet high in folic acid. Identify alcoholics or other high-risk people with poor dietary habits, and try to arrange for appropriate counseling.
• Teach the patient to meet daily folic acid requirements by including a food from each food group in every meal. If the patient has a severe deficiency, explain that diet only reinforces folic acid supplementation and isn't therapeutic by itself. Urge compliance with the prescribed course of therapy. Advise the patient not to stop taking the supplements when he begins to feel better.
• Warn the patient to guard against infections, and tell him to report signs of infection promptly, especially pulmonary and urinary tract infections, because his weakened condition may increase susceptibility.

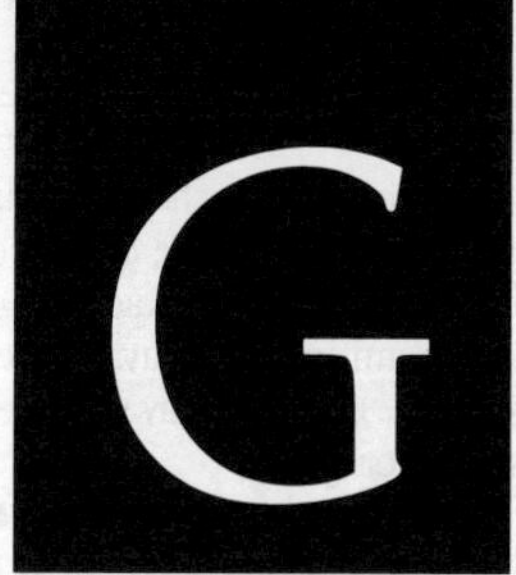

Gallbladder and bile duct cancers

Usually discovered coincidentally in patients with cholecystitis (about 90% have gallstones), gallbladder and bile duct cancers account for less than 1% of all cancer cases. The predominant type is adenocarcinoma (responsible for 85% to 95% of cases). Squamous cell carcinoma accounts for between 5% and 15%. Mixed-tissue types are rare.

Gallbladder cancer is most prevalent in women over age 60. And because it's usually discovered after cholecystectomy and at an advanced stage, the prognosis is poor. If the cancer invades gallbladder musculature, the survival rate is less than 5% – even after extensive surgery. Although some long-term survivals (4 to 5 years) have been reported, few patients survive more than 6 months after surgery. In most patients – with or without surgery – the disease progresses rapidly. Patients seldom live a year after diagnosis.

Carcinoma of the extrahepatic bile duct causes less than 1% of all cancer deaths in the United States. This disease affects more men than women (ratio of 5:2) between ages 60 and 70. The usual site is the bifurcation in the common bile duct. About 50% of patients also have gallstones. And carcinoma at the distal end of the common duct is commonly confused with carcinoma of the pancreas. Metastasis affects local lymph nodes, the liver, the lungs, and the peritoneum. Patients typically die of hepatic failure. No staging protocol exists for this type of cancer.

Causes

Whereas tumors of the biliary system are usually related to cholelithiasis, bile duct cancer seems to accompany infestation by liver flukes or other parasites.

The cause of extrahepatic bile duct cancer isn't known; however, statistics show an unexplained increase of this cancer in patients with sclerosing cholangitis, portal bacteremia, viral infections, or ulcerative colitis. Suspected causes include failure of an immune mechanism or chronic use of certain drugs by the colitis patient.

Complications

Cholangitis from obstructed bile ducts may develop as disease progresses. Typically, lymph node metastases appear in up to 70% of patients at diagnosis. Direct extension to the liver is also common (affecting up to 90% of patients). Direct extension to the cystic and the common bile ducts, stomach, colon, duodenum, and jejunum also occurs and produces obstructions. Metastases further spread by portal or hepatic veins to the peritoneum, ovaries, and lower lung lobes.

Assessment

The patient history may reveal pain centered in the epigastric area or in the right upper quadrant. The patient may describe the pain as sporadic rather than continuous. Like a patient with cholecystitis, he may report weight loss and fatigue, resulting from anorexia, nausea, and vomiting. He also may report pruritus.

Inspection may identify scleral or gingival jaundice (usually associated with advanced disease in gallbladder cancer patients).

Palpation in the right upper quadrant will reveal gallbladder enlargement.

Diagnostic tests

- *Liver function tests*–to evaluate bilirubin, urine bile and bilirubin, and urobilinogen balances–show elevated levels in more than half of gallbladder cancer patients. Serum alkaline phosphatase levels are consistently elevated.
- *Liver-spleen scan* detects abnormalities.
- *Cholecystography* may demonstrate stones or calcification (the "porcelain" gallbladder).
- *Magnetic resonance imaging* may show areas of tumor growth.
- *Cholangiography* may outline a common bile duct obstruction.

The following tests help to confirm extrahepatic bile duct carcinoma:

- *Liver function studies* indicate biliary obstruction; elevated bilirubin (5 to 30 mg/dl), alkaline phosphatase, and blood cholesterol levels; prolonged prothrombin time; and response to vitamin K.
- *Endoscopic retrograde cholangiopancreatography* identifies the tumor site and permits tissue specimen retrieval for biopsy.

Treatment

The treatment of choice for gallbladder cancer, surgery includes cholecystectomy, common bile duct exploration, T-tube drainage, and wedge excision of hepatic tissue.

As a rule, surgery can relieve obstruction and jaundice, resulting from extrahepatic bile duct cancer. The procedure depends on the cancer site and may include cholecystoduodenostomy or T-tube drainage of the common bile duct.

Radiation therapy may be palliative, and adjuvant chemotherapy (infrequently used) may produce some good results.

Key nursing diagnoses and patient outcomes

Altered nutrition: Less than body requirements. Based on this nursing diagnosis, you'll establish these patient outcomes. The patient will:

- consume an adequate daily diet, either by eating nutritionally balanced meals and snacks or through alternative nutritional programs, such as total parenteral nutrition
- not show signs and symptoms of malnutrition.

Anxiety related to threat of death because of poor prognosis. Based on this nursing diagnosis, you'll establish these patient outcomes. The patient will:

- express feelings about the diagnosis and prognosis
- use support systems to assist with coping
- accept the outcome and have decreased physical symptoms of anxiety.

Pain related to tumor growth. Based on this nursing diagnosis, you'll establish these outcomes. The patient will:

- express feelings of comfort after analgesic administration
- identify factors that intensify pain and then modify behavior accordingly.

The patient or caregiver will:

- learn appropriate pain relief methods and carry them out.

Nursing interventions

Listen to the patient's fears and concerns. Stay with him when his stress and anxiety increase. Encourage him to identify actions and care measures that promote comfort and relaxation.

After biliary resection

- Provide meticulous skin care, using strict aseptic technique when caring for the incision and surrounding tissue.

• Give pain medications as ordered. Place the patient in low Fowler's position to promote comfort.
• Prevent respiratory problems by encouraging the patient to cough and breathe deeply despite the high incision, which will make him prefer taking shallow breaths. Provide analgesics. Also show the patient how to splint the abdomen with a pillow or an abdominal binder. This will ease discomfort and promote greater respiratory efforts.
• Secure the T tube and nasogastric (NG) tube to minimize tension and to prevent them from being pulled out.
• Encourage deep-breathing and coughing exercises.

During radiation therapy

• Encourage the patient to eat high-calorie, well-balanced meals.
• Offer fluids, such as ginger ale, to minimize nausea and vomiting.

During chemotherapy

• Give supportive care when adverse reactions occur, and prepare the patient to cope with them.

Monitoring

• Monitor the patient's pain level and the effectiveness of analgesics.
• Check the patient's intake and output carefully. Watch for electrolyte imbalances. Monitor I.V. solutions to avoid overloading the cardiovascular system.
• If the patient has an NG tube and a T tube in place after surgery, monitor and record the amount and color of drainage at each shift. These tubes may remain for 24 to 72 hours to relieve distention and to promote drainage of blood, bile, and serosanguineous fluid.
• Watch for radiation's adverse effects, such as nausea, vomiting, hair loss, malaise, and diarrhea; promote comfort measures and offer reassurance as appropriate.
• Watch for complications, such as infection.

Patient teaching

• Offer information and support to help the patient and his family deal with their initial fears and reactions to the diagnosis.
• Explain postoperative procedures. Prepare the patient for intubation with an NG tube, a T tube, or I.V. tubes.
• Before surgery, teach coughing and deep-breathing exercises that the patient should perform postoperatively.
• Discuss ordered treatments, such as radiation therapy and chemotherapy, with the patient and his family. Make sure they understand the implications of treatments. Describe potential adverse effects, and advise the patient to notify the doctor if effects persist.
• If appropriate, direct the patient and his family to hospital and community services, such as cancer support groups and hospice care.

Gastric cancer

Although gastric cancer is common throughout the world in people of all races, its incidence exhibits unexplained geographic, cultural, and gender differences. For example, mortality from this disorder is high in Japan, Iceland, Chile, and Austria. Incidence is also higher in men over age 40.

Over the past 25 years in the United States, the incidence of gastric cancer has fallen 50%, with the resulting death rate now one-third of what it was 30 years ago. This decrease has been attributed, without proof, to the improved, well-balanced diets most Americans enjoy.

Gastric cancer occurs more commonly in some parts of the stomach than in others. (See *Sites of gastric cancer,* page 314.)

This adenocarcinoma rapidly infiltrates the regional lymph nodes, omentum, liver, and lungs by way of the walls of the stomach, duodenum, and esophagus; the lym-

Sites of gastric cancer

The illustration below shows how frequently gastric cancer occurs in different parts of the stomach.

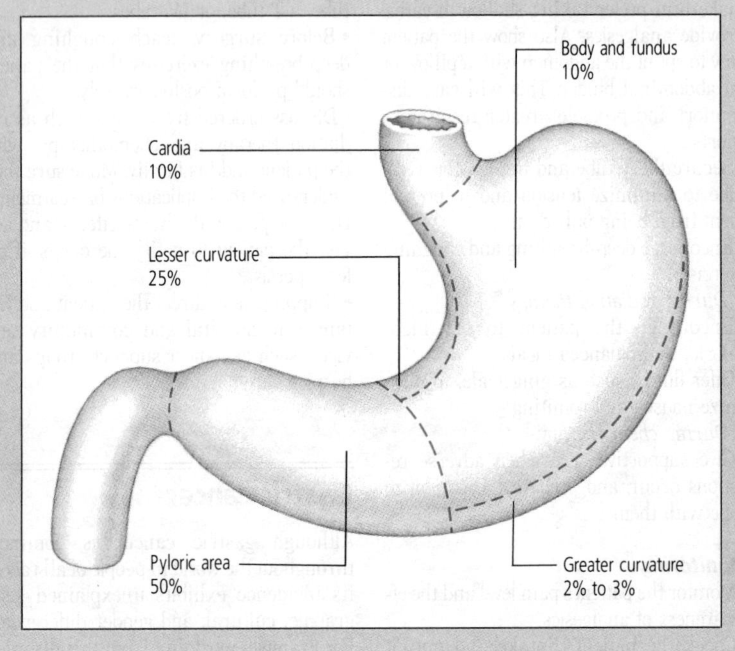

phatic system; adjacent organs; the bloodstream; and the peritoneal cavity.

The patient's prognosis depends on the stage of the disease at the time of diagnosis. Overall, the 5-year survival rate is about 15%.

Causes

Although the cause of gastric cancer is unknown, predisposing factors, such as gastritis with gastric atrophy, increase the risk. Genetic factors have also been implicated. People with type A blood have a 10% increased risk, and the disease occurs more commonly in people with a family history of such cancer.

Dietary factors also seem to have an effect. For instance, certain types of food preparation and preservation (especially smoked foods, pickled vegetables, and salted fish and meat) and physical properties of some foods increase the risk. Furthermore, high alcohol consumption and smoking increase the chances of developing gastric cancer.

Complications

Malnutrition occurs when the stomach can't digest protein, and GI obstruction develops as the tumor enlarges. Iron deficiency anemia results as the tumor causes ulceration and bleeding. If the patient has pernicious anemia, the tumor can interfere with the production of intrinsic factor needed for vitamin B_{12} absorption. As the cancer metastasizes to other structures, related complications appear.

Assessment

In the early stages, the patient may complain of pain in his back or in the epigastric or retrosternal areas that's relieved with nonprescription medications. (He may not report this symptom because he doesn't realize its significance.) The patient typically reports a vague feeling of fullness, heaviness, and moderate abdominal distention after meals.

Depending on cancer progression, the patient may report weight loss, resulting from appetite disturbance, nausea, and vomiting. He may report coffee-ground vomitus if the tumor is located in the cardia. He also may complain of weakness and fatigue. If the tumor is located in the proximal area of the stomach, he may experience dysphagia.

Palpation of the abdomen may disclose a mass. You may also be able to palpate enlarged lymph nodes, especially the supraclavicular and axillary nodes. Other assessment findings depend on the extent of the disease and the location of metastasis.

Diagnostic tests

- *Barium X-rays of the GI tract with fluoroscopy* show changes that suggest gastric cancer. Changes include a tumor or filling defect in the outline of the stomach, loss of flexibility and distensibility, and abnormal gastric mucosa with or without ulceration.
- *Gastroscopy with fiber-optic endoscope* helps rule out other diffuse gastric mucosal abnormalities by allowing direct visualization. Gastroscopic biopsy permits evaluation of gastric mucosal lesions. Photography during gastroscopy provides a permanent record of gastric lesions that can later be used to judge disease progression and the effect of treatment.
- *Gastric acid stimulation test* determines whether the stomach secretes acid properly.
- *Blood studies* monitor the course of the disease, complications, and the effectiveness of treatment. These studies include a complete blood count (CBC), chemistry profiles, arterial blood gas analysis, liver function studies, and a carcinoembryonic antigen radioimmunoassay.

Certain other studies may rule out specific organ metastases. These include computed tomography scans, chest X-rays, liver and bone scans, and liver biopsy. (See *Staging gastric cancer*, page 316.)

Treatment

Surgery to remove the tumor often is the treatment of choice. Excision of the lesion with appropriate margins is possible in more than one-third of patients. Even in a patient whose disease isn't considered surgically curable, resection eases symptoms and improves the potential benefits of the chemotherapy and radiation therapy that usually follow surgery.

The nature and extent of the lesion determine the type of surgery. Surgical procedures include gastroduodenostomy, gastrojejunostomy, partial gastric resection, and total gastrectomy. If metastasis has occurred, the omentum and spleen may have to be removed.

Chemotherapy for GI tumors may help control signs and symptoms and prolong survival. Gastric adenocarcinomas respond to several agents, including fluorouracil, carmustine, doxorubicin, and mitomycin. Antiemetics can control nausea, which intensifies as the tumor grows. In the more advanced stages, the patient may need sedatives and tranquilizers to control overwhelming anxiety. Opioid analgesics can relieve severe and unremitting pain.

If the patient has a nonresectable or partially resectable tumor, radiation therapy is effective if combined with chemotherapy. The patient should receive this therapy on an empty stomach but not preoperatively

Staging gastric cancer

Both prognosis and treatment of gastric cancer depend on its type and stage. Using the TNM (tumor, node, metastasis) system, the American Joint Committee on Cancer describes the following stages of gastric cancer.

Primary tumor
TX—primary tumor can't be assessed
T0—no evidence of primary tumor
Tis—carcinoma in situ: intraepithelial tumor doesn't penetrate the lamina propria
T1—tumor penetrates the lamina propria or submucosa
T2—tumor penetrates the muscularis propria or subserosa
T3—tumor penetrates the serosa (visceral peritoneum) without invading adjacent structures
T4—tumor invades adjacent structures

Regional lymph nodes
NX—regional lymph nodes can't be assessed
N0—no evidence of regional lymph node metastasis
N1—involvement of perigastric lymph nodes within 3 cm of the edge of the primary tumor
N2—involvement of the perigastric lymph nodes more than 3 cm from the edge of the primary tumor, or in lymph nodes along the left gastric, common hepatic, splenic, or celiac arteries

Distant metastasis
MX—distant metastasis can't be assessed
M0—no evidence of distant metastasis
M1—distant metastasis

Staging categories
Gastric cancer stages progress from mild to severe as follows:
Stage 0—Tis, N0, M0
Stage IA—T1, N0, M0
Stage IB—T1, N1, M0; T2, N0, M0
Stage II—T1, N2, M0; T3, N0, M0
Stage IIIA—T2, N2, M0; T3, N1, M0; T4, N0, M0
Stage IIIB—T3, N2, M0; T4, N1, N0
Stage IV—T4, N2, M0; any T, any N, M1

because it may damage viscera and impede healing.

Treatment with antispasmodics and antacids may help relieve GI distress.

Key nursing diagnoses and patient outcomes

Altered nutrition: Less than body requirements, related to adverse GI effects. Based on this nursing diagnosis, you'll establish these patient outcomes. The patient will:
• eat a high-protein, high-calorie diet daily
• regain any weight lost and keep his weight within the normal range
• not develop malnutrition.

Fatigue related to anemia. Based on this nursing diagnosis, you'll establish these patient outcomes. The patient will:
• express an understanding of the relationship between fatigue, activity tolerance, and gastric cancer
• employ measures to prevent and decrease fatigue
• regain his normal energy level when treatment is complete.

Anxiety related to potential threat of death from cancer diagnosis. Based on this nursing diagnosis, you'll establish these patient outcomes. The patient will:
• express his feelings about his diagnosis and prognosis
• use support systems to assist with coping
• cope with gastric cancer without showing signs of severe anxiety.

Nursing interventions

- Provide a high-protein, high-calorie diet to help the patient avoid or recover from the weight loss, malnutrition, and anemia associated with gastric cancer. This diet also helps the patient tolerate surgery, radiotherapy, and chemotherapy; helps prevent wound dehiscence; and promotes wound healing. Plus, it provides enough protein, fluid, and potassium to aid glycogen and protein synthesis.
- Give the patient dietary supplements, such as vitamins and iron, and provide small, frequent meals. If the patient has an iron deficiency, give him iron-rich foods, such as spinach and dried fruit.
- To stimulate a poor appetite, administer steroids or antidepressants, as ordered. Wine or brandy also may help stimulate his appetite.
- If the patient can't tolerate oral foods, provide parenteral nutrition.
- Administer an antacid to relieve heartburn and acid stomach and a histamine$_2$-receptor antagonist, such as cimetidine or famotidine, to decrease gastric secretions. Give opioid analgesics, as ordered, to relieve pain.
- Prepare the patient for surgery, as indicated.
- During radiation or chemotherapy treatment, offer orange juice, grapefruit juice, ginger ale, or other fluids to minimize nausea and vomiting. Provide comfort measures and reassurance as needed.
- Throughout treatment, listen to the patient's fears and concerns, and offer reassurance when appropriate. Stay with him during periods of severe anxiety.
- Encourage the patient to identify actions and care measures that promote comfort and relaxation. Try to perform these measures, and encourage the patient and his family to do so, too.
- Whenever possible, include the patient and his family in decisions related to the patient's care.
- If all treatments fail, keep the patient comfortable and free from unnecessary pain, and provide psychological support. Encourage him to express his feelings and fears and to ask questions about his illness. Answer such questions honestly; evasive answers will make him retreat and feel isolated.
- Also talk with family members, and answer their questions. Advise them to let the patient talk about his future; encourage them to maintain a realistic outlook.

Monitoring

- Monitor the patient's nutritional intake. Weigh him regularly and report excessive weight loss to the doctor. Watch for signs and symptoms of malnutrition.
- Watch for signs of anemia and vitamin B_{12} malabsorption. Monitor CBC and serum vitamin B_{12} levels.
- During radiation therapy, watch for adverse reactions, such as nausea, vomiting, alopecia, malaise, and diarrhea.
- During chemotherapy, watch for complications, such as infection, and for expected adverse reactions, such as nausea, vomiting, mouth ulcers, and alopecia.
- Watch for surgical complications, such as infection.

Patient teaching

- Provide preoperative teaching for the patient scheduled for surgery.
- Stress the importance of sound nutrition. Explain that the patient may need vitamins to prevent B_{12} deficiency and iron to prevent or treat anemia.
- Explain the ordered treatments to the patient and his family. Describe the adverse effects the treatment may cause, and tell the patient to notify the doctor if these effects persist.
- Prepare the patient for chemotherapy's adverse effects, such as nausea and vomiting, and suggest measures, such as drinking plenty of fluids, that may help relieve these problems.
- Encourage the patient to follow his normal routine as much as possible after recovering from surgery and during radia-

tion therapy and chemotherapy. Leading a near-normal life will help foster feelings of independence and control and will reduce complications of immobility.

- Caution the patient to avoid crowds and people with known infections because chemotherapy and radiation therapy diminish the body's natural resistance to infection.
- Encourage the patient to learn and practice relaxation and pain management techniques to help control anxiety and discomfort.
- If appropriate, direct the patient and his family to hospital and community support personnel and services. These include social workers, psychologists, cancer support groups, home health care agencies, and hospices.

Gastric surgery

If chronic ulcer disease doesn't respond to medication, dietary therapy, and rest, gastric surgery may be necessary to remove diseased tissue and prevent recurrence of ulcers. This surgery may also be used to excise a malignancy or relieve an obstruction. In an emergency, it may be performed to control severe GI hemorrhage resulting from a perforated ulcer.

Gastric surgery can take various forms, depending on the location and extent of the disorder. For example, a partial gastrectomy may be performed to reduce the amount of acid-secreting mucosa. A bilateral vagotomy may relieve ulcer symptoms and eliminate vagal nerve stimulation of gastric secretions. A pyloroplasty may improve drainage and prevent obstruction. Most commonly, though, two gastric surgeries are combined, such as vagotomy with gastroenterostomy or vagotomy with antrectomy.

Procedure

Surgery begins with an upper abdominal incision, such as an upper paramedial incision, to expose the stomach and part of the intestine. Total gastrectomy, the removal of the entire stomach, requires a more extensive incision.

The rest of the procedure varies, depending on the type of surgery. (See *Understanding common gastric surgeries.*) To complete the operation, the surgeon inserts abdominal drains and closes the incision.

Complications

Gastric surgery carries the risk of serious complications, including hemorrhage, obstruction, dumping syndrome, paralytic ileus, perforation, vitamin B_{12} deficiency, anemia, and atelectasis.

Key nursing diagnoses and patient outcomes

Altered nutrition: Less than body requirements. Based on this nursing diagnosis, you'll establish these patient outcomes. The patient will:

- maintain adequate nutrition with I.V. therapy or total parenteral nutrition (TPN) until oral feedings can resume
- regain and retain normal complete blood count, serum protein electrophoresis, and serum calcium and potassium levels
- tolerate oral feedings without experiencing dumping syndrome.

Ineffective breathing pattern related to guarded respirations caused by discomfort from chest or abdominal incision, or both. Based on this nursing diagnosis, you'll establish these patient outcomes. The patient will:

- recover and retain his normal respiratory rate
- maintain adequate ventilation
- not develop respiratory complications, such as pneumonia and atelectasis.

Risk for fluid volume deficit related to nasogastric (NG) drainage and potential for hemorrhage. Based on this nursing diagnosis, you'll establish these patient outcomes. The patient will:

- have vital signs within the normal range

Understanding common gastric surgeries

Besides treating chronic ulcers, gastric surgeries help remove obstructions and neoplasms. Be sure you're familiar with these commonly performed gastric surgeries.

Vagotomy with gastroenterostomy
The surgeon resects the vagus nerves and creates a stoma for gastric drainage. He'll perform selective, truncal, or parietal cell vagotomy, depending on the degree of gastric acid reduction required.

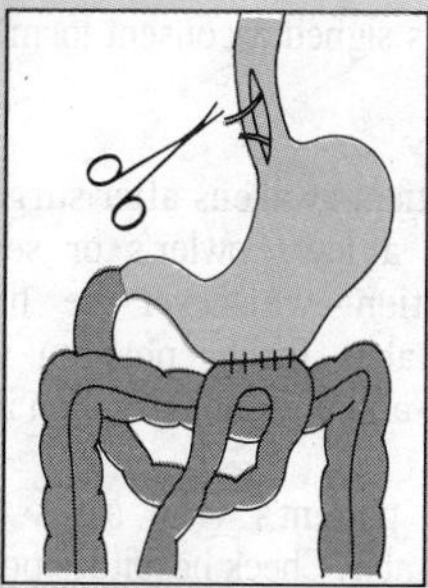

Vagotomy with antrectomy
After resecting the vagus nerves, the surgeon removes the antrum. Then he anastomoses the remaining stomach segment to the jejunum and closes the duodenal stump.

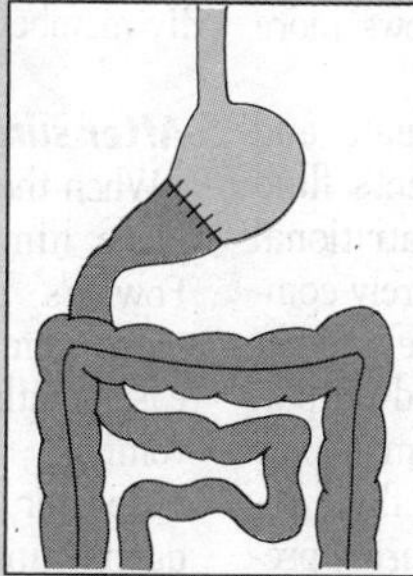

Vagotomy with pyloroplasty
In this procedure, the surgeon resects the vagus nerves and refashions the pylorus to widen the lumen and aid gastric emptying.

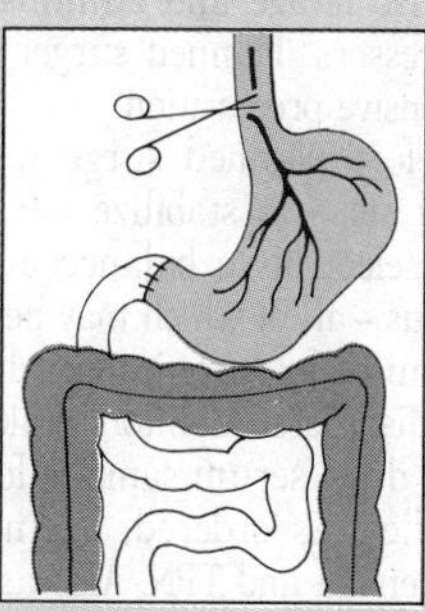

Billroth I
In this partial gastrectomy with a gastroduodenoscopy, the surgeon excises the distal third to half of the stomach and anastomoses the remaining stomach to the duodenum.

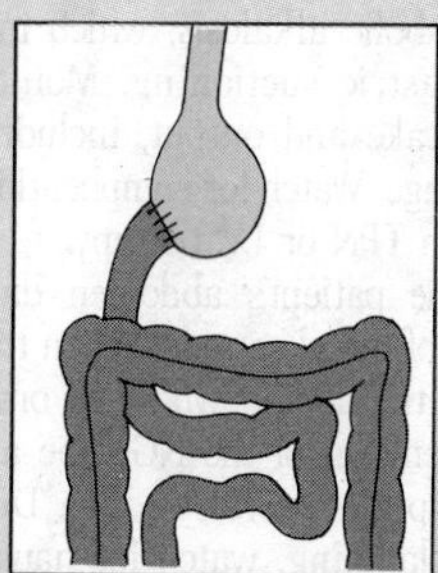

Billroth II
In this partial gastrectomy with a gastrojejunostomy, the surgeon removes the distal segment of the stomach and antrum. Then he anastomoses the remaining stomach and the jejunum and closes the duodenal stump.

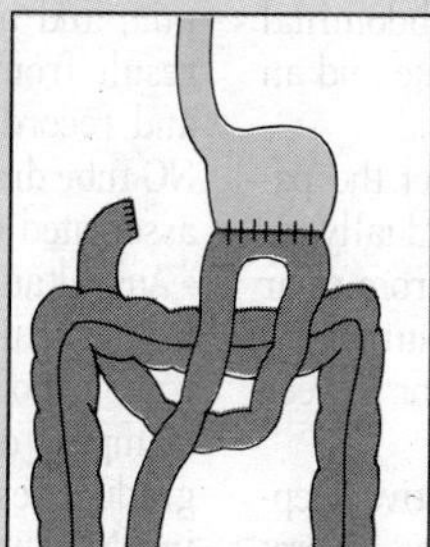

Total gastrectomy
The surgeon removes the entire stomach and attaches the lower end of the esophagus to the jejunum (esophagojejunostomy) at the entrance to the small intestine.

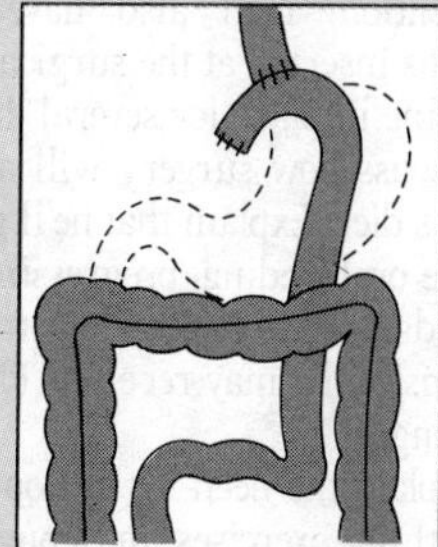

- not show signs of incisional bleeding
- maintain fluid and electrolyte balance.

Nursing interventions

When preparing a patient for gastric surgery or managing him afterwards, expect to implement these interventions.

Before surgery

- Be aware that the extent of preoperative preparation depends on the nature of the surgery. If emergency surgery is necessary, preparation may be limited to immunohematologic studies and measures to control acute hemorrhage, such as cool gastric lavage and administration of vasopressors. Planned surgery allows more extensive preparation.
- Before planned surgery, evaluate and take steps to stabilize the patient's fluid and electrolyte balance and nutritional status – all of which may be severely compromised by chronic ulcer disease or other GI disorders. Monitor intake and output, and draw serum samples for hematologic studies. As ordered, begin I.V. fluid replacement and TPN. Also as ordered, prepare the patient for abdominal X-rays. On the night before surgery, administer cleansing laxatives and enemas, as necessary. On the morning of surgery, insert an NG tube.
- As time permits, discuss postoperative care measures with the patient. Explain that the NG tube will remain in place for 2 to 3 days to remove fluid, blood, and air from the abdominal cavity and to prevent distention; he'll also have abdominal drains inserted at the surgical site and an I.V. line in place for several days.
- Discuss how surgery will affect the patient's diet. Explain that he'll gradually resume oral feeding, progressing from clear liquids to solid foods. If gastric surgery is extensive, he may receive TPN for 1 week or longer.
- Explain the need for postoperative deep-breathing exercises and coughing to prevent pulmonary complications. Stress the importance of performing these measures even though incisional pain may make the patient reluctant to do so.
- Remember that the patient will have fears about the surgery and concerns about its effect on his life-style, even if he doesn't express them. Take the time to reassure him. Point out that other, more conservative treatments haven't worked and that surgery is now necessary to relieve his symptoms and prevent more serious, possibly even life-threatening, complications. Explain that with successful surgery, he should be able to lead a near-normal life with few activity restrictions.
- Be sure the patient or a responsible family member has signed a consent form.

After surgery

- When the patient awakens after surgery, place him in a low Fowler's or semi-Fowler's position – whichever he finds more comfortable. Either position will ease breathing and prevent aspiration if he vomits.
- Monitor the patient's vital signs frequently until stable. Check hospital's policy for specific guidelines. Watch especially for hypotension, bradycardia, and respiratory changes, which may signal hemorrhage and shock. Periodically check the wound site, NG tube, and abdominal drainage tubes for bleeding.
- Maintain tube feedings or TPN and I.V. fluid and electrolyte replacement therapy, as ordered. Monitor blood studies daily. Watch for signs of dehydration, hyponatremia, and metabolic alkalosis, which may result from gastric suctioning. Monitor and record intake and output, including NG tube drainage. Watch for complications associated with TPN or I.V. therapy.
- Auscultate the patient's abdomen daily for the return of bowel sounds. When they return, notify the doctor, who will order clamping or removal of the NG tube and gradual resumption of oral feeding. During NG tube clamping, watch for nausea and vomiting; if they occur, unclamp the

tube immediately and reattach it to suction.

- Throughout recovery, have the patient cough, deep-breathe, and change position frequently. Provide incentive spirometry, as necessary. Teach him to splint his incision while coughing to help reduce pain. Assess his breath sounds frequently to detect atelectasis.
- Assess for other complications, including vitamin B_{12} deficiency, anemia (especially common in patients who have undergone total gastrectomy), and dumping syndrome, a potentially serious digestive complication marked by weakness, nausea, flatulence, and palpitations within 30 minutes after a meal.

Home care instructions

- Instruct the patient to notify the doctor immediately if he develops any signs of life-threatening complications, such as hemorrhage, obstruction, or perforation.
- Explain dumping syndrome and ways to avoid it. Advise the patient to eat small, frequent meals evenly spaced throughout the day. He should chew his food thoroughly and drink fluids between meals rather than with them. He should decrease intake of carbohydrates and salt while increasing fat and protein. After a meal, he should lie down for 20 to 30 minutes.
- Advise the patient to avoid or limit foods high in fiber, such as fresh fruits and vegetables and whole-grain breads.
- If the doctor has prescribed a GI anticholinergic to decrease motility and acid secretion, instruct the patient to take the drug 30 minutes to 1 hour before meals.
- If the patient is being discharged on tube feedings, make sure that he and his family understand how to give the feedings.
- Encourage the patient and his family to help speed healing and lessen the risk of recurrence by identifying and eliminating sources of emotional stress at home and in the workplace. Instruct the patient to balance activity and rest and to schedule a realistic pattern of work and sleep. Suggest that he learn and apply stress management techniques, such as progressive relaxation and meditation. If the patient finds self-management difficult, encourage him to seek professional counseling.
- Advise the patient to avoid smoking because it alters pancreatic secretions that neutralize gastric acid in the duodenum.

Gastritis

An inflammation of the gastric mucosa, gastritis may be acute or chronic. Acute gastritis, the most common stomach disorder, produces mucosal reddening, edema, hemorrhage, and erosion. Chronic gastritis is common among elderly patients and patients with pernicious anemia. It's often present as chronic atrophic gastritis, in which all stomach mucosal layers are inflamed, with reduced numbers of chief and parietal cells. However, acute or chronic gastritis can occur at any age.

Causes

Acute gastritis has numerous causes, including:

- chronic ingestion of irritating foods, such as hot peppers (or an allergic reaction to them), or alcohol
- drugs, such as aspirin and other nonsteroidal anti-inflammatory agents (in large doses), cytotoxic agents, caffeine, corticosteroids, antimetabolites, phenylbutazone, and indomethacin
- ingested poisons, especially ammonia, mercury, carbon tetrachloride, or corrosive substances
- endotoxins released from infecting bacteria, such as staphylococci, *Escherichia coli,* or salmonella.

Acute gastritis also may develop in acute illnesses, especially when the patient has major trauma; burns; severe infection; hepatic, renal, or respiratory failure; or major surgery.

Chronic gastritis usually involves an underlying pathology that results in atrophy of the gastric mucosa. It is associated with pernicious anemia (Type A) and infection with *Helicobacter pylori* (Type B). Individuals with Type A chronic gastritis are at risk for developing gastric cancer.

Complications

Although gastritis usually resolves when the causative agent is removed, persistent or untreated disease can lead to hemorrhage, shock, obstruction, perforation, peritonitis, and gastric cancer.

Assessment

The patient history may reveal one or more causative agents. After exposure to the offending substance, the patient with acute gastritis typically reports rapid onset of symptoms, such as epigastric discomfort, indigestion, cramping, anorexia, nausea, hematemesis, and vomiting. The symptoms may last from a few hours to a few days.

The patient with chronic gastritis may describe similar symptoms or he may only experience mild epigastric discomfort. Or his complaints may be vague. For example, he may report an intolerance for spicy or fatty foods or have mild epigastric pain that's relieved by eating. Patients with chronic atrophic gastritis are often asymptomatic.

On inspection, the patient may appear normal or exhibit signs of distress, such as fatigue, grimacing, or restlessness, depending on severity of symptoms. If gastric bleeding has occurred, the patient may appear pale, and his vital signs may reveal tachycardia and hypotension. Inspection and palpation may disclose abdominal distention, tenderness, and guarding. Auscultation may reveal increased bowel sounds.

Diagnostic tests

- *Gastroscopy* (commonly with biopsy) confirms gastritis when done before lesions heal (usually within 24 hours). This test is contraindicated after ingestion of a corrosive agent.
- *Laboratory analyses* can detect occult blood in vomitus or stools (or both) if the patient has gastric bleeding.
- *Hemoglobin and hematocrit levels* are decreased if the patient has developed anemia from bleeding.

Treatment

An immediate therapeutic priority is to eliminate the cause of gastritis. For example, bacterial gastritis is treated with antibiotics; ingested poisons are neutralized with the appropriate antidote. Once the associated disease is treated or the offending agent is eradicated or neutralized, the gastric mucosa usually will begin to heal.

Treatment for acute gastritis is symptomatic and supportive. Healing usually occurs within a few hours to a few days after the cause has been eliminated. Histamine antagonists, such as cimetidine, ranitidine, or famotidine, may be ordered to block gastric secretion. Antacids may be used as buffering agents.

For critically ill patients, antacids administered hourly, with or without histamine antagonists, may reduce the frequency of acute gastritis episodes. Some patients also require analgesics. Until healing occurs, the patient's oxygen needs, blood volume, and fluid and electrolyte balance must be monitored and maintained.

When gastritis causes massive bleeding, treatment includes blood replacement; iced saline lavage, possibly with norepinephrine; angiography with vasopressin infused in 0.9% sodium chloride solution; and, sometimes, surgery.

A last resort, surgery is performed only if more conservative treatments fail. Vagotomy and pyloroplasty have been used with limited success. Rarely, partial or total gastrectomy may be required.

Because patients with chronic gastritis may be asymptomatic or have only vague complaints, no specific treatment may be necessary, except for avoiding aspirin and spicy foods. If symptoms develop or persist, antacids may be taken. If pernicious anemia is the underlying cause, vitamin B_{12} may be administered parenterally.

Key nursing diagnoses and patient outcomes

Altered nutrition: Less than body requirements, related to adverse GI effects. Based on this nursing diagnosis, you'll establish these patient outcomes. The patient will:

• not develop signs and symptoms of malnutrition
• resume or maintain adequate nutritional intake daily
• regain any weight lost and maintain his weight within a normal range.

Risk for fluid volume deficit related to vomiting. Based on this nursing diagnosis, you'll establish these patient outcomes. The patient will:

• not demonstrate signs and symptoms of dehydration during acute episodes of gastritis
• maintain normal fluid balance.

Pain related to inflammation of gastric mucosa. Based on this nursing diagnosis, you'll establish these patient outcomes. The patient will:

• express feelings of comfort after analgesic administration
• identify factors that increase pain, such as specific foods or stress
• become pain free with treatment for gastritis and elimination of potential risk factors.

Nursing interventions

• If the patient is vomiting, give antiemetics.
• Administer I.V. fluids, as ordered, to maintain fluid and electrolyte balance.
• When the patient can tolerate oral feedings, provide a bland diet that takes into account his food preferences. Restart feedings slowly.
• Offer smaller, more frequent servings to reduce the amount of irritating gastric secretions.
• Help the patient identify specific foods that cause gastric upset, and eliminate them from his diet.
• Administer antacids and other prescribed medications, as ordered.
• If pain or nausea interferes with the patient's appetite, administer pain medications or antiemetics about 1 hour before meals.
• If surgery is necessary, prepare the patient preoperatively and provide appropriate postoperative care.
• Provide emotional support to the patient to help him manage his symptoms.

Monitoring

• Monitor the patient's fluid intake and output and electrolyte levels.
• If the patient has received nothing by mouth, watch for returning symptoms as you reintroduce food.
• Assess the patient for the presence of bowel sounds.
• Monitor the patient's response to antacids and other prescribed medications.
• Monitor the patient's compliance to treatment and elimination of risk factors in his life-style.

Patient teaching

• Teach the patient about the disorder. Explain the relationship between his symptoms and the causative agents so that he'll understand the need to modify his diet or life-style. Be attentive to his questions, and inform him about diagnostic tests and treatments.
• If the patient is scheduled for surgery, reinforce the doctor's explanation of the procedure and provide preoperative teaching.
• Give the patient a list of irritating foods to avoid, such as spicy or highly seasoned foods, alcohol, and caffeine. Be sure he understands that these changes are lifelong measures to prevent recurrence of gastri-

tis. If necessary, refer him to the dietitian for further instruction.
- If the patient smokes, encourage him to quit by pointing out that this habit can cause or aggravate symptoms by irritating the gastric mucosa. Refer him to a smoking-cessation program.
- If appropriate, help the patient identify the need for stress reduction. Teach him stress-reduction techniques, such as meditation, deep breathing, progressive relaxation, and guided imagery.
- Urge the patient to seek immediate attention for recurring symptoms, such as hematemesis, nausea, or vomiting.
- To prevent recurrence, stress the importance of taking prophylactic medications as ordered. To reduce gastric irritation, advise the patient to take steroids with milk, food, or antacids. Instruct him to take antacids between meals and at bedtime and to avoid aspirin-containing compounds.
- Teach family members the importance of supporting the patient as he makes the necessary dietary and life-style changes.

Gastroenteritis

A self-limiting disorder, gastroenteritis (intestinal flu, traveler's diarrhea, viral enteritis, food poisoning) is an inflammation of the stomach and small intestine. The bowel reacts to any of the varied causes of gastroenteritis with hypermotility, producing severe diarrhea and secondary depletion of intracellular fluid.

A major cause of morbidity and mortality in underdeveloped nations, gastroenteritis occurs in persons of all ages. In the United States, this disorder ranks second to the common cold as a cause of lost work time and fifth as the cause of death among young children. It also can be life-threatening in elderly and debilitated patients.

Causes

Gastroenteritis has many possible causes, including:
- bacteria, such as *Staphylococcus aureus, Salmonella, Shigella, Clostridium botulinum, C. perfringens,* and *Escherichia coli*
- amoebae, especially *Entamoeba histolytica*
- parasites, such as *Ascaris, Enterobius,* and *Trichinella spiralis*
- viruses, such as adenoviruses, echoviruses, and coxsackieviruses
- ingestion of toxins, such as poisonous plants or toadstools
- drug reactions from antibiotics
- food allergens.

Complications

In most patients, the disorder resolves with no sequelae. However, persistent or untreated gastroenteritis can cause severe dehydration and loss of crucial electrolytes, which can lead to shock, vascular collapse, renal failure and, rarely, death. Typically, infants, elderly patients, and debilitated patients are at greatest risk because of their immature or impaired immune systems.

Assessment

Patient history commonly reveals the acute onset of diarrhea accompanied by abdominal pain and discomfort. The patient may complain of cramping, nausea, and vomiting. He may also report malaise, fatigue, anorexia, fever, abdominal distention, and rumbling in his lower abdomen. If diarrhea is severe, he may experience rectal burning, tenesmus, and bloody mucoid stools.

Investigate the patient's history to try to determine the cause of his signs and symptoms. Ask about ingestion of contaminated food or water. The cause may be apparent if the patient reports that others who ingested the same food or water have similar signs and symptoms. Also ask about the health of other family members and about his recent travels. (See *Preventing traveler's diarrhea.*)

Inspection may reveal slight abdominal distention. On palpation, the patient's skin turgor may be poor, a sign of dehydration. Auscultation may disclose hyperactive bowel sounds and, if the patient is dehydrated, orthostatic hypotension or generalized hypotension. Temperature may be normal or elevated.

Diagnostic tests

Laboratory studies identify the causative bacteria, parasites, or amoebae. These studies include Gram stain, stool culture (by direct rectal swab), or blood culture.

Treatment

Medical management is usually supportive, consisting of bed rest, nutritional support, increased fluid intake and, occasionally, antidiarrheal therapy. If gastroenteritis is severe or affects a young child or an elderly or debilitated patient, hospitalization may be required. Treatment may include I.V. fluid and electrolyte replacement and administration of antidiarrheals, antiemetics, and antimicrobials.

Antidiarrheals, such as bismuth subsalicylate, are typically used as the first line of defense against diarrhea. If necessary, other antidiarrheals, such as camphorated opium tincture (paregoric), diphenoxylate with atropine, and loperamide, may be ordered.

Antiemetics (oral, I.M., or rectal suppository), such as prochlorperazine or trimethobenzamide, may be prescribed for severe vomiting. However, these medications should be avoided in patients with viral or bacterial gastroenteritis.

Specific antibiotic administration is restricted to patients who have bacterial gastroenteritis, as identified by diagnostic testing.

Preventing traveler's diarrhea

If the patient travels, especially to developing nations, discuss precautions that he can take to reduce his chances of getting traveler's diarrhea. Inform him that traveler's diarrhea is caused by inadequate sanitation and occurs after ingestion of bacteria-contaminated food or water. These organisms attach to the lining of the small intestine, where they release a toxin that causes diarrhea and cramps.

To minimize this risk, advise him to:

- drink water (or brush his teeth with water) only if it's chlorinated. Chlorination protects the water supply from bacterial contaminants, such as *Escherichia coli.*
- avoid beverages in glasses that may have been washed in contaminated water.
- refuse ice cubes if they may have been made from contaminated water.
- drink only beverages made with boiled water, such as coffee or tea, or those contained in bottles or cans.
- sanitize impure water by adding 2% tincture of iodine (5 drops/liter of clear water; 10 drops/liter of cloudy water) or by adding liquid laundry bleach (about 2 drops/liter of clear water; 4 drops/liter of cloudy water).
- avoid uncooked vegetables, fresh fruits with no peel, salads, unpasteurized milk, and other dairy products.
- beware of foods offered by street vendors.

If traveler's diarrhea occurs despite precautions, bismuth subsalicylate, diphenoxylate with atropine, or loperamide can be used to relieve symptoms.

Key nursing diagnoses and patient outcomes

Diarrhea related to inflammatory process in GI tract. Based on this nursing diagnosis, you'll establish these patient outcomes. The patient will:

• demonstrate a positive response to antidiarrheals
• not develop complications of diarrhea, such as skin breakdown in the anal area or dehydration
• regain normal bowel patterns when gastroenteritis is resolved.

Risk for fluid volume deficit related to adverse GI effects. Based on this nursing diagnosis, you'll establish these patient outcomes. The patient will:
• not show signs and symptoms of dehydration
• maintain normal fluid balance.

Pain related to inflammatory process in GI tract. Based on this nursing diagnosis, you'll establish these patient outcomes. The patient will:
• express feelings of comfort with treatment to alleviate gastroenteritis
• become pain free when gastroenteritis is resolved.

Nursing interventions

• Plan your care to allow uninterrupted rest periods for the patient. Rest usually helps to relieve the patient's symptoms, increase his resistance, and conserve his strength.
• If the patient is nauseated, advise him to avoid quick movements, which can increase the severity of nausea.
• If the patient can tolerate oral fluids, replace lost fluids and electrolytes with broth, ginger ale, and lemonade, as tolerated. Vary his diet to make eating more enjoyable, and allow some choice of foods. Warn him to avoid milk and milk products, which may provoke recurrence.
• If dehydration occurs, administer oral and I.V. fluids, as ordered. If necessary, a potassium supplement may be added to the I.V. solution. If the patient is receiving a potassium supplement, be especially alert for the development of hyperkalemia.
• Administer medications, as ordered. Correlate dosages and routes with the patient's meals and activities (for example, give antiemetics 30 to 60 minutes before meals).
• To ease anal irritation caused by diarrhea, clean the area carefully and apply a repellent cream, such as petroleum jelly. Warm sitz baths and application of witch hazel compresses can also soothe irritation.
• Wash your hands thoroughly after giving care to avoid spreading infection, and use standard precautions whenever handling vomitus or stools.
• If food poisoning is probable, contact public health authorities so they can interview patients and food handlers and take samples of the suspected contaminated food.

Monitoring

• Monitor the patient's fluid status carefully. Assess vital signs at least every 4 hours, weigh him daily, monitor for fluid and electrolyte balance, and record intake and output.
• Watch for signs of dehydration, such as dry skin and mucous membranes, fever, and sunken eyes.
• Monitor the patient's response to therapy.

Patient teaching

• Teach the patient about gastroenteritis, describing its symptoms and varied causes. Explain why a stool specimen may be necessary for diagnosis. Discuss the purpose of prescribed treatments.
• Instruct the patient to wait until his diarrhea subsides and then to start drinking unsweetened fruit juice, tea, bouillon, or other clear broths and eating bland soft foods, such as cooked cereal, rice, or applesauce. Tell him to avoid foods that are spicy, greasy, or high in roughage, such as whole-grain products or raw fruits or vegetables. Explain that these foods can precipitate recurrent diarrhea.
• Review the proper use of prescribed drugs, making sure the patient understands their desired effects and possible adverse reactions.
• Teach preventive measures. If the patient expects to travel, advise him to pay close

attention to what he eats and drinks, especially in developing nations. Review proper hygiene measures to prevent recurrence. Instruct the patient to thoroughly cook foods, especially pork; to refrigerate perishable foods, such as milk, mayonnaise, potato salad, and cream-filled pastry; to always wash his hands with warm water and soap before handling food, especially after using the bathroom; to clean utensils thoroughly; and to eliminate flies and roaches in the home.

Gastroesophageal reflux

Popularly known as heartburn, gastroesophageal reflux is the backflow of gastric or duodenal contents, or both, into the esophagus and past the lower esophageal sphincter (LES), without associated belching or vomiting. Reflux may or may not cause symptoms or pathologic changes. Persistent reflux may cause reflux esophagitis, an inflammation of the esophageal mucosa. The prognosis varies with the underlying cause.

Causes

Normally, gastric contents don't back up into the esophagus because the LES creates enough pressure around the lower end of the esophagus to close it. (The sphincter relaxes after each swallow to allow food into the stomach.) Reflux occurs when LES pressure is deficient or pressure within the stomach exceeds LES pressure. Any of the following predisposing factors may lead to reflux:

- nasogastric intubation for more than 4 days
- any agent that lowers LES pressure: food; alcohol; cigarettes; anticholinergics, such as atropine, belladonna, and propantheline; and other drugs, such as morphine, diazepam, calcium channel blockers, and meperidine.
- hiatal hernia with incompetent sphincter
- any condition or position that increases intra-abdominal pressure.

Complications

Reflux esophagitis, the primary complication of gastric reflux, can lead to other sequelae, including esophageal stricture, esophageal ulcer, and replacement of the normal squamous epithelium with columnar epithelium (Barrett's epithelium). A patient with severe reflux esophagitis may also develop anemia from chronic low-grade bleeding of inflamed mucosa.

Pulmonary complications may develop if the patient experiences reflux of gastric contents into his throat and subsequent aspiration. Reflux aspiration may lead to chronic pulmonary disease.

Assessment

Typically, the patient complains of heartburn, which worsens with vigorous exercise, bending, or lying down. He may report relief from antacids or sitting upright. If asked, he may recall regurgitating without associated nausea or belching. This symptom is often described as a feeling of warm fluid traveling up the throat, followed by a sour or bitter taste in the mouth if the fluid reaches the pharynx.

Although heartburn is the most common feature of reflux, the patient may report any of these signs and symptoms:

- a feeling of fluid accumulation in the throat without a sour or bitter taste. This is caused by hypersecretion of saliva.
- odynophagia, possibly followed by a dull substernal ache. This symptom may indicate severe, long-term reflux dysphagia from esophageal spasm, stricture, or esophagitis.
- bright red or dark brown blood in vomitus.
- chronic pain that may mimic angina pectoris, radiating to the neck, jaw, and arm. This pain may be associated with esophageal spasm and result from reflux esophagitis.

Factors affecting LES pressure

Various dietary and life-style elements can increase or decrease LES pressure. Take these into account as you plan the patient's treatment program.

What increases LES pressure
- Protein
- Carbohydrate
- Nonfat milk
- Low-dose ethanol

What decreases LES pressure
- Fat
- Whole milk
- Orange juice
- Tomatoes
- Antiflatulent (such as simethicone)
- Chocolate
- High-dose ethanol
- Cigarette smoking
- Lying on either side
- Sitting

- nocturnal hypersalivation, a rare symptom that the patient says awakens him with coughing, choking, and a mouthful of saliva.

Diagnostic tests

Although a careful history and physical examination are essential to the diagnosis, the following tests help to confirm it:

- *Esophageal acidity test,* a standard test for acid reflux, is the most sensitive and accurate measure of gastroesophageal reflux.
- *Gastroesophageal scintillation testing* may also detect reflux.
- *Esophageal manometry* evaluates the resting pressure of the LES and determines sphincter competence.
- *Acid perfusion test* confirms esophagitis.
- *Esophagoscopy* and *biopsy* allow visualization and tissue sampling of the esophagus. These tests help to evaluate the extent of the disease and confirm pathologic changes in the mucosa.
- *Barium swallow with fluoroscopy* reveals normal findings except in patients with advanced disease. In children, *barium esophagography* under fluoroscopic control may show reflux.

Treatment

Effective management relieves symptoms by reducing reflux through gravity, strengthening the LES with drug therapy, neutralizing gastric contents, and reducing intra-abdominal pressure. Treatment should also include reviewing how the patient's life-style or dietary habits may affect his LES pressure and reflux symptoms. (See *Factors affecting LES pressure.*) In mild cases, diet therapy may reduce symptoms sufficiently so that no other treatment is required. Positional therapy, which relieves symptoms by reducing intra-abdominal pressure, may be useful in uncomplicated cases.

For intermittent reflux, antacids given 1 hour and 3 hours after meals and at bedtime may be effective. For more intensive therapy, hourly antacid administration may be necessary. Depending on the patient's bowel status, a nondiarrheal, magnesium-free antacid may be prescribed. Drug therapy may also include cholinergic drugs, such as bethanechol, to increase LES pressure, histamine-receptor antagonists, such as cimetidine or ranitidine, to reduce gastric acidity, or a proton pump inhibitor, such as omeprazole (Prilosec). Metoclopramide has also been used with beneficial results. Recently, the FDA approved the prokinetic drug cisapride (Propulsid) for the treatment of gastroesophageal reflux.

Surgery is usually reserved for patients with refractory symptoms or serious complications. Indications include pulmonary aspiration, hemorrhage, esophageal obstruction or perforation, intractable pain, incompetent LES, or associated hiatal hernia. Surgical procedures reduce reflux by creating an artificial closure at the gastroesophageal junction. Several surgical approaches are available, including Belsey Mark IV operation, Hill posterior gastropexy, and Nissen operation; all involve wrapping the gastric fundus around the esophagus. Other surgery includes a vagotomy or pyloroplasty (which may be combined with an antireflux regimen) to modify gastric contents.

Key nursing diagnoses and patient outcomes

Risk for aspiration related to backflow of stomach or duodenal contents, or both. Based on this nursing diagnosis, you'll establish these patient outcomes. The patient will:

- identify measures to prevent aspiration
- not aspirate
- have no adventitious breath sounds on auscultation and have clear, odorless respiratory secretions.

Knowledge deficit related to gastroesophageal reflux. Based on this nursing diagnosis, you'll establish these patient outcomes. The patient will:

- express an interest in learning about the disorder
- seek information from a knowledgeable source
- communicate an understanding of the disorder and its treatment.

Pain related to irritation of the esophagus. Based on this nursing diagnosis, you'll establish these patient outcomes. The patient will:

- express feelings of pain relief with antacid therapy
- identify contributing factors that cause or worsen gastroesophageal reflux, such as eating certain foods
- comply with the prescribed treatment regimen and avoid or minimize contributing factors in his life-style.

Nursing interventions

- Develop a diet for the patient that takes his food preferences into account while helping to minimize his reflux symptoms. If he's obese, place him on a weight reduction diet, as ordered.
- To reduce intra-abdominal pressure, have the patient sleep in a reverse Trendelenburg position (with the head of the bed elevated 6″ to 12″ [15 to 31 cm]). He should also avoid lying down immediately after meals and late-night snacks.
- After surgery, provide care as you would for any patient who has undergone laparotomy. Pay particular attention to the patient's respiratory status because the surgery is performed close to the diaphragm. Administer prescribed analgesics, oxygen, and I.V. fluids. If a thoracic approach was used, give chest physiotherapy, as needed.
- Offer the patient emotional and psychological support to help him cope with pain and discomfort.

Monitoring

- Monitor the patient's response to therapy and compliance with treatment.
- If surgery was performed, monitor his intake and output and vital signs. If a thoracic approach was used, watch and record chest tube drainage.
- Monitor for complications of the disease and of surgery, if appropriate.

Patient teaching

- Teach the patient about the causes of gastroesophageal reflux, and review his antireflux regimen of medication, diet, and positional therapy.
- Discuss recommended dietary changes. Advise the patient to sit upright after meals and snacks and to eat small, frequent meals. Explain that he should eat at least 2 to 3 hours before lying down. Tell him to avoid highly seasoned food, acidic juices, bedtime snacks, alcoholic beverages, and foods high in fat or carbohydrates because these reduce LES pressure.
- Instruct the patient to avoid situations or activities that increase intra-abdominal pressure, such as bending, coughing, vigorous exercise, obesity, constipation, and

wearing tight clothing. Tell him to avoid using any substance that reduces sphincter control, including cigarettes, alcoholic beverages, fatty foods, and certain drugs.
- Encourage compliance with his drug regimen. Review the desired drug actions and potential adverse effects.

Gastrostomy

In a gastrostomy, an opening is created in the stomach to allow food and fluid administration. It's usually performed in a patient who requires prolonged nutritional support, such as an elderly, debilitated, or comatose patient who can't eat or swallow properly. It may also be performed in a patient with extensive oral or esophageal cancer, obstruction, or trauma.

Gastrostomy feedings are preferred over long-term nasogastric feedings because the incidence of regurgitation is lower. A gastrostomy may be permanent if the underlying condition can't be reversed, such as an impermeable stricture of the esophagus from lye burns or an inoperable malignant tumor.

Procedure

After the patient receives a local anesthetic, the surgeon makes a vertical abdominal incision directly over the stomach. He then inserts a gastrostomy tube into the anterior gastric wall and aspirates the gastric contents. The tube is clamped and several purse-string sutures are inserted to hold it in place. A sterile dressing is applied around the tube.

A gastrostomy may also be placed by percutaneous endoscopic gastrostomy (PEG). The use of endoscopy for tube placement eliminates the need for laparotomy and general anesthesia.

Complications

After a gastrostomy, possible complications include local skin irritation, excoriation, or breakdown; infection; and accidental displacement of the gastrostomy tube.

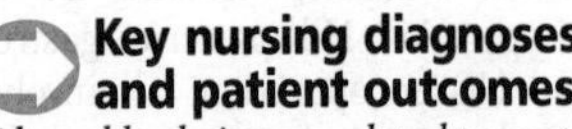

Key nursing diagnoses and patient outcomes

Altered body image related to gastrostomy. Based on this nursing diagnosis, you'll establish these patient outcomes. The patient will:
- communicate his feelings about body image changes caused by insertion of a gastrostomy tube
- express positive feelings about himself.

Altered nutrition: Less than body requirements, related to intolerance to gastrostomy tube feedings postoperatively. Based on this nursing diagnosis, you'll establish these patient outcomes. The patient will:
- not have signs of feeding intolerance, such as abdominal distention or diarrhea
- feel comfortable after a feeding is administered
- maintain adequate nutrition.

Impaired skin integrity related to leaking around the gastrostomy tube postoperatively. Based on this nursing diagnosis, you'll establish these patient outcomes. The patient will:
- report any leaking around the tube
- have a clean, irritation-free gastrostomy site.

The patient or caregiver will:
- demonstrate skill in caring for the gastrostomy site.

Nursing interventions

When preparing for or managing a patient with a gastrostomy, expect to implement these nursing interventions.

Before surgery

- Explain to the patient (if appropriate) and his family the purpose of a gastrostomy tube, how and where it's inserted, and what it looks like. Answer questions and address concerns to allay anxiety.
- Tell the patient (if appropriate) and family if the gastrostomy is expected to be permanent. Provide emotional support.

• If the patient is receiving nasogastric feedings, withhold them after midnight on the day of surgery. But don't remove the nasogastric tube unless the surgeon orders it – he may want it left in place to decompress the stomach during surgery or until gastrostomy tube feedings are started.

After surgery

• Take the patient's vital signs frequently until he's fully recovered from the anesthesia.
• Prepare the patient for the first fluid administration soon after surgery. At this time, assess for tube patency and leaking around the tube. Ensure the patient's privacy, and place him in semi-Fowler's position before the instillation.
• Prepare the patient for further gastrostomy instillations in the same manner. Check tube patency by aspirating gastric fluids with a syringe and administering 30 to 60 ml of water at room temperature through the tube. Expect to gradually increase the amount given as the patient tolerates it and if no leaking occurs. After instillation, clamp the tube, and follow the institution's protocol for covering and securing the tube and dressing the site.
• Administer intermittent (bolus) tube feedings, as ordered. Keep the patient in semi-Fowler's position for at least 30 minutes after each feeding to facilitate digestion and prevent aspiration. Record the amount and contents of each feeding as well as the patient's tolerance.
• If continuous feedings are ordered, periodically check for residual stomach contents and give feedings according to the surgeon's guidelines. To maintain patency, flush the gastrostomy tube with water at least once every 8 hours.
• Monitor the gastrostomy site for signs of skin irritation and infection.
• Wash the area around the tube daily with soap and water or 0.9% sodium chloride, and apply a bland ointment, such as zinc oxide or petroleum jelly, to protect the skin from irritation. Keep the gastrostomy site clean and dry.

Home care instructions

• Tell the patient or caregiver to notify the doctor if signs of infection (such as redness, swelling, purulent drainage) occur, if problems with administering feedings arise, or if they observe leaking around the tube.
• Teach the patient or caregiver how to care for the gastrostomy tube. If the gastrostomy is permanent, show the patient or caregiver how to change the tube every 2 to 3 days. Tell them that the tube may be removed after several weeks and reinserted only for feedings, and that in between feedings, the gastrostomy opening will be protected by a small gauze pad held in place by adhesive.
• Provide skin care instructions, stressing the importance of keeping the skin around the tube clean and dry to prevent skin breakdown.
• Teach the patient or caregiver how to prepare and administer the type of gastrostomy tube feedings ordered. If continuous feedings are to be administered, make sure the patient or caregiver understands how to operate the pump used for this procedure.
• Help arrange for visiting nurse follow-up after discharge.

Genital warts

A common sexually transmitted disease (STD), genital warts are papillomas that consist of fibrous tissue overgrowth from the dermis and thickened epithelial coverings. Also known as venereal warts and condylomata acuminata, these growths are rare before puberty or after menopause. In people under age 25, genital warts are the fastest-growing STD.

Causes

Genital warts result from infection with one of the more than 60 known strains of human papillomavirus. Transmitted by sexual contact, the virus incubates from 1 to 6 months (the average is 2 months) before warts erupt.

Complications

During pregnancy, genital warts in the vaginal and cervical walls may grow so large that they impede vaginal delivery. Other complications include possible genital tract dysplasia or cancer. (Studies show an association between human papillomavirus types 11, 16, and 18 and cervical dysplasia and cancer.)

Assessment

The patient's health history may include reported unprotected sexual contact with a partner with a known infection, a new partner, or many partners.

On examination, you'll observe warts growing on the moist genital surfaces, such as the subpreputial sac, the urethral meatus and, less commonly, the penile shaft or scrotum in male patients and the vulva and vaginal and cervical walls in female patients. In both sexes, papillomas spread to the perineum and the perianal area. On inspection, you may find warts that begin as tiny red or pink swellings. These warts may grow as large as 4″ (10 cm) and may become pedunculated. Multiple swellings have a cauliflower-like appearance. Most patients report no symptoms; a few complain of itching or pain. Infected lesions become malodorous.

Diagnostic tests

Dark-field microscopy of wart-cell scrapings shows marked epidermal cell vascularization. This differentiates genital warts from condylomata lata associated with second-stage syphilis.

Another test involves applying 5% acetic acid (white vinegar) to the warts, which will turn white if they're papillomas.

Treatment

Genital warts occasionally resolve spontaneously. To remove small warts, the doctor usually recommends topical drug therapy. Medications of choice include 10% to 25% podophyllum resin in tincture of benzoin (contraindicated in pregnancy), trichloroacetic acid, and bichloroacetic acid. (Treatment aims to remove exophytic warts and ameliorate signs and symptoms, not to eradicate the human papillomavirus.)

Warts that grow larger than 1″ (2.5 cm) usually are removed by carbon dioxide laser, cryosurgery, electrocautery, or fluorouracil cream debridement. Conventional surgery may be recommended to remove perianal warts.

Rarely, immune therapy may be prescribed. This involves excising the warts and using them to prepare a vaccine to stimulate antibodies. Interferon therapy is under evaluation.

Key nursing diagnoses and patient outcomes

Altered sexuality patterns related to presence of genital warts. Based on this nursing diagnosis, you'll establish these patient outcomes. The patient will:
- express feelings about changes in sexuality patterns
- resume normal sexuality patterns using precautions to avoid spreading the human papillomavirus.

Body image disturbance related to presence of genital warts. Based on this nursing diagnosis, you'll establish these patient outcomes. The patient will:
- acknowledge a change in body image
- have the genital warts removed
- express positive feelings about himself.

Knowledge deficit related to human papillomavirus as an STD. Based on this diagnosis, you'll establish these patient outcomes. The patient will:
- express an interest in learning about human papillomavirus and its role in causing genital warts

• learn about human papillomavirus from an appropriate source
• communicate an understanding of human papillomavirus, including how it's contracted, its role in genital wart formation, and precautions to prevent infecting sexual partners.

Nursing interventions

• Use standard precautions when examining the patient, collecting a specimen, or performing associated procedures.
• Provide a nonthreatening, nonjudgmental atmosphere that encourages the patient to verbalize his feelings about perceived changes in sexual identity and behavior.

Monitoring

• Monitor the patient for signs and symptoms of genital tract cancer.
• Monitor for infection.

Patient teaching

• Tell the patient to remove podophyllum resin with soap and water 4 to 6 hours after applying it to warts.
• Recommend sexual abstinence or condom use during intercourse until healing is complete.
• Advise the patient to inform his sexual partners about the risk of genital warts and of their need for evaluation.
• Urge the patient to be tested for human immunodeficiency virus infection and other STDs.
• Emphasize that genital warts can recur and that the virus can mutate, causing infection with warts of a different strain.
• Remind the patient to report for weekly treatments until all warts are removed. Then instruct him to schedule a checkup 3 months after all warts are gone.
• Encourage female patients to have a Papanicolaou test every 6 months.

Glaucoma

A group of disorders, glaucoma is characterized by high intraocular pressure (IOP) that damages the optic nerve. Glaucoma may occur as a primary or congenital disease or secondary to other causes, such as injury, infection, surgery, or prolonged topical corticosteroid use.

Primary glaucoma has two forms: *open-angle* (also known as chronic, simple, or wide-angle) glaucoma and *angle-closure* (also known as acute or narrow-angle) glaucoma. Angle-closure glaucoma attacks suddenly and may cause permanent vision loss in 48 to 72 hours.

One of the leading causes of blindness, glaucoma affects about 2% of Americans over age 40 and accounts for about 12% of newly diagnosed blindness in the United States. The incidence is highest among blacks. In the United States, early detection and effective treatment contribute to the good prognosis for preserving vision.

Causes

Open-angle glaucoma results from degenerative changes in the trabecular meshwork. These changes block the flow of aqueous humor from the eye, which causes IOP to increase. The result is optic nerve damage. Affecting about 90% of all patients who have glaucoma, open-angle glaucoma commonly occurs in families.

Angle-closure glaucoma results from obstruction to the outflow of aqueous humor caused by an anatomically narrow angle between the iris and the cornea. This causes IOP to increase suddenly. Angle-closure glaucoma attacks may be triggered by trauma, pupillary dilation, stress, or any ocular change that pushes the iris forward (a hemorrhage or a swollen lens, for example).

Secondary glaucoma can proceed from such conditions as uveitis, trauma, drug use (such as corticosteroids), venous occlusion, or diabetes. In some instances, new

How glaucoma progresses

Because open-angle glaucoma begins insidiously and takes a slowly progressive course, the patient may report no symptoms. Later in the disease, the patient may complain of a dull, morning headache; mild aching in the eyes; loss of peripheral vision; seeing halos around lights; and reduced visual acuity (especially at night) that's uncorrected by glasses.

In contrast, angle-closure glaucoma typically has a rapid onset and constitutes an emergency. The patient may complain of pain and pressure over the eye, blurred vision, decreased visual acuity, seeing halos around lights, and nausea and vomiting (from increased IOP).

blood vessels (neovascularization) may form, blocking the passage of aqueous humor.

Complications

If untreated, glaucoma can progress from gradual vision loss to total blindness.

Assessment

Inspection may reveal unilateral eye inflammation, a cloudy cornea, and a moderately dilated pupil that's nonreactive to light. Palpation may also disclose increased IOP discovered by applying gentle fingertip pressure to the patient's closed eyelids. With angle-closure glaucoma, one eye may feel harder than the other. (See *How glaucoma progresses.*)

Diagnostic tests

• *Tonometry* (with an applanation, a Schiøtz', or a pneumatic tonometer) measures IOP and provides a baseline for reference. Normal IOP ranges from 8 to 21 mm Hg. However, patients whose pressures fall within the normal range can develop signs and symptoms of glaucoma, and patients who have abnormally high IOP may have no clinical effects.

• *Slit-lamp examination* allows the doctor to see the effects of glaucoma on the anterior eye structures, including the cornea, iris, and lens.

• *Gonioscopy* determines the angle of the eye's anterior chamber. This enables the doctor to distinguish between open-angle and angle-closure glaucoma. The angle is normal in open-angle glaucoma. In older patients, however, partial closure of the angle may occur (allowing two forms of glaucoma to coexist).

• *Ophthalmoscopy* facilitates visualization of the fundus. In open-angle glaucoma, cupping of the optic disk may be seen earlier than in angle-closure glaucoma.

• *Perimetry or visual field tests* determine the extent of peripheral vision loss, which helps evaluate deterioration in open-angle glaucoma.

• *Fundus photography* monitors and records optic disk changes.

Treatment

For open-angle glaucoma, initial treatment aims to reduce pressure by decreasing aqueous humor production with medications. These include beta blockers, such as timolol (used cautiously in asthmatic patients or patients with bradycardia) or betaxolol. Other drug treatments include epinephrine to decrease production of and increase outflow of aqueous humor (contraindicated in angle-closure glaucoma) and miotic eyedrops, such as pilocarpine, to promote aqueous humor outflow.

Patients who don't respond to drug therapy may benefit from argon laser trabeculoplasty or from a surgical filtering procedure called trabeculectomy.

To perform *argon laser trabeculoplasty,* the ophthalmologist focuses an argon laser beam on the trabecular meshwork of an open angle. This produces a thermal burn that changes the meshwork surface and facilitates the outflow of aqueous humor.

To perform a *trabeculectomy,* the surgeon dissects a flap of sclera to expose the trabecular meshwork. He removes a small tissue block and performs a peripheral iridectomy, which produces an opening for aqueous outflow under the conjunctiva and creates a filtering bleb. Postoperatively, subconjunctival injections of fluorouracil may be given to maintain the fistula's patency.

An emergency, angle-closure glaucoma requires immediate treatment to lower high IOP. Initial preoperative drug therapy aims to lower IOP with acetazolamide, pilocarpine (which constricts the pupil, forces the iris away from the trabeculae, and allows fluid to escape), and I.V. mannitol or oral glycerin (which forces fluid from the eye by making the blood hypertonic). If these medications fail to decrease the pressure, laser iridotomy or surgical peripheral iridectomy must be performed promptly to save the patient's vision.

An *iridectomy* relieves pressure by excising part of the iris to reestablish the outflow of aqueous humor. A few days later, the surgeon performs a prophylactic iridectomy on the other eye. This prevents an episode of acute glaucoma in the normal eye.

If the patient has severe pain, treatment may include narcotic analgesics. After peripheral iridectomy, treatment includes cycloplegic eyedrops to relax the ciliary muscle and to decrease inflammation and thereby prevent adhesions.

Key nursing diagnoses and patient outcomes

Fear related to potential for blindness. Based on this nursing diagnosis, you'll establish these patient outcomes. The patient will:

- identify sources of fear
- seek knowledge about glaucoma from an appropriate source to help reduce his fears
- express an understanding that compliance with the prescribed treatment regimen can prevent further vision loss.

High risk for injury related to visual disturbances. Based on this nursing diagnosis, you'll establish these patient outcomes. The patient will:

- take precautions to prevent injury when visual disturbances occur during periods of elevated IOP
- not suffer injury because of visual impairment.

Sensory or perceptual alterations (visual) related to increased IOP. Based on this nursing diagnosis, you'll establish these patient outcomes. The patient will:

- identify types of visual changes that can occur when his IOP increases beyond a safe level
- seek medical attention when visual changes occur
- regain and maintain normal vision with treatment.

Nursing interventions

- For the patient with angle-closure glaucoma, give medications, as ordered, and prepare him physically and psychologically for laser iridotomy or surgery.
- Remember to administer cycloplegic eyedrops *in the affected eye only.* In the unaffected eye, these drops may precipitate an attack of angle-closure glaucoma and threaten the patient's residual vision.
- After trabeculectomy, give medications, as ordered, to dilate the pupil. Also apply topical corticosteroids, as ordered, to rest the pupil.
- After surgery, protect the affected eye by applying an eye patch and eye shield, positioning the patient on his back or unaffected side, and following general safety measures.
- Administer pain medication, as ordered.
- Encourage ambulation immediately after surgery.
- Encourage the patient to express his concerns related to having a chronic condition.

Monitoring

- Monitor the patient's ability to see clearly. Question him regularly about the occurrence of visual changes.
- Monitor the patient's IOP regularly.
- Monitor the patient's compliance with treatment and lifelong follow-up care.

Patient teaching

- Stress the importance of meticulous compliance with prescribed drug therapy to maintain low IOP and prevent optic disk changes that cause vision loss.
- Explain all procedures and treatments, especially surgery, to help reduce the patient's anxiety.
- Inform the patient that lost vision can't be restored but that treatment can usually prevent further loss.
- Instruct the family how to modify the patient's environment for safety. For example, suggest keeping pathways clear and reorienting the patient to room layouts, if necessary.
- Teach the patient the signs and symptoms that require immediate medical attention, such as sudden vision change or eye pain.
- Discuss the importance of glaucoma screening for early detection and prevention. Point out that all persons over age 35 should have an annual tonometric examination.

Glomerulonephritis, acute poststreptococcal

Also called acute glomerulonephritis, acute poststreptococcal glomerulonephritis is relatively common. This disorder, a bilateral inflammation of the glomeruli, follows a Streptococcaceae infection elsewhere in the body. Most common in boys ages 3 to 7, it can occur at any age. Up to 95% of children and 70% of adults recover fully; the rest, especially elderly patients, may progress to chronic renal failure within months.

Causes

Acute poststreptococcal glomerulonephritis results from the entrapment and collection of antigen-antibody complexes (produced as an immunologic mechanism in response to a group A beta-hemolytic streptococcus) in the glomerular capillary membranes, inducing inflammatory damage and impeding glomerular function. Sometimes the immune complement further damages the glomerular membrane. The damaged and inflamed glomeruli lose the ability to be selectively permeable, allowing red blood cells (RBCs) and proteins to filter through as the glomerular filtration rate (GFR) falls. Uremic poisoning may result.

Complications

Renal function progressively deteriorates in 33% to 50% of adults who contract sporadic acute poststreptococcal glomerulonephritis, usually in the form of glomerulosclerosis accompanied by hypertension. The more severe the disorder, the more likely it is that complications will follow.

Assessment

In most cases, acute poststreptococcal glomerulonephritis begins within 1 to 3 weeks after an untreated streptococcal infection in the respiratory tract. The patient – or the patient's parents – may report decreased urination, dark brown or rust-colored urine, and fatigue. The patient also may experience shortness of breath, dyspnea, and orthopnea. These symptoms of pulmonary edema point to congestive heart failure (CHF) resulting from hypervolemia.

Assessment findings may show oliguria (with output less than 400 ml/24 hours) and mild to moderate periorbital edema. Findings also may reveal mild to severe hypertension resulting from either sodium or water retention (caused by decreased GFR) or inappropriate renin release.

An elderly patient may complain of vague, nonspecific symptoms, such as nausea, malaise, and arthralgia. Auscultation reveals bibasilar crackles if CHF is present.

Diagnostic tests

Abnormal blood values (elevated electrolyte, blood urea nitrogen [BUN], and creatinine levels and decreased serum protein levels) and the presence of RBCs, white blood cells, mixed cell casts, and protein in the urine indicate renal failure. (Proteinuria in an elderly patient usually isn't as pronounced.) Urine frequently contains high levels of fibrin-degradation products and C3 protein.

Elevated antistreptolysin-O titers (in 80% of patients), elevated streptozyme and anti-DNase B titers, and low serum complement levels verify recent streptococcal infection. A throat culture may show group A beta-hemolytic streptococci.

Kidney-ureter-bladder X-rays show bilateral kidney enlargement. A renal biopsy may be necessary to confirm the diagnosis or assess renal tissue status.

Treatment

Therapy aims to relieve symptoms and prevent complications. Vigorous supportive care includes bed rest, fluid and dietary sodium restrictions, and correction of electrolyte imbalances (possibly with dialysis, although this seldom is necessary).

Treatment may include loop diuretics, such as metolazone or furosemide, to reduce extracellular fluid overload, and vasodilators, such as hydralazine, nifedipine, or propranolol. If the patient has a documented staphylococcal infection, antibiotics are recommended for 7 to 10 days; otherwise, their use is controversial.

Key nursing diagnoses and patient outcomes

Altered urinary elimination related to changes in renal function. Based on this nursing diagnosis, you'll establish these patient outcomes. The patient will:
- identify abnormal changes in his urine elimination pattern and seek medical attention
- communicate an understanding of the treatment prescribed to restore renal function
- regain and maintain his normal urine elimination pattern.

Fluid volume excess related to inability of kidneys to excrete fluid adequately. Based on this nursing diagnosis, you'll establish these patient outcomes. The patient will:
- not show signs and symptoms of severe fluid retention, such as CHF
- adhere to fluid and sodium restrictions to minimize fluid retention
- regain and maintain normal kidney function and normal fluid balance.

Risk for injury related to potential for permanent kidney damage. Based on this nursing diagnosis, you'll establish these patient outcomes. The patient will:
- express an understanding of the prescribed treatment and the need for compliance to minimize or prevent kidney damage
- regain and maintain normal kidney function.

Nursing interventions

- Acute poststreptococcal glomerulonephritis usually resolves within 2 weeks, so nursing care primarily is supportive.
- Provide bed rest during the acute phase. Perform passive range-of-motion exercises for the patient on bed rest. Allow the patient to resume normal activities *gradually* as symptoms subside.
- Consult the dietitian about a diet high in calories and low in protein, sodium, potassium, and fluids.

• Protect the debilitated patient against secondary infection by providing good nutrition and good hygienic technique and preventing contact with infected people.
• Provide emotional support for the patient and his family. Encourage the patient to verbalize his concerns about his inability to perform in his expected role. Assure him that the activity restrictions are temporary.

Monitoring

• Check the patient's vital signs and electrolyte values. Assess renal function daily through serum creatinine and BUN levels and urine creatinine clearance tests. Immediately report signs of acute renal failure (oliguria, azotemia, and acidosis).
• Monitor intake and output and daily weight. Report peripheral edema or the formation of ascites.

Patient teaching

• Stress to the patient or his parents that follow-up examinations are necessary to detect chronic renal failure. Emphasize the need for regular blood pressure, urine protein, and renal function assessments during the convalescent months to detect recurrence. Explain that after acute poststreptococcal glomerulonephritis, gross hematuria may recur during nonspecific viral infections and abnormal urinary findings may persist for years.
• If the patient is scheduled for dialysis, explain the procedure fully.
• Advise a patient with a history of chronic upper respiratory tract infections to report signs and symptoms of infection, such as fever and sore throat, immediately.
• Encourage a pregnant patient with a history of acute poststreptococcal glomerulonephritis to have frequent medical evaluations because pregnancy further stresses the kidneys and increases the risk of chronic renal failure.
• Explain to the patient taking diuretics that he may experience orthostatic hypotension and dizziness when he changes positions quickly.

Glomerulonephritis, chronic

A slowly progressive disease, chronic glomerulonephritis is characterized by inflammation of the glomeruli, which results in sclerosis, scarring and, eventually, renal failure. This condition normally remains subclinical until the progressive phase begins. By the time it produces symptoms, chronic glomerulonephritis usually is irreversible.

Causes

Common causes of chronic glomerulonephritis include primary renal disorders, such as membranoproliferative glomerulonephritis, membranous glomerulopathy, focal glomerulosclerosis, rapidly progressive glomerulonephritis and, less often, poststreptococcal glomerulonephritis. Systemic disorders that may cause chronic glomerulonephritis include systemic lupus erythematosus, Goodpasture's syndrome, and hemolytic-uremic syndrome.

Complications

Chronic glomerulonephritis can cause contracted, granular kidneys and lead to end-stage renal failure. It also can produce severe hypertension, leading to cardiovascular complications, including cardiac hypertrophy and congestive heart failure (CHF), which may speed the development of advanced renal failure, eventually necessitating dialysis or kidney transplantation.

Assessment

This disorder usually develops insidiously and without symptoms, often over many years. But when it becomes suddenly progressive, your assessment may reveal edema and hypertension.

In late stages, the patient may complain of nausea, vomiting, pruritus, dyspnea, malaise, fatigue, and mild to severe edema. Your assessment may show severe hypertension and associated cardiac complications.

Diagnostic tests

• *Urinalysis* shows proteinuria, hematuria, cylindruria, and red blood cell casts.
• *Blood studies* reveal rising blood urea nitrogen (BUN) and serum creatinine levels in advanced renal insufficiency as well as a decrease in hemoglobin.
• *X-rays* exhibit symmetrically contracted kidneys with normal pelves and calyces.
• *Renal biopsy* establishes the underlying disease and provides data to plan therapy.

Treatment

Appropriate treatment is essentially nonspecific and symptomatic. Goals include controlling hypertension with antihypertensives and a sodium-restricted diet, correcting fluid and electrolyte imbalances through restrictions and replacement, reducing edema with loop diuretics, such as furosemide, and preventing CHF. Treatment also may include antibiotics for symptomatic urinary tract infections (UTIs), dialysis, or kidney transplantation.

Key nursing diagnoses and patient outcomes

Altered urinary elimination related to progressive deterioration of renal function. Based on this nursing diagnosis, you'll establish these patient outcomes. The patient will:
• express an understanding of the disease; its symptoms, complications, and treatments; and adjustments to life-style caused by altered urine elimination
• have an equal fluid intake and urine output.

The patient or caregiver will:
• skillfully perform measures to treat altered urine elimination.

Fluid volume excess related to inability of kidneys to excrete fluid adequately. Based on this nursing diagnosis, you'll establish these patient outcomes. The patient will:
• adhere to fluid and sodium restrictions to minimize fluid retention
• not show signs and symptoms of severe fluid retention, such as CHF.
• control fluid retention by adhering to the prescribed treatment regimen.

Risk for injury related to hypertensive effects on the cardiovascular system. Based on this nursing diagnosis, you'll establish these patient outcomes. The patient will:
• understand the relationship between chronic glomerulonephritis and hypertension
• maintain normal blood pressure with antihypertensives and diet modifications
• not show signs and symptoms of cardiovascular dysfunction.

Nursing interventions

• Ask the dietitian to help the patient plan low-sodium, high-calorie meals with adequate protein.
• Provide good skin care to help prevent complications of pruritus, edema, and friability.
• Prepare the patient with severe renal dysfunction for dialysis.
• Help the patient adjust to his illness by encouraging him to express his feelings and ask questions.

Monitoring

• Monitor renal function and renal deterioration regularly through serum creatinine, BUN, and urine creatinine clearance levels.
• Monitor the patient's response to therapy and need for dialysis.
• Monitor vital signs, intake and output, and daily weight to evaluate fluid reten-

tion. Observe for signs of fluid, electrolyte, and acid-base imbalances.
• Monitor the patient for cardiovascular dysfunction.

Patient teaching

• Instruct the patient to take prescribed antihypertensives and diuretics as scheduled, even if he feels better. Advise him to take diuretics in the morning so his nightly sleep won't be disturbed.
• Teach the patient the signs of infection, particularly those of UTI, and warn him to report them immediately. Tell him to avoid contact with people who have communicable illnesses.
• Urge compliance with the prescribed diet.
• Stress the importance of keeping all follow-up examinations to assess renal function.

Gonorrhea

A common sexually transmitted disease (STD), gonorrhea usually starts as an infection of the genitourinary (GU) tract, especially the urethra and cervix. It also can begin in the rectum, pharynx, or eyes. Left untreated, gonorrhea spreads through the blood to the joints, tendons, meninges, and endocardium; in women, it also can lead to chronic pelvic inflammatory disease (PID) and sterility.

Gonorrhea is especially prevalent among people between ages 15 and 29, with the highest incidence occurring between ages 20 and 24. It's also prevalent in those with multiple partners. With adequate treatment, the prognosis is excellent, although reinfection is common.

Causes

Transmission of *Neisseria gonorrhoeae,* the organism that causes gonorrhea, occurs almost exclusively through sexual contact with an infected person. A child born of an infected mother, however, can contract gonococcal ophthalmia neonatorum during passage through the birth canal. Also, a patient with gonorrhea can contract gonococcal conjunctivitis by touching his eyes with a contaminated hand.

Complications

Gonorrhea can lead to PID, acute epididymitis, septic arthritis, dermatitis, and perihepatitis. Severe gonococcal conjunctivitis can lead to corneal ulceration and, possibly, blindness. Rare complications include meningitis, osteomyelitis, pneumonia, and adult respiratory distress syndrome.

Assessment

The patient may report unprotected sexual contact (vaginal, oral, or anal) with an infected person, an unknown partner, or multiple sex partners. He also may have a history of STD.

After a 3- to 6-day incubation period, a male patient may complain of dysuria, although both sexes can remain asymptomatic. A patient with a rectal infection may complain of anal itching, burning, and tenesmus and pain with defecation, or he may be asymptomatic. A patient with a pharyngeal infection may be asymptomatic or may complain of a sore throat.

Assessment of a patient with gonorrhea reveals a low-grade fever. If the disease has become systemic or if the patient has developed PID or acute epididymitis, the fever is higher. Other assessment findings vary with the infection site. (See *Assessing infection sites in gonorrhea.*)

Diagnostic tests

A culture from the infection site (the urethra, cervix, rectum, or pharynx), grown on a Thayer-Martin medium, usually establishes the diagnosis. A culture of conjunctival scrapings confirms gonococcal conjunctivitis. In a male patient, a Gram stain that shows gram-negative diplococci may confirm gonorrhea.

Diagnosis of gonococcal arthritis requires identification of gram-negative diplococci on smears made from joint fluid and skin lesions. Complement fixation and immunofluorescent assays of serum reveal antibody titers four times the normal rate.

Treatment

For uncomplicated gonorrhea in adults, the recommended treatment is 250 mg of ceftriaxone given I.M. in a single dose plus 100 mg of doxycycline hyclate given twice daily by mouth for 7 days. As an alternative to doxycycline – which helps combat gonorrhea and also treats the frequently coexisting chlamydial or mycoplasmal infection – the patient can receive 500 mg of oral tetracycline four times daily for 7 days. For patients who can't take doxycycline or tetracycline, such as pregnant women, treatment consists of 500 mg of oral erythromycin for 7 days.

If the infection was acquired from a person proven to have susceptible non-penicillinase-producing gonorrhea, the patient can receive 1 g of probenecid by mouth (to block penicillin excretion) plus either 3.5 g of ampicillin by mouth in a single dose or 3 g of amoxicillin by mouth in a single dose. This is followed by a 7-day course of doxycycline or tetracycline.

Disseminated gonococcal infection requires 1 g of ceftriaxone given I.M. or I.V. every 24 hours for 7 days. Adult gonococcal ophthalmia requires 1 g of ceftriaxone given I.M. in a single dose.

Because many strains of antibiotic-resistant gonococci exist, follow-up cultures are necessary 4 to 7 days after treatment and again in 6 months. (For a pregnant patient, final follow-up must occur before delivery.)

Routine instillation of 1% silver nitrate drops or erythromycin ointment into the eyes of neonates has greatly reduced the incidence of gonococcal ophthalmia neonatorum.

Assessing infection sites in gonorrhea

Inspection of a male patient's urethral meatus reveals a purulent discharge. In a female patient, this discharge may be expressed from the urethra, and the meatus may appear red and edematous. Inspection of the cervix with a speculum discloses a greenish yellow discharge, the most common sign in females. Vaginal inspection reveals engorgement, redness, swelling, and a profuse purulent discharge.

If the patient has a rectal infection, inspection may reveal a purulent discharge or rectal bleeding. In an ocular infection, inspection may reveal a purulent discharge from the conjunctiva; in a pharyngeal infection, redness and a purulent discharge.

If the infection has become systemic, papillary skin lesions – possibly pustular, hemorrhagic, or necrotic – may appear on the hands and feet.

Palpation of the patient with PID reveals tenderness over the lower quadrant, abdominal rigidity and distention, and adnexal tenderness (usually bilateral). In a patient with perihepatitis, palpation discloses right upper quadrant tenderness.

Your assessment of a patient with a systemic infection may reveal pain and a cracking noise when moving an involved joint. Asymmetrical involvement of only a few joints – typically the knees, ankles, and elbows – may differentiate gonococcal arthritis from other forms of arthritis.

Key nursing diagnoses and patient outcomes

Altered sexuality patterns related to infection of the GU tract. Based on this nursing diagnosis, you'll establish these patient outcomes. The patient will:

• express an understanding of the need to abstain from sexual activity until the infection clears up
• resume normal sexuality patterns when gonorrhea has been eradicated.

Risk for infection related to recurrence. Based on this nursing diagnosis, you'll establish these patient outcomes. The patient will:
• understand how gonorrhea is contracted and what precautions to take to prevent a recurrence
• take precautions when engaging in sexual activity to prevent reinfection
• not become reinfected with gonorrhea.

Pain related to inflammation caused by infection. Based on this nursing diagnosis, you'll establish these patient outcomes. The patient will:
• comply with the prescribed therapy to eradicate gonorrhea and its symptoms, including pain
• become pain free when gonorrhea resolves.

Nursing interventions

• Use standard precautions when obtaining specimens for laboratory examination and when caring for the patient. Dispose of all soiled dressings and contaminated instruments according to institution's policy.
• Isolate the patient with an eye infection.
• If the patient has gonococcal arthritis, apply moist heat to ease pain in affected joints. Administer analgesics, as ordered.
• If the doctor or laboratory hasn't already done so, report all cases of gonorrhea to the local public health authorities so that they can follow up with the patient's sexual partners. Examine and test all people exposed to gonorrhea.

Monitoring

• Before treatment, determine if the patient has any drug sensitivities. During treatment, watch closely for signs of a drug reaction.
• Monitor the patient for complications.

Patient teaching

• Tell the patient that until cultures prove negative, he's still infectious and should avoid sexual contact.
• Urge the patient to inform his sexual partners of his infection so that they can seek treatment.
• Advise the partner of an infected person to receive treatment even if she doesn't have a positive culture. Also advise her to avoid sexual contact with anyone until treatment is complete because reinfection is extremely common.
• Counsel the patient and his sexual partners to be tested for human immunodeficiency virus and hepatitis B infection.
• Instruct the patient to be careful when coming into contact with his bodily discharges so that he doesn't contaminate his eyes.
• Tell the patient to take anti-infective drugs for the length of time prescribed.
• To prevent reinfection, tell the patient to avoid sexual contact with anyone *suspected* of being infected, to use condoms during intercourse, to wash genitalia with soap and water before and after intercourse, and to avoid sharing washcloths.
• Advise returning for follow-up testing.

Goodpasture's syndrome

In this disorder, hemoptysis and rapidly progressive glomerulonephritis result from the deposition of antibodies against the alveolar and glomerular basement membranes (GBMs). Goodpasture's syndrome may occur at any age but most commonly strikes men between ages 20 and 30. The prognosis improves with aggressive immunosuppressant and antibiotic therapy and with dialysis or kidney transplantation.

Causes

The cause of Goodpasture's syndrome is unknown. Although some cases have been associated with exposure to hydrocarbons or type 2 influenza, many have no precipitating events. The high incidence of human leukocyte antigen–DR2 in patients with this disorder suggests a genetic predisposition.

Abnormal production and deposition of antibodies against the GBM and alveolar basement membrane activate the complement and inflammatory responses, resulting in glomerular and alveolar tissue damage.

Complications

Renal failure, requiring dialysis or transplantation, and severe pulmonary complications, such as pulmonary edema and hemorrhage, may occur.

Assessment

Initially, the patient with Goodpasture's syndrome may complain of malaise, fatigue, and pallor – signs and symptoms associated with severe iron deficiency anemia.

Your assessment may reveal hematuria and signs of peripheral edema associated with renal involvement. You may also note signs of pulmonary involvement, such as dyspnea and hemoptysis, ranging from a cough with blood-tinged sputum to frank pulmonary hemorrhage. The patient may have had subclinical pulmonary bleeding for months or years before developing overt hemorrhage and signs of renal disease.

Diagnostic tests

Measurement of circulating anti-GBM antibodies by radioimmunoassay, as well as linear staining of GBM and alveolar basement membrane by immunofluorescence, confirm the diagnosis.

Immunofluorescence of alveolar basement membrane shows linear deposition of immunoglobulins, as well as C3 and fibrinogen. Immunofluorescence of GBM also shows linear deposition of immunoglobulins. This finding, along with circulating anti-GBM antibodies, distinguishes Goodpasture's from other pulmonary-renal syndromes, such as Wegener's granulomatosis, polyarteritis, and systemic lupus erythematosus.

Lung biopsy shows interstitial and intra-alveolar hemorrhage with hemosiderin-laden macrophages. Chest X-rays reveal pulmonary infiltrates in a diffuse, nodular pattern, and renal biopsy frequently shows focal necrotic lesions and cellular crescents.

Serum creatinine and blood urea nitrogen (BUN) levels typically increase to two to three times normal. Urinalysis may reveal red blood cells and cellular casts, which typify glomerular inflammation. Tests may also show granular casts and proteinuria.

Treatment

Plasmapheresis may be used to remove antibodies, and immunosuppressants to suppress antibody production. Patients with renal failure may benefit from dialysis or kidney transplantation. Aggressive ultrafiltration helps relieve pulmonary edema that may aggravate pulmonary hemorrhage. High-dose I.V. corticosteroids also help control pulmonary hemorrhage.

Key nursing diagnoses and patient outcomes

Altered urinary elimination related to renal dysfunction. Based on this nursing diagnosis, you'll establish these outcomes. The patient will:
• communicate an understanding of the treatment to correct altered urine elimination.

The patient or caregiver will:
• demonstrate skill in treating altered urine elimination.

Fatigue related to iron deficiency anemia. Based on this nursing diagnosis, you'll establish these patient outcomes. The patient will:
• be able to explain the relationship between fatigue, activity level, and Goodpasture's syndrome

• employ measures to prevent and decrease fatigue
• regain his normal energy level.

Impaired gas exchange related to pulmonary complications. Based on this nursing diagnosis, you'll establish these patient outcomes. The patient will:
• maintain clear sputum
• not experience further deterioration of pulmonary function with effective treatment of Goodpasture's syndrome
• perform activities of daily living without shortness of breath.

Nursing interventions

• Elevate the head of the bed and administer humidified oxygen to promote adequate oxygenation.
• Encourage the patient to conserve his energy. If he's bedridden, perform range-of-motion exercises. Assist with activities of daily living, and provide frequent rest periods.
• Assist with plasmapheresis, as ordered.
• Administer blood transfusions to treat severe iron deficiency anemia, and administer corticosteroids, as ordered.
• If appropriate, prepare the patient for dialysis or kidney transplantation to manage renal failure.

Monitoring

• Assess respiratory rate and breath sounds regularly, and note the quantity and quality of the patient's sputum.
• Monitor the patient's vital signs, arterial blood gas levels, hematocrit, and coagulation studies.
• Monitor the patient's daily intake and output, daily weight, creatinine clearance, and BUN and serum creatinine levels, and observe his signs and symptoms to determine his renal function.
• Watch closely for signs of a transfusion reaction or an adverse reaction to the corticosteroids.

Patient teaching

• Stress the importance of conserving energy, especially if the patient develops iron deficiency anemia.
• Teach the patient to follow an appropriate diet – usually a low-protein diet if renal disease is significant. Explain that his fluid intake may also be restricted. Stress the importance of complying with these measures to prevent further deterioration of renal tissue.
• If the patient has a sore, dry mouth, advise him to suck on sugarless hard candy.
• Teach the patient and his family the signs of respiratory or genitourinary bleeding. Tell them to report any such signs to the doctor at once.
• If the patient needs dialysis or kidney transplantation, refer him to a renal support group.

Gout

Also known as gouty arthritis, this metabolic disease is marked by monosodium urate deposits that cause red, swollen, and acutely painful joints. Gout may affect any joint but mostly affects those in the feet, especially the great toe, ankle, and midfoot.

Primary gout typically occurs in men over age 30 and in postmenopausal women who take diuretics. It follows an intermittent course that may leave patients symptom-free for years between attacks.

In asymptomatic patients, serum urate levels rise but produce no symptoms. In symptom-producing gout, the first acute attack strikes suddenly and peaks quickly. Although it may involve only one or a few joints, this attack causes extreme pain. Mild, acute attacks usually subside quickly yet tend to recur at irregular intervals. Severe attacks may persist for days or weeks.

Intercritical periods are the symptom-free intervals between attacks. Most patients have a second attack between 6 months and 2 years after the first; in some patients, however, the second attack is delayed for 5 to 10 years. Delayed attacks, which may be polyarticular, are more common in untreated patients. These attacks tend to last longer and produce more symptoms than initial episodes. A migratory attack strikes various joints and the Achilles tendon sequentially and may be associated with olecranon bursitis.

Eventually, *chronic polyarticular gout* sets in. This final, unremitting stage of the disease (also known as tophaceous gout) is marked by persistent painful polyarthritis. An increased concentration of uric acid leads to urate deposits – called tophi – in cartilage, synovial membranes, tendons, and soft tissue.

Tophi form in the fingers, hands, knees, feet, ulnar sides of the forearms, pinna of the ear, Achilles tendon and, rarely, in such internal organs as the kidneys and myocardium. Renal involvement may adversely affect renal function.

Patients who receive treatment for gout have a good prognosis.

Causes

Although the underlying cause of primary gout remains unknown, in many patients the disease results from decreased renal excretion of uric acid. In a few patients, gout is linked to a genetic defect in purine metabolism that causes overproduction of uric acid (hyperuricemia).

Secondary gout develops during the course of another disease, such as obesity, diabetes mellitus, hypertension, polycythemia, leukemia, myeloma, sickle cell anemia, and renal disease. Secondary gout can also follow treatment with such drugs as hydrochlorothiazide or pyrazinamide.

Complications

Potential complications include renal disorders, such as renal calculi; circulatory problems, such as atherosclerotic disease, cardiovascular lesions, cerebrovascular accident, coronary thrombosis, and hypertension; and infection that develops with tophi rupture and nerve entrapment.

Assessment

Patient history may reveal a sedentary lifestyle and a history of hypertension and renal calculi. The patient may report waking during the night with pain in his great toe or another location in the foot. He may complain that initially moderate pain has grown intense so that eventually he can't bear the weight of bed sheets or the vibrations of a person walking across the room. He may report accompanying chills and a mild fever.

Inspection typically reveals a swollen, dusky red or purple joint with limited movement. You may also notice tophi, especially in the outer ears, hands, and feet. Late in the chronic stage of gout, the skin over the tophi may ulcerate and release a chalky white exudate or pus. Chronic inflammation and tophaceous deposits prompt secondary joint degeneration. Then erosions, deformity, and disability may develop.

Palpation may reveal warmth over the joint and extreme tenderness. The vital signs assessment may disclose fever and hypertension. If the patient has a fever, possible occult infection must be investigated.

Diagnostic tests

• *Needle aspiration* of synovial fluid (arthrocentesis) or of tophaceous material for examination under polarized light microscopy reveals needlelike intracellular crystals of sodium urate. Monosodium urate monohydrate crystals in synovial fluid that's been taken from an inflamed joint or tophus establishes the diagnosis. If test results identify calcium pyrophosphate crystals, the patient probably has pseudogout, a disease similar to gout. (See *Understanding pseudogout,* page 346.)
• *Serum uric acid levels* may be normal. However, the higher the level (especially

Understanding pseudogout

Also known as calcium pyrophosphate disease, pseudogout results when calcium pyrophosphate crystals collect in periarticular joint structures.

Signs and symptoms

Like true gout, pseudogout causes sudden joint pain and swelling – most commonly of the knee, wrist, ankle, or other peripheral joints.

Pseudogout attacks are self-limiting and triggered by stress, trauma, surgery, severe dieting, thiazide therapy, or alcohol abuse. Associated symptoms resemble those of rheumatoid arthritis.

Establishing a diagnosis

Diagnosis of pseudogout hinges on joint aspiration and synovial biopsy to detect calcium pyrophosphate crystals. X-rays show calcium deposits in the fibrocartilage and linear markings along the bone ends. Blood tests may detect an underlying endocrine or metabolic disorder.

Relief for pressure and inflammation

Management of pseudogout may include aspirating the joint to relieve pressure; instilling corticosteroids and administering analgesics, salicylates, phenylbutazone, or other NSAIDS to treat inflammation; and, if appropriate, treating the underlying disorder.

Without treatment, pseudogout leads to permanent joint damage in about half of those it affects – most of whom are elderly patients.

when it's above 10 mg/dl), the more likely a gout attack.

• *Urine uric acid levels* are high in about 20% of gout patients.

• *X-ray studies* initially produce normal results. However, in chronic gout, X-ray findings show damage to the articular cartilage and subchondral bone. Outward displacement of the overhanging margin from the bone contour characterizes gout.

Treatment

Correct management has three goals:

• First, terminate the acute attack.

• Next, treat hyperuricemia to reduce urine uric acid levels.

• Finally, prevent recurrent gout and renal calculi.

Treatment of an acute attack consists of bed rest; immobilization and protection of the inflamed, painful joints; and local application of cold. Analgesics, such as acetaminophen, relieve the pain associated with mild attacks. Acute inflammation, however, requires nonsteroidal anti-inflammatory drugs (NSAIDs) or I.M. corticotropin. Colchicine, oral or parenteral, or intra-articular corticosteroids are occasionally necessary to treat acute attacks.

Treatment of chronic gout involves decreasing the serum uric acid level to less than 6.5 mg/dl. This may be accomplished with various medications after a 24-hour urinalysis determines whether the patient overexcretes or underexcretes uric acid. If he overexcretes uric acid, he may be given allopurinol (in reduced doses if he has decreased renal function). If he underexcretes uric acid, he may be treated with probenecid or sulfinpyrazone (if he has no history of renal calculi). Taken once or twice daily, colchicine effectively prevents acute gout attacks, although it doesn't affect uric acid levels.

Adjunctive therapy emphasizes avoiding alcohol (especially beer and wine) and sparing use of purine-rich foods, such as anchovies, liver, sardines, kidneys, sweetbreads, and lentils. Obese patients should begin a weight-loss program because weight reduction will decrease uric acid levels and stress on painful joints as well.

Key nursing diagnoses and patient outcomes

Risk for injury related to complications. Based on this nursing diagnosis, you'll establish these patient outcomes. The patient will:

- communicate an understanding of the treatment for gout and of the importance of compliance to minimize or prevent complications
- not exhibit signs and symptoms of renal or cardiovascular dysfunction or infection
- not develop an injury related to gout.

Impaired physical mobility related to pain and joint changes. Based on this nursing diagnosis, you'll establish these patient outcomes. The patient will:

- seek assistance in performing activities of daily living as needed, but especially during acute gout attacks
- not show evidence of complications caused by impaired physical mobility, such as skin breakdown or contractures
- attain the highest degree of mobility possible within the restrictions imposed by gout.

Pain related to monosodium urate deposits in joints. Based on this nursing diagnosis, you'll establish these patient outcomes. The patient will:

- express feelings of comfort after analgesic administration
- modify his life-style, particularly dietary intake, to reduce his uric acid level
- become pain free with compliance with the prescribed treatment regimen.

Nursing interventions

- Give pain medication, as needed, especially during acute attacks. Apply cold packs to inflamed joints to ease discomfort and reduce swelling.
- Administer anti-inflammatory medication and other drugs, as ordered. Also administer sodium bicarbonate or other agents to alkalinize the patient's urine, as ordered.
- To promote sleep, administer pain medication at times that allow for maximum rest. Provide the patient with sleep aids, such as an extra pillow, a bath, or a back rub.
- Encourage bed rest, but use a bed cradle to keep bed linens off sensitive, inflamed joints.
- Encourage the patient to perform techniques that promote rest and relaxation.
- Provide a nutritious diet; avoid purine-rich foods.
- Before and after surgery, administer colchicine to help prevent gout attacks, as ordered.
- Urge the patient to perform as much self-care as his immobility and pain allow. Provide adequate time to perform these activities.
- Provide emotional support during diagnostic tests and procedures.
- To diffuse anxiety and promote coping mechanisms, encourage the patient to express his concerns about his condition. Listen supportively. Include him and his family in care-related decisions and all phases of care. Answer the patient's questions about his disorder.

Monitoring

- Monitor the patient's condition after joint aspiration for signs of improvement and complications, such as infection.
- Monitor the patient's pain level and his response to pain-control measures, including analgesics.
- Watch for adverse reactions when administering anti-inflammatory medication and other drugs. Be alert for GI disturbances with colchicine administration.
- When forcing fluids, record intake and output accurately. Monitor serum uric acid levels regularly.
- Watch for acute gout attacks 24 to 96 hours after surgery. Even minor surgery can trigger an attack.

Patient teaching

- Urge the patient to drink plenty of fluids (up to 2 liters a day) to prevent renal calculi.

- Explain all treatments, tests, and procedures. Warn the patient before his first needle aspiration that it will be extremely painful.
- Make sure the patient understands the rationale for evaluating serum uric acid levels periodically.
- Teach the patient relaxation techniques. Encourage him to perform them regularly.
- Instruct the patient to avoid purine-rich foods because they raise the urate level.
- Discuss the principles of gradual weight reduction with an obese patient. Explain the advantages of a diet containing moderate amounts of protein and little fat.
- If the patient receives allopurinol, probenecid, or other drugs, instruct him to report any adverse reactions immediately. (Reactions may include nausea, vomiting, drowsiness, dizziness, urinary frequency, and dermatitis.) Warn the patient taking probenecid or sulfinpyrazone to avoid aspirin or other salicylates. Their combined effect causes urate retention.
- Inform the patient that long-term colchicine therapy is essential during the first 3 to 6 months of treatment with uricosuric drugs or allopurinol. Stress the importance of compliance.
- Urge the patient to control hypertension, especially if he has tophaceous renal deposits. Keep in mind that diuretics aren't advised for the gout patient; alternative antihypertensives are preferred.

Granulocytopenia and lymphocytopenia

Granulocytopenia is characterized by a marked reduction in the number of circulating granulocytes. Although this implies that all granulocytes (neutrophils, basophils, and eosinophils) are reduced, granulocytopenia usually refers to decreased neutrophils – a condition known as neutropenia (a deficiency in the number of mature neutrophils.) Its severest form is known as agranulocytosis.

A rare disorder, lymphocytopenia (lymphopenia) is a deficiency of circulating lymphocytes (leukocytes produced mainly in lymph nodes).

Causes

Granulocytopenia may result from diminished production of granulocytes in bone marrow, increased peripheral destruction of granulocytes, or greater use of granulocytes. Diminished production of granulocytes in bone marrow generally stems from radiation therapy or drug therapy. Drug-induced granulocytopenia usually develops slowly and typically correlates with the dosage and duration of therapy. Granulocyte production also decreases in such conditions as aplastic anemia and malignant bone marrow diseases and in some hereditary disorders.

Infections such as mononucleosis may cause granulocytopenia because of increased use of granulocytes.

Similarly, lymphocytopenia may result from decreased production, increased destruction, or loss of lymphocytes. Decreased lymphocyte production may result from a genetic or thymic abnormality or from an immunodeficiency disorder, such as thymic dysplasia or ataxia-telangiectasia. Increased lymphocyte destruction may be caused by radiation therapy, chemotherapy, or human immunodeficiency virus (HIV) infection. Loss of lymphocytes may follow postoperative thoracic duct drainage, intestinal lymphangiectasia, or impaired intestinal lymphatic drainage (as in Whipple's disease). Lymphocyte depletion can also result from elevated plasma corticoid levels (due to stress, corticotropin or steroid therapy, or congestive heart failure). Other disorders associated with lymphocyte depletion include Hodgkin's disease, leukemia, aplastic anemia, sarcoidosis, myasthenia gravis, lupus erythematosus, protein-calorie malnutrition, renal failure, terminal cancer, tuberculosis and, in infants, severe combined immunodeficiency disease (SCID).

Complications

Localized infection can quickly become systemic (as in bacteremia) or can spread throughout an organ (as in pneumonia).

Assessment

Typically, patients with granulocytopenia experience slowly progressive fatigue and weakness. However, if they develop an infection, they can exhibit sudden onset of fever and chills and mental status changes. Overt signs of infection (pus formation) are usually absent. If granulocytopenia results from an idiosyncratic drug reaction, signs of infection develop abruptly, without causing slowly progressive fatigue and weakness.

In a patient with lymphocytopenia, palpation may reveal enlarged lymph nodes, spleen, and tonsils and signs of an associated disease.

Diagnostic tests

Marked reduction in neutrophils (less than 500/mm³ leads to severe bacterial infections) and a white blood cell (WBC) count below 2,000/mm³, with few observable granulocytes on the complete blood count (CBC), confirm granulocytopenia.

Bone marrow examination shows a scarcity of granulocytic precursor cells beyond the most immature forms, but this may vary, depending on the cause.

A lymphocyte count below 1,500/mm³ in adults or below 3,000/mm³ in children indicates lymphocytopenia. Evaluation of the patient's clinical status, bone marrow and lymph node biopsies, or other appropriate diagnostic tests can help identify the cause and establish the diagnosis.

Treatment

Effective management of granulocytopenia must identify and eliminate the cause and control infection until the bone marrow can generate more leukocytes. This often means drug or radiation therapy must be stopped and antibiotic treatment begun immediately, even before test results are known. Treatment may also include antifungal preparations. Administration of granulocyte- or granulocyte-macrophage colony-stimulating factor (G-CSF or GM-CSF) is a newer treatment used to stimulate bone marrow production of neutrophils. Spontaneous restoration of leukocyte production in bone marrow generally occurs within 1 to 3 weeks.

Treatment of lymphocytopenia includes eliminating the cause and managing the underlying disorder. For an infant with SCID, therapy may include bone marrow transplantation.

Key nursing diagnoses and patient outcomes

Risk for infection related to decrease in WBC. Based on this nursing diagnosis, you'll establish these patient outcomes. The patient will:

- remain free from evidence of infection
- demonstrate knowledge of measures to prevent infection
- verbalize appropriate signs and symptoms to report to the health care team.

Fatigue related to decreased WBC. Based on this nursing diagnosis, you'll establish these patient outcomes. The patient will:

- explain the relationship between fatigue and activity level
- demonstrate measures to prevent and modify fatigue.

Knowledge deficit related to neutropenia. Based on this nursing diagnosis, you'll establish these patient outcomes. The patient will:

- show knowledge of treatment regimen
- verbalize appropriate measures to prevent infection.

Nursing interventions

- Monitor vital signs frequently. Obtain cultures from blood, throat, urine, mouth,

nose, rectum, vagina, and sputum, as ordered. Give antibiotics, as scheduled.
• Explain the necessity of infection-prevention procedures.
• Maintain adequate nutrition and hydration. Make sure the patient with mouth ulcerations receives a high-calorie liquid diet. Offer a straw to make drinking less painful.
• Provide good oral hygiene for comfort and healing.
• Ensure adequate rest. Provide good skin and perineal care.
• Monitor the CBC and differential count, blood culture results, serum electrolyte levels, fluid intake and output, and daily weight.
• To help detect granulocytopenia and lymphocytopenia in the early, most treatable stages, monitor the WBC count of any patient receiving radiation or chemotherapy.
• Advise a patient with known or suspected sensitivity to a drug that can cause granulocytopenia or lymphocytopenia to alert medical personnel to this sensitivity in the future.

Patient teaching

• Reinforce the doctor's explanation of the disease.
• Teach the patient and family members how to institute and maintain infection control precautions.

Guillain-Barré syndrome

An acute, rapidly progressive, and potentially fatal form of polyneuritis, Guillain-Barré syndrome causes segmented demyelination of peripheral nerves. The syndrome occurs equally in both sexes, usually between ages 30 and 50. It affects about 2 of every 100,000 people.

The clinical course of Guillain-Barré syndrome has three phases. The *acute phase* begins when the first definitive symptom develops; it ends 1 to 3 weeks later, when no further deterioration is noted. The *plateau phase* lasts for several days to 2 weeks and is followed by the *recovery phase*, which is believed to coincide with remyelination and axonal process regrowth. The recovery phase extends over 4 to 6 months; however, patients with severe disease may take 2 to 3 years to recover. What's more, the recovery may not be complete. The syndrome is also known as infectious polyneuritis, Landry-Guillain-Barré syndrome, or acute idiopathic polyneuritis.

Causes

The precise cause of Guillain-Barré syndrome is unknown, but it's thought to be a cell-mediated immunologic attack on peripheral nerves in response to a virus. Risk factors include surgery, rabies or swine influenza vaccination, viral illness, Hodgkin's or some other malignant disease, and lupus erythematosus.

The major pathologic effect is segmental demyelination of the peripheral nerves that prevents normal transmission of electrical impulses along the sensorimotor nerve roots.

Complications

Because of the patient's inability to use his muscles, complications can occur. These include thrombophlebitis, pressure ulcers, contractures, muscle wasting, aspiration, respiratory tract infections, and life-threatening respiratory and cardiac compromise.

Assessment

Most patients seek treatment when the syndrome is in the acute stage. Typically, the history reveals that the patient experienced a minor febrile illness (usually an upper respiratory tract infection or, less often, GI infection) 1 to 4 weeks before his current symptoms.

The patient may report feelings of tingling and numbness (paresthesia) in the legs. If the syndrome has progressed further, he may report that the tingling and numbness began in the legs and progressed to the arms, the trunk and, finally, the face. The paresthesia usually precedes muscle weakness but tends to vanish quickly; in some patients, it may never occur. Some patients may also report stiffness and pain in the calves, such as a severe charley horse, and in the back.

Neurologic examination uncovers muscle weakness (the major neurologic sign) and sensory loss, usually in the legs. If the syndrome has progressed, the weakness and sensory loss may also be present in the arms. Keep in mind that the syndrome progresses rapidly and that symptoms may progress beyond the legs in 24 to 72 hours.

If the cranial nerves are affected—as they often are—the patient may have difficulty talking, chewing, and swallowing. Subsequent cranial nerve testing may reveal paralysis of the ocular, facial, and oropharyngeal muscles.

Remember that muscle weakness sometimes develops in the arms first (descending type), rather than in the legs (ascending type) or the arms and legs simultaneously. Remember, too, that in milder forms of the syndrome, muscle weakness may affect only the cranial nerves or may not occur at all. Neurologic examination may reveal a loss of position sense and diminished or absent deep tendon reflexes.

Diagnostic tests

- *Cerebrospinal fluid (CSF) analysis* may show a normal white blood cell count, an elevated protein count and, in severe disease, increased CSF pressure. The CSF protein level begins to rise several days after the onset of signs and symptoms, peaking in 4 to 6 weeks, probably resulting from widespread inflammatory disease of the nerve roots.
- *Electromyography* may demonstrate repeated firing of the same motor unit instead of widespread sectional stimulation.
- *Electrophysiologic testing* may reveal marked slowing of nerve conduction velocities.

Treatment

In Guillain-Barré syndrome, treatment is primarily supportive and may require endotracheal intubation or tracheotomy if the patient has difficulty clearing secretions. Mechanical ventilation is necessary if the patient has respiratory difficulties.

Continuous electrocardiogram monitoring is necessary to identify cardiac arrhythmias. Propranolol may be administered to treat tachycardia and hypotension. Atropine may be administered to treat bradycardia. Marked hypotension may require volume replacement.

Plasmapheresis produces a temporary reduction in circulating antibodies. It's usually reserved for the most severely affected patients or those whose illness is progressing very rapidly. It's most effective if performed during the first few days of the illness.

Key nursing diagnoses and patient outcomes

Risk for injury related to an inability to move muscles. Based on this nursing diagnosis, you'll establish these patient outcomes. The patient will:

- remain safe and free of injury during immobility.

Impaired mobility related to an inability to move muscles. Based on this nursing diagnosis, you'll establish these outcomes. The patient will:

- not develop complications from immobility, such as contractures, venous stasis, thrombus formation, or skin breakdown
- regain mobility with no permanent deficits.

The caregiver will:

- carry out the patient's physical regimen.

Ineffective breathing pattern related to weakness or paralysis of respiratory muscles. Based on this nursing diagnosis, you'll establish these patient outcomes. The patient will:
• maintain adequate ventilation naturally or with mechanical support
• regain and maintain normal arterial blood gas (ABG) measurements when Guillain-Barré syndrome disappears
• recover normal breathing patterns when the syndrome resolves.

Nursing interventions

• Turn and reposition the patient, and encourage coughing and deep breathing. Begin respiratory support at the first sign of dyspnea (in adults, this means a vital capacity less than 800 ml or decreasing partial pressure of oxygen in arterial blood [PaO_2]).
• If respiratory failure becomes imminent, establish an emergency airway with an endotracheal tube. Be prepared to begin and maintain mechanical ventilation.
• Give meticulous skin care to prevent skin breakdown and contractures. Establish a strict turning schedule and reposition the patient every 2 hours. Use alternating pressure pads at points of contact.
• Perform passive range-of-motion exercises within the patient's pain limits, possibly using a Hubbard tank. (Exercising little-used muscles will cause pain.) Remember that the proximal muscle group of the thighs, shoulders, and trunk will be the most tender and will cause the most pain on passive movement and turning. When the patient's condition stabilizes, change to gentle stretching and active assistance exercises.
• To prevent aspiration, test the gag reflex, and elevate the head of the bed before giving the patient anything to eat. If the gag reflex is absent, give nasogastric feedings until this reflex returns.
• As the patient regains strength and can tolerate a vertical position, apply toe-to-groin elastic bandages or an abdominal binder to prevent postural hypotension, if necessary.
• To prevent thrombophlebitis, apply antiembolism stockings or compression boots and give prophylactic anticoagulants, as ordered.
• If the patient has facial paralysis, give eye and mouth care every 4 hours. Protect the corneas with isotonic eyedrops and conical eye shields.
• Offer the bedpan every 3 to 4 hours. Encourage adequate fluid intake (2,000 ml/day) unless contraindicated. If urine retention develops, begin intermittent catheterization, as ordered. Because the abdominal muscles are weak, the patient may need manual pressure on the bladder (Credé's method) before he can urinate.
• To prevent or relieve constipation, offer prune juice and a high-bulk diet. If necessary, give daily or alternate-day suppositories (glycerin or bisacodyl) or enemas, as ordered.
• Administer medications as ordered. Analgesics may be prescribed to relieve muscle stiffness and spasm.
• If the patient can't communicate because of paralysis, tracheostomy, or intubation, try to establish some form of communication – for example, have the patient blink his eyes, once for yes and twice for no.
• Provide diversions for the patient, such as television, family visits, or listening to tapes.
• Provide emotional support to the patient and his family. Listen to their concerns. Stay with the patient during periods of severe stress.

Monitoring

• Monitor the patient's muscle function daily for pattern and degree of loss and later for return of muscle function.
• Monitor the patient's vital signs and level of consciousness.
• Continually assess the patient's respiratory function. Auscultate for breath sounds regularly. If respiratory muscles are weak, take serial vital capacity recordings. Use a

respirometer with a mouthpiece or a face mask for bedside testing.

• Obtain baseline ABG measurements, as ordered. Monitor pulse oximetry readings. Because neuromuscular disease results in primary hypoventilation with hypoxemia and hypercapnia, watch for PaO_2 below 70 mm Hg, which signals respiratory failure. Be alert for confusion and tachypnea – signs of rising partial pressure of carbon dioxide in arterial blood.

• Inspect the patient's skin regularly for evidence of skin breakdown.

• As the patient regains strength and can tolerate a vertical position, be alert for postural hypotension. Monitor blood pressure and pulse rate during tilting periods.

• Inspect the patient's legs regularly for signs of thrombophlebitis (localized pain, tenderness, erythema, edema, positive Homans' sign).

• Watch for urine retention. Measure and record intake and output every 8 hours.

• Monitor for other complications, such as infection and cardiac compromise.

Patient teaching

• Explain the syndrome and its signs and symptoms to the patient and his family. Explain the diagnostic tests that will be performed.

• Discuss the treatments that are ordered, and tell the patient why they're necessary. For example, if the patient loses his gag reflex, tell him tube feedings are necessary to maintain nutritional status.

• Advise the family to help the patient maintain mental alertness, fight boredom, and avoid depression. Suggest that they plan frequent visits, read books to the patient, or borrow library books on tape for him.

• Before discharge, prepare an appropriate home care plan. Teach the patient how to transfer from bed to wheelchair or from wheelchair to toilet or tub, and how to walk short distances with a walker or a cane.

• Instruct the family how to help the patient eat, compensating for facial weakness, and how to help him avoid skin breakdown.

• Emphasize the importance of establishing a regular bowel and bladder elimination routine.

• Tell the patient to schedule physical therapy sessions.

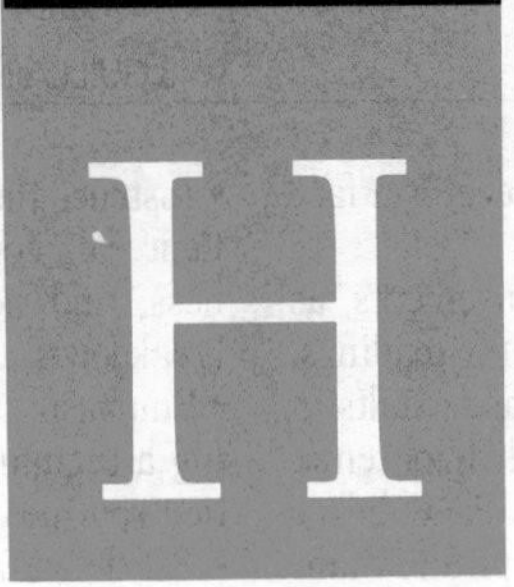

Haemophilus influenzae infection

Although *Haemophilus influenzae* can affect many organ systems, it most frequently attacks the respiratory system. It's a common cause of epiglottitis, laryngotracheobronchitis, pneumonia, bronchiolitis, otitis media, and meningitis. Less often, it causes bacterial endocarditis, conjunctivitis, facial cellulitis, septic arthritis, and osteomyelitis.

H. influenzae infection predominantly affects children, although it's becoming more common in adults, especially if they have a history of alcoholism and are over age 50. It infects about half of all children before age 1 and virtually all children by age 3, although a vaccine has reduced this number. The vaccine is administered at ages 2, 4, 6, and 15 months.

Causes

A small, gram-negative, pleomorphic aerobic bacillus, *H. influenzae* appears predominantly in coccobacillary exudates. It's usually found in the pharynx and less often in the conjunctiva and genitourinary tract. Transmission occurs by direct contact with secretions or by airborne droplets.

Complications

The microorganism can cause subdural effusions and permanent neurologic sequelae from meningitis; complete upper airway obstruction from epiglottitis; and pericarditis, pleural effusion, and respiratory failure from pneumonia.

Assessment

The patient may report a recent viral infection. He commonly complains of a generalized malaise and is likely to have a high fever. Other symptoms vary. For example, with acute epiglottitis, the patient may complain of a sore throat, severe dysphagia, and dyspnea. With pneumonia, he may report a productive cough, dyspnea, and pleuritic chest pain. With meningitis, he may experience headache, vomiting, photophobia, and diplopia.

Your inspection findings will vary with the site of infection. For example, a child with acute epiglottitis appears restless and irritable and may exhibit use of accessory muscles to breathe. Typically, he attempts to relieve severe respiratory distress by hyperextending his neck, sitting up, and leaning forward with his mouth open, tongue protruding, and nostrils flaring. (See *Preventing respiratory obstruction in acute epiglottitis.*)

You also may observe stridor and inspiratory retractions. The trachea appears normal. The pharyngeal mucosa may look reddened (rarely with soft yellow exudate) but usually appears normal or shows only slight, diffuse redness. The epiglottis appears red with considerable edema. Severe pain makes swallowing difficult or impossible.

Your inspection of a patient with pneumonia may reveal shaking chills, tachypnea, a productive cough, and impaired or asymmetrical chest movement caused by pleuritic pain.

With meningitis, you may note an altered level of consciousness (LOC) progressing to seizures and coma as the disease advances. You also may observe positive Brudzinski's and Kernig's signs and exaggerated and symmetrical deep tendon reflexes. If the patient is a young child, he's less likely to exhibit the nuchal rigidity you may see in other patients. With severe meningeal irritation, you may observe opisthotonos.

If the patient has advanced pneumonia, chest percussion may reveal dullness over areas of lung consolidation.

In epiglottitis or pneumonia, auscultation may detect gurgles; in lung consolidation and upper airway obstruction, decreased breath sounds.

Diagnostic tests

Isolation of the organism, usually with a blood culture, confirms infection with *H. influenzae.* A positive nasopharyngeal culture isn't diagnostic because this may be a normal finding in healthy people. Other laboratory findings include polymorphonuclear leukocytosis (15,000 to 30,000/mm^3) and, in young children with severe infection, leukopenia (2,000 to 3,000/mm^3).

Treatment

H. influenzae type B infections may be rapidly fatal without prompt, effective treatment. Formerly, ampicillin produced excellent results, but strains of *H. influenzae* resistant to this antibiotic have developed. Because of this, therapy for serious infections must include other agents until the infection's susceptibility to ampicillin is ensured. Many doctors now use cefotaxime or ceftriaxone initially. As an alternative, they may prescribe a combination of chloramphenicol and ampicillin. If the strain proves susceptible to ampicillin, the doctor discontinues chloramphenicol.

The outpatient with a less serious infection may receive ampicillin or amoxicillin.

NURSING ALERT

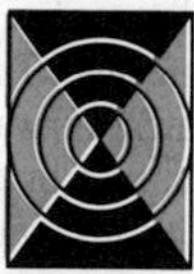

Preventing respiratory obstruction in acute epiglottitis

If a child develops symptoms of acute epiglottitis, *don't* attempt to examine his throat or obtain a throat culture— either could lead to a fatal respiratory obstruction. Only an experienced professional, such as an anesthetist or anesthesiologist, should perform such a procedure, and only with emergency airway equipment nearby.

Key nursing diagnoses and patient outcomes

Activity intolerance related to malaise. Based on this nursing diagnosis, you'll establish these patient outcomes. The patient will:

- express an understanding of his illness, particularly as it relates to his activity intolerance
- demonstrate skill in conserving energy while carrying out his daily activities
- regain a normal activity level after the infection resolves.

Hyperthermia related to infection with H. influenzae *bacillus.* Based on this nursing diagnosis, you'll establish these patient outcomes. The patient will:

- regain and maintain a normal temperature
- not experience complications of high fever, such as seizures and delirium.

Impaired gas exchange related to H. influenzae*-induced pneumonia.* Based on

this nursing diagnosis, you'll establish these patient outcomes. The patient will:
• maintain a patent airway and adequate ventilation, as shown by normal arterial blood gas (ABG) values and a normal respiratory rate
• exhibit improved respiratory function because of bronchial hygiene measures
• regain normal respiratory function after the infection heals.

Nursing interventions

• Maintain droplet precautions. Use proper hand-washing technique, properly dispose of respiratory secretions, place soiled tissues in a plastic bag, and decontaminate all equipment.
• Maintain adequate respiratory function. Provide cool humidification and oxygenation therapy for respiratory infection, as needed; use croup tents for children and face tents for adults.
• Keep emergency equipment readily available, especially for the patient with meningitis or epiglottitis. This includes an oral airway, a tracheotomy tray, endotracheal tubes, a hand-held resuscitation bag, suction and oxygen equipment, and a laryngoscope with blades of various sizes. The patient may need a smaller endotracheal tube because of laryngeal edema.
• Suction the patient as needed, using sterile technique.
• Give analgesics or anxiolytics, as ordered.
• Administer racemic epinephrine to the oropharynx.
• Provide sufficient oral or I.V. fluids, or both, as ordered.
• Provide a quiet, calm environment. Organize physical care measures, and perform them quickly to avoid disrupting the patient's rest.
• Avoid fluid overload in a patient with meningitis because of the danger of cerebral edema.
• Frequently reorient the patient with an altered LOC.
• Maintain adequate nutrition and elimination.
• Position the patient carefully. Elevate the head of the bed, turn him often, and assist with range-of-motion exercises.

Monitoring

• Frequently monitor the patient's respiratory status. Watch for increasing restlessness and tachycardia, cyanosis, dyspnea, and retractions. These may indicate the need for emergency tracheotomy.
• Monitor ABG values. Be sure to assess the patient's LOC or degree of lethargy; these may indicate the severity of hypoxemia.
• For the patient with meningitis, assess neurologic function often, watching for deterioration. Be alert for a temperature increase up to 102° F (38.9° C), deteriorating LOC, nuchal rigidity, seizures, and altered respirations. These signs may herald an impending crisis.
• Check the patient's history for drug allergies before administering antibiotics. Monitor his complete blood count for signs of bone marrow depression when therapy includes ampicillin or chloramphenicol.
• Monitor intake (including I.V. infusions) and output. Watch for signs of dehydration, such as decreased skin turgor, parched lips, concentrated urine, decreased urine output, and increased pulse rate.

Patient teaching

• Inform the parents of a child infected with *H. influenzae* about the high risk of acquiring this infection at day-care centers.
• Encourage parents to have their young children receive the *H. influenzae* vaccine to prevent these infections.
• Make sure the patient or his parents understand the importance of taking the prescribed antibiotic until the entire prescription is finished. The patient shouldn't stop taking the drug because he begins to feel better.

• Provide support and a careful explanation of procedures (especially intubation, tracheotomy, and suctioning) to the patient and his family or to the patient's parents.
• If the patient undergoes a tracheotomy, explain to him and his family that this measure usually is used for 4 to 7 days.
• Teach the patient with pneumonia how to cough and perform deep-breathing exercises to clear secretions.
• To control the spread of infection, teach him to dispose of secretions properly and to use proper hand-washing technique.
• For home treatment of a respiratory infection, suggest using a room humidifier or breathing moist air from a shower or bath, as necessary.

Hantavirus pulmonary syndrome

Mainly occurring in the southwestern United States, *Hantavirus* pulmonary syndrome, which causes flulike symptoms and rapidly progresses to respiratory failure, is known for its high mortality. The *Hantavirus* strain that causes disease in Asia and Europe is distinctly different from the one currently found in North America.

Causes

A member of the Bunyaviridae family, the genus *Hantavirus* is responsible for *Hantavirus* pulmonary syndrome. Disease transmission is associated with exposure to infected rodents, which are the primary reservoir for this virus. *Hantavirus* infections have been documented in people whose activities are associated with rodent contact, such as farming, hiking, or camping in rodent-infested areas and occupying rodent-infested dwellings.

Infected rodents shed the virus in their feces, urine, and saliva. Human infection may occur from inhalation, ingestion (of contaminated food or water, for example), contact with rodent excrement, or rodent bites.

Complications

Hantavirus pulmonary syndrome can very quickly progress to respiratory failure, possibly leading to death.

Assessment

Noncardiogenic pulmonary edema distinguishes this syndrome. Common complaints include myalgia, fever, headache, nausea, vomiting, and cough. Respiratory distress typically follows the onset of a cough. Fever, hypoxia and, in some patients, serious hypotension typify the hospital course.

Other signs and symptoms include increased respiratory and heart rates.

Diagnostic tests

Diagnosis currently rests mainly on clinical suspicion in conjunction with a process of elimination developed by the Centers for Disease Control and Prevention (CDC) with the Council of State and Territorial Epidemiologists. (See *Screening for* Hantavirus *pulmonary syndrome.*)

Laboratory studies usually reveal an elevated white blood cell count with a predominance of neutrophils, myeloid precursors, and atypical lymphocytes. Tests also show an elevated hematocrit level, a decreased platelet count, an elevated partial thromboplastin time, and a normal fibrinogen level. Usually, laboratory findings demonstrate only minimal abnormalities in renal function, with serum creatinine levels no higher than 2.5 mg/dl.

Chest X-rays eventually show bilateral diffuse infiltrates in almost all patients (findings consistent with adult respiratory distress syndrome).

Treatment

Treatment consists of maintaining adequate oxygenation, monitoring vital signs, and intervening to stabilize the heart rate and blood pressure. Drug therapy includes

Screening for *Hantavirus* pulmonary syndrome

The CDC has developed a screening procedure to identify potential and actual cases of *Hantavirus* pulmonary syndrome.

Potential cases
For a diagnosis of possible *Hantavirus* pulmonary syndrome, a patient must have one of the following:
• a febrile illness (temperature of 101° F [38.3° C] or more) occurring in a previously healthy person and characterized by unexplained adult respiratory distress syndrome
• bilateral interstitial pulmonary infiltrates that develop within 1 week of hospitalization and cause respiratory compromise that requires supplemental oxygen
• an unexplained respiratory illness that results in death and autopsy findings that demonstrate noncardiogenic pulmonary edema without an identifiable specific cause of death.

Exclusions
Of the patients who meet the criteria for having potential *Hantavirus* pulmonary syndrome, the CDC excludes those who have any of the following:
• a predisposing underlying medical condition (for example, severe underlying pulmonary disease, solid tumors or hematologic cancers, congenital or acquired immunodeficiency disorders) or a medical condition such as rheumatoid arthritis or organ transplantation that requires immunosuppressive drug therapy (for example, steroids or cytotoxic chemotherapy)
• an acute illness that provides a likely explanation for the respiratory illness—for example, a recent major trauma, burn, or surgery; a recent seizure disorder or history of aspiration; bacterial sepsis; another respiratory disorder such as respiratory syncytial virus in young children; influenza; or pneumonia caused by *Legionella.*

Confirmed cases
Cases of confirmed *Hantavirus* pulmonary syndrome must include the following:
• at least one serum or tissue specimen that shows evidence of *Hantavirus* infection
• in a patient with a compatible clinical illness, serologic evidence (presence of *Hantavirus*-specific immunoglobulin M or rising titers of immunoglobulin G), polymerase chain reaction for *Hantavirus* ribonucleic acid, or a positive immunohistochemistry test for the *Hantavirus* antigen.

administration of vasopressors, such as dopamine or epinephrine, for hypotension. Fluid volume replacement may also be necessary, although precautions must be taken not to overhydrate the patient.

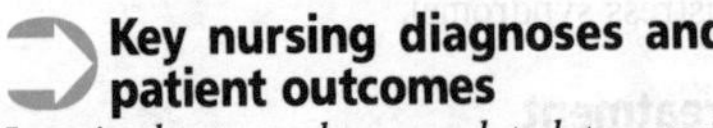

Key nursing diagnoses and patient outcomes

Impaired gas exchange related to respiratory failure. Based on this nursing diagnosis, you'll establish these patient outcomes. The patient will:
• exhibit arterial blood gas values within normal limits
• remain free from hypoxemia.

Ineffective breathing pattern related to respiratory distress. Based on this nursing diagnosis, you'll establish these patient outcomes. The patient will:
• maintain a patent airway
• exhibit eupnea
• remain free of respiratory difficulties.

Risk for fluid volume deficit related to viral progression. Based on this nursing

diagnosis, you'll establish these patient outcomes. The patient will:
• maintain fluid balance
• tolerate fluid volume replacement.

Nursing interventions

• Assess the patient's respiratory status and arterial blood gas values often.
• Monitor serum electrolyte levels and correct imbalances as appropriate.
• Maintain a patent airway by suctioning. Ensure adequate humidification, and check mechanical ventilator settings frequently.
• If the patient is hypoxic, assess his neurologic status frequently as well as his heart rate and blood pressure.
• Administer drug therapy and monitor the patient's response.
• Provide I.V. fluid therapy based on results of hemodynamic monitoring.
• Report cases of *Hantavirus* pulmonary syndrome to your state health department.
• Provide patients with prevention guidelines for rodent control.

Patient teaching

• Teach the patient about his disorder, and answer any questions he might have.
• Fully discuss all treatments, procedures, and diagnostic tests with the patient, and explain why they have been ordered.

Head injuries

Injuries to the head may result in a concussion, a cerebral contusion, or a skull fracture. The most common head injury, a *concussion* results from a blow to the head – a blow hard enough to jostle the brain and make it strike the skull, causing temporary neural dysfunction, but not hard enough to cause a cerebral contusion. Most concussion victims recover completely within 48 hours. Repeated concussions, however, exact a cumulative toll on the brain.

More serious than a concussion, a *cerebral contusion* is an ecchymosis of brain tissue that results from a severe blow to the head. A contusion disrupts normal nerve functions in the bruised area and may cause loss of consciousness, hemorrhage, edema, and even death.

A *skull fracture* is always considered serious and at times may be life-threatening. Because the main concern isn't the fracture itself but possible damage to the brain, the injury is considered a neurosurgical condition. Signs and symptoms reflect the severity and extent of the head injury.

Skull fractures may be simple (closed) or compound (open) and may or may not displace bone fragments. They're also described as linear, comminuted, or depressed. A linear, or hairline, fracture doesn't displace structures and seldom requires treatment. A comminuted fracture splinters or crushes the bone into several fragments. A depressed fracture pushes the bone toward the brain; it's considered serious only if it compresses underlying structures.

Skull fractures also are classified according to location, such as cranial vault or basilar. A basilar fracture occurs at the base of the skull and involves the cribriform plate and the frontal sinuses. Because of the danger of cranial complications and meningitis, basilar fractures are often more serious than cranial vault fractures.

Causes

A traumatic blow to the head causes a head injury. The blow is usually sudden and forceful, such as a fall, motor vehicle accident, or punch to the head. If the blow causes an acceleration-deceleration or coup-contrecoup injury, then a cerebral contusion results. Acceleration-deceleration or coup-contrecoup injuries can occur directly beneath the site of impact when the brain rebounds against the skull from the force of a blow (a beating with a blunt instrument, for example), when the force of the blow drives the brain against the opposite side of the skull, or when the head is hurled forward and stopped abruptly (as when a driver's head strikes the windshield). The brain continues moving and slaps against the skull (acceleration) and rebounds (deceleration).

Complications

A *concussion* usually causes no significant anatomic brain injury. Seizures, persistent vomiting, or both may occur. Rarely, a concussion leads to intracranial hemorrhage (subdural, epidural, or parenchymal).

A *cerebral contusion* can cause intracranial hemorrhage or hematoma if the injury causes the brain to strike against bony prominences inside the skull (especially the sphenoidal ridges). Residual headaches and vertigo may complicate recovery. Secondary effects, such as brain swelling, may accompany serious contusions, resulting in increased intracranial pressure (ICP) and herniation.

Skull fractures can lead to infection, intracerebral hemorrhage and hematoma, brain abscess, and increased ICP from edema. Recovery from the injury can be further complicated by residual effects of the injury, such as seizure disorders, hydrocephalus, and organic mental syndrome.

Assessment

The patient's history (obtained from the patient, his family, eyewitnesses, or emergency personnel) reveals a traumatic injury to the head. A period of unconsciousness may follow the trauma. If unconscious, the patient may appear pale and motionless. If conscious, he may appear drowsy or easily disturbed by any form of stimulation, such as noise or light.

If the patient has a concussion, a family member or friend may report behavioral changes, saying that the patient is behaving out of character. The patient usually complains of dizziness, nausea, and severe headache. He may also exhibit anterograde and retrograde amnesias. In retrograde amnesia, the patient not only can't recall what happened immediately after the injury but also has difficulty recalling events that led up to it. Typically, he repeats the same questions. The presence of anterograde amnesia and the duration of retrograde amnesia reliably correlate with the injury's severity. A conscious patient with a cerebral contusion may become agitated and even violent. If he has a skull fracture, he may complain of a persistent, localized headache. Depending on the type and location of the fracture, he may appear dazed, anxious, or agitated.

Your assessment findings will vary, depending on the type and location of the head injury. Your examination should focus on evaluating the patient's level of consciousness, pupillary responses, and strength of extremities. Vital signs aren't good indicators of neurologic status and don't correlate specifically with the type of injury unless the brain stem is involved.

Because scalp wounds usually accompany a cerebral contusion or skull fracture, scalp inspection may reveal abrasions, contusions, lacerations, or avulsions. If the scalp was lacerated or torn away, profuse bleeding may occur, although it isn't heavy enough to induce hypovolemic shock. However, the patient may be in shock from other injuries or from medullary failure in the case of a severe head injury.

Other inspection findings in a patient with a skull fracture may include bleeding in the nose, pharynx, or ears; under the conjunctivae; under the periorbital skin (raccoon's eyes); and behind the eardrum. You also may note Battle's sign. Inspection of the ears and nose may reveal cerebrospinal fluid (CSF) and brain tissue leakage. (Leakage may be found on the patient's pillowcase or bed linens.) Basilar fractures of the skull often produce hemorrhage from these areas. Red-tinged CSF drainage strongly suggests brain injury.

Palpation of the skull may reveal tenderness or hematomas in a patient with a concussion. It may reveal palpable fractures, areas of swelling, and possibly hematoma formation in a patient with a skull fracture. A vault fracture commonly causes soft-tissue swelling near the site, making other fractures hard to detect without X-rays.

A neurologic assessment usually produces normal findings in a patient with a concussion and abnormal findings in a patient with a cerebral contusion or skull fracture. A patient with a cerebral contusion may display hemiparesis, decorticate or decerebrate posturing, and unequal pupillary response. With effort, you may be able to rouse an unconscious patient temporarily. If the acute stage has passed, you may find that the patient has returned to a relatively alert state, perhaps with temporary aphasia, slight hemiparesis, or unilateral numbness.

If the patient has a skull fracture, you may note an altered level of consciousness (LOC) along with other classic signs of brain injury. These include agitation and irritability, abnormal deep tendon reflexes, altered pupillary and motor responses, hemiparesis, dizziness, seizures, and projectile vomiting. Loss of consciousness may last for hours, days, weeks, or indefinitely. Many findings, however, will vary with the location and severity of the fracture. For example, a linear fracture associated only with a concussion won't produce loss of consciousness; a sphenoidal fracture may produce vision loss; a temporal fracture may trigger unilateral hearing loss or facial paralysis.

Diagnostic tests

Skull X-rays will locate a fracture, if present, unless the fracture is of the cranial vault. (These fractures aren't visible or palpable.) Cerebral angiography locates vascular disruptions from internal pressure or injury that result from a cerebral contusion or skull fracture. A computed tomography scan will disclose intracranial hemorrhage from ruptured blood vessels, ischemic or necrotic tissue, cerebral edema, areas of petechial hemorrhage, a shift in brain tissue, and subdural, epidural, and intracerebral hematomas that may have occurred from the head injury. Magnetic resonance imaging and a radioisotope scan may also disclose intracranial hemorrhage from ruptured blood vessels in a patient with a skull fracture.

Treatment

Treatment depends on the type of injury. Most patients with a concussion require no treatment except bed rest, observation, and acetaminophen for headache.

However, a patient with a cerebral contusion may require immediate emergency treatment, including establishment of a patent airway and, if necessary, a tracheotomy or endotracheal intubation. Treatment also may consist of I.V. fluids (dextrose 5% in 0.45% sodium chloride solution), I.V. mannitol to reduce ICP, and restricted fluid intake to decrease intracerebral edema. The patient's ICP may be reduced by maintaining his level of partial pressure of carbon dioxide in arterial blood ($Paco_2$) between 25 and 30 mm Hg, which will constrict cerebral blood vessels. If necessary, additional treatments for the patient with a cerebral contusion may include blood transfusion and craniotomy.

Specific treatment for a skull fracture depends on the type of fracture. In general, if the patient hasn't lost consciousness, he should be observed in the emergency department for at least 4 hours. After this period, a patient with stable vital signs can be discharged. He should receive an instruction sheet for 24 to 48 hours of observation at home.

Although a simple linear skull fracture can tear an underlying blood vessel or cause a CSF leak, most linear fractures require only supportive treatment. Such treatment includes mild analgesics (acetaminophen) and wound management (local injection of procaine, shaving the scalp around the wound, and cleaning and debriding the wound).

More severe vault fractures, especially depressed fractures, usually require a craniotomy to elevate or remove fragments that have been driven into the brain and to extract foreign bodies and necrotic tissue. This reduces the risk of infection and further brain damage. Cranioplasty follows the use of tantalum mesh or acrylic plates to replace the removed skull section. The patient commonly requires antibiotics and, in profound hemorrhage, blood transfusions.

A basilar fracture calls for immediate prophylactic antibiotics to prevent meningitis from CSF leakage. The patient also needs close observation for secondary hematomas and hemorrhages; surgery may be necessary. Also, a patient with a basilar or vault fracture requires I.V. or I.M. dexamethasone to reduce cerebral edema and minimize brain tissue damage.

For status epilepticus, which may result from head injury, the patient may receive an anticonvulsant; usually, 10 to 15 mg/kg of I.V. phenytoin sodium is given at a rate of not more than 50 mg/minute or according to hospital policy.

Key nursing diagnoses and patient outcomes

Anxiety related to the threat of permanent neurologic injury or death. Based on this nursing diagnosis, you'll establish these patient outcomes. The patient will:

- express his feelings of anxiety
- use available support systems to help cope with his anxiety
- demonstrate that he experiences fewer physical symptoms caused by anxiety.

Risk for injury related to complications of head injury. Based on this nursing diagnosis, you'll establish these patient outcomes. The patient will:

- avoid permanent neurologic deficit because of the head injury
- exhibit normal neurologic findings after the head injury heals.

Pain related to altered brain or skull tissue. Based on this nursing diagnosis, you'll establish these patient outcomes. The patient will:

- maintain normal ICP
- express pain relief with treatment
- obtain complete pain relief after the head injury heals.

Nursing interventions

- Maintain a patent airway. Assist with endotracheal intubation or tracheotomy, as necessary.
- Administer medications as ordered. However, don't administer narcotics or sedatives because they may depress respirations, raise $PaCO_2$ levels, and lead to increased ICP. They also can mask changes in neurologic status. Give acetaminophen for pain, as ordered.
- Protect the patient from injury according to his condition. Use side rails, assist the unsteady patient with walking, stay with the patient while he uses the bathroom, and place the confused patient where he can be easily observed.
- Insert an indwelling urinary catheter, if ordered.
- If the patient is unconscious, insert a nasogastric tube to prevent aspiration – but only after a basilar skull fracture has been ruled out. Otherwise, the tube may be inserted into the cranial vault.
- If the patient has CSF leakage or is unconscious, elevate the head of the bed 30 degrees; otherwise, leave it flat. Remember that such a patient is at risk for jugular compression, leading to increased ICP, when he's not positioned on his back. So be sure to keep his head properly aligned. Enforce bed rest.
- Position the patient so that secretions drain properly. If you detect CSF leakage from the nose, place a gauze pad under the nostrils. If CSF leaks from the ear, position the patient so his ear drains naturally; don't pack the ear or nose. If the patient requires suctioning, suction him through the mouth, not the nose, to avoid introducing bacteria into CSF.
- Monitor the patient's intake and output as needed to help maintain a normovolemic state.
- To decrease the patient's anxiety, speak calmly to him and explain your actions,

even if he's unconscious. Don't make any sudden, unexpected moves. Touch the patient gently.
• After the patient is stabilized, clean and dress any superficial scalp wounds. Be sure to wear sterile gloves. (If the skin has been broken, the patient may need tetanus prophylaxis.) Assist with suturing if needed. Carefully cover scalp wounds with a sterile dressing; control any bleeding as necessary.
• If the patient develops temporary aphasia, provide an alternative means of communication.
• Institute seizure precautions, but don't restrain the patient.
• Prepare the patient for a craniotomy, as indicated. (See the entry "Craniotomy.")

Monitoring

• Initially, monitor vital signs continuously and check for additional injuries. Abnormal respirations could indicate a breakdown in the brain's respiratory center and possibly an impending tentorial herniation – a neurologic emergency.
• Continue to check vital signs and neurologic status, including LOC and pupil size, every 15 minutes. If the patient's condition worsens or fluctuates, arrange for a neurosurgical consultation.
• Observe the patient for headache, dizziness, irritability, and anxiety. If his condition worsens, perform a complete neurologic evaluation and notify the doctor.
• Monitor fluid and electrolyte levels and replace them as necessary.
• Monitor the patient's oxygenation status through serial arterial blood gas studies, as ordered – especially if he's intubated.
• Carefully observe the patient for CSF leakage. Check the bed sheets for a blood-tinged spot surrounded by a lighter ring (halo sign).
• Observe the patient for agitated behavior, which may stem from hypoxia or increased ICP.
• Monitor the elderly patient especially closely. He may have brain atrophy and therefore more space for cerebral edema; ICP may increase, yet cause no signs.
• If the patient remains stable after 4 or more hours of observation, he can be discharged in the care of a responsible adult.

Patient teaching

• Explain to the patient who is discharged from the emergency department that a responsible adult, such as a family member or friend, should continue to observe his condition at home for the next 24 to 48 hours. If this isn't possible, the patient may be hospitalized briefly. Be sure to provide a head injury instruction sheet.
• Instruct the caregiver to awaken the patient every 2 hours throughout the night and to ask him his name, where he is, and whether he can identify the person. Tell the caregiver to return the patient to the hospital if he is difficult to arouse, is disoriented, or has seizures.
• Advise the caregiver to keep the sleep area quiet so the patient can sleep between the 2-hour intervals.
• Tell the patient to return to the hospital immediately if he experiences a persistent or worsening headache, forceful or constant vomiting, blurred vision, any change in personality, abnormal eye movements, a staggering gait, or twitching.
• Instruct the patient not to take anything stronger than acetaminophen for a headache. Warn him not to take aspirin because it may heighten the risk of bleeding.
• If vomiting occurs, instruct the patient to eat lightly until it stops. (Occasional vomiting is normal after a concussion.)
• Teach the patient to recognize symptoms of postconcussion syndrome – headache, dizziness, vertigo, anxiety, and fatigue. Tell him that the syndrome may persist for several weeks.
• Tell the patient with a cerebral contusion not to cough, sneeze, or blow his nose because these activities can increase ICP.
• Teach the patient and his family how to care for his scalp wound, if applicable.

Emphasize the need to return for suture removal and follow-up evaluation.

Heart failure

When the myocardium can't pump effectively enough to meet the body's metabolic needs, heart failure occurs. Pump failure usually occurs in a damaged left ventricle (left ventricular failure) primarily, or secondary to left ventricular failure. Usually, however, left and right ventricular failure develop simultaneously. Heart failure is classified as high-output or low-output, acute or chronic, left-sided or right-sided, and forward or backward. (See *Categorizing heart failure.*)

For many patients, the symptoms of heart failure restrict the ability to perform activities of daily living, severely affecting quality of life. Advances in diagnostic and therapeutic techniques have greatly improved the outlook for these patients, but the prognosis still depends on the underlying cause and its response to treatment.

Causes

Heart failure frequently results from a primary abnormality of the heart muscle (such as an infarction) that impairs ventricular function to the point that the heart can no longer pump sufficient blood. Heart failure can also result from causes not related to myocardial function. These include:

- mechanical disturbances in ventricular filling during diastole, which result from blood volume that's insufficient for the ventricle to pump. This occurs in mitral stenosis secondary to rheumatic heart disease or constrictive pericarditis and atrial fibrillation.
- systolic hemodynamic disturbances – such as excessive cardiac work load caused by volume overloading or pressure overload – that limit the heart's pumping ability. These disturbances can result from mitral or aortic insufficiency, which causes volume overloading, and aortic stenosis or systemic hypertension, which results in increased resistance to ventricular emptying.

In addition, certain conditions can predispose the patient to heart failure, particularly if he has some form of underlying heart disease. These include:

- arrhythmias – such as tachyarrhythmias, which can reduce ventricular filling time; bradycardia, which can reduce cardiac output; and arrhythmias that disrupt the normal atrial and ventricular filling synchrony
- pregnancy and thyrotoxicosis because of the increased demand for cardiac output
- pulmonary embolism because it elevates pulmonary artery pressures that can cause right ventricular failure
- infections because increased metabolic demands further burden the heart
- anemia because to meet the oxygen needs of the tissues, cardiac output must increase
- increased physical activity, emotional stress, increased sodium or water intake, or failure to comply with the prescribed treatment regimen for the underlying heart disease.

Complications

Pulmonary congestion can lead to pulmonary edema, a life-threatening condition. (See the entry "Pulmonary edema.") Decreased perfusion to major organs, especially the brain and kidneys, can cause these organs to fail. Myocardial infarction can occur because the oxygen demands of the overworked heart can't be sufficiently met.

Assessment

The patient's history reveals a disorder or condition that can precipitate heart failure. The patient often complains of shortness of breath, which occurs in early stages during activity, and, in late stages, also at rest. He may report that dyspnea

Categorizing heart failure

Although heart failure is usually classified by the site of failure (left ventricle, right ventricle, or both), it may also be classified by level of cardiac output, stage, and direction (high-output or low-output, acute or chronic, or forward or backward). These classifications represent different clinical aspects of heart failure, not distinct diseases.

Left ventricular failure

Failure of the left ventricle to pump blood to the vital organs and periphery is usually caused by myocardial infarction (MI). Decreased left ventricular output causes fluid to accumulate in the lungs, precipitating dyspnea, orthopnea, and paroxysmal nocturnal dyspnea.

Right ventricular failure

Resulting from failure of the right ventricle to pump sufficient blood to the lungs, this type usually is caused by disorders that increase pulmonary vascular resistance, such as pulmonary embolism, pulmonic stenosis, and pulmonary hypertension. Right ventricular failure produces congestive hepatomegaly, ascites, and edema.

High-output failure

Failure with an elevated cardiac output occurs when tissue demands for oxygenated blood exceed the heart's ability to supply it. High-output failure occurs in arteriovenous fistula, hyperthyroidism, anemia, sickle cell anemia, beriberi, Paget's disease of the bone, and thyrotoxicosis.

Low-output failure

Failure with decreased cardiac output is caused by decreased pumping ability of the myocardium. Low-output failure occurs in coronary artery disease, hypertension, primary myocardial disease, and valvular disease.

Acute failure

This failure occurs suddenly, as in MI or ruptured cardiac valve. The sudden reduction in cardiac output results in systemic hypotension without peripheral edema. Acute failure may occur in a chronic condition, such as when a patient with chronic heart failure experiences acute heart failure with MI. It may also occur in any condition that stresses an already diseased heart.

Chronic failure

This type of heart failure occurs gradually and is sustained for long periods. The arterial blood pressure doesn't drop, but peripheral edema is present. Chronic failure may occur in cardiomyopathy or multivalvular disease or in a healed, extensive MI.

Forward failure

The heart fails to expel enough blood into the arterial system. Sodium and water retention result from decreased renal perfusion and excessive proximal tubular sodium reabsorption or excessive distal tubular reabsorption, through activation of the renin-angiotensin-aldosterone system.

Backward failure

When backward failure occurs, one ventricle fails to empty its contents normally, and end-diastolic ventricular pressures rise. The pressures and volume in the atrium and venous system behind the failing ventricle also rise, and sodium and water retention occur because of the elevated systemic venous and capillary pressures and the resulting transudation of fluid into the interstitial space.

worsens at night when he lies down. He may use two or three pillows to elevate his head to sleep or may have to sleep sitting up in a chair. He may relate that his shortness of breath wakes him up soon after he falls asleep, causing him to sit bolt upright to catch his breath. Often he may remain dyspneic, coughing and wheezing even when he sits up. This is referred to as paroxysmal nocturnal dyspnea.

The patient may report that his shoes or rings have become too tight, a result of peripheral edema. He may also report increasing fatigue, weakness, insomnia, anorexia, nausea, and a sense of abdominal fullness (particularly in right ventricular failure).

Inspection may reveal a dyspneic, anxious patient in respiratory distress. In mild cases, dyspnea may occur while the patient is lying down or active; in severe cases, it's not related to position. The patient may have a cough that produces pink, frothy sputum. You may note cyanosis of the lips and nail beds, pale skin, diaphoresis, dependent peripheral and sacral edema, and jugular vein distention. Ascites may also be present, especially in patients with right ventricular failure. If heart failure is chronic, the patient may appear cachectic.

When palpating the pulse, you may note that the skin feels cool and clammy. The pulse rate will be rapid, and pulsus alternans may be present. Hepatomegaly and, possibly, splenomegaly also may be present.

Percussion reveals dullness over lung bases that are fluid-filled.

Auscultation of the blood pressure may detect decreased pulse pressure, reflecting reduced stroke volume. Heart auscultation may disclose an S_3 and S_4. Lung auscultation reveals moist, bibasilar crackles. If pulmonary edema is present, you'll hear crackles throughout the lung, accompanied by rhonchi and expiratory wheezing.

Diagnostic tests

- *Electrocardiography* reflects heart strain or enlargement, or ischemia. It may also reveal atrial enlargement, tachycardia, and extrasystoles.
- *Chest X-rays* show increased pulmonary vascular markings, interstitial edema, or pleural effusion and cardiomegaly.
- *Pulmonary artery pressure monitoring* typically demonstrates elevated pulmonary artery and capillary wedge pressures, left ventricular end-diastolic pressure in left ventricular failure, and elevated right atrial or central venous pressure in right ventricular failure.

Treatment

The aim of therapy is to improve pump function by reversing the compensatory mechanisms producing the clinical effects. Heart failure can usually be controlled quickly by treatment consisting of:

- diuresis (with diuretics, such as furosemide, hydrochlorothiazide, spironolactone, ethacrynic acid, bumetanide, or triamterene) to reduce total blood volume and circulatory congestion
- prolonged bed rest
- oxygen administration to increase oxygen delivery to the myocardium and other vital organ tissues
- inotropic drugs, such as digoxin, to strengthen myocardial contractility; sympathomimetics, such as dopamine and dobutamine, in acute situations; or amrinone, to increase contractility and cause arterial vasodilation
- vasodilators to increase cardiac output or angiotensin-converting enzyme inhibitors to decrease afterload
- antiembolism stockings to prevent venostasis and possible thromboembolism formation.

After recovery, the patient usually must continue taking digitalis, diuretics, and potassium supplements and must remain under medical supervision. If the patient with valve dysfunction has recurrent acute heart failure, surgical replacement may be necessary.

Key nursing diagnoses and patient outcomes

Decreased cardiac output related to reduced stroke volume caused by mechanical, structural, or electrophysiologic heart problems. Based on this nursing diagnosis, you'll establish these patient outcomes. The patient will:
- maintain a normal pulse rate and blood pressure
- avoid dizziness, syncope, arrhythmias, and chest pain
- express an understanding of why he must comply with the prescribed diet, take medications as ordered, and maintain an appropriate activity level.

Fluid volume excess related to blood pooling in the pulmonary system or the systemic circulation caused by myocardial damage. Based on this nursing diagnosis, you'll establish these patient outcomes. The patient will:
- restrict fluid intake, as ordered, so that it doesn't exceed fluid output
- regain and maintain baseline weight
- regain and maintain central venous and pulmonary artery pressures within normal limits (if available).

Ineffective breathing pattern related to fatigue caused by pulmonary congestion. Based on this nursing diagnosis, you'll establish these patient outcomes. The patient will:
- regain his baseline respiratory rate and maintain stable respirations
- regain and maintain arterial blood gas values within normal limits
- exhibit an ability to conserve energy while performing activities of daily living.

Nursing interventions

- Place the patient in Fowler's position and give supplemental oxygen, as ordered, to ease his breathing.
- Organize all activities to provide maximum rest periods.
- To prevent deep vein thrombosis due to vascular congestion, assist the patient with range-of-motion exercises. Enforce bed rest, and apply antiembolism stockings.
- Report changes in the patient's condition immediately.

Monitoring

- Weigh the patient daily to help detect fluid retention and observe for peripheral edema. Monitor I.V. intake and urine output (especially if the patient is receiving diuretics).
- Assess the patient's vital signs (for increased respiratory and heart rates and for narrowing pulse pressure) and mental status. Auscultate the heart for abnormal sounds and the lungs for crackles or rhonchi.
- Frequently monitor blood urea nitrogen and serum creatinine, potassium, sodium, chloride, and magnesium levels.
- Provide continuous cardiac monitoring during acute and advanced disease stages to identify and manage arrhythmias promptly.
- Watch for calf pain and tenderness.

Patient teaching

- Advise the patient to avoid foods high in sodium content, such as canned and commercially prepared foods and dairy products, to curb fluid overload.
- Teach the patient that he must replace the potassium lost through diuretic therapy by taking a prescribed potassium supplement and eating potassium-rich foods, such as bananas, apricots, and orange juice.
- Stress the need for regular medical checkups and periodic blood tests to monitor drug levels.
- Stress the importance of taking digitalis exactly as prescribed. Tell the patient to watch for and immediately report signs of toxicity, such as anorexia, vomiting, confusion, slow or irregular pulse rate and, in elderly patients, flulike symptoms.
- Tell the patient to notify the doctor if his pulse rate is unusually irregular or less

than 60 beats/minute; if he experiences dizziness, blurred vision, shortness of breath, persistent dry cough, palpitations, increased fatigue, paroxysmal nocturnal dyspnea, swollen ankles, or decreased urine output; or if he gains 3 to 5 lb (1.4 to 2.3 kg) in 1 week.

Heart valve replacement

Severe valvular stenosis or insufficiency often requires excision of the affected valve and replacement with a mechanical or biological prosthesis. The mitral and aortic valves are most commonly affected because of the high pressure generated by the left ventricle during contraction.

Indications for valve replacement depend on the patient's symptoms and the affected valve. For example, if the patient has severe symptoms that can't be managed with drugs and dietary restrictions, a commissurotomy may be performed. If this is not successful, valve replacement may be done. In aortic insufficiency, valve replacement is usually done once symptoms – palpitations, dizziness, dyspnea on exertion, angina, and murmurs – have developed or if the chest X-ray and electrocardiogram (ECG) reveal left ventricular hypertrophy. In aortic stenosis, which may be asymptomatic, valve replacement may be performed if cardiac catheterization reveals significant stenosis. In mitral stenosis, it's indicated if the patient develops fatigue, dyspnea, hemoptysis, arrhythmias, pulmonary hypertension, or right ventricular hypertrophy. In mitral insufficiency, surgery is usually done when the patient's symptoms – dyspnea, fatigue, and palpitations – interfere with his activities or if insufficiency is acute, as in papillary muscle rupture.

Diseased or damaged mitral or aortic valves may be replaced by either mechanical or biological heart valves. (See *Comparing prosthetic valves.*)

Procedure

After performing a medial sternotomy and initiating cardiopulmonary bypass, the surgeon cannulates the coronary arteries and perfuses them with a cold cardioplegic solution. For aortic valve replacement, he clamps the aorta above the right coronary artery; for mitral valve replacement, he incises the left atrium to expose the mitral valve.

After excising the diseased valve, the surgeon sutures around the margin of the valve annulus (the ring or encircling structure, which is left intact after valve excision). He then threads the suture material through the sewing ring of the prosthetic valve and, using a valve holder, positions the prosthesis and secures the sutures. Once he's satisfied with prosthetic placement, he removes the patient from the bypass machine. As the heart fills with blood, the surgeon vents the aorta and ventricle for air. Finally, he places epicardial pacemaker leads, inserts a chest tube(s), closes the incision, and applies a sterile dressing.

Complications

Although valve replacement surgery carries a low mortality, it can cause serious complications. Hemorrhage may result from unligated vessels, anticoagulant therapy (with mechanical prosthetic valve replacement), or coagulopathy resulting from cardiopulmonary bypass during surgery. Cerebrovascular accident (CVA) may result from thrombus formation due to turbulent blood flow through the prosthetic valve or from poor cerebral perfusion during cardiopulmonary bypass. Bacterial endocarditis can develop within days of implantation or months later. Valve dysfunction or failure may occur as the prosthetic device wears out. (This may occur 5 to 10 years after insertion of a biological prosthetic valve and 15 to 20 years after insertion of a mechanical prosthetic valve.)

Key nursing diagnoses and patient outcomes

Altered protection related to decreased blood clotting caused by anticoagulation therapy. Based on this nursing diagnosis, you'll establish these patient outcomes. The patient will:

- report for regular prothrombin time (PT) measurements and adjust his anticoagulant dosage, as directed
- incorporate bleeding precautions into his daily routine
- avoid bleeding episodes.

Risk for infection related to potential for bacterial endocarditis. Based on this nursing diagnosis, you'll establish these patient outcomes. The patient will:

- express his understanding of signs and symptoms of infection and why he must seek medical attention if these occur
- maintain a temperature and white blood cell count within a normal range
- incorporate into his daily life precautions to prevent or minimize infection
- avoid infection.

Risk for fluid volume deficit related to hemorrhage caused by valve replacement complications. Based on this nursing diagnosis, you'll establish these patient outcomes. The patient will:

- maintain normal cardiac output, as shown by stable vital signs, alertness, and orientation to time, person, and place
- avoid excessive chest tube drainage
- avoid signs and symptoms of dehydration or hemorrhage
- maintain a normal postoperative fluid balance.

Nursing interventions

When caring for a patient undergoing a heart valve replacement, your major roles include instruction and monitoring the patient's vital functions.

Before surgery

- As necessary, reinforce and supplement the doctor's explanation of the procedure.

Comparing prosthetic valves

Both mechanical and biological prosthetic valves are commonly used. The mechanical valve, such as the Starr caged-ball valve (by Baxter-Edwards),

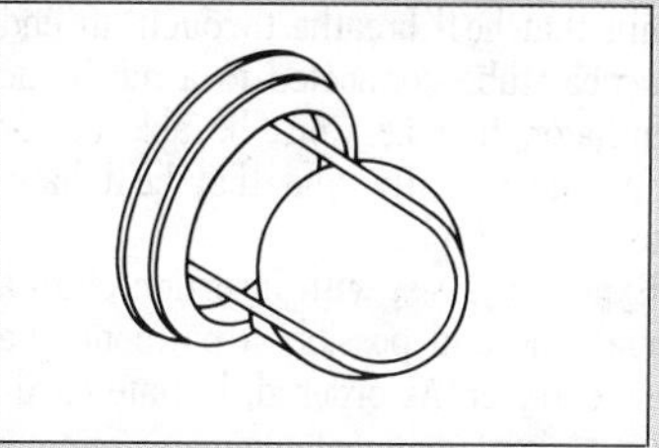

can withstand considerable stress. However, its large size sometimes makes it difficult to implant. And because blood flow is turbulent through the valve, the patient usually requires long-term anticoagulant therapy to prevent thrombus formation.

The biological prosthetic heart valve such as the Carpentier valve (by Baxter-Edwards) doesn't obstruct blood flow

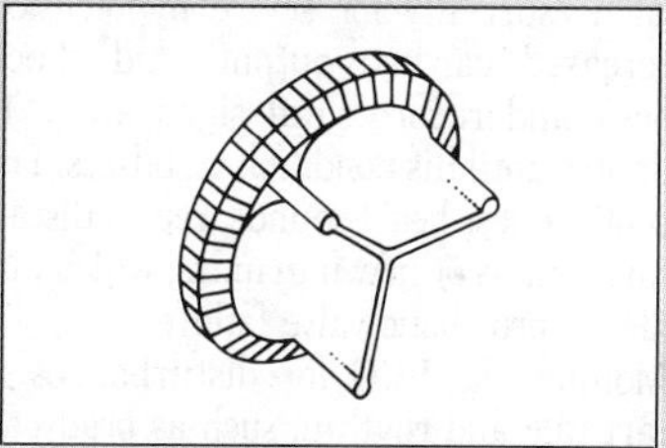

as much as a mechanical valve and is less likely to cause thrombus formation. In addition, a biological prosthetic valve doesn't require prolonged anticoagulant therapy. However, the valve is difficult to insert and less durable (prone to degeneration or calcification, especially in patients with renal disease) than its mechanical counterpart. Despite these drawbacks, the doctor will probably select a biological prosthetic valve for implantation if the patient appears unlikely to comply with anticoagulant therapy. Other types of biological prosthetic heart valves include human and animal valves.

Listen to the patient's concerns and encourage him to ask questions.
• Tell the patient he'll awaken from surgery in an intensive care unit or recovery room. Mention that he'll be connected to a cardiac monitor and have I.V. lines, an arterial line, and possibly a pulmonary artery catheter or left atrial catheter in place. Explain that he'll breathe through an endotracheal tube connected to a mechanical ventilator, that he won't be able to communicate verbally, and that he'll have a chest tube in place.
• Expect to assist with insertion of an arterial line and possibly a pulmonary artery catheter. As ordered, initiate cardiac monitoring.
• Make sure the patient has signed a consent form and necessary laboratory studies and blood typing and crossmatching have been done.

After surgery

• Closely monitor the patient's hemodynamic status for signs of compromise. Watch especially for severe hypotension, decreased cardiac output, and shock. Check and record vital signs every 15 minutes until his condition stabilizes. Frequently assess heart sounds; report distant heart sounds or new murmurs, which may indicate prosthetic valve failure.
• Monitor the ECG for disturbances in heart rate and rhythm, such as bradycardia, ventricular tachycardia, and heart block. Such disturbances may signal injury of the conduction system, which may occur during valve replacement from proximity of the atrial and mitral valves to the atrioventricular node. Arrhythmias also may result from myocardial irritability or ischemia, fluid and electrolyte imbalance, hypoxemia, or hypothermia. If you detect serious abnormalities, notify the doctor and be prepared to assist with temporary epicardial pacing.
• To ensure adequate myocardial perfusion, maintain the patient's mean arterial pressure within the guidelines set by the doctor (for adults, usually between 70 and 100 mm Hg). Also monitor pulmonary artery and left atrial pressures, as ordered.
• Frequently assess the patient's peripheral pulses, capillary refill time, and skin temperature and color, and auscultate for heart sounds. Evaluate tissue oxygenation by assessing breath sounds, chest excursion, and symmetry of chest expansion. Report any abnormalities. Check arterial blood gas values every 2 to 4 hours, and adjust ventilator settings as needed.
• Maintain chest tube drainage at the prescribed negative pressure (usually −10 to −40 cm H_2O for adults). Assess chest tubes every hour for signs of hemorrhage, excessive drainage (greater than 200 ml/hour), and sudden decrease or cessation of drainage.
• As ordered, administer analgesic, anticoagulant, antibiotic, antiarrhythmic, inotropic, and pressor medications, as well as I.V. fluids and blood products. Monitor intake and output and assess for electrolyte imbalances, especially hypokalemia. Once anticoagulant therapy begins, evaluate its effectiveness by monitoring PT daily.
• Throughout the patient's recovery period, observe him carefully for complications. Watch especially for symptoms of CVA (altered level of consciousness, pupillary changes, weakness and loss of movement in the extremities, ataxia, aphasia, dysphagia, sensory disturbances), pulmonary embolism (dyspnea, cough, hemoptysis, chest pain, pleural friction rub, cyanosis, hypoxemia), and impaired renal perfusion (decreased urine output and elevated blood urea nitrogen and serum creatinine levels).
• After weaning the patient from the ventilator and removing the endotracheal tube, promote chest physiotherapy. Start him on incentive spirometry and encourage him to cough, turn frequently, and deep-breathe. Gradually increase his activities.

Home care instructions

• Tell the patient to immediately report chest pain, fever, or redness, swelling, or drainage at the incision site.

• Explain that postpericardiotomy syndrome – fever, muscle and joint pain, weakness, and chest discomfort – often develops after open-heart surgery. Tell the patient to notify the doctor if these symptoms occur.

• Make sure the patient understands the dose, schedule, and adverse effects of all prescribed drugs.

• Advise the patient to carry medical identification with information and instructions on his anticoagulant and antibiotic therapy.

• Encourage the patient to follow his prescribed diet, especially the sodium and fat restrictions.

• Provide tips for maintaining a balance between activity and rest. Tell the patient to try to sleep at least 8 hours a night, schedule a short rest period each afternoon, and rest frequently during tiring physical activity. As appropriate, tell him he can climb stairs, engage in sexual activity, take baths and showers, and do light housework and other chores. Tell him to avoid lifting heavy objects (greater than 20 lb or so), driving a car, doing heavy work, or performing activities that require him to raise his arms over his head until the doctor gives permission. If the doctor has prescribed an exercise program, encourage the patient to follow it carefully.

• Instruct the patient to tell his dentist and his other doctors that he has a prosthetic valve before he undergoes extensive dental work or surgery. He'll probably need to take prophylactic antibiotics.

Hemodialysis

This procedure removes toxic wastes and other impurities from the blood of a patient with renal failure. In hemodialysis, blood is removed from the body through a surgically created access site, pumped through a filtration unit to remove toxins, and then returned to the body. The extracorporeal dialyzer works through a combination of osmosis, diffusion, and filtration. (See *How hemodialysis works,* page 372.) By extracting by-products of protein metabolism – notably urea and uric acid – as well as creatinine and excess water, hemodialysis helps restore or maintain acid-base and electrolyte balance and prevent complications associated with uremia.

Hemodialysis can be performed in an emergency in acute renal failure or as chronic long-term therapy in end-stage renal disease. In chronic renal failure, the frequency and duration of treatments depend on the patient's condition. Rarely, hemodialysis is done to treat acute poisoning or drug overdose.

Specially trained nurses usually perform the procedure in a kidney center or satellite unit. Home dialysis, another option, is more convenient for the patient and allows greater flexibility and comfort. However, only 30% of patients needing dialysis meet the medical and training requirements to undergo the procedure at home.

Procedure

Hemodialysis begins with connection of the blood lines from the dialyzer to the needles that have been placed in the venous access site. After all connections have been made, blood samples are drawn for laboratory analysis.

The dialyzer's pump is then switched on, and hemodialysis begins at a blood flow rate of 90 to 120 ml/minute. If heparin is being used to prevent blood coagulation problems, a loading dose of 1,000 to 3,000 units is injected in the port on the arterial line. Blood pressure and vital signs are checked periodically; if stable, the blood flow rate is gradually increased to about 300 ml/minute and maintained at this level for the duration of treatment, unless complications arise. Depending on the pa-

How hemodialysis works

Within the dialyzer, the patient's blood flows between coils, plates, or hollow fibers of semipermeable material, depending on the machine being used. Simultaneously, the dialysis solution—an aqueous solution typically containing low concentrations of sodium, potassium, calcium, magnesium cations, and chloride anions and high concentrations of acetate (which the body readily converts to bicarbonate) and glucose—is pumped around the other side under hydrostatic pressure.

Pressure and concentration gradients between blood and the dialysis solution remove toxic wastes and excess water. Because blood has higher concentrations of hydrogen ions and other electrolytes than dialysis solution, these solutes diffuse across the semipermeable material into the solution. Conversely, glucose and acetate are more highly concentrated in the dialysis solution and so diffuse back across the semipermeable material into the blood. Through this mechanism, hemodialysis removes excess water and toxins, reverses acidosis, and corrects electrolyte imbalances.

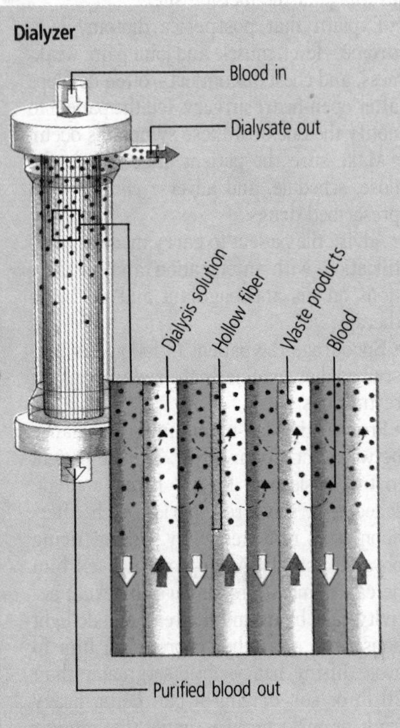

tient's condition, dialysis continues for 3 to 5 hours.

To end the treatment, more blood samples are taken and checked, the blood remaining in the dialyzer is returned to the patient, and the needles are removed from the venous access site.

Complications

Life-threatening complications may occur during or after hemodialysis, such as dialysis disequilibrium syndrome, air embolism, excessive bleeding, infections (sepsis, hepatitis), and acquired immunodeficiency syndrome. More common but less serious complications include hypotension, headache, nausea, malaise, vomiting, dizziness, fever, muscle cramps, and chronic anemia. Complications of chronic hemodialysis include arteriosclerotic cardiovascular disease, congestive heart failure, stroke, gastric ulcers, and bone problems secondary to altered calcium metabolism.

Key nursing diagnoses and patient outcomes

Risk for infection related to regular exposure of the patient's blood to the external environment. Based on this nursing diagnosis, you'll establish these patient outcomes. The patient will:

- understand the signs and symptoms of infection and notify the doctor if they occur
- practice infection control measures daily

• avoid infection, as shown by a normal temperature and white blood cell count and absence of signs and symptoms of infection.

Impaired gas exchange related to altered blood flow during dialysis. Based on this nursing diagnosis, you'll establish these patient outcomes. The patient will:
• maintain arterial blood gas values within the normal range
• avoid signs and symptoms of hypoxia, such as dyspnea, chest pain, cyanosis, and a weak, rapid pulse
• maintain adequate ventilation.

Risk for fluid volume deficit related to rapid fluid removal and electrolyte changes during dialysis. Based on this nursing diagnosis, you'll establish these patient outcomes. The patient will:
• maintain vital signs within the normal range
• avoid signs and symptoms of hypovolemic shock
• maintain an adequate fluid volume throughout dialysis.

Nursing interventions

When caring for a patient who is receiving hemodialysis, your primary responsibilities include instruction and monitoring the patient for complications.

Before the procedure

• If this is the patient's first hemodialysis session, make him understand the purpose of the treatment and what to expect during and after the procedure. Explain that he'll undergo surgery first to create vascular access. (See *Hemodialysis access sites,* page 374.)
• After vascular access has been created and the patient is ready for dialysis, weigh him and take his vital signs. Be sure to measure blood pressure in the nonaccessed arm while he's both in a supine position and standing.
• As ordered, prepare the hemodialysis equipment, following the manufacturer's guidelines and hospital protocol. Maintain strict aseptic technique so as not to introduce pathogens into the patient's bloodstream during treatment.
• Place the patient in a supine position and make him as comfortable as possible. Keep the venous access site well supported and resting on a sterile drape or sterile barrier shield.

During the procedure

• Follow Occupational Safety and Health Administration guidelines by wearing appropriate gloves and protective eye shields throughout the procedure.
• Monitor the patient throughout dialysis. Once every 30 minutes, check and record vital signs to detect possible complications. Fever may indicate infection from pathogens in the dialysate or equipment; notify the doctor, who may prescribe an antipyretic, an antibiotic, or both. Hypotension may indicate hypovolemia or a decreased hematocrit level; give blood or I.V. fluid supplements, as ordered. Rapid respirations may signal hypoxemia; give supplemental oxygen, as ordered.
• Approximately every hour, draw a blood sample for analysis of clotting time. Using the dialyzing unit's bed scale or a portable scale, measure the patient's weight regularly to ensure adequate ultrafiltration during treatment. Also periodically check the dialyzer's blood lines to make sure all connections are secure, and monitor the lines for clotting.
• Assess the patient for headache, muscle twitching, backache, nausea or vomiting, and seizures, which may indicate disequilibrium syndrome caused by rapid fluid removal and electrolyte changes. If this syndrome occurs, notify the doctor immediately; he may reduce the blood flow rate or stop dialysis. Muscle cramps also may result from rapid fluid and electrolyte shifts. As ordered, relieve cramps by injecting 0.9% sodium chloride solution into the venous return line.
• Observe the patient carefully for signs of internal bleeding: apprehension; restless-

Hemodialysis access sites

Hemodialysis requires vascular access. The site and type of access selected will vary, depending on the expected duration of dialysis, the surgeon's preference, and the patient's condition.

Arteriovenous fistula

To create a fistula, the surgeon makes an incision into the patient's wrist, then a small incision in the side of an artery and another in the side of a vein. He sutures the edges of these incisions together to make a common opening 1" to 3" (3 to 7 cm) long.

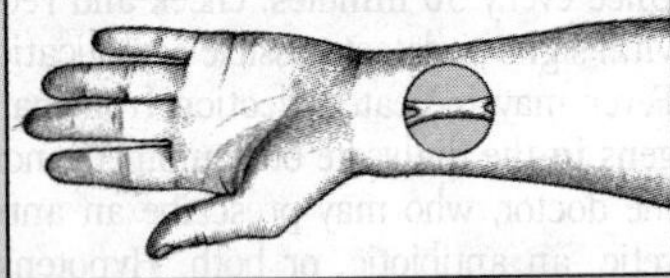

Arteriovenous shunt

To create a shunt, the surgeon makes an incision in the patient's wrist or (rarely) an ankle. He then inserts a 6" to 10" (15.2 to 25.4 cm) transparent Silastic cannula into an artery and another into a vein. Finally, he tunnels the cannulas out through stab wounds and connects them with a short piece of Teflon tubing.

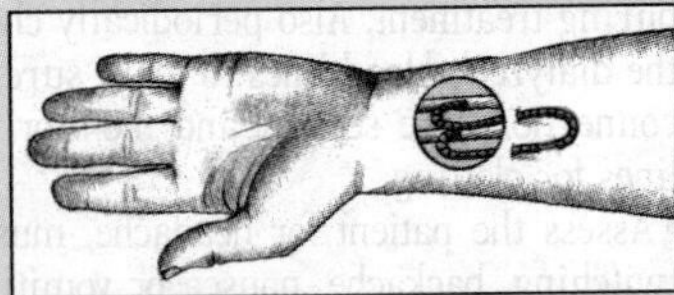

Arteriovenous graft

To create a graft, the surgeon makes an incision in the patient's forearm, upper arm, or thigh. He then tunnels a natural or synthetic graft under the skin and sutures the distal end to an artery and the proximal end to a vein.

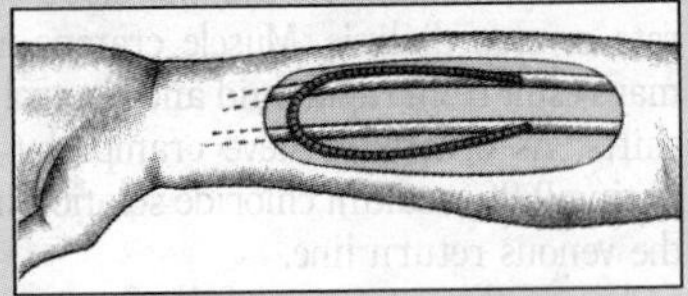

Subclavian vein catheterization

Using the Seldinger technique, the surgeon inserts an introducer needle into the subclavian vein. He then inserts a guide wire through the introducer needle and removes the needle. Using the guide wire, he then threads a 5" to 12" (12.7 to 30.5 cm) plastic or Teflon catheter (with a Y hub) into the vein.

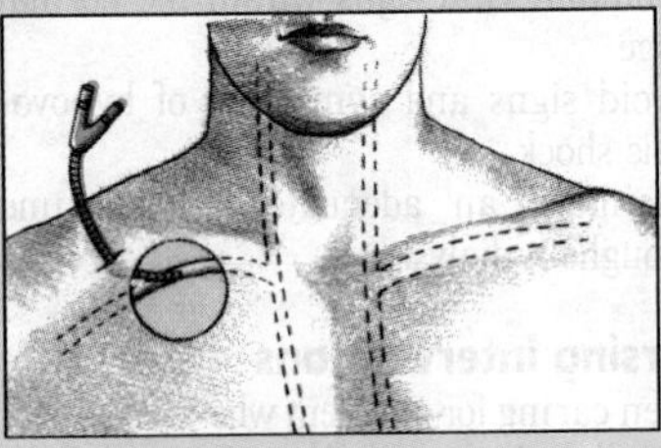

Femoral vein catheterization

Using the Seldinger technique, the surgeon inserts an introducer needle into the left or right femoral vein. He then inserts a guide wire through the introducer needle and removes the needle. Using the guide wire, he threads a 5" to 12" plastic or Teflon catheter into the vein. He may use a single catheter with a Y hub or two catheters, one for inflow and another placed about ½" (1 cm) distal to the first for outflow.

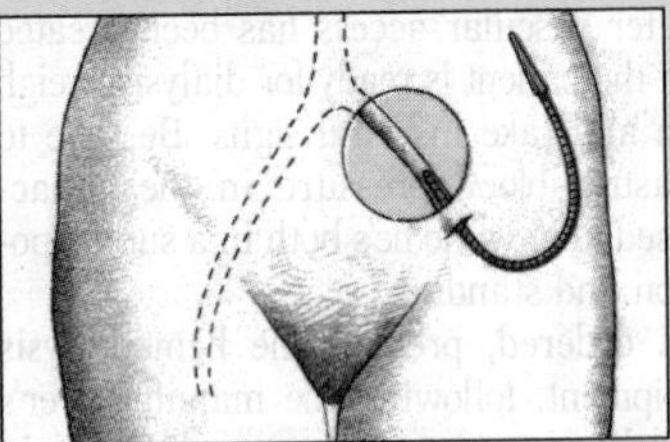

ness; pale, cold, clammy skin; excessive thirst; hypotension; rapid, weak, thready pulse; increased respirations; and decreased body temperature. Report these signs immediately and prepare to decrease heparinization. The doctor also may order blood transfusions.

• Be especially alert for signs of air embolism – a potentially fatal complication characterized by sudden hypotension, dyspnea, chest pain, cyanosis, and a weak, rapid pulse. If these signs develop, turn the patient onto his left side and lower the head of the bed (to help keep air bubbles on the right side of his body, where they can be absorbed by the pulmonary artery); call the doctor immediately.

After the procedure

• Monitor the venous access site for bleeding. If bleeding is excessive, maintain pressure on the site and notify the doctor.

• To prevent clotting and other blood flow problems, make sure the arm used for venous access isn't used for any other procedure, including I.V. line insertion, blood pressure monitoring, and venipuncture. At least four times a day, assess circulation at the access site by auscultating for bruits and palpating for thrills.

• Keep an accurate record of the patient's food and fluid intake, and encourage him to comply with prescribed restrictions, such as limited protein, potassium, and sodium intake; increased caloric intake; and decreased fluid intake.

Home care instructions

• Teach the patient how to care for the venous access site. Tell him to keep the incision clean and dry to prevent infection and to clean it with hydrogen peroxide solution daily until healing is complete and the sutures are removed (usually 10 to 14 days after surgery).

• Tell him to notify the doctor of pain, swelling, redness, or drainage in the accessed arm. Teach him how to use a stethoscope to auscultate for bruits.

• Explain that once the access site has healed, he may use the arm freely. Inform him that exercise is beneficial because it helps stimulate vein enlargement. Remind the patient not to allow any treatments or procedures on the accessed arm, including blood pressure measurement and needle punctures. Also tell him to avoid putting excessive pressure on the arm; for instance, he shouldn't sleep on it, wear constricting clothing, or lift heavy objects. Instruct him to avoid showering, bathing, or swimming for several hours after dialysis.

• Teach him exercises for the affected arm to promote venous dilation and enhance blood flow. Instruct him to perform the following exercise regimen: One week after surgery, squeeze a small rubber ball or other soft object for 15 minutes, four times a day. Two weeks after surgery, apply a tourniquet on the upper arm above the fistula site, making sure it's snug but not tight. With the tourniquet in place, squeeze the rubber ball for 5 minutes; repeat four times daily. After the incision has healed completely, perform the exercise with the arm submerged in warm water.

• If the patient will perform hemodialysis at home, make sure he thoroughly understands all aspects of the procedure. Give him the phone number of the dialysis center and encourage him to call if he has any questions. Also encourage him to arrange for another person to be present during dialysis in case any problems arise.

• Encourage the patient to contact the American Association of Kidney Patients or the National Kidney Foundation for information and support.

Hemophilia

A hereditary bleeding disorder, hemophilia results from deficiency of specific clotting factors. Hemophilia A (classic hemophilia), which affects more than 80% of all hemophiliacs, results from deficiency of factor VIII; hemophilia B (Christmas disease), which affects 15% of hemophiliacs, results from deficiency of factor IX. However, other evidence suggests that hemophilia may actually result from nonfunctioning factors VIII and IX, rather than from their deficiency.

Hemophilia, which is the most common X-linked genetic disease, occurs in about 1.25 per 10,000 live male births.

The severity and prognosis of bleeding disorders vary with the degree of deficiency and the site of bleeding. The overall prognosis is best in mild hemophilia, which doesn't cause spontaneous bleeding and joint deformities. Advances in treatment have greatly improved the prognosis, and many hemophiliacs live normal life spans.

Causes

Hemophilia A and B are inherited as X-linked recessive traits. Therefore, female carriers have a 50% chance of transmitting the gene to each daughter, who would then be a carrier, and a 50% chance of transmitting the gene to each son, who would be born with hemophilia.

Hemophilia produces abnormal bleeding, which may be mild, moderate, or severe, depending on the degree of factor deficiency. After a person with hemophilia forms a platelet plug at a bleeding site, the lack of clotting factors impairs formation of a stable fibrin clot. Immediate hemorrhage isn't prevalent, but delayed bleeding is common.

Complications

Bleeding into joints and muscles causes pain, swelling, extreme tenderness and, possibly, permanent deformity. Bleeding near peripheral nerves may cause peripheral neuropathies, pain, paresthesia, and muscle atrophy. If bleeding impairs blood flow through a major vessel, it can cause ischemia and gangrene. Pharyngeal, lingual, intracardial, intracerebral, and intracranial bleeding may all lead to shock and death.

Assessment

Varying assessment findings depend on the severity of the patient's condition. A patient with undiagnosed hemophilia typically presents with pain and swelling in a weight-bearing joint, such as the hip, knee, and ankle.

Mild hemophilia frequently goes undiagnosed until adulthood because the patient with a mild deficiency doesn't bleed spontaneously or after minor trauma but has prolonged bleeding if challenged by major trauma or surgery. Postoperative bleeding continues as a slow ooze or ceases and starts again, up to 8 days after surgery.

Moderate hemophilia causes symptoms similar to those of severe hemophilia but produces only occasional spontaneous bleeding episodes.

Severe hemophilia causes spontaneous bleeding. Often, the first sign of severe hemophilia is excessive bleeding after circumcision. Later, spontaneous bleeding or severe bleeding after minor trauma may produce large subcutaneous and deep I.M. hematomas.

The patient history may reveal prolonged bleeding after surgery (including dental extractions) or trauma or joint pain if episodes of spontaneous bleeding into muscles or joints have occurred. The history may disclose signs of internal bleeding, such as abdominal, chest, or flank pain, episodes of hematuria or hematemesis, and tarry stools. It should also reveal any activity or movement limitations that the patient has experienced in the past and any need for assistive devices, such as splints, canes, or crutches.

Inspection may reveal hematomas on the extremities or the torso or both and, if bleeding has occurred in joints, joint swelling. Joint range of motion (ROM) may be limited, and the patient may complain of pain when this assessment is done if bleeding has occurred into the joints.

Diagnostic tests

Specific coagulation factor assays can diagnose the type and severity of hemophilia. A positive family history can also help diagnose hemophilia.

Characteristic findings in hemophilia A are:

- factor VIII assay 0% to 25% of normal prolonged activated partial thromboplastin time (APTT)
- normal platelet count and function, bleeding time, and prothrombin time.

Characteristic findings in hemophilia B are:

- deficient factor IX assay
- baseline coagulation results similar to those of hemophilia A, with normal factor VIII.

In hemophilia A or B, the degree of factor deficiency determines severity:

- mild hemophilia – factor levels 5% to 25% of normal
- moderate hemophilia – factor levels 1% to 5% of normal
- severe hemophilia – factor levels less than 1% of normal.

Blood studies are the key diagnostic tool for assessing hemophilia, but additional tests may be ordered periodically to evaluate complications caused by bleeding. For example, a computed tomography scan would be used for suspected intracranial bleeding, arthroscopy or arthrography for certain joint problems, and endoscopy for GI bleeding.

Treatment

Hemophilia is incurable, but treatment can prevent crippling deformities and prolong life. Correct treatment quickly stops bleeding by increasing plasma levels of deficient clotting factors to help prevent disabling deformities that result from repeated bleeding into muscles, joints, and organs.

In hemophilia A, cryoprecipitated antihemophilic factor (AHF), lyophilized AHF, or both, given in doses large enough to raise clotting factor levels above 25% of normal, can permit normal hemostasis. Before surgery, AHF is administered to raise clotting factors to hemostatic levels. Levels are then kept within a normal range until the wound has healed. Fresh-frozen plasma can also be given, but it does have some drawbacks. (See *Reviewing factor replacement products,* page 378.)

Inhibitors to factor VIII develop after multiple transfusions in 10% to 20% of patients with severe hemophilia. This renders the patient resistant to factor VIII infusions. Desmopressin may be given to stimulate the release of stored factor VIII, raising the level in the blood.

In hemophilia B, administration of factor IX concentrate during bleeding episodes increases factor IX levels.

A patient with hemophilia who undergoes surgery needs careful management by a hematologist with expertise in hemophilia care. The patient will require deficient factor replacement before and after surgery. Such replacement may be necessary even for minor surgery, such as a dental extraction. In addition, aminocaproic acid is frequently used for oral bleeding to inhibit the active fibrinolytic system present in the oral mucosa.

Key nursing diagnoses and patient outcomes

Activity intolerance related to bleeding episodes. Based on this nursing diagnosis, you'll establish these patient outcomes. The patient will:

- demonstrate safety precautions while performing activities of daily living
- avoid or seek assistance in performing activities that may cause a bleeding episode
- avoid injury when performing activities.

Altered peripheral tissue perfusion related to impaired blood flow through a ma-

Reviewing factor replacement products

Each of these agents replaces a specific clotting factor.

Cryoprecipitate
- Factor VIII (70 to 100 units/bag); doesn't contain factor IX
- Can be stored frozen for up to 12 months, but must be used within 6 hours after it thaws
- Given through a blood filter; compatible only with 0.9% sodium chloride solution

Lyophilized factor VIII or IX
- Derived from monoclonal antibodies
- May be freeze-dried and labeled with exact units of factor VIII or IX contained in the vial (vials range from 200 to 1,500 units of factor VIII or IX each and contain 20 to 40 ml after reconstitution with diluent); can be stored for 2 years at temperatures ranging from 36° to 46° F (2° to 8° C), or for 6 months at room temperature not exceeding 88° F (31° C)
- No blood filter needed; usually given by slow I.V. push through a butterfly infusion set

Fresh-frozen plasma
- Factor VIII (about 0.75 unit/ml) and factor IX (about 1 unit/ml); impractical for most hemophiliacs because a large volume is needed to raise factors to hemostatic levels; a poor source of factor VIII because freezing the plasma destroys the factor (in contrast, fresh plasma [not frozen] is a good source of factor VIII)
- Can be stored frozen for up to 12 months, but must be used within 2 hours after it thaws
- Given through a blood filter; compatible only with 0.9% sodium chloride solution

jor vessel caused by bleeding. Based on this nursing diagnosis, you'll establish these patient outcomes. The patient will:
- implement measures to stop bleeding or seek medical attention at the first sign of bleeding
- maintain adequate tissue perfusion when bleeding occurs, as shown by a palpable pulse and normal skin color and temperature at and beyond the bleeding site.

Risk for fluid volume deficit related to bleeding. Based on this nursing diagnosis, you'll establish these patient outcomes. The patient will:
- quickly regain or maintain a normal fluid balance during a bleeding episode
- avoid signs and symptoms of fluid volume deficit during or after a bleeding episode.

Nursing interventions

- Provide emotional support, and listen to the patient's fears and concerns. Reassure him when possible. Remember that people who may have been exposed to the human immunodeficiency virus (HIV) through contaminated blood products need special support and infection control.
- If the newly diagnosed patient has difficulty adjusting to his diagnosis, reassure him that his feelings are normal. Point out areas of his life where he can maintain control. Arrange for others with the same problem to speak with the patient and his family.
- Give the patient private time with his family and friends to help overcome feelings of social isolation.

During bleeding episodes:
- If the patient has surface cuts or epistaxis, apply pressure – often the only treatment needed. With deeper cuts, pressure may stop the bleeding temporarily. Cuts deep enough to require suturing may also require factor infusions to prevent further bleeding. (See *Managing bleeding in hemophilia.*)
- Give the deficient clotting factor or plasma, as ordered. The body uses up AHF in 48 to

Managing bleeding in hemophilia

Bleeding in hemophilia may occur spontaneously or stem from an injury. Inform the patient and his family about possible types of bleeding and their associated signs and symptoms. Accordingly, advise them what actions to take and when to call for medical help.

Bleeding site	Signs and symptoms	Interventions
Intracranial	Change in personality or wakefulness (level of consciousness), headache, nausea	Instruct the patient or his family to notify the doctor immediately and treat symptoms as an emergency.
Joints (hemarthroses) Most often affects the knees, followed by elbows, ankles, shoulders, hips, and wrists	Joint pain and swelling, joint tingling and warmth (at onset of hemorrhage)	Tell the patient to begin antihemophilic factor (AHF) infusions and then to notify the doctor.
Muscles	Pain and reduced function of affected muscle; tingling, numbness, or pain in a large area away from the affected site (referred pain)	Urge the patient to notify the doctor and to start an AHF infusion if the patient is reasonably certain that bleeding results from recent injury (otherwise, call the doctor for instructions).
Subcutaneous tissue or skin	Pain, bruising, and swelling at the site (delayed oozing may also occur after an injury)	Show the patient how to apply appropriate topical agents, such as ice packs or absorbable gelatin sponges (Gelfoam), to stop bleeding.
Kidney	Pain in the lower back near the waist, decreased urine output	Instruct the patient to notify the doctor and to start AHF infusion if bleeding results from a known recent injury.
Heart (cardiac tamponade)	Chest tightness, shortness of breath, swelling (usually occurs in patients who are very young or who have severe disease)	Instruct the patient to contact the doctor or to go to the nearest emergency department at once.

72 hours, so repeat infusions, as ordered, until the bleeding stops.

• Apply cold compresses or ice bags and raise the injured part.

• To prevent recurrence of bleeding, restrict activity for 48 hours after bleeding is under control.

• Control pain with an analgesic, such as acetaminophen, propoxyphene, codeine, or meperidine, as ordered. Avoid I.M. injections because they may cause hematoma formation at the injection site. Aspirin and aspirin-containing medications are con-

traindicated because they decrease platelet adherence and may increase the bleeding.
• If the patient can't tolerate activities because of blood loss, provide rest periods between activities.

If the patient has bled into a joint:
• Immediately elevate the joint.
• To restore joint mobility, if ordered, begin ROM exercises at least 48 hours after the bleeding is controlled. Tell the patient to avoid weight bearing until bleeding stops and swelling subsides.
• Administer analgesics for the pain associated with hemarthrosis. Also, apply ice packs and elastic bandages to alleviate the pain.

Monitoring

• Watch for signs and symptoms of decreased tissue perfusion, such as restlessness, anxiety, confusion, pallor, cool and clammy skin, chest pain, decreased urine output, hypotension, and tachycardia. Monitor the patient's blood pressure and pulse and respiratory rates. Observe him frequently for bleeding from the skin, mucous membranes, and wounds.
• During bleeding episodes, assess the patient for adverse reactions to blood products, such as flushing, headache, tingling, fever, chills, urticaria, and anaphylaxis.
• After a bleeding episode or surgery, watch closely for signs and symptoms of further bleeding, such as increased pain and swelling, fever, and evidence of shock. Closely monitor the patient's laboratory values, particularly his APTT.

Patient teaching

• Teach the patient the benefits of regular exercise. Explain that strong muscles help protect the joints and that this, in turn, reduces the incidence of hemarthrosis. Instruct him to perform isometric exercises, which can also help prevent muscle weakness and recurrent joint bleeding.
• Advise parents to protect their child from injury while avoiding unnecessary restrictions that impair his normal development. For example, for a toddler, padded patches can be sewn into the knees and elbows of clothing to protect these joints during frequent falls. An older child must be prevented from joining in contact sports, such as football, but he can be encouraged to swim or to play golf.
• Tell the patient to avoid such activities as heavy lifting and using power tools because they increase the risk of injury that can result in serious bleeding problems.
• If an injury occurs, direct the parents to apply cold compresses or ice bags and elevate the injured part or to apply light pressure to the bleeding. To prevent recurrence of bleeding after treatment, instruct the parents to restrict the child's activity for 48 hours after bleeding is under control.
• Advise the parents to notify the doctor immediately after even a minor injury, especially to the head, neck, or abdomen. Such injuries may require special blood factor replacement.
• Instruct parents to watch for signs of internal bleeding, such as severe pain or swelling in a joint or muscles, stiffness, decreased joint movement, severe abdominal pain, blood in urine, tarry stools, and severe headache.
• Explain to the patient and, if appropriate, his parents the importance of avoiding aspirin, combination medications that contain aspirin, and over-the-counter (OTC) anti-inflammatory agents, such as ibuprofen compounds. Teach the patient and his parents how to recognize OTC medications that contain aspirin. Tell them to use acetaminophen instead.
• Stress the importance of good dental care, including regular, careful toothbrushing to prevent the need for dental surgery. Have the child use a soft toothbrush to avoid gum injury. Emphasize that poor dental hygiene can lead to bleeding from inflamed gums.
• Tell the parents to check with the doctor before allowing dental extractions or any other surgery. Advise them to get the

names of other doctors they can contact in case their regular doctor isn't available.
• Teach the patient the importance of protecting his veins for lifelong therapy.
• As necessary, encourage the patient to remain independent and be self-sufficient. Refer him for counseling as necessary.
• Tell the parents to make sure the child wears a medical identification bracelet at all times.
• Refer new patients to a hemophilia treatment center for evaluation. The center will devise a treatment plan for such patients' primary doctors and is a resource for other medical and school personnel, dentists, or others involved in their care. Explain that these centers also offer carrier testing, prenatal diagnosis, and other genetic counseling services.

For patients receiving blood components:
• Train the parents to administer blood factor components at home to avoid frequent hospitalization. Teach them proper venipuncture and infusion techniques, and urge them not to delay treatment during bleeding episodes. Tell parents to keep blood factor concentrate and infusion equipment available at all times, even on vacation.
• Review possible adverse reactions, such as blood-borne infection and factor inhibitor development, that can result from replacement factor procedures.
• If the patient develops flushing, headache, or tingling from replacement factors, inform him or his parents that these reactions occur most often with freeze-dried concentrate. Slowing the infusion rate may cause symptoms to abate.
• If fever and chills occur, indicating an allergy to white blood cell antigens, instruct the patient or his parents that this reaction occurs most often with plasma infusions. Acetaminophen may relieve the patient's discomfort.
• Tell the patient that urticaria is the most common reaction to cryoprecipitate or plasma. This hypersensitivity sign results from an allergy to a plasma protein. The wheals usually subside after administration of diphenhydramine or another antihistamine. Ideally, the patient who develops urticaria frequently should receive an antihistamine about 45 minutes before a clotting factor infusion.
• Review the signs and symptoms of anaphylaxis: rapid or difficult breathing, wheezing, hoarseness, stridor, and chest tightness. (The same plasma proteins that cause urticaria may cause anaphylaxis.) Teach the patient to administer epinephrine and then to contact the doctor at once.
• Tell the patient or the parents to watch for early signs of hepatitis: headache, fever, decreased appetite, nausea, vomiting, abdominal tenderness, and pain over the liver. Explain that the patient who receives blood components risks hepatitis, which may appear 3 weeks to 6 months after treatment with blood components.
• Inform the patient that all donated blood and plasma are screened for antibodies to HIV, which causes acquired immunodeficiency syndrome. Also, all freeze-dried products are heat-treated to kill HIV.
• For more information, refer the patient and his family to the National Hemophilia Foundation.

Hemorrhoidectomy

In hemorrhoidectomy, the surgeon removes hemorrhoidal varicosities through cauterization or excision. The most effective treatment for intolerable hemorrhoidal pain, excessive bleeding, or large prolapse, it's used when diet, drugs, sitz baths, and compresses fail to provide symptomatic relief.

Procedure

After administering a local anesthetic, the surgeon digitally dilates the rectal sphincter. He then removes the hemorrhoidal var-

Ligating hemorrhoidal tissue

Removal of large internal hemorrhoids often requires ligation. In this surgical technique, the doctor inserts an anoscope to dilate the rectal sphincter, then uses grasping forceps to pull the hemorrhoid into position. He then inserts a ligator through the anoscope and slips a small rubber band over the pedicle of the hemorrhoid to bind it and cut off blood flow. Next, he excises the hemorrhoid or allows it to slough off naturally, which usually occurs within 5 to 7 days.

Grasping the hemorrhoid

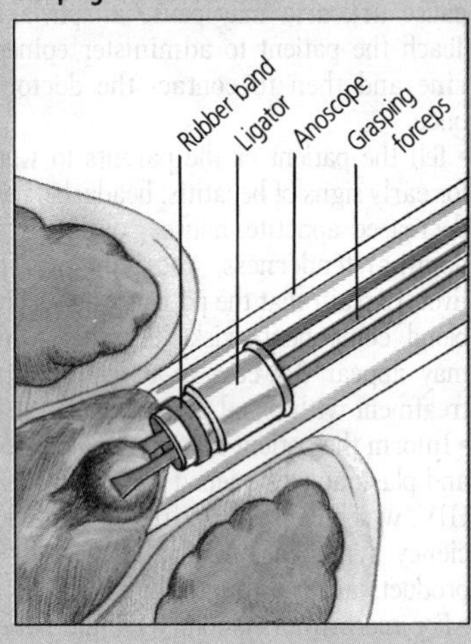

Ligating the hemorrhoid

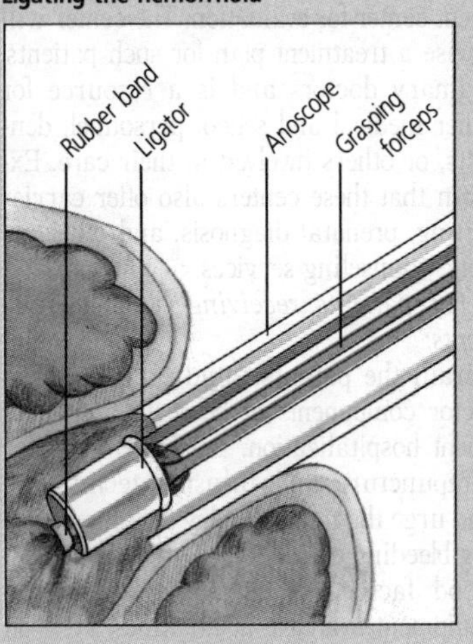

icosities, either by clamping and cauterization or by ligation and excision. (See *Ligating hemorrhoidal tissue.*) He may place a small, lubricated tube in the patient's anus to drain fluid, blood, and flatus, or he may elect to pack the area with petroleum gauze.

Complications

A relatively quick and simple surgery, hemorrhoidectomy carries only one potentially serious complication: hemorrhage due to the rich vascularity of the region that could be severe enough to cause hypovolemic shock. This risk is greatest during the first 24 hours after surgery and then again after 7 to 10 days when the sutures slough off. Because of this risk, hemorrhoidectomy is contraindicated in patients with blood dyscrasias or certain GI cancers, or during the first trimester of pregnancy.

Key nursing diagnoses and patient outcomes

Risk for infection related to normal bacterial flora at the surgical site. Based on this nursing diagnosis, you'll establish these patient outcomes. The patient will:

- maintain a normal temperature and white blood cell count
- maintain a clean surgical site with no purulent drainage
- avoid excessive postoperative anal pain and tenderness.

Risk for fluid volume deficit related to hemorrhage caused by excision of highly vascular hemorrhoidal tissue. Based on this nursing diagnosis, you'll establish these patient outcomes. The patient will:
• maintain normal vital signs
• avoid excessive bleeding, as shown by a dry perianal dressing
• maintain a normal fluid volume balance.

Pain related to hemorrhoidectomy. The patient will:
• express pain relief after analgesic administration
• participate in diversional activities to minimize pain
• report a decrease in pain 24 hours after surgery and complete pain relief after healing occurs.

Nursing interventions

With a hemorrhoidectomy patient, your major roles are preparing the patient for surgery, monitoring his progress after surgery, and preparing him for discharge.

Before surgery

• Tell the patient that this operation will remove his hemorrhoids and relieve pain and bleeding.
• Explain the details of postoperative care, including frequent dressing changes and regular perianal cleansing. Reassure him that the nursing staff will respect his need for privacy as much as possible during these procedures.
• Prepare the patient for surgery by administering an enema (usually 2 to 4 hours before surgery). Check the institution's policy for shaving and cleaning the perianal area.
• Ensure that the patient or a responsible family member has signed a consent form.

After surgery

• Position the patient comfortably in bed; support his buttocks with pillows, if necessary. Encourage him to shift his position regularly and to assume a prone position for 15 minutes every few hours to reduce edema at the surgical site.
• Keep alert for acute hemorrhage and hypovolemic shock. Monitor vital signs every 2 to 4 hours, check and record intake and output, and assess for signs of fluid volume deficit, such as poor skin turgor, dry mucous membranes, and feelings of faintness, weakness, and confusion.
• Check the dressing regularly, and immediately report any excessive bleeding or drainage. If bleeding is excessive, you may be asked to insert a balloon-tipped catheter into the rectum and inflate it to exert pressure on the hemorrhagic area and reduce blood loss.
• Ensure that the patient voids within the first 24 hours after surgery. If necessary, help stimulate voiding with measures such as massages and warm sitz baths; catheterize him only if other measures fail to induce urination.
• Using warm water and a mild soap, clean the perianal area to prevent infection and irritation. Gently pat the area dry. Apply a wet dressing (a 1:1 solution of cold water and witch hazel) or a commercially available product to the perianal area.
• As needed, provide analgesics and sitz baths or warm compresses to reduce local pain, swelling, and inflammation and to prevent rectoanal spasms.
• As soon as the patient can resume oral feeding, administer a bulk-forming or stool-softening laxative, as ordered, to ease defecation. Explain that he needs to pass stools shortly after surgery to dilate the anus and prevent the formation of strictures from scar tissue during wound healing. If he experiences pain during defecation, administer analgesics, as ordered.

Home care instructions

• Before discharge, teach the patient proper perianal hygiene: wiping gently with soft, white toilet paper (the dyes used in colored paper may cause irritation); cleaning with mild soap and warm water; and applying a sanitary pad.

- Encourage the patient to take sitz baths three to four times daily and after each bowel movement to reduce swelling and discomfort.
- Instruct the patient to report increased rectal bleeding, purulent drainage, fever, constipation, or rectal spasm.
- Stress the importance of regular bowel habits. Provide tips on avoiding constipation, including regular exercise and adequate intake of dietary fiber and fluids (8 to 10 glasses of water a day).
- Warn against overusing stool-softening laxatives. Explain that a firm stool is necessary to dilate the anal canal and prevent stricture formation.

Hemorrhoids

Often painful, hemorrhoids are varicosities in the superior or inferior hemorrhoidal venous plexus. Dilation and enlargement of the superior plexus produce mucosa-covered, internal hemorrhoids that bulge into the rectal lumen and may prolapse during defecation. Dilation and enlargement of the inferior plexus produce skin-covered, external hemorrhoids that may protrude from the rectum. External hemorrhoids are more likely to be thrombotic than internal hemorrhoids. Generally, the incidence of hemorrhoids peaks between ages 20 and 50 and affects both sexes.

Causes

Hemorrhoids probably result from increased intravenous pressure in the hemorrhoidal plexus. Predisposing factors include occupations that require prolonged standing or sitting; straining due to constipation, diarrhea, coughing, sneezing, or vomiting; heart failure; hepatic disease, such as cirrhosis, amoebic abscesses, or hepatitis; alcoholism; anorectal infections; loss of muscle tone due to old age, rectal surgery, or episiotomy; anal intercourse; and pregnancy.

Complications

Local infection or thrombosis of hemorrhoids may occur. Rarely, hemorrhoids cause severe or recurrent bleeding, leading to secondary anemia with significant pallor, fatigue, and weakness.

Assessment

Typically, the patient notices and reports intermittent rectal bleeding after defecation. He may report bright red blood on his stools or toilet paper – a sign that the fragile mucosa covering the hemorrhoid was injured during defecation. He also may complain of anal itching (the result of poor anal hygiene) or describe a vague feeling of anal discomfort when bleeding occurs.

If the hemorrhoids are thrombosed, the patient usually complains of rectal pain, which may be accompanied by anal pruritus and mucus discharge. If external hemorrhoids are thrombosed, he may be aware of a large subcutaneous lump in the anal area.

Inspection of the anal area confirms the presence of external hemorrhoids. If the external hemorrhoids are thrombosed, they appear on inspection as blue swellings at the anus. Although internal hemorrhoids usually aren't seen on inspection, they will be obvious if they have prolapsed.

Palpation reveals anal tenderness. Digital rectal examination may detect internal hemorrhoids.

Diagnostic tests

Anoscopy and flexible sigmoidoscopy confirm internal hemorrhoids and rule out other possible causes of symptoms, such as rectal polyps or anal fistulas.

Treatment

Hemorrhoids generally require only conservative treatment, designed to ease pain, combat swelling and congestion, and regulate bowel habits. To reduce local pain and swelling, local anesthetic agents (lotions, creams, or suppositories), astringents, or cold compresses may be applied, followed by warm sitz baths or thermal packs. A steroid preparation, such as hydrocortisone, can relieve itching or inflammation.

Stool softeners help prevent straining during defecation. If the patient has a mildly prolapsed internal hemorrhoid, manual reduction may be attempted. Rarely, the patient with chronic, profuse bleeding may require a blood transfusion.

Several procedures also may be used to treat hemorrhoids. A sclerosing solution may be injected to induce scar formation and decrease prolapse. Other surgical techniques are cryosurgery, hemorrhoidectomy, and ligation. Cryosurgery uses a probe to freeze the hemorrhoid, causing necrosis. Although the procedure may be performed on an outpatient basis, it isn't widely used because it causes foul-smelling, profuse drainage and large, painful skin tags.

Hemorrhoidectomy, the most effective treatment, is indicated for patients with severe bleeding, intolerable pain, pruritus, and large prolapse. This surgery, which removes the hemorrhoid through cauterization or excision, can now be performed on an outpatient basis.

Key nursing diagnoses and patient outcomes

Constipation related to avoiding painful defecation. Based on this nursing diagnosis, you'll establish these patient outcomes. The patient will:

- express an understanding of how hemorrhoids relate to constipation
- take measures to prevent constipation
- not become constipated.

Risk for infection related to tearing of the outer hemorrhoid covering during defecation. Based on this nursing diagnosis, you'll establish these patient outcomes. The patient will:

- take measures to prevent tearing of the hemorrhoid covering, such as avoiding constipation and not straining during defecation
- not have signs and symptoms of anal infection, such as foul-smelling anal drainage and pain.

Pain related to a thrombosed hemorrhoid. Based on this nursing diagnosis, you'll establish these patient outcomes. The patient will:

- use measures to minimize or alleviate anal pain
- express pain relief after receiving a local anesthetic or using a nonpharmacologic measure, such as cold compresses or a warm sitz bath.

Nursing interventions

- Administer local anesthetics as prescribed.
- As needed, provide warm sitz baths or cold compresses to reduce local pain, swelling, and inflammation.
- Provide the patient with a high-fiber diet and encourage adequate fluid intake and exercise to prevent constipation.
- Prepare the patient for a hemorrhoidectomy, if indicated. (See the entry "Hemorrhoidectomy.")

Monitoring

- Monitor the patient's pain level and the effectiveness of the prescribed medication.
- Check for signs and symptoms of anal infection, such as increased pain and foul-smelling anal drainage.
- Assess the patient for constipation.

Patient teaching

- Teach the patient about hemorrhoidal development, predisposing factors, and tests.
- If conservative treatment is ordered, teach the patient measures to relieve hemorrhoidal discomfort. Suggest that he apply cold packs to the anorectal region for 3 to 4 hours at the onset of pain, followed by warm sitz baths. Recommend nonprescription remedies, such as witch hazel

soaks or dibucaine ointment. Advise him to use dibucaine ointment only temporarily; if his pain continues for more than 5 days, he must notify the doctor. Point out that this ointment may mask worsening symptoms and cause him to delay seeking attention for a more serious disorder.
• Encourage the patient to eat a high-fiber diet to promote regular bowel movements. Advise him to increase the amount of raw vegetables, fruits, and whole grain cereals in his diet. To avoid venous congestion, remind him not to sit on the toilet longer than necessary.
• Emphasize the need for good anal hygiene. Caution against vigorous wiping with washcloths and using harsh soaps. Encourage the use of medicated astringent pads and toilet paper made without dyes or perfumes.

Hemothorax

This disorder occurs when blood enters the pleural cavity – from damaged intercostal, pleural, or mediastinal vessels (or occasionally from the lung's parenchymal vessels). Depending on the amount of blood and the underlying cause of bleeding, hemothorax can cause varying degrees of lung collapse. About 25% of patients with chest trauma (blunt or penetrating) experience hemothorax. Pneumothorax (air in the pleural cavity) commonly accompanies hemothorax.

Causes

Hemothorax usually results from either blunt or penetrating chest trauma. Less often, it occurs because of thoracic surgery, pulmonary infarction, neoplasm, dissecting thoracic aneurysm, or anticoagulant therapy.

Complications

Hemothorax may result in mediastinal shift, ventilatory compromise, lung collapse and, without successful intervention, cardiopulmonary arrest.

Assessment

The patient history typically reflects recent trauma. In addition, the patient may complain of chest pain and sudden difficulty breathing, which may be mild to severe, depending on the amount of blood in the pleural cavity.

Inspection typically discloses a patient with tachypnea, dusky skin color, diaphoresis, and hemoptysis (bloody, frothy sputum). If hemothorax progresses to respiratory failure, the patient may show restlessness, anxiety, cyanosis, and stupor. As the chest rises and falls, you may notice that the affected side may expand and stiffen; the unaffected side may rise with the patient's gasping respirations.

Percussion may disclose dullness over the affected side of the chest; auscultation may detect decreased or absent breath sounds over the affected side, tachycardia, and hypotension.

Diagnostic tests

• *Thoracentesis* performed for diagnosis and therapy may yield blood or serosanguineous fluid. Fluid specimens may be sent to the laboratory for analysis.
• *Chest X-rays* display pleural fluid and detect mediastinal shift.
• *Arterial blood gas (ABG) analysis* documents respiratory failure.
• *Hemoglobin levels* may be decreased, depending on blood loss.

Treatment

In hemothorax, treatment aims to stabilize the patient's condition, stop the bleeding, evacuate blood from the pleural cavity, and reexpand the affected lung. Mild hemothorax usually clears in 10 to 14 days, requiring only observation for further bleeding. In severe hemothorax, treatment includes thoracentesis to remove blood and other fluids from the pleural cavity and then insertion of a chest tube into the sixth intercostal space in the posterior axillary line. The diameter of a typical chest tube is large to prevent clots from blocking it. Suction may also be used. If the chest tube isn't effective, the surgeon may need to perform a thoracotomy to evacuate blood and clots and control bleeding.

With symptomatic anemia (usually hemoglobin level below 9 and hematocrit under 27%), analogous blood transfusion may be given. Autotransfusion may be considered if the patient is unable or unwilling to receive donor blood. (See *Understanding autotransfusion,* page 388.)

Other treatment measures include oxygen therapy, I.V. therapy to restore fluid volume, and administration of analgesics.

Key nursing diagnoses and patient outcomes

Altered cerebral tissue perfusion related to hypotension. Based on this nursing diagnosis, you'll establish these patient outcomes. The patient will:

- avoid permanent neurologic deficit caused by altered cerebral tissue perfusion
- remain awake, alert, and oriented to time, person, and place
- regain and maintain normal blood pressure.

Anxiety related to situational crisis. Based on this nursing diagnosis, you'll establish these patient outcomes. The patient will:

- identify sources of his anxiety and express his feelings of anxiety
- use available support systems to help cope with his anxiety
- report fewer physical symptoms related to anxiety.

Impaired gas exchange related to lung dysfunction. Based on this nursing diagnosis, you'll establish these patient outcomes. The patient will:

- quickly regain normal lung function with emergency treatment
- maintain adequate gas exchange after treatment, shown by normal ABG values and lack of signs and symptoms of hypoxia
- exhibit nonlabored respirations, as shown by equal rise and fall of the chest wall with inspiration and expiration.

Nursing interventions

- Listen to the patient's fears and concerns and offer reassurance. Stay with him during periods of stress and anxiety. Encourage him to identify actions and care measures that promote comfort and relaxation. Perform these measures and encourage the patient and his family to do so also. Include the patient and his family in care-related decisions whenever possible.
- As ordered, give oxygen by face mask or nasal cannula.
- Administer blood transfusions, as ordered, using a large-bore needle.
- To correct shock, give I.V. fluids and blood transfusions, as ordered. Use a central venous pressure line to monitor treatment progress.
- Give pain medication, as ordered, and record its effectiveness.
- Assist with thoracentesis, as indicated. (See the entry "Thoracentesis.")
- Assist with chest tube insertion and provide appropriate care of tube. (See the entry "Chest drainage.")
- Prepare the patient for surgery, as indicated.

Monitoring

- Check the patient's ABG values often. Also monitor hemoglobin levels and hematocrit, white blood cell count, and coagulation studies to determine blood replacement needs.
- Watch for complications signaled by pallor and gasping respirations.
- Monitor the patient's vital signs diligently. Watch for increasing pulse and respiratory rates and falling blood pressure, which may indicate shock or massive bleeding.
- Monitor chest tube drainage. Immediately report a chest tube that's warm and full of blood and a rapidly rising, bloody

Understanding autotransfusion

Used most often in patients with chest wounds—especially those that involve hemothorax—autotransfusion collects, filters, and reinfuses a patient's own blood. The procedure may also be used when two or three units of pooled blood can be recovered—for example, in cardiac or orthopedic surgery.

Autotransfusion eliminates the patient's risk for transfusion reaction or blood-borne disease and is contraindicated in patients with sepsis or cancer.

How autotransfusion works

A large-bore chest tube connected to a closed drainage system is used to collect the patient's blood from a wound or chest cavity. This blood passes through a filter, which catches most potential thrombi, including clumps of fibrin and damaged red blood cells (RBCs). The filtered blood passes into a collection bag. From the bag, the blood is reinfused immediately, or it is processed in a commercial cell washer that reduces anticoagulated whole blood to washed RBCs for later infusion.

A continuous autotransfusion system is available, in which there is no bag and the blood is taken directly out of the drainage system and pumped intravenously directly into the patient's vein.

Assisting with autotransfusion

- Set up the blood collection system as you would any closed chest drainage system. Follow the manufacturer's instructions for attaching the collection bag.
- If ordered, inject an anticoagulant (heparin or acid-citrate-dextrose solution) into the self-sealing port on the connector of the patient's drainage tubing.
- During reinfusion, monitor the patient for complications, such as blood clotting, hemolysis, coagulopathies, thrombocytopenia, particulate and air emboli, sepsis, and citrate toxicity (from the acid-citrate-dextrose solution).

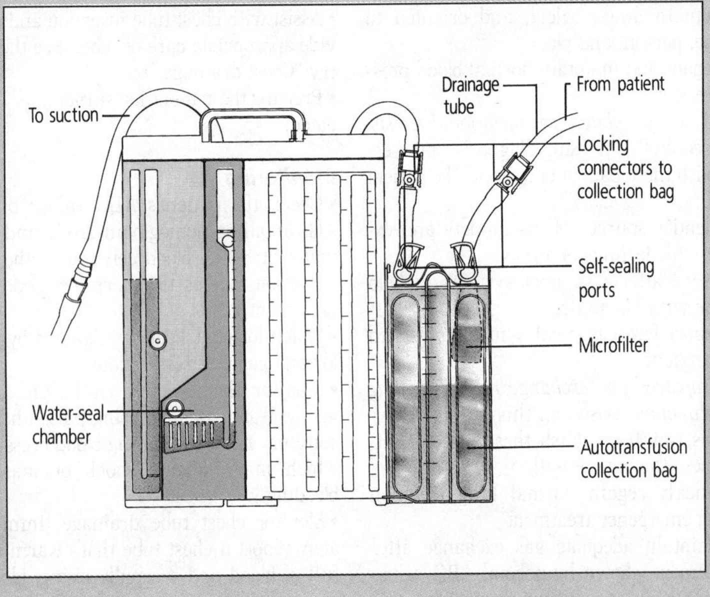

fluid level in the drainage collection chamber. The patient may need emergency surgery.

Patient teaching

- Explain all procedures to the patient and his family to allay their fears. Encourage the patient to ask questions about his care. Answer all questions as honestly as you can.
- If appropriate, provide preoperative and postoperative teaching. Explain and prepare the patient and his family for mechanical ventilation if necessary.
- Encourage the patient to perform deep-breathing exercises every hour whenever he's awake to promote gas exchange.
- Instruct the patient not to cough during thoracentesis.
- Discuss the rationale for chest tube therapy with the patient and his family.

Hepatic encephalopathy

A neurologic syndrome, hepatic encephalopathy (hepatic coma, portal-systemic encephalopathy) develops as a complication of aggressive fulminant hepatitis or chronic hepatic disease. Most common in patients with cirrhosis, this syndrome may be acute and self-limiting or chronic and progressive. In advanced stages, the prognosis is extremely poor despite vigorous treatment.

Causes

Most experts attribute this syndrome to ammonia intoxication of the brain, but the precise etiology is unknown. Normally, the ammonia produced by protein breakdown in the bowel is metabolized to urea in the liver. When portal blood shunts past the liver, ammonia directly enters the systemic circulation and is carried to the brain. Such shunting may result from the collateral venous circulation that develops in portal hypertension or from surgically created portal-systemic shunts. Cirrhosis further compounds this problem because impaired hepatocellular function prevents conversion of ammonia that reaches the liver.

Other factors that may lead to rising ammonia levels include excessive protein intake, sepsis, excessive accumulation of nitrogenous body wastes (from constipation or GI hemorrhage), and bacterial action on protein and urea to form ammonia.

Certain other factors heighten the brain's sensitivity to ammonia intoxication: fluid and electrolyte imbalance (especially metabolic alkalosis), hypoxia, azotemia, impaired glucose metabolism, infection, and administration of sedatives, narcotics, and general anesthetics.

Complications

Hepatic encephalopathy can lead to irreversible coma and death.

Assessment

Clinical features vary, depending on the severity of neurologic involvement. The disorder usually progresses through four stages, but the patient's symptoms can fluctuate from one stage to another.

In the *prodromal stage,* early symptoms are typically overlooked because they're so subtle. The patient's history, obtained from the patient or from a family member or caregiver, may reveal slight personality changes, such as agitation, belligerence, disorientation, or forgetfulness. The patient may also have trouble concentrating or thinking clearly. He may report feeling fatigued or drowsy. He may have slurred or slowed speech. On inspection, you may observe a slight tremor.

In the *impending stage,* the patient undergoes continuing mental changes. He may be confused and disoriented as to time, place, and person. Inspection continues to reveal tremor that has progressed to asterixis (liver flap, flapping tremor). The hallmark of hepatic encephalopathy, asterixis refers to quick, irregular extensions and flexions of the wrists and fingers, when the wrists are held out straight and the hands flexed upward. On inspection, you may observe lethargy and aberrant behavior. Some patients demonstrate apraxia. When asked, the patient can't reproduce a simple design, such as a star.

In the *stuporous stage,* the patient shows marked mental confusion. On inspection, he appears drowsy and stuporous. Yet he can still be aroused and is often noisy and abusive when aroused. Hyperventilation, muscle twitching, and asterixis are also evident.

In the *comatose stage,* the patient can't be aroused and is obtunded with no asterixis. Seizures, though uncommon, may occur. Palpation may reveal hyperactive reflexes and demonstrate a positive Babinski's sign. The patient often has fetor hepaticus (musty odor of the breath and urine). Fetor hepaticus may occur in other stages also. Eventually this stage progresses to coma; it's usually fatal.

Diagnostic tests

- *Serum ammonia levels in venous and arterial samples* are elevated and, together with characteristic clinical features, highly suggest hepatic encephalopathy.
- *EEG* shows slowing waves as the disease progresses.

Treatment

Therapy aims to eliminate the underlying cause of the disorder and lower serum ammonia levels to stop progression of encephalopathy. In mild cases, treating the underlying cause of the encephalopathy may reverse the symptoms. In most patients, though, the toxic products, often ammonia, must also be eliminated from the body.

Treatments to eliminate ammonia from the GI tract include administration of neomycin to suppress bacterial flora (preventing them from converting amino acids into ammonia); sorbitol-induced catharsis to produce osmotic diarrhea; continuous aspiration of blood from the stomach; reduction of dietary protein intake; and administration of lactulose to reduce serum ammonia levels.

Lactulose traps ammonia in the bowel and promotes its excretion. It's effective because bacterial enzymes change lactulose to lactic acid, thereby rendering the colon too acidic for bacterial growth. At the same time, the resulting increase in free hydrogen ions prevents diffusion of ammonia through the mucosa; lactulose promotes conversion of systemically absorbable ammonia to ammonium, which is poorly absorbed and can be excreted. Lactulose syrup may be given orally. In acute hepatic coma, lactulose may be administered by retention enema. Lactulose therapy requires careful monitoring of fluid and electrolyte balance.

Neomycin can be administered orally or by retention enema. Although neomycin is nonabsorbable at recommended dosages of 3 to 4 g/day, an amount that exceeds 4 g/day may produce irreversible hearing loss and nephrotoxicity.

Treatment may also include potassium supplements (80 to 120 mEq/day, given orally or I.V.) to correct alkalosis (from increased ammonia levels), especially if the patient is taking diuretics. Salt-poor albumin may be used to maintain fluid and electrolyte balance, replace depleted albumin levels, and restore plasma.

Other treatments that have been tried, usually with little success, are hemodialysis and exchange transfusions.

Key nursing diagnoses and patient outcomes

Altered thought processes related to neurologic dysfunction. Based on this nursing diagnosis, you'll establish these patient outcomes. The patient will:

- remain safe and protected in his environment
- be observed by a family member or caregiver for signs of confusion

• comply with prescribed treatments to prevent further mental deterioration.

Risk for injury related to impaired cerebral function. Based on this nursing diagnosis, you'll establish these patient outcomes. The patient will:
• be observed by a family member or caregiver to ensure his safety when he's confused or combative
• avoid injury caused by mental changes.

Risk for caregiver role strain related to constant patient care requirements. Based on this nursing diagnosis, you'll establish these outcomes. The caregiver will:
• report any signs and symptoms of excessive stress resulting from patient care demands
• seek assistance from family or community resources to help provide care for the patient
• avoid undue stress.

Nursing interventions

• Continually orient the patient to place and time. Remember to keep a daily record of the patient's handwriting to monitor the progression of neurologic involvement.
• Promote rest, comfort, and a quiet atmosphere. Instruct the patient to avoid stressful exercise.
• Administer medications, as ordered.
• Ask the dietary department to provide the specified low-protein diet, with carbohydrates supplying most of the calories. Provide good mouth care. As ordered, provide parenteral nutrition to the semicomatose or comatose patient.
• Use appropriate safety measures to protect the patient from injury. Avoid physical restraints, if possible.
• Don't give the semicomatose or comatose patient sedatives because they deepen the coma. Protect the comatose patient's eyes from corneal injury by using artificial tears or eye patches.
• Provide emotional support for the patient's family in the terminal stage of encephalopathy.

Monitoring

• Frequently assess and record the patient's level of consciousness.
• Monitor the patient's intake, output, and fluid and electrolyte balance. Check his weight and measure abdominal girth daily.
• Watch for and immediately report laboratory indicators or clinical signs of anemia (decreased hemoglobin level), alkalosis (increased serum bicarbonate), GI bleeding (melena, hematemesis), and infection. Monitor the patient's serum ammonia level for signs of improvement.
• Assess the patient for the desired effects of medication and watch for adverse reactions.

Patient teaching

• Teach the patient, if he still can understand, and his family about the disease and its treatment. Repeat explanations of each treatment before you perform it. Be sure to explain all procedures even if the patient is comatose.
• If the patient has chronic encephalopathy, be sure he and his family understand the mental and physical effects that the illness will eventually have on the patient. Alert them to signs of complications or worsening symptoms. Advise them when to notify the doctor.
• As the patient begins to recover, inform him about the low-protein diet. Emphasize that recovery from so severe an illness takes time. Review how to use medications.

Hepatitis

A fairly common systemic disease, viral hepatitis is marked by hepatic cell destruction, necrosis, and autolysis, leading to anorexia, jaundice, and hepatomegaly. In most patients, hepatic cells eventually regenerate with little or no residual damage, allowing ready recovery. However, old age and serious underlying disorders make complications more likely. The prognosis is poor if edema and hepatic encephalopathy develop.

More than 70,000 cases are reported annually in the United States. Today, five types of viral hepatitis are recognized:

- *Type A* (infectious or short-incubation hepatitis). The incidence of this type is rising among homosexuals and in persons with immunosuppression related to human immunodeficiency virus (HIV) infection.
- *Type B* (serum or long-incubation hepatitis). In moderate prevalence areas, the lifetime risk of becoming infected is 20% to 60%; infections occur in patients of all age groups.
- *Type C.* This type accounts for about 20% of all viral hepatitis and for most posttransfusion hepatitis cases.
- *Type D* (also called delta hepatitis). This type is responsible for most cases of fulminant hepatitis, which has an extremely high mortality rate. In the United States, type D is associated with transfusion and transplantation from an infectious donor and injecting drug use. Other routes include hemodialysis and needlestick injuries.
- *Type E* (formerly grouped with Type C under the name type non-A, non-B hepatitis). Type E primarily occurs among patients who have ingested contaminated drinking water, uncooked shellfish, or uncooked fruits and vegetables when traveling to developing countries.

Causes

The five major forms of viral hepatitis result from infection with the causative viruses: A, B, C, D, or E.

Type A hepatitis is highly contagious and is usually transmitted by the fecal-oral route, commonly within institutions or families. However, it may also be transmitted parenterally. Hepatitis A usually results from ingestion of contaminated food, milk, or water. Outbreaks of this type are often traced to ingestion of seafood from polluted water.

Type B hepatitis, once thought to be transmitted only by the direct exchange of contaminated blood, is now known to be transmitted also by contact with contaminated human secretions and feces. As a result, nurses, doctors, laboratory technicians, and dentists are frequently exposed to type B hepatitis, often from wearing defective gloves. Transmission of this type also occurs during intimate sexual contact and through perinatal transmission.

Although specific viruses defined as type C hepatitis have been isolated, only a small percentage of patients have tested positive for them – reflecting, perhaps, poor specificity of the test. Usually, this type is transmitted through transfused blood from asymptomatic donors.

Type D hepatitis is found primarily in patients with an acute or a chronic episode of hepatitis B. Type D infection requires the presence of the hepatitis B surface antigen; the type D virus depends on the double-shelled type B virus to replicate. For this reason, type D infection can't outlast a type B infection.

Type E hepatitis is a form of hepatitis that is transmitted enterically, much like type A. No commercially available serologic test for diagnosis exists in the United States.

Complications

Life-threatening fulminant hepatitis is the most feared complication. Developing in about 1% of patients, it causes unremitting liver failure with encephalopathy. It progresses to coma and commonly leads to death within 2 weeks. (See *Recognizing fulminant hepatitis.*)

Major complications may be specific to the type of hepatitis:

- Chronic active hepatitis may occur as a late complication of hepatitis B.
- During the prodromal stage of acute hepatitis B, a syndrome resembling serum sickness, characterized by arthralgia or arthritis, rash, and angioedema, may oc-

LIFE-THREATENING COMPLICATIONS

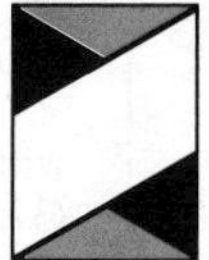

Recognizing fulminant hepatitis

A rare but severe form of hepatitis, fulminant hepatitis rapidly causes massive liver necrosis. It usually occurs in patients with hepatitis B, hepatitis D, or enteric type E hepatitis. Although the mortality is extremely high (more than 80% of patients lapse into deep coma), patients who survive may recover completely.

Assessment

In a patient with viral hepatitis, suspect fulminant hepatitis if you assess confusion, somnolence, ascites, and edema. Suggestive diagnostic test results include rapid liver shrinkage, a rapidly rising bilirubin level, and a markedly prolonged prothrombin time.

As the disease progresses swiftly to the terminal phase, the patient may experience cerebral edema, brain-stem compression, GI bleeding, sepsis, respiratory failure, cardiovascular collapse, and renal failure.

Emergency interventions

- Notify the doctor immediately. Then prepare to transfer the patient to the intensive care unit.
- Provide supportive care, such as maintaining fluid volume, supporting ventilation through mechanical means, controlling bleeding, and correcting hypoglycemia.
- Restrict protein intake, as ordered.
- Expect to administer oral lactulose or neomycin and, possibly, massive doses of glucocorticoids.
- If necessary and if the patient meets the criteria, prepare the patient for a liver transplant.

cur. This syndrome may cause misdiagnosis of hepatitis B as rheumatoid arthritis or lupus erythematosus.

- Type D hepatitis can cause a mild or asymptomatic form of type B hepatitis to flare into severe, progressive chronic active hepatitis and cirrhosis.
- Weeks to months after apparent recovery from acute hepatitis A, relapsing hepatitis may develop.

Rarely, hepatitis may lead to pancreatitis, myocarditis, atypical pneumonia, aplastic anemia, transverse myelitis, or peripheral neuropathy.

Assessment

Investigate the patient's history for the source of transmission. For example, you may learn that he was recently exposed to individuals with hepatitis A or B; underwent recent blood transfusions or used I.V. drugs; or had hemodialysis for renal failure. Look for evidence of recent ear piercing or tattooing (significant because contaminated instruments can transmit hepatitis); travel to a foreign country where hepatitis is endemic; or living conditions that are, or were, overcrowded.

Be sure to ask about alcohol consumption, which holds paramount significance in suspected cirrhosis. Remember, the alcoholic often deliberately underestimates how much he drinks, so you may need to interview family members as well.

Also check the patient's employment history; you may turn up occupational exposure. For instance, he may work in a hospital or laboratory, where the risk of viral exposure from contaminated instruments or waste could be high. Also probe

CHECKLIST

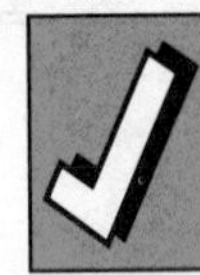

Diagnosing viral hepatitis

In suspected viral hepatitis, a hepatitis profile is routinely performed. This study identifies antibodies specific to the causative virus, establishing the type of hepatitis:

- ☐ *Type A.* Detection of an antibody to hepatitis A (anti-HAV) confirms the diagnosis.
- ☐ *Type B.* The presence of hepatitis B surface antigens (HBsAgs) and hepatitis B antibodies (anti-HBs) confirms the diagnosis.
- ☐ *Type C.* Diagnosis depends on serologic testing for the specific antibody 1 or more months after the onset of acute illness. Until then, the diagnosis is principally established by obtaining negative test results for hepatitis A, B, and D.
- ☐ *Type D.* Detection of intrahepatic delta antigens or immunoglobulin (Ig) M antidelta antigens in acute disease (or IgM and IgG in chronic disease) establishes the diagnosis.
- ☐ *Type E.* Detection of hepatitis E antigens supports the diagnosis; however, the diagnosis may also consist of ruling out hepatitis C.

the patient's background for possible exposure to toxic chemicals, such as carbon tetrachloride, which can cause nonviral hepatitis.

Assessment findings are similar for the different types of hepatitis. Typically, signs and symptoms progress in several stages. In the prodromal (preicteric) stage, the patient generally complains of easy fatigue and anorexia, possibly with mild weight loss. He may also report generalized malaise, depression, headache, weakness, arthralgia, myalgia, photophobia, and nausea with vomiting. He may describe changes in his senses of taste and smell.

Vital signs assessment may reveal fever, with a temperature of 100° to 102° F (37.8° to 38.9° C). As the prodromal stage draws to a close, usually within 1 to 5 days before the onset of the clinical jaundice stage, inspection of urine and stool specimens may reveal dark-colored urine and clay-colored stools.

If the patient has progressed to the clinical jaundice stage, he may report pruritus, abdominal pain or tenderness, and indigestion. Early in this stage, he may complain of anorexia; later, his appetite may return. Inspection of the sclerae, mucous membranes, and skin may show jaundice, which can last for 1 to 2 weeks. Jaundice indicates that the damaged liver can't remove bilirubin from the blood; however, its presence doesn't indicate disease severity. Occasionally, hepatitis occurs without jaundice.

During the clinical jaundice stage, skin inspection may detect rashes, erythematous patches, or hives, especially if the patient has hepatitis B or C. Palpation may disclose abdominal tenderness in the right upper quadrant, an enlarged and tender liver and, in some cases, splenomegaly and cervical adenopathy.

If you assess the patient during the recovery or posticteric stage, you'll find most symptoms are decreasing or have subsided. On palpation, you may notice a decrease in liver enlargement. The recovery phase generally lasts from 2 to 12 weeks – sometimes longer in patients with hepatitis B, C, or E.

Diagnostic tests

A hepatitis profile is routinely performed to diagnose viral hepatitis. (See *Diagnosing viral hepatitis.*) Additional findings from liver function studies support the diagnosis:

- *Serum aspartate aminotransferase (formerly SGOT)* and *serum alanine aminotransferase (formerly SGPT) levels* are increased in the prodromal stage of acute viral hepatitis.

• *Serum alkaline phosphatase levels* are slightly increased.

• *Serum bilirubin levels* are elevated. Levels may continue to be high late in the disease, especially if the patient has severe disease.

• *Prothrombin time* is prolonged (more than 3 seconds longer than normal indicates severe liver damage).

• *White blood cell counts* commonly reveal transient neutropenia and lymphopenia followed by lymphocytosis.

• *Liver biopsy* is performed if chronic hepatitis is suspected. (This study is performed for acute hepatitis only if the diagnosis is questionable.)

Treatment

No specific drug therapy has been developed for hepatitis. Instead, the patient is advised to rest in the early stages of the illness and combat anorexia by eating small, high-calorie, high-protein meals. (Protein intake should be reduced if signs of precoma – lethargy, confusion, mental changes – develop.) Large meals are usually better tolerated in the morning because many patients experience nausea late in the day.

In acute viral hepatitis, hospitalization usually is required only for those patients with severe symptoms or complications. Parenteral nutrition may be required if the patient has persistent vomiting and can't maintain oral intake.

Antiemetics (trimethobenzamide or benzquinamide) may be given a half hour before meals to relieve nausea and prevent vomiting; phenothiazines have a cholestatic effect and should be avoided. For severe pruritus, the resin cholestyramine, which sequesters bile salts, may be given.

Key nursing diagnoses and patient outcomes

Activity intolerance related to fatigue and malaise. Based on this nursing diagnosis, you'll establish these patient outcomes. The patient will:

• express an understanding of how hepatitis relates to fatigue and why he must comply with activity restrictions

• seek assistance, when needed, to perform self-care activities

• regain energy needed to perform activities of daily living as hepatitis subsides.

Altered nutrition: Less than body requirements, related to adverse GI reactions. Based on this nursing diagnosis, you'll establish these patient outcomes. The patient will:

• eat a nutritionally balanced, high-protein diet (unless protein is restricted)

• regain any lost weight and maintain weight within a normal range

• avoid signs and symptoms of malnutrition.

Risk for injury related to potential for permanent liver damage. Based on this nursing diagnosis, you'll establish these patient outcomes. The patient will:

• exhibit normal liver function test results after hepatitis resolves

• avoid signs and symptoms of fulminant hepatitis, cirrhosis, or chronic hepatitis.

Nursing interventions

• Observe appropriate isolation precautions to prevent disease transmission. (See *Taking isolation precautions for hepatitis A,* page 396.) Be sure that visitors also observe these precautions.

• Provide rest periods throughout the day. Schedule treatments and tests so the patient can rest between activities.

• Because inactivity may make the patient anxious, include diversional activities as part of his care. Suggest television programs of interest to him. Gradually add activities to his schedule as he begins to recover.

• To help the patient maintain an adequate diet, don't overload his meal tray. Too much food may only diminish his appetite. Also take care not to overmedicate him, which may cause loss of appetite. Determine his

Taking isolation precautions for hepatitis A

To prevent transmission of hepatitis, you'll need to observe isolation precautions—and discuss them with your patient to promote his cooperation. According to the most recent recommendations from the Centers for Disease Control and Prevention (CDC), standard precautions are observed.

- The patient may have a private room (necessary for a patient with fecal incontinence or poor hygiene). Staff members will wear gowns (when soiling is likely) and gloves (for contact with blood, body fluids, secretions, excretions, or contaminated items).
- All hospital personnel will wash their hands after touching body fluids, blood, secretions, and contaminated items, regardless of whether gloves were worn. Hands will be washed immediately after gloves are removed and when otherwise indicated to avoid transmission to other patients or environments.
- Hospital staff will wear masks or goggles during procedures and patient care activities that are likely to generate splashes or sprays of body fluids, secretions, or excretions.
- Staff members will dispose of needles and syringes in prominently labeled, puncture-resistant containers and won't recap needles and syringes. They'll dispose of dressings and tissues in the hospital's designated area for contaminated refuse.
- Hospital staff members will dispose of any contaminated bed linens in isolation bags and label any fecal specimens as "Biohazard."
- Whenever hospital staff members transport the patient, they'll use added protection (moisture-resistant pads for a fecally incontinent patient, for example). The personnel in the area to which the patient will be taken will be notified of his arrival, so that they can take the necessary precautions.
- At home, the patient should use meticulous hygiene after a bowel movement—starting with thorough hand washing, for example. Furthermore, he shouldn't handle food or share food or hand towels.
- After discussing isolation measures, educate the patient about the mode of transmission, incubation period, diagnostic tests, prophylaxis, and those at high risk for his type of hepatitis.

food preferences and try to include favorite foods in his meal plan.

- Administer supplemental vitamins and commercial feedings, as ordered. If symptoms are severe and the patient can't tolerate oral intake, provide I.V. therapy and parenteral nutrition, as ordered.
- Provide adequate fluid intake. The patient should consume at least 4 liters of liquid daily to maintain adequate hydration. To help him meet or exceed this goal, provide him with fruit juices, soft drinks, ice chips, and water.
- Administer antiemetics, as ordered.
- Report all cases of hepatitis to health officials. Ask the patient to name anyone he came in contact with recently.

Monitoring

- Observe the patient for both desired and adverse effects of medications.
- Record the patient's weight daily, and keep accurate intake and output records. Observe feces for color, consistency, and amount. Also note the frequency of defecation.

• Watch for signs of complications, such as changes in level of consciousness, ascites, edema, dehydration, respiratory problems, myalgia, and arthralgia.

Patient teaching

• Teach the patient about the disease, its signs and symptoms, and recommended treatments.
• Explain all necessary diagnostic tests. Review any special preparation that may be required. Point out that the findings from these tests, together with his symptoms, help to establish his diagnosis.
• Stress that complete recovery takes time. Point out that the liver takes 3 weeks to regenerate and up to 4 months to return to normal functioning. Advise the patient to avoid contact sports until his liver returns to its normal size. Instruct him to check with his doctor before performing any strenuous activity.
• Review measures to prevent spread of the disease. Stress the importance of thorough and frequent hand washing. Tell the patient not to share food, eating utensils, or toothbrushes. If he has hepatitis A or E, warn him not to contaminate food or water with fecal matter, because the disease is transmitted via the fecal-oral route. If he has hepatitis B, C, or D, explain that transmission occurs through exchange of blood or body fluids that contain blood. Therefore, while he is infected, he shouldn't donate blood or have sexual relations. Also advise him to take extra care to avoid cutting himself.
• Emphasize the importance of rest and good nutrition in promoting liver regeneration. Instruct the patient to eat a high-calorie, high-protein diet. Advise him to eat several small meals rather than three large meals. Also stress the importance of drinking adequate fluids every day.
• Tell the patient who is recuperating at home to weigh himself every day and to report any weight loss greater than 5 lb (2.3 kg) to his doctor.
• Warn the patient to abstain from alcohol while he has this disease. If necessary, explain that because alcohol is detoxified in the liver, its consumption could put undue stress on the liver during the illness.
• Explain to the patient and his family that anyone exposed to the disease through contact with him should receive prophylaxis as soon as possible after exposure. Immune globulin is given for hepatitis A. It may also be given for hepatitis C and E, but its effectiveness for these forms of hepatitis has not been proven. Hepatitis B vaccine is given for hepatitis B or D.
• Tell the patient to check with the doctor before taking any medication – even nonprescription drugs – because some medications can precipitate a relapse.
• Stress the need for continued medical care. Advise the patient to see the doctor again about 2 weeks after the diagnosis is made. Mention that he'll probably have follow-up visits every month for up to 6 months after diagnosis. Also explain that if chronic hepatitis develops, he'll always have to visit the doctor regularly so the disease can be monitored.

Hernia repair

A hernia may be corrected by herniorrhaphy or hernioplasty. Herniorrhaphy, the surgery of choice for inguinal and other abdominal hernias, returns the protruding intestine to the abdominal cavity and repairs the abdominal wall defect. Hernioplasty, a related surgery used to correct more extensive hernias, reinforces the weakened area around the repair with plastic, steel or tantalum mesh, or wire.

Typically, herniorrhaphy and hernioplasty are elective surgeries that can be done quickly and produce few complications. However, emergency herniorrhaphy may be necessary to reduce a strangulated hernia and prevent ischemia and gangrene.

Procedure

With the patient under general or spinal anesthesia, the surgeon makes an incision over the area of herniation. He manipulates the herniated tissue back to its proper position and then repairs the defect in the muscle or fascia. If necessary, he reinforces the area of the defect with wire, mesh, or another material. Then he closes the incision and applies a dressing.

If the hernia is uncomplicated, it can be repaired laparoscopically.

Complications

A hernia repair is a relatively simple surgical procedure that causes no serious complications postoperatively. Occasionally, a patient may experience a wound infection or develop a transient difficulty voiding after surgery.

Key nursing diagnoses and patient outcomes

Risk for infection related to normal bacterial flora at the incision site. Based on this nursing diagnosis, you'll establish these patient outcomes. The patient will:

- maintain a normal temperature and white blood cell count
- maintain a clean surgical incision with no purulent drainage
- avoid increased pain and tenderness at the surgical site
- remain free from infection.

Pain related to abdominal surgery. Based on this nursing diagnosis, you'll establish these patient outcomes. The patient will:

- express pain relief after analgesic administration
- engage in diversional activities to reduce pain
- experience decreasing pain 24 hours after surgery and complete pain relief after healing occurs.

Urinary retention related to a surgical complication. Based on this nursing diagnosis, you'll establish these patient outcomes. The patient will:

- void within 12 hours after hernia repair
- maintain a fluid output equal to intake
- avoid signs and symptoms of bladder distention.

Nursing interventions

When caring for a patient undergoing a hernia repair, your major roles include instructing him, preparing him for surgery, and monitoring him for postoperative complications.

Before surgery

- Explain the surgery to the patient, gearing your discussion to his age and level of comprehension. Tell him that the surgery will relieve the discomfort of hernia.
- If the patient is having elective surgery, assure him that recovery is usually rapid; if no complications occur, he may return home the day of surgery and usually can resume normal activities within 4 to 6 weeks.
- If the patient is having emergency surgery for a strangulated or incarcerated hernia, explain that he may be hospitalized for several days with a nasogastric tube in place.
- Ensure that the patient or a responsible family member has signed a consent form.
- Prepare the patient for surgery by shaving the surgical site and administering a cleansing enema and a sedative, as ordered.

After surgery

- Take steps to reduce pressure on the incision site. For example, teach the patient how to get up from a lying or sitting position without straining his abdomen. Instruct him how to splint his incision when he coughs or sneezes, and reassure him that coughing or sneezing won't cause the hernia to recur.
- As ordered, administer a stool softener to prevent straining during defecation. Encourage early ambulation but warn against bending, lifting, or other strenuous activities.

• Make sure the patient voids within 12 hours after surgery. If swelling interferes with normal urination, insert an indwelling urinary catheter.
• Provide comfort measures. Administer analgesics, as ordered. After inguinal hernia repair, apply an ice bag to the patient's scrotum to reduce swelling and pain. If appropriate, apply a scrotal bridge or truss; for best results, apply it in the morning before the patient gets out of bed.
• Regularly check the dressing for drainage and the incision site for inflammation or swelling. Assess the patient for other symptoms of infection. Report possible infection to the doctor, and expect to administer antibiotics, as ordered.

Home care instructions

• Instruct the patient to avoid lifting, bending, and pushing or pulling movements for 8 weeks after surgery or until his doctor allows them.
• Tell the patient to watch for and report signs of infection, including fever, chills, diaphoresis, malaise, lethargy, and pain, inflammation, swelling, and drainage at the incision site. Instruct him to keep the incision clean and covered until the sutures are removed.
• Stress the importance of regular follow-up examinations to evaluate wound healing and the success of hernia repair.
• If the patient's job involves heavy lifting or other strenuous activity, discuss the possible need for a job change.

Herniated disk

Also known as a herniated nucleus pulposus or a slipped disk, a herniated disk occurs when all or part of the nucleus pulposus – an intervertebral disk's gelatinous center – extrudes through the disk's weakened or torn outer ring (annulus fibrosus). The resultant pressure on spinal nerve roots or on the spinal cord itself causes back pain and other symptoms of nerve root irritation.

About 90% of herniations affect the lumbar (L) and lumbosacral spine; 8% occur in the cervical (C) spine and 1% to 2% in the thoracic spine. The most common site for herniation is the L4-L5 disk space. Other sites include L5-S1, L2-L3, L3-L4, C6-C7, and C5-C6.

Lumbar herniation usually develops in people ages 20 to 45 and cervical herniation in those age 45 or older. Herniated disks affect more men than women.

Causes

Herniated disks may result from severe trauma or strain, or they may be related to intervertebral joint degeneration. In an elderly person with degenerative disk changes, minor trauma may cause herniation. A person with a congenitally small lumbar spinal canal or with osteophytes along the vertebrae may be more susceptible to nerve root compression with a herniated disk. This person is also more likely to exhibit neurologic symptoms.

Complications

Neurologic deficits (most common) and bowel and bladder problems (with lumbar herniations) are complications of herniated disk.

Assessment

Initially, the patient may seek relief for usually unilateral, low back pain radiating to the buttocks, legs, and feet. Typically, he may report a previous traumatic injury or back strain.

When herniation follows trauma, the patient may tell you that the pain began suddenly, subsided in a few days, and then recurred at shorter intervals and progressive intensity. He may then describe sciatic pain that began as a dull ache in the buttocks and that grows with Valsalva's maneuver, coughing, sneezing, or bending. He may also complain of accompanying muscle spasms and may add that the pain subsides with rest.

Inspection may reveal a patient with limited ability to bend forward and a posture favoring the affected side. In later stages, you may observe muscle atrophy. Palpation may disclose tenderness over the affected region.

Tissue tension assessment may reveal radicular pain from straight leg raising (with lumbar herniation) and increased pain from neck movement (with cervical herniation).

Thorough assessment of the patient's peripheral vascular status – including posterior tibial and dorsalis pedis pulses and skin temperature of the arms and legs – may help to rule out ischemic disease as the cause of leg pain or numbness.

Diagnostic tests

- *X-ray studies* of the spine are essential to show degenerative changes and to rule out other abnormalities. Films may not show a herniated disk because even marked disk prolapse may show up as normal on an X-ray.
- *Myelography* pinpoints the level of the herniation.
- *Computed tomography scan* detects bone and soft-tissue abnormalities. It can also show spinal canal compression that results from herniation.
- *Magnetic resonance imaging* defines tissues in areas usually obscured by bone on other imaging tests, such as those done with X-rays.
- *Electromyography* confirms nerve involvement by measuring the electrical activity of muscles innervated by the herniated disk.
- *Neuromuscular tests* can detect sensory and motor loss as well as leg muscle weakness.

Treatment

Unless neurologic impairment progresses rapidly, initial treatment is conservative, consisting of bed rest (possibly with pelvic traction) for several weeks; supportive devices (such as a brace); heat or ice applications; and exercise. Nonsteroidal anti-inflammatory drugs reduce inflammation and edema at the injury site. Steroidal drugs, such as dexamethasone, may be prescribed or administered epidurally for the same purpose. Muscle relaxants (diazepam or methocarbamol) may help also.

A herniated disk that fails to respond to conservative treatment may require surgery. The most common procedure, laminectomy, involves removing a portion of the lamina and the protruding nucleus pulposus. If laminectomy doesn't alleviate pain and disability, the patient may undergo spinal fusion to stabilize the spine. Laminectomy and spinal fusion may be performed concurrently.

Chemonucleolysis, an alternative to surgery, is seldom performed because of its limited success. This procedure involves injection of the enzyme chymopapain into the herniated disk to dissolve the nucleus pulposus and relieve pressure on the nerve root.

Percutaneous automated diskectomy is another alternative. Guided by X-ray visualization, the doctor suctions out the disk portion that causes pain. Typically used for smaller, less severe disk abnormalities, this procedure succeeds about 50% of the time.

Key nursing diagnoses and patient outcomes

Impaired physical mobility related to pain and neurologic impairment. Based on this nursing diagnosis, you'll establish these patient outcomes. The patient will:

- maintain normal muscle strength and joint range of motion
- avoid complications, such as contractures, venous stasis, thrombus formation, and skin breakdown
- regain physical mobility with treatment.

Chronic pain related to nerve root irritation. Based on this nursing diagnosis,

you'll establish these patient outcomes. The patient will:
• express pain relief after analgesic administration
• comply with prescribed treatments
• become pain free with treatment.

Impaired home maintenance management related to pain and physical limitations. Based on this nursing diagnosis, you'll establish these patient outcomes. The patient will:
• report any areas of home maintenance need
• seek assistance from available resources
• regain the ability to perform self-care and home maintenance activities with treatment.

Nursing interventions

• Offer supportive care, careful patient teaching, and emotional encouragement to help the patient cope with the discomfort and frustration of chronic back pain and impaired mobility.
• With the patient and doctor, plan a pain-control regimen, using such methods as relaxation, transcutaneous nerve stimulation, distraction, heat or ice application, traction, bracing, or positioning. Give pain medications and muscle relaxants, as ordered.
• Encourage the patient to express his concerns about his disorder. Listen and offer support and encouragement. Include the patient and his family in all phases of care. Answer questions as honestly as you can.
• Urge the patient to perform as much self-care as his immobility and pain allow. Provide him with adequate time to perform these activities at his own pace.
• Help the patient identify and perform care and activities that promote rest and relaxation.
• Use antiembolism stockings, as prescribed, and encourage the patient to move his legs, as allowed. Provide high-topped sneakers or a footboard to prevent footdrop. Work closely with the physical therapy department to ensure a consistent regimen of leg- and back-strengthening exercises. Give plenty of fluids to prevent urinary stasis. Remind the patient to cough, breathe deeply, or blow into bottles or an incentive spirometer to avoid pulmonary complications. Provide thorough skin care. Supply a fracture bedpan for the patient on complete bed rest.
• If the patient will undergo myelography, question him carefully about allergies to iodides, iodine-containing substances, or seafood. Such allergies may indicate sensitivity to a radiopaque contrast agent used in the test. Monitor intake and output. Watch for seizures and an allergic reaction.
• Prepare the patient for a laminectomy or spinal fusion, as indicated. (For more information, see the entry "Laminectomy" later in this book.)
• After microdiskectomy, encourage the patient to increase activity quickly. If a blood drainage system (Hemovac) is in use, check the tubing frequently for patency and a secure vacuum seal. Empty the system at the end of each shift, as ordered, and record the amount and color of drainage. Immediately report colorless moisture on dressings (which may indicate cerebrospinal fluid leakage) or excessive drainage. Administer analgesics, as ordered, especially 30 minutes or so before the patient's first postoperative attempts at sitting or walking. Assist the patient during his first attempt to walk. Provide a straight-backed chair and allow him to sit in it briefly.
• Before chemonucleolysis, make sure the patient is not allergic to meat tenderizers (chymopapain is a similar substance). Such an allergy contraindicates the use of this enzyme, which can produce severe anaphylaxis in a sensitive patient.
• After chemonucleolysis, enforce bed rest, as ordered. Administer analgesics and apply heat, as needed. Urge the patient to cough and breathe deeply. Assist with special exercises.

Monitoring

- Assess the patient's pain status and his response to the pain-control regimen.
- During conservative treatment, watch for deterioration in neurologic status (especially in the first 24 hours after admission), which may indicate an urgent need for surgery.
- Perform neurovascular checks of the patient's legs (color, motion, temperature, sensation).
- Monitor vital signs, and check for bowel sounds and abdominal distention.

Patient teaching

- Teach the patient about treatments, which may include bed rest and pelvic traction; local heat application to decrease pain; an exercise program; medications to decrease pain, inflammation, and muscle spasms; and surgery.
- Before myelography, reinforce previous explanations of the need for this test, and tell the patient to expect some pain. Assure him that he'll receive a sedative before the test, if needed, to keep him as calm and comfortable as possible. After the test, urge the patient to remain in bed with his head elevated (especially if metrizamide was used) and to drink plenty of fluids.
- Before discharge, teach proper body mechanics: bending at the knees and hips (never at the waist), standing straight, and carrying objects close to the body. Tell the patient to lie down when he's tired and to sleep on his side (never on his abdomen) on an extra-firm mattress or a bed board.
- Urge the patient to maintain an ideal body weight to prevent lordosis caused by obesity.
- Discuss all prescribed medications with the patient. Name possible adverse reactions, and advise the patient which adverse reactions require immediate medical attention. If the patient takes a prescribed muscle relaxant, caution him about its possible effects, such as drowsiness. Warn him to avoid activities that require alertness until his tolerance to the drug's sedative effect builds.
- As necessary, refer the patient to an occupational therapist or a home health nurse to help him manage activities of daily living.
- If surgery is required, explain all preoperative and postoperative procedures and treatments to the patient and his family.
- Teach the patient relaxation techniques to promote rest and relaxation. Urge him to do them regularly.

Herpes simplex

A common infection, herpes simplex virus (HSV) occurs subclinically in about 85% of patients. In the rest, it causes localized lesions. HSV may be latent for years, but after the initial infection, the patient becomes a carrier susceptible to recurrent attacks. The outbreaks may be provoked by fever, menses, stress, heat, cold, lack of sleep, sun exposure, and contact with reactivated disease (for example, by kissing or by sharing cosmetics). In recurrent infections, the patient usually has no constitutional signs and symptoms.

Generally not serious in an otherwise healthy adult, HSV infection in an immunocompromised patient, such as one with acquired immunodeficiency syndrome (AIDS), can produce severe illness. In fact, serious HSV infections are a prominent feature of AIDS.

HSV infection occurs worldwide equally in males and females. Lower socioeconomic groups are infected more often, probably because of crowded living conditions.

Causes

Herpesvirus hominis, a widespread infectious agent, causes two serologically distinct HSV types. Seen most commonly in children, *type 1* (HSV-1) is transmitted primarily by contact with oral secretions. It mainly affects oral, labial, ocular, or skin tissues. *Type 2* (HSV-2), transmitted primarily by contact with genital secretions, mainly affects genital structures, typically in adolescents and young adults.

In homosexual men, HSV-2 anal and perianal infection is common. However, with changing sexual practices, some studies report an increasing incidence of genital HSV-1 and oral HSV-2 infections. Although HSV most frequently occurs in the structures mentioned, it may infect any epithelial tissue. The incubation period varies, depending on the infection site. The average incubation for generalized infection is 2 to 12 days; for localized genital infection, 3 to 7 days.

Complications

Primary (or initial) HSV infection during pregnancy can lead to abortion, premature labor, microcephaly, and uterine growth retardation. Congenital herpes transmitted during vaginal birth may produce a subclinical neonatal infection or severe infection with seizures, chorioretinitis, skin vesicles, and hepatosplenomegaly.

Blindness may result from ocular infection. Females with HSV may be at increased risk for cervical cancer. Urethral stricture may result from recurrent genital herpes.

Perianal ulcers, colitis, esophagitis, pneumonitis, and various neurologic disorders, resulting from HSV infection, are serious complications in patients with AIDS and other immunocompromised conditions.

Assessment

In a patient with suspected herpes simplex, the history may reveal oral, vaginal, or anal sexual contact with an infected person or other direct contact with lesions. With recurrent infection, the patient may identify various precipitating factors. (See *Detecting herpes simplex,* page 404.)

Diagnostic tests

Confirmation of HSV infection requires isolating the virus from local lesions and a histologic biopsy. In primary infection, a rise in antibodies and moderate leukocytosis may support the diagnosis.

Treatment

Symptomatic and supportive therapy is the rule. Generalized primary infection usually requires antipyretic and analgesic medications to reduce fever and pain. Anesthetic mouthwashes, such as viscous lidocaine, may reduce the pain of gingivostomatitis, enabling the patient to consume food and fluids and thus promote hydration. (Avoid offering alcohol-based mouthwashes, which can increase discomfort.) A bicarbonate-based mouth rinse may be used for oral care. Drying agents, such as calamine lotion, may soothe labial and skin lesions. Avoid using petroleum jelly–based salves or dressings because they promote viral spread and slow healing.

Refer patients with eye infections to an ophthalmologist. Topical corticosteroids are contraindicated in active infection, but ophthalmic medications, such as idoxuridine, trifluridine, and vidarabine, may be effective.

Acyclovir is a major agent for combating genital herpes, particularly primary infection. The drug may reduce symptoms, viral shedding, and healing time. And although it's mostly ineffective in treating recurrent attacks, it may be prescribed to treat and suppress HSV in immunocompromised patients and those with severe and frequent recurrences. Acyclovir therapy also may help treat perioral herpes, especially primary infection. The drug is available in topical, oral, and I.V. form (usually reserved for severe infection).

Key nursing diagnoses and patient outcomes

Altered oral mucous membrane related to oral lesions. Based on this nursing diag-

Detecting herpes simplex

Assessment findings in herpes simplex include the following:

Primary perioral HSV
In primary perioral HSV, the patient may have generalized or localized infection. The patient with generalized infection usually reports a sore throat, fever, increased salivation, halitosis, anorexia, and severe mouth pain. If pain prevents adequate fluid intake, you also may note such signs of dehydration as poor skin turgor. After a brief prodromal tingling and itching, typical primary lesions erupt.

Examination of the pharyngeal and oral mucosa may disclose edema and small vesicles on an erythematous base. These vesicles eventually rupture, leaving a painful ulcer that is followed by yellow crusting. Vesicles most commonly occur on the tongue, gingiva, and cheeks, but any part of the oral mucosa may be involved. Palpation reveals tender cervical adenopathy. A generalized infection usually runs its course in 4 to 10 days.

Primary genital HSV
With primary genital HSV, the patient usually complains first of malaise, dysuria, dyspareunia, and, in females, leukorrhea. Then fluid-filled vesicles appear.

In examining a female patient, you may detect vesicles on the cervix (the primary infection site) and, possibly, on the labia, perianal skin, vulva, and vagina. In male patients, vesicles develop on the glans penis, foreskin, and penile shaft. Extragenital lesions may be seen on the mouth or anus. Ruptured vesicles appear as extensive, shallow, painful ulcers, with redness, marked edema, and characteristic oozing, yellow centers. Lesions may persist for several weeks. Palpation may reveal tender inguinal adenopathy.

Recurrent perioral or genital HSV
The patient with recurrent perioral or genital HSV also may report prodromal symptoms (pain, tingling, or itching) at the site. Typically, the disease course is shorter than that of the primary infection. Recurrent perioral infection usually triggers no systemic symptoms, but the outer lip may be affected and painful. A male patient with recurrent genital herpes usually has less severe systemic symptoms and less local involvement. A female patient may have more symptoms and report severe discomfort. Palpation may reveal tender cervical adenopathy.

Primary ocular infection
The patient with a primary ocular infection may report localized signs and symptoms, such as photophobia and excessive tearing. Follicular conjunctivitis or blepharitis with vesicles on the eyelid, eyelid edema, and chemosis also may occur. Systemic signs and symptoms may include lethargy and fever. The infection usually is unilateral and heals within 2 to 3 weeks. Recurrent ocular infections may cause decreased visual acuity and even permanent vision loss. Palpation may reveal regional adenopathy.

nosis, you'll establish these patient outcomes. The patient will:

- comply with prescribed treatments to alleviate oral lesions
- exhibit healing of oral lesions.

Risk for infection related to herpes simplex recurrence. Based on this nursing diagnosis, you'll establish these patient outcomes. The patient will:

- express an understanding of how herpes simplex can recur

• take precautions to prevent recurrences
• avoid herpes simplex recurrences.

Pain related to the infection. Based on this nursing diagnosis, you'll establish these patient outcomes. The patient will:
• express pain relief with treatment
• become pain free once lesions heal.

Nursing interventions

• Observe standard precautions. For the patient with extensive cutaneous, oral, or genital lesions, institute contact precautions.
• Instruct caregivers with active oral or cutaneous infections not to care for a patient in a high-risk group until the caregiver's lesions crust and dry. Also, insist that the caregiver wear protective coverings, including a mask and gloves.
• Administer pain medications and prescribed antiviral agents, as ordered.
• Provide supportive care, as indicated, such as oral hygiene, nutritional supplements, and antipyretics for fever.
• As appropriate, refer the patient to a support group, such as the Herpes Resource Center.

Monitoring

• Observe the patient's response to treatment measures.
• Assess the patient for complications associated with herpes simplex.
• Monitor the patient with oral lesions for signs and symptoms of nutritional deficits and dehydration. Weigh the patient regularly.

Patient teaching

• Instruct the patient with cold sores not to kiss infants or people with eczema. Tell the patient with genital herpes to wash his hands carefully after using the bathroom or touching his genitalia, to avoid spreading the infection to infants or other susceptible people.
• Instruct the patient with oral lesions to use lip balm with sunscreen to avoid reactivating lesions.
• Encourage the patient to get adequate rest and nutrition and to keep his lesions dry, except for applying prescribed medications.
• Teach the patient how to apply medications, using aseptic technique.
• Urge the patient with genital herpes to avoid sexual intercourse during the active disease stage before lesions completely heal.
• Instruct the patient with genital herpes to inform any sexual partner of his condition. Advise patients and partners to be screened for other sexually transmitted diseases, including human immunodeficiency virus infection.
• If the patient is pregnant, explain the potential risk to the infant during vaginal delivery. Answer her questions about cesarean delivery if she has an HSV outbreak when labor begins and if her membranes haven't ruptured.
• Advise the female patient with genital herpes to have a Papanicolaou test yearly if results have been normal. If results have been abnormal, advise her to be tested more frequently.
• Instruct the patient with herpetic whitlow not to share towels or eating utensils with uninfected people. Educate hospital staff members and other susceptible people about the risk of contracting the disease.
• Accept the patient's feelings of powerlessness as normal. Help him to identify and develop coping mechanisms, strengths, and resources for support.
• Provide a nonthreatening, nonjudgmental atmosphere to encourage the patient with genital herpes to voice his feelings about perceived changes in sexuality and behavior. Provide him and his partner with current information about the disease and treatment options. Offer to refer them for appropriate counseling, as needed.

Herpes zoster

An acute unilateral and segmental inflammation of the dorsal root ganglia, herpes zoster (shingles) produces localized vesicular skin lesions confined to a dermatome. The patient with shingles may have severe neuralgic pain in the areas bordering the inflamed nerve root ganglia. (See *Tracing the path of herpes zoster,* pages 408 and 409.)

The infection, found primarily in adults over age 50, seldom recurs. The prognosis is good, and most patients recover completely unless the infection spreads to the brain. Herpes zoster is more severe in the immunocompromised patient but seldom is fatal.

Causes

The varicella-zoster virus, a herpesvirus, causes shingles. For unknown reasons and by an unidentified process, the disease erupts when the virus reactivates after dormancy in the cerebral ganglia (extramedullary ganglia of the cranial nerves) or the ganglia of posterior nerve roots. Although the process is unclear, the virus may multiply as it reactivates, and antibodies remaining from the initial infection may neutralize it. Without opposition from effective antibodies, the virus continues to multiply in the ganglia, destroys neurons, and spreads down the sensory nerves to the skin.

Herpes zoster may be more prevalent in people who had chicken pox at a very young age, especially before age 1 – but this is still a hypothesis.

Complications

Herpes zoster ophthalmicus may result in vision loss. Complications of generalized infection may involve acute urine retention and unilateral paralysis of the diaphragm. In postherpetic neuralgia (most common in elderly patients), intractable neurologic pain may persist for years, and scars may be permanent. In rare cases, herpes zoster may be complicated by generalized central nervous system (CNS) infection, muscle atrophy, motor paralysis (usually transient), acute transverse myelitis, and ascending myelitis.

Assessment

The typical patient reports no history of exposure to others with the varicella-zoster virus. He may complain of fever, malaise, pain that mimics appendicitis, pleurisy, musculoskeletal pain, or other conditions. In 2 to 4 days, he may report severe, deep pain; pruritus; and paresthesia or hyperesthesia (usually affecting the trunk and occasionally the arms and legs). Pain – described as intermittent, continuous, or debilitating – usually lasts from 1 to 4 weeks.

During examination of the patient within 2 weeks after his initial symptoms, you may observe small, red, nodular skin lesions spread unilaterally around the thorax or vertically over the arms or legs. Or instead of nodules, you may see vesicles filled with clear fluid or pus. About 10 days after they appear, these vesicles dry, forming scabs. The lesions are most vulnerable to infection after rupture; some even become gangrenous.

During palpation, you may detect enlarged regional lymph nodes.

Herpes zoster may involve the cranial nerves (especially the trigeminal and geniculate ganglia or the oculomotor nerve). With geniculate involvement, you may observe vesicle formation in the external auditory canal and ipsilateral facial palsy. The patient may complain of hearing loss, dizziness, and loss of taste. With trigeminal involvement, the patient may complain of eye pain. He also may have corneal and scleral damage and impaired vision. Rarely, oculomotor involvement causes conjunctivitis, extraocular weakness, ptosis, and paralytic mydriasis.

Diagnostic tests

Vesicular fluid and infected tissue analyses typically show eosinophilic intranuclear inclusions and varicella virus. Differentiation of herpes zoster from localized herpes simplex requires staining antibodies from vesicular fluid and identification under fluorescent light. Usually, though, the locations of herpes simplex and herpes zoster lesions are distinctly different.

With CNS involvement, results of a lumbar puncture indicate increased pressure, and cerebrospinal fluid analysis demonstrates increased protein levels and, possibly, pleocytosis.

Treatment

Primary therapeutic goals include relief of itching with antipruritics (such as calamine lotion) and relief of neuralgic pain with analgesics (such as aspirin, acetaminophen, or possibly codeine). A similar goal involves preventing secondary infection by applying a demulcent and skin protectant (such as collodion or tincture of benzoin) to unbroken lesions.

If bacteria infect ruptured vesicles, treatment includes an appropriate systemic antibiotic. Herpes zoster affecting trigeminal and corneal structures calls for instillation of idoxuridine ointment or another antiviral agent.

To help a patient cope with the intractable pain of postherpetic neuralgia, a systemic corticosteroid, such as cortisone or corticotropin, may be ordered to reduce inflammation. The doctor also may order tranquilizers, sedatives, or tricyclic antidepressants with phenothiazines.

In an immunocompromised patient at high risk for complications and in a patient with an infection of the ophthalmic branch of the trigeminal nerve, acyclovir may be prescribed. This drug halts the progressing rash, reduces the duration of viral shedding and acute pain, and prevents visceral complications.

As a last resort for pain relief, transcutaneous peripheral nerve stimulation, patient-controlled analgesia, or a small dose of radiotherapy may be considered.

Key nursing diagnoses and patient outcomes

Impaired skin integrity related to skin lesions. Based on this nursing diagnosis, you'll establish these patient outcomes. The patient will:
- demonstrate skill in performing the prescribed skin-care regimen
- avoid complications of skin lesions, such as infection and skin breakdown
- demonstrate healing of skin lesions and regain normal skin integrity.

Pain related to inflamed nerve root ganglia. Based on this nursing diagnosis, you'll establish these patient outcomes. The patient will:
- express pain relief after analgesic administration
- comply with prescribed treatments to eliminate the infection and alleviate pain
- avoid chronic pain.

Sensory/perceptual alterations (tactile) related to paresthesia or hyperesthesia. Based on this nursing diagnosis, you'll establish these patient outcomes. The patient will:
- take precautions to prevent injury to the affected area
- regain normal sensory function once the infection heals.

Nursing interventions

- Administer topical therapies as directed. If the doctor orders calamine, apply it liberally to the patient's lesions. Avoid blotting contaminated swabs on unaffected skin areas. Be prepared to administer drying therapies, such as oxygen, if the patient has severe disseminated lesions. Use silver sulfadiazine, as ordered, to soften and debride infected lesions.
- Give analgesics exactly as scheduled to minimize severe neuralgic pain. For a patient with postherpetic neuralgia, consult

(Text continues on page 410.)

Tracing the path of herpes zoster

The herpes zoster virus infects the nerves that innervate the skin, eyes, and ears. Each nerve (tagged for its corresponding vertebral source) emanates from the spine, banding and branching around the body to innervate a skin area called a dermatome. The herpes zoster rash erupts along the course of the affected nerve fibers, covering

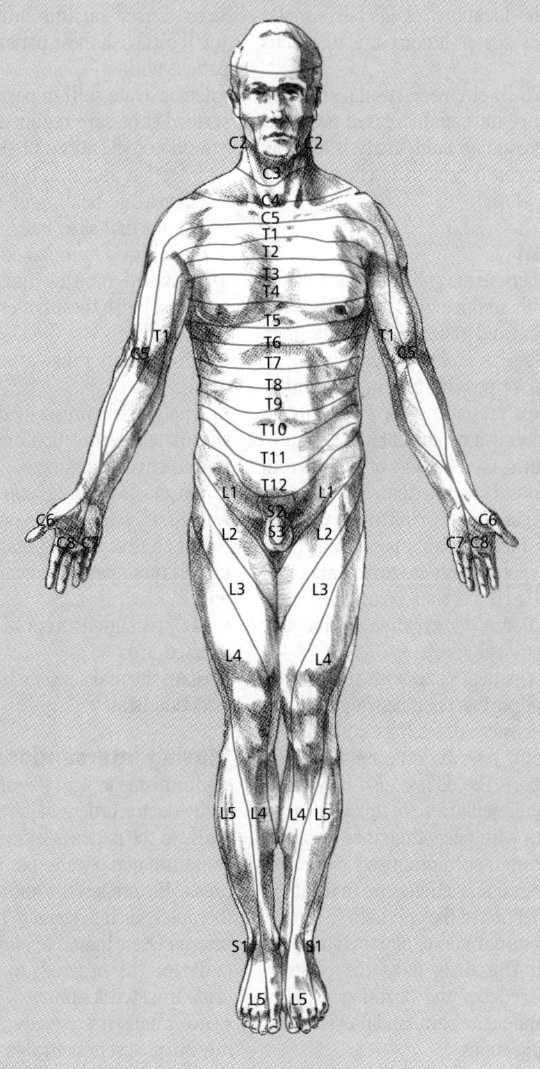

the skin in one or several of the dermatomes (as shown).

The thoracic (T) and lumbar (L) dermatomes are the most commonly affected, but others, such as those covering the cervical (C) and sacral (S) areas, can also be affected. Dermatome levels can vary and overlap.

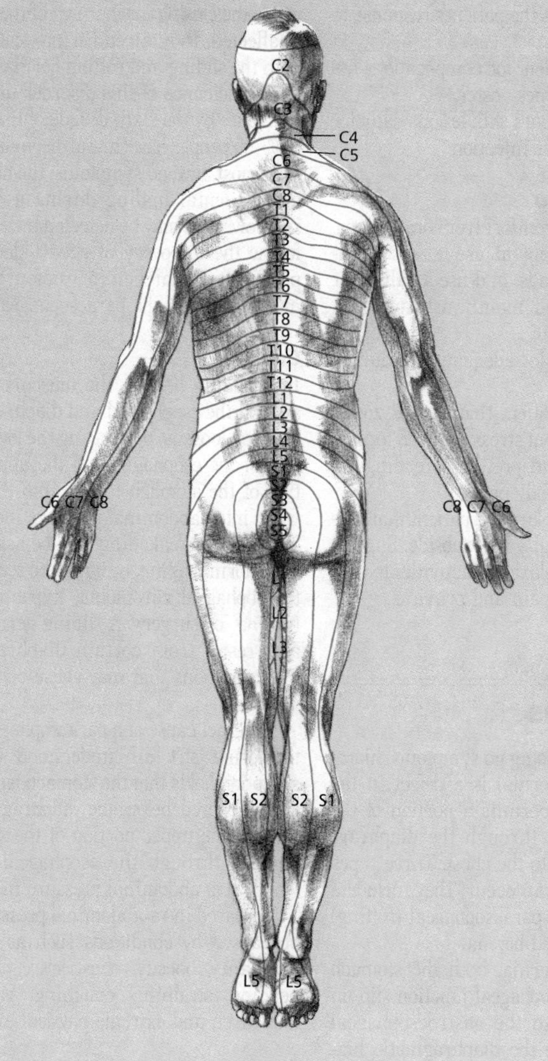

with a pain specialist, and follow his recommendations to maximize pain relief without risking tolerance to the analgesic.
• Maintain meticulous hygiene to prevent spreading the infection to other parts of the patient's body.

Monitoring

• Regularly assess the patient's response to treatment.
• Monitor the patient for complications associated with herpes zoster.
• Inspect the patient's skin lesions daily for signs of healing or infection.

Patient teaching

• To decrease discomfort from oral lesions, instruct the patient to use a soft toothbrush, eat soft foods, and use a saline- or bicarbonate-based mouthwash and oral anesthetics.
• Stress the need for adequate rest during the acute phase.
• Reassure the patient that herpes zoster isn't contagious, but stress the need for meticulous hygiene to prevent spreading infection to other body parts.
• Repeatedly reassure the patient that herpetic pain eventually will subside. Suggest diversionary or relaxation activities to take his mind off the pain and pruritus.

Hiatal hernia

Commonly producing no symptoms, hiatal hernia (hiatus hernia) is a defect in the diaphragm that permits a portion of the stomach to pass through the diaphragmatic opening into the chest. Three types of hiatal hernia can occur. They include a sliding hernia, a paraesophageal (rolling) hernia, or a mixed hernia.

In a sliding hernia, both the stomach and the gastroesophageal junction slip up into the chest, so the gastroesophageal junction is above the diaphragmatic hiatus. This type of hernia causes symptoms if the lower esophageal sphincter (LES) is incompetent, which permits gastric reflux and heartburn.

In a paraesophageal or rolling hernia, a part of the greater curvature of the stomach rolls through the diaphragmatic defect. This type of hernia usually doesn't cause gastric reflux and heartburn because the closing mechanism of the LES is unaffected. In a mixed hernia, features of both the sliding and rolling hernias occur.

The incidence of this disorder increases with age. By the sixth decade of life, about 60% of people have hiatal hernias. However, most have no symptoms; the hernia is an incidental finding during a barium swallow. Or it may be detected by tests that follow the discovery of occult blood. The prevalence is higher in women than in men (especially the paraesophageal type).

Causes

In a sliding hernia, the muscular collar around the esophageal and diaphragmatic junction loosens, permitting the lower portion of the esophagus and the upper portion of the stomach to rise into the chest when intra-abdominal pressure increases. This muscle weakening may be associated with normal aging, or it may be secondary to esophageal carcinoma, kyphoscoliosis, trauma, or surgery. A sliding hernia may also result from certain diaphragmatic malformations that may cause congenital weakness.

The exact cause of a paraesophageal hiatal hernia isn't fully understood. One assumption holds that the stomach isn't properly anchored below the diaphragm, permitting the upper portion of the stomach to slide through the esophageal hiatus when intra-abdominal pressure increases.

Increased intra-abdominal pressure can be caused by conditions such as ascites, pregnancy, obesity, constrictive clothing, bending, straining, coughing, Valsalva's maneuver, and extreme physical exertion.

Complications

If the hiatal hernia is associated with gastroesophageal reflux, the esophageal mucosa may become irritated, leading to esophagitis, esophageal ulceration, hemorrhage, peritonitis, and mediastinitis. Aspiration of refluxed fluids may lead to respiratory distress, aspiration pneumonia, or cardiac dysfunction from pressure on the heart and lungs.

Other complications include esophageal stricture and incarceration, in which a large portion of the stomach is caught above the diaphragm. Incarceration may lead to perforation, gastric ulcer, and strangulation and gangrene of the herniated stomach portion.

Assessment

When a sliding hernia causes symptoms, the patient typically complains of heartburn, indicating an incompetent LES and gastroesophageal reflux. The patient history usually reveals that heartburn occurs from 1 to 4 hours after eating and is aggravated by reclining, belching, or conditions that increase intra-abdominal pressure. Heartburn may be accompanied by regurgitation or vomiting. The patient may complain of retrosternal or substernal chest pain (typically after meals or at bedtime), reflecting reflux of gastric contents, distention of the stomach, and spasm.

Keep in mind that the patient with a paraesophageal hernia is usually asymptomatic. Because this type of hernia doesn't disturb the closing mechanism of the LES, it doesn't usually cause gastric reflux and reflux esophagitis. Symptoms, when present, usually stem from incarceration of a stomach portion above the diaphragmatic opening. The symptomatic patient may report a feeling of fullness after eating or, if the hernia interferes with breathing, a feeling of breathlessness or suffocation. He may also complain of chest pain resembling angina pectoris.

During the history, be attentive for the following signs and symptoms of possible complications:

• dysphagia, especially after ingestion of very hot or cold foods, alcoholic beverages, or a large amount of food (may indicate esophagitis, esophageal ulceration, or stricture)
• bleeding, which may be mild or massive, frank or occult (may indicate esophagitis or erosion of the gastric pouch).

Severe pain and shock are signs of incarceration, in which a large portion of the stomach is caught above the diaphragm (usually occurs in paraesophageal hernia). Incarceration requires immediate surgery because it can lead to perforation or strangulation and gangrene of the herniated stomach portion.

Diagnostic tests

• *Chest X-ray* occasionally shows an air shadow behind the heart in a large hernia and infiltrates in the lower lung lobes if the patient has aspirated the refluxed fluids.
• *Barium swallow with fluoroscopy* is the most specific test for detecting a hiatal hernia. The hernia may appear as an outpouching containing barium at the lower end of the esophagus. (Small hernias are difficult to recognize.) This study also shows diaphragmatic abnormalities.
• *Serum hemoglobin* and *hematocrit levels* may be decreased in patients with paraesophageal hernia.
• *Endoscopy* and *biopsy* differentiate between hiatal hernia, varices, and other small gastroesophageal lesions. These tests also identify the mucosal junction and the edge of the diaphragm indenting the esophagus and can rule out cancer that otherwise may remain undetected.
• *Esophageal motility studies* reveal esophageal motor or lower esophageal pressure abnormalities before surgical repair of the hernia.
• *pH studies* assess for reflux of gastric contents.

• *Acid perfusion test* indicates that heartburn results from esophageal reflux when perfusion of hydrochloric acid through a nasogastric tube provokes this symptom.

Treatment

The goals of treatment are to relieve symptoms by minimizing or correcting the incompetent LES (if present) and to manage and prevent complications. Medical therapy to reduce gastroesophageal reflux consists of medications, activity modifications, and dietary measures.

Antacids, which help neutralize refluxed fluids, are probably the best treatment for intermittent reflux. Intensive antacid therapy may call for hourly administration; however, the choice of antacids should take into account the patient's bowel function. Histamine-receptor antagonists, such as cimetidine, also modify the acidity of the fluid refluxed into the esophagus.

Drug therapy to strengthen LES tone may consist of a cholinergic agent, such as bethanechol. Metoclopramide has also been used to stimulate smooth-muscle contraction, increase LES tone, and decrease reflux after eating.

Other measures to reduce intermittent reflux include restricting any activity that increases intra-abdominal pressure and discouraging smoking because it stimulates gastric acid production. Modifying the diet to include smaller, more frequent meals and to eliminate spicy or irritating foods also may help to reduce reflux.

Rarely, surgery is required when symptoms persist despite medical treatment or if complications develop. Indications for surgery include esophageal stricture, significant bleeding, pulmonary aspiration, or incarceration or strangulation of the herniated stomach portion. Techniques vary greatly, but most forms of surgery create an artificial closing mechanism at the gastroesophageal junction to strengthen the barrier function of the LES. The surgeon may use an abdominal or a thoracic approach.

Rare postsurgical complications may include mucosal erosion, ulcers, and bleeding of the gastric pouch; pressure on the left lung due to the size and placement of the pouch; and formation of a volvulus.

Generally, a sliding hernia without an incompetent sphincter produces no reflux or symptoms and therefore requires no treatment. A large rolling hernia, however, should be surgically repaired (even if it produces no symptoms) because of the high risk of complications, especially strangulation.

Key nursing diagnoses and patient outcomes

Risk for aspiration of refluxed stomach fluids. Based on this nursing diagnosis, you'll establish these patient outcomes. The patient will:
• comply with the prescribed drug regimen to reduce gastroesophageal reflux
• modify diet and activity as prescribed to reduce gastroesophageal reflux
• avoid aspiration of refluxed stomach fluids.

Impaired swallowing related to esophagitis, esophageal ulceration, or stricture. Based on this nursing diagnosis, you'll establish these patient outcomes. The patient will:
• remain adequately nourished, as shown by a stable weight and absence of signs and symptoms of malnutrition
• regain ability to swallow normally through medical or surgical therapy.

Pain related to esophageal irritation caused by refluxed stomach fluids. Based on this nursing diagnosis, you'll establish these patient outcomes. The patient will:
• express pain relief after taking medications as prescribed
• take precautions to minimize reflux of stomach contents.

Nursing interventions

• Prepare the patient for diagnostic tests, as needed.

• Administer prescribed antacids and other medications.
• To reduce intra-abdominal pressure and prevent aspiration, have the patient sleep in a reverse Trendelenburg position (with the head of the bed elevated 6″ to 12″ [15 to 31 cm]). Advise him to avoid lying down immediately after meals and late-night snacks.
• If surgery is necessary, prepare the patient and provide appropriate preoperative and postoperative care.

Monitoring

• Assess the patient's response to treatment.
• Observe for complications, especially significant bleeding, pulmonary aspiration, or incarceration or strangulation of the herniated stomach portion.
• After endoscopy, watch for signs of perforation (falling blood pressure, rapid pulse, shock, and sudden pain) caused by the endoscope.

Patient teaching

• To enhance compliance, teach the patient about her disorder. Explain significant symptoms, diagnostic tests, and prescribed treatments.
• Review prescribed medications, explaining their desired actions and possible adverse effects. Tell the patient that he'll need medications for hiatal hernia treatment indefinitely, even after surgical repair.
• Teach the patient dietary changes to reduce reflux. For example, instruct him to eat small, frequent, bland meals to reduce stomach bulk and acid secretion. Advise him to avoid beverages and foods that intensify his symptoms, such as alcohol and spicy foods.
• Explain how gravity can help to prevent reflux. Encourage the patient to delay lying down for 2 hours after eating. Suggest that he elevate the head of his bed on 6″ (15-cm) blocks at home. Instruct him to avoid activities that increase intra-abdominal pressure, such as coughing, wearing constrictive clothing, and straining.

Histoplasmosis

This fungal infection has several other names, including Ohio Valley disease, Central Mississippi Valley disease, Appalachian Mountain disease, and Darling's disease. In the United States, histoplasmosis occurs in three forms: primary acute histoplasmosis, progressive disseminated histoplasmosis (acute disseminated or chronic disseminated disease), and chronic pulmonary (cavitary) histoplasmosis. The last form produces cavitations in the lung similar to those seen in pulmonary tuberculosis.

A fourth form, African histoplasmosis, occurs only in Africa and is caused by the fungus *Histoplasma capsulatum* var. *duboisii*.

Histoplasmosis occurs worldwide, especially in the temperate areas of Asia, Africa, Europe, North America, and South America. In the United States, it's most prevalent in the central and eastern states, especially in the Mississippi and Ohio river valleys.

Probably because of occupational exposure, histoplasmosis is more common in men than in women. Fatal disseminated disease occurs more frequently in infants and elderly men.

The incubation period ranges from 5 to 18 days, although chronic pulmonary histoplasmosis may progress slowly for many years. The prognosis varies with each form. The primary acute form is benign, but the progressive disseminated form is fatal in about 90% of patients. Without proper chemotherapy, chronic pulmonary histoplasmosis is fatal in about 50% of patients within 5 years.

Causes

Histoplasmosis is caused by *H. capsulatum,* which is found in the feces of birds and bats and in soil contaminated by their feces, such as that near roosts, chicken coops, barns, and caves and underneath bridges.

Transmission occurs through inhalation of *H. capsulatum* or *H. capsulatum* var. *duboisii* spores or through the invasion of spores after minor skin trauma.

Complications

Possible complications include vascular or bronchial obstruction, acute pericarditis, pleural effusion, mediastinal fibrosis or granuloma, intestinal ulceration, Addison's disease, endocarditis, and meningitis.

Assessment

The patient may have a history of an immunocompromised condition or exposure to contaminated soil in an endemic area.

The severity of symptoms depends on the size of the inhaled inoculum and the immune condition of the host. Also, symptoms vary with the form of the disease. For example, a patient with *primary acute histoplasmosis* may be asymptomatic, or he may complain of a mild respiratory illness similar to a severe cold or influenza. He also may report malaise, headache, myalgia, anorexia, cough, and chest pain. A patient with *progressive disseminated histoplasmosis* may complain of anorexia, weight loss and, possibly, pain, hoarseness, and dysphagia. A patient with *chronic pulmonary histoplasmosis* may have symptoms that mimic pulmonary tuberculosis. He may complain of a productive cough, dyspnea, and occasional hemoptysis. He'll eventually experience weight loss and breathlessness.

During your assessment, you'll usually note a fever, which may rise as high as 105° F (40.6° C), although its severity and duration can vary.

Inspection findings vary with the form of histoplasmosis. A patient with primary acute histoplasmosis usually won't reveal any characteristic signs. If the patient has progressive disseminated histoplasmosis, though, you may observe ulceration of the oropharynx, tachypnea in later stages, and pallor from anemia. You also may observe jaundice and ascites. In the patient with late-stage chronic pulmonary histoplasmosis, inspection may reveal shortness of breath, extreme weakness, and cyanosis.

Palpation may reveal hepatosplenomegaly and lymphadenopathy, characteristic findings in the progressive disseminated form of the disease.

Diagnostic tests

Miliary calcification in the lung or spleen and a positive histoplasmin skin test indicate exposure to histoplasmosis. Rising complement fixation and agglutination titers (more than 1:32) strongly suggest histoplasmosis.

Diagnosis requires a morphologic examination of tissue biopsy and culture of *H. capsulatum* from sputum in acute primary and chronic pulmonary histoplasmosis. A diagnosis of progressive disseminated histoplasmosis requires biopsy and culture of bone marrow, lymph nodes, blood, and infection sites. Cultures take several weeks to grow these organisms.

Faster diagnosis is possible with stained biopsies, using Gomori's stains (methenamine silver) or periodic acid–Schiff reaction. Findings must rule out tuberculosis and other diseases that produce similar symptoms.

The diagnosis of histoplasmosis caused by *H. capsulatum* var. *duboisii* calls for an examination of tissue biopsy and culture of the affected site.

Treatment

Treatment includes antifungal therapy, surgery, and supportive care.

Antifungal therapy plays the most important role. Except for asymptomatic primary acute histoplasmosis (which resolves spontaneously) and the African form, histoplasmosis requires high-dose or long-term (10-week) therapy with amphotericin B or ketoconazole.

Surgery includes lung resection to remove pulmonary nodules, a shunt for increased intracranial pressure, and cardiac repair for constrictive pericarditis.

Supportive care includes oxygen for respiratory distress, glucocorticoids for adrenal insufficiency, and parenteral fluids for dysphagia caused by oral or laryngeal ulcerations. Histoplasmosis doesn't necessitate isolation.

Key nursing diagnoses and patient outcomes

Activity intolerance related to hypoxia and malaise. Based on this nursing diagnosis, you'll establish these patient outcomes. The patient will:
• communicate controllable factors that reduce his activity tolerance
• demonstrate skill in conserving energy while carrying out daily activities
• seek support from his family and community services to assist with activities of daily living, as needed.

Altered nutrition: Less than body requirements, related to adverse GI effects of histoplasmosis. Based on this nursing diagnosis, you'll establish these patient outcomes. The patient will:
• regain any lost weight and maintain weight within a normal range
• eat nutritionally balanced meals
• avoid complications, such as malnutrition or vitamin deficiency.

Ineffective breathing pattern related to lung tissue changes. Based on this nursing diagnosis, you'll establish these patient outcomes. The patient will:
• maintain normal tissue oxygenation, as shown by normal arterial blood gas values.
• maintain adequate ventilation and maximum lung expansion.
• exhibit normal, unlabored respirations.

Nursing interventions

• Provide supportive nursing care for the patient with histoplasmosis.
• Administer drugs, as ordered. Because amphotericin B may cause pain, chills, fever, nausea, and vomiting, give appropriate antipyretics, antihistamines, analgesics, and antiemetics, as ordered. Small doses of meperidine or morphine sulfate may help reduce shaking chills. Give these drugs in the early morning or late evening so they don't sedate the patient for the entire day.
• Provide oxygen therapy if needed. Plan rest periods.
• Obtain chest X-ray results to determine if the patient has pulmonary or pleural effusion.
• Consult with the dietitian and patient concerning food preferences. Provide an appetizing, nutritious diet. The patient may benefit from small, frequent feedings. If he has oropharyngeal ulceration, he may need soft, bland foods. If the ulcerations are severe, he may need I.V. therapy.
• Make sure a patient with chronic pulmonary or progressive disseminated histoplasmosis receives psychological support to help him cope with long-term treatment. As needed, refer him to a social worker or an occupational therapist. Help the parents of a child with this disease arrange for a visiting teacher.
• Notify local public health authorities.

Monitoring

• Assess the patient's respiratory status every shift. Note diminished breath sounds or pleural friction rub, and evaluate for effusion.
• Check the patient's cardiovascular status every shift. Report any muffled heart sounds, jugular vein distention, pulsus paradoxus, or other signs of cardiac tamponade to the doctor immediately.
• Monitor the patient's neurologic status every shift and report any changes in level of consciousness or nuchal rigidity.

• Observe for signs and symptoms of hypoglycemia and hyperglycemia, which indicate adrenal dysfunction.
• Test all stools for blood and report its presence.

Patient teaching

• Teach the patient about drug therapy, including adverse effects.
• Inform the patient about the need for follow-up care on a regular basis for at least a year.
• Tell the patient to report to the doctor cardiac and pulmonary signs that could indicate effusions.
• To help prevent histoplasmosis, teach people in endemic areas to watch for early signs of this infection and to seek treatment promptly. Instruct people who risk occupational exposure to contaminated soil to wear face masks.

Hodgkin's disease

A neoplastic disorder, Hodgkin's disease is characterized by painless, progressive enlargement of the lymph nodes, spleen, and other lymphoid tissue. This enlargement results from proliferation of lymphocytes, histiocytes, eosinophils, and Reed-Sternberg cells. The latter cells are the special histologic feature of Hodgkin's disease.

Hodgkin's disease occurs in all races but is slightly more common in whites. Its incidence peaks in two age-groups – 15 to 38 and after age 50. It occurs most commonly in young adults – except in Japan, where it occurs exclusively among people over age 50. It has a higher incidence in men than in women. A family history of Hodgkin's disease increases the likelihood of acquiring the disorder.

Untreated, Hodgkin's disease follows a variable but relentlessly progressive and ultimately fatal course. However, recent advances in therapy make Hodgkin's disease potentially curable, even in advanced stages. Appropriate treatment yields a 5-year survival rate of about 90%.

Causes

Although the cause of Hodgkin's disease is unknown, some studies point to genetic, viral, or environmental factors.

Complications

Hodgkin's disease can cause multiple organ failure.

Assessment

Most commonly, the patient's history will reveal painless swelling of one of the cervical lymph nodes or sometimes the axillary or inguinal lymph nodes. The history may also reveal a persistent fever and night sweats. The patient may complain of weight loss despite an adequate diet, with resulting fatigue and malaise. As the disease advances, the patient may become increasingly susceptible to infection.

Inspection during the advanced stages of the disease may reveal edema of the face and neck, and jaundice.

Palpation may identify enlarged, rubbery lymph nodes in the neck. These nodes enlarge during periods of fever and then revert to normal size.

Diagnostic tests

Tests must first rule out other disorders that enlarge the lymph nodes.

Lymph node biopsy confirms the presence of Reed-Sternberg cells, abnormal histiocyte proliferation, and nodular fibrosis and necrosis.

Lymph node biopsy also helps determine lymph node and organ involvement, as do bone marrow, liver, mediastinal, and spleen biopsies; routine chest X-rays; abdominal computed tomography, lung, and bone scans; lymphangiography; and laparoscopy.

Hematologic tests show mild to severe normocytic anemia; normochromic anemia (in 50% of patients); and elevated, normal, or reduced white blood cell count and differential, showing any combination of neutrophilia, lymphocytopenia, monocytosis, and eosinophilia. Elevated serum alkaline phosphatase levels indicate liver or bone involvement.

A staging laparotomy is necessary for patients under age 55 and for those without obvious stage III or stage IV disease, lymphocyte predominance subtype histology, or medical contraindications. (See *Stages of Hodgkin's disease,* page 418.)

Treatment

Depending on the stage of the disease, the patient may receive chemotherapy, radiation therapy, or both. Correct treatment allows longer survival and may even induce a cure in many patients.

A patient with stage I or stage II disease receives radiation therapy alone; a patient with stage III disease receives radiation therapy and chemotherapy. For stage IV, the patient receives chemotherapy alone, sometimes inducing a complete remission. As an alternative, he may receive chemotherapy and radiation therapy to involved sites.

Chemotherapy consists of various combinations of drugs. The well-known MOPP protocol (mechlorethamine, vincristine [Oncovin], procarbazine, and prednisone) was the first to provide significant cures for generalized Hodgkin's disease. Another useful combination is ABVD (doxorubicin [Adriamycin], bleomycin, vinblastine, and dacarbazine). Treatment with these drugs may require concomitant administration of antiemetics, sedatives, and antidiarrheals to combat adverse GI effects.

Other treatments include autologous bone marrow transplantation and immunotherapy, which by itself hasn't proved effective.

Key nursing diagnoses and patient outcomes

Altered nutrition: Less than body requirements, related to GI effects of disease and treatment. Based on this nursing diagnosis, you'll establish these patient outcomes. The patient will:
- eat a nutritionally balanced diet
- regain lost weight and maintain weight within a normal range
- avoid complications, such as malnutrition and vitamin deficiency.

Fatigue related to the disease and adverse effects of chemotherapy or radiation therapy. Based on this nursing diagnosis, you'll establish these patient outcomes. The patient will:
- report controllable factors that cause fatigue
- demonstrate skill in conserving energy while carrying out daily activities
- regain a normal energy level after completing treatment.

Fear related to the threat of death. Based on this nursing diagnosis, you'll establish these patient outcomes. The patient will:
- express his feelings of fear
- use available support systems to cope with his fear
- have fewer physical symptoms of fear.

Nursing interventions

- Provide a well-balanced, high-calorie, high-protein diet. If the patient is anorexic, provide frequent, small meals. Consult with the dietitian to incorporate foods the patient enjoys into his diet.
- Offer the patient grapefruit juice, orange juice, or ginger ale to alleviate nausea and vomiting.
- Perform comfort measures that promote relaxation. Provide for periods of rest if the patient tires easily.
- Provide supportive care as indicated for any adverse effects of chemotherapy or radiation therapy.
- Throughout therapy, listen to the patient's fears and concerns. Encourage him to express his feelings, and stay with him during periods of extreme stress and anxiety. Provide emotional support to the patient and his family.

Stages of Hodgkin's disease

Treatment of Hodgkin's disease depends on the stage it has reached—that is, the number, location, and degree of involved lymph nodes. The Ann Arbor classification system, adopted in 1971, divides Hodgkin's disease into four stages.

Stage I
Hodgkin's disease appears in a single lymph node region (I) or a single extralymphatic organ (IE).

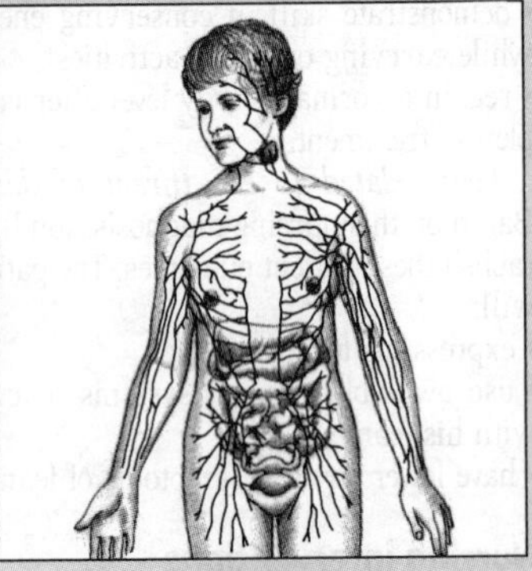

Stage II
The disease appears in two or more nodes on the same side of the diaphragm (II) and possibly in an extralymphatic organ (IIE).

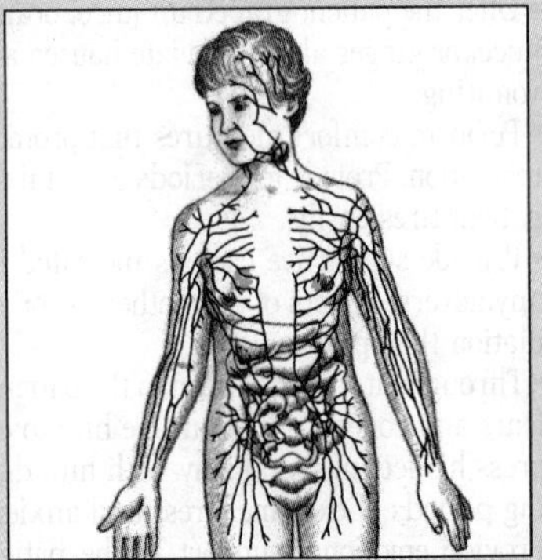

Stage III
Hodgkin's disease spreads to both sides of the diaphragm (III) and perhaps to an extralymphatic organ (IIIE), the spleen (IIIS), or both (IIIES).

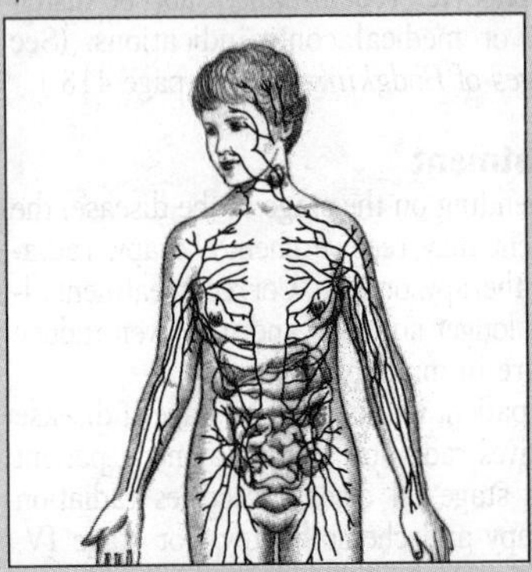

Stage IV
The disease disseminates, involving one or more extralymphatic organs or tissues, with or without lymph node involvement.

Doctors subdivide each stage into categories. Category A includes patients without defined signs and symptoms, and category B includes patients who experience such defined signs as recent unexplained weight loss, fever, and night sweats.

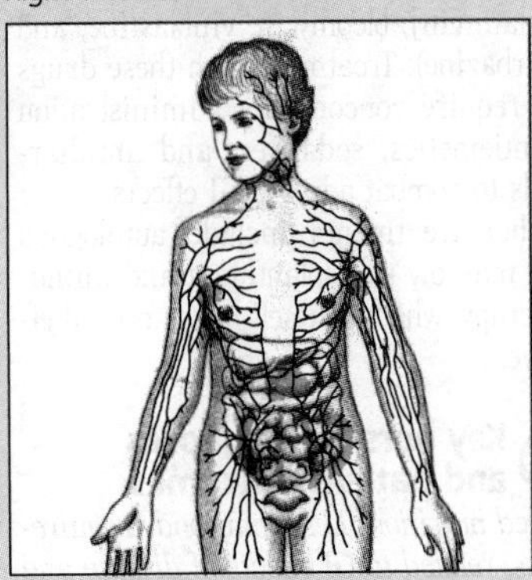

• Involve the patient and his family in all aspects of his care.

Monitoring

• Assess the patient for nutritional deficiencies and malnutrition. Weigh him regularly.

• Watch for complications during chemotherapy, including anorexia, nausea, vomiting, alopecia, and mouth ulcers.

• Stay alert for adverse effects of radiation therapy, such as hair loss, nausea, vomiting, and anorexia.

• Observe for signs of hypothyroidism, sterility, and other neoplastic disease, including late-onset leukemia and malignant lymphoma. Although these problems are complications of treatment, they also indicate the success of treatment.

Patient teaching

• Explain all procedures and treatments associated with the plan of care.

• Because sudden withdrawal of prednisone is life-threatening, advise the patient taking this medication not to change his drug dosage or discontinue the drug without contacting his doctor.

• If the patient is a woman of childbearing age, advise her to delay pregnancy until long-term remission occurs. Radiation therapy and chemotherapy can cause genetic mutations and spontaneous abortions.

• Stress the importance of maintaining good nutrition (aided by eating small, frequent meals of the patient's favorite foods) and drinking plenty of fluids.

• Instruct the patient to pace his activities to counteract therapy-induced fatigue. Teach him how to use relaxation techniques to promote comfort and reduce anxiety.

• Stress the importance of good oral hygiene to prevent stomatitis. To control pain and bleeding, teach the patient to use a soft toothbrush, a cotton swab, or an anesthetic mouthwash, such as viscous lidocaine (as prescribed); to apply petroleum jelly to his lips; and to avoid astringent mouthwashes.

• Advise the patient to avoid crowds and any person with a known infection. Emphasize that he should notify the doctor if he develops any infections.

• Because enlarged lymph nodes may indicate disease recurrence, teach the patient the importance of checking his lymph nodes.

• Make sure the patient understands the possible adverse effects of his treatments. Tell him to notify the doctor if these signs and symptoms persist.

• When appropriate, refer the patient and his family to community organizations, such as psychological counseling services, support groups, and hospices.

• Advise the patient to seek follow-up care after he has completed the initial treatment.

Huntington's disease

In this disease (also called Huntington's chorea, hereditary chorea, chronic progressive chorea, or adult chorea), degeneration in the cerebral cortex and basal ganglia causes chronic progressive chorea (dancelike movements) and mental deterioration, ending in dementia.

Huntington's disease usually strikes people between ages 25 and 55 (the average age is 35); however, 2% of cases occur in children, and 5%, as late as age 60. Death usually results 10 to 15 years after onset, from heart failure or pneumonia. Because the disease is hereditary, it's prevalent in areas where affected families have lived for several generations.

Causes

In 1993, after decades of research, scientists discovered the gene that causes Huntington's disease. Because the disease is transmitted as an autosomal dominant trait, either sex can transmit and inherit it. Each child of a parent with this disease has a 50% chance of inheriting it; however, the child who doesn't inherit it can't pass it on to his own children.

Complications

Potential complications include choking, aspiration, pneumonia, heart failure, and infections.

Assessment

Assessment findings vary, depending on disease progression. The patient history usually shows a family history of the disorder, along with emotional and mental changes.

The onset of Huntington's disease is insidious. The patient eventually becomes totally dependent through intellectual decline, emotional disturbances, and loss of musculoskeletal control.

In the early stages, the patient is described as being clumsy, irritable, or impatient and subject to fits of anger and periods of suicidal depression, apathy, or elation. As the disease progresses, family members may report that the patient's judgment and memory have became impaired. Hallucinations, delusions, and paranoid thinking may occur. (In late stages, emotional symptoms may subside, but eventually dementia does occur.) The family describes a gradual loss of intellectual ability, although the patient seems to be aware that his symptoms result from the disease. (Keep in mind that the dementia doesn't always progress at the same rate as the chorea.)

The patient may be described as having a ravenous appetite, especially for sweets. In late stages, the patient may note loose bladder and bowel control.

Inspection usually reveals choreic movements. These movements are rapid, often violent, and purposeless. In the early stages, they're unilateral and more prominent in the face and arms than in the legs. As the disease progresses, the choreic movements progress from mild fidgeting to grimacing, tongue smacking, dysarthria (indistinct speech), athetoid movements (especially of the hands) related to emotional state, and torticollis. In later stages, the movements involve the entire body musculature. Writhing and twitching are constant, speech becomes unintelligible, chewing and swallowing are difficult, and ambulation is impossible. In these late stages, the patient may appear emaciated and exhausted.

Diagnostic tests

Positron emission tomography and deoxyribonucleic acid analysis can detect Huntington's disease, but no reliable confirming test exists. However, the recent discovery of the causative gene has opened the way for development of further tests to detect and predict the disease. Computed tomography scan, a secondary study, shows brain atrophy.

Treatment

Because no cure currently exists for Huntington's disease, treatment is supportive, protective, and based on the patient's symptoms. Tranquilizers, as well as chlorpromazine, haloperidol, or imipramine, help control choreic movements, but they can't stop mental deterioration. They also alleviate discomfort and depression. However, tranquilizers increase patient rigidity. To control choreic movements without rigidity, choline may be prescribed.

Psychotherapy to decrease anxiety and stress may also be helpful. The patient may require institutionalization because of mental deterioration.

Key nursing diagnoses and patient outcomes

Altered health maintenance related to progressive physical and mental deterioration. Based on this nursing diagnosis, you'll establish these patient outcomes. The patient will:

- avoid injury resulting from a physical or mental deficit

• receive adequate care from a family member or caregiver.

Chronic low self-esteem related to physical and mental disabilities. Based on this nursing diagnosis, you'll establish these patient outcomes. The patient will:
• express his feelings about how the disease has affected his self-esteem
• describe at least two positive qualities about himself
• take steps to optimize his physical and emotional wellness.

Impaired physical mobility related to neurologic dysfunction. Based on this nursing diagnosis, you'll establish these patient outcomes. The patient will:
• use assistive devices and seek help when performing physical activities
• maintain normal muscle strength and joint range of motion
• avoid complications of impaired physical mobility, such as skin breakdown, contractures, venous stasis, or thrombus formation.

Nursing interventions

• Provide psychological support to the patient and his family, and listen to their fears and concerns. Stay with the patient during especially stressful periods. Answer questions honestly.
• Identify the patient's self-care deficits each time he's admitted to the hospital. Then provide physical support by attending to his basic needs, such as hygiene, skin care, bowel and bladder care, and nutrition. Increase this support as mental and physical deterioration make him increasingly immobile.
• Administer medications as ordered.
• Encourage the patient to remain as independent as possible. To help him do this, give short, explicit directions. Provide demonstrations, and give the patient ample time to perform the tasks that he's capable of performing.
• To help improve the patient's body image, allow him to participate in his care as much as possible. Encourage his efforts to adapt to the changes that he's experiencing.
• If the patient has difficulty speaking, provide him with communication aids, such as an alphabet board. Allow him sufficient time to communicate.
• Take suicide precautions. Control the patient's environment to protect him from suicide or other self-inflicted injury. Pad the side rails of the bed, but avoid restraints, which may cause the patient to injure himself with violent, uncontrolled movements.
• If the patient has difficulty walking, provide a walker to help him maintain his balance. If his choreic movements are violent enough to cause injury, pad the bed rails and be sure the patient is secure if he's sitting in a chair or wheelchair.
• If the patient is confined to bed, turn him every 2 hours. Post a turning schedule at the bedside.
• Minimize the patient's risk of infection by washing your hands before providing care and helping the patient wash his hands before and after meals and after using the bathroom, bedpan, or urinal.
• Elevate the head of the bed whenever the patient eats to reduce the risk of aspiration. Stay with him while he's eating, and instruct him to eat only small amounts of food at one time.
• Provide the incontinent patient with bladder elimination devices, such as an indwelling urinary catheter and body-worn drainage devices as appropriate. If the patient has bowel incontinence, provide incontinence aids, such as pad and pants or bed protector pads.

Monitoring

• Observe the patient for desired and adverse effects of medications.
• Stay alert for possible suicide attempts.
• Monitor the patient's temperature and white blood cell count to detect and correct infection early.
• Assess the patient for signs of neurologic deterioration.

Patient teaching

- Teach the patient and his family about the disease and its genetic cause. Explain the diagnostic tests and any required treatments.
- Teach the family how to perform home care.
- Encourage affected families to receive genetic counseling. All affected family members should realize that each of their offspring has a 50% chance of inheriting this disease.
- Refer the patient and his family to appropriate community organizations, such as home health care agencies, the social service department, psychiatric counseling, and long-term care facilities.
- For more information about this degenerative disease, refer the patient and family to the Huntington's Disease Society of America.

Hydronephrosis

An abnormal dilation of the renal pelvis and the calyces of one or both kidneys, hydronephrosis is caused by an obstruction of urine flow in the genitourinary tract. Although a partial obstruction and hydronephrosis may not produce symptoms initially, the pressure built up behind the area of obstruction eventually results in symptoms of renal dysfunction.

Causes

Almost any type of obstructive uropathy can lead to hydronephrosis. The most common causes are benign prostatic hyperplasia, urethral strictures, and calculi. Less common causes include strictures or stenosis of the ureter or bladder neck, congenital abnormalities, and abdominal tumors.

If the obstruction is in the urethra or bladder, hydronephrosis usually is bilateral; if the obstruction is in a ureter, hydronephrosis usually is unilateral. Obstructions distal to the bladder cause the bladder to dilate and act as a buffer zone, delaying hydronephrosis. Total and prolonged obstruction of urine flow with dilation of the collecting system ultimately causes complete cortical atrophy and cessation of glomerular filtration.

Complications

The most common complication of an obstructed kidney is life-threatening infection (pyelonephritis) caused by urinary stasis that exacerbates renal damage. If hydronephrosis results from acute obstructive uropathy, the patient may develop paralytic ileus. Untreated bilateral hydronephrosis can lead to renal failure, a life-threatening condition.

Assessment

The patient's history and chief complaint will vary, depending on the cause of the obstruction. For example, a patient may have no symptoms or complain of only mild pain and slightly decreased urine flow. Or he may report severe, colicky renal pain or dull flank pain that radiates to the groin and gross urinary abnormalities, such as hematuria, pyuria, dysuria, alternating oliguria and polyuria, and anuria.

A patient with hydronephrosis also may report nausea, vomiting, abdominal fullness, pain on urination, dribbling, and urinary hesitancy. Pain on only one side, usually in the flank area, may signal a unilateral obstruction.

Diagnostic tests

Excretory urography, retrograde pyelography, and renal function studies confirm the diagnosis. Visualization tests show concave (early stage) or convex (later stage) calyces as dilation progresses.

If the disease is extensive, tests will show atrophied distal and proximal tubules and obstructions. Urine studies will confirm the inability to concentrate urine, a decreased glomerular filtration rate and, possibly, pyuria if infection is present.

Treatment

Treatment should preserve renal function and prevent infection by surgical removal of the obstruction. Surgery includes dilatation for a urethral stricture or prostatectomy for benign prostatic hyperplasia.

If renal function has already been affected, therapy may include a diet low in protein, sodium, and potassium. This diet is designed to stop the progression of renal failure before surgery.

Inoperable obstructions may necessitate decompression and drainage of the kidney, using a nephrostomy tube placed temporarily or permanently in the renal pelvis. Concurrent infection requires appropriate antibiotic therapy.

Key nursing diagnoses and patient outcomes

Altered urinary elimination related to urinary tract obstruction. Based on this nursing diagnosis, you'll establish these patient outcomes. The patient will:

- recognize and report changes in his urine elimination pattern
- seek immediate medical attention if his urine elimination pattern changes
- avoid complications of urinary tract obstruction
- regain a normal urine elimination pattern with treatment
- show how to safely manage catheters placed to relieve or bypass the obstruction.

Risk for infection related to urinary stasis. Based on this nursing diagnosis, you'll establish these patient outcomes. The patient will:

- maintain a normal temperature and normal serum and urine white blood cell counts
- exhibit clear urine with no foul odor
- avoid urinary tract or kidney infection.

Pain related to urinary tract irritation and inflammation caused by obstruction. Based on this nursing diagnosis, you'll establish these patient outcomes. The patient will:

What happens in postobstructive diuresis

Polyuria—urine output that exceeds 2,000 ml in 8 hours—and excessive electrolyte losses characterize postobstructive diuresis. Although usually self-limiting, this condition can cause vascular collapse, shock, and death if not treated with fluid and electrolyte replacement.

Prolonged pressure of retained urine damages renal tubules, limiting their ability to concentrate urine. Removing the obstruction relieves the pressure, but tubular function may not significantly improve for days or weeks, depending on the patient's condition.

Although diuresis typically abates in a few days, it persists if serum creatinine levels remain high. When these levels approach the normal range (0.7 to 1.4 mg/dl), diuresis usually subsides.

- express pain relief after analgesic administration
- become pain free once the obstruction and disease resolve.

Nursing interventions

- Administer prescribed pain medication.
- Keep in mind that postobstructive diuresis may cause the patient to lose excessive dilute urine over hours or days. If this occurs, give I.V. fluids at a constant rate, as ordered, and an amount of I.V. fluid equal to a percentage of hourly urine, to safely replace intravascular volume. (See *What happens in postobstructive diuresis.*)
- Consult with a dietitian to provide a diet consistent with the treatment plan.
- If a nephrostomy tube has been inserted, irrigate the tube only as ordered, and don't clamp it. If a nephrostomy tube is placed percutaneously and is small, irrigation may be dangerous and should only be done if the tube is not draining. Give meticulous skin care to the area around the tube; if urine

leaks, provide a protective skin barrier to decrease excoriation.
• Prepare the patient for surgery, as indicated. (See the entry "Prostatectomy.")
• Allow the patient to express his fears and anxieties, and help him find effective coping strategies.

Monitoring

• Check renal function studies daily, including blood urea nitrogen, serum creatinine, and serum potassium levels. As appropriate, arrange for specific gravity tests at the bedside.
• Postoperatively, closely monitor intake and output, vital signs, and fluid and electrolyte status. Watch for a rising pulse rate and cold, clammy skin, which may signal impending hemorrhage and shock.
• If a nephrostomy tube has been inserted, check it frequently for bleeding and patency. Observe for signs of infection.

Patient teaching

• Explain hydronephrosis to the patient and his family. Also explain the purpose of diagnostic tests and how they're performed.
• If the patient is scheduled for surgery, explain the procedure and postoperative care.
• If the patient will be discharged with a nephrostomy tube in place, teach him how to care for it, including how to thoroughly clean the skin around the insertion site.
• If the patient must take antibiotics after discharge, tell him to take all of the prescribed medication, even if he feels better.
• To prevent the progression of hydronephrosis to irreversible renal disease, urge an older male patient (especially a patient with a family history of benign prostatic hyperplasia or prostatitis) to have routine medical checkups. Teach him to recognize and report symptoms of hydronephrosis, such as colicky pain or hematuria, or urinary tract infection.

Hyperaldosteronism

In this disorder, hypersecretion of the mineralocorticoid aldosterone by the adrenal cortex causes excessive reabsorption of sodium and water and excessive renal excretion of potassium.

The disorder may be classified as primary, resulting from a stimulus inside the adrenal gland, or secondary, resulting from an extraadrenal stimulus. Incidence of hyperaldosteronism is two times greater in women than in men and highest between ages 30 and 50.

Causes

Primary hyperaldosteronism (Conn's syndrome) is uncommon. In 70% of patients it results from a small, unilateral aldosterone-producing adrenal adenoma. In the remaining 30%, the cause is either unclear, adrenocortical hyperplasia (in children), or carcinoma. Excessive ingestion of English black licorice or a similar substance can produce a syndrome similar to primary hyperaldosteronism due to the mineralocorticoid action of glycyrrhizic acid, which is present in licorice.

Secondary hyperaldosteronism results from extraadrenal pathology, which stimulates the adrenal gland to increase production of aldosterone. For example, conditions that reduce renal blood flow (renal artery stenosis) and extracellular fluid volume or that produce a sodium deficit activate the renin-angiotensin-aldosterone system and, subsequently, increase aldosterone secretion. Thus, secondary hyperaldosteronism may result from conditions that induce hypertension through increased renin production (such as Wilms' tumor), from ingestion of oral contraceptives, and from pregnancy. However, this type may also result from disorders unrelated to hypertension that may or may not cause edema. For example, nephrotic syndrome, hepatic cirrhosis with ascites, and congestive heart failure (CHF) commonly induce edema; Bartter's syndrome and salt-losing nephritis don't.

Complications

Hyperaldosteronism can produce neuromuscular irritability, tetany, paresthesia, and seizures. Cardiac complications include arrhythmias, ischemic heart disease, left ventricular hypertrophy, CHF, and death. Metabolic alkalosis, nephropathy, and azotemia may also occur.

Assessment

The patient may complain of headache, visual disturbances, muscle weakness, fatigue, polyuria, and polydipsia. Inspection may detect intermittent flaccid paralysis, resulting from hypokalemia and, possibly, tetany, which may be caused by metabolic alkalosis and lead to hypocalcemia. Secondary hyperaldosteronism rarely occurs without edema.

Palpation may reveal a weak pulse, signs of muscle tonicity, and positive Chvostek's and Trousseau's signs. Auscultation of the apical pulse may detect cardiac arrhythmias. Auscultation of blood pressure reveals hypertension.

Diagnostic tests

Persistently low serum potassium levels in a nonedematous patient who isn't taking diuretics, who doesn't have obvious GI losses (from diarrhea), and who has a normal sodium intake suggest hyperaldosteronism. If hypokalemia develops in a hypertensive patient shortly after starting treatment with potassium-wasting diuretics (such as thiazides), and it persists after the diuretic has been discontinued and potassium replacement therapy has been instituted, evaluation for hyperaldosteronism is necessary. The test results below confirm hyperaldosteronism:

- A low plasma renin level after volume depletion by diuretic administration when the patient is sitting or standing and a high plasma aldosterone level after volume expansion by salt loading confirm primary hyperaldosteronism in a hypertensive patient without edema.
- An elevated serum bicarbonate level with ensuing alkalosis commonly results from hydrogen and potassium ion loss in the distal renal tubules.

Other test findings show markedly increased urine aldosterone levels, increased plasma aldosterone levels, and increased plasma renin levels (in secondary hyperaldosteronism).

A suppression test differentiates between primary and secondary hyperaldosteronism. The patient receives corticotropin, 80 units I.M. b.i.d. for 2 days. Small doses of dexamethasone are also given to supplement physiologic levels of glucocorticoid activity. Plasma and urine cortisol levels are measured. These levels increase in normal patients, while patients with secondary adrenal insufficiency exhibit small increases. Patients with primary adrenal insufficiency have nearly undetectable levels.

Other helpful diagnostic evidence includes increased plasma volume of 30% to 50% above normal; electrocardiogram signs of hypokalemia (ST-segment depression and U waves); chest X-ray showing left ventricular hypertrophy from chronic hypertension; and localization of tumor shown on computed tomography scan, ultrasonography, or magnetic resonance imaging.

Treatment

Although treatment for primary hyperaldosteronism may include unilateral adrenalectomy, hyperaldosteronism may be controlled without surgery through administration of the potassium-sparing diuretic spironolactone and sodium restriction. Bilateral adrenalectomy reduces blood pressure for most patients with idiopathic primary hyperaldosteronism. However, some degree of hypertension usually persists, requiring treatment with spironolactone or another antihypertensive drug. Such patients also require lifelong adrenal hormone replacement.

Treatment of secondary hyperaldosteronism must include correction of the underlying cause.

Key nursing diagnoses and patient outcomes

Altered urinary elimination related to polyuria. Based on this nursing diagnosis, you'll establish these patient outcomes. The patient will:

- express an understanding of how hyperaldosteronism causes polyuria
- comply with the treatment regimen, including restricting sodium intake and taking medications as prescribed
- exhibit cessation of polyuria with treatment.

Decreased cardiac output related to arrhythmias caused by hypokalemia. Based on this nursing diagnosis, you'll establish these patient outcomes. The patient will:

- maintain a normal heart rate and rhythm
- maintain adequate cardiac output as shown by normal blood pressure and intact mental status.

Knowledge deficit related to hyperaldosteronism and its treatment. Based on this nursing diagnosis, you'll establish these patient outcomes. The patient will:

- express a desire to learn about hyperaldosteronism and its treatment
- actively participate in a learning situation that addresses hyperaldosteronism and its treatment
- express an understanding of hyperaldosteronism and its treatment.

Nursing interventions

- Give potassium replacements, as ordered, and keep I.V. calcium gluconate available.
- Provide comfort measures to relieve headache. For example, administer analgesics, apply ice packs, and decrease environmental stimuli.
- Consult a dietitian to plan a low-sodium, high-potassium diet.
- Schedule activities to encourage rest, prevent fatigue, and decrease myocardial oxygen demand. Gradually increase activity as tolerated.
- Prepare the patient for adrenalectomy, as indicated. (See the entry "Adrenalectomy.")
- Encourage the patient to verbalize his feelings about his illness. Offer emotional support, and help him identify his strengths and use them to develop coping strategies. Refer him to a mental health professional, if necessary.

Monitoring

- Measure and record the patient's vital signs, fluid intake, urine output, and weight.
- Monitor serum electrolyte levels.
- Assess the patient for signs of tetany (muscle twitching and Chvostek's sign) and for hypokalemia-induced arrhythmias, paresthesia, or weakness.

Patient teaching

- Advise the patient that he'll need long-term adrenal hormone replacement. Tell him and his family to identify and report signs of drug overdose or underdose.
- Encourage the patient to wear a medical identification bracelet and to carry his medications with him at all times.
- Instruct the patient to follow a low-sodium, high-potassium diet.
- If the patient is taking spironolactone, tell him to watch for and report signs of hyperkalemia. Warn a male patient that impotence and gynecomastia may follow long-term use.

Hyperlipoproteinemia

Marked by increased plasma concentrations of one or more lipoproteins, hyperlipoproteinemia affects lipid transport in serum. Primary hyperlipoproteinemia oc-

Classifying hyperlipoproteinemia

Type	Causes and incidence	Diagnostic findings
Type I Frederickson's hyperlipoproteinemia, fat-induced hyperlipemia, idiopathic familial hyperlipoproteinemia	• Deficient or abnormal lipoprotein lipase, resulting in decreased or absent lipolytic activity after heparin administration • Relatively rare • Present at birth	• Chylomicrons (VLDL, LDL, HDL) in plasma 14 hours or more after last meal • High elevated serum chylomicron and triglyceride levels; slightly elevated serum cholesterol levels • Decreased serum lipoprotein lipase levels • Leukocytosis
Type II Familial hyperbetalipoproteinemia, essential familial hypercholesterolemia	• Deficient cell surface receptor that regulates LDL degradation and cholesterol synthesis, resulting in increased levels of plasma LDL over joints and pressure points • Onset between ages 10 and 30	• Increased plasma concentrations of LDL • Elevated serum LDL and cholesterol levels • Increased LDL levels detected by amniocentesis
Type III Familial broad-beta hyperlipoproteinemia, xanthoma tuberosum	• Primary defect involving deficient LDL receptor • Uncommon: usually occurring after age 20, possibly earlier in men	• Abnormal serum beta-lipoprotein levels • Elevated cholesterol and triglyceride levels • Slightly elevated glucose tolerance
Type IV Endogenous hypertriglyceridemia, hyperbetalipoproteinemia	• Primary defect unknown; usually occurs with increased prevalence of obesity, diabetes, hypertension • Relatively common, especially in middle-aged men	• Elevated VLDL levels • Moderately increased plasma triglyceride levels • Normal or slightly elevated serum cholesterol levels • Mildly abnormal glucose tolerance • Family history • Early CAD
Type V Mixed hypertriglyceridemia, mixed hyperlipemia	• Defective triglyceride clearance causes pancreatitis; usually secondary to another disorder, such as obesity or nephrosis • Uncommon: usually occurring in late adolescence or early adulthood	• Chylomicrons in plasma • Elevated plasma VLDL levels • Elevated serum cholesterol and triglyceride levels

curs as at least five distinct metabolic disorders, all of which may be inherited. Hyperlipoproteinemia may also occur secondary to other conditions, such as diabetes mellitus. (See *Classifying hyperlipoproteinemia.*) The disorder produces varied clinical changes. These include relatively mild signs and symptoms that can be corrected by dietary management to potentially fatal pancreatitis.

Causes

The primary hyperlipoproteinemias result from genetic disorders. Types I and III are transmitted as autosomal recessive traits; Types II, IV, and V are transmitted as autosomal dominant traits. Secondary hyperlipoproteinemia results from another metabolic disorder, such as diabetes mellitus; consumption of alcohol; or ingestion of oral contraceptives.

Complications

Sequelae of hyperlipoproteinemia include coronary artery disease (CAD) and pancreatitis.

Assessment

The history of a patient with Type I disease typically reveals recurrent attacks of severe abdominal pain similar to pancreatitis, usually preceded by fat intake. The patient may also report malaise and anorexia.

Inspection may reveal papular or eruptive xanthomas (pinkish yellow cutaneous deposits of fat) over pressure points and extensor surfaces. Ophthalmoscopic examination typically reveals lipemia retinalis (reddish white retinal vessels). Palpation may detect abdominal spasm, rigidity, or rebound tenderness, and hepatosplenomegaly, with liver or spleen tenderness. Fever may be present.

A patient with Type II disease may have a history of premature and accelerated coronary atherosclerosis, with symptoms typically developing when the patient is in his twenties or thirties. Inspection commonly reveals tendinous xanthomas (firm masses) on the Achilles tendons and tendons of the hands and feet, tuberous xanthomas, xanthelasma, and juvenile corneal arcus (opaque ring surrounding the corneal periphery).

Typically, a patient with Type III disease doesn't complain of clinical symptoms until after age 20 when severe atherosclerosis may develop. The patient's history may include such aggravating factors as obesity, hypothyroidism, and diabetes mellitus.

Inspection may reveal tuberoeruptive xanthomas (soft, inflamed, pedunculated lesions) over the elbows and knees and palmar xanthomas on the hands, particularly the fingertips (orange or yellow discolorations of the palmar and digital creases).

A patient with Type IV disease may have a history of atherosclerosis and early CAD. Patient history also may include factors, such as excessive alcohol consumption, poorly controlled diabetes mellitus, and ingestion of birth control pills containing estrogen, which can precipitate severe hypertriglyceridemia. Hypertension and hyperuricemia may also be present. Inspection commonly reveals the presence of obesity. Although not characteristic, xanthomas may be noted during exacerbations.

The history of a patient with Type V disease may reveal abdominal pain associated with pancreatitis and complaints related to peripheral neuropathy. Inspection may note eruptive xanthomas on the extensor surface of the arms and legs. Ophthalmoscopic examination may reveal lipemia retinalis. Palpation may detect hepatosplenomegaly.

Diagnostic tests

Serum lipid profiles – elevated levels of total cholesterol, triglycerides, very-low-density lipoproteins (VLDL), low-density lipoproteins (LDL), or high-density lipoproteins (HDL) – indicate hyperlipoproteinemia.

Treatment

Primary treatment focuses on dietary management, including weight reduction, restriction of cholesterol and saturated animal fat intake, and inclusion of polyunsaturated vegetable oils, which reduce concentration of plasma LDL.

The second therapeutic aim is to eliminate aggravating factors, such as diabetes mellitus, alcoholism, or hypothyroidism.

The patient should also reduce other risk factors that may predispose him to atherosclerosis. As appropriate, self-care measures may include cessation of smoking, treatment of hypertension, maintenance of a good exercise and physical fitness program and, if the patient has diabetes mellitus, control of blood glucose levels.

Treatment may be supplemented by drug therapy (cholestyramine, gemfibrozil, lovastatin, clofibrate, nicotinic acid) to lower plasma concentrations of lipoproteins, either by decreasing their production or by increasing their removal from plasma.

Type I hyperlipoproteinemia requires long-term weight reduction, with fat intake restricted to less than 20 g/day. A 20- to 40-g/day, medium-chain triglyceride diet may be ordered to supplement caloric intake. The patient should also avoid alcoholic beverages to decrease plasma triglyceride levels. The prognosis is good with treatment; without treatment, death can result from pancreatitis.

For Type II hyperlipoproteinemia, dietary management to restore normal lipid levels and decrease the risk of atherosclerosis includes restriction of cholesterol intake to under 300 mg/day for adults and under 150 mg/day for children. Additional measures include restricting triglyceride intake to under 100 mg/day for both children and adults. The diet should also be high in polyunsaturated fats.

If these measures don't bring cholesterol levels to within normal range, bile acid–binding resins, such as cholestyramine, are added to the regimen. (See *Using bile acid sequestrants.*) The regimen also may be supplemented with nicotinic acid or lovastatin.

If the patient can't tolerate drug therapy, surgical creation of an ileal bypass may be necessary. This surgery accelerates the loss of bile acids in the stool and often causes heterozygotes to show a moderate to marked lowering of plasma cholesterol levels.

NURSING ALERT

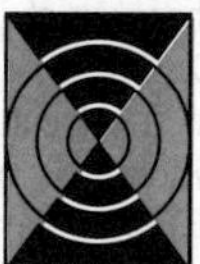

Using bile acid sequestrants

Before giving your patient a bile acid sequestrant, such as cholestyramine, to lower cholesterol levels, make sure he isn't taking one of the following drugs, whose absorption may be affected by bile acid sequestrants:
- beta-adrenergic blockers
- digitoxin
- diuretics
- fat-soluble vitamins
- folic acid
- thiazides
- thyroxine
- warfarin.

For severely affected homozygote children, portacaval shunt may be used as a last resort to reduce plasma cholesterol levels. A continuous-flow blood cell centrifuge to perform plasma exchanges at monthly intervals may be used to lower cholesterol levels.

For Type III hyperlipoproteinemia, dietary management includes restriction of cholesterol intake to under 300 mg/day; carbohydrates must also be restricted, and polyunsaturated fats are increased. Clofibrate and gemfibrozil help lower blood lipid levels. Weight reduction is helpful. With strict adherence to the prescribed diet, the prognosis is good.

For Type IV hyperlipoproteinemia, weight reduction may normalize blood lipid levels without additional treatment. Long-term dietary management includes restricted cholesterol intake, increased polyunsaturated fats, and avoidance of alcoholic beverages. Some patients respond to drug therapy, for example, gemfibrozil or nicotinic acid. Clofibrate may also be helpful in treating certain patients. The prognosis remains uncertain, however, because of predisposition to premature CAD.

The most effective treatment for Type V hyperlipoproteinemia is weight reduction and long-term maintenance of a low-fat diet. Alcoholic beverages and oral contraceptives must be avoided. Nicotinic acid, clofibrate, gemfibrozil, and a 20- to 40-g/day, medium-chain triglyceride diet may prove helpful. The prognosis is uncertain because of the risk of pancreatitis. Increased fat intake may cause recurrent bouts of illness, possibly leading to pseudocyst formation, hemorrhage, and death.

Key nursing diagnoses and patient outcomes

Risk for injury related to the cardiovascular and pancreatic effects of hyperlipoproteinemia. Based on this nursing diagnosis, you'll establish these patient outcomes. The patient will:

- express an understanding of the effects of uncorrected hyperlipoproteinemia
- comply with prescribed treatments, as shown by a consistently normal lipid profile
- exhibit few or no changes in cardiovascular and pancreatic function.

Knowledge deficit related to hyperlipoproteinemia and its treatment. Based on this nursing diagnosis, you'll establish these patient outcomes. The patient will:

- express a need to learn about hyperlipoproteinemia and its treatment and express the desire to do so
- participate actively in a learning situation that addresses hyperlipoproteinemia and its treatment
- express an understanding of hyperlipoproteinemia and its treatment.

Pain related to pancreatitis. Based on this nursing diagnosis, you'll establish these patient outcomes. The patient will:

- express pain relief after analgesic administration
- comply with prescribed treatments to reduce pancreatic effects of hyperlipoproteinemia and thus decrease pain severity and frequency
- become pain free with treatment.

Nursing interventions

- Administer antilipemics as ordered, taking measures to prevent or minimize adverse reactions.
- Urge the patient to adhere to his diet (usually 1,000 to 1,500 calories/day) and to avoid excess sugar and alcoholic beverages, to minimize the intake of saturated fats (higher in meats, coconut oil), and to increase the intake of polyunsaturated fats (vegetable oils).
- Assist the patient with additional lifestyle changes. Stress the need for medically supervised exercise and cessation of smoking. Refer him to safe, effective programs and support groups, as needed.
- Encourage the patient to verbalize fears related to premature CAD. Offer support and provide a clear explanation of the treatment regimen. Refer the patient for additional counseling, if needed.
- Provide supportive care as necessary, such as controlling pain in pancreatitis and administering cardiovascular drugs in CAD.
- Prepare the patient for surgery, if indicated.

Monitoring

- Check the patient's lipid profile regularly.
- Observe the patient for therapeutic and adverse effects of antilipemic therapy. Document and report any adverse reactions.
- Monitor the patient for signs and symptoms of CAD and pancreatitis.

Patient teaching

- For the 2 weeks preceding serum cholesterol and serum triglyceride tests, instruct the patient to maintain a steady weight and to adhere strictly to the prescribed diet. He should also fast for 12 hours before the test.

• Caution women with elevated serum lipids to avoid oral contraceptives or drugs that contain estrogen.
• Provide the patient with written information about foods high in cholesterol and saturated fats. Refer him to a dietitian, if necessary.
• Teach the patient about the varying components of the lipid profile and the ramifications of each. Discuss various means of lowering VLDL and LDL levels while increasing HDL levels.
• Make sure the patient understands his prescribed medication regimen. Provide verbal and written information on drug name, action, dosage, adverse reactions, monitoring requirements, and signs and symptoms requiring medical evaluation.

Bone resorption in primary hyperparathyroidism

Primary hyperparathyroidism is marked by characteristic bone changes that are revealed by X-rays.

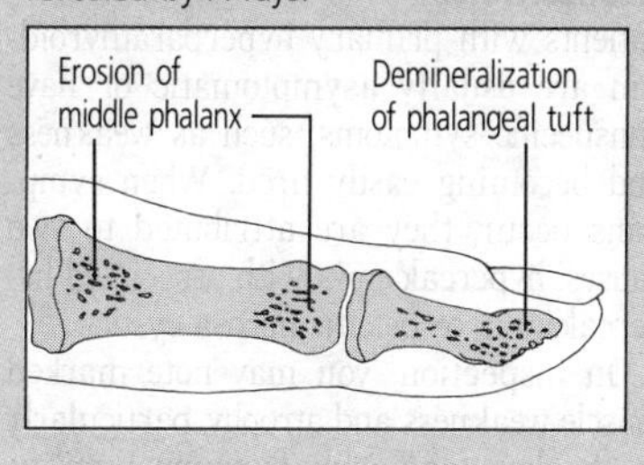

Hyperparathyroidism

Characterized by overactivity of one or more of the four parathyroid glands, hyperparathyroidism results in excessive secretion of parathyroid hormone (PTH). Increased PTH levels act directly on the bone and kidney tubules, causing an increase of calcium in the extracellular fluid that can't be compensated for by renal excretion or uptake into the soft tissues or skeleton. (See *Bone resorption in primary hyperparathyroidism.*)

Hyperparathyroidism increases dramatically in both men and women after age 50 and is two to four times more common in women. The disorder is classified as primary or secondary, based on its etiology.

Causes

In primary hyperparathyroidism, one or more of the parathyroid glands enlarges, increasing PTH secretion and elevating serum calcium levels. The cause of primary hyperparathyroidism is unknown. A genetic factor may be involved. Also, patients with thyroid carcinoma who have had neck irradiation have developed primary hyperparathyroidism.

In secondary hyperparathyroidism, excessive compensatory production of PTH stems from a hypocalcemia-producing abnormality outside the parathyroid gland, which causes a resistance to the metabolic action of PTH. Rickets, chronic renal failure, vitamin D deficiency, osteomalacia due to laxative abuse or phenytoin, or an excessive intake of thiazide diuretics, vitamin D, and calcium supplements may cause hypocalcemia.

Complications

Untreated hyperparathyroidism damages the skeleton and kidneys from hypercalcemia. Bone and articular problems, such as chondrocalcinosis; occasional severe osteopenia, especially of the vertebrae; erosions of the juxta-articular surface; subchondrial fractures; traumatic synovitis; and pseudogout, may occur.

Renal complications include renal calculi, renal colic, nephrolithiasis, urinary tract infections, renal insufficiency and, eventually, renal failure.

Other possible complications include peptic ulcers, cholelithiasis, pancreatitis, cardiac arrhythmias, vascular damage, hypertension, and heart failure. Severe hypercalcemia may cause parathyroid poisoning, which includes central nervous system (CNS) changes, renal failure, rapid precipitation of calcium throughout the soft tissues and, possibly, coma.

Assessment

Patients with primary hyperparathyroidism are usually asymptomatic or have nonspecific symptoms, such as weakness and becoming easily tired. When symptoms occur, they are attributed to two causes: hypercalcemia with associated hypercalciuria or osteitis fibrosa cystica.

On inspection, you may note marked muscle weakness and atrophy, particularly in the legs, and joint hyperextensibility. With CNS involvement, alterations in level of consciousness, such as disorientation, stupor, and coma, may appear. Skeletal deformities of the long bones are visible. Palpation may detect hyporeflexia, and auscultation of blood pressure may reveal hypertension.

Diagnostic tests

- *Serum PTH, calcium, and phosphorus levels,* and *urine cyclic adenosine monophosphate determinations* are the tests used most often to detect hyperparathyroidism.
- *Radioimmunoassay* confirms diagnosis by showing increased concentration of PTH, with accompanying hypercalcemia.
- *X-rays* reveal diffuse bone demineralization, bone cysts, subperiosteal resorption in long bones, and a "salt and pepper" appearance of the skull.
- *X-ray spectrophotometry* or other microscopic examinations of the bone demonstrate increased bone turnover.
- *Esophagography, thyroid scan, parathyroid thermography, ultrasonography, thyroid angiography, computed tomography scan,* and *magnetic resonance imaging* can help locate parathyroid lesions.
- *Supportive laboratory tests* reveal decreased serum phosphorus; elevated urine and serum calcium, chloride, uric acid, creatinine, alkaline phosphatase, and basal acid secretion; and serum immunoreactive gastrin levels.

In diagnosing secondary hyperparathyroidism, laboratory test findings show normal or slightly decreased serum calcium levels and variable serum phosphorus levels, especially when hyperparathyroidism is due to rickets, osteomalacia, or renal disease. Other laboratory values and physical examination findings identify the cause of secondary hyperparathyroidism.

Treatment

Primary hyperparathyroidism may be treated by surgical removal of the adenoma or, depending on the extent of hyperplasia, all but half of one gland (the remaining part is necessary to maintain normal PTH levels). Although surgery may relieve bone pain within 3 days, renal damage may be irreversible.

Preoperatively – or if surgery isn't feasible or necessary – other treatments can decrease calcium levels. Such treatments include forcing fluids; limiting dietary intake of calcium; promoting sodium and calcium excretion through forced diuresis using 0.9% sodium chloride solution (up to 6 liters in life-threatening circumstances), furosemide, or ethacrynic acid; and administering oral sodium or potassium phosphate, calcitonin, or plicamycin.

To prevent postoperative magnesium and phosphate deficiencies, the patient receives I.V. magnesium and phosphate or sodium phosphate solution given orally or by retention enema. In addition, during the first 4 or 5 days after surgery, when serum calcium falls to low-normal levels, supplemental calcium may be necessary; vitamin D or calcitriol may also be used to raise serum calcium levels.

Treatment of secondary hyperparathyroidism aims to correct the underlying cause of parathyroid hypertrophy and includes vitamin D therapy or, in the patient with renal disease, aluminum hydroxide for hyperphosphatemia. The patient with renal failure requires dialysis – possibly for the rest of his life – to lower calcium levels. In the patient with chronic secondary hyperparathyroidism, the enlarged glands may not revert to normal size and function even after calcium levels have been controlled.

Glucocorticoids are effective inhibitors of bone resorption and may be particularly useful in treating hypercalcemia associated with certain cancers.

Key nursing diagnoses and patient outcomes

Activity intolerance related to bone pain and neuromuscular deficits. Based on this nursing diagnosis, you'll establish these patient outcomes. The patient will:
- regain and maintain normal muscle mass and strength
- maintain maximum joint range of motion
- perform self-care activities as tolerated.

Risk for injury related to the effects of hypercalcemia. Based on this nursing diagnosis, you'll establish these patient outcomes. The patient will:
- express an understanding of how hypercalcemia affects her body
- comply with prescribed treatments, as shown by normal serum calcium levels, to minimize organ damage
- maintain normal body functions.

Pain related to musculoskeletal changes caused by persistently elevated serum calcium levels. Based on this nursing diagnosis, you'll establish these patient outcomes. The patient will:
- express pain relief after analgesic administration
- use comfort measures to relieve pain
- become pain free when calcium levels return to normal.

Nursing interventions

- Obtain baseline serum potassium, calcium, phosphate, and magnesium levels before treatment because these values may change abruptly once treatment begins.
- Provide at least 3 liters of fluid a day, including cranberry or prune juice, to increase urine acidity and help prevent calculus formation.
- Take safety precautions to minimize the risk of injury from a fall. Help the patient walk, keep the bed in the lowest position, and raise the side rails. Lift the immobilized patient carefully to minimize bone stress.
- Schedule care to allow the patient with muscle weakness as much rest as possible. Gradually increase activity according to his tolerance. Moderate weight-bearing activities are more beneficial than exercising in a bed or chair.
- Provide comfort measures to alleviate bone pain. Help the patient to turn, and reposition him every 2 hours. Support the affected extremities with pillows. Use extreme care when lifting the patient. Provide analgesics as ordered.
- Administer antacids, as appropriate, to prevent peptic ulcers. Consult a dietitian to plan a diet with adequate calories.
- Encourage the patient to verbalize his feelings about body image changes and rejection by others. Offer emotional support, and help him to develop coping strategies. Refer him to a mental health professional for additional counseling, if necessary.

Monitoring

- Monitor the patient's serum potassium, calcium, phosphate, and magnesium levels regularly.
- During hydration aimed at reducing the serum calcium level, monitor and record intake and output and strain urine to check for renal calculi.
- Auscultate the lungs regularly. Check for signs of pulmonary edema in the patient receiving large amounts of 0.9% sodium chloride solution, especially if he has pulmonary or cardiac disease.
- Check for elevated serum calcium levels if the patient is receiving digitalis.

• Assess the patient for parathyroid poisoning, musculoskeletal changes, and renal impairment.
• Observe the patient for signs of pain and monitor him for the effectiveness of analgesics and comfort measures.

Patient teaching
• Before discharge, advise the patient of possible adverse reactions to drug therapy.
• Teach him and his family to identify and report signs of tetany, respiratory distress, and renal dysfunction.
• Emphasize the need for periodic blood tests.
• If the patient didn't have surgery to correct his hyperparathyroidism, warn him to avoid calcium-containing antacids and thiazide diuretics.
• Encourage the patient to wear a medical identification bracelet.

Hyperpituitarism

Also called acromegaly and gigantism, hyperpituitarism is a chronic, progressive disease marked by hormonal dysfunction and startling skeletal overgrowth. Although the prognosis depends on the causative factor, this disease usually reduces life expectancy.

Hyperpituitarism appears in two forms: acromegaly (rare) and gigantism. Acromegaly occurs after epiphyseal closure, causing bone thickening and transverse growth and visceromegaly. This form of hyperpituitarism occurs equally among men and women, usually between ages 30 and 50.

Gigantism begins before epiphyseal closure and causes proportional overgrowth of all body tissues. As the disease progresses, loss of other trophic hormones, such as thyroid-stimulating hormone, luteinizing hormone, follicle-stimulating hormone, and corticotropin, may cause dysfunction of the target organs.

Gigantism affects infants and children, causing them to grow to as much as three times the normal height for their age. As adults, they may eventually reach a height of more than 8′ (2.4 m).

Causes

In most patients, the source of excessive growth hormone (GH) secretion is a GH-producing adenoma of the anterior pituitary gland, usually macroadenoma (eosinophilic or mixed-cell). However, the etiology of the tumor itself is unclear. Occasionally, hyperpituitarism occurs in more than one family member, suggesting a genetic cause.

Complications

Prolonged effects of excessive GH secretion include arthritis, carpal tunnel syndrome, osteoporosis, kyphosis, hypertension, arteriosclerosis, heart enlargement, and congestive heart failure. Acromegaly may result in blindness and severe neurologic disturbances due to tumor compression of surrounding tissues. Both gigantism and acromegaly may also cause signs of glucose intolerance and clinically apparent diabetes mellitus because of the insulin-antagonistic character of GH.

Assessment

The onset of acromegaly is gradual. The patient may report soft-tissue swelling and hypertrophy of the face and extremities at first. Then as the disease progresses, he may complain of diaphoresis, oily skin, fatigue, heat intolerance, weight gain, headaches, decreased vision, decreased libido, impotence, oligomenorrhea, infertility, joint pain (possibly from osteoarthritis), hypertrichosis, and sleep disturbances (related to obstructive sleep apnea).

Observation reveals an enlarged jaw, thickened tongue, enlarged and weakened hands, coarsened facial features, oily or leathery skin, and a prominent supraorbital ridge. You may also notice a deep, hollow-sounding voice, caused by laryngeal hypertrophy, and enlarged paranasal sinuses and tongue. Additional observations include irritability, hostility, and other psychological disturbances.

Inspection may reveal cartilaginous and connective tissue overgrowth, causing a characteristic hulking appearance and thickened ears and nose. Prognathism (projection of the jaw) becomes marked and may interfere with chewing. The fingers are thick, and the tips appear "tufted" or shaped like arrowheads on X-ray.

Gigantism develops abruptly, producing some of the same skeletal abnormalities seen in acromegaly. In infants, inspection reveals a highly arched palate, muscular hypotonia, slanting eyes, and exophthalmos. On palpation, patients commonly exhibit a characteristic moist, doughy, weak handshake.

Diagnostic tests

The following tests support a diagnosis of hyperpituitarism:

- *GH radioimmunoassay* shows increased plasma GH levels. However, because GH isn't secreted at a steady rate, a random sampling may be misleading.
- *Glucose suppression test* offers more reliable information. Glucose normally suppresses GH secretion; therefore, a glucose infusion that fails to suppress the hormone level to below the accepted norm of 5 mg strongly suggests hyperpituitarism when combined with characteristic clinical features.
- *Skull X-ray, computed tomography scan, magnetic resonance imaging,* or *pneumoencephalography* may be used to locate the pituitary tumor.
- *Bone X-rays* show a thickening of the cranium (especially of frontal, occipital, and parietal bones) and of the long bones, as well as osteoarthritis in the spine.

Treatment

Treatment aims to curb overproduction of GH by removing the underlying tumor. Removal occurs by cranial or transsphenoidal hypophysectomy or pituitary radiation therapy. In acromegaly, surgery is mandatory when a tumor is compressing surrounding healthy tissue. Postoperative therapy commonly requires replacement of thyroid, cortisone, and gonadal hormones. Adjunctive treatment may include bromocriptine, which inhibits GH synthesis, and a long-acting analogue of somatostatin, which lowers GH levels in at least two-thirds of patients with acromegaly.

Key nursing diagnoses and patient outcomes

Altered growth and development related to abnormal increase in growth and development. Based on this nursing diagnosis, you'll establish these patient outcomes. The patient will:

- seek medical treatment early to minimize the effects of hyperpituitarism
- stop excessive growth with treatment.

Body image disturbance related to physical changes. Based on this nursing diagnosis, you'll establish these patient outcomes. The patient will:

- acknowledge how his body image has changed
- express positive feelings about himself
- exhibit an ability to cope with his altered body image.

Risk for injury related to long-term effects of excessive GH. Based on this nursing diagnosis, you'll establish these patient outcomes. The patient will:

- comply with prescribed medical or surgical treatment to reduce his GH level
- avoid complications of hyperpituitarism.

Nursing interventions

- Prepare the patient for surgery or radiation, as indicated. Provide supportive care if adverse effects occur. (See the entry "Hypophysectomy.")
- The grotesque body changes and sexual dysfunction that occur in this disorder can cause severe psychological stress. Provide emotional support to help the patient cope with an altered body image. Encour-

age him to verbalize his feelings, and discuss fear of rejection by others. Provide a positive, but realistic, assessment of his situation. Encourage him to develop other interests that support a positive self-image and de-emphasize appearance. Refer him and his family for counseling to help them deal with body image changes and sexual dysfunction.
• Be sensitive to any mood changes the patient may experience. Reassure him and his family that these changes result from hormonal imbalances caused by the disease and can be lessened with treatment.
• If the patient has skeletal manifestations, such as arthritis of the hands or osteoarthritis of the spine, administer analgesics and provide comfort measures. To preserve joint function, perform or assist with range-of-motion exercises. Apply heat or cold as ordered. Use pillows and splints to support painful extremities.
• If muscle weakness occurs, help the patient walk and perform such tasks as cutting food. Also take other safety precautions to prevent injury.
• Provide meticulous skin care. Keep the skin dry, and use oil-free skin cleansers and lotions.
• Remember that the tumor may cause visual problems. If the patient has hemianopia, stand where he can see you.

Monitoring
• Evaluate GH levels regularly to assess the effectiveness of therapy.
• Check the strength of the patient's hand clasp to assess muscle weakness, especially in late-stage acromegaly.
• Assess the patient for complications of hyperpituitarism, and report any suggestive findings.
• Monitor serum glucose levels. Observe for signs of hyperglycemia, such as sweating, fatigue, polyuria, and polydipsia.

Patient teaching
• If the patient is scheduled for surgery or radiation therapy, teach him about the procedure.
• If the patient is taking bromocriptine, explain that nausea, light-headedness, and postural hypotension are common at the beginning of therapy but will usually subside. Other adverse effects include constipation and nasal congestion.
• Advise the patient to wear a medical identification bracelet at all times.
• Instruct the patient to have follow-up examinations at least once a year for the rest of his life because a slight chance exists that the tumor may recur.

Hypersplenism

A syndrome marked by exaggerated splenic activity and, possibly, splenomegaly, hypersplenism causes peripheral blood cell deficiency as the spleen traps and destroys these cells.

In this disorder, the spleen's normal filtering and phagocytic functions accelerate indiscriminately, automatically removing antibody-coated, aging, and abnormal cells, even though some cells may be functionally normal. The spleen may also temporarily sequester normal platelets and red blood cells (RBCs), withholding them from circulation. In this manner, the enlarged spleen may trap as much as 90% of the body's platelets and up to 45% of its RBC mass.

Causes
Hypersplenism may be idiopathic (primary) or secondary to an extrasplenic disorder, such as malaria or polycythemia vera. (See *What causes splenomegaly.*)

Complications
Infection, anemia, and hemorrhage can complicate hypersplenism.

Assessment

Typically, the patient with hypersplenism has a history of frequent infections. He may also complain of weakness, easy bruising, a sore mouth and, rarely, abdominal pain. The patient history may reveal disorders, such as rheumatoid arthritis, in which hypersplenism occurs as a secondary disorder. Vital signs may disclose fever and a rapid pulse rate, and inspection of the oral mucosa may reveal lacerations. Palpation may reveal a tender and enlarged spleen. Auscultation may detect palpitations.

Other assessment findings include the signs and symptoms of the underlying problem when hypersplenism is a secondary disorder.

Diagnostic tests

Diagnosis requires evidence of abnormal splenic destruction or sequestration of RBCs or platelets and splenomegaly.

The most definitive test measures the accumulation of erythrocytes in the spleen and liver after I.V. infusion of chromium-labeled RBCs or platelets. A high spleen-liver ratio of radioactivity indicates splenic destruction or sequestration.

The complete blood count (CBC) shows decreased hemoglobin levels (as low as 4 g/dl), white blood cell (WBC) count (below 4,000/mm³), platelet count (below 125,000/mm³), and an elevated reticulocyte count.

Biopsy, scan, and angiography of the spleen may be useful; biopsy is risky, however, and should be avoided if possible.

Treatment

Appropriate treatment depends on the problem's cause. Secondary hypersplenism necessitates treatment of the underlying disease. Splenectomy is indicated in a transfusion-dependent patient who fails to respond to other therapy. Splenectomy seldom cures the patient, but it does correct the effects of cytopenia. Occasionally, splenectomy may hasten blood cell destruction in the bone marrow and liver.

What causes splenomegaly

An enlarged spleen may develop in any of the disorders listed below.

Infectious disorders
Acute (abscesses, subacute bacterial endocarditis), chronic (tuberculosis, malaria, Felty's syndrome)

Congestive disorders
Cirrhosis, thrombosis

Hyperplastic disorders
Hemolytic anemia, polycythemia vera

Infiltrative disorders
Gaucher's disease, Niemann-Pick disease

Cystic or neoplastic disorders
Cysts, leukemia, lymphoma, myelofibrosis, Hodgkin's disease, multiple myeloma

Key nursing diagnoses and patient outcomes

Altered protection related to potential hemorrhage caused by trapped platelets in the spleen. Based on this nursing diagnosis, you'll establish these patient outcomes. The patient will:
- exhibit adequate tissue perfusion, as shown by normal body function and stable vital signs
- avoid signs of hemorrhage
- regain a normal platelet count with treatment.

Fatigue related to anemia. Based on this nursing diagnosis, you'll establish these patient outcomes. The patient will:
- express an understanding of how fatigue and a decreased activity level relate to hypersplenism
- incorporate measures into his daily routine to minimize fatigue

• regain a normal energy level with treatment.

Risk for infection related to a reduced WBC count. Based on this nursing diagnosis, you'll establish these patient outcomes. The patient will:
• maintain a normal temperature
• avoid signs and symptoms of infection
• regain a normal WBC count with treatment.

Nursing interventions

• Prepare the patient for a splenectomy, if indicated. (See the entry "Splenectomy.")
• If the patient has pain, administer analgesics as ordered, and provide distractions to help him cope with discomfort.
• If the patient tolerates activities poorly because of decreased tissue perfusion, provide rest periods between activities.
• Perform all procedures using aseptic technique to help prevent infection.
• Institute bleeding precautions when the patient's platelet count drops below normal.
• Administer transfusions of blood or blood products (fresh-frozen plasma, platelets), as ordered, to replace deficient blood elements. Manage symptoms or complications of any underlying disorder as ordered.
• Provide emotional support as necessary. Listen to the patient's fears and concerns. Reassure him when possible.

Monitoring

• Check the patient's CBC and platelet counts regularly.
• Watch for signs and symptoms of decreased tissue perfusion, such as restlessness, anxiety, confusion, pallor, cool and clammy skin, chest pain, decreased urine output, hypotension, and tachycardia. Monitor the patient's vital signs at least every 4 hours and observe him frequently for bleeding.
• Watch for adverse reactions to blood products, such as flushing, headache, tingling, fever, chills, urticaria, and anaphylaxis.
• Monitor the patient's activity tolerance and degree of fatigue.
• Check for signs and symptoms of infection, and take the patient's temperature regularly.

Patient teaching

• Reinforce the doctor's explanation of the disease as necessary. Be sure the patient understands the problem and the care required.
• If splenectomy will be performed, teach the patient about the surgery.
• Explain the need to prevent infection, and teach the patient the value of good hand-washing technique. Also teach him how to recognize infection, and urge him to report all signs and symptoms (such as fever and weakness), even if they seem minor.
• Explain the need to maintain a quiet, safe home environment, free of potentially infectious visitors.
• Teach the patient to take bleeding precautions when his platelet count is depressed.
• Explain the laboratory tests that will be performed repeatedly to monitor his status. These include serial CBCs, platelet counts, and chemistries performed to assess blood counts and help identify fluid shifts into the abdomen.

Hypertension

This disorder is marked by an intermittent or sustained elevation of diastolic or systolic blood pressure. Generally, a sustained systolic pressure of 140 mm Hg or more or a diastolic pressure of 90 mm Hg or more qualifies as hypertension.

Aside from characteristic high blood pressure, hypertension is classified according to its cause, severity, and type. The two major types are *essential* (also

LIFE-THREATENING COMPLICATIONS

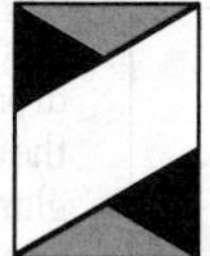

Dangers of malignant hypertension

A medical emergency, malignant hypertension is characterized by marked blood pressure elevation, papilledema, retinal hemorrhages and exudates, and manifestations of hypertensive encephalopathy, such as severe headache, vomiting, visual disturbances, transient paralysis, seizures, stupor, and coma. Cardiac decompensation and acute renal failure may also develop in this disorder.

The average age at diagnosis is 40, and the disorder affects more men than women. Before the availability of effective antihypertensives, most patients died within 2 years. Even with effective treatment, however, at least half the patients die within 5 years.

Causes

What causes malignant hypertension remains a mystery. However, studies do show that dilation of cerebral arteries and generalized arteriolar fibrinoid necrosis contribute to the disorder. The cerebral arteries dilate because markedly high arterial pressure prevents normal regulation of cerebral blood flow. The resulting excess in cerebral blood flow produces encephalopathy.

Treatment

Emergency treatment aims to quickly reduce blood pressure and identify the underlying cause.

- Diazoxide given rapidly I.V. can begin to reduce blood pressure in 1 to 3 minutes. Nitroprusside and trimethaphan, given by continuous infusion, may be tried. Other drugs for maintaining long-term control of blood pressure include hydralazine and methyldopa.
- With suspected pheochromocytoma, drugs that release additional catecholamines—such as methyldopa, reserpine, and guanethidine—are contraindicated.
- Furosemide and digitalis glycosides may be used to treat associated heart failure.

called primary or idiopathic) *hypertension,* the most common (90% to 95% of cases), and *secondary hypertension,* which results from renal disease or another identifiable cause. *Malignant hypertension* is a severe, fulminant form of hypertension that commonly arises from both types. (See *Dangers of malignant hypertension.*) Hypertension affects more than 60 million adults in North America. Blacks are twice as likely as whites to be affected and four times as likely to die of the disorder.

Essential hypertension usually begins insidiously as a benign disease, slowly progressing to an accelerated or malignant state. If untreated, even mild hypertension can cause significant complications and a high mortality rate. In many cases, however, treatment with stepped care offers patients an improved prognosis. (See *Stepped care for hypertension,* page 440.)

Causes

The cause of essential hypertension is unknown. Family history, race, stress, obesity, a diet high in sodium or saturated fat, use of tobacco or oral contraceptives, sedentary life-style, and aging have all been studied to determine their role in the development of hypertension.

Secondary hypertension may result from renovascular disease; renal parenchymal disease; pheochromocytoma; primary hyperaldosteronism; Cushing's syndrome; diabetes mellitus; dysfunction of the thyroid, pituitary, or parathyroid gland; coarctation of the aorta; pregnancy; and neurologic disorders. Use of oral contraceptives may be the most common cause of secondary hypertension, probably because these drugs activate the renin-angiotensin-aldosterone system.

Stepped care for hypertension

Recently, the National Institutes of Health revised its stepped care approach to hypertension. The latest guidelines follow.

Step 1
Initial therapy to reduce high blood pressure includes life-style modifications, such as weight reduction, increased physical activity, and moderation of sodium and alcohol intake as well as smoking cessation.

Step 2
If blood pressure isn't adequately reduced by life-style modifications, therapy with a single drug should be started. Diuretics and beta blockers are preferred because they've been shown to reduce cardiovascular illness and mortality in long-term controlled clinical trials.

If the patient has other underlying medical problems, alternative drugs (such as ACE inhibitors, calcium channel blockers, $alpha_1$-receptor blockers, and labetalol) may be substituted.

Step 3
If initial therapy fails to control blood pressure sufficiently in 1 to 3 months and the patient is compliant and not experiencing significant adverse reactions, three options for subsequent therapy should be considered: increased drug dose, substitution of another drug, or addition of a second agent from a different class.

Step 4
Although some patients may respond adequately to therapy with a single drug, frequently a second or third agent and, if not already prescribed, a diuretic must be added if the desired blood pressure reduction hasn't been achieved.

Complications

Hypertension is a major cause of cerebrovascular accident (CVA), cardiac disease, and renal failure. Complications occur late in the disease and can attack any organ system. Cardiac complications may include coronary artery disease, angina, myocardial infarction (MI), heart failure, arrhythmias, and sudden death. Neurologic complications include cerebral infarctions and hypertensive encephalopathy. Hypertensive retinopathy can cause blindness. Renovascular hypertension can lead to renal failure.

Assessment

In many cases, the hypertensive patient has no symptoms, and the disorder is revealed incidentally during evaluation for another disorder or during a routine blood pressure screening program. When symptoms do occur, they reflect the effect of hypertension on the organ systems.

The patient may report awakening with a headache in the occipital region, which subsides spontaneously after a few hours. This symptom usually is associated with severe hypertension. He may also complain of dizziness, palpitations, fatigue, and impotence.

With vascular involvement, the patient may complain of nosebleeds, bloody urine, weakness, and blurred vision. Complaints of chest pain and dyspnea may indicate cardiac involvement.

Inspection may reveal peripheral edema in late stages when heart failure is present. Ophthalmoscopic evaluation may reveal hemorrhages, exudates, and papilledema in late stages if hypertensive retinopathy is present.

Palpation of the carotid artery may disclose stenosis or occlusion. Palpation of the abdomen may reveal a pulsating mass, suggesting an abdominal aneurysm. Enlarged kidneys may point to polycystic disease, a cause of secondary hypertension.

Systolic or diastolic pressure, or both, may be elevated. A rise in diastolic blood pressure from a sitting to a standing position suggests essential hypertension, whereas a fall in blood pressure from the sitting to the standing position indicates secondary hypertension.

An abdominal bruit may be heard just to the right or left of the umbilicus midline, or in the flanks if renal artery stenosis is present. Bruits may also be heard over the abdominal aorta and femoral arteries.

Diagnostic tests

The following tests may elicit predisposing factors and help identify the cause of hypertension:

- *Urinalysis* may show protein, red blood cells, or white blood cells, suggesting renal disease, or glucose, suggesting diabetes mellitus.
- *Excretory urography* may reveal renal atrophy, indicating chronic renal disease; one kidney that is more than 5/8″ (1.6 cm) shorter than the other suggests unilateral renal disease.
- *Serum potassium* levels less than 3.5 mEq/liter may indicate adrenal dysfunction (primary hyperaldosteronism).
- *Blood urea nitrogen* levels that are normal or elevated to more than 20 mg/dl and *serum creatinine* levels that are normal or elevated to more than 1.5 mg/dl suggest renal disease.

Other tests that help detect cardiovascular damage and other complications include electrocardiography, which may show left ventricular hypertrophy or ischemia, and chest X-rays, which may demonstrate cardiomegaly.

Treatment

Although essential hypertension has no cure, drugs and modifications in diet and life-style can control it. Generally, nondrug treatment, such as life-style modification, is tried first, especially in early, mild cases. If this is ineffective, treatment progresses in a stepwise manner to include various types of antihypertensives. This stepped-care approach may need modification. For instance, most blacks respond poorly to beta-adrenergic blockers; however, for unclear reasons, they respond well to a combination of a diuretic and an angiotensin-converting enzyme (ACE) inhibitor. Many elderly patients can be treated with diuretics alone.

Treatment of secondary hypertension includes correcting the underlying cause and controlling hypertensive effects.

Severely elevated blood pressure (hypertensive crisis) may be refractory to medications and may be fatal.

Key nursing diagnoses and patient outcomes

Risk for injury related to complications of hypertension. Based on this nursing diagnosis, you'll establish these patient outcomes. The patient will:

- keep regular appointments for blood pressure evaluation to detect persistent or serious elevations
- seek medical attention immediately for any abnormal signs or symptoms
- avoid dysfunction of any organ system, especially the cardiovascular and renal systems.

Knowledge deficit related to hypertension and its treatment. Based on this nursing diagnosis, you'll establish these patient outcomes. The patient will:

- acknowledge the need to learn about hypertension and its control and express a desire to do so
- participate in a learning situation to gain

EXPERT GERIATRIC CARE

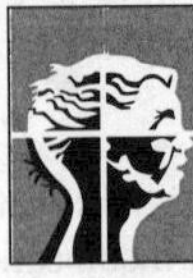

Managing hypertension in the elderly

Because of age-related changes in blood vessels, specifically vasoconstriction, many elderly patients have an elevated blood pressure. To manage hypertension in elderly patients, you should:
- avoid aggressive treatment with antihypertensives because of the increased risk of adverse effects, namely orthostatic hypertension; also, lower doses may be needed
- watch for signs of low blood pressure in patients receiving antihypertensive therapy, such as dizziness, confusion, syncope, restlessness, or drowsiness
- aim to achieve a blood pressure level that is high enough to provide optimum circulation yet low enough to prevent serious, but related, complications.

knowledge about hypertension and its treatment
- express an understanding of hypertension and the methods used to control it.

Noncompliance related to the lifelong need for antihypertensive therapy and the misconception that such therapy is needed only during symptomatic periods. Based on this nursing diagnosis, you'll establish these patient outcomes. The patient will:
- express an understanding of the need for lifelong therapy even when he lacks overt signs and symptoms
- comply with prescribed treatments, as shown by normal blood pressure and absence of organ dysfunction.

Nursing interventions

- If a patient is hospitalized with hypertension, find out if he was taking prescribed antihypertensive medication. If he wasn't, ask why. If he can't afford the medication, refer him to the appropriate social service department.
- When routine blood pressure screening reveals elevated pressure, make sure the sphygmomanometer cuff size is appropriate for the patient's upper arm circumference. Take the pressure in both arms in lying, sitting, and standing positions. Ask the patient if he smoked, drank a beverage containing caffeine, or was emotionally upset before the test. Advise him to return for blood pressure testing at frequent and regular intervals.
- To help identify hypertension and prevent untreated hypertension, participate in public education programs dealing with the disorder and ways to reduce risk factors. Encourage public participation in blood pressure screening programs. Routinely screen all patients, especially those at risk (blacks and people with family histories of hypertension, CVA, or MI).

Monitoring

- Check the patient's blood pressure regularly.
- Assess the patient for complications of uncontrolled hypertension at each follow-up visit.
- Monitor the patient's compliance with prescribed treatment.
- Periodically reevaluate the patient's knowledge level about hypertension and correct any misconceptions about the disease. (See *Managing hypertension in the elderly.*)

Patient teaching

- Teach the patient to use a self-monitoring blood pressure cuff and to record the reading at least twice weekly in a journal for review by the doctor at every office appointment. Tell the patient to take his blood pressure at the same hour each time with relatively the same type of activity preceding the measurement.
- Tell the patient and family to keep a record of drugs used in the past, noting es-

pecially which ones were or weren't effective. Suggest recording this on a card so the patient can show it to his doctor.

• To encourage compliance with antihypertensive therapy, suggest establishing a daily routine for taking medication. Warn him that uncontrolled hypertension may cause CVA and MI. Tell him to report adverse effects of drugs. Advise him to avoid high-sodium antacids and over-the-counter cold and sinus medications containing harmful vasoconstrictors.

• Help the patient examine and modify his life-style. Suggest stress-reduction groups, dietary changes, and an exercise program, particularly aerobic walking, to improve cardiac status and reduce obesity and serum cholesterol levels.

• Encourage a change in dietary habits. Help the obese patient plan a reducing diet. Tell him to avoid high-sodium foods (pickles, potato chips, canned soups, cold cuts), table salt, and foods high in cholesterol and saturated fat.

Hyperthyroidism

Thyroid hormone overproduction results in a metabolic imbalance in this disorder, also called Graves' disease, Basedow's disease, Parry's disease, and thyrotoxicosis.

The most common form of hyperthyroidism is Graves' disease, which increases thyroxine (T_4) production, enlarges the thyroid gland (goiter), and causes multiple systemic changes. The incidence of Graves' disease peaks between ages 30 and 40, especially in persons with family histories of thyroid abnormalities; only 5% of hyperthyroid patients are below age 15. With treatment, most patients can lead normal lives. However, thyrotoxic crisis or thyroid storm – an acute exacerbation of hyperthyroidism – is a medical emergency that may lead to life-threatening cardiac, hepatic, or renal failure. (See *Thyrotoxic crisis*, page 445.)

Besides Graves' disease, other forms include toxic adenoma (Plummer's disease), toxic multinodular goiter, thyrotoxicosis factitia, functioning metastatic thyroid carcinoma, thyroid-stimulating hormone (TSH)–secreting pituitary tumor, and subacute thyroiditis.

Causes

Although the origin of hyperthyroidism is unclear, in view of its various manifestations, there may not be a single cause. For example, many experts believe that Graves' disease results from genetic and immunologic factors. Increased incidence in monozygotic twins suggests an inherited factor, probably an autosomal recessive gene. Graves' disease occasionally coexists with abnormal iodine metabolism and other endocrine abnormalities, such as diabetes mellitus, thyroiditis, and hyperparathyroidism. It's also associated with production of autoantibodies (long-acting thyroid stimulator [LATS], LATS-protector, and human thyroid adenylate cyclase stimulators), possibly caused by a defect in suppressor-T-lymphocyte function that allows the formation of these autoantibodies.

In a patient with latent hyperthyroidism, excessive intake of iodine and, possibly, stress can induce clinical hyperthyroidism. Also, in a patient with inadequately treated hyperthyroidism, stressful conditions (such as surgery, infection, toxemia of pregnancy, and diabetic ketoacidosis) can precipitate thyrotoxic crisis.

Toxic adenoma (Plummer's disease), a small, benign nodule in the thyroid gland, secretes thyroid hormone and is the second most common cause of hyperthyroidism. The cause of toxic adenoma is unknown.

Toxic multinodular goiter is seen in elderly patients with long-standing goiter. There are multiple functioning nodules in the gland. This disorder is often seen in elderly patients who have other health problems. Hyperthyroidism in these patients can often be precipitated by the administration of iodides. The goiter is driven to excess hormone production by a high level of circulating iodide. Treatment is difficult because the typical patient cannot tolerate a subtotal thyroidectomy. Ideal therapy is administration of antithyroid drugs followed by a subtotal thyroidectomy.

Thyrotoxicosis factitia results from chronic ingestion of thyroid hormone for thyrotropin suppression in patients with thyroid cancer. It also may result from thyroid hormone abuse.

Functioning metastatic thyroid carcinoma causes excessive production of thyroid hormone. TSH–secreting pituitary tumors also cause increased production of thyroid hormone.

Subacute thyroiditis results from a virus-induced granulomatous inflammation of the thyroid. It is associated with fever, pain, pharyngitis, and tenderness of the thyroid gland.

Complications

Because thyroid hormones have widespread effects on almost all body tissues, the complications of hypersecretion may be far-reaching and varied. Cardiovascular complications are most common in elderly patients and include arrhythmias, especially atrial fibrillation; cardiac insufficiency; cardiac decompensation; and resistance to the usual therapeutic dose of digitalis glycosides. Additional complications include muscle weakness and atrophy; paralysis; osteoporosis; vitiligo and skin hyperpigmentation; corneal ulcers; myasthenia gravis; impaired fertility; decreased libido; and gynecomastia.

Assessment

The patient's history may disclose that the onset of symptoms followed a period of acute physical or emotional stress. A family history of Graves' disease is also common. The patient may report classic symptoms of nervousness, heat intolerance, weight loss despite increased appetite, excessive sweating, diarrhea, tremor, and palpitations. Symptoms suggesting nervous system involvement generally dominate in younger patients, whereas cardiovascular and myopathic symptoms are more common in older patients.

The patient may complain of difficulty concentrating; trouble climbing stairs; dyspnea on exertion and possibly at rest; anorexia; nausea and vomiting; and menstrual abnormalities. (See *Nursing care in thyrotoxicosis,* pages 446 and 447.)

On inspection, the patient typically appears anxious and restless. You may note fine tremor of the fingers and tongue, shaky handwriting, clumsiness, emotional instability, and mood swings (occasional outbursts to overt psychosis). The skin appears flushed, and the hair is fine and soft. Premature graying and increased hair loss occur commonly in both sexes. The nails appear fragile, and the distal nail may be separated from the nail bed (onycholysis).

Inspection also reveals pretibial myxedema over the dorsum of the legs or feet, which produces raised, thickened skin that may be itchy, hyperpigmented, and usually well demarcated from normal skin. Lesions typically appear plaquelike or nodular. Generalized or localized muscle atrophy and acropachy (soft-tissue swelling with underlying bone changes where new bone formation occurs) may also be seen.

Inspection of the eyes detects infrequent blinking, a characteristic stare, and lid lag, resulting from sympathetic overstimulation. Another characteristic finding is exophthalmos, which results from accumulated mucopolysaccharides and fluids in the retro-orbital tissues that force the eyeball outward. The conjunctiva and cornea may appear reddened. The patient may have an impaired upward gaze, convergence, and strabismus due to ocular muscle weakness (exophthalmic ophthalmoplegia).

On palpation, the thyroid gland may feel asymmetrical, lobular, and enlarged to three or four times its normal size. The liver may also feel enlarged. The skin is warm and moist with a velvety texture, and tachycardia with a full bounding pulse is palpable. Hyperreflexia is present.

LIFE-THREATENING COMPLICATIONS

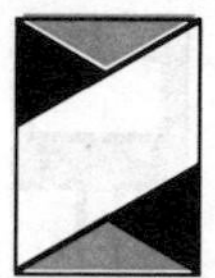

Thyrotoxic crisis

Also known as thyroid storm, thyrotoxic crisis is an acute manifestation of hyperthyroidism, usually occurring in patients with preexisting (though often unrecognized) thyrotoxicosis. Left untreated, it's invariably fatal.

Onset is almost always abrupt, evoked by a stressful event, such as trauma, surgery, or infection. Other, less common, precipitators include:

- insulin-induced hypoglycemia or diabetic ketoacidosis
- cerebrovascular accident
- myocardial infarction
- pulmonary embolism
- sudden discontinuation of antithyroid drug therapy
- initiation of ^{131}I therapy
- preeclampsia, and
- subtotal thyroidectomy with excess intake of synthetic thyroid hormone.

Pathophysiology

The thyroid gland secretes the thyroid hormones T_3 and T_4. When it overproduces them in response to any of the above factors, systemic adrenergic activity increases. This results in epinephrine overproduction and severe hypermetabolism, leading rapidly to cardiac, GI, and sympathetic nervous system decompensation.

Assessment findings

Initially, the patient may have marked tachycardia, vomiting, and stupor. Untreated, he may experience vascular collapse, hypotension, coma, and death. Other findings may include irritability and restlessness; visual disturbance, such as diplopia; tremor and weakness; angina; or shortness of breath, a cough, and swollen extremities. Palpation may disclose warm, moist flushed skin and a high fever (beginning insidiously and rising rapidly to a lethal level).

Emergency interventions

If you suspect your patient may be experiencing thyrotoxic crisis, take these steps:

- Notify the patient's doctor immediately and prepare to transfer the patient to the intensive care unit.
- Monitor the patient's vital signs, ECG pattern, and cardiopulmonary status continuously.
- Expect to administer an antithyroid drug, such as propylthiouracil or beta blockers, such as propranolol, to block sympathetic effects; a corticosteroid to inhibit the conversion of T_3 to T_4 and to replace depleted cortisol; and an iodide to block the release of the thyroid hormones.
- Closely monitor the patient's temperature. If indicated, employ cooling measures and administer acetaminophen, as ordered. Never administer aspirin because it may further increase the patient's metabolic rate.
- Provide supportive care, such as administering vitamins, nutrients, fluids, and sedatives, as necessary.

Auscultation of the heart may detect paroxysmal supraventricular tachycardia and atrial fibrillation (especially in elderly patients) and, occasionally, a systolic murmur at the left sternal border. Wide pulse pressures may be audible when taking blood pressure readings. Auscultation of the abdomen may detect increased bowel sounds. In Graves' disease, an audible bruit over the thyroid gland indicates thy-

(Text continues on page 448.)

NURSING PRIORITY

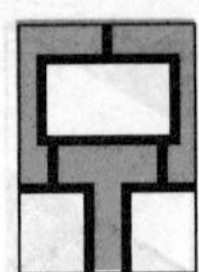

Nursing care in thyrotoxicosis

- History of hyperthyroidism, recent physical stress, infection, or acute emotional shock; family history of Graves' disease; abrupt onset of classic signs and symptoms
- Physical findings including agitation and restlessness progressing to manic or psychotic behavior, fine tremors, tachypnea and respiratory distress, fever as high as 106° F (41° C), tachyarrhythmias, and signs and symptoms of dehydration
- Results of serum triiodothyronine and serum thyroxine tests

Decreased cardiac output related to arrhythmias

- Monitor vital signs frequently.
- Evaluate electrocardiogram continuously.
- Monitor intake and output and neurologic status frequently.

Administer oxygen therapy.

Limit patient's activities.

Establish peripheral I.V. line for fluid and drug administration.

Administer antiarrhythmic agents as ordered.

Is patient's cardiac output adequate?

NO

Notify doctor immediately.

Expect to increase antiarrhythmic dosage or change to new antiarrhythmic agent.

Be prepared to assist with emergency defibrillation and cardiopulmonary resuscitation measures.

Continue to monitor patient's response to therapy closely.

YES

Continue supportive care.

Patient's cardiac output is adequate, as exhibited by:
- hemodynamic stability
- normal cardiac rate and rhythm
- no signs or symptoms of decreased cardiac output.

KEY

- Assessment
- Nursing diagnoses
- Interventions
- Evaluation

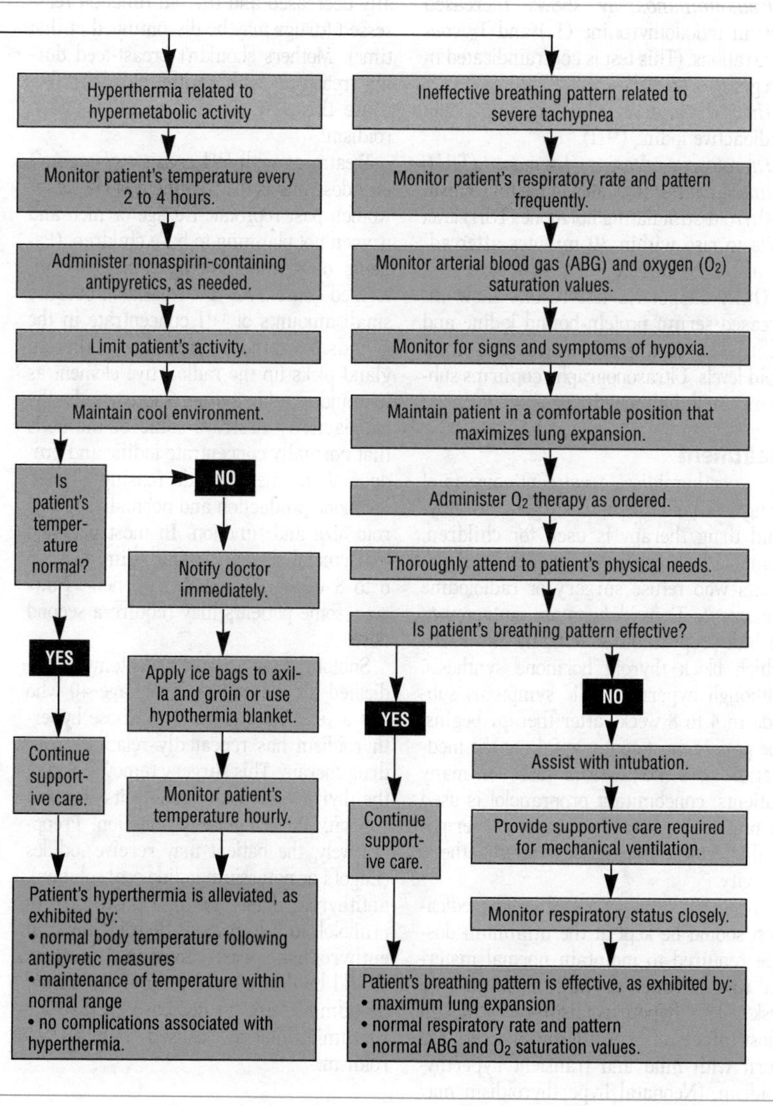
Hyperthermia related to hypermetabolic activity
Monitor patient's temperature every 2 to 4 hours.
Administer nonaspirin-containing antipyretics, as needed.
Limit patient's activity.
Maintain cool environment.
Is patient's temperature normal?
NO
Notify doctor immediately.
Apply ice bags to axilla and groin or use hypothermia blanket.
Monitor patient's temperature hourly.
YES
Continue supportive care.
Patient's hyperthermia is alleviated, as exhibited by:
• normal body temperature following antipyretic measures
• maintenance of temperature within normal range
• no complications associated with hyperthermia.
Ineffective breathing pattern related to severe tachypnea
Monitor patient's respiratory rate and pattern frequently.
Monitor arterial blood gas (ABG) and oxygen (O_2) saturation values.
Monitor for signs and symptoms of hypoxia.
Maintain patient in a comfortable position that maximizes lung expansion.
Administer O_2 therapy as ordered.
Thoroughly attend to patient's physical needs.
Is patient's breathing pattern effective?
YES
Continue supportive care.
NO
Assist with intubation.
Provide supportive care required for mechanical ventilation.
Monitor respiratory status closely.
Patient's breathing pattern is effective, as exhibited by:
• maximum lung expansion
• normal respiratory rate and pattern
• normal ABG and O_2 saturation values.

rotoxicity, but occasionally, it may also be present in other disorders associated with a hyperplastic thyroid.

Diagnostic tests

The following laboratory test results confirm the diagnosis of hyperthyroidism:

• *Radioimmunoassay* shows increased serum triiodothyronine (T_3) and T_4 concentrations. (This test is contraindicated in pregnant patients.)

• *Thyroid scan* reveals increased uptake of radioactive iodine (^{131}I).

• *Thyrotropin-releasing hormone (TRH) stimulation test* indicates hyperthyroidism if thyroid-stimulating hormone (TSH) level fails to rise within 30 minutes after administration of TRH.

Other supportive test results show increased serum protein-bound iodine and decreased serum cholesterol and total lipid levels. Ultrasonography confirms subclinical ophthalmopathy.

Treatment

In hyperthyroidism, treatment consists of drugs, radioiodine, and surgery. Antithyroid drug therapy is used for children, young adults, pregnant women, and patients who refuse surgery or radioiodine treatment. Thyroid hormone antagonists include propylthiouracil and methimazole, which block thyroid hormone synthesis. Although hypermetabolic symptoms subside in 4 to 8 weeks after therapy begins, the patient must continue taking the medication for 6 months to 2 years. In many patients, concomitant propranolol is used to manage tachycardia and other peripheral effects of excessive hypersympathetic activity.

During pregnancy, antithyroid medication should be kept at the minimum dosage required to maintain normal maternal thyroid function and to minimize the risk of fetal hypothyroidism – even though most infants of hyperthyroid mothers are born with mild and transient hyperthyroidism. (Neonatal hyperthyroidism may even require treatment with antithyroid drugs and propranolol for 2 to 3 months.) Because exacerbation of hyperthyroidism sometimes occurs in the puerperium, continuous control of maternal thyroid function is essential. About 3 to 6 months postpartum, antithyroid drugs can be gradually decreased and thyroid function reassessed (drugs may be discontinued at that time). Mothers shouldn't breast-feed during treatment with antithyroid drugs because this may cause neonatal hypothyroidism.

Treatment with ^{131}I consists of a single oral dose and is the treatment of choice for women past reproductive age or men and women not planning to have children. (Patients of reproductive age must give informed consent for this treatment because small amounts of ^{131}I concentrate in the gonads.) During treatment, the thyroid gland picks up the radioactive element as it would regular iodine. Subsequently, the radioactivity destroys some of the cells that normally concentrate iodine and produce thyroxine, thus decreasing thyroid hormone production and normalizing thyroid size and function. In most patients, hypermetabolic symptoms diminish in 6 to 8 weeks after such treatment. However, some patients may require a second dose.

Subtotal (partial) thyroidectomy is indicated for the patient under age 40 who has a very large goiter and whose hyperthyroidism has repeatedly relapsed after drug therapy. This surgery removes part of the thyroid gland, decreasing its size and capacity for hormone production. Preoperatively, the patient may receive iodides (Lugol's or potassium iodide oral solution), antithyroid drugs, or high doses of propranolol, to help prevent thyroid storm. If euthyroidism isn't achieved, surgery should be delayed and propranolol should be administered to decrease cardiac arrhythmias that are caused by hyperthyroidism.

Therapy for hyperthyroid ophthalmopathy includes local applications of topical medications but may require high doses of corticosteroids. A patient with severe exophthalmos that causes pressure on the optic nerve may require surgical decompression to lessen pressure on the orbital contents.

Treatment of thyrotoxic crisis includes administration of an antithyroid drug such as propylthiouracil, I.V. propranolol to block sympathetic effects, a corticosteroid to inhibit the conversion of T_3 to T_4 and to replace depleted cortisol, and an iodide to block release of the thyroid hormones. Supportive measures include nutrients, vitamins, fluid administration, and sedatives, as necessary.

Key nursing diagnoses and patient outcomes

Altered nutrition: Less than body requirements, related to hypermetabolism. Based on this nursing diagnosis, you'll establish these patient outcomes. The patient will:

- eat a nutritionally balanced diet containing enough calories to prevent further weight loss
- regain lost weight and maintain weight within a normal range
- not have signs and symptoms of malnutrition or nutritional deficits.

Altered thought processes related to emotional lability. Based on this nursing diagnosis, you'll establish these patient outcomes. The patient will:

- remain safe and protected in his environment
- receive emotional support and understanding from his family and friends
- regain emotional stability with hyperthyroidism treatment.

Decreased cardiac output related to supraventricular tachycardia. Based on this nursing diagnosis, you'll establish these patient outcomes. The patient will:

- regain and maintain a normal heart rate and electorcardiogram (ECG) pattern with hyperthyroidism treatment
- maintain adequate cardiac output, as shown by normal blood pressure, alertness, and orientation to time, person, and place.

Nursing interventions

- Prepare the patient for surgery, as indicated. (See the entry "Thyroidectomy.")
- Administer prescribed antithyroid medications, as ordered.
- If iodide is part of the treatment, mix it with milk, juice, or water to prevent GI distress, and give it through a straw to prevent tooth discoloration.
- Give antidiarrheal preparations, as ordered. Provide meticulous skin care to minimize perianal skin breakdown.
- Consult a dietitian to ensure a nutritious diet with adequate calories and fluids. Offer frequent, small meals.
- If the patient has exophthalmos or other ophthalmopathy, moisten the conjunctivae often with isotonic eyedrops.
- Avoid excessive palpation of the thyroid – this can precipitate thyroid storm.
- Minimize physical and emotional stress. Try to balance rest and activity periods. Keep the patient's room cool and quiet and the lights dim. Encourage the patient to dress in loose-fitting, cotton clothing.
- Reassure the patient and his family that mood swings and nervousness will probably subside with treatment. Encourage the patient to verbalize feelings about changes in body image. Help him identify and develop coping strategies. Offer emotional support. Refer him and his family to a mental health counselor, if necessary.

Monitoring

- Monitor and record the patient's vital signs, weight, fluid intake, and urine output. Measure neck circumference daily to check for progression of thyroid enlargement.
- Evaluate serum electrolyte levels, and check for hyperglycemia and glycosuria. Monitor the ECG for arrhythmias and ST-segment changes.

• Assess the patient for signs of heart failure, such as dyspnea, jugular vein distention, pulmonary crackles, and peripheral or sacral edema.
• Check for signs of hypotension (dizziness and decreased urine output) if the patient is taking propranolol.
• If the patient is taking propylthiouracil and methimazole, monitor complete blood count results periodically to detect leukopenia, thrombocytopenia, and agranulocytosis.
• Monitor the patient for thyrotoxic crisis and report any suspicious signs or symptoms to the doctor immediately.
• Check stools for frequency and characteristics.

Patient teaching
• Stress the importance of regular medical follow-up after discharge because hypothyroidism may develop 2 to 4 weeks postoperatively and after ^{131}I therapy. Advise the patient that he'll need lifelong thyroid hormone replacement. Encourage him to wear a medical identification bracelet and to carry his medication with him at all times.
• Tell the patient who has had ^{131}I therapy not to expectorate or cough freely because his saliva is radioactive for 24 hours. Stress the need for repeated measurement of serum T_4 levels. Be sure he understands that he must not resume antithyroid drug therapy.
• Instruct the patient taking propylthiouracil and methimazole to take these drugs with meals to minimize GI distress and to avoid over-the-counter cough preparations because many contain iodine.
• Tell the patient taking propranolol to rise slowly after sitting or lying down to prevent a feeling of faintness.
• Instruct the patient taking antithyroid drugs or radioisotope therapy to identify and report symptoms of hypothyroidism.
• Advise the patient with exophthalmos or other ophthalmopathy to wear sunglasses or eye patches to protect his eyes from light. If he has severe lid retraction, warn him to avoid sudden physical movements that might cause the lid to slip behind the eyeball. Instruct him to report signs of decreased visual acuity.

Hypertrophic cardiomyopathy

Also called idiopathic hypertrophic subaortic stenosis, this primary disease of cardiac muscle is characterized by left ventricular hypertrophy and disproportionate, asymmetrical thickening of the intraventricular septum, particularly in the anterosuperior part. It's also distinguished by a dynamic left ventricular outflow tract pressure gradient. This is related to the narrowing of the subaortic area caused by the septal hypertrophy in the mitral valve area. The obstruction produced may change between examinations and even from beat to beat.

In hypertrophic cardiomyopathy, cardiac output may be low, normal, or high, depending on whether stenosis is obstructive or nonobstructive. Eventually, left ventricular dysfunction – a result of rigidity and decreased compliance – causes pump failure. If cardiac output is normal or high, the stenosis may go undetected for years, but low cardiac output may lead to potentially fatal congestive heart failure.

The course of this disorder varies. Some patients demonstrate progressive deterioration, whereas others remain stable for several years.

Causes
About half of all cases are transmitted as an autosomal dominant trait.

Complications
Pulmonary hypertension and heart failure may occur secondary to left ventricular stiffness. Sudden death is also possible and

usually results from ventricular arrhythmias, such as ventricular tachycardia and premature ventricular contractions.

Assessment

Generally, clinical features don't appear until the disease is well advanced. At that point, atrial dilation and sometimes atrial fibrillation abruptly reduce blood flow to the left ventricle. Most patients are asymptomatic but have a family history of hypertrophic cardiomyopathy. In some instances, death occurs without warning, particularly in children and young adults. Patients who have symptoms complain of dyspnea on exertion. They often have anginal pain, fatigue, and syncope.

Inspection of the carotid artery may show a rapidly rising carotid arterial pulse. Palpation of peripheral arteries reveals a characteristic double impulse (pulsus biferiens). Palpation of the chest reveals a double or triple apical impulse. Percussion may reveal bibasilar crackles if heart failure is present. Auscultation reveals a harsh systolic murmur, heard after S_1 at the apex near the left sternal border. The murmur is intensified by standing and with Valsalva's maneuver. An S_4 may also be audible.

Diagnostic tests

- *Echocardiography,* the most useful test, shows left ventricular hypertrophy and a thick intraventricular septum. The septum may have a ground-glass appearance. Poor septal contraction, abnormal motion of the anterior mitral leaflet during systole, and narrowing or occlusion of the left ventricular outflow tract may also be seen in obstructive hypertrophic cardiomyopathy. The left ventricular cavity appears small, with vigorous posterior wall motion but reduced septal excursion.
- *Cardiac catheterization* reveals elevated left ventricular end-diastolic pressure and possibly mitral insufficiency. In a rare form of the disease, the left atrium appears to have a slipper-foot shape and the left ventricle takes on a spade shape.
- *Electrocardiography* usually shows left ventricular hypertrophy, ST-segment and T-wave abnormalities, Q waves in leads II, III, aV_F, and in V_4 to V_6 (due to hypertrophy, not infarction), left anterior hemiblock, left axis deviation, and ventricular and atrial arrhythmias.
- *Chest X-rays* may show a mild to moderate increase in heart size.
- *Thallium scan* usually reveals myocardial perfusion defects.

Treatment

The goals of treatment are to relax the ventricle and to relieve outflow tract obstruction. Propranolol, a beta-adrenergic blocking agent, is the drug of choice. It slows the heart rate and increases ventricular filling by relaxing the obstructing muscle, thereby reducing angina, syncope, dyspnea, and arrhythmias. However, propranolol may aggravate symptoms of cardiac decompensation.

Calcium channel blockers may reduce elevated diastolic pressures and severity of outflow tract gradients and increase exercise tolerance. Disopyramide can be used to reduce left ventricular contractility and the outflow gradient.

Atrial fibrillation, a medical emergency in hypertrophic cardiomyopathy, necessitates cardioversion. It also calls for heparin administration prior to cardioversion and continuing until fibrillation subsides because of the high risk for systemic embolism.

If heart failure occurs, amiodarone may be used unless an atrioventricular block exists. This drug seems to be effective in reducing ventricular and supraventricular arrhythmias, as well. Vasodilators (such as nitroglycerin), diuretics, and sympathetic stimulators (such as isoproterenol) are contraindicated.

If drug therapy fails, surgery is indicated. Ventricular myotomy (resection of the hypertrophied septum) alone or combined with mitral valve replacement may ease outflow tract obstruction and relieve symptoms. However, ventricular myotomy may cause complications, such as complete heart block and a ventricular septal defect, and is experimental.

Key nursing diagnoses and patient outcomes

Activity intolerance related to imbalance between oxygen supply and demand. Based on this nursing diagnosis, you'll establish these patient outcomes. The patient will:

- maintain his blood pressure, pulse, and respiratory rate within prescribed limits during exertion
- demonstrate skill in conserving energy while carrying out his daily activities
- express an understanding of hypertrophic cardiomyopathy and identify the symptoms of activity intolerance.

Decreased cardiac output related to ventricular dysfunction. Based on this nursing diagnosis, you'll establish these patient outcomes. The patient will:

- remain hemodynamically stable, as evidenced by the absence of cardiac arrhythmias and by the maintenance of his blood pressure, pulse, and respiratory rate within a safe range
- not experience complications related to decreased cardiac output, such as chest pain, ischemic changes on electrocardiogram, or decreased tissue perfusion to vital organs.

Fluid volume excess related to left ventricular stiffness. Based on this nursing diagnosis, you'll establish these patient outcomes. The patient will:

- comply with the treatment prescribed to minimize fluid retention
- tolerate fluid and sodium restrictions without physical or emotional discomfort
- identify the signs and symptoms of acute fluid volume excess and verbalize the importance of seeking medical treatment if they should occur.

Nursing interventions

- Alternate periods of rest with required activities of daily living and treatments. Provide personal care as needed to prevent fatigue.
- Provide active or passive range-of-motion exercises to prevent muscle atrophy if the patient is on bed rest.
- If propranolol is to be discontinued, don't stop the drug abruptly; doing so may cause rebound effects, resulting in myocardial infarction or sudden death.
- Therapeutic restrictions and an uncertain prognosis usually cause profound anxiety and depression, so offer support and let the patient express his feelings. Be flexible with visiting hours. If hospitalization is prolonged, try to obtain permission for the patient to spend occasional weekends away from the hospital.
- Allow the patient and his family to express their fears and concerns. As needed, help them identify effective coping strategies.

Monitoring

- Monitor the patient's cardiopulmonary status and vital signs frequently.
- Monitor the patient for signs and symptoms of such complications as pulmonary hypertension or heart failure. Monitor the patient's weight, intake and output, and vital signs regularly.
- To determine the patient's tolerance for an increased dose of propranolol, take his pulse to check for bradycardia and have him stand and walk around slowly to check for orthostatic hypotension.

Patient teaching

- Remind the patient and his family that propranolol therapy may cause depression. Notify the doctor if symptoms appear.
- Instruct the patient to take his medication as ordered. Tell him to notify any doctor caring for him that he shouldn't be given nitroglycerin, digitalis glycosides, or diuretics because they can worsen obstruction.

• Inform the patient that before dental work or surgery, he'll need antibiotic prophylaxis for subacute bacterial endocarditis.

• Because syncope or sudden death may follow well-tolerated exercise, warn the patient against strenuous physical activity, such as running. Urge his family to learn cardiopulmonary resuscitation.

Hypoglycemia

Potentially dangerous, hypoglycemia is an abnormally low blood glucose level. It occurs when glucose burns up too rapidly, when the glucose release rate falls behind tissue demands, or when excessive insulin enters the bloodstream. When the brain is deprived of glucose, as with oxygen deprivation, its functioning becomes deranged. With prolonged glucose deprivation, tissue damage – or even death – may occur.

Hypoglycemia may be classified as reactive, pharmacologic, or fasting. *Reactive hypoglycemia* results from the reaction to the disposition of meals. Blood glucose levels typically fall 2 to 4 hours after a meal.

Pharmacologic hypoglycemia results in response to a drug that does one of the following: increases the amount of insulin circulating in the blood, enhances insulin action, or impairs the liver's glucose-producing capacity. Blood glucose levels may fall slowly or rapidly.

Fasting hypoglycemia causes discomfort during periods of abstinence from food. Blood glucose levels fall gradually. Signs and symptoms don't occur until 5 hours or more after a meal. This rare type of hypoglycemia occurs most often during the night.

Manifestations of hypoglycemia tend to be vague and depend on how quickly the patient's glucose levels drop. Gradual onset of hypoglycemia produces predominantly central nervous system (CNS) signs and symptoms; a more rapid decline in plasma glucose levels results predominantly in adrenergic signs and symptoms. (See *Acute hypoglycemia,* pages 454 and 455.)

Causes

Reactive hypoglycemia may take several forms. Most commonly, it results from alimentary hyperinsulinism caused by dumping syndrome. Fructose or galactose ingestion may cause hypoglycemia in patients with fructose intolerance or galactosemia. Reactive hypoglycemia may also occur secondary to imminent onset of Type II diabetes mellitus or impaired glucose tolerance. In some patients, reactive hypoglycemia may have no known cause (idiopathic reactive).

Pharmacologic hypoglycemia most commonly results from the use of insulin or oral sulfonylureas. Other causes include the use of beta blockers and excessive alcohol ingestion.

Fasting hypoglycemia most commonly results from hepatic disease or a tumor. Insulinomas, small islet cell tumors in the pancreas, secrete excessive amounts of insulin, which inhibits hepatic glucose production. These tumors are usually benign (in 90% of patients). Extrapancreatic tumors, though uncommon, can also cause hypoglycemia by increasing glucose utilization and inhibiting glucose output. Such tumors occur primarily in the mesenchyma, liver, adrenal cortex, GI system, and lymphatic system. They may be benign or malignant.

Among nonendocrine causes of fasting hypoglycemia are severe hepatic diseases, including hepatitis, cancer, cirrhosis, and liver congestion associated with heart failure. All of these conditions reduce the uptake and release of glycogen from the liver.

Some endocrine causes include destruction of pancreatic islet cells; adrenocortical insufficiency, which contributes to hypoglycemia by reducing the production of cortisol and cortisone needed for gluconeogenesis; and pituitary insufficiency,

(Text continues on page 456.)

LIFE-THREATENING COMPLICATIONS

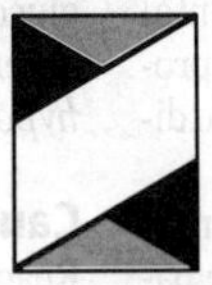

Acute hypoglycemia

Normally, homeostatic mechanisms maintain blood glucose levels within narrow limits (60 to 120 mg/dl). The body burns available glucose and stores the rest as glycogen in the liver and muscles. When the glucose level drops, the liver converts glycogen back to glucose (glycogenolysis) or makes new glucose from noncarbohydrate sources, such as amino acids or fatty acids (gluconeogenesis).

Hormones maintain the delicate balance between glucose production and use. But this balance is upset when a patient has hypoglycemia. The flowchart below shows the events that lead to CNS and autonomic nervous system reactions associated with hypoglycemia.

Signs and symptoms

Acute hypoglycemia initially causes signs and symptoms of mild cerebral dysfunction, such as headache, dizziness, restlessness, and decreased mental capacity. If left untreated, the blood glucose level continues to drop, producing such adrenergic signs and symptoms as hunger, weakness, diaphoresis, tachycardia, pallor, anxiety, tremor, and possibly rebound hyperglycemia. If hypoglycemia continues, any beneficial effects of rebound hyperglycemia quickly dissipate and coma, seizures, and permanent brain damage or even death may follow.

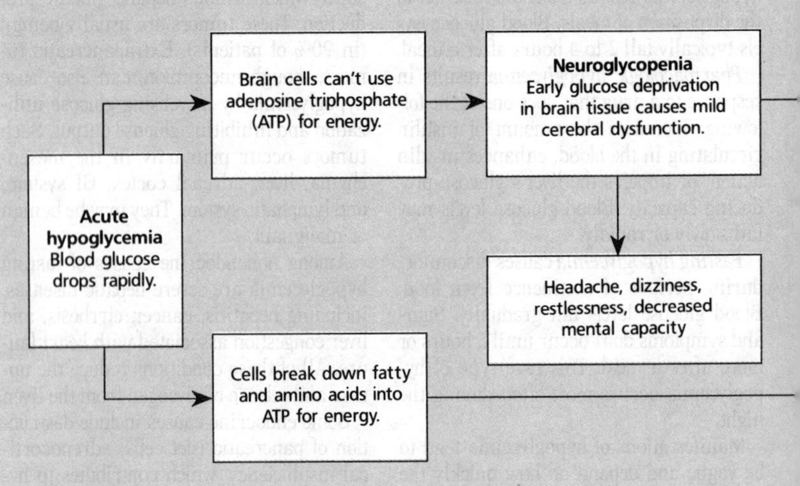

Emergency interventions

The patient's signs and symptoms determine which interventions to take.

For severe hypoglycemia (suggested by confusion or coma), expect to administer 25 or 50 g of 50% glucose solution by I.V. bolus, followed by continuous glucose infusion until the patient can eat a meal.

For mild hypoglycemia (suggested by adrenergic but no CNS symptoms), administer a readily available source of glucose, such as five to six pieces of hard candy; 4 to 6 oz of apple juice, orange juice, cola, or other soft drink; or 1 tbs of honey or grape jelly. When symptoms subside, give the patient a snack to prevent hypoglycemia recurrence (unless the next meal will be served within the hour).

Notify the doctor if hypoglycemic episodes don't respond to treatment, if they recur frequently, or if they're severe.

AUTONOMIC NERVOUS SYSTEM STIMULATION

Pancreas
Sympathetic nerves and epinephrine rapidly stimulate glucagon secretion; epinephrine inhibits insulin secretion.

Adrenal glands
Sympathetic nerves stimulate epinephrine secretion (rapid response). Hypothalamus stimulates pituitary gland to secrete corticotropin, which acts on the adrenal cortex to cause cortisol secretion (delayed response).

Stomach
Hypothalamus stimulates hunger; parasympathetic nerves increase gastric juices and stomach contractions.

Liver
Sympathetic nerves directly stimulate glycogenolysis; epinephrine, glucagon, cortisol, and growth hormone increase gluconeogenesis; glucagon also stimulates glycogenolysis.

Muscle
Hypothalamus stimulates pituitary to secrete growth hormone (delayed response), which – along with epinephrine and cortisol – inhibits glucagon use.

→ **Adrenergic changes**
Hunger, weakness, diaphoresis, tachycardia, pallor, anxiety, tremor, rebound hyperglycemia

which reduces corticotropin and growth hormone levels.

Complications

Prolonged or severe hypoglycemia (blood glucose levels of 20 mg/dl or less) can cause permanent brain damage and may be fatal.

Assessment

The history of a patient with suspected hypoglycemia should note the pattern of food intake for the preceding 24 hours, as well as drug and alcohol use. The medical or surgical history may note the existence of causative factors, such as gastrectomy or hepatic disease.

A patient with reactive hypoglycemia may report adrenergic symptoms, such as diaphoresis, anxiety, hunger, nervousness, and weakness, indicating a rapid decline in his blood glucose levels. A patient with fasting hypoglycemia may report signs and symptoms of CNS disturbance, such as dizziness, headache, clouding of vision, restlessness, and mental status changes, indicating a slow decline in blood glucose levels. With prolonged glucose deprivation, the patient's history (obtained from family or friends, if necessary) may reveal seizures, decreasing level of consciousness (LOC), and coma. A patient with pharmacologic hypoglycemia may experience a rapid or slow decline in blood glucose levels.

Inspection may reveal adrenergic signs, such as diaphoresis, pallor, and tremor; or CNS signs, such as restlessness, loss of fine-motor skills, and altered LOC. Palpation may detect tachycardia.

Diagnostic tests

Glucometer readings provide quick screening methods for determining blood glucose levels. Laboratory testing confirms the diagnosis by showing decreased blood glucose values of less than 40 mg/dl before a meal or less than 50 mg/dl after a meal.

In addition, a 5-hour glucose tolerance test may be administered to provoke reactive hypoglycemia. Following a 12-hour fast, laboratory testing to detect plasma insulin and plasma glucose levels may identify fasting hypoglycemia.

A C-peptide assay helps diagnose fasting hypoglycemia. It also differentiates fasting hypoglycemia caused by an insulinoma from fasting hypoglycemia caused by insulin injections.

Treatment

For *severe hypoglycemia* (producing confusion or coma), initial treatment is usually I.V. administration of a bolus of 25 or 50 g of glucose as a 50% solution. This is followed by a constant infusion of glucose until the patient can eat a meal. A patient who experiences adrenergic reactions without CNS symptoms may receive oral carbohydrate (parenteral therapy isn't required).

Reactive hypoglycemia requires dietary modification to help delay glucose absorption and gastric emptying. Usually, this includes small, frequent meals; avoidance of simple carbohydrates; and ingestion of high-protein meals with added fiber. The patient may also receive anticholinergic drugs to slow gastric emptying and intestinal motility and to inhibit vagal stimulation of insulin release.

For *fasting hypoglycemia,* surgery and drug therapy may be required. In patients with insulinoma, removal of the tumor is the treatment of choice. Drug therapy may include diazoxide or octreotide for inoperable insulinomas. Hormone replacement therapy may be needed for pituitary or adrenal gland insufficiency. In many cases of recurrent hypoglycemia, the only treatment needed is avoidance of fasting.

Key nursing diagnoses and patient outcomes

Anxiety related to frequent or severe hypoglycemic episodes. Based on this nurs-

ing diagnosis, you'll establish these patient outcomes. The patient will:
- identify and express his feelings of anxiety
- request information about hypoglycemia
- exhibit fewer physical signs of anxiety.

Risk for injury related to neurologic damage from a hypoglycemic episode. Based on this nursing diagnosis, you'll establish these patient outcomes. The patient will:
- comply with treatments to prevent hypoglycemia-induced injury
- exhibit normal neurologic function after hypoglycemic episodes
- avoid neurologic damage.

Knowledge deficit related to hypoglycemia and its treatment. Based on this nursing diagnosis, you'll establish these patient outcomes. The patient will:
- express a need for information about hypoglycemia and its treatment
- participate in learning situations that address hypoglycemia and its treatment
- articulate an understanding of hypoglycemia and its treatment.

Nursing interventions

- Administer medications, as prescribed.
- Avoid delays in meal times and provide a proper diet. Arrange to have a dietitian visit the patient to teach him about proper diet.
- Correct hypoglycemic episodes quickly. Implement measures to protect the unconscious patient, such as maintaining a patent airway.
- Prepare the insulinoma patient for surgery, if indicated. Provide the same preoperative and postoperative care as for a patient undergoing abdominal surgery.

Monitoring

- Watch for and report signs of hypoglycemia in high-risk patients. If possible, measure blood glucose before correcting hypoglycemia to verify its presence and severity.
- Monitor any infusion of hypertonic glucose to avoid hyperglycemia, circulatory overload, and cellular dehydration.
- Measure blood glucose levels, as ordered.
- Assess the effects of drug therapy, and watch for adverse reactions.

Patient teaching

- Explain the purpose, preparation, and procedure for any diagnostic tests.
- Emphasize the importance of preventing or promptly treating hypoglycemic episodes to avoid severe complications. Be sure the patient understands the key danger with hypoglycemia: Once it occurs, he may quickly lose his ability to think clearly. If this should happen while he's driving a car or operating machinery, a serious accident could result.
- Inform the patient that he should note what early symptoms he typically experiences with hypoglycemia. Family, friends, and coworkers should also be able to recognize the warning signs so that immediate treatment can be initiated.
- Review with the patient and family the treatment measures they should follow if the patient has a hypoglycemic episode. If the patient is conscious, he should consume a readily available source of glucose, such as five to six pieces of hard candy; 4 to 6 oz of apple juice, orange juice, cola, or other soft drink; or 1 tbs of honey or grape jelly. If the patient is unconscious, he should be given a subcutaneous injection of glucagon. Teach the patient's family how to administer glucagon. Advise the patient and family to notify the doctor if hypoglycemic episodes don't respond to treatment or if they occur frequently.
- Emphasize the importance of carefully following the prescribed diet to prevent a rapid drop in blood glucose levels. Advise the patient to eat small meals throughout the day, and mention that bedtime snacks also may be necessary to keep blood glucose at an even level. Instruct the patient to avoid alcohol and caffeine because they may trigger severe hypoglycemic episodes.

- If the patient is obese and has impaired glucose tolerance, suggest ways he can restrict his caloric intake and lose weight. If necessary, help him find a weight-loss support group.
- Warn the patient with fasting hypoglycemia not to postpone or skip meals and snacks. Instruct the patient to call his doctor for instructions if he doesn't feel well enough to eat.
- Discuss life-style and personal habits to help the patient identify precipitating factors, such as poor diet, stress, or noncompliance with diabetes mellitus treatment. Explain ways that he can change or avoid each precipitating factor identified. If necessary, teach him stress-reduction techniques, and encourage him to join a support group.
- Teach the patient about precautions to take when exercising; for example, tell him to consume extra calories and not to exercise alone or when his blood glucose level is likely to drop.
- Inform the patient that he should carry a source of fast-acting carbohydrate, such as hard candy, with him at all times. Advise him to wear a medical identification bracelet or to carry a medical identification card that describes his condition and its emergency treatment measures.
- For the patient with pharmacologic hypoglycemia from insulin or oral antidiabetic agents, review the essentials of managing diabetes mellitus, if indicated.
- If warranted, teach the patient about prescribed drug therapy or surgery.
- Because hypoglycemia is a chronic disorder, encourage the patient to see his doctor regularly.
- Encourage the patient and family to discuss their concerns about the patient's condition and treatment.

Hypoparathyroidism

A deficiency in parathyroid hormone (PTH) secretion by the parathyroid glands or decreased action of peripheral PTH creates hypoparathyroidism. Because the parathyroid glands primarily regulate calcium balance, hypoparathyroidism causes hypocalcemia, which produces neuromuscular symptoms ranging from paresthesia to tetany.

PTH normally maintains serum calcium levels by increasing bone resorption and GI absorption of calcium. It also maintains the inverse relationship between serum calcium and phosphate levels by inhibiting phosphate reabsorption in the renal tubules. Abnormal PTH production in hypoparathyroidism disrupts this delicate balance.

Hypoparathyroidism may be acute or chronic and is classified as idiopathic, acquired, or reversible. The idiopathic and reversible forms are most common in children, and the clinical effects are usually correctable with replacement therapy. The acquired form, which is irreversible, is most common in older patients who have undergone thyroid gland surgery.

Causes

Idiopathic hypoparathyroidism may result from an autoimmune genetic disorder or the congenital absence of the parathyroid glands.

Acquired hypoparathyroidism typically results from accidental removal of or injury to one or more parathyroid glands during thyroidectomy or other neck surgery. It may also result from ischemic infarction of the parathyroid glands during surgery, hemochromatosis, sarcoidosis, amyloidosis, tuberculosis, neoplasms, trauma, or massive thyroid irradiation (rare).

Reversible hypoparathyroidism may result from hypomagnesemia-induced impairment of hormone synthesis, from suppression of normal gland function due to hypercalcemia, or from delayed maturation of parathyroid function.

Complications

In hypoparathyroidism, complications are related to long-standing hypocalcemia. Decreased calcium levels can cause reduced contractility and, eventually, heart failure. Lens calcification leads to cataract formation that persists despite calcium replacement therapy. Papillary edema from increased intracranial pressure, irreversible calcification of basal ganglion, and bone deformity also occur. Laryngospasm, respiratory stridor, anoxia, paralysis of the vocal cords, and death may occur in severe cases of tetany. Hypoparathyroidism that develops during childhood results in mental retardation, stunted growth, and malformed teeth.

Assessment

The patient's history may reveal recent neck surgery or irradiation or long-term hypomagnesemia from GI malabsorption or alcoholism.

The patient may report symptoms that reflect altered neuromuscular irritability. (See *Acute tetany,* page 460.) The patient may also complain of personality changes, ranging from irritability and anxiety to depression, delirium, and frank psychosis.

On inspection, you may find dry skin, brittle hair, alopecia, transverse and longitudinal ridges in the fingernails, loss of eyelashes and fingernails, and stained, cracked, and decayed teeth from weakened enamel.

Palpation may elicit Chvostek's and Trousseau's signs, which indicate latent tetany. Chvostek's sign may appear in other disorders, but only a hypocalcemic patient exhibits Trousseau's sign. You may also palpate increased deep tendon reflexes resulting from neuromuscular irritability. Auscultation of the apical pulse may detect cardiac arrhythmias.

Diagnostic tests

- *Radioimmunoassay* for PTH shows diminished serum PTH concentration.
- *Blood and urine tests* reveal decreased serum and urine calcium levels, increased serum phosphate levels (above 5.4 mg/dl), and reduced urine creatinine levels.
- *X-rays* indicate greater bone density and malformation.
- *Electrocardiogram (ECG) changes* disclose increased QT and ST intervals due to hypocalcemia.

Treatment

Because calcium absorption from the small intestine depends on the presence of activated vitamin D, treatment initially includes vitamin D, with or without supplemental calcium. Such therapy is usually lifelong, except in patients with reversible hyperthyroidism. If the patient can't tolerate the pure form of vitamin D, alternatives include dihydrotachysterol if renal function is adequate, and calcitriol if renal function is severely compromised.

Key nursing diagnoses and patient outcomes

Altered thought processes related to hypocalcemia-induced neurologic dysfunction. Based on this nursing diagnosis, you'll establish these patient outcomes. The patient will:

- remain safe and protected in his environment
- regain and maintain normal thought patterns through hypoparathyroidism treatment.

Risk for injury related to acute and long-term calcium deficiency. Based on this nursing diagnosis, you'll establish these patient outcomes. The patient will:

- regain and maintain normal serum calcium and phosphorus levels
- not exhibit signs and symptoms of tetany
- avoid complications of long-term hypocalcemia.

Ineffective breathing pattern related to hyperventilation caused by neuromuscular

LIFE-THREATENING COMPLICATIONS

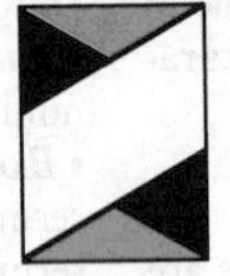

Acute tetany

Acute (overt) tetany results from a sudden or severe drop in the serum calcium level. Remember that a calcium deficit increases neuronal membrane permeability and allows sodium to enter cells more easily than usual. In turn, this promotes spontaneous depolarization, causing neuromuscular irritability. The more severe the calcium deficit, the greater the neuromuscular irritability.

Signs and symptoms

In acute tetany, the patient may report tingling that begins in the fingertips, around the mouth and, occasionally, in the feet. Tingling spreads and becomes more severe, causing muscle tension and spasms. Pain varies with the degree of muscle tension but rarely affects the face, legs, and feet. The patient may also complain of throat constriction and dysphagia. Smooth muscle hyperactivity leads to GI upset, exhibited as nausea, vomiting, abdominal pain, or constipation or diarrhea.

During a tetany episode, you may note that the patient's hands, forearms and, less commonly, feet contort in a specific pattern, with thumb adduction followed by metacarpophalangeal joint flexion, interphalangeal joint extension, and wrist and elbow joint flexion. In severe cases, he may also have signs of laryngospasm, respiratory stridor, anoxia, and convulsions.

Emergency interventions

If you suspect acute tetany, take the following steps:

- Notify the doctor at once and have another staff member bring emergency equipment to the bedside.
- Maintain a patent airway, and have a tracheotomy tray and an endotracheal tube available. Take seizure precautions.
- Insert an I.V. line and prepare to administer 10% calcium gluconate or 10% calcium chloride I.V. *stat* to raise the serum ionized calcium level.
- If the patient can do so, have him breathe into a paper bag so that he inhales his own carbon dioxide.
- Be prepared to administer anticonvulsant agents, such as phenytoin or phenobarbitol, to control seizures until the serum calcium level rises. Avoid use of phenothiazine drugs because of possible inducement of severe dyskinesia.
- Monitor serum calcium and phosphorus levels closely.
- Be aware that hyperventilation, which may result from anxiety, can worsen tetany. Keep the patient calm, and give a sedative, if prescribed.
- Monitor ECG in a patient taking a digitalis glycoside because calcium potentiates the drug's action on the heart.

irritability. Based on this nursing diagnosis, you'll establish these patient outcomes. The patient will:

- receive appropriate respiratory support to maintain adequate ventilation
- maintain adequate gas exchange, as shown by normal arterial blood gas values
- avoid hyperventilation once serum calcium levels return to normal.

Nursing interventions

- Maintain a patent I.V. line. Keep emergency equipment available, including I.V. calcium gluconate and calcium chloride, an airway, a tracheotomy tray, and an en-

dotracheal tube. Maintain seizure precautions.
• Hyperventilation, which may result from anxiety during a tetany episode, can worsen tetany. So can recent blood transfusions because anticoagulant in stored blood binds calcium. Keep the patient calm, and give a sedative, if prescribed. Help the patient with mild tetany rebreathe his own exhaled air by breathing into a paper bag.
• Provide meticulous skin care. Use alcohol-free skin care products and an emollient lotion after bathing.
• Institute safety precautions to minimize the risk of injury from falls. Provide support for walking.
• Encourage the patient to verbalize his feelings about body image changes and rejection by others. Offer emotional support, and help him identify his strengths and use them to develop coping strategies. Refer him to a mental health professional for additional counseling, if necessary.

Monitoring

• Check the patient's serum calcium and phosphorus levels regularly.
• Monitor the patient's ECG for increasing QT-interval changes, heart block, and signs of decreasing cardiac output. Closely observe the patient who is receiving both digitalis and calcium, because calcium potentiates the effect of digitalis. Stay alert for signs of digitalis toxicity (arrhythmias, nausea, fatigue, and visual changes).
• Assess the patient for tetany and long-term complications of chronic hypocalcemia.

Patient teaching

• Discuss the importance of long-term management and follow-up care, especially periodic checks of the patient's serum calcium levels.
• Advise the patient that long-term replacement therapy will be necessary. Instruct him to take the medication as ordered and not to discontinue it abruptly.
• Instruct the patient to take calcium supplements with or after meals and to chew the tablets well.
• Encourage the patient to wear a medical identification bracelet and to carry his medication with him at all times.
• Teach the patient and his family to identify and report signs and symptoms of hypercalcemia, tetany, and respiratory distress.
• Teach the patient protective measures to decrease stress and to avoid fatigue and infection.
• Advise the patient to follow a high-calcium, low-phosphorus diet. Discuss foods high in calcium; for example, dairy products, salmon, egg yolks, shrimp, and green, leafy vegetables. Caution him to avoid high-phosphate foods, such as spinach, rhubarb, and asparagus.

Hypophysectomy

New microsurgical methods have dramatically reversed the high mortality once associated with removal of pituitary and sella turcica tumors. Hypophysectomy is now the treatment of choice for pituitary tumors, which can cause acromegaly, gigantism, and Cushing's disease. And it can be used as a palliative measure for patients with metastatic breast or prostate cancer to relieve pain and reduce the hormonal secretions that spur neoplastic growth.

Hypophysectomy may be performed *transfrontally* (approaching the sella turcica through the cranium) or *transsphenoidally* (entering from the inner aspect of the upper lip through the sphenoid sinus). The transfrontal approach carries a high risk of mortality and such complications as smell and taste loss and permanent, severe diabetes insipidus. For these reasons, this approach is rarely used. In the commonly used transsphenoidal approach, powerful microscopes and improved ra-

Adenectomy: Alternative to hypophysectomy

Both adenectomy and hypophysectomy can be used to remove pituitary tumors. In hypophysectomy, the doctor removes the tumor and all or part of the pituitary gland. However, for a tumor confined to the sella turcica, the doctor may be able to perform an adenectomy, in which he removes the lesion while leaving the pituitary intact. Both surgeries involve the transsphenoidal approach shown here.

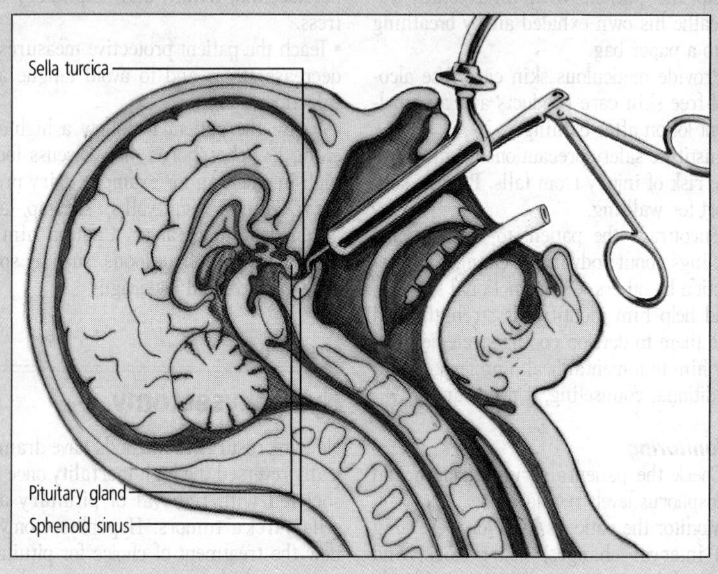

diologic techniques allow microadenoma removal. Laser surgery, an alternative approach, is experimental. (See *Adenectomy: Alternative to hypophysectomy*.)

Procedure

In transsphenoidal hypophysectomy, with the patient under general anesthesia, the doctor makes an incision in the superior gingival tissue of the maxilla. After dissecting membranes and tissues, he places a speculum blade in the developed space slightly anterior to the sphenoid sinus to avoid lateral compression of the opened anterior walls of the sinus. (Some doctors prefer the septal passage approach for the speculum.) Then he evaluates the deeper anatomy using an operating microscope with binocular vision and high-power lighting.

Using a microdrill, the doctor penetrates the sphenoid bone to visualize the anterior sella floor. He can then resect and aspirate a soft tumor downward. Before wound closure, he may apply hemostatic agents, such as oxidized cellulose cotton. Or he may use the patient's own subcutaneous fat or a muscle plug from the thigh as intrasellar graft tissue. The sella floor may be sealed off with a small piece of bone or cartilage.

Finally, the doctor inserts nasal catheters with petroleum gauze packed around them. He closes the initial incision with stitches inside the inner lip.

Complications

Transient diabetes insipidus is a common postsurgical problem; in some cases, it's followed by transient syndrome of inappropriate antidiuretic hormone, which necessitates careful patient monitoring for 24 to 48 hours. Other potential complications include infection, cerebrospinal fluid (CSF) leakage, hemorrhage, and visual defects. Total pituitary gland removal causes a hormonal deficiency that calls for close monitoring and replacement therapy; usually, though, the anterior pituitary is preserved.

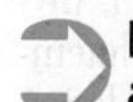

Key nursing diagnoses and patient outcomes

Risk for fluid volume deficit related to lack of vasopressin release. Based on this nursing diagnosis, you'll establish these patient outcomes. The patient will:

- maintain normal serum osmolality and serum sodium levels
- maintain normal vital signs and skin integrity
- not exhibit signs and symptoms of hypertonic dehydration, such as chorea, confusion, coma, seizures, and paralysis.

Altered protection related to glucocorticoid deficiency caused by corticotropin hormone loss. Based on this nursing diagnosis, you'll establish these patient outcomes. The patient will:

- comply with life-long hormonal replacement therapy
- express an understanding of why he must seek medical attention during illness, injury, and severe stress
- protect himself by wearing a medical identification bracelet
- not have signs and symptoms of adrenal crisis, such as nausea, vomiting, and orthostatic blood pressure changes.

Risk for injury related to complications of hypophysectomy. Based on this nursing diagnosis, you'll establish these patient outcomes. The patient will:

- use appropriate measures to prevent injury, such as avoiding coughing, sneezing, and blowing his nose after surgery until healing is complete
- demonstrate good oral hygiene technique
- avoid injury, as shown by absence of CSF leakage and signs and symptoms of infection.

Nursing interventions

When caring for a hypophysectomy patient, your major roles include instruction and care tailored to the patient's condition.

Before surgery

- Explain to the patient that this surgery will remove a tumor from his pituitary gland. Tell him he will receive a general anesthetic and, after surgery, will remain in the intensive care unit for 48 hours for careful monitoring. Mention that he'll have a nasal catheter and packing in place for 1 to 2 days after surgery, as well as an indwelling urinary catheter.
- Arrange for appropriate tests and examinations, as ordered. For example, if the patient has acromegaly, he'll need a thorough cardiac evaluation because he's at risk for incipient myocardial ischemia. If he has Cushing's disease, he'll need blood pressure checks and serum potassium determinations. For any patient, arrange visual field tests to serve as a baseline.
- Review the patient's preoperative medication regimen, if appropriate. If he is hypothyroid, he may need hormone replacement therapy. If he has a prolactin-secreting tumor, find out if he's been taking bromocriptine for 6 weeks before surgery to help shrink the tumor.
- Make sure the patient or a responsible family member has signed a consent form.

After surgery

- Keep the patient on bed rest for 24 hours, then encourage ambulation. Keep the head of his bed elevated to avoid placing tension or pressure on the suture line. Tell him not to sneeze, cough, blow his nose, or bend over for several days to avoid disturbing the muscle graft.

- Give mild analgesics, as ordered, for headache caused by CSF loss during surgery or for paranasal pain. Paranasal pain typically subsides when the catheters and packing are removed – usually 24 to 48 hours after surgery.
- Expect the patient to develop transient diabetes insipidus, usually within 24 hours after surgery. Be alert for increased thirst and greater urine volume with a low specific gravity. If diabetes insipidus occurs, replace fluids and administer aqueous vasopressin, as ordered. Or give sublingual desmopressin acetate, as ordered. With these measures, diabetes insipidus usually resolves within 72 hours.
- Arrange for visual field testing as soon as possible because visual defects may signal hemorrhage. Collect a serum sample to measure pituitary hormone levels and evaluate the need for hormone replacement. As ordered, give prophylactic antibiotics.

Home care instructions

- Teach the patient how to recognize diabetes insipidus and instruct him to report signs and symptoms immediately. Explain that he may need to limit fluid intake or take prescribed medications.
- If ordered, tell the patient not to brush his teeth for 2 weeks to avoid suture line disruption. Mention that he can use a mouthwash.
- The patient may need hormonal replacement therapy because of decreased pituitary secretion of thyroid-stimulating hormone. If he needs cortisol or thyroid hormone replacement, teach him to recognize the signs of excessive or insufficient dosage. Advise him to wear a medical identification bracelet.
- Tell the patient with hyperprolactinemia that he'll need follow-up visits for several years because relapse is possible. Explain that he may be placed on bromocriptine if relapse occurs.

Hypopituitarism

A complex syndrome marked by metabolic dysfunction, sexual immaturity, and growth retardation (when it occurs in childhood), hypopituitarism results from a deficiency of the hormones secreted by the anterior pituitary gland. The disorder is also known as panhypopituitarism and dwarfism.

Panhypopituitarism refers to a generalized condition caused by partial or complete failure of the gland to produce all six of the vital hormones: corticotropin, thyroid-stimulating hormone (TSH), luteinizing hormone (LH), follicle-stimulating hormone (FSH), growth hormone (GH), and prolactin. Partial hypopituitarism and complete hypopituitarism occur in adults and children; in children, these diseases may cause dwarfism and pubertal delay.

Total loss of all hormones is fatal unless treated, but the prognosis is good with adequate replacement therapy and correction of the underlying causes.

Causes

The most common cause of primary hypopituitarism is tumor. Other causes include congenital defects (hypoplasia or aplasia of the pituitary gland); pituitary infarction (most often from postpartum hemorrhage); partial or total hypophysectomy by surgery, irradiation, or chemical agents; and, rarely, granulomatous disease, such as tuberculosis. Occasionally, primary hypopituitarism has no identifiable cause.

Secondary hypopituitarism stems from a deficiency of releasing hormones produced by the hypothalamus. The process may be idiopathic or may result from infection, trauma, or tumor.

LIFE-THREATENING COMPLICATIONS

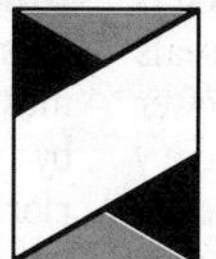

Identifying pituitary apoplexy

Five to ten percent of patients with pituitary tumors develop pituitary apoplexy, a life-threatening condition caused by hemorrhage into the tumor. Pituitary apoplexy usually occurs suddenly when rapid adenoma growth causes infarction or rupture of the tumor's thin-walled vessels. Patients with acromegaly or Cushing's disease have a higher-than-average incidence of pituitary apoplexy.

Assessment findings

Suspect pituitary apoplexy if your patient exhibits the following signs or symptoms:

- sudden, severe headache
- blurred vision
- diplopia
- blindness (from optic chiasma compression)
- eye deviation and pupil dilation (from oculomotor nerve paralysis)
- altered level of consciousness (possibly progressing to unconsciousness)
- nausea and vomiting
- hyperpyrexia
- nuchal rigidity.

Emergency interventions

Because this complication is life-threatening, take the following steps immediately:

- Notify the patient's doctor.
- Prepare the patient for emergency diagnostic tests, including a WBC count (which may be elevated), CT scan (which may show suprasellar extension), and a lumbar puncture (which may reveal an elevated cerebrospinal fluid [CSF] pressure, and CSF that is xanthochromic or frankly bloody and has an elevated protein concentration).
- Prepare to transfer the patient to the intensive care unit.
- Be aware that treatment is controversial, but it may involve corticosteroid administration. If visual deterioration continues, the doctor may order surgical evacuation of the hematoma in an attempt to preserve vision.

Complications

Any combination of deficits in the production of the six major hormones may occur. If the process is an evolving one (due to a hypothalamic destructive lesion), additional hormonal deficiencies may occur over time. Hypopituitarism can result in GH deficiency, TSH or corticotropin deficiency, and gonadotropin and prolactin deficiency. Pituitary apoplexy is a medical emergency. (See *Identifying pituitary apoplexy.*) The patient's inability to cope with minor stressors can lead to high fever, shock, coma, and death. In secondary hypopituitarism, damage to the posterior pituitary from infection, trauma, or tumor is occasionally extensive enough to cause diabetes insipidus.

Assessment

Physical findings depend on the specific pituitary hormones that are deficient, the patient's age, and the disorder's severity. Typically, clinical features develop slowly and don't become apparent until 75% of the pituitary gland is destroyed. Assessment findings related to specific hormonal deficiencies include the following:

- *GH deficiency.* Physical signs of GH deficiency may not be apparent in neonates, but by age 6 months, growth retardation is obvious. In children, inspection reveals chubbiness from fat deposits in the lower trunk, short stature, delayed secondary tooth eruption, and delayed puberty. Growth continues at less than half the normal rate – sometimes extending into the patient's twenties or thirties – to an average height of 4′ (122 cm), with normal proportions.

Inspection of adults with GH deficiency finds more subtle signs, such as fine wrinkles near the mouth and eyes.

• *Gonadotropin (FSH and LH) deficiency.* In women, history discloses amenorrhea; dyspareunia related to reduced vaginal secretions; infertility; and reduced libido. Inspection may reveal breast atrophy, sparse or absent axillary and pubic hair, and dry skin. Men report weakness, impotence, and reduced libido. Inspection may show decreased muscle strength, testicular softening and shrinkage, and retarded secondary sexual hair growth.

• *TSH deficiency.* Patients may report cold intolerance, constipation, increased or decreased menstrual flow, and lethargy. Children will have severe growth retardation despite treatment. Inspection may show dry, pale, puffy skin and slow thought processes. Palpation may detect bradycardia.

• *Corticotropin deficiency.* Patient history discloses fatigue, nausea, vomiting, anorexia, and weight loss. During inspection you may note depigmentation of the skin and nipples. Vital signs during periods of stress may reflect fever and hypotension.

• *Prolactin deficiency.* Patients commonly report absent postpartum lactation, amenorrhea, sparse or absent growth of pubic and axillary hair, and symptoms of thyroid and adrenocortical failure.

• *Panhypopituitarism.* All six pituitary hormones are at least partially deficient. This may result in a host of mental and physical abnormalities, including lethargy, psychosis, orthostatic hypotension, bradycardia, and anemia.

Diagnostic tests

In suspected hypopituitarism, evaluation must confirm hormonal deficiency caused by impairment or destruction of the anterior pituitary gland. It must also rule out disease of the target organs (adrenals, gonads, and thyroid gland) or the hypothalamus. Low serum levels of thyroxine, for example, indicate diminished thyroid gland function, but further tests are necessary to identify the source of this dysfunction as the thyroid, pituitary, or hypothalamus.

• Radioimmunoassay showing decreased plasma levels of some or all pituitary hormones (except corticotropin, which requires more sophisticated testing), accompanied by target-organ hypofunction, suggests pituitary failure and eliminates target gland disease. Failure of thyrotropin-releasing hormone administration to increase TSH or prolactin concentrations rules out hypothalamic dysfunction as the cause of hormonal deficiency.

• Gonadotropin-releasing hormone administered I.V. can distinguish between pituitary and hypothalamic causes of gonadotropin deficiency.

• Administering a dopamine antagonist, such as metoclopramide, evaluates prolactin secretory reserve. In patients with hypopituitarism, increased levels of prolactin indicate a lesion in the hypothalamus or pituitary stalk.

• Clomiphene, an estrogen antagonist, can also be used as a diagnostic agent.

• Diagnosis of dwarfism requires measurement of GH levels in the blood after administration of regular insulin to induce hypoglycemia, or of levodopa, which causes hypotension. These drugs should provoke increased GH secretion. Persistently low GH levels, despite provocative testing, confirm GH deficiency.

• Computed tomography (CT) scans, magnetic resonance imaging, or cerebral angiography confirm the presence of intrasellar or extrasellar tumors.

The following provocative tests are also used, but both require careful medical supervision because they may precipitate an adrenal crisis:

- Oral administration of metyrapone pinpoints the source of low hydroxycorticosteroid levels. The drug blocks cortisol synthesis, which should stimulate pituitary secretion of corticotropin.
- Insulin administration induces hypoglycemia and stimulates corticotropin secretion. Persistently low levels of corticotropin indicate pituitary or hypothalamic failure.

Treatment

Replacement of hormones normally secreted by the target glands is the most effective treatment for hypopituitarism and panhypopituitarism. Hormonal replacement includes cortisol, the most important drug; thyroxine; and androgens or cyclic estrogen. Prolactin doesn't need replacement. The patient of reproductive age may benefit from FSH and human chorionic gonadotropin to boost fertility.

Somatropin or somatrem, identical to GH but the product of recombinant DNA technology, has replaced GHs derived from human sources. It's effective for treating dwarfism, stimulating growth increases of 4″ to 6″ to (10.2 to 15.2 cm) in the first year of treatment. The growth rate tapers off in subsequent years. However, after pubertal changes occur, the effects of GH therapy are limited.

Occasionally, a child becomes unresponsive to GH therapy, even with larger doses, perhaps because of antibody formation against the hormone. In such patients, small doses of androgen may again stimulate growth, but extreme caution is necessary to prevent premature closure of the epiphyses. Children with hypopituitarism may also need adrenal and thyroid hormone replacement and, as they approach puberty, sex hormones.

Key nursing diagnoses and patient outcomes

Altered protection related to lack of anterior pituitary gland hormone release when needed. Based on this nursing diagnosis, you'll establish these patient outcomes. The patient will:

- use protective measures, such as complying with hormonal replacement therapy, using stress-reduction techniques, and seeking immediate medical treatment if signs or symptoms of hormonal insufficiency occur
- maintain follow-up care, such as keeping doctors' appointments and having periodic blood tests to monitor the effectiveness of hormonal replacement therapy
- maintain adequate glucocorticoid and thyroid hormone levels through replacement therapy.

Risk for infection related to suppressed inflammatory response caused by chronic steroid therapy. Based on this nursing diagnosis, you'll establish these patient outcomes. The patient will:

- use precautions in his daily life to prevent or minimize infection
- maintain a normal temperature and white blood cell count
- avoid infection.

Hypothermia related to hypometabolism caused by TSH deficiency. Based on this nursing diagnosis, you'll establish these patient outcomes. The patient will:

- regain and maintain a normal body temperature
- avoid permanent tissue damage from hypothermia.

Nursing interventions

- For the patient with panhypopituitarism, determine food preferences and encourage him to maintain an adequate caloric intake. Offer frequent small meals and keep accurate records of weight loss or gain.
- Provide meticulous skin care, and use good hand-washing technique to prevent infection. Combat skin dryness with al-

cohol-free skin care products and an emollient lotion after bathing.
- Keep the patient warm if his body temperature is low. Provide extra clothing and blankets, and adjust room temperature, if possible.
- Keep dextrose 50% in water available for I.V. administration to correct hypoglycemia rapidly.
- To prevent postural hypotension, keep the patient supine during levodopa testing.
- Institute safety precautions for patients with impaired visual acuity to decrease the risk of injury.
- Support the family in setting realistic goals for the child, based on his age and abilities.
- Provide strong emotional support for the patient who is coping with changes in body appearance and sexual functioning. Encourage verbalization of feelings, and discuss fear of rejection by others. Provide a positive, realistic assessment of the patient's situation. Encourage him to develop interests that support a positive self-image and de-emphasize appearance.
- Refer the family for psychological counseling or to appropriate community resources. Emotional stress increases as the child becomes older and more aware of his condition.

Monitoring
- Monitor laboratory test results for hormonal deficiencies until the patient completes hormone replacement therapy.
- Assess the patient with panhypopituitarism for anorexia. Regularly monitor his weight.
- Record the patient's vital signs every 4 to 8 hours, and monitor intake and output. Observe eyelids, nail beds, and skin for pallor, which indicates anemia. Check neurologic status. Observe for signs of pituitary apoplexy, a medical emergency.
- During insulin testing, monitor the patient closely for signs of hypoglycemia (initially, slow cerebration, tachycardia, and nervousness; later, seizures).

Patient teaching
- Teach the patient and his family about the limitations imposed by the disease. If the patient has dwarfism, explain that these children often look younger than their chronological age and that they may grow in height more slowly than their peers.
- Review the treatment regimen with the patient and his family, especially long-term hormonal replacement therapy. Discuss the importance of taking the medication as ordered and of keeping regular follow-up appointments for blood studies.
- Instruct the patient to wear a medical identification bracelet.
- Teach the patient and his family measures to conserve the patient's energy, manage stressful situations, and prevent infections. Stress the importance of adequate rest to avoid fatigue, a balanced diet with adequate calories and fluids, good personal hygiene and hand-washing technique, and avoidance of people with colds or other infections.
- Emphasize the importance of identifying and reporting emergency situations. If necessary, teach the family to administer steroids parenterally.

Hypothyroidism

In this disorder, metabolic processes slow down because of a deficiency of the thyroid hormones triiodothyronine (T_3) or thyroxine (T_4).

Hypothyroidism is classified as primary or secondary. Primary hypothyroidism stems from a disorder of the thyroid gland. Secondary hypothyroidism is caused by a failure to stimulate normal thyroid function or by a failure of target tissues to respond to normal blood levels of thyroid hormones. Either type may progress to myxedema, which is clinically much more severe and considered a medical emer-

LIFE-THREATENING COMPLICATIONS

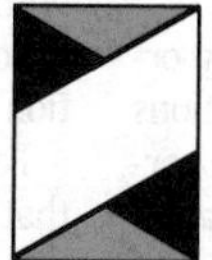

What to do in myxedema coma

A medical emergency, myxedema coma often has a fatal outcome. Progression is usually gradual, but when stress aggravates severe or prolonged hypothyroidism, coma may develop abruptly. Examples of severe stress are infection, exposure to cold, and trauma. Other precipitating factors include thyroid medication withdrawal and the use of sedatives, narcotics, or anesthetics.

Signs and symptoms

Patients in myxedema coma have significantly depressed respirations, so their $PaCO_2$ levels may rise. Decreased cardiac output and worsening cerebral hypoxia may also occur. The patient is stuporous and hypothermic, and his vital signs reflect bradycardia and hypotension.

Emergency interventions

If your patient becomes comatose, begin these interventions as soon as possible:

- Maintain airway patency with ventilatory support if necessary.
- Maintain circulation through I.V. fluid replacement.
- Provide continuous ECG monitoring.
- Monitor arterial blood gas measurements to detect hypoxia and metabolic acidosis.
- Warm the patient by wrapping him in blankets. Don't use a warming blanket because it might increase peripheral vasodilation, causing shock.
- Monitor body temperature until stable with a low-reading thermometer.
- Replace thyroid hormone by administering large I.V. levothyroxine doses, as ordered. Monitor vital signs because rapid correction of hypothyroidism can cause adverse cardiac effects.
- Monitor intake and output and daily weight. With treatment, urine output should increase and body weight decrease; if not, report this to the doctor.
- Replace fluids and other substances, such as glucose. Monitor serum electrolyte levels.
- Administer corticosteroids, as ordered.
- Check for possible sources of infection, such as blood, sputum, or urine, which may have precipitated coma. Treat infections or any other underlying illness.

gency. (See *What to do in myxedema coma.*)

The disorder is most prevalent in women; in the United States, incidence is rising significantly in persons ages 40 to 50.

Causes

Hypothyroidism results from a variety of abnormalities that lead to insufficient synthesis of thyroid hormones. Common causes of hypothyroidism include thyroid gland surgery (thyroidectomy), inflammation from irradiation therapy, chronic autoimmune thyroiditis (Hashimoto's disease), or inflammatory conditions, such as amyloidosis and sarcoidosis.

The disorder may also result from pituitary failure to produce thyroid-stimulating hormone (TSH), hypothalamic failure to produce thyrotropin-releasing hormone, inborn errors of thyroid hormone synthesis, inability to synthesize thyroid hormones because of iodine deficiency (usually dietary), or the use of antithyroid medications, such as propylthiouracil.

Complications

Thyroid hormones affect almost every organ system in the body, so complications of hypothyroidism vary according to organs involved, as well as to the duration and severity of the condition.

Cardiovascular complications may include hypercholesterolemia with associated arteriosclerosis and ischemic heart disease. Poor peripheral circulation, heart enlargement, congestive heart failure, and pleural and pericardial effusions may also occur.

GI complications include achlorhydria, pernicious anemia, and adynamic colon, resulting in megacolon and intestinal obstruction.

Anemia due to the generalized suppression of erythropoietin may result in bleeding tendencies and iron deficiency anemia. Other complications include conductive or sensorineural deafness, psychiatric disturbances, carpal tunnel syndrome, benign intracranial hypertension, and impaired fertility.

Assessment

The patient history may reveal vague and varied symptoms that developed slowly over time. The patient may report energy loss, fatigue, forgetfulness, sensitivity to cold, unexplained weight gain, and constipation. As the disorder progresses, signs and symptoms may include anorexia, decreased libido, menorrhagia, paresthesia, joint stiffness, and muscle cramping.

Inspection reveals characteristic alterations in the patient's overall appearance and behavior. These changes include decreased mental stability (slight mental slowing to severe obtundation) and a thick, dry tongue, causing hoarseness and slow, slurred speech.

You'll probably note dry, flaky, inelastic skin; puffy face, hands, and feet; periorbital edema; and drooping upper eyelids. Hair may be dry and sparse with patchy hair loss and loss of the outer third of the eyebrow. Nails may be thick and brittle with visible transverse and longitudinal grooves. You may also find ataxia, intention tremor, and nystagmus.

Palpation may detect rough, doughy skin that feels cool; a weak pulse and bradycardia; muscle weakness; sacral or peripheral edema; and delayed reflex relaxation time (especially in the Achilles tendon). The thyroid tissue itself may not be easily palpable unless a goiter is present.

Auscultation may show absent or decreased bowel sounds, hypotension, a gallop or distant heart sounds, and adventitious breath sounds. Percussion and palpation may detect abdominal distention or ascites.

Diagnostic tests

Hypothyroidism is confirmed when radioimmunoassay with radioactive iodine (^{131}I) shows low serum levels of thyroid hormones and when a thorough history and physical examination show characteristic signs and symptoms. A differential diagnosis requires additional tests and may reveal the following results:

- *Serum TSH levels* determine the primary or secondary nature of the disorder. An increased serum TSH level with hypothyroidism is due to thyroid insufficiency; a decreased TSH level, hypothalamic or pituitary insufficiency.
- *Serum antithyroid antibodies* are elevated in autoimmune thyroiditis.
- *Radioisotope scanning* of the thyroid tissue identifies ectopic thyroid tissue.
- *Skull X-ray, computed tomography scan,* and *magnetic resonance imaging* help locate pituitary or hypothalamic lesions that may be the underlying cause of hypothyroidism.

Treatment

In hypothyroidism, treatment consists of gradual thyroid hormone replacement with synthetic hormone or thyroprotein derived from animal thyroids. Synthetic hormones include levothyroxine (T_4), liothyronine (T_3), dessicated thyroid USP, liotrix (T_3 and T_4), and thyroglobulin (T_3 and T_4). Levothyroxine is available in pure form, is stable, and is inexpensive. It is converted to T_3 intracellularly, so both hormones become available even though only one is administered. It usually takes about 2 months to reach equilibrium on a full dosage of levothyroxine.

Rapid treatment may be necessary for patients with myxedema coma and those about to undergo emergency surgery (because of sensitivity to central nervous system depression). In these patients, both I.V. administration of levothyroxine and hydrocortisone therapy are warranted.

In underdeveloped areas, prophylactic iodine supplements have successfully lowered the incidence of iodine-deficient goiter.

Key nursing diagnoses and patient outcomes

Activity intolerance related to slow metabolism and low energy level. Based on this nursing diagnosis, you'll establish these patient outcomes. The patient will:

- express an understanding of the need to increase his activity level gradually
- maintain blood pressure and heart and respiratory rates within prescribed limits whenever he's active
- regain and maintain his normal activity level.

Altered cardiopulmonary tissue perfusion related to arteriosclerosis and myocardial ischemic changes. Based on this nursing diagnosis, you'll establish these patient outcomes. The patient will:

- not have chest pain when he's at rest
- maintain a normal heart rate and rhythm and avoid ischemic changes on an electrocardiogram (ECG)
- maintain adequate cardiopulmonary tissue perfusion.

Body image disturbance related to changes in weight, skin, and hair. Based on this nursing diagnosis, you'll establish these patient outcomes. The patient will:

- express his feelings about body image changes
- comply with treatments to improve his body image
- regain a positive body image and express positive feelings about himself.

Nursing interventions

- Administer thyroid hormone therapy, as prescribed.
- Increase the patient's activity level gradually, and provide frequent rest periods to avoid fatigue and decrease myocardial oxygen demand.
- Apply antiembolism stockings and elevate the patient's legs to assist venous return.
- Encourage the patient to cough and breathe deeply to prevent pulmonary complications. Maintain fluid restrictions and a low-sodium diet.
- Provide a high-bulk, low-calorie diet, and encourage activity to combat constipation and promote weight loss. Administer cathartics and stool softeners, as needed.
- If needed, reorient the patient to person, place, and time, and use alternative communication techniques if he has impaired hearing. Explain all procedures slowly and carefully, and avoid sedation, if possible. Provide a consistent environment to decrease confusion and frustration. Offer support and encouragement to the patient and his family.
- Provide meticulous skin care. Turn and reposition the patient every 2 hours if he's on extended bed rest. Use alcohol-free skin care products and an emollient lotion after bathing.
- Provide extra clothing and blankets for a patient with decreased cold tolerance. Dress the patient in layers, and adjust room temperature, if possible.
- Encourage the patient to verbalize his feelings and fears about changes in body image and possible rejection by others. Help him identify his strengths and use them to develop coping strategies, and encourage him to develop interests that foster a positive self-image and de-emphasize appearance.

Monitoring

- Monitor and record vital signs, fluid intake, urine output, and daily weight.
- Assess the patient's cardiovascular status. Auscultate heart and breath sounds, and watch for chest pain or dyspnea. Observe for dependent and sacral edema.
- Monitor the patient for constipation. Auscultate bowel sounds, check for abdominal distention, and check bowel movement frequency.
- Observe the patient's mental and neurologic status. Check for disorientation, decreased level of consciousness, and hearing loss.
- During thyroid replacement therapy, watch for symptoms of hyperthyroidism, such as restlessness, sweating, and excessive weight loss.

Patient teaching

- Help the patient and his family understand the patient's physical and mental changes (such as mood changes and altered thought processes). Stress that these problems will probably subside with proper treatment. Urge the family to encourage and accept the patient and to help him adhere to his treatment regimen. If necessary, refer the patient and his family to a mental health professional for additional counseling.
- Teach the patient and his family to identify the signs and symptoms of life-threatening myxedema. Stress the importance of obtaining prompt medical care for respiratory problems and chest pain.
- Explain long-term hormone replacement therapy. Emphasize that the patient needs lifelong administration if this medication is necessary, that he should take it exactly as prescribed, and that he should never abruptly discontinue it. Advise the patient always to wear a medical identification bracelet and to carry his medication with him.
- Advise the patient and his family to keep accurate records of daily weight and intake and output.
- Instruct the patient to eat a well-balanced diet that's high in fiber and fluids to prevent constipation, to restrict sodium to prevent fluid retention, and to limit calories to minimize weight gain.
- Tell the patient to schedule activities to avoid fatigue and to get adequate rest.

Hypovolemic shock

Potentially life-threatening, hypovolemic shock stems from reduced intravascular blood volume, which leads to decreased cardiac output and inadequate tissue perfusion. The subsequent tissue anoxia prompts a shift in cellular metabolism from aerobic to anaerobic pathways. This results in an accumulation of lactic acid, which produces metabolic acidosis.

Causes

Hypovolemic shock most commonly results from acute blood loss – about 20% of total volume. Massive blood loss may result from GI bleeding, internal or external hemorrhage, or any condition that reduces circulating intravascular volume or other body fluids.

Other causes include intestinal obstruction, peritonitis, acute pancreatitis, ascites and dehydration from excessive perspiration, severe diarrhea or protracted vomiting, diabetes insipidus, diuresis, and inadequate fluid intake.

Complications

Without immediate treatment, hypovolemic shock can cause adult respiratory distress syndrome, acute tubular necrosis and renal failure, disseminated intravascular coagulation, multisystem organ failure, and death.

Assessment

The patient's history will include conditions that reduce blood volume, such as GI hemorrhage, trauma, and severe diarrhea and vomiting. A patient with cardiac disease may report anginal pain.

Inspection may reveal pale skin, decreased sensorium, and rapid, shallow respirations. Urine output usually falls below 25 ml/hour. Palpation may disclose rapid, thready peripheral pulses and cold, clammy skin. Auscultation of blood pressure usually detects a mean arterial pressure below 60 mm Hg and a narrowing pulse pressure. In patients with chronic hypotension, the mean pressure may fall below 50 mm Hg before signs of shock appear. (See *Abnormal hemodynamic values in hypovolemic shock.*)

Orthostatic vital signs and the tilt test may also detect shock.

Diagnostic tests

Characteristic laboratory findings include:

- low hematocrit and decreased hemoglobin levels and red blood cell and platelet counts
- elevated serum potassium, sodium, lactate dehydrogenase, creatinine, and blood urea nitrogen levels
- increased urine specific gravity (greater than 1.020) and urine osmolality
- decreased urine creatinine levels
- decreased pH and Pao_2 and increased $Paco_2$
- X-rays, gastroscopy, aspiration of gastric contents through a nasogastric tube, and tests for occult blood identify internal bleeding sites. Coagulation studies may detect coagulopathy from disseminated intravascular coagulation.

Treatment

Emergency treatment relies on prompt and adequate blood and fluid replacement to restore intravascular volume and to raise blood pressure and maintain it above 60 mm Hg. Rapid infusion of 0.9% sodium chloride or lactated Ringer's solution and, possibly, albumin or other plasma expanders may expand volume adequately until whole blood can be matched.

CHECKLIST

Abnormal hemodynamic values in hypovolemic shock

Hemodynamic monitoring helps you evaluate the patient's cardiovascular status in hypovolemic shock. Look for values below the following normal ranges.

- ☐ CVP below the normal range of 5 to 15 cm H_2O
- ☐ Right atrial pressure below the normal mean of 1 to 6 mm Hg
- ☐ Pulmonary artery pressure below the normal mean of 10 to 20 mm Hg
- ☐ Pulmonary artery wedge pressure below the normal mean of 6 to 12 mm Hg
- ☐ Cardiac output below the normal range of 4 to 8 liters/minute.

Treatment may also include application of a pneumatic antishock garment, oxygen administration, control of bleeding, dopamine or another inotropic drug and, possibly, surgery. To be effective, dopamine or other inotropic drugs must be used with vigorous fluid resuscitation.

Key nursing diagnoses and patient outcomes

Altered cardiopulmonary, cerebral, or renal tissue perfusion related to reduced cardiac output caused by blood loss. Based on this nursing diagnosis, you'll establish these outcomes. The patient will:

- not develop chest pain, cardiac arrhythmias, or shortness of breath
- stay alert and oriented to time, person, and place
- maintain urine output of at least 30 ml hourly
- regain or maintain normal GI function

• regain normal peripheral pulses, color, and temperature.

Decreased cardiac output related to diminished venous return caused by blood loss. Based on this nursing diagnosis, you'll establish these outcomes. The patient will:
• regain normal cardiac output as evidenced by normal blood, central venous, right atrial, pulmonary artery, and pulmonary capillary wedge pressure readings
• identify early signs and symptoms of decreased cardiac output (dizziness, syncope, cool or clammy skin, fatigue, and dyspnea), and express the importance of seeking immediate medical attention if they occur.

Fluid volume deficit related to blood loss. Based on this nursing diagnosis, you'll establish these outcomes. The patient will:
• recover and maintain normal fluid volume as evidenced by stable vital signs and adequate urine output
• recover normal hemoglobin levels, hematocrit, red blood cell and platelet counts, arterial blood gas (ABG) and electrolyte levels, and urine specific gravity
• identify causes of fluid volume deficit and express the rationale for following a prescribed diet, taking medications, maintaining his activity level, and obtaining follow-up medical care.

Nursing interventions

• Check for a patent airway and adequate circulation. If the patient experiences cardiac or respiratory arrest, start CPR.
• Begin an I.V. infusion with 0.9% sodium chloride or lactated Ringer's solution delivered through a large-bore (14G to 18G) catheter.
• Help insert a central venous line and pulmonary artery catheter for hemodynamic monitoring.
• Insert an indwelling urinary catheter. If output falls below 30 ml/hour in an adult, increase the fluid infusion rate, but watch for signs of fluid overload, such as elevated pulmonary capillary wedge pressure (PCWP). Notify the doctor if urine output doesn't increase.
• If the doctor orders an osmotic diuretic to increase renal blood flow and urine output, determine how much fluid to give by checking blood pressure, urine output, and central venous pressure (CVP) or PCWP.
• Draw an arterial blood sample to measure ABG levels. Administer oxygen by face mask or airway to ensure adequate tissue oxygenation. Adjust the oxygen flow rate as ABG measurements indicate.
• Obtain and record the patient's blood pressure, pulse and respiratory rates, and peripheral pulse rates. When systolic blood pressure drops below 80 mm Hg, increase the oxygen flow rate, and notify the doctor immediately because systolic blood pressure below 80 mm Hg usually results in inadequate coronary artery blood flow, cardiac ischemia, arrhythmias, and further complications of low cardiac output.
• Also notify the doctor, and increase the infusion rate if the patient experiences a progressive drop in blood pressure accompanied by a thready pulse. This usually signals inadequate cardiac output from reduced intravascular volume.
• Draw venous blood for a complete blood count, electrolyte measurements, type and crossmatching, and coagulation studies.

Monitoring

• Record blood pressure, pulse and respiratory rates, and peripheral pulse rates every 15 minutes until stable. Monitor cardiac rhythm continuously.
• Monitor the patient's CVP, right atrial pressure, pulmonary artery pressure, pulmonary artery wedge pressure, and cardiac output at least hourly or as ordered.
• Measure the patient's urine output hourly.
• Monitor the patient's ABG and electrolyte levels frequently as ordered.
• During therapy, assess skin color and temperature, and note any changes. Cold, clammy skin may signal continuing peripheral vascular constriction, indicating progressive shock.

• Watch for signs of impending coagulopathy (petechiae, bruising, bleeding or oozing from gums or venipuncture sites).

Patient teaching
• Explain all procedures and their purposes to ease the patient's anxiety.
• Discuss the risks associated with blood transfusions to the patient and his family.

Hysterectomy

A surgical procedure that involves the removal of the uterus, a hysterectomy may be performed abdominally, vaginally, or through a laparoscope. In a laparoscopic hysterectomy, the surgeon uses the laparoscope to perform preparatory steps before removing the uterus through the vagina. (See *Advantages of laparoscopic hysterectomy.*)

A hysterectomy may be classified in one of the following ways: subtotal, total, panhysterectomy, or radical. Rarely performed today, a *subtotal hysterectomy* involves the removal of the entire uterus except the cervix. In a *total hysterectomy,* both the uterus and the cervix are removed. In a *panhysterectomy,* the entire uterus as well as the ovaries and the fallopian tubes are removed. And, in a *radical hysterectomy,* the uterus, ovaries, fallopian tubes, adjoining ligaments and lymph nodes, upper one-third of the vagina, and surrounding tissues are all removed. Because of the extensiveness of the procedure, a radical hysterectomy requires an abdominal approach.

Common indications for a hysterectomy include malignant or benign tumors in or on the uterus, cervix, or adnexa; uterine bleeding and hemorrhage; uterine rupture or perforation; life-threatening pelvic infection; endometriosis unresponsive to conservative treatment; and pelvic floor relaxation or prolapse.

Advantages of laparoscopic hysterectomy

Although not appropriate for all patients, the laparoscopic approach to hysterectomy is gaining wide acceptance—especially as an alternative to abdominal hysterectomy. Technologic advancements have made this approach a viable option.

Among the benefits of the laparoscopic approach are the avoidance of a large abdominal incision (used in traditional abdominal hysterectomy), reduced tissue trauma, fewer sutures required (reducing the chance of reaction to suture material), and dramatically improved postoperative recuperation. This results in shorter hospital stays, lower cost, and decreased pain and morbidity as compared with traditional hysterectomy procedures.

Procedure

After the patient has received general anesthesia, the surgeon makes the incision. For an abdominal approach, the surgeon makes a midline vertical incision from the umbilicus to the symphysis pubis or a horizontal incision in the lower abdomen. He then excises and removes the uterus and necessary accompanying structures. Afterward, he closes the incision and applies a dressing and perineal pad.

For a vaginal approach, the surgeon makes an incision inside the vagina above, but near, the cervix. After excising the uterus, the surgeon removes it through the vaginal canal. He then closes the opening to the peritoneal cavity with sutures and applies a perineal pad.

In a laparoscopic approach, the surgeon makes an incision in the umbilicus. He then infuses nitrous oxide or carbon dioxide into the abdominal cavity. This lifts the abdominal wall away from the abdominal organs, making viewing easier. The patient is then placed in the Trendelenburg position, which causes the small intestine to fall out of the pelvis, thus creating room for the instruments. The surgeon then inserts the laparoscope, which allows him to view the pelvic cavity. If he's using an operative laparoscope, no other incisions are required because this device contains an operative channel through which he can pass instruments. But, if he's not using an operative laparoscope, he'll make several other small abdominal incisions through which he'll pass the instruments to excise the uterus. After excising the uterus and any accompanying structures, the surgeon removes them vaginally. He then closes the incision and applies a dressing and perineal pad.

Complications

Potential complications include wound infection, urine retention, abdominal distention, thromboembolism, atelectasis, pneumonia, hemorrhage, and ureteral or bowel injury. After an abdominal hysterectomy, the patient may also experience wound dehiscence, pulmonary embolism, or a paralytic ileus. In general, fewer complications occur after a vaginal or laparoscopic hysterectomy.

Regardless of the type of hysterectomy performed, the patient may also experience psychological complications, such as depression (the most common), loss of libido, and a perceived loss of femininity.

Key nursing diagnoses and patient outcomes

Impaired adjustment related to psychological complications, such as depression. Based on this nursing diagnosis, you'll establish these patient outcomes. The patient will:
- verbalize how the hysterectomy has affected her emotionally
- seek psychological counseling if depression becomes severe or prolonged
- regain her emotional stability.

Ineffective breathing pattern related to abdominal pain after an abdominal hysterectomy. Based on this nursing diagnosis, you'll establish these patient outcomes. The patient will:
- use incentive spirometer regularly to maintain respiratory effort
- maintain normal ventilation through the appropriate use of pain medication
- not demonstrate any signs and symptoms of respiratory complications, such as pneumonia or atelectasis
- regain a normal breathing pattern.

Urinary retention related to manipulation of the patient's bladder during surgery. Based on this nursing diagnosis, you'll establish these patient outcomes. The patient will:
- void normally after surgery
- maintain urine output equal to her intake
- not develop signs and symptoms of urine retention, such as a feeling of fullness, a palpable bladder, or inadequate urine output.

Nursing interventions

When caring for a patient who has had a hysterectomy, your primary responsibilities include instructing the patient and monitoring for postoperative complications.

Before surgery

- Explore expectations about menstrual and reproductive status after surgery and answer any questions the patient may have about the procedure and her physical recovery.
- Review the surgical approach and the extent of the excision. To prepare the patient for a hysterectomy, tell her to expect a cleansing enema the evening before surgery. Administer prophylactic antibiotics as ordered.
- Make sure that preoperative laboratory tests have been performed and review the results.
- Instruct the patient on postoperative care measures. Explain that she'll be asked to turn, cough, and perform deep-breathing exercises often. Show her how to use an incentive spirometer. Inform the patient that

after surgery she'll lie in a supine position or a low Fowler's or semi-Fowler's position to prevent pelvic congestion. Tell her she'll be encouraged to get out of bed and walk as soon as possible to prevent venous stasis.

- If she's having an abdominal hysterectomy, explain that urine retention commonly occurs after surgery, requiring an indwelling urinary catheter or a suprapubic tube. Also explain that a nasogastric (NG) or rectal tube may be in place to prevent abdominal distention.
- Tell the patient scheduled for a laparoscopic, vaginal, or abdominal hysterectomy to expect abdominal cramping and moderate amounts of drainage postoperatively and that she'll have a perineal pad in place.
- Ensure that the patient has signed a consent form.

After surgery

- Encourage the patient to cough, deep-breathe, and turn frequently (at least every 2 hours). Monitor her respiratory status for abnormalities that suggest complications, such as pneumonia.
- Administer and regulate I.V. fluids as ordered until the patient can resume oral intake. Monitor intake and output and vital signs regularly.
- Auscultate for bowel sounds regularly. Give the patient nothing by mouth until peristalsis has returned and the doctor has ordered that she may resume oral intake.
- Provide analgesics to relieve cramps (after a vaginal or laparoscopic hysterectomy) or abdominal pain (after an abdominal hysterectomy).
- Keep the patient in a supine position or a low Fowler's or semi-Fowler's position, but be sure to change her position every 2 hours. Begin ambulation as soon as ordered. Encourage the patient to perform the prescribed exercises to prevent venous stasis.
- Provide indwelling urinary catheter or suprapubic catheter care, if appropriate.
- Assess the patient's vaginal drainage and change her perineal pad frequently. Notify the doctor if the patient saturates more than one pad every 4 hours.
- If the patient has had an abdominal or laparoscopic hysterectomy, assess the abdominal incisions for drainage and bleeding.
- If the patient has had a vaginal or laparoscopic hysterectomy, provide perineal care.
- Assist with suture or clip removal (usually by the fifth postoperative day) in the patient with an abdominal or laparoscopic hysterectomy. Reassure the patient with a vaginal hysterectomy that vaginal sutures are usually absorbed.

Home care instructions

- If the patient has had a vaginal or laparoscopic hysterectomy, instruct her to report severe cramping, heavy bleeding, or hot flashes to her doctor immediately.
- If the patient has had an abdominal hysterectomy, tell her to avoid heavy lifting, rapid walking, or dancing, which can cause pelvic congestion. Encourage her to walk a little more each day and to avoid sitting for a prolonged period. Tell her that swimming is permissible but that tub baths, douching, and sexual activity should be avoided until after her 6-week checkup.
- Advise the patient to eat a high-protein, high-residue diet to avoid constipation, which may increase abdominal pressure. Her doctor may also order increased fluids (3,000 ml/day).
- Advise the patient to express her feelings about her altered body image and to contact the doctor if she has questions about any changes.
- Explain to the patient and her family that she may feel depressed or irritable temporarily because of abrupt hormonal fluctuations. Encourage family members to respond calmly and with understanding.
- If the patient has had a panhysterectomy or radical hysterectomy, instruct her to discuss the potential for exogenous hormonal and calcium supplementation with her doctor.

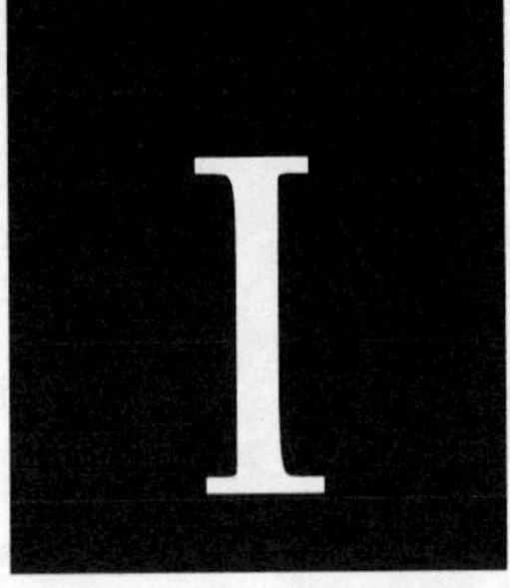

Idiopathic thrombocytopenic purpura

Thrombocytopenia that results from immunologic platelet destruction is known as idiopathic thrombocytopenic purpura (ITP). This form of thrombocytopenia may be acute (postviral thrombocytopenia) or chronic (Werlhof's disease, purpura hemorrhagica, essential thrombocytopenia, or autoimmune thrombocytopenia). The acute form usually affects children between ages 2 and 6; the chronic form mainly affects adults under age 50, especially women between ages 20 and 40. The prognosis for the acute form is excellent: nearly four out of five patients recover completely without specific treatment. The prognosis for the chronic form is good: transient remissions lasting weeks or even years are common, especially among women.

Causes

ITP is an autoimmune disorder. Antibodies that reduce the life span of platelets have been found in nearly all patients. The spleen probably helps to remove platelets modified by the antibody. The acute form usually follows a viral infection, such as rubella or chicken pox, and can result from immunization with a live vaccine. The chronic form seldom follows infection and is often linked with other immunologic disorders, such as systemic lupus erythematosus.

Human immunodeficiency virus (HIV) infection has become a common cause of ITP and should be considered in the differential diagnosis. ITP can be the initial symptom of HIV infection, a symptom indicating acquired immunodeficiency syndrome (AIDS), or a complication of AIDS. It is also often a precursor to lymphoma.

Complications

As with other purpuric conditions, hemorrhage can severely complicate ITP. A major complication during the initial phase of the disease, cerebral hemorrhage is most likely to occur if the patient's platelet count falls below 500/mm³. As well, potentially fatal purpuric lesions may occur in vital organs, such as the brain and kidneys.

Assessment

The patient's history usually reveals clinical features common to all forms of thrombocytopenia: epistaxis, oral bleeding, and the development of purpura and petechiae. A female patient may complain of menorrhagia. In the acute form, the sudden onset of bleeding usually follows a recent viral illness, although bleeding can occur up to 21 days after the virus strikes. In the chronic form, the onset of bleeding is insidious.

Inspection typically reveals petechiae or ecchymoses in the skin or bleeding into mucous membranes (GI, urinary, vaginal, or respiratory). Palpation may reveal splenomegaly.

The patient's platelet count determines the type of abnormal bleeding he experiences. For example, a platelet count between 30,000 and 50,000/mm³ causes bruising with minor trauma. A platelet count between 15,000 and 30,000/mm³ produces spontaneous bruising and petechiae, mostly on the arms and legs. A platelet count below 15,000/mm³ triggers spontaneous bruising or, after minor trauma, mucosal bleeding, generalized purpura, epistaxis, hematuria, and GI or intracranial bleeding.

Diagnostic tests

A platelet count less than 20,000/mm³ and prolonged bleeding time suggest ITP. Platelet size and morphologic appearance may be abnormal; anemia may be present if bleeding has occurred.

As in thrombocytopenia, bone marrow studies show an abundance of megakaryocytes (platelet precursors) and a shortened circulating platelet survival time (several hours or days rather than the usual 7 to 10 days).

Highly sensitive tests that quantitate platelet-associated immunoglobulin G (IgG) may help to establish the diagnosis; however, because these tests are nonspecific, their usefulness is limited. Half of all patients with thrombocytopenia show an increased IgG level on the platelet.

Treatment

Acute ITP may be allowed to run its course without intervention, or it may be treated with glucocorticoids or immune globulin. Treatment with plasmapheresis or plateletpheresis with transfusion has been attempted with limited success.

For chronic ITP, corticosteroids are the treatment of choice to suppress phagocytic activity, promote capillary integrity, and enhance platelet production. Patients who fail to respond spontaneously within 1 to 4 months or who require high doses of corticosteroids to maintain platelet counts require splenectomy.

Splenectomy may be up to 85% successful in adults when splenomegaly accompanies the initial thrombocytopenia. Before splenectomy, the patient may require blood, blood components, and vitamin K to correct anemia and coagulation defects. After splenectomy, he may need blood and component replacement and platelet concentrate. Normally, however, platelets multiply spontaneously after splenectomy.

Alternative treatments include immunosuppressants (cytoxan or vincristine sulfate, for example) and high-dose I.V. immune globulin in adults (85% effective).

The use of immunosuppressants requires weighing the risks against the benefits. Immune globulin treatment has a rapid effect, raising platelet counts within 1 to 5 days, but the beneficial effect lasts only about 1 to 2 weeks. Immune globulin is usually administered to prepare severely thrombocytic patients for emergency surgery.

Key nursing diagnoses and patient outcomes

Risk for fluid volume deficit related to bleeding caused by low platelet count. Based on this nursing diagnosis, you'll establish these patient outcomes. The patient will:

- comply with the treatment regimen prescribed to boost his platelet count
- incorporate bleeding precautions into his daily routine
- not develop a fluid volume deficit as a result of bleeding.

Risk for infection related to immunosuppression caused by corticosteroid or immunosuppressant therapy. Based on this nursing diagnosis, you'll establish these patient outcomes. The patient will:

- maintain a white blood cell count within normal limits
- take precautions to minimize or prevent infection

• remain free from infection.

Risk for injury related to adverse effects of ITP on vital organs. Based on this nursing diagnosis, you'll establish these patient outcomes. The patient will:
• maintain normal function in all organs, particularly his brain and kidneys
• remain safe when his platelet count drops below normal
• not experience an injury related to a low platelet count.

Nursing interventions

• Patient care for ITP is essentially the same as for thrombocytopenia, but a key difference is the use of platelet support. Although thrombocytopenia responds well to treatment with platelet replacement, ITP is not usually treated with platelets because the body often rejects them.
• Provide emotional support. Encourage the patient to discuss any concerns about his disease and its treatment. Reassure him that any petechiae and ecchymoses will heal as the disease resolves.
• Protect all areas of petechiae and ecchymoses from further injury.
• Provide rest periods between activities if the patient tires easily.
• Guard against bleeding by protecting the patient from trauma. Keep the bed's side rails raised and pad them if possible. Promote the use of an electric razor and a soft toothbrush. Avoid invasive procedures, such as venipuncture or urinary catheterization, if possible. When venipuncture is unavoidable, exert pressure on the puncture site for at least 20 minutes or until the bleeding stops.
• During active bleeding, maintain the patient on strict bed rest. Keep the head of the bed elevated to prevent gravity-related pressure increases, possibly leading to intracranial bleeding.
• Before splenectomy, administer transfusions as ordered and according to hospital protocol. Prepare the patient for surgery, as indicated. (See the entry "Splenectomy.")

Monitoring

• Monitor the patient's platelet count daily.
• Watch for bleeding (petechiae, ecchymoses, surgical or GI bleeding, menorrhagia). Identify the amount of bleeding or the size of ecchymoses at least every 24 hours. Test stool, urine, and vomitus for blood.
• If the patient is receiving corticosteroid therapy, monitor his fluid and electrolyte balance and watch for infection, pathologic fractures, and mood changes.
• Take the patient's vital signs immediately before a transfusion and monitor them closely after the transfusion has begun. Observe the patient for possible adverse reactions.
• Closely monitor the patient receiving immunosuppressants (commonly given before splenectomy) for signs of bone marrow depression, infection, mucositis, GI tract ulceration, and severe diarrhea or vomiting.
• Monitor the patient for complications of ITP.

Patient teaching

• Teach the patient about his disorder.
• Explain the importance of reporting bleeding (such as epistaxis or gingival, urinary tract, or uterine bleeding) or signs of internal bleeding (tarry stools or coffee-ground vomitus).
• Advise the patient to avoid straining during defecation or coughing because both can lead to increased intracranial pressure, possibly causing cerebral hemorrhage. Provide a stool softener, if necessary, because constipation and the passage of hard stools are likely to tear the rectal mucosa and cause bleeding.
• Explain the purpose of any diagnostic tests. Also explain the function of platelets, and tell the patient how the results of platelet counts can help identify symptoms of abnormal bleeding.
• Warn the patient that the lower his platelet count falls, the more precautions he'll need to take. In severe thrombocytopenia,

even minor bumps or scrapes can result in bleeding.
- Caution the patient to avoid taking aspirin in any form as well as other drugs that impair coagulation. Teach him how to recognize aspirin compounds and nonsteroidal anti-inflammatory drugs listed on labels of nonprescription remedies.
- If the patient experiences frequent nosebleeds, instruct him to use a humidifier at night. Suggest also that he moisten his inner nostrils twice a day with an anti-infective ointment.
- Teach the patient to monitor his condition by examining his skin for ecchymoses and petechiae. Show him how to test his stools for occult blood.
- Advise the patient to carry medical identification stating that he has ITP.

Immunoglobulin A deficiency

The most common immunoglobulin deficiency, selective immunoglobulin A (IgA) deficiency affects as many as 1 in 800 persons. IgA is the major immunoglobulin in human saliva, nasal and bronchial fluids, and intestinal secretions; its role is to guard against bacterial and viral infections. Consequently, selective IgA deficiency usually leads to chronic sinopulmonary infections, GI diseases, and other disorders.

Some patients, however, remain healthy throughout their lives; a few survive to age 70. These patients may have no signs or symptoms because they have extra amounts of low molecular weight immunoglobulin M (IgM), which takes over IgA function and helps maintain immunity.

The age of onset varies. The prognosis is good for patients who receive correct treatment, especially if they have no associated disorders.

What causes IgA deficiency?

Although the patterns aren't clearly established, IgA deficiency may be linked with autosomal dominant or recessive inheritance. An increased incidence is found in families with hypogammaglobulinemia.

Several other theories about the cause of IgA deficiency exist. Patients with IgA deficiency have a normal number of peripheral blood lymphocytes carrying IgA receptors and a normal amount of other immunoglobulins, which suggests that their B cells may not be secreting IgA. In an occasional patient, suppressor T cells appear to inhibit IgA. Patients with rheumatoid arthritis or systemic lupus erythematosus are also IgA-deficient, pointing to a link between IgA deficiency and autoimmune disorders. A transient form of the deficiency seems to result from certain drugs, such as anticonvulsants. And toxoplasmosis, rubella, and cytomegalovirus have produced IgA deficiency through congenital intrauterine infections.

Causes

The exact cause of IgA deficiency is unknown. However, several theories exist. (See *What causes IgA deficiency?*)

Complications

Mild to severe chronic pulmonary disease (such as asthma) and chronic diarrheal diseases commonly result from IgA deficiency. A patient who develops significant levels of antibodies to IgA may have a severe anaphylactic reaction if he receives a transfusion of normal blood or blood products.

Assessment

Some IgA-deficient patients have no signs or symptoms. Among those who do develop symptoms, the most common complaint is chronic sinopulmonary infection. The patient may also complain of symptoms of other disorders. These include respiratory allergy, often triggered by infection; GI tract diseases, such as spruelike disease, ulcerative colitis, and regional enteritis; autoimmune diseases, such as rheumatoid arthritis, systemic lupus erythematosus, chronic hepatitis, and immunohemolytic anemia; and malignant tumors, such as squamous cell carcinoma of the lungs, reticulum cell sarcoma, and thymoma.

Diagnostic tests

Hematologic analyses of the IgA-deficient patient show serum IgA levels below 5 mg/dl. Although the patient usually has no IgA in his secretions, such levels are occasionally normal. The patient has normal immunoglobulin E levels; his IgM levels may be normal or elevated in serum and secretions. Normally absent low molecular weight IgM may be present.

Tests may also detect autoantibodies and antibodies against immunoglobulin G (rheumatoid factor), IgM, and cow's milk. Cell-mediated immunity and secretory component (the glycopeptide that transports IgA) are usually normal, and most circulating B cells appear normal.

Treatment

Selective IgA deficiency has no known cure. Treatment aims to control symptoms of associated diseases, such as respiratory tract and GI infections, and is the same as for a patient with normal IgA. In severe recurrent infection, the patient may receive IgA-free gamma globulin preparation.

Key nursing diagnoses and patient outcomes

Altered protection related to IGA deficiency. Based on this nursing diagnosis, you'll establish these patient outcomes. The patient will:
• identify the signs and symptoms requiring early medical treatment
• practice good health habits
• not develop any complications related to IgA deficiency.

Diarrhea related to GI tract infection. Based on this nursing diagnosis, you'll establish these patient outcomes. The patient will:
• regain normal bowel consistency and pattern
• not develop complications of diarrhea, such as fluid volume deficit and skin irritation in the anal area
• take precautions to prevent a recurrence.

Risk for infection. Based on this nursing diagnosis, you'll establish these patient outcomes. The patient will:
• maintain a normal white blood cell (WBC) count
• not exhibit any signs and symptoms of infection, especially sinopulmonary infection
• incorporate infection control measures into his daily routine.

Nursing interventions

• Consult the dietitian to develop a nutritious diet that minimizes adverse effects of GI tract diseases, diarrhea, anemias, and autoimmune diseases.
• If the patient needs a transfusion with blood products, minimize the risk for an adverse reaction by using washed red blood cells. Or, avoid the reaction by cross-matching the patient's blood with that of an IgA-deficient donor.

Monitoring

• Monitor the patient for signs and symptoms of infection. Obtain a WBC count and culture any drainage, as appropriate.
• If the patient has GI disease, monitor his nutritional status.
• Monitor the patient's fluid volume, especially when he experiences GI distress or has an infection. Weigh the patient regularly, and monitor his intake and output.

Patient teaching

• Because IgA deficiency is lifelong, teach the patient steps to prevent infection. Also

teach him to recognize early signs of infection; tell him to seek treatment immediately if such signs occur.
• Advise the patient to use acetaminophen instead of aspirin and other nonsteroidal anti-inflammatory drugs for mild pain relief.

Incision and drainage

Called an I & D, incision and drainage involves draining accumulated pus from an infected area through a surgically created incision. It's indicated when an infection fails to resolve spontaneously. For example, in a furuncle or carbuncle, inflammation traps bacteria within a small, localized area. Because antibiotics can't reach this area, an I & D is required to drain it.

The timing of an I & D is critical. If induration is just beginning, more pus is likely to form, so the procedure should be postponed. In that case, the area should be treated with moist heat until the pus consolidates, thereby allowing an I & D to be most effective.

Procedure

The surgeon begins by anesthetizing the area. If the infected area is superficial and nearly ready to rupture, he may simply aspirate the pus with needle and syringe. If the area is large, he may make an incision directly over the suppurative area, spreading its edges to allow drainage of pus.

After culturing the pus and allowing it to drain, the surgeon leaves the cavity open to promote healing. If the cavity is large, he may pack it with gauze to provide further drainage and to assist debridement. Finally, he applies a sterile dressing.

Complications

I & D is a minor surgical procedure with no serious complications. At worst, I & D may fail to relieve the infection.

Key nursing diagnoses and patient outcomes

Impaired skin integrity related to the open wound resulting from an I & D. Based on this nursing diagnosis, you'll establish these patient outcomes. The patient will:
• not develop complications from an open wound, such as infection or delayed healing
• regain normal skin integrity.

Pain related to inflammation from the infectious process and the incision used to facilitate drainage. Based on this nursing diagnosis, you'll establish these patient outcomes. The patient will:
• express relief from pain following administration of an analgesic
• become pain free when healing is complete.

Nursing interventions

When caring for a patient with an I & D, your major responsibilities include teaching the patient, assisting with the procedure, and watching for signs of infection.

Before surgery

• Explain that the surgeon will make an incision in the infected area to drain pus. Inform the patient that he'll receive a local anesthetic before the procedure and that he'll receive analgesics afterward to relieve pain.
• Assemble sterile equipment to perform the procedure and specimen tubes to collect culture samples. Prepare the skin with antiseptic solution, and cover the area with sterile drapes.

After surgery

• Frequently change the patient's dressings, using sterile technique. Record the appearance and amount of drainage, and check for signs of infection.
• Give analgesics, as ordered, and assess any complaints of excessive pain. Typically, local pain lessens soon after the I & D. Watch for any signs of systemic infection:

fever, malaise, and chills. Check culture results.

Home care instructions

- Tell the patient to report inflammation, warmth, swelling, excessive pain, or a change in the appearance of drainage.
- Warn the patient not to pierce any lesions. Doing so could spread the infection.
- If the doctor orders warm soaks to promote further drainage, teach the patient to perform this procedure.
- If the patient must change the dressings at home, stress the importance of maintaining sterile technique and correctly disposing of soiled dressings.

Influenza

Also called the grippe or the flu, influenza is an acute, highly contagious infection of the respiratory tract.

Although it affects all age-groups, the highest incidence occurs in schoolchildren. The greatest severity is in young children, elderly people, and those with chronic diseases. In these groups, influenza may even lead to death.

Influenza occurs sporadically or in epidemics (usually during the colder months). Epidemics usually peak within 2 to 3 weeks after initial cases and subside within a month. The catastrophic pandemic of 1918 was responsible for an estimated 20 million deaths. The most recent pandemics – in 1957, 1968, and 1977 – began in mainland China.

Causes

Influenza results from three types of myxoviruses. Type A, the most prevalent, strikes every year, with new serotypes causing epidemics every 3 years. Type B also strikes annually but only causes epidemics every 4 to 6 years. Type C is endemic and causes only sporadic cases.

The infection is transmitted by inhaling a respiratory droplet from an infected person or by indirect contact, such as drinking from a contaminated glass. The virus then invades the epithelium of the respiratory tract, causing inflammation and desquamation.

One remarkable feature of the influenza virus is its capacity for antigenic variation – that is, its ability to mutate into different strains so that no immunologic resistance is present in those at risk. Antigenic variation is characterized as *antigenic drift* (minor changes that occur yearly or every few years) and *antigenic shift* (major changes that lead to pandemics).

Complications

The most common complication of influenza is pneumonia, which can be either primary influenza viral pneumonia or pneumonia secondary to bacterial infection. Influenza also may cause myositis, exacerbation of chronic obstructive pulmonary disease, Reye's syndrome and, rarely, myocarditis, pericarditis, transverse myelitis, and encephalitis.

Assessment

The patient's history usually reveals recent exposure to a person with influenza. Most patients say that they didn't receive the influenza vaccine during the past season.

After an incubation period of 24 to 48 hours, flu symptoms appear. The patient may report sudden onset of chills, fever (101° to 104° F [38.3° to 40° C]), headache, malaise, myalgia (particularly in the back and limbs), photophobia, a nonproductive cough and, occasionally, laryngitis, hoarseness, rhinitis, and rhinorrhea. These signs usually subside in 3 to 5 days, but cough and weakness may persist. Some patients (especially elderly people) may feel tired and listless for several weeks.

Inspection initially may reveal red, watery eyes; erythema of the nose and throat without exudate; and clear nasal discharge.

As the disease progresses, respiratory findings become more apparent. The patient frequently coughs and looks tired. If pulmonary complications occur, tachypnea, cyanosis, and shortness of breath may be noted. With bacterial pneumonia, you'll see purulent or bloody sputum.

Palpation may reveal cervical adenopathy and tenderness, especially in children. Auscultation may disclose transient crackles. With pneumonia, breath sounds may be diminished in areas of consolidation.

Diagnostic tests

At the start of an influenza epidemic, many patients are misdiagnosed with other respiratory disorders. Because signs and symptoms of influenza aren't pathognomonic, isolation of the virus through inoculation of chicken embryos (with nasal secretions from infected patients) is essential at the first sign of an epidemic. In addition, nose and throat cultures and increased serum antibody titers help confirm the diagnosis.

Once an epidemic is confirmed, diagnosis requires only observation of clinical signs and symptoms. Uncomplicated cases show decreased white blood cells with an increase in lymphocytes.

Treatment

The patient with uncomplicated influenza needs bed rest, adequate fluid intake, acetaminophen or aspirin to relieve fever and muscle pain, and guaifenesin or another expectorant to relieve nonproductive coughing. Prophylactic antibiotics aren't recommended; they have no effect on the influenza virus. (See *Using drugs to relieve flu symptoms,* pages 486 and 487.)

The antiviral agent amantadine has effectively reduced the duration of influenza A infection. In influenza complicated by pneumonia, the patient needs supportive care (fluid and electrolyte replacement, oxygen, and assisted ventilation) and treatment of bacterial superinfection with appropriate antibiotics. No specific therapy exists for cardiac, central nervous system, or other complications.

Key nursing diagnoses and patient outcomes

Fatigue related to infectious process. Based on this nursing diagnosis, you'll establish these patient outcomes. The patient will:
- explain the relationship between influenza and fatigue and express an understanding of how his activity level can affect his level of fatigue
- employ measures to minimize fatigue
- regain his normal energy level after the influenza has resolved.

Risk for fluid volume deficit related to fever and potential for pneumonia. Based on this nursing diagnosis, you'll establish these patient outcomes. The patient will:
- not exhibit signs and symptoms of dehydration
- maintain an adequate intake, either orally or I.V.
- maintain a normal fluid volume, as evidenced by normal vital signs and an output that equals his intake.

Hyperthermia related to infectious process. Based on this nursing diagnosis, you'll establish these patient outcomes. The patient will:
- not experience complications associated with hyperthermia, such as seizures or dehydration
- demonstrate a drop in temperature following the use of antipyretic agents
- regain and maintain a normal temperature after the influenza has resolved.

Nursing interventions

- Administer analgesics, antipyretics, and decongestants, as ordered.
- Follow droplet and standard precautions.
- Provide cool, humidified air, but change the water daily to prevent *Pseudomonas* superinfection.

Using drugs to relieve flu symptoms

Drug	Adverse reactions	Special considerations
Antihistamines		
azatadine (Optimine) **brompheniramine** (Dimetane) **chlorpheniramine** (Chlor-Trimeton, Teldrin) **clemastine** (Tavist) **dexchlorpheniramine** (Polaramine)	• Watch for fever, hallucinations, severe drowsiness, severe dry mouth or throat, sore throat, unusual bleeding or bruising, and unusual fatigue or weakness. • Other reactions include anorexia; blurred vision; insomnia; irritability; mild drowsiness; mild dry nose, mouth, or throat; thickened bronchial secretions; and tremors.	• Reduce GI distress by giving antihistamines with food; give sugarless gum or hard candy or ice chips to relieve dry mouth; increase fluid intake (if allowed) or humidify air to decrease adverse effect of thickened secretions. • Warn him to avoid drinking alcoholic beverages while taking antihistamines. Remind him that some nonprescription cough and cold medications also contain alcohol. • Note that some antihistamines may mask ototoxicity from high doses of salicylates.
astemizole (Hismanal) **terfenadine** (Seldane)	• Watch for sweating; visual disturbances; wheezing; and yellow skin, mucous membranes, and sclera. • Other reactions include dizziness, dry mouth and throat, mild drowsiness, and nausea.	• Be aware that astemizole and terfenadine usually cause less drowsiness than other antihistamines. • Caution the patient not to alter his dosage schedule without checking with his doctor. • Give the patient sugarless gum or hard candy or ice chips to help relieve mouth dryness.
Antitussives		
codeine	• Watch for confusion, dizziness, respiratory difficulty, and sedation. • Other reactions include constipation, drowsiness, dry mouth, and nausea.	• Monitor the patient's cough type and frequency. • Advise the patient against taking this drug with alcohol or nonprescription cough and cold medications that contain alcohol or antihistamines. • Caution the ambulatory patient against activities that require alertness. • Give the patient sugarless gum or hard candy or ice chips to help relieve mouth dryness.
dextromethorphan (Comtrex, Coricidin Cough Syrup, Robitussin-DM)	• Watch for insomnia, irritability, nervousness, and unusual excitement. • Other reactions include dizziness, drowsiness, and GI upset.	• Monitor the patient for dizziness and drowsiness. • Perform percussion and chest vibration during drug therapy. • Monitor cough type and frequency. • Give the patient sugarless gum or hard candy or ice chips to help relieve mouth dryness.

Using drugs to relieve flu symptoms *(continued)*

Drug	Adverse reactions	Special considerations
Antiviral		
amantadine (Symadine, Symmetrel)	• Watch for insomnia, irritability, orthostatic hypotension, and skin reaction. • Other reactions include anxiety, confusion, constipation, depression, dizziness, dry mouth, light-headedness, nausea, and urine retention.	• Administer the drug after meals to enhance absorption. Give the drug several hours before bedtime to avoid insomnia. • Advise the patient to report adverse reactions, especially dizziness, depression, anxiety, nausea, and urine retention. • Tell the patient not to stand or change positions too quickly to avoid orthostatic hypotension. • Elderly patients are more susceptible to neurologic adverse effects. Taking the drug in two daily doses rather than a single dose may reduce adverse effects.
Expectorants		
guaifenesin (Novahistine DMX, Robitussin, Triaminic)	• Watch for nausea and vomiting. • Other reactions include diarrhea, drowsiness, and mild GI upset.	• If not contraindicated, encourage the patient to drink as much water as possible to help thin his mucus. • Monitor cough type and frequency, and encourage deep-breathing exercises. • If the patient is continuing drug therapy at home, advise him to avoid unintentional double-dosing by checking with his doctor before taking any other cough or cold remedies.

• Encourage the patient to rest in bed and drink plenty of fluids. Administer I.V. fluids, as ordered.
• Administer oxygen therapy if warranted.
• Help the patient to gradually return to his normal activities.

Monitoring

• Regularly monitor the patient's vital signs, including his temperature.
• Monitor the patient's fluid intake and output for signs of dehydration.
• Watch for signs and symptoms of developing pneumonia, such as crackles, increased fever, chest pain, dyspnea, and coughing accompanied by purulent or bloody sputum.

Patient teaching

• Influenza usually doesn't require hospitalization. Teach the home patient about supportive care measures and signs and symptoms of serious complications.
• Advise the patient to use mouthwash or warm saline gargles to ease sore throat.
• Teach the patient the importance of increased fluids to prevent dehydration.
• Suggest a warm bath or a heating pad to relieve myalgia.
• Advise the patient to use a vaporizer to provide cool, moist air, but tell him to

clean the reservoir and change the water every 8 hours.

- Teach the patient how to dispose of tissues properly, and demonstrate proper hand-washing technique to prevent the virus from spreading.
- Advise parents of children with fever and the flu not to give aspirin because of the risk of Reye's syndrome.
- Discuss influenza immunization. Suggest that high-risk patients and health care workers get an annual inoculation at the start of flu season (late autumn). Explain that each year's vaccine is based on the previous year's virus and usually is about 75% effective.

Tell a patient receiving the vaccine about possible adverse reactions (discomfort at the vaccination site, fever, malaise and, rarely, Guillain-Barré syndrome).

The vaccine also shouldn't be given to anyone who's allergic to eggs, feathers, or chickens because it's made from chicken embryos. (Amantadine is an effective alternative for these people.)

Inguinal hernia

When part of an internal organ protrudes through an abnormal opening in the containing wall of its cavity, a hernia results. In an inguinal hernia – the most common type – the large or small intestine, omentum, or bladder protrudes into the inguinal canal.

Inguinal hernias can be classified as reducible (if the hernia can be manipulated back into place with relative ease); incarcerated (if the hernia can't be reduced because adhesions have formed in the hernial sac); or strangulated (if part of the herniated intestine becomes twisted or edematous, causing serious complications).

Inguinal hernias can be direct or indirect, depending on where the abnormal opening in the inguinal canal occurs. When indirect, it causes the abdominal viscera to protrude through the inguinal ring and follow the spermatic cord (in males) or round ligament (in females). If direct, it results from a weakness in the fascial floor of the inguinal canal. Indirect hernias, the more common form, can develop at any age but are especially prevalent in infants under age 1. This form is three times more common in males.

Causes

Inguinal hernias result from abdominal muscles weakened by congenital malformation, traumatic injury, or aging or from increased intra-abdominal pressure due to heavy lifting, exertion, pregnancy, obesity, excessive coughing, or straining during defecation.

Inguinal hernia is a common congenital malformation that may occur in males during the seventh month of gestation. Normally, at this time, the testicle descends into the scrotum, preceded by the peritoneal sac. If the sac closes improperly, it leaves an opening through which the intestine can slip, causing a hernia.

Complications

Inguinal hernia may lead to incarceration or strangulation. Strangulation may seriously interfere with normal blood flow and peristalsis, possibly leading to intestinal obstruction and necrosis.

Assessment

The patient history may reveal precipitating factors, such as weight lifting, recent pregnancy, or excessive coughing. Usually, the patient reports the appearance of a lump in the inguinal area when he stands or strains. He may also complain of sharp, steady groin pain, which tends to worsen when tension is placed on the hernia and improve when the hernia is reduced.

If the patient has a large hernia, inspection may reveal an obvious swelling in the inguinal area. If he has a small hernia, the affected area may simply appear full.

As part of your inspection, have the patient lie down. If the hernia disappears, it is reducible. Also ask him to perform Valsalva's maneuver; while he does so, inspect the inguinal area for characteristic bulging.

Auscultation should reveal bowel sounds. The absence of bowel sounds may indicate incarceration or strangulation. Palpation helps to determine the size of an obvious hernia. It also can disclose the presence of a hernia in a male patient.

Diagnostic tests

Although assessment findings are the cornerstone of diagnosis, suspected bowel obstruction requires X-rays and a white blood cell count (may be elevated).

Treatment

The choice of therapy depends on the type of hernia. For a reducible hernia, temporary relief may result from moving the protruding organ back into place. To keep the abdominal contents from protruding through the hernial sac, a truss may be applied. (A truss is a firm pad, with a belt attached, that is placed over the hernia to keep it reduced.) Although a truss can't cure a hernia, the device is especially helpful for an elderly or debilitated patient for whom any surgery is potentially hazardous.

Herniorrhaphy is the preferred surgical treatment for infants, adults, and otherwise healthy elderly patients. This procedure replaces hernial sac contents into the abdominal cavity and seals the opening. Another effective procedure is hernioplasty, which reinforces the weakened area with steel mesh, fascia, or wire.

A strangulated or necrotic hernia requires bowel resection. Rarely, an extensive resection may require a temporary colostomy.

Key nursing diagnoses and patient outcomes

Activity intolerance related to presence of an inguinal hernia. Based on this nursing diagnosis, you'll establish these patient outcomes. The patient will:

- skillfully perform activities to minimize or prevent enlargement of inguinal hernia
- regain his normal activity level, either by wearing a truss or by undergoing surgical repair of the hernia.

Altered GI tissue perfusion related to hernia incarceration. Based on this nursing diagnosis, you'll establish these patient outcomes. The patient will:

- communicate that he knows the signs and symptoms of incarceration and the importance of seeking immediate medical attention if they should occur
- regain and then maintain normal GI function.

Pain related to the presence of an inguinal hernia. Based on this nursing diagnosis, you'll establish these patient outcomes. The patient will:

- avoid activities that cause or increase pain
- express relief of pain when wearing a truss
- become pain free after surgical repair of the hernia.

Nursing interventions

- Apply a truss only after a hernia has been reduced. For best results, apply it in the morning before the patient gets out of bed. Apply powder for protection because the truss may be irritating.
- Don't try to reduce an incarcerated hernia; doing so may perforate the bowel. If severe intestinal obstruction arises because of hernial strangulation, tell the doctor immediately. A nasogastric tube may be inserted promptly to empty the stomach and relieve pressure on the hernial sac.
- Prepare the patient for surgery, as indicated. (See the entry "Hernia repair.")

Monitoring

- If the patient is wearing a truss, inspect his skin daily.

• Watch for and immediately report signs of incarceration and strangulation.

Patient teaching

• Explain what an inguinal hernia is and how it is usually treated. Point out that elective surgery is the treatment of choice and far safer than waiting until hernial complications develop, necessitating emergency surgery. Warn the patient that a strangulated hernia can require extensive bowel resection, involving a protracted hospital stay and possibly a colostomy.

• Teach the patient who will not undergo surgery to watch for signs of incarceration or strangulation. Tell him that severe pain, nausea, vomiting, and diarrhea may indicate complications. Warn him and his family that shock, high fever, and bloody stools are signs of complete obstruction and must be reported at once. Tell them that immediate surgery is needed if complications occur.

• If the patient uses a truss, instruct him to bathe daily and apply liberal amounts of cornstarch or baby powder to prevent skin irritation. Warn against applying the truss over clothing, which reduces its effectiveness and may cause slippage. Point out that wearing a truss doesn't cure a hernia and may be uncomfortable.

• If surgery is scheduled, provide preoperative teaching. Reinforce the doctor's explanation of the surgery and its possible complications.

Intestinal obstruction

Commonly a medical emergency, intestinal obstruction is the partial or complete blockage of the small- or large-bowel lumen. Complete obstruction in any part of the bowel, if untreated, can cause death within hours from shock and vascular collapse. Intestinal obstruction is most likely after abdominal surgery or in persons with congenital bowel deformities.

Causes

Intestinal obstruction results from either mechanical or nonmechanical (neurogenic) blockage of the lumen. Causes of mechanical obstruction include adhesions and strangulated hernias (usually associated with small-bowel obstruction); carcinomas (usually associated with large-bowel obstruction); foreign bodies, such as fruit pits, gallstones, or worms; compression of the bowel wall from stenosis; intussusception; volvulus of the sigmoid or cecum; tumors; or atresia.

Nonmechanical obstruction usually results from paralytic ileus (the most common intestinal obstruction). Paralytic ileus is a physiologic form of intestinal obstruction that usually develops in the small bowel after abdominal surgery. Other nonmechanical causes of obstruction include electrolyte imbalances; toxicity, such as that associated with uremia or generalized infection; neurogenic abnormalities, such as spinal cord lesions; and thrombosis or embolism of mesenteric vessels.

Although intestinal obstruction may occur in several forms, the underlying pathophysiology is similar.

Complications

Intestinal obstruction can lead to perforation, peritonitis, septicemia, secondary infection, metabolic alkalosis or acidosis, hypovolemic or septic shock and, if untreated, death.

Assessment

Investigation of the patient's history often reveals predisposing factors, such as surgery (especially abdominal surgery), radiation therapy, or gallstones. The history may also disclose certain illnesses, such as Crohn's disease, diverticular disease, or ulcerative colitis, that can lead to obstruction. Family history may reveal colorectal cancer among one or more relatives.

Hiccups are a common complaint in all types of bowel obstruction. Other specific assessment findings depend on the cause of obstruction – mechanical or nonmechanical – and its location in the bowel. (See *Monitoring for colon cancer.*)

In mechanical obstruction of the small bowel, the patient may complain of colicky pain, nausea, vomiting, and constipation. If obstruction is complete, he may report vomiting of fecal contents. This results from vigorous peristaltic waves that propel bowel contents toward the mouth instead of the rectum.

Inspection of this patient may reveal a distended abdomen, the hallmark of all types of mechanical obstruction. Auscultation may detect bowel sounds, borborygmi, and rushes (occasionally loud enough to be heard without a stethoscope). Palpation may disclose abdominal tenderness. Rebound tenderness may be noted in patients with obstruction that results from strangulation with ischemia.

In mechanical obstruction of the large bowel, a history of constipation is common, with a more gradual onset of signs and symptoms than in small-bowel obstruction. Several days after constipation begins, the patient may report the sudden onset of colicky abdominal pain, producing spasms that last less than 1 minute and recur every few minutes.

The patient history may reveal constant hypogastric pain, nausea and, in the later stages, vomiting. He may describe his vomitus as orange-brown and foul smelling, which is characteristic of large-bowel obstruction. On inspection, the abdomen may appear dramatically distended, with visible loops of large bowel. Auscultation may reveal loud, high-pitched borborygmi.

Partial obstruction usually causes similar signs and symptoms, in a milder form. Leakage of liquid stools around the partial obstruction is common.

In nonmechanical obstruction, such as paralytic ileus, the patient usually describes diffuse abdominal discomfort instead of colicky pain. Typically, he also reports frequent vomiting, which may consist of gastric and bile contents and, rarely, fecal contents. He may also complain of constipation and hiccups.

If obstruction results from vascular insufficiency or infarction, the patient may complain of severe abdominal pain. On inspection, the abdomen is distended. Early in the disease, auscultation discloses decreased bowel sounds; this sign disappears as the disorder progresses.

NURSING ALERT

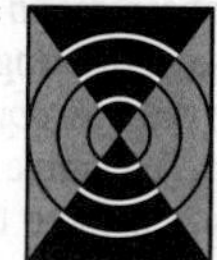

Monitoring for colon cancer

If a patient with an intestinal obstruction tells you that he's had a recent change in his bowel or bladder habits or that he's noticed blood in his stools, inform the doctor immediately. Such symptoms suggest that colon cancer may be causing the obstruction.

Diagnostic tests

Various tests help to establish the diagnosis and pinpoint complications.

- *Abdominal X-rays* confirm intestinal obstruction and reveal the presence and location of intestinal gas or fluid. In small-bowel obstruction, a typical "stepladder" pattern emerges, with alternating fluid and gas levels apparent in 3 to 4 hours. In large-bowel obstruction, barium enema reveals a distended, air-filled colon or a closed loop of sigmoid with extreme distention (in sigmoid volvulus).
- *Serum sodium, chloride,* and *potassium levels* may fall because of vomiting.
- *White blood cell counts* may be normal or slightly elevated if necrosis, peritonitis, or strangulation occurs.
- *Serum amylase level* may increase, possibly from irritation of the pancreas by a bowel loop.

• *Hemoglobin concentration* and *hematocrit* may increase, indicating dehydration.
• *Sigmoidoscopy, colonoscopy,* or a *barium enema* may help determine the cause of obstruction; however, these tests are contraindicated if perforation is suspected.

Treatment

Surgery is usually the treatment of choice. One important exception is paralytic ileus, in which nonoperative therapy is usually attempted first. The type of surgery depends on the cause of blockage. For example, if a tumor is obstructing the intestine, a colon resection with anastomosis is performed; if adhesions are obstructing the lumen, these are lysed.

Surgical preparation includes correction of fluid and electrolyte imbalances; decompression of the bowel to relieve vomiting and distention; treatment of shock and peritonitis; and administration of broad-spectrum antibiotics. Often, decompression is begun preoperatively with passage of a nasogastric (NG) tube attached to continuous suction. This tube relieves vomiting, reduces abdominal distention, and prevents aspiration. In strangulating obstruction, preoperative therapy also usually requires blood replacement and I.V. fluids.

Postoperative care involves careful patient monitoring and interventions geared to the type of surgery. Total parenteral nutrition may be ordered if the patient has a protein deficit from chronic obstruction, postoperative or paralytic ileus, or infection.

Nonsurgical treatment may be attempted in some patients with partial obstruction, particularly those who suffer recurrent partial obstruction or who developed it after surgery or a recent episode of diffuse peritonitis.

Nonsurgical treatment usually includes decompression with an NG tube attached to low-pressure continuous suction; correction of fluid and electrolyte deficits; administration of broad-spectrum antibiotics; and occasionally total parenteral nutrition. A long nasointestinal tube also may be used for decompression.

Throughout nonsurgical treatment, the patient's condition must be closely monitored. If he fails to improve or his condition deteriorates, surgery is required.

Another indication for nonsurgical treatment is nonmechanical obstruction from adynamic ileus (paralytic ileus). Most of these cases occur postoperatively and disappear spontaneously in 2 to 3 days. However, if the disorder doesn't resolve within 48 hours, treatment consists of decompression with an NG tube attached to low-pressure continuous suction. Oral intake is restricted until bowel function resumes; then the diet is gradually advanced.

In the patient with paralytic ileus, decompression occasionally responds to colonoscopy or rectal tube insertion. When paralytic ileus develops secondary to another illness, such as severe infection or electrolyte imbalance, the primary problem must also be treated. Again, if conservative treatment fails, surgery is required.

In both surgical and nonsurgical treatment, drug therapy includes antibiotics and analgesics or sedatives, such as meperidine or phenobarbital (but not opiates because they inhibit GI motility).

Key nursing diagnoses and patient outcomes

Altered nutrition: Less than body requirements related to inability to eat. Based on this nursing diagnosis, you'll establish these patient outcomes. The patient will:
• receive adequate nutrition either I.V. or with the aid of total parenteral nutrition until the obstruction is alleviated
• maintain his weight within a normal range
• resume his oral intake after the obstruction is alleviated.

Risk for fluid volume deficit related to inability to ingest oral fluids. Based on

this nursing diagnosis, you'll establish these patient outcomes. The patient will:
- maintain an adequate fluid volume balance, as evidenced by normal vital signs and an I.V. intake that equals his output
- not demonstrate any signs and symptoms of dehydration
- ingest fluids orally after the obstruction is alleviated.

Pain related to the pressure and irritation resulting from an intestinal obstruction. Based on this nursing diagnosis, you'll establish these patient outcomes. The patient will:
- express relief of pain following analgesic administration
- become pain free after the obstruction is alleviated.

Nursing interventions

- Because intestinal obstruction may be fatal and often causes overwhelming pain and distress, patients require skillful supportive care and keen observation.
- Allow the patient nothing by mouth, as ordered, but be sure to provide frequent mouth care to help keep mucous membranes moist. If surgery won't be performed, he may be allowed a small amount of ice chips. Avoid using lemon-glycerin swabs, which can increase mouth dryness.
- Insert an NG tube to decompress the bowel, as ordered. Attach the tube to low-pressure, intermittent suction. Irrigate the tube with 0.9% sodium chloride solution if necessary to maintain patency.
- If ordered, assist with insertion of a weighted nasointestinal tube, such as a Miller-Abbott, Cantor, or Harris tube. Help the patient turn from side to side (or walk around, if he can) to facilitate passage of the tube.
- Begin and maintain I.V. therapy, as ordered. Provide I.V. fluids to keep levels within normal ranges. Provide blood replacement therapy as necessary.
- Administer analgesics, broad-spectrum antibiotics, and other medications, as ordered.
- Keep in mind that analgesics may be withheld until a diagnosis is confirmed. To ease discomfort, help the patient to change positions frequently.
- If you suspect bladder compression, catheterize the patient for residual urine immediately after he has voided.
- Keep the patient in semi-Fowler's or Fowler's position as much as possible. These positions help to promote pulmonary ventilation and ease respiratory distress from abdominal distention.
- If surgery is scheduled, prepare the patient as required. (See the entries "Bowel resection with anastomosis" or "Bowel resection with ostomy.")

Monitoring

- Look for signs of dehydration (thick, swollen tongue; dry, cracked lips; dry oral mucous membranes).
- Monitor NG tube drainage for color, consistency, and amount.
- If a weighted tube has been inserted, check periodically to make sure it's advancing.
- Monitor intake and output. Maintain fluid and electrolyte balance by monitoring electrolyte, blood urea nitrogen, and creatinine levels.
- Monitor vital signs frequently. A drop in blood pressure may indicate reduced circulating blood volume due to blood loss from a strangulated hernia. Remember, as much as 10 liters of fluid can collect in the small bowel, drastically reducing plasma volume. Observe closely for signs of shock (pallor, rapid pulse, and hypotension).
- When administering medication, monitor the patient for the desired effects and for adverse reactions.
- Continually assess the patient's pain. Remember, colicky pain that suddenly becomes constant could signal perforation.
- Watch for signs of metabolic alkalosis (changes in sensorium; slow, shallow respirations; hypertonic muscles; tetany) or acidosis (shortness of breath on exertion; disorientation; and, later, deep, rapid breathing,

weakness, and malaise). Watch for signs and symptoms of secondary infection, such as fever and chills.

• Monitor urine output carefully to assess renal function, circulating blood volume, and possible urine retention due to bladder compression by the distended intestine. Also measure abdominal girth frequently to detect progressive distention.

• Listen for bowel sounds, and watch for other signs of resuming peristalsis (passage of flatus and mucus through the rectum).

Patient teaching

• Teach the patient about his disorder, focusing on his type of intestinal obstruction, its cause, and signs and symptoms. Listen to his questions and take time to answer them.

• Explain necessary diagnostic tests and treatments. Make sure the patient understands that these procedures are necessary to relieve the obstruction and reduce pain. Instruct him in pretest guidelines; for example, advise him to lie on his left side for about a half hour before X-rays are taken.

• Prepare the patient and his family for the possibility of surgery. Provide preoperative teaching, and reinforce the doctor's explanation of the surgery. Demonstrate techniques for coughing and deep breathing, and teach the patient how to use incentive spirometry.

• Tell the patient what to expect postoperatively.

• Review the proper use of prescribed medications, focusing on their correct administration, desired effects, and possible adverse effects.

• Emphasize the importance of following a structured bowel regimen, particularly if the patient had a mechanical obstruction from fecal impaction. Encourage him to eat a high-fiber diet and to exercise daily.

• Reassure the patient who had an obstruction from paralytic ileus that recurrence is unlikely. However, remind him to report any recurrence of abdominal pain, abdominal distention, nausea, or vomiting.

Intussusception

Considered a pediatric emergency, intussusception occurs when a portion of the bowel telescopes or invaginates into an adjacent bowel portion. (See *What happens in intussusception.*) This disorder can lead to bowel obstruction and other serious complications. Treatment should not be delayed.

Intussusception is most common in infants and occurs three times more often in males than in females; approximately 87% of children with intussusception are younger than age 2, and about 70% of these children are between 4 and 11 months old.

Causes

In infants, intussusception usually arises from unknown causes. In older children, polyps, hemangioma, lymphosarcoma, lymphoid hyperplasia, Meckel's diverticulum, or alterations in intestinal motility may trigger the process. In adults, intussusception most commonly results from benign or malignant tumors (65% of patients); other possible causes include polyps, Meckel's diverticulum, gastroenterostomy with herniation, or an appendiceal stump.

In addition, studies suggest that intussusception may be linked to viral infections because seasonal peaks are observed – in the spring and summer, coinciding with peak incidence of enteritis, and in midwinter, coinciding with peak incidence of respiratory tract infections.

Complications

Without prompt treatment, strangulation of the intestine may occur, with gangrene, shock, perforation, and peritonitis. These complications can be fatal.

Assessment

If the patient is an infant or child, the history may reveal intermittent attacks of colicky pain. Typically, this pain causes the child to scream, draw his legs up to his abdomen, turn pale and diaphoretic, and possibly grunt. Parents may report that the child vomits–initially, stomach contents, and later, bile-stained or fecal material. Parents may describe the child's "currant jelly" stools, which contain a mixture of blood and mucus.

Inspection and palpation may reveal a distended, tender abdomen, with some guarding over the intussusception site. A sausage-shaped abdominal mass may be palpable in the right upper quadrant or in the midepigastrium if the transverse colon is involved. Rectal examination may show bloody mucus.

In the adult patient, the history may reveal nonspecific, chronic, and intermittent symptoms, such as colicky abdominal pain and tenderness, vomiting, diarrhea (occasionally constipation), bloody stools, and weight loss. He may describe abdominal pain that's localized in the right lower quadrant, radiates to the back, and increases with eating. The abdomen may be distended. Palpation may help pinpoint the tender area in the right lower quadrant.

In the adult patient, excruciating pain, abdominal distention, and tachycardia are signs that severe intussusception has led to strangulation.

Diagnostic tests

The following tests help to confirm the diagnosis.

- *Barium enema* confirms colonic intussusception when it shows the characteristic coiled-spring sign; it also delineates the extent of intussusception.
- *Upright abdominal X-rays* may show a soft-tissue mass and signs of complete or partial obstruction, with dilated loops of bowel.
- *White blood cell count* up to 15,000/mm³ indicates obstruction; more than 15,000/mm³, strangulation; more than 20,000/mm³, bowel infarction.

What happens in intussusception

In intussusception, a bowel segment invaginates and is propelled along by peristalsis, pulling in more bowel. In this illustration, a portion of the cecum invaginates and is propelled into the large intestine. Intussusception typically produces edema, hemorrhage from venous engorgement, incarceration, and obstruction.

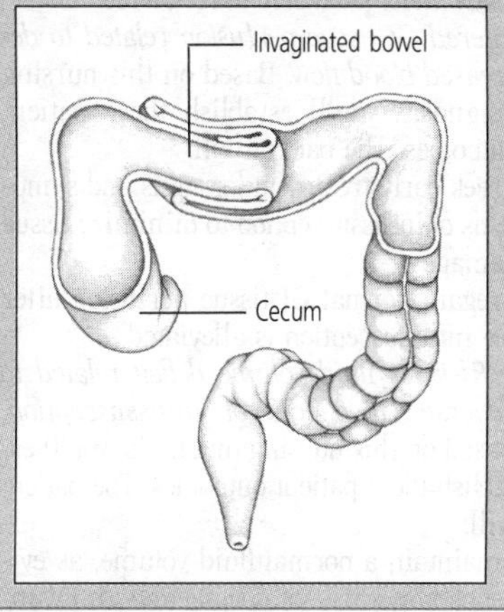

Treatment

In children, therapy may include hydrostatic reduction or surgery. Surgery is indicated for children with recurrent intussusception, for those who show signs of shock or peritonitis, and for those in whom symptoms have been present longer than 24 hours. In adults, surgery is always the treatment of choice.

During hydrostatic reduction, the radiologist drips a barium solution into the rectum through a catheter from a height of not more than 3′ (0.9 m); fluoroscopy traces the progress of the barium. If the procedure is successful, the barium backwashes into the ileum and the mass disappears. If not, the procedure is stopped and the patient is prepared for surgery.

During surgery, manual reduction is attempted first. After compressing the bowel above the intussusception, the doctor attempts to milk the intussusception back through the bowel. However, if manual reduction fails or if the bowel is gangrenous or strangulated, the doctor will perform a resection of the affected bowel segment.

Key nursing diagnoses and patient outcomes

Altered GI tissue perfusion related to decreased blood flow. Based on this nursing diagnosis, you'll establish these patient outcomes. The patient will:

- seek early treatment for signs and symptoms of intussusception to minimize tissue damage
- regain normal GI tissue perfusion after the intussusception is alleviated.

Risk for fluid volume deficit related to adverse GI effects of intussusception. Based on this nursing diagnosis, you'll establish these patient outcomes. The patient will:

- maintain a normal fluid volume, as evidenced by stable vital signs and an I.V. intake that equals his output
- not exhibit signs and symptoms of dehydration
- stop vomiting or having diarrhea.

Pain related to intestinal pressure and ischemia. Based on this nursing diagnosis, you'll establish these patient outcomes. The patient will:

- express relief from pain following administration of an analgesic
- become pain free.

Nursing interventions

- Offer reassurance and emotional support to the patient and, if the patient is a child, to his parents. Because this condition is considered a pediatric emergency, parents are often unprepared for their child's hospitalization and possible surgery. Similarly, the child is unprepared for an abrupt separation from his parents and familiar environment.
- Administer I.V. fluids, as ordered. If the patient is in shock, give blood or plasma, as ordered.
- A nasogastric (NG) tube is inserted to decompress the bowel. Replace volume lost as ordered.
- Prepare the patient for hydrostatic reduction, and answer questions to allay fears.
- Prepare the patient for surgery, if necessary, and provide postoperative care in the same manner as for the patient with a bowel resection and anastomosis. (See the entry "Bowel resection with anastomosis.")

Monitoring

- Monitor vital signs frequently. A change in temperature may indicate sepsis; infants may become hypothermic at the onset of infection. Rising pulse rate and falling blood pressure may signal peritonitis.
- Check intake and output, and watch for signs of dehydration and bleeding.
- Monitor the amount and type of drainage from the NG tube.
- Monitor the patient who has undergone hydrostatic reduction for passage of stools and barium, a sign that the reduction has been successful. Keep in mind that a few patients have a recurrence of intussusception; this usually occurs within the first 36 to 48 hours after the hydrostatic reduction.

Patient teaching

- Depending on the patient's age, explain what happens in intussusception to him or his parents. Review required diagnostic tests and treatments. If hydrostatic reduction by barium enema will be attempted, be sure the patient or his parents understand the procedure. Let them know that surgery will be necessary if the procedure isn't successful.
- If surgery is required, provide preoperative teaching. Reinforce the doctor's ex-

planation of the surgery and its possible complications.
• To minimize the stress of hospitalization, encourage parents to participate in their child's care as much as possible. Be flexible about visiting hours.

Iron deficiency anemia

A common disease worldwide, iron deficiency anemia affects 10% to 30% of the adult population of North America. It's most prevalent among premenopausal women, infants (particularly premature or low-birthweight infants), children, adolescents (especially girls), alcoholics, and elderly people (especially those unable to cook). The prognosis after replacement therapy is favorable.

Causes

Iron deficiency anemia stems from an inadequate supply of iron for optimal formation of red blood cells (RBCs), which produces smaller (microcytic) cells with less color on staining. Body stores of iron, including plasma iron, decrease, as does transferrin, which binds with and transports iron. Insufficient body stores of iron lead to a depleted RBC mass and, in turn, to a decreased hemoglobin concentration (hypochromia) and decreased oxygen-carrying capacity of the blood. (See *Understanding iron absorption and storage.*)

Iron deficiency can result from any of the following:
• inadequate dietary intake of iron, as in prolonged unsupplemented breast- or bottle-feeding of infants; during periods of stress, such as rapid growth in children and adolescents; and in elderly patients existing on a poorly balanced diet
• iron malabsorption, as in chronic diarrhea, partial or total gastrectomy, and malabsorption syndromes such as celiac disease
• blood loss secondary to drug-induced GI bleeding (from anticoagulants, aspirin, steroids) or due to heavy menses, hemorrhage from trauma, GI ulcers, malignant tumors, and varices
• pregnancy, in which the mother's iron supply is diverted to the fetus for erythropoiesis
• intravascular hemolysis-induced hemoglobinuria or paroxysmal nocturnal hemoglobinuria
• mechanical erythrocyte trauma caused by a prosthetic heart valve or vena cava filter.

Understanding iron absorption and storage

Essential to erythropoiesis, iron is abundant throughout the body. Two-thirds of total-body iron is found in hemoglobin; the other third, mostly in the reticuloendothelial system (liver, spleen, and bone marrow), with small amounts in muscle, serum, and body cells.

Adequate dietary ingestion of iron and recirculation of iron released from disintegrating red cells maintain iron supplies. The duodenum and upper part of the small intestine absorb dietary iron. Such absorption depends on gastric acid content, the amount of reducing substances (ascorbic acid, for example) present in the alimentary canal, and dietary iron intake. If iron intake is deficient, the body gradually depletes its iron stores, causing decreased hemoglobin and eventually signs and symptoms of iron deficiency anemia.

Complications

Possible complications of this disorder include infection and pneumonia. Lead poisoning may result from increased intestinal absorption of lead when combined with pica, another symptom of this disorder. Another complication is bleeding, which may be identified by ecchymotic areas on the skin, hematuria, and gingival bleeding. Plummer-Vinson syndrome can occur in severe cases.

The most significant complication of iron deficiency anemia stems from overreplacement of iron with oral or I.M. supplements. Hemochromatosis (excessive iron deposits in tissue) can result, affecting the liver, heart, pituitary gland, and joints. Iron poisoning can occur in children when toxic levels are allowed to build up during therapy.

Assessment

Iron deficiency anemia may persist for years without signs and symptoms. The characteristic history of fatigue, inability to concentrate, headache, and shortness of breath (especially on exertion) may not develop until long after iron stores and circulating iron become low. The patient may report increased frequency of infections and pica, an uncontrollable urge to eat strange things, such as clay, starch, ice and, in children, lead. A female patient may give a history of menorrhagia.

In chronic iron deficiency anemia, the patient history may include complaints of dysphagia and neuromuscular effects, such as vasomotor disturbances, numbness and tingling of the extremities, and neuralgic pain. Inspection may reveal a red, swollen, smooth, shiny, and tender tongue (glossitis). The corners of the mouth may be eroded, tender, and swollen (angular stomatitis). Inspection may also reveal spoon-shaped, brittle nails.

A patient with advanced iron deficiency anemia may develop tachycardia because decreased oxygen perfusion causes the heart to compensate with increased cardiac output.

Diagnostic tests

Blood studies and stores in bone marrow may confirm iron deficiency anemia. However, the results of these tests can be misleading because of complicating factors, such as infection, pneumonia, blood transfusion, and iron supplements. Characteristic blood study results include:

- low hemoglobin levels (males, less than 12 g/dl; females, less than 10 g/dl)
- low hematocrit (males, less than 47 ml/dl; females, less than 42 ml/dl)
- low serum iron levels, with high binding capacity
- low serum ferritin levels
- low RBC count, with microcytic and hypochromic cells (in early stages, RBC count may be normal, except in infants and children)
- decreased mean corpuscular hemoglobin in severe anemia.

Bone marrow studies reveal depleted or absent iron stores (done by staining) and normoblastic hyperplasia.

GI studies, such as guaiac stool tests, barium swallow and enema, endoscopy, and sigmoidoscopy, rule out or confirm the diagnosis of bleeding causing the iron deficiency.

Diagnosis must rule out other forms of anemia, such as those that result from thalassemia minor, cancer, and chronic inflammatory, hepatic, and renal disease.

Treatment

First, the underlying cause of anemia must be determined. Then, iron replacement therapy can begin. The treatment of choice is an oral preparation of iron or a combination of iron and ascorbic acid (which enhances iron absorption). In rare cases, iron may have to be administered I.M.—for instance, if the patient is noncompliant with the oral preparation, if he needs more iron than he can take orally, if malabsorption prevents adequate iron absorption, or if a maximum rate of hemoglobin regeneration is desired.

Total-dose I.V. infusions of supplemental iron can be administered to pregnant and elderly patients with severe iron deficiency anemia. The patient should receive this painless infusion of iron dextran in 0.9% sodium chloride solution over 8 hours. To minimize the risk of an allergic reaction to iron, an I.V. test dose of 0.5 ml should be given first.

Key nursing diagnoses and patient outcomes

Altered nutrition: Less than body requirements related to dietary deficiency of iron. Based on this nursing diagnosis, you'll establish these patient outcomes. The patient will:

- express his understanding of foods rich in iron
- increase his daily dietary intake of iron to meet the recommended daily allowance
- express relief from the signs and symptoms of iron deficiency anemia.

Fatigue related to decreased tissue oxygenation caused by decreased hemoglobin. Based on this nursing diagnosis, you'll establish these patient outcomes. The patient will:

- employ measures to prevent and modify fatigue
- perform all self-care activities without undue fatigue
- regain his normal energy level.

Risk for poisoning with iron related to overreplacement of iron supplements. Based on this nursing diagnosis, you'll establish these patient outcomes. The patient will:

- verbalize his understanding of the signs and symptoms of iron poisoning and the importance of reporting such signs and symptoms
- not take more than the prescribed amount of iron each day
- not develop iron poisoning.

Nursing interventions

- Administer iron supplements as ordered. Use the Z-track injection method when administering iron I.M. to prevent skin discoloration, scarring, and irritating iron deposits in the skin.
- Provide oxygen therapy as necessary to help prevent and reduce hypoxia.
- Because a sore mouth and tongue make eating painful, ask the dietitian to give the patient nonirritating foods. If these symptoms make talking difficult, supply a pad and pencil or some other communication aid. Provide diluted mouthwash or, in especially severe conditions, swab the patient's mouth with tap water or warm saline solution. Oral anesthetic diluted in saline solution may also be used.
- As ordered, administer analgesics for headache and other discomfort.
- Provide frequent rest periods to decrease physical exhaustion. Plan activities so that the patient has sufficient rest between them.
- Provide good nutrition and meticulous care of I.V. sites, such as those used for blood transfusions, to help prevent infection.

Monitoring

- Monitor the patient's complete blood count and serum iron and ferritin levels regularly.
- Assess the family's dietary habits for iron intake, noting the influence of childhood eating patterns, cultural food preferences, and family income on adequate nutrition.
- Monitor the patient for signs and symptoms of decreased perfusion to vital organs: dyspnea, chest pain, dizziness, and signs of neuropathy, such as tingling in the extremities.
- Monitor the patient's compliance with the prescribed iron supplement therapy.
- Monitor the effectiveness of prescribed analgesics.
- Evaluate the patient's drug history. Certain drugs, such as pancreatic enzymes and vitamin E, may interfere with iron metabolism and absorption; aspirin, steroids, and other drugs may cause GI bleeding.
- Monitor the patient's pulse rate often; tachycardia indicates that his activities are too strenuous.
- If the patient receives iron I.V., monitor the infusion rate carefully. Stop the infusion and begin supportive treatment immediately if the patient shows signs of an allergic reaction. Also, watch for dizziness

NURSING ALERT

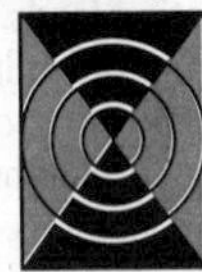

Recognizing iron overdose

Excessive iron replacement may cause signs and symptoms such as diarrhea, fever, severe stomach pain, nausea, and vomiting.

Notify the doctor promptly if the patient experiences these signs and symptoms, and administer prescribed treatments. For this acute condition, treatment may include iron-binding agents (deferoxamine), induced vomiting to produce systemic alkalinization, and anticonvulsants.

and headache and for thrombophlebitis around the I.V. site.

• Monitor the patient for iron replacement overdose. (See *Recognizing iron overdose.*)

Patient teaching

• Reinforce the doctor's explanation of the disorder, and answer any questions. Be sure the patient understands the prescribed treatments and possible complications.

• Ask about possible exposure to lead in the home (especially for children) or on the job. Teach the patient and his family about the dangers of lead poisoning, especially if the patient reports pica.

• Advise the patient not to stop therapy even if he feels better because replacement of iron stores takes time.

• Inform the patient that milk or an antacid interferes with absorption but that vitamin C can increase absorption. Instruct him to drink liquid supplemental iron through a straw to prevent staining his teeth.

• Tell the patient to report any adverse effects of iron therapy, such as nausea, vomiting, diarrhea, and constipation, which may require a dosage adjustment or supplemental stool softeners.

• Teach the basics of a nutritionally balanced diet – red meats, green vegetables, eggs, whole wheat, iron-fortified bread, and milk. However, explain that no food in itself contains enough iron to *treat* iron deficiency anemia; an average-sized person with anemia would have to eat at least 10 lb (4.5 kg) of steak daily to receive therapeutic amounts of iron.

• Warn the patient to guard against infections because his weakened condition may increase his susceptibility. Stress the importance of meticulous wound care, periodic dental checkups, good hand-washing technique, and other measures to prevent infection. Also tell him to report any signs of infection, including temperature elevation and chills.

• Because an iron deficiency may recur, explain the need for regular checkups and compliance with prescribed treatments.

Irritable bowel syndrome

A common condition, irritable bowel syndrome (spastic colon, spastic colitis, mucous colitis) is marked by chronic or periodic diarrhea alternating with constipation. It is accompanied by straining during defecation and abdominal cramps.

Irritable bowel syndrome occurs mostly in women, with symptoms first emerging before age 40. The prognosis is good.

Causes

Although the precise etiology is unclear, irritable bowel syndrome involves a change in bowel motility, reflecting an abnormality in the neuromuscular control of intestinal smooth muscle.

Contributing or aggravating factors include anxiety and stress. Initial episodes occur early in life; psychological stress probably causes most exacerbations. Irritable bowel syndrome may also result from dietary factors, such as fiber, fruits, coffee, alcohol, or foods that are cold, highly seasoned, or laxative. Other possible triggers include hormones, laxative abuse, and allergy to certain foods or drugs.

Complications

Irritable bowel syndrome is associated with a higher-than-normal incidence of diverticulitis and colon cancer. Although complications are usually few, the disorder may lead (rarely) to chronic inflammatory bowel disease.

Because symptoms mimic those of acute abdomen, misdiagnosis occasionally results in unnecessary surgery.

Assessment

Typically, the patient reports a history of chronic constipation, diarrhea, or both. She may complain of lower abdominal pain (usually in the left lower quadrant) that is often relieved by defecation or passage of gas. She may report bouts of diarrhea, which typically occur during the day. This symptom alternates with constipation or normal bowel function.

The patient may describe her stools as small with visible mucus. Or, she may have small, pasty, and pencil-like stools instead of diarrhea. Other common complaints include dyspepsia, abdominal bloating, heartburn, faintness, and weakness.

During history taking, investigate possible contributing psychological factors, such as a recent stressful life change, that may have triggered or aggravated symptoms.

On inspection, the patient may seem anxious and fatigued but otherwise normal. Auscultation may reveal normal bowel sounds. Palpation typically discloses a relaxed abdomen. Occasionally, percussion reveals tympany over a gas-filled bowel.

Diagnostic tests

Because no definitive test exists to confirm irritable bowel syndrome, the diagnosis typically involves studies to rule out other, more serious, disorders, such as diverticulitis or colon cancer. The most frequently performed tests include the following.

- *Barium enema* may reveal colonic spasm and a tubular appearance of the descending colon. It also rules out certain other disorders, such as diverticula, tumors, and polyps.
- *Sigmoidoscopy* may disclose spastic contractions.
- *Stool examination* for occult blood, parasites, and pathogenic bacteria is negative.

Treatment

The aim of therapy is to control symptoms through dietary changes, stress management, and life-style modifications. Medications are reserved for severe symptoms and, if used, are discontinued as the patient learns to control her symptoms through diet and stress reduction.

The type of dietary therapy depends on the patient's symptoms. If she has diarrhea, an elimination diet may help determine whether her symptoms result from food intolerance. In this type of diet, certain foods, such as citrus fruits, coffee, corn, dairy products, tea, and wheat, are sequentially eliminated. Then, each food is gradually reintroduced to identify which foods, if any, trigger the patient's symptoms.

Other dietary changes include elimination of sorbitol, an artificial sweetener that may cause diarrhea, abdominal distention, and bloating. Also helpful is dietary elimination of nonabsorbable carbohydrates, such as beans and cabbage, and lactose-containing foods, all of which can cause flatulence.

To control diarrhea, bran may be added to increase dietary bulk. By increasing the time the stool remains in the bowel, bran helps to promote stool formation.

If the patient has constipation and abdominal pain, her diet should contain at least 15 to 20 g daily of bulky foods, such as wheat bran, oatmeal, oat bran, rye cereals, prunes, dried apricots, and figs. These foods help to minimize the effect of nonpropulsive colonic contractions that may trap stool or retard its passage, causing abdominal pain. The patient should also increase her water intake to at least eight 8-oz glasses a day.

Counseling to help the patient understand the relationship between stress and her illness is essential, as is instruction in stress-management techniques.

Drug therapy, if required, may include:
- anticholinergic, antispasmodic drugs, such as propantheline bromide, to reduce intestinal hypermotility
- antidiarrheals, such as loperamide, to control diarrhea
- laxatives for constipation
- antiemetics, such as metoclopramide, to relieve heartburn, epigastric discomfort, and after-meal fullness
- simethicone to relieve belching and bloating from gas in the stomach and intestines
- mild tranquilizers, such as diazepam, prescribed for a short time to help reduce psychological stress associated with irritable bowel syndrome
- tricyclic antidepressants, if depression accompanies the disorder.

Key nursing diagnoses and patient outcomes

Constipation related to change in bowel function. Based on this nursing diagnosis, you'll establish these patient outcomes. The patient will:
- take steps to prevent constipation
- comply with prescribed treatment for irritable bowel syndrome
- regain and maintain normal bowel function.

Diarrhea related to change in bowel function. Based on this nursing diagnosis, you'll establish these patient outcomes. The patient will:
- avoid foods that cause diarrhea
- adhere to the medication regimen prescribed for irritable bowel syndrome
- regain and maintain normal bowel function.

Pain related to intestinal hypermotility. Based on this nursing diagnosis, you'll establish these patient outcomes. The patient will:
- express relief from pain following administration of anticholinergic, antispasmodic medication
- experience relief from intestinal hypermotility, as evidenced by normal bowel sounds
- become pain free.

Nursing interventions

Because the patient with irritable bowel syndrome isn't hospitalized, nursing interventions almost always focus on patient teaching.

Patient teaching

- Explain the disorder to the patient, and reassure her that irritable bowel syndrome can be relieved. Point out, however, that the condition is chronic with no known cure.
- Help the patient understand ordered diagnostic tests. Review all pretest guidelines. Explain that diagnostic tests cannot specifically diagnose irritable bowel syndrome but can rule out other disorders.
- Review the patient's dietary plan, then suggest ways to implement it. Help her schedule meals; the GI tract works best if meals are eaten at regular intervals. Show her how to keep a daily record of her symptoms and food intake, carefully noting which foods trigger symptoms. Advise her to eat slowly and carefully to prevent swallowing air, which causes bloating, and to increase her intake of dietary fiber.
- Encourage the patient to drink eight to ten 8-oz glasses of water or other compatible fluids daily. Point out that this will help regulate the consistency of her stools and promote balanced hydration. Caution her to avoid beverages associated with GI

discomfort, such as carbonated or caffeinated drinks, fruit juices, and alcohol.

- Discuss the proper use of prescribed drugs, reviewing their desired effects and possible adverse effects.
- Help the patient to implement life-style changes that will reduce stress. Teach her to set priorities in her daily activities and, if possible, to delegate some responsibilities to other family members. Encourage her to schedule more time for rest and relaxation. Provide instruction in relaxation techniques, such as guided imagery or deep-breathing exercises, and advise her to perform them regularly. If appropriate, instruct her to seek professional counseling for stress management.
- Remind the patient that regular exercise is important to relieve stress and promote regular bowel function; even a 20- or 30-minute walk each day is helpful.
- Discourage smoking. If the patient smokes, warn her that this habit can aggravate her symptoms by altering bowel motility.
- Explain the need for regular physical examinations. For patients over age 40, emphasize the need for colorectal cancer screening, including annual proctosigmoidoscopy and rectal examinations.

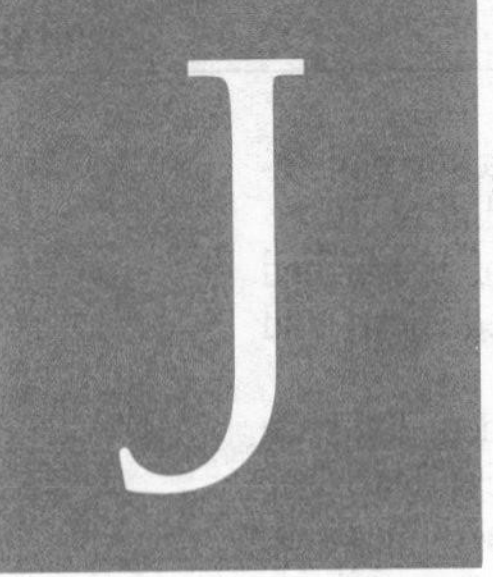

Joint replacement

Called an arthroplasty, the total or partial replacement of a joint with a synthetic prosthesis restores mobility and stability and relieves pain. In fact, recent improvements in surgical techniques and prosthetic devices have made joint replacement an increasingly common treatment for patients with severe chronic arthritis, degenerative joint disorders, and extensive joint trauma. All joints except the spine can be replaced with a prosthesis; hip and knee replacements are the most common. The benefits of joint replacement include not only improved, pain-free mobility but also an increased sense of independence and self-worth. (See *Arthroplasty variations.*)

Procedure

The joint replacement procedure varies slightly depending on the joint and its condition. In a total hip replacement, for instance, the patient is usually placed in a lateral position and given a regional or general anesthetic. The surgeon then makes an incision to expose the hip joint. As necessary, he incises or excises the hip capsule, then dislocates the joint to expose the acetabulum and the head of the femur.

Next, the surgeon reams and shapes the acetabulum to accept the socket part of the ball-and-socket hip prosthesis and secures the device in place. Polymethyl methacrylate adhesive is used to secure the device in place if the prosthesis is cemented. He then repeats this process on the head of the femur for the ball portion of the prosthesis.

Once the parts of the prosthesis are in place, the surgeon fits them together to restore the joint. Then he closes the incision in layers and applies a dressing.

Complications

If infection occurs at the implant site, the implant almost always needs to be removed.

Other serious complications include hypovolemic shock, fat embolism, thromboembolism, and pulmonary embolism. In fact, pulmonary embolism is the most common cause of postoperative mortality following a joint replacement.

Less serious complications include dislocation or loosening of the prosthesis, heterotrophic ossification (formation of bone in the periprosthetic space), avascular necrosis, and dead bone caused by loss of blood supply. Respiratory complications, such as atelectasis and pneumonia, commonly affect elderly patients because of their decreased activity tolerance.

Key nursing diagnoses and patient outcomes

Risk for injury related to increased chance of fat embolism from intramedullary reaming and seating of prostheses. Based on this nursing diagnosis, you'll establish these patient outcomes. The patient will:
• not develop any signs and symptoms of fat embolism

• demonstrate normal neurologic, respiratory, and cardiac function following joint replacement.

Risk for infection related to surgical intervention within the joint space. Based on this nursing diagnosis, you'll establish these patient outcomes. The patient will:
• maintain his temperature and white blood cell count within the normal range following the joint replacement
• not demonstrate any signs and symptoms of infection, such as persistent fever, pain, or stiffness and loss of joint range of motion
• take prophylactic antibiotics before dental or other surgical procedures to decrease the chance of organisms migrating to the joint prostheses.

Impaired gas exchange related to high risk of pulmonary embolism. Based on this nursing diagnosis, you'll establish these patient outcomes. The patient will:
• maintain adequate ventilation and lung perfusion, as evidenced by normal arterial blood gas analyses and normal respiratory function on physical examination
• not demonstrate any signs and symptoms of pulmonary embolism, such as sudden shortness of breath, chest pain, anxiety, and restlessness
• take measures to prevent pulmonary embolism.

Nursing interventions

When caring for a patient receiving a joint replacement, your primary responsibilities will include instructing the patient and monitoring for postoperative complications.

Before surgery

• Because of joint replacement's complexity, patient preparation begins long before the day of surgery, with extensive testing. By the time the patient enters the hospital for surgery, the doctor will have explained the procedure to him in detail. However, the patient and his family still may have questions about the surgery and its expected outcome. Answer them as completely as you can.
• Discuss postoperative recovery. Mention that the patient will probably be out of bed the 1st or 2nd day after surgery. Explain that a physical therapist will see him either preoperatively or soon after surgery to begin an exercise program to maintain joint mobility. As appropriate, show him range-of-motion (ROM) exercises or demonstrate the continuous passive motion (CPM) device that he'll use during recovery (most often used in knee replacements).
• Prepare the patient for an extended period of rehabilitation. Point out that he may not experience pain relief immediately after surgery and that, in fact, pain actually may worsen for several weeks. Reassure him that pain will diminish dramatically once edema subsides. Reassure him that analgesics will be available as needed.

Arthroplasty variations

Arthroplasty is a surgical technique intended to restore motion to a stiffened joint. Joint replacement is one option. Other options include joint resection or interpositional reconstruction.

Joint resection involves careful excision of bone portions, creating a ¾" (2-cm) gap in one or both bone surfaces of the joint. Fibrous scar tissue eventually fills in the gap. Although this surgery restores mobility and relieves pain, it decreases joint stability.

Interpositional reconstruction involves reshaping the joint and placing a prosthetic disk between the reshaped bony ends. The prosthesis used for this procedure may be composed of metal, plastic, fascia, or skin. However, with repeated injury and surgical reshaping, total joint replacement may be necessary.

LIFE-THREATENING COMPLICATIONS

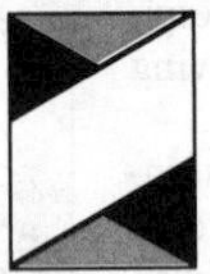

Fat embolism

This life-threatening complication can occur after total-joint surgery, typically during insertion of the prosthesis into the femoral shaft. The insertion alters the pressure in the bone marrow, forcing marrow fat globules into the patient's venous circulation. Signs and symptoms usually occur within 24 to 48 hours after surgery.

Signs and symptoms

If the fat emboli are small and few, the patient may experience only vague symptoms, such as a slight fever and disorientation.

However, if the embolus is large or if multiple emboli exist, the patient may experience severe respiratory symptoms, such as dyspnea, "air hunger," tachypnea, and wheezing. He may also develop central nervous system symptoms, such as confusion, impaired consciousness, sleepiness, restlessness, disorientation, agitation, and possibly coma.

If untreated, the emboli will lodge in the pulmonary capillaries, causing an acute pulmonary disorder similar to acute respiratory distress syndrome. Ultimately, death will occur.

Emergency intervention

- At the first sign of any change in the patient's mental or respiratory status, notify the doctor immediately.
- Administer oxygen or mechanical respiratory support with positive end-expiratory pressure to correct hypoxemia, as indicated.
- Be prepared to administer anti-inflammatory steroids to decrease lung edema and inflammation caused by the infarcted tissue response. Diuretics may be given to decrease pulmonary edema, and low molecular weight dextran may be administered for its fibrinolytic action to prevent disseminated intravascular coagulation. Heparin may or may not be given.
- Monitor the patient's vital signs, intake and output, arterial blood gas levels, complete blood counts (which may show thrombocytopenia and decreased hemoglobin), electrocardiogram, and lung scan results.
- Provide reassurance and support for the patient to help decrease his anxiety level.

- Ensure that the patient or a responsible family member has signed a consent form.

After surgery

- When the patient returns from surgery, keep him on bed rest for the prescribed period. Maintain the affected joint in proper alignment.
- Assess the patient's level of pain, and provide analgesics as ordered. If you're administering narcotic analgesics, be alert for signs of toxicity or oversedation.
- During the recovery period, monitor for complications of joint replacement. In particular, watch for hypovolemic shock from massive blood loss during surgery. Assess the patient's vital signs frequently, and report hypotension, narrowed pulse pressure, tachycardia, decreased level of consciousness, rapid and shallow respirations, or cold, pale, clammy skin.
- Also watch for signs of a fat embolism, a potentially fatal complication. (See *Fat embolism.*)

• Inspect the incision site and dressing frequently for signs of infection. Change the dressing as ordered, maintaining strict aseptic technique. Assess neurovascular and motor status distal to the site of joint replacement regularly. Immediately report any abnormalities.
• Be sure to reposition the patient often to enhance comfort and prevent pressure sores. Encourage frequent coughing and deep breathing to prevent pulmonary complications and adequate fluid intake to prevent urinary stasis and constipation.
• As ordered, have the patient begin exercising the affected joint soon after surgery. (Some doctors routinely order physical therapy to begin on the day of surgery.) The doctor may prescribe CPM, which involves the use of a machine or a system of suspended ropes and pulleys, or a series of active or passive ROM exercises.
• If joint displacement occurs, notify the doctor. If traction is used to correct displacement, periodically check the weights and other equipment.

Home care instructions

• Reinforce the doctor's and physical therapist's instructions for the patient's exercise regimen. Remind him to stick closely to the prescribed schedule and not to rush rehabilitation, no matter how good he feels.
• Review prescribed limitations on activity. Depending on the location and extent of surgery, the doctor may order the patient to avoid bending or lifting, extensive stair climbing, or sitting for prolonged periods (including long car trips or plane flights). He also will caution against overusing the joint – especially weight-bearing joints.
• If the patient has undergone hip replacement, instruct him to keep his hips abducted and not to cross his legs when sitting, to reduce the risk of dislocating the prosthesis. Tell him to avoid flexing his hips more than 90 degrees when arising from a bed or chair. Encourage him to sit in chairs with high arms and a firm seat and to sleep only on a firm mattress. Before the patient with a knee or hip replacement is discharged, make sure that he has a properly sized pair of crutches or a cane and knows how to use them properly.
• If the patient has undergone shoulder joint replacement, instruct him to keep his arm in a sling until postoperative swelling subsides, then to slowly begin the prescribed exercise program when healing is complete – usually about 6 weeks after surgery. If the patient will be using a shoulder CPM, instruct him in its use.
• Caution the patient to promptly report signs of possible infection, such as persistent fever and increased pain, tenderness, and stiffness in the joint and surrounding area. Remind him that infection may develop even several months after joint replacement.
• Stress the importance of taking prophylactic antibiotics before any dental or surgical procedures. Explain that this is necessary to prevent organisms from migrating to the joint replacement site and causing an infection.
• Tell the patient to report a sudden increase of pain, which may indicate dislodgment of the prosthesis.

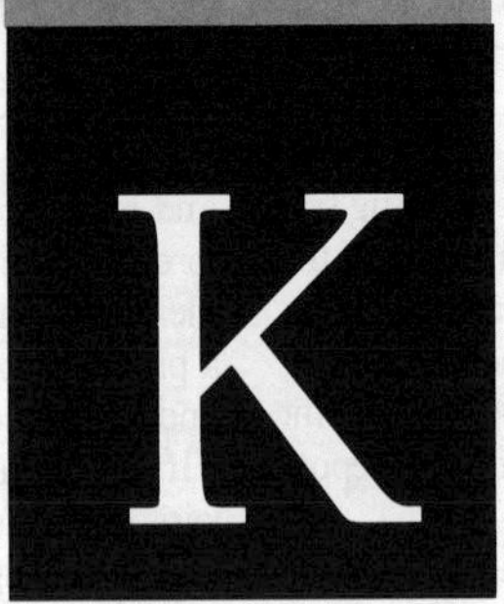

Kaposi's sarcoma

Initially, this cancer of vascular and lymphatic endothelial cell origin was described as a rare sarcoma occurring mostly in elderly Italian and Jewish men. In recent years, the incidence of Kaposi's sarcoma has risen dramatically along with the incidence of acquired immunodeficiency syndrome (AIDS). Currently, it's the most common AIDS-related cancer.

Characterized by obvious, colorful lesions, Kaposi's sarcoma causes structural and functional damage. When associated with AIDS, it progresses aggressively, involving the lymph nodes, the viscera, and possibly GI structures.

Causes

The exact cause of Kaposi's sarcoma is unknown, but the disease is related to immunosuppression. Genetic or hereditary predisposition is also suspected.

Complications

Disease progression can cause severe pulmonary involvement, resulting in respiratory distress, and GI involvement, leading to digestive problems.

Assessment

The health history typically reveals that the patient has AIDS. If the sarcoma advances beyond the early stages or if a lesion breaks down, the patient may report pain. Usually, however, the lesions remain painless unless they impinge on nerves or organs.

On inspection, you may observe several lesions in various shapes, sizes, and colors (ranging from red-brown to dark purple). The lesions occur most commonly on the skin, buccal mucosa, hard and soft palates, lips, gums, tongue, tonsils, conjunctiva, and sclera. In advanced disease, the lesions may join, becoming one large plaque. Untreated lesions may appear as large, ulcerative masses. You may notice that the patient has dyspnea, especially if pulmonary involvement occurs.

Palpation and inspection may also disclose edema from lymphatic obstruction.

Auscultation may uncover wheezing and hypoventilation. The most common extracutaneous sites are the lungs and GI tract (esophagus, oropharynx, and epiglottis).

Diagnostic tests

Usually, the patient will undergo a tissue biopsy to determine the lesion's type and stage. Then, a computed tomography scan may be performed to evaluate metastasis. (See *Laubenstein's stages in Kaposi's sarcoma.*)

Treatment

Radiation therapy, chemotherapy, and drug therapy with biological response modifiers are treatment options. Occasionally, intralesional injection is performed with vinblastine or bleomycin. Radiation therapy offers palliation of symptoms, including pain from obstructing lesions in the oral cavity or extremities and edema caused by lymphatic blockage. It may also be used for cosmetic improvement.

Chemotherapy includes combinations of doxorubicin, vinblastine, vincristine, and etoposide. The biological response modifier interferon alfa-2b may be prescribed in AIDS-related Kaposi's sarcoma. It reduces the number of skin lesions but is ineffective in advanced disease.

Key nursing diagnoses and patient outcomes

Altered nutrition: Less than body requirements related to GI dysfunction. Based on this nursing diagnosis, you'll establish these patient outcomes. The patient will:

- consume a nutritionally balanced diet high in calories and protein
- regain and maintain his weight within a normal range
- not become malnourished or develop a nutritional deficiency.

Body image disturbance related to cutaneous lesions. Based on this nursing diagnosis, you'll establish these patient outcomes. The patient will:

- express his feelings about how his body has changed
- participate in decisions about his care
- express positive feelings about himself.

Impaired gas exchange related to respiratory dysfunction. Based on this nursing diagnosis, you'll establish these patient outcomes. The patient will:

- maintain adequate ventilation, as evidenced by normal arterial blood gases and a normal respiratory assessment
- not develop signs and symptoms of respiratory distress.

Nursing interventions

- Listen to the patient's fears and concerns, and answer his questions honestly. Stay with him during periods of severe stress and anxiety. Allow him to participate in care decisions whenever possible, and encourage him to participate in self-care measures as much as he can.

Laubenstein's stages in Kaposi's sarcoma

The following staging system was proposed by L.J. Laubenstein for use in evaluating and treating patients who have AIDS and Kaposi's sarcoma:
Stage I—locally indolent cutaneous lesions
Stage II—locally aggressive cutaneous lesions
Stage III—mucocutaneous and lymph node involvement
Stage IV—visceral involvement.

Within each stage, a patient may have different symptoms classified as a stage subtype—A or B—as follows:
Subtype A—no systemic signs or symptoms
Subtype B—one or more systemic signs and symptoms, including 10% weight loss, fever of unknown origin that exceeds 100° F (37.8° C) for more than 2 weeks, chills, lethargy, night sweats, anorexia, and diarrhea.

- If the patient has painful lesions, help him into a more comfortable position.
- Administer pain medications. Suggest distractions, and help the patient with relaxation techniques.
- Supply the patient with high-calorie, high-protein meals. If he can't tolerate regular meals, provide him with frequent, smaller meals. Consult with the dietitian, and plan meals around the patient's treatment. If he can't take food by mouth, administer I.V. fluids. Give antiemetics and sedatives, as ordered.
- Provide rest periods if the patient tires easily.
- To help the patient adjust to changes in his appearance, urge him to share his feelings. Give encouragement.

Monitoring

- Inspect the patient's skin every shift. Look for new lesions and skin breakdown.
- Be alert for adverse effects of radiation therapy or chemotherapy – such as anorexia, nausea, vomiting, and diarrhea – and take steps to prevent or alleviate them.
- Monitor the patient for signs and symptoms of GI or respiratory dysfunction.

Patient teaching

- Offer emotional support to help the patient and family cope with the diagnosis and prognosis. Provide opportunities for them to discuss their concerns.
- Reinforce the doctor's explanation of treatments. Be sure the patient understands which adverse reactions to expect and how to manage them. For example, during radiation therapy, instruct the patient to keep irradiated skin dry to avoid possible breakdown and subsequent infection.
- Explain infection prevention techniques and, if necessary, demonstrate basic hygiene measures to prevent infection. These measures are especially important if the patient also has AIDS.
- Stress the need for ongoing treatment and care.
- As appropriate, refer the patient to the social service department for information about support groups.

Kidney cancer

About 85% of kidney cancers – also called nephrocarcinoma, renal cell carcinoma, hypernephroma, and Grawitz's tumor – originate in the kidneys. Others are metastases from various primary-site cancers.

Most kidney tumors are large, firm, nodular, encapsulated, unilateral, and solitary. They may affect either kidney; occasionally they're bilateral or multifocal.

The incidence of kidney cancer is rising, possibly from exposure to environmental carcinogens and increased longevity. Even so, kidney cancer accounts for only about 2% of all adult cancers. Twice as common in men as in women, kidney cancer typically strikes after age 40, with peak incidence between ages 50 and 60. Renal pelvic tumors and Wilms' tumor occur most commonly in children.

Kidney cancer can be separated histologically into clear cell, granular cell, and spindle cell types. Sometimes the prognosis is considered better for the clear cell type than for the other types; in general, however, the prognosis depends more on the cancer's stage than on its type. (See *Staging kidney cancer.*)

Overall prognosis has improved considerably, with the 5-year survival rate about 50% and the 10-year survival rate at 18% to 23%. Left untreated, kidney cancer is fatal.

Causes

Although the cause of kidney cancer is unknown, some studies implicate particular factors, including heavy cigarette smoking. Patients who receive regular hemodialysis also may be at increased risk.

Complications

Hemorrhage, respiratory problems from metastasis to the lungs, neurologic problems from brain metastasis, and GI problems from liver metastasis are possible complications.

Assessment

The patient may complain of hematuria and often a dull, aching flank pain. He also may report weight loss, although this is uncommon. Rarely, his temperature may be elevated. Palpation may reveal a smooth, firm, nontender abdominal mass.

Diagnostic tests

Renal ultrasound and a computed tomography scan or magnetic resonance imag-

Staging kidney cancer

Using the tumor, node, metastasis (TNM) system, the American Joint Committee on Cancer has established the following stages for kidney cancer.

Primary tumor

TX—primary tumor can't be assessed
T0—no evidence of primary tumor
T1—tumor 2.5 cm or less in greatest dimension and limited to the kidney
T2—tumor greater than 2.5 cm in greatest dimension and limited to the kidney
T3—tumor extends into major veins or invades adrenal gland or perinephric tissues, but not beyond Gerota's fascia
T3a—tumor extends into adrenal gland or perinephric tissues, but not beyond Gerota's fascia
T3b—tumor grossly extends into renal veins or vena cava
T4—tumor extends beyond Gerota's fascia

Regional lymph nodes

NX—regional lymph nodes can't be assessed
N0—no evidence of regional lymph node metastasis
N1—metastasis in a single lymph node, 2 cm or less in greatest dimension
N2—metastasis in a single lymph node, between 2 and 5 cm in greatest dimension, or metastases to several lymph nodes, none more than 5 cm in greatest dimension
N3—metastasis in a lymph node, more than 5 cm in greatest dimension

Distant metastasis

MX—distant metastasis can't be assessed
M0—no known distant metastasis
M1—distant metastasis

Staging categories

Kidney cancer progresses from mild to severe as follows:
Stage I—T1, N0, M0
Stage II—T2, N0, M0
Stage III—T1, N1, M0; T2, N1, M0; T3a, N0, M0; T3a, N1, M0; T3b, N0, M0; T3b, N1, M0
Stage IV—T4, any N, M0; any T, N2, M0; any T, N3, M0; any T, any N, M1

ing can separate between simple cysts and renal cancer. In many cases, these tests eliminate the need for renal angiography. Other tests that aid diagnosis and help in staging include excretory urography, nephrotomography, and kidney-ureter-bladder radiography.

Additional relevant tests include liver function studies, which show increased alkaline phosphatase, bilirubin, and transaminase levels and prolonged prothrombin time. Such results may point to liver metastasis. If the tumor hasn't metastasized, these abnormal values reverse after tumor resection.

Treatment

Radical nephrectomy, with or without regional lymph node dissection, offers the only chance of cure. It's the treatment of choice in localized cancer or with tumor extension into the renal vein and vena cava. Preoperative embolization of the affected kidney is often done to simplify nephrectomy and minimize blood loss. Nephrectomy won't help in disseminated disease.

Because this disease resists radiation, this treatment is used only when the cancer has spread into the perinephric region or the lymph nodes or when the primary tumor or metastatic sites can't be completely excised. Then the patient usually needs high radiation doses.

Chemotherapy and hormonal therapy have no effect on kidney cancer. Immunotherapy with lymphokine-activated killer T cells plus recombinant interleukin-2 shows promise but is expensive and causes many adverse reactions. Interferon is somewhat effective in treating advanced disease.

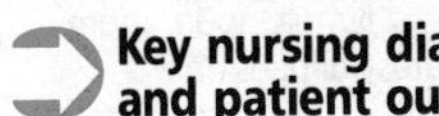

Key nursing diagnoses and patient outcomes

Fear related to the diagnosis of kidney cancer. Based on this nursing diagnosis, you'll establish these patient outcomes. The patient will:
- verbalize his feelings about having cancer
- use available support systems to help him cope with his kidney cancer
- manifest no physical signs or symptoms of fear.

Pain related to tumor pressure in the kidney. Based on this nursing diagnosis, you'll establish these patient outcomes. The patient will:
- express relief from pain following analgesic administration
- employ distraction techniques to minimize pain
- become pain free after a nephrectomy is performed.

Nursing interventions

- Administer prescribed analgesics as needed by the patient. Provide comfort measures, such as positioning and distractions, to help the patient cope with his discomfort.
- Prepare the patient for a nephrectomy. (See the entry "Nephrectomy.")
- Provide symptomatic treatment for adverse effects of chemotherapeutic drugs.
- Encourage the patient to express his anxieties and fears, and remain with him during periods of severe stress and anxiety.

Monitoring

- Watch the patient for signs and symptoms of pulmonary, neurologic, and liver dysfunction.
- Monitor laboratory test results for anemia, polycythemia, and abnormal blood chemistry values that may point to bone or hepatic involvement or be a consequence of radiation therapy or chemotherapy.
- Watch for adverse effects of radiation or chemotherapy.
- Monitor the patient's degree of pain, and assess the effectiveness of analgesics.

Patient teaching

- Tell the patient what to expect from surgery and other treatments.
- Explain the possible adverse effects of radiation and drug therapy. Teach the patient how to prevent and minimize them.
- When preparing the patient for discharge, stress the importance of compliance with any prescribed outpatient treatment. This includes an annual follow-up chest X-ray to rule out lung metastasis and excretory urography to be performed every 6 to 12 months to check for contralateral tumors.
- If appropriate, refer the patient and his family to hospital and community services, such as cancer support groups and hospice care.

Kidney transplant

Ranking among the most commonly performed and most successful of all organ transplants, kidney transplant represents an alternative to dialysis for many patients with otherwise unmanageable end-stage renal disease. It also may be necessary to sustain life in a patient who has suffered traumatic loss of kidney function or in whom dialysis is contraindicated. Kidney transplant, however, isn't performed on all patients who seemingly could benefit from it. For instance, severely debilitated, diabetic, or elderly patients or those with human immunodeficiency virus infection or psychiatric disorders aren't considered good candidates.

In this transplant, a healthy kidney harvested from a living relative or cadaver donor is implanted in the recipient's iliac fossa and anastomosed in place. The recipient's own kidneys usually aren't removed unless they're chronically infected, greatly enlarged, cancerous, or causing intractable hypertension. Because the recipient's own kidneys often secrete erythropoietin fluid, they're left in place to increase circulating hematocrit levels, to ease dialysis management, and to reduce blood transfusion requirements in case of transplant rejection.

Procedure

With the patient under general anesthesia, the surgeon makes a curvilinear incision in the right or left lower quadrant, extending from the symphysis pubis to the anterior superior iliac spine and up to just below the thoracic cage. He exposes the iliac fossa with a self-retaining retractor, then performs segmental separation, ligature, and division of perivascular tissue. Next, he clamps the iliac vein and artery in preparation for anastomosis to the donor kidney's renal vein and artery.

Meanwhile, the donor kidney is prepared for transplantation. If a cadaver kidney is being used, it's removed from cold storage or a perfusion preparation machine.

If the kidney is from a living donor, it's harvested in an adjacent operating room via nephrectomy and placed in cold lactated Ringer's solution. Before transplantation, the donor kidney's renal artery is flushed with cold heparinized lactated Ringer's solution to prevent clogging. Then, the surgeon positions the kidney in a sling over the implantation site. (He never holds the kidney in his hands because this would warm it and possibly cause necrosis.)

The surgeon then implants the kidney in the retroperitoneal area of the iliac fossa, where it's protected by the hip bone. If a donor's left kidney is being used, the surgeon implants it in the recipient's right side; conversely, he implants a donor's right kidney in the recipient's left side. Doing so permits the renal pelvis to rest anteriorly and allows the new kidney's ureter to rest in front of the iliac artery, where the ureter is more accessible.

Once the kidney is in place, the surgeon anastomoses its renal vein to the recipient's iliac vein and the renal artery to the recipient's internal iliac artery (see *Understanding kidney transplant,* page 514). He then removes the venous and arterial clamps and checks for patency of the anastomoses. Next, he attaches the donor kidney's ureter to the recipient's bladder, taking care to ensure a watertight closure. When the transplant is complete, the surgeon sutures the incision and sends the patient to the recovery room.

Complications

The major impediment to transplantation is rejection of the donated organ. However, careful tissue matching between donor and recipient decreases this risk. (See *Managing transplant rejection,* page 515.)

Kidney transplantation may also be associated with vascular complications – such as stenosis of the renal artery, vascular leakage, and thrombosis at the surgical site – or genitourinary tract complications – such as ureteral leakage, ureteral fistula, ureteral obstruction, calculus formation, bladder neck contracture, scrotal swelling, and graft rupture. Other potential complications include infection, hematomas, abscesses, and lymphoceles.

Key nursing diagnoses and patient outcomes

Risk for infection related to immunosuppression following transplantation. Based on this nursing diagnosis, you'll establish these patient outcomes. The patient will:

Understanding kidney transplant

In kidney transplant, the donated organ is implanted in the iliac fossa. The organ's vessels are then connected to the internal iliac vein and internal iliac artery, as shown in the illustration. Typically, the patient's own kidneys are left in place.

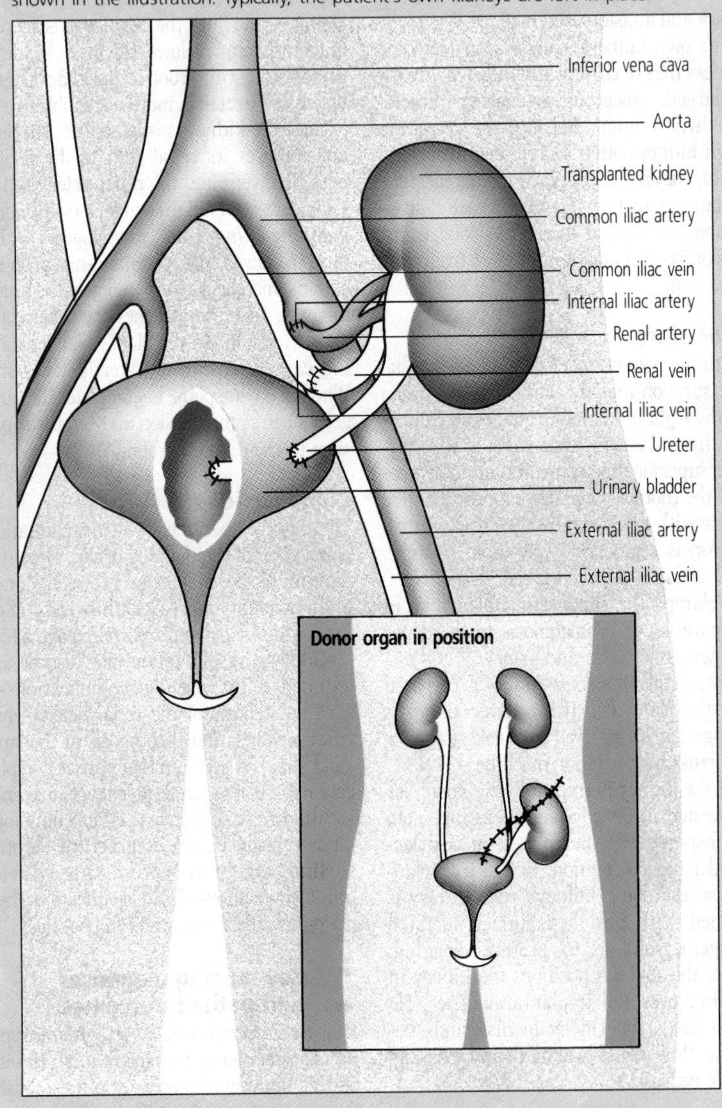

Managing transplant rejection

Transplant rejection can occur immediately after surgery or not until years later. But whenever rejection occurs, it demands prompt intervention.

Hyperacute rejection

In hyperacute rejection, the patient's circulating antibodies attack the donor kidney several minutes to hours after transplantation. Renal perfusion plummets, and the organ rapidly becomes ischemic and dies.

If the patient experiences hyperacute rejection, prepare him for removal of the rejected kidney. Provide emotional support to help lessen his disappointment. Also provide support for the donor, if possible, who may feel dejected.

Acute rejection

This type of rejection may occur 1 week to 6 months after transplantation of a living donor kidney or 1 week to 2 years after transplantation of a cadaver kidney, although it most commonly occurs 7 to 14 days after transplantation. This form of rejection is caused by an antigen-antibody reaction, which produces acute tubular necrosis.

Most transplant patients have at least one or two episodes of acute rejection, which can be stopped with early recognition and immediate administration of increased dosages of immunosuppressant drugs. If treatment is unable to reverse the process, the transplanted kidney eventually stops functioning.

Be alert for the characteristic indicators of acute rejection: signs of infection (fever, rapid pulse, elevated white blood cell count, lethargy), oliguria or anuria, hypertension, or a weight gain of more than 3 lb (1.4 kg) in a day.

If the patient displays signs of acute rejection, reassure him that this complication is common and often reversible. As ordered, prepare him for dialysis.

Chronic rejection

This irreversible complication can start several months or even years after transplantation. It's caused by long-term antibody destruction of the donor kidney. Typically, it's detected by serial laboratory studies that show a declining glomerular filtration rate with rising BUN and serum creatinine levels.

If the patient is experiencing chronic rejection, inform him that complete destruction of the donor kidney may not occur for several years. Prepare him for a renal scan, renal biopsy, and other tests, as ordered. Administer increased dosages of immunosuppressant drugs and adjust his dietary and fluid regimen, as ordered. When necessary, prepare him for dialysis or another transplant, as ordered.

- verbalize his understanding of the early signs and symptoms of infection and the importance of notifying the doctor if they should occur
- incorporate infection control measures into his daily routine
- remain free of infection, as evidenced by a normal temperature and white blood cell count and the absence of infection symptoms.

Anxiety related to the possibility of organ rejection. Based on this nursing diagnosis, you'll establish these patient outcomes. The patient will:

- express his feelings of anxiety
- perform stress-reduction exercises
- demonstrate fewer physical symptoms of anxiety.

Noncompliance with treatment related to the long-term need for immunosuppression. Based on this nursing diagnosis, you'll establish these patient outcomes. The patient will:

- express an understanding of the need for long-term immunosuppressant therapy
- comply with prescribed immunosuppressant therapy
- not demonstrate signs and symptoms of rejection.

Nursing interventions

When caring for a patient undergoing a kidney transplant, your major responsibilities will include instructing the patient and monitoring for postoperative complications, including tissue rejection.

Before surgery

- Prepare the patient thoroughly for transplantation and a prolonged recovery period, and offer him ongoing emotional support.
- Encourage the patient to express his feelings. If he's concerned about rejection of the donor kidney, explain that if this happens and cannot be reversed, he will resume dialysis and wait for another suitable donor organ. Reassure him that transplant rejection is common and normally isn't life-threatening.
- Describe routine preoperative measures, such as a thorough physical examination and a battery of laboratory tests to detect any infection (followed by antibiotic therapy to clear it up), electrolyte studies, abdominal X-rays, an electrocardiogram (ECG), a cleansing enema, and shaving of the operative area.
- Tell the patient that he'll undergo dialysis the day before surgery to clean his blood of unwanted fluid and electrolytes. Also point out that he may need dialysis for a few days after surgery if his transplanted kidney doesn't start functioning immediately.
- Review the transplant procedure itself, supplementing and clarifying the doctor's explanation as necessary. Tell the patient that he'll receive a general anesthetic before surgery and that the procedure should take about 4 hours.
- Next, explain what the patient can expect after he awakens from anesthesia, including the presence of I.V. lines, an indwelling urinary catheter, an arterial line, and possibly a respirator. Describe routine postoperative care, including frequent checks of vital signs, monitoring of intake and output, and respiratory therapy. Prepare him for postoperative pain, and reassure him that analgesics will be available. If possible, arrange for him to tour the postanesthesia room and intensive care unit.
- Teach the patient the proper methods for performing coughing, turning, deep breathing and, if ordered, incentive spirometry.
- Discuss the immunosuppressant drugs that the patient will be taking, and explain their possible adverse effects. Point out that these drugs increase his susceptibility to infection.
- As ordered, begin giving immunosuppressant drugs, such as azathioprine, cyclosporine, muromonab-CD3 (Orthoclone OKT3), and corticosteroids. You may begin oral azathioprine as early as 5 days before surgery.
- In contrast, you'll usually begin slow I.V. infusion of cyclosporine 4 to 12 hours before surgery; when doing so, closely monitor the patient for anaphylaxis, especially during the first 30 minutes of administration. If anaphylaxis occurs, give epinephrine, as ordered.
- Administer blood transfusions as ordered.
- Ensure that the patient or a responsible family member has signed a form consenting to transplantation.

After surgery

- Keep in mind that you're caring for a patient whose immune system has been suppressed by medication and who therefore runs a high risk for contracting an infection. Take precautions to reduce this risk. For instance, use strict aseptic technique when changing dressings and performing catheter care. Also, limit the patient's contact with staff, other patients, and visitors and to avoid exposure to persons with any type of infection. Monitor the patient's white blood cell (WBC) count; if it drops precipitously, notify the doctor, who may order isolation.

• Throughout the recovery period, watch for signs and symptoms of tissue rejection. Observe the transplant site for redness, tenderness, and swelling. Does the patient have a fever or an elevated WBC count? Decreased urine output with increased proteinuria? Sudden weight gain or hypertension? Elevated serum creatinine and blood urea nitrogen (BUN) levels? Report any of these adverse effects immediately.

• Assess the patient for pain, and provide analgesics as ordered. Look for a significant decrease in pain after 24 hours.

• Carefully monitor urine output; promptly report output of less than 100 ml/hour. In a living donor transplant, urine flow usually begins immediately after revascularization and connection of the ureter to the recipient's bladder. In a cadaver kidney transplant, however, anuria may persist for anywhere from 2 days to 2 weeks; dialysis will be necessary during this period.

• Connect the patient's indwelling urinary catheter to a closed drainage system to prevent overextension of the bladder. Observe his urine color; it should be slightly blood tinged for several days and then should gradually clear. Irrigate the catheter as ordered, using strict aseptic technique.

• Assess for pain related to bladder spasms, which may continue briefly after removal of the catheter.

• Review daily the results of renal function tests, such as creatinine clearance and BUN, hematocrit, and hemoglobin levels. Also review results of tests that assess renal perfusion, such as urine creatinine, urea, sodium, potassium, pH, and specific gravity. Monitor for hematuria and proteinuria.

• Assess the patient's fluid and electrolyte balance. Watch particularly for signs of hyperkalemia, such as weakness and pulse irregularities and peaked T waves on ECG. If these signs develop, notify the doctor and give calcium carbonate I.V. as ordered. Weigh the patient daily, and report any rapid gain—a possible sign of fluid retention.

• Periodically auscultate for bowel sounds, and notify the doctor when they return. He'll order gradual resumption of a normal diet, perhaps with some restrictions. For instance, he may order a low-sodium diet if the patient is receiving corticosteroids, to prevent fluid retention.

Home care instructions

• Instruct the patient to carefully measure and record intake and output to monitor kidney function. Teach him how to collect 24-hour urine samples. Tell him to notify the doctor if output falls below 20 oz (600 ml) during any 24-hour period. Tell him to drink at least 1 qt (or liter) of fluid a day unless the doctor gives him other instructions.

• Have the patient weigh himself at least twice a week and report any rapid gain. Explain that such gain may indicate fluid retention.

• Direct the patient to watch for and promptly report signs and symptoms of infection or transplant rejection, including redness, warmth, tenderness, or swelling over the kidney; fever exceeding 100° F (37.8° C); decreased urine output; and elevated blood pressure.

• Because the patient has an increased risk of infection, advise him to avoid crowds and contact with persons with known or suspected infections for at least 3 months after surgery.

• Stress strict compliance with all prescribed medication regimens. Remind the patient that he needs to continue immunosuppressant therapy for as long as he has the transplanted kidney, to prevent rejection.

• If ordered, instruct the patient to take an antacid immediately before a corticosteroid to combat its ulcerogenic effects. Also instruct him to report any adverse reactions.
• Encourage a program of regular, moderate exercise. Tell the patient to begin slowly and increase the amount of exercise gradually.
• Recommend that the patient avoid excessive bending, heavy lifting, or contact sports for at least 3 months or until the doctor grants permission for such activities.
• Also warn against activities or positions that place pressure on the new kidney–for example, long car trips and lap-style seat belts.
• Advise the patient to wait at least 6 weeks before resuming sexual relations. Because pregnancy poses an added risk to a new kidney, provide the female patient with information on birth control.
• Stress the importance of regular follow-up doctor's visits to evaluate the patient's renal function and transplant acceptance.

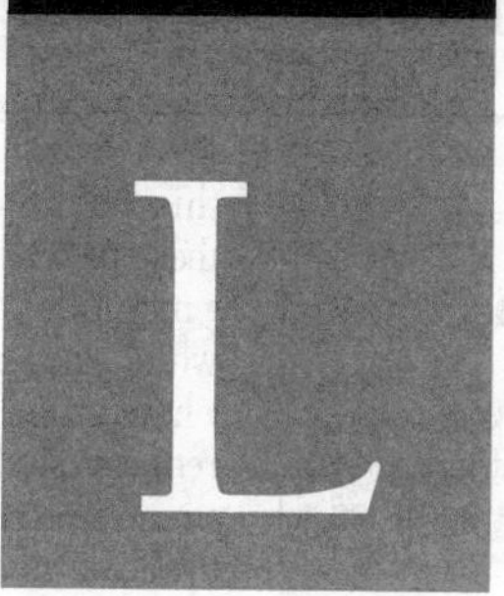

Laminectomy and spinal fusion

In laminectomy, the surgeon removes one or more of the bony laminae that cover the vertebrae. Most commonly performed to relieve pressure on the spinal cord or spinal nerve roots resulting from a herniated disk, laminectomy also may be done to treat compression fracture, dislocation of vertebrae, or a spinal cord tumor.

After removal of several laminae, spinal fusion – grafting of bone chips between vertebral spaces – is often performed to stabilize the spine. It also may be done apart from laminectomy in some patients with vertebrae seriously weakened by trauma or disease. Usually, spinal fusion is done when more conservative treatments – including prolonged bed rest, traction, or the use of a back brace – prove ineffective. (See *Alternative to laminectomy,* page 520.)

Procedure

The patient is given a general anesthetic and placed in a prone position. To perform a laminectomy, the surgeon makes a midline vertical incision and strips the fascia and muscles off the bony laminae. He then removes one or more sections of laminae to expose the spinal defect. For a herniated disk, the surgeon removes part or all of the disk. For a spinal cord tumor, he incises the dura and explores the cord for metastasis. He then dissects the tumor and removes it, using suction, forceps, or dissecting scissors.

To perform spinal fusion, the surgeon exposes the affected vertebrae, then inserts bone chips obtained from the patient's iliac crest, from a bone bank, or both. For optimum strength, he will use wire, spinal plates, rods, or screws to secure these bone grafts into several vertebrae surrounding the area of instability. Then he closes the incision and applies a dressing. After completion of the operation, external traction (such as a halo device, if surgery involved the cervical spine) may be applied.

Complications

This complex and delicate surgery carries the risk of several potentially serious complications. The most common include herniation relapse, arachnoiditis, chronic neuritis caused by adhesions and scarring, and problems associated with prolonged immobility, such as urine retention, paralytic ileus, and pulmonary complications. And even though surgery may relieve pressure on the nerves, reducing pain and improving mobility, it can't reverse existing nerve or muscle damage from chronic disorders.

Key nursing diagnoses and patient outcomes

Risk for injury related to potential for reherniation. Based on this nursing diagnosis, you'll establish these patient outcomes. The patient will:

Alternative to laminectomy

Percutaneous automated diskectomy represents an alternative to the traditional surgical treatment of a herniated disk.

Percutaneous automated diskectomy

In this technique, the doctor uses a suction technique and X-ray visualization to remove only the disk portion that's causing pain. Typically used for smaller, less severe disk abnormalities, percutaneous automated diskectomy has an unimpressive 50% success rate, perhaps because it doesn't involve direct visualization of the operative site. One report indicates a high incidence of postoperative diskitis with this method.

Nursing care of the patient after diskectomy is similar to that after laminectomy; he's generally allowed out of bed in 24 to 48 hours, and he is encouraged to ambulate without assistance as soon as possible.

- demonstrate proper logrolling technique postoperatively to decrease back pressure and to minimize the risk of disrupting a hematoma
- avoid physical strain, such as from heavy lifting or harsh coughing; also, when performing permitted activities, he will demonstrate proper body mechanics
- not develop signs and symptoms of reherniation.

Pain related to surgical trauma and nerve inflammation. Based on this nursing diagnosis, you'll establish these patient outcomes. The patient will:

- verbalize the need for an analgesic
- report a reduction in pain
- exhibit relaxed facial expression and muscle tone
- exhibit vital signs within normal limits.

Risk for infection related to possible cerebrospinal fluid (CSF) leakage. Based on this nursing diagnosis, you'll establish these patient outcomes. The patient will:

- maintain a normal temperature and white blood cell count
- have an incision that will remain free of redness, swelling, and drainage
- remain free of infection.

Sensory/perceptual alterations (tactile) related to chronic neuritis from adhesions and tissue scarring. Based on this nursing diagnosis, you'll establish these patient outcomes. The patient will:

- verbalize the importance of calling his doctor immediately if he experiences pain when he moves his arms or legs or if he notices sensory changes in his arms or legs
- remain free of abnormal tactile sensations.

Impaired physical mobility related to imposed physical limitations, pain, and possible impaired neurologic function. Based on this nursing diagnosis, you'll establish these patient outcomes. The patient will:

- remain free of any complications of immobility
- maintain proper body alignment
- participate in measures such as exercise to regain mobility
- return to optimal level of functioning.

Nursing interventions

When caring for a patient undergoing a laminectomy and spinal fusion, your primary responsibilities will include educating the patient and monitoring for postoperative complications.

Before surgery

- Try to ease the patient's fears by answering his questions clearly.
- Discuss postoperative recovery and rehabilitation. Point out that surgery won't relieve back pain immediately and that pain may even worsen after the operation. Explain that relief will come only after chronic nerve irritation and swelling subside, which may take up to several weeks. Reassure him that analgesics and muscle

relaxants will be available during recovery.

• Tell the patient that he'll return from surgery with a dressing over the incision and that he'll be kept on bed rest for the duration prescribed by the doctor. Explain that he'll be turned often to prevent pressure sores and pulmonary complications. Show him the logrolling method of turning, and explain that he'll use this method later to get in and out of bed by himself.

• Just before surgery, perform a baseline assessment of motor function and sensation in the patient's lower trunk, legs, and feet as well as upper extremities and fingers for cervical involvement. Carefully document the results for comparison with postoperative findings.

• Check to be sure the patient or responsible person has signed the consent form.

After surgery

• After surgery, keep the head of the patient's bed flat or elevated no higher than 45 degrees for at least 24 hours. Urge the patient to remain in the supine position for the prescribed period to prevent any strain on the involved vertebrae. When he's able to assume a side-lying position, make sure he keeps his spine straight, with his knees flexed and drawn up toward his chest. Insert a pillow between his knees to relieve pressure on the spine from hip adduction.

• Inspect the dressing frequently for bleeding or CSF leakage; report either immediately. The surgeon will probably perform the initial dressing change himself; you may be asked to perform subsequent changes.

• Assess motor and neurologic function in the patient's trunk and lower extremities as well as upper extremeties and fingers for cervical involvement, and compare the results with baseline findings. Also evaluate circulation in his legs and feet, and report any abnormalities. Give analgesics and muscle relaxants, as ordered.

• Every 2 to 4 hours, assess urine output and auscultate for the return of bowel sounds. If the patient doesn't void within 8 to 12 hours after surgery, notify the doctor and prepare to insert an indwelling urinary catheter to relieve retention. If the patient can void normally, assist him in getting on and off a bedpan while maintaining proper alignment.

Home care instructions

• Teach the patient and his caregiver proper incision care measures. Tell them to check the incision site often for signs of infection – increased pain and tenderness, redness, swelling, and changes in the amount and character of drainage – and to report any such signs immediately. Instruct the patient to avoid soaking his stitches in a bathtub until healing is complete. Also advise him to shower with his back facing away from the stream of water.

• Make sure the patient understands the importance of resuming activity gradually after surgery. As ordered, instruct him to start with short walks and to slowly progress to longer distances. Review any prescribed exercises, such as pelvic tilts, leg raises, and toe pointing. Advise him to rest frequently and avoid overexertion.

• Review any prescribed activity restrictions. Usually, the doctor will prohibit sitting for prolonged periods, lifting heavy objects or bending over, and climbing long flights of stairs. He may also impose other restrictions, depending on the patient's condition.

• Teach the patient proper body mechanics to lessen strain and pressure on his spine. Instruct him to lie on his back, with his knees propped up with pillows, or on his side, with his knees drawn up and a pillow placed between his legs. Warn him against lying on his stomach or on his back with legs flat. When sitting, he should place his feet on a low stool to elevate his knees above hip level. He should use a firm, straight-backed chair and sit up straight with his lower back pressed flat against the chair back. When standing for prolonged periods, he should alternate placing each foot on a low stool to straighten his lower back and relieve strain. When bending, he should keep his spine straight and bend at his knees and hips rather than at his waist.

• Instruct the patient to sleep only on a firm mattress. If necessary, advise him to purchase a new one or to insert a bed board between his existing mattress and box spring.

Laparoscopy and laparotomy

Laparoscopy and laparotomy allow examination of the pelvic cavity and, when necessary, the repair or removal of diseased or injured structures. A laparoscopy, also known as a pelvic peritoneoscopy, involves the insertion of a laparoscope (a type of endoscope) through the abdominal wall close to the umbilicus. Recent advances in surgical equipment and techniques have made it possible for some abdominal surgical procedures, such as cholecystectomy and hysterectomy, to be performed using the laparascopic approach.

In addition, a laparoscopy may be performed for tubal ligations, aspiration of ovarian cysts, ovarian biopsy, graafian follicle aspiration to retrieve ova for in vitro fertilization, cauterization of endometrial implants, lysis of adhesions, oophorectomy, and salpingectomy.

Laparoscopy may also help detect abnormalities such as cysts, adhesions, fibroids, and infection; identify the cause of pelvic pain; diagnose endometriosis, ectopic pregnancy, or pelvic inflammatory disease; and evaluate pelvic masses or the fallopian tubes of infertile patients.

A laparotomy–a general term for any surgical incision made into the abdominal wall–is used when the extent of abdominal injury or disease is unknown (referred to as an exploratory laparotomy), when extensive surgical repair is indicated, or for pelvic conditions untreatable by laparoscopy (such as the removal of very large endometrial implants). Laparotomy also allows resection of ovarian cysts containing endometrial tissue, thereby averting the risk for rupture.

Procedure

For a laparoscopy, the patient receives a regional or general anesthesia and is placed in a lithotomy position. The surgeon then inserts a needle below the umbilicus and infuses carbon dioxide into the pelvic cavity. This distends the abdomen and permits better visualization of the organs. Next, the surgeon makes an infraumbilical incision and inserts a trocar and cannula. He then removes the trocar and inserts the laparoscope through the cannula. The surgeon looks through the laparoscope to visualize the pelvic cavity. If he needs additional instruments, they may be inserted through a second small incision close to the infraumbilical incision. Or, in certain instances, the instruments may be passed through the laparoscope. Laparoscopes allow passage of such instruments as laser beams and cryosurgical and electrocautery devices. At the end of the procedure, the surgeon removes the carbon dioxide gas, sutures the incisions, and applies a dressing.

For a laparotomy, the patient receives a general anesthesia. The surgeon then makes an abdominal incision and explores the abdominal cavity and performs any necessary repairs or excisions. After the procedure, he sutures the incision and applies a sterile dressing.

Complications

Potential complications of a laparoscopy include infection, bleeding, abdominal cramps, and referred shoulder pain as a result of phrenic nerve irritation. Possible complications of a laparotomy include infection or other complications associated with the specific procedure performed.

Key nursing diagnoses and patient outcomes

Pain related to shoulder discomfort caused by phrenic nerve irritation. Based on this nursing diagnosis, you'll establish these patient outcomes. The patient will:

- express relief from pain following analgesic administration
- use diversional activities to minimize pain
- become pain free within 48 hours of the procedure.

Risk for fluid volume deficit related to bleeding. Based on this nursing diagnosis, you'll establish these patient outcomes. The patient will:

- exhibit normal vital signs and have an intake equal to his output
- not demonstrate signs or symptoms of hypovolemic shock
- maintain a normal fluid balance.

Nursing interventions

When caring for a patient undergoing a laparoscopy or laparotomy, your primary responsibilities will include instructing the patient and monitoring for complications in the immediate postoperative period.

Before surgery

- Describe the specific laparoscopy or laparotomy procedure to the patient, and answer her questions.
- If the patient is having a laparoscopic procedure, tell her that she may be discharged the same day, as soon as she's recovered from the anesthesia. Tell the patient not to eat, drink, or smoke for 6 to 8 hours before the procedure.
- If the patient is having a laparotomy, prepare her as you would for for any abdominal surgery.
- Ensure that the patient has signed a consent form and that preoperative laboratory work (complete blood count, blood chemistry studies, urinalysis) has been completed.

After surgery

- Monitor the patient's vital signs and intake and output, as ordered.
- Check abdominal dressings frequently for drainage. Notify the surgeon if drainage is excessive. Also check for vaginal bleeding if applicable.
- Monitor the patient closely for complications.
- Monitor the patient for abdominal pain and, if the patient has had a laparoscopy, for abdominal cramps or shoulder pain. Provide analgesics, as ordered. If the patient recovering from a laparoscopy complains of bloating or abdominal fullness, explain that the feeling will subside as the gas in her abdomen is absorbed into the bloodstream, exchanged in the lungs, and exhaled.
- Provide additional care for the patient who has undergone a laparotomy as you would for any patient who has undergone abdominal surgery.

Home care instructions

- Instruct the patient how to change the incision bandage. Stress the importance of reporting any signs of wound infection or hematoma. If appropriate, also stress the importance of reporting bright-red vaginal bleeding.
- Tell the patient to shower (not to bathe in a tub) until the incision has healed.
- Instruct the patient to wait until the day after laparoscopy to change the bandage. Also tell her to eat lightly after laparoscopy to minimize any residual abdominal gas.
- After laparoscopy, advise the patient that she may resume normal activities after 2 days and tell her to avoid strenuous work and sports for 1 week or as ordered. If the patient has had a laparotomy, encourage her to follow the prescribed activity restrictions.
- Encourage the patient to follow specific discharge instructions related to the abdominal procedure performed and to maintain follow-up doctor's visits.

Laryngeal cancer

Squamous cell carcinoma constitutes about 95% of laryngeal cancers. Rare laryngeal cancer forms – adenocarcinoma and sarcoma – account for the rest. The disease affects men about five times more often than women, and most victims are between ages 50 and 65.

A tumor on the true vocal cord seldom spreads because underlying connective tissues lack lymph nodes. On the other hand, a tumor on another part of the larynx tends to spread early. Laryngeal cancer is classified by its location:

- supraglottis (false vocal cords)
- glottis (true vocal cords)
- subglottis (rare downward extension from vocal cords).

Causes

The cause of laryngeal cancer is unknown. Major risk factors include smoking and alcoholism. Minor risk factors include chronic inhalation of noxious fumes, familial disposition, and a history of frequent laryngitis and vocal straining.

Complications

Untreated, laryngeal cancer causes increasing swallowing difficulty and pain.

Assessment

Varied assessment findings in laryngeal cancer depend on the tumor's location and its stage. (See *Staging laryngeal cancer.*)

Stage 0 is asymptomatic. In stage I disease, the patient may complain of local throat irritation or hoarseness that lasts about 2 weeks. In stages II and III, he usually reports hoarseness. He may also have a sore throat, and his voice volume may be reduced to a stage whisper. In stage IV, he typically reports pain radiating to his ear, dysphagia, and dyspnea. In advanced (stage IV) disease, palpation may detect a neck mass or enlarged cervical lymph nodes.

Diagnostic tests

The usual workup includes laryngoscopy, xeroradiography, biopsy, laryngeal tomography and computed tomography scans, and laryngography to visualize and define the tumor and its borders. Chest X-ray findings can help detect metastases.

Treatment

Early lesions may respond to laser surgery or radiation therapy; advanced lesions to laser surgery, radiation therapy, and chemotherapy. Treatment aims to eliminate cancer and preserve speech. If speech preservation isn't possible, speech rehabilitation may include esophageal speech or prosthetic devices. (See *Alternative speech methods,* page 526.) Surgical techniques to construct a new voice box are experimental.

In early disease, laser surgery destroys precancerous lesions; in advanced disease, it can help clear obstructions. Other surgical procedures vary with tumor size and include cordectomy, partial or total laryngectomy, supraglottic laryngectomy, and total laryngectomy with laryngoplasty.

Radiation therapy alone or combined with surgery can create complications, including airway obstruction, pain, and loss of taste (xerostomia).

Chemotherapy is minimally beneficial in treating laryngeal cancer.

Key nursing diagnoses and patient outcomes

Impaired swallowing related to presence of tumor. Based on this nursing diagnosis, you'll establish these patient outcomes. The patient will:

- consume a nutritionally balanced diet containing sufficient calories
- maintain his weight within a normal range
- not exhibit signs or symptoms of aspiration pneumonia.

Impaired verbal communication related to presence of tumor. Based on this nurs-

Staging laryngeal cancer

Review the following classification system developed by the American Joint Committee on Cancer. This tumor, node, metastasis (TNM) system helps define the advancement of your patient's laryngeal cancer and direct treatment. The T stages cover supraglottic, glottic, and subglottic tumors.

Primary tumor

TX—primary tumor can't be assessed
T0—no evidence of primary tumor
Tis—carcinoma in situ
Supraglottic tumor stages
T1—tumor confined to one subsite in supraglottis; vocal cords retain normal motion
T2—tumor extends to other sites in supraglottis, or to glottis; vocal cords retain motion
T3—tumor confined to larynx, but vocal cords lose motion; or tumor extends to the postcricoid area, the pyriform sinus, or the preepiglottic space and vocal cords lose motion; or both
T4—tumor extends through thyroid cartilage, extends to tissues beyond the larynx (such as the oropharynx or soft tissues of the neck), or both
Glottic tumor stages
T1—tumor confined to vocal cords, which retain normal motion; may involve anterior or posterior commissures
T2—tumor extends to supraglottis or subglottis or both; vocal cords may lose motion
T3—tumor confined to larynx, but vocal cords lose motion
T4—tumor extends through thyroid cartilage, extends to tissue beyond the larynx (such as the oropharynx or soft tissues of the neck), or both
Subglottic tumor stages
T1—tumor confined to the subglottis
T2—tumor extends to vocal cords; vocal cords may lose motion
T3—tumor confined to larynx with vocal cord fixation
T4—tumor extends through cricoid or thyroid cartilage, extends to tissues beyond the larynx (such as the oropharynx or soft tissues of the neck), or both

Regional lymph nodes

NX—regional lymph nodes can't be assessed
N0—no evidence of regional lymph node metastasis
N1—metastasis in a single ipsilateral lymph node, 3 cm or less in greatest dimension
N2—metastasis in one or more ipsilateral lymph nodes, or in bilateral or contralateral nodes, larger than 3 cm but less than 6 cm in greatest dimension
N3—metastasis in a node larger than 6 cm in greatest dimension

Distant metastasis

MX—distant metastasis can't be assessed
M0—no evidence of distant metastasis
M1—distant metastasis

Staging categories

Laryngeal cancer progresses from mild to severe as follows:
Stage 0—Tis, N0, M0
Stage I—T1, N0, M0
Stage II—T2, N0, M0
Stage III—T3, N0, M0; T1, N1, M0; T2, N1, M0; T3, N1, M0
Stage IV—T4, N0 or N1, M0; any T, N2 or N3, M0; any T, any N, M1

ing diagnosis, you'll establish these patient outcomes. The patient will:

- communicate his needs and desires without undue frustration
- use an alternate method of communication as necessary
- use available resources to help him maximize his communication skills.

Alternative speech methods

During convalescence, your patient may work with a speech pathologist, who can teach him new ways to speak using various communication techniques—some of which are outlined below.

Esophageal speech

By drawing air in through the mouth, trapping it in the upper esophagus, and releasing it slowly while forming words, the patient can again communicate by voice. With training and practice, a highly motivated patient can master esophageal speech in about a month. Recognize that speech will sound choppy at first, but with increasing skill, words will flow more smoothly and understandably.

Because esophageal speech requires strength, an elderly patient or one with asthma or emphysema may find it too physically demanding to learn. And because it also requires frequent sessions with a speech pathologist, a chronically ill patient may find learning esophageal speech overwhelming.

Artificial larynges

The throat vibrator and the Cooper-Rand device are basic artificial larynges. Both types vibrate to produce speech that's easy to understand, although it sounds monotonous and mechanical.

Tell the patient to operate a throat vibrator by holding it in place against his neck. A pulsating disk in the device vibrates the throat tissue as the patient forms words with his mouth. The throat vibrator may be difficult to use immediately after surgery, when the patient's neck wounds are still sore.

The Cooper-Rand device vibrates sounds piped into the patient's mouth through a thin tube, which the patient positions in the corner of his mouth. Easy to use, this device may be preferred soon after surgery.

Surgically implanted prostheses

Most surgical implants generate speech by vibrating when the patient manually closes the tracheostomy, forcing air upward. One such device is the Blom-Singer voice prosthesis. Only hours after it's inserted through an incision in the stoma, the patient can speak in a normal voice. The surgeon may implant the device when radiation therapy ends or within a few days (or even years) after laryngectomy.

To speak, the patient covers his stoma while exhaling. Exhaled air travels through the trachea, passes through an airflow port on the bottom of the prosthesis, and exits through a slit at the esophageal end of the prosthesis. This creates the vibrations needed to produce sound.

Not all patients are eligible for tracheoesophageal puncture, the procedure needed to insert the prosthesis. Considerations include the extent of the laryngectomy; pharyngoesophageal muscle status; stomal size and location; and the patient's mental and emotional status, visual and auditory acuity, hand-eye coordination, bimanual dexterity, and self-care skills.

Ineffective airway clearance related to presence of tumor. Based on this nursing diagnosis, you'll establish these patient outcomes. The patient will:
- cough effectively and expectorate any sputum
- maintain a patent airway
- maintain arterial blood gas values within a normal range.

Nursing interventions

- Provide supportive psychological, preoperative, and postoperative care to minimize complications and speed recovery.

• Encourage the patient to voice his concerns before surgery.
• Help the patient choose a temporary, alternative way to communicate, such as writing or using sign language or an alphabet board. If appropriate, arrange for a well-adjusted laryngectomee to visit him.

After partial laryngectomy:
• Give I.V. fluids and, usually, tube feedings for the first 2 days after surgery; then, resume oral fluids. Keep the tracheostomy tube (inserted during surgery) in place until tissue edema subsides.
• Make sure the patient doesn't use his voice until the doctor gives permission (usually 2 to 3 days postoperatively). Then, caution the patient to whisper until he heals completely.

After total laryngectomy:
• As soon as the patient returns to his room from surgery, position him on his side and elevate his head 30 to 45 degrees. When you move him, remember to support the back of his neck. This will prevent tension on sutures and possible wound dehiscence.
• If the patient has a laryngectomy tube in place, care for it as you would a tracheostomy tube. Shorter and thicker than a tracheostomy tube, the laryngectomy tube stays in place until the stoma heals (about 7 to 10 days).
• To prevent crusting of the laryngectomy stoma, provide adequate room humidification. Remove crusts with petroleum jelly, antimicrobial ointment, and moist gauze.
• Provide frequent mouth care. Clean the patient's tongue and the sides of his mouth with a soft toothbrush or a terry washcloth, and rinse his mouth with a deodorizing mouthwash.
• Suction gently. Unless ordered otherwise, do not attempt deep suctioning, which could penetrate the suture line. Suction through both the tube and the patient's nose because the patient can no longer blow air through his nose. Suction his mouth gently.
• After inserting a drainage catheter (usually connected to a blood drainage system or a GI drainage system), don't stop suction without the doctor's consent. After removing the catheter, check the dressings for drainage.
• Give analgesics, as ordered. Keep in mind that opioid analgesics depress respiration and inhibit coughing.
• If the doctor orders nasogastric (NG) tube feeding, check tube placement and elevate the patient's head to prevent aspiration. Be ready to perform suctioning after NG tube removal or oral fluid intake because the patient may have difficulty swallowing.
• Support the patient through inevitable grieving. If his depression becomes severe, consider referring him for appropriate counseling.

Monitoring

• If the patient will undergo chemotherapy (typically with methotrexate or bleomycin), assess bone marrow and pulmonary function before treatment begins. Once treatment is under way, reassess these functions. Also, monitor for renal toxicity related to chemotherapy.
• Postoperatively, monitor vital signs. Be especially alert for fever, which indicates infection. Record fluid intake and output, and watch for dehydration. Also, be alert for and report postoperative complications. (See *Managing complications of laryngeal surgery,* page 528.)
• If the patient has had a total laryngectomy, watch the stoma for crusting and secretions, which can cause skin breakdown.
• Monitor the patient's emotional state, especially after a total laryngectomy.

Patient teaching

• Before partial or total laryngectomy, instruct the patient in good oral hygiene practices. If appropriate, instruct a male

Managing complications of laryngeal surgery

Once your patient returns from surgery, you'll need to monitor his recovery, watching carefully for complications such as fistula formation, a ruptured carotid artery, and stenosis of the tracheostomy site.

Fistula formation
Warning signs of fistula formation include redness, swelling, and secretions on the suture line. The fistula may form between the reconstructed hypopharynx and the skin. This eventually heals spontaneously, although the process may take weeks or months.

Feed the patient who has a fistula through a nasogastric tube. Otherwise, food will leak through the fistula and delay healing.

Ruptured carotid artery
Bleeding, a cardinal sign of a ruptured carotid artery, may occur in a patient who received preoperative radiation therapy or in a patient with a fistula that constantly bathes the carotid artery in oral secretions.

If rupture occurs, apply pressure to the site. Call for help immediately, and take the patient to the operating room for carotid ligation.

Tracheostomy stenosis
Constant shortness of breath alerts you to this complication, which may occur weeks to months after laryngectomy.

Management includes fitting the patient with successively larger tracheostomy tubes until he can tolerate insertion of a full-sized one.

patient to shave off his beard to facilitate postoperative care.
• Explain postoperative procedures, such as suctioning, NG tube feeding, and laryngectomy tube care. Carefully discuss the effects of these procedures (breathing through the neck and speech alteration, for example).
• Prepare the patient for other functional losses. Forewarn him that he won't be able to smell aromas, blow his nose, whistle, gargle, sip, or suck on a straw.
• Reassure the patient that speech rehabilitation measures (including laryngeal speech, esophageal speech, an artificial larynx, and various mechanical devices) may help him communicate again.
• Encourage the patient to take advantage of services and information offered by the American Speech-Learning-Hearing Association, the International Association of Laryngectomees, the American Cancer Society, or the local chapter of the Lost Chord Club.

Legionnaires' disease

An acute bronchopneumonia, Legionnaires' disease is produced by a gram-negative bacillus. This disease was named for 221 persons (34 of whom died) who became ill while attending an American Legion convention in Philadelphia in July 1976. Outbreaks, usually occurring in late summer and early fall, may be epidemic or confined to a few cases. The disease may range from a mild illness (with or without pneumonitis) to serious multilobar pneumonia with mortality as high as 15%.

A less severe, self-limiting form of the illness, Pontiac fever subsides within a few days but leaves the patient fatigued for several weeks. This disorder mimics Legionnaires' disease but produces few or no respiratory symptoms, no pneumonia, and no fatalities.

Legionnaires' disease is more common in men than in women and is most likely to affect:

- middle-aged or elderly people
- immunocompromised patients (particularly those receiving corticosteroids after transplantation) or those with lymphoma or other disorders associated with impaired humoral immunity
- patients with a chronic underlying disease, such as diabetes, chronic renal failure, or chronic obstructive pulmonary disease
- alcoholics
- cigarette smokers (three to four times more likely to contract Legionnaires' disease than nonsmokers).

Causes

Legionnaires' disease results from infection with *Legionella pneumophila,* an aerobic, gram-negative bacillus that's probably transmitted by air. The organism's natural habitat seems to be water – either hot or cold. In the past, air-conditioning systems were thought to be the main source of transmission. However, public health officials have identified water distribution systems as the primary reservoir for the organism.

Complications

Patients in whom pneumonia develops also may experience hypoxia and acute respiratory failure. Other complications include hypotension, delirium, seizures, congestive heart failure, arrhythmias, renal failure, and shock that usually is fatal.

Assessment

The patient history may include presence at a suspected source of infection. Onset of Legionnaires' disease may be gradual or sudden. After a 2- to 10-day incubation period (or a 1- to 2-day incubation period in Pontiac fever), the patient may report nonspecific prodromal symptoms, including diarrhea, anorexia, malaise, diffuse myalgia and generalized weakness, headache, and recurrent chills.

With Legionnaires' disease, the patient typically reports a cough – initially nonproductive but eventually productive. He also may complain of dyspnea and chest pain or sometimes nausea, vomiting, and abdominal pain.

With Pontiac fever, the patient may complain of myalgia, malaise, chills, headache, a nonproductive cough, and nausea. An unremitting fever may develop within 12 to 48 hours, and the patient's temperature may reach 105° F (40.6° C).

Inspection may reveal grayish or rust-colored, nonpurulent, and occasionally blood-streaked sputum. You also may note tachypnea, bradycardia (in about 50% of patients), and neurologic signs, especially an altered level of consciousness.

Chest percussion may disclose dullness over areas of secretions and consolidation or pleural effusions. Auscultation may reveal fine crackles, developing into coarse crackles as the disease progresses.

Diagnostic tests

- *Chest X-ray* typically shows patchy, localized infiltration, which progresses to multilobar consolidation (usually involving the lower lobes) and pleural effusion. In fulminant disease, chest X-ray reveals opacification of the entire lung.
- *Laboratory tests* include various blood studies and cultures. Blood test findings may include leukocytosis; increased erythrocyte sedimentation rate; a moderate increase in liver enzyme (alkaline phosphatase, alanine aminotransferase [formerly SGPT], and aspartate aminotransferase [formerly SGOT]) levels; and decreased partial pressure of oxygen in arterial blood and, initially, decreased partial pressure of carbon dioxide in arterial blood.

Bronchial washings, blood and pleural fluid cultures, and *transtracheal aspirate* studies rule out other pulmonary infections.

- Definitive tests include *direct immunofluorescence* of *L. pneumophila* and *indirect fluorescent serum antibody testing.* These tests compare findings from initial blood studies with findings from those done at least 3 weeks later. A convalescent serum sample showing a fourfold or greater rise in antibody titer for *L. pneumophila* confirms the diagnosis.

Treatment

Antibiotic treatment begins as soon as Legionnaires' disease is suspected and diagnostic material is collected. Treatment needn't await test results. Erythromycin is the drug of choice. If erythromycin is ineffective alone, rifampin can be added to the regimen. If erythromycin is contraindicated (for example, in a patient allergic to the drug), rifampin alone or rifampin with doxycycline or co-trimoxazole may be used.

Supportive therapy includes administration of antipyretics, fluid replacement, circulatory support with pressor drugs if necessary, and oxygen administration by mask or nasal cannula or by mechanical ventilation with positive end-expiratory pressure.

Key nursing diagnoses and patient outcomes

Risk for injury related to complications caused by Legionnaires' disease. Based on this nursing diagnosis, you'll establish these patient outcomes. The patient will:

- comply with prescribed treatment to minimize his risk for complications and to decrease their severity if they should occur
- remain free of complications associated with Legionnaires' disease.

Hyperthermia related to Pontiac fever caused by Legionnaires' disease. Based on this nursing diagnosis, you'll establish these patient outcomes. The patient will:

- demonstrate a temperature within the normal range after the administration of antipyretic medications
- not develop complications associated with hyperthermia, such as dehydration and seizures
- regain and maintain a normal temperature without antipyretic agents after Legionnaires' disease has been resolved.

Impaired gas exchange related to pulmonary dysfunction. Based on this nursing diagnosis, you'll establish these patient outcomes. The patient will:

- regain and maintain adequate ventilation.
- regain and maintain arterial blood gas values within a normal range
- not develop any complications associated with impaired gas exchange, such as altered tissue perfusion and pneumonia.

Nursing interventions

- Provide respiratory care, such as suctioning, repositioning, postural drainage, chest physiotherapy, or aggressive oxygen therapy, as indicated by the patient's condition and as ordered.
- Provide mechanical ventilation or other respiratory therapy if ordered.
- Keep the patient comfortable and protected from drafts. Give tepid sponge baths or use cooling blankets to lower his fever.
- Provide mouth care frequently. If necessary, apply soothing cream to irritated nostrils.
- Replace fluids and electrolytes as needed. Nausea and vomiting may require administration of antiemetics, as ordered. If renal failure develops, prepare the patient for dialysis.
- Administer antipyretics and antibiotic therapy, as ordered.
- Report case to local public health officials, according to your state's guidelines.

Monitoring

- Monitor the patient's respiratory status. Evaluate chest wall expansion, depth and pattern of respirations, cough, and chest pain. Watch the patient for restlessness, which may indicate hypoxemia.
- Continually evaluate vital signs, arterial blood gas levels, hydration, and color of lips and mucous membranes. Be alert for signs of shock.
- Monitor the patient's level of consciousness for signs of neurologic deterioration. As needed, institute seizure precautions.

• Monitor the effectiveness of antipyretic medications.

Patient teaching

• Provide pulmonary hygiene instructions. Explain the purpose of postural drainage, and tell the patient how to perform coughing and deep-breathing exercises. Emphasize the need to practice these measures until he recovers completely.
• Teach the patient how to dispose of soiled tissues to prevent disease transmission.

Leukemia, acute

Beginning as a malignant proliferation of white blood cell (WBC) precursors, or blasts, in bone marrow or lymph tissue, acute leukemia results in an accumulation of these cells in peripheral blood, bone marrow, and body tissues. (See *Forms of acute leukemia*.)

Acute leukemia ranks 20th among causes of cancer-related death in people of all ages. In the United States, an estimated 11,000 persons develop acute leukemia annually. The disease is more common in males, in whites (especially those of Jewish ancestry), in children between ages 2 and 5, and in those who live in urban and industrialized areas.

Untreated, acute leukemia is invariably fatal, usually because of complications resulting from leukemic cell infiltration of bone marrow or vital organs. With treatment, the prognosis varies.

In acute lymphoblastic (lympocytic) leukemia (ALL), treatment induces remissions in 90% of children (average survival time: 5 years) and in 65% of adults (average survival time: 1 to 2 years). Children between ages 2 and 8 have the best survival rate – about 50% – with intensive therapy.

In acute myeloblastic (myelogenous) leukemia (AML), the average survival time is only 1 year after diagnosis, even with aggressive treatment. Remissions lasting 2 to 10 months occur in 50% of children; adults survive only about 1 year after diagnosis of AML, even if they receive treatment.

Forms of acute leukemia

The most common forms of acute leukemia include:

• acute lymphoblastic (lymphocytic) leukemia, characterized by abnormal growth of lymphocyte precursors (lymphoblasts)
• acute myeloblastic (myelogenous) leukemia, which causes rapid accumulation of myeloid precursors (myeloblasts)
• acute monoblastic (monocytic) leukemia, or Schilling's type, which results in a marked increase in monocyte precursors (monoblasts).

Other variants are acute myelomonocytic leukemia and acute erythroleukemia.

Causes

The exact cause of acute leukemia is unknown; however, radiation (especially prolonged exposure), certain chemicals and drugs, viruses, genetic abnormalities, and chronic exposure to benzene are likely contributing factors.

In children, Down's syndrome, ataxia, and telangiectasia may increase the risk, as may such congenital disorders as albinism and congenital immunodeficiency syndrome.

Although the pathogenesis isn't clearly understood, immature, nonfunctioning WBCs appear to accumulate first in the tissue where they originate. (Lymphocytes originate in lymph tissue; granulocytes originate in bone marrow.) These immature WBCs then spill into the bloodstream. From there, they infiltrate other tissues.

Complications

Acute leukemia increases the risk for infection and, eventually, organ malfunction through encroachment or hemorrhage.

Assessment

The patient's history usually shows a sudden onset of high fever and abnormal bleeding, such as bruising after minor trauma, nosebleeds, gingival bleeding, purpura, ecchymoses, petechiae, and prolonged menses. He may also report fatigue and night sweats. More insidious symptoms include weakness, lassitude, recurrent infections, and chills.

The patient with ALL, AML, or acute monoblastic leukemia may also complain of abdominal or bone pain. When assessing this patient, you may note tachycardia and, during auscultation, decreased ventilation, palpitations, and a systolic ejection murmur.

Inspection of any patient with acute leukemia may reveal pallor. On palpation, you may note lymph node enlargement as well as liver or spleen enlargement.

Diagnostic tests

Bone marrow aspiration showing a proliferation of immature WBCs confirms acute leukemia. If the aspirate is dry or free of leukemic cells but the patient has other typical signs of leukemia, a bone marrow biopsy – usually of the posterior superior iliac spine – must be performed.

Blood counts show thrombocytopenia and neutropenia, and a WBC differential determines the cell type. Lumbar puncture detects meningeal involvement. A computed tomography scan shows the affected organs, and cerebrospinal fluid analysis detects abnormal WBC invasion of the central nervous system.

Treatment

Systemic chemotherapy aims to eradicate leukemic cells and induce remission. It's used when fewer than 5% of blast cells in the marrow and peripheral blood are normal. The specific chemotherapeutic and radiation treatment varies with the diagnosis.

- For meningeal infiltration, the patient receives an intrathecal instillation of methotrexate or cytarabine and cranial irradiation.
- For ALL, the treatment is vincristine, prednisone, high-dose cytarabine, and daunorubicin. Because ALL carries a 40% risk of meningeal infiltration, the patient also receives intrathecal methotrexate or cytarabine. If brain or testicular infiltration has occurred, the patient also needs radiation therapy.
- For AML, treatment consists of a combination of I.V. daunorubicin and cytarabine. If these fail to induce remission, treatment involves some or all of the following: a combination of cyclophosphamide, vincristine, prednisone, or methotrexate; high-dose cytarabine alone or with other drugs; amsacrine; etoposide; and azacitidine and mitoxantrone.
- For acute monoblastic leukemia, the patient receives cytarabine and thioguanine with daunorubicin or doxorubicin.

Treatment may also include antibiotic, antifungal, and antiviral drugs and granulocyte injections to control infection as well as transfusions of platelets to prevent bleeding and of red blood cells to prevent anemia. Bone marrow transplantation is performed in some patients.

Key nursing diagnoses and patient outcomes

Fatigue related to hematologic abnormalities. Based on this nursing diagnosis, you'll establish these patient outcomes. The patient will:

- explain the relationship between fatigue and his activity level
- incorporate measures to modify his level of fatigue into his daily routine.

Risk for infection related to abnormal WBC count. Based on this nursing diagnosis, you'll establish these patient outcomes. The patient will:

• maintain his temperature within a normal range
• not exhibit signs or symptoms of infection
• remain free from infection.

Risk for injury related to thrombocytopenia. Based on this nursing diagnosis, you'll establish these patient outcomes. The patient will:
• incorporate bleeding precautions into his daily routine
• not become injured
• regain a normal platelet count.

Nursing interventions

• Develop a plan of care for the leukemic patient that emphasizes comfort, minimizes the adverse effects of chemotherapy, promotes preservation of veins, manages complications, and provides teaching and psychological support. Because so many of these patients are children, be especially sensitive to their emotional needs and to those of their families when developing your plan.
• Before treatment begins, help establish an appropriate rehabilitation program for the patient during remission.
• After drug instillation, place the patient in Trendelenburg's position for 30 minutes. Make sure he receives enough fluids, and keep him supine for 4 to 6 hours.
• Take steps to prevent hyperuricemia, a possible result of rapid, chemotherapy-induced leukemic cell lysis. Make sure the patient receives about ½ gal (2 liters) of fluid daily, and give acetazolamide, sodium bicarbonate tablets, and allopurinol, as ordered.
• To control infection, place the patient in a private room and impose isolation precautions if necessary (although the benefits of these precautions are controversial). Coordinate care so that the patient doesn't come into contact with staff members who also care for patients with infections or infectious diseases. Don't use an indwelling urinary catheter or give I.M. injections; they provide an avenue for infection.
• Keep the patient's skin and perianal area clean, apply mild lotions or creams to keep the skin from drying and cracking, and thoroughly clean the skin before all invasive skin procedures. Change I.V. tubing according to your hospital's policy. Use strict aseptic technique and a metal scalp vein needle (metal butterfly needle) when starting an I.V. line. If the patient is receiving total parenteral nutrition, provide scrupulous central venous catheter care.
• If bleeding occurs, apply ice compresses and pressure and elevate the extremity. Avoid giving the patient aspirin or aspirin-containing drugs or rectal suppositories, taking a rectal temperature, or performing a digital rectal examination.
• Prepare the patient for a bone marrow transplant, as indicated. (See the entry "Bone marrow transplant.")
• Administer prescribed pain medications as needed. Provide comfort measures, such as position changes and distractions, to alleviate the patient's discomfort.
• Control mouth ulceration by providing frequent mouth care and saline rinses.
• Minimize stress by providing a calm, quiet atmosphere that's conducive to rest and relaxation. Especially if the patient is a child, be flexible with patient care and visiting hours so that he has time to be with his family and friends and to play and do schoolwork.
• Establish a trusting relationship to promote communication. Allow the patient and his family to express their anger, anxiety, and depression.
• Let the patient and his family participate in his care as much as possible.
• If the patient doesn't respond to treatment and has reached the terminal phase of the disease, he'll need supportive nursing care. Take steps to manage pain, fever, and bleeding; make sure the patient is comfortable; and provide emotional support for him and his family. If the patient wishes, provide for religious counseling. Discuss the option of home or hospice care.

Monitoring

- Monitor the patient's complete blood count and platelet count for signs of improvement.
- Watch for signs of meningeal infiltration (confusion, lethargy, and headache). If it develops, the patient will need intrathecal chemotherapy.
- After drug instillation, check the lumbar puncture site often for bleeding.
- Check the patient's urine pH often; it should be above 7.5. Watch for a rash or other hypersensitivity reactions to allopurinol.
- If the patient receives daunorubicin or doxorubicin, watch for early indications of cardiotoxicity, such as arrhythmias and signs of heart failure.
- Screen staff members and visitors for contagious diseases, and watch for and report any signs of infection in the patient.
- Monitor the patient's temperature every 4 hours. If his temperature rises over 101° F (38.3° C) and his WBC count decreases, he will need prompt antibiotic therapy.
- Monitor the patient for bleeding.
- Monitor the effectiveness of administered analgesics.
- Check the patient's oral cavity daily for ulceration and his rectal area daily for induration, swelling, erythema, skin discoloration, and drainage.

Patient teaching

- Explain the course of the disease to the patient.
- Teach the patient and his family how to recognize signs and symptoms of infection (fever, chills, cough, sore throat). Tell them to report an infection to the doctor.
- Explain to the patient that his blood may not have enough platelets for proper clotting, and teach him the signs of abnormal bleeding (bruising, petechiae). Explain that he can apply pressure and ice to the area to stop such bleeding. Also, teach him steps he can take to prevent bleeding. Urge him to report excessive bleeding or bruising to the doctor.
- Inform the patient that drug therapy is tailored to his type of leukemia. Explain that he'll probably need a combination of drugs; teach him about the ones he'll receive. Make sure he understands their adverse effects and the measures he can take to prevent or alleviate those effects.
- Explain that if the chemotherapy causes weight loss and anorexia, the patient will need to eat and drink high-calorie, high-protein foods and beverages. If he loses his appetite, advise him to eat small, frequent meals. If the chemotherapy and adjunctive prednisone instead cause weight gain, he'll need dietary counseling.
- Instruct the patient to use a soft toothbrush and to avoid hot, spicy foods and commercial mouthwashes, which can irritate the mouth ulcers that result from chemotherapy.
- If the patient receives cranial irradiation, explain what the treatment is and how it will help him. Be sure to discuss potential adverse effects and the steps he can take to minimize those effects.
- If the patient needs a bone marrow transplant, reinforce the doctor's explanation of the treatment, its possible benefits, and the potential adverse effects. Teach him about total-body irradiation and the chemotherapy that he'll undergo before transplantation. Tell the patient what to expect after the transplantation.
- Advise the patient to limit his activities and to plan rest periods during the day.
- Refer the patient to the social service department, home health care agencies, and support groups such as the American Cancer Society.

Leukemia, chronic granulocytic

Also called chronic myelogenous (or myelocytic) leukemia, chronic granulocytic leukemia is characterized by the abnormal overgrowth of granulocytic precursors (myeloblasts, promyelocytes, metamyelocytes, and myelocytes) in bone marrow, peripheral blood, and body tissues.

The disease is most common in young and middle-aged adults, slightly more common in men than in women, and rare in children. In the United States, between 3,000 and 4,000 cases of chronic granulocytic leukemia develop annually, accounting for about 20% of all leukemias.

The clinical course of chronic granulocytic leukemia proceeds in two distinct phases: the insidious chronic phase, characterized by anemia and bleeding abnormalities, and eventually the acute phase (blast crisis), in which myeloblasts, the most primitive granulocytic precursors, proliferate rapidly. The disease is always fatal. Average survival time is 3 to 4 years after onset of the chronic phase and 3 to 6 months after onset of the acute phase.

Causes

Although the exact causes remain unknown, almost 90% of patients with this leukemia have the Philadelphia chromosome, an abnormality in which the long arm of chromosome 22 translocates to chromosome 9. Radiation and carcinogenic chemicals may induce this abnormality.

Myeloproliferative diseases also may increase the incidence of chronic granulocytic leukemia. Some researchers suspect that an unidentified virus causes this leukemia.

Complications

Complications include infection, hemorrhage, and pain.

Assessment

The patient history may reveal renal calculi or gouty arthritis (from increased uric acid excretion). The patient may relate symptoms of anemia: fatigue, weakness, dyspnea, decreased exercise tolerance, and headache. Evidence of bleeding and clotting disorders may include bleeding gums, nosebleeds, easy bruising, and hematuria. Additionally, the patient may report recent weight loss and anorexia.

The patient's vital signs may include a low-grade fever and tachycardia. Inspection may reveal pallor and difficulty breathing, and ophthalmoscopic examination may disclose retinal hemorrhage.

Palpation may uncover hepatosplenomegaly with abdominal discomfort and pain (in splenic infarction from leukemic cell infiltration) and sternal and rib tenderness (from leukemic infiltration of the periosteum).

Auscultation may disclose hypoventilation, especially if the patient has dyspnea.

Complete blood count findings in chronic granulocytic leukemia

Serum analysis shows white blood cell (WBC) abnormalities: leukocytosis (WBC count over 50,000/mm^3, rising as high as 250,000/mm^3); occasionally leukopenia (WBC count under 5,000/mm^3); neutropenia (neutrophil count under 1,500/mm^3) despite high WBC count; and increased circulating myeloblasts.

Additional findings may include a decreased hemoglobin level (below 10 g/dl), low hematocrit (less than 30%), and thrombocytosis (more than 1 million thrombocytes/mm^3).

Diagnostic tests

- *Chromosomal studies* of peripheral blood or bone marrow showing the Philadelphia chromosome and low leukocyte alkaline phosphatase levels confirm chronic granulocytic leukemia.
- *Serum uric acid* level may exceed 8 mg/dl.

For other blood test results, see *Complete blood count findings in chronic granulocytic leukemia.*

• *Bone marrow aspirate*—or *biopsy* (performed only if the aspirate is dry)—may be hypercellular, showing bone marrow infiltration by a significantly increased number of myeloid elements; in the acute phase, myeloblasts predominate.
• *Computed tomography scan* may identify the organs affected by this leukemia.

Treatment

In the chronic phase, treatment strives to control leukocytosis and thrombocytosis. Commonly used drugs include busulfan and hydroxyurea. Aspirin may be given to prevent a cerebrovascular accident if the patient's platelet count exceeds 1 million/mm^3.

Bone marrow transplantation may be tried. During the chronic phase, more than 60% of patients who receive a transplant achieve remission.

Ancillary treatments may include the following:
• local splenic irradiation or splenectomy to increase the platelet count and to decrease adverse effects associated with splenomegaly
• leukapheresis (selective leukocyte removal) to reduce the WBC count
• allopurinol to prevent secondary hyperuricemia or colchicine to relieve gouty attacks caused by elevated serum levels of uric acid
• prompt antibiotic treatment of infections that may result from chemotherapy-induced bone marrow suppression.

During the acute phase of this leukemia, either lymphoblastic or myeloblastic disease may develop. Treatment is similar to that for acute lymphoblastic leukemia. Remission, if achieved, is commonly short lived.

Despite vigorous treatment, chronic granulocytic leukemia rapidly advances after onset of the acute phase.

Key nursing diagnoses and patient outcomes

Altered protection related to anemia and bleeding abnormalities. Based on this nursing diagnosis, you'll establish these patient outcomes. The patient will:
• verbalize an understanding of the precautionary measures that he needs to incorporate into his daily life
• not develop any complications associated with chronic granulocytic leukemia, such as infection and bleeding.

Anticipatory grieving related to probability of death within a few months or years of diagnosis. Based on this nursing diagnosis, you'll establish these patient outcomes. The patient will:
• express his feelings about his diagnosis and prognosis
• use available support systems to help him cope
• accept the probable outcome of his illness and make appropriate decisions about his immediate future.

Pain related to changes in tissue function or structure. Based on this nursing diagnosis, you'll establish these patient outcomes. The patient will:
• receive adequate analgesic medication to control his pain
• express relief of pain following administration of analgesic medication.

Nursing interventions

Take the following steps during the chronic phase of chronic granulocytic leukemia when the patient is hospitalized.
• If the patient has persistent anemia, plan your care to minimize his fatigue. Schedule laboratory tests and physical care with frequent rest periods in between. Assist the patient with walking, if necessary.
• To minimize bleeding and infection risks, provide the patient with a soft-bristled toothbrush, an electric razor, and other safety devices.
• To minimize the abdominal discomfort of splenomegaly, provide small, frequent meals. For the same reason, prevent con-

stipation with a stool softener or laxative, as needed. Maintain adequate fluid intake, and ask the dietary department to provide a high-bulk diet.
• To prevent atelectasis, help the patient perform coughing and deep-breathing exercises.
• Listen to the patient's fears and concerns, and provide emotional support. Stay with him during periods of severe stress, and answer his questions honestly. Encourage his participation in care decisions whenever possible.
• Administer ordered pain medications as necessary. Provide comfort measures and distractions to help the patient cope with his discomfort. Instruct the patient in relaxation techniques.
• Take measures that will reduce or prevent adverse effects of treatment. For example, the patient who is undergoing chemotherapy should rinse his mouth with a saline mouthwash to reduce the severity of ulcers.
• After bone marrow transplantation, institute infection-control measures and administer antibiotics and packed red blood cells as ordered.

For more information about nursing interventions during the acute phase, see the entry "Leukemia, acute."

Monitoring

• Regularly check the patient's skin and mucous membranes for pallor, petechiae, and bruising.
• Monitor the patient's pain level, and evaluate the effectiveness of administered analgesics.
• Watch the patient for adverse reactions to treatment, such as stomatitis, nausea, vomiting, diarrhea, and infection.
• Monitor the patient's ability to cope with his diagnosis and prognosis.

Patient teaching

• At the time of diagnosis, repeat and reinforce the doctor's explanation of the disease and its treatment to the patient and his family.
• Take extra care to provide sound patient teaching because the patient with chronic granulocytic leukemia typically receives outpatient chemotherapy throughout the chronic phase.
• Explain diagnostic test procedures to the patient. Be sure he understands why the tests are necessary.
• Explain expected adverse effects of chemotherapy, especially bone marrow suppression (bleeding, infection). Inform the patient that he'll receive a combination of drugs tailored to his leukemia type.
• Teach the patient the signs and symptoms of infection to watch for and report: any temperature over 100° F (37.8° C), chills, redness or swelling anywhere on the skin, sore throat, or cough.
• Instruct the patient to watch for signs of thrombocytopenia and to apply ice and pressure immediately to any external bleeding site. Unless his doctor tells him to do otherwise, advise him to avoid using aspirin and aspirin-containing compounds, which may increase his bleeding risk.
• Urge the patient to obtain adequate rest to minimize fatigue from anemia.
• To minimize the toxic effects of chemotherapy, encourage the patient to eat foods high in calories and protein. Explain that these foods will help him maintain his strength and prevent body tissues from breaking down. Suggest that he eat small, frequent meals throughout the day, especially if he has little appetite.
• If the patient will undergo bone marrow transplantation, reinforce the doctor's explanation of the procedure, its possible outcome, and potential adverse effects. Be sure the patient fully understands the therapy. Teach him about total-body irradiation, which usually takes place before the procedure, and discuss any chemotherapy that he will undergo.
• As appropriate, refer the patient and his family to the social service department, home health care agencies, hospices, and

support groups such as the American Cancer Society.

Leukemia, chronic lymphocytic

A generalized, progressive disease, chronic lymphocytic leukemia is marked by the uncontrollable spread of abnormal, small lymphocytes in lymphoid tissue, blood, and bone marrow. Once these cells infiltrate bone marrow, lymphoid tissue, and organ systems, clinical signs begin to appear.

This disease occurs most commonly in elderly people; nearly all those afflicted are men over age 50. According to the American Cancer Society, chronic lymphocytic leukemia accounts for almost one-third of new leukemia cases annually.

Chronic lymphocytic leukemia is the most benign and the most slowly progressive form of leukemia. However, the prognosis is poor if anemia, thrombocytopenia, neutropenia, bulky lymphadenopathy, and severe lymphocytosis develop. Gross bone marrow replacement by abnormal lymphocytes is the most common cause of death, usually within 4 to 5 years of diagnosis.

Causes

Although the cause of the disease is unknown, researchers suspect hereditary factors because a higher incidence has been recorded within families. Undefined chromosomal abnormalities and certain immunologic defects, such as ataxia-telangiectasia or acquired agammaglobulinemia, are also suspected. The disease doesn't seem to result from radiation exposure.

Complications

The most common complication is infection, which can be fatal. In the end stage of the disease, possible complications include anemia, progressive splenomegaly, leukemic cell replacement of the bone marrow, and profound hypogammaglobulinemia, which usually terminates with fatal septicemia.

Assessment

In the early stages of the disease, the patient usually complains of fatigue, malaise, fever, weight loss, and frequent infections.

Inspection may reveal macular or nodular eruptions, evidence of skin infiltration. On palpation, you may note enlargement of lymph nodes, liver, and spleen, along with bone tenderness and edema from lymph node obstruction.

As the disease progresses, you may note anemia, pallor, weakness, dyspnea, tachycardia, palpitations, bleeding, and infection from bone marrow involvement. You may also see signs of opportunistic fungal, viral, or bacterial infections, which commonly occur in late stages of the disease.

Diagnostic tests

Typically, chronic lymphocytic leukemia is an incidental finding during a routine blood test that reveals numerous abnormal lymphocytes. In the early stages, the patient has a mildly but persistently elevated white blood cell (WBC) count. Granulocytopenia is the rule, although the WBC count climbs as the disease progresses.

Blood studies also reveal a hemoglobin count under 11g/dl, hypogammaglobulinemia, and depressed serum globulin levels. Other common developments include neutropenia (less than 1,500/mm^3), lymphocytosis (more than 10,000/mm^3), and thrombocytopenia (less than 150,000/mm^3).

Bone marrow aspiration and biopsy show lymphocytic invasion. A computed tomography scan identifies affected organs.

Treatment

Systemic chemotherapy includes alkylating agents, usually chlorambucil or cyclophosphamide, and sometimes corticosteroids (prednisone) when autoimmune hemolytic anemia or thrombocytopenia occurs.

When chronic lymphocytic leukemia causes obstruction or organ impairment or enlargement, local radiation therapy can reduce organ size and splenectomy can help relieve the symptoms. Allopurinol can prevent hyperuricemia, a relatively uncommon finding.

Radiation therapy can help relieve symptoms. It's generally used to treat enlarged lymph nodes, painful bony lesions, or massive splenomegaly.

Key nursing diagnoses and patient outcomes

Anticipatory grieving related to threat of death. Based on this nursing diagnosis, you'll establish these patient outcomes. The patient will:

- verbalize his feelings about his diagnosis of chronic lymphocytic leukemia
- maintain control by making decisions about his care
- use appropriate coping behaviors to deal with the threat of death.

Fatigue related to decreased hemoglobin. Based on this nursing diagnosis, you'll establish these patient outcomes. The patient will:

- explain the relationship between fatigue and his activity level
- employ measures to prevent and modify fatigue
- regain a normal hemoglobin level.

Risk for infection related to abnormal lymphocytes. Based on this nursing diagnosis, you'll establish these patient outcomes. The patient will:

- incorporate infection control measures into his daily routine
- maintain a normal temperature and remain free from signs and symptoms of infection
- remain free from infection.

Nursing interventions

- Help establish an appropriate rehabilitation program for the patient during remission.
- To control infection, place the patient in a private room and impose isolation precautions if necessary (although the benefits of these precautions are controversial). Coordinate care so that the patient doesn't come into contact with staff members who also care for patients with infections or infectious diseases. Don't use an indwelling urinary catheter or give I.M. injections; they provide an avenue for infection.
- Clean the patient's skin daily with mild soap and water, and provide frequent soaks if ordered. Keep the patient's perianal area clean, apply mild lotions or creams to keep the skin from drying and cracking, and thoroughly clean the skin before all invasive skin procedures. Change I.V. tubing according to your hospital's policy. Use strict aseptic technique and a metal scalp vein needle (metal butterfly needle) when starting an I.V. line. If the patient is receiving total parenteral nutrition, provide scrupulous central venous catheter care.
- If bleeding occurs, apply ice compresses and pressure and elevate the extremity. Don't give the patient aspirin or aspirin-containing drugs, and don't administer rectal suppositories, take a rectal temperature, or perform a digital rectal examination.
- Take measures to prevent or alleviate adverse effects of treatment. For instance, you can control mouth ulceration by providing frequent mouth care and saline rinses.
- Administer blood component therapy as necessary.
- Administer prescribed pain medications as appropriate. Provide comfort measures, such as position changes and distractions, to help alleviate the patient's discomfort.
- Establish a trusting relationship to promote communication. Allow the patient and his family to express their anger, anxiety, and depression. Let the family partic-

ipate in the patient's care as much as possible.

• The patient with chronic lymphocytic leukemia is likely to be elderly and may feel frightened. Take the time to listen to his fears. Try to keep his spirits up by concentrating on little things, such as improving his personal appearance, providing a pleasant environment, and asking questions about his family. If possible, provide opportunities for favorite activities.

• Minimize stress by maintaining a calm, quiet atmosphere that's conducive to rest and relaxation.

• If the patient doesn't respond to treatment and has reached the terminal phase of the disease, he'll need supportive nursing care. Take steps to manage pain, fever, and bleeding; make sure the patient is comfortable; and provide emotional support for him and his family. If the patient wishes, provide for religious counseling. Discuss the option of home or hospice care.

Monitoring

• Monitor the patient's hematologic studies for evidence of improvement.

• Watch the patient closely for signs and symptoms of infection. Take the patient's temperature regularly. Screen staff members and visitors for contagious diseases. If the patient does develop any signs of infection – a temperature over 100° F (37.8° C), chills, or redness or swelling of any body part – report them at once.

• Be alert for signs of thrombocytopenia (easy bruising and nosebleeds, bleeding gums, and black, tarry stools) and anemia (pale skin, weakness, fatigue, dizziness, and palpitations). Also monitor the patient for bleeding.

• Monitor the patient for adverse effects of treatment, for example by checking his oral cavity regularly for ulcerations.

• Check the rectal area daily for induration, swelling, erythema, skin discoloration, and drainage.

• Monitor the effectiveness of administered analgesics and other comfort measures used to minimize or alleviate pain.

Patient teaching

• Describe the disease course, diagnostic tests, and treatments and their adverse effects.

• Teach the patient and his family how to recognize signs and symptoms of infection (fever, chills, cough, sore throat).

• Warn the patient about to be discharged to avoid coming into contact with obviously ill people, especially children with common contagious childhood diseases.

• Explain that if the chemotherapy causes weight loss and anorexia, the patient will need to eat and drink high-calorie, high-protein foods and beverages. If he loses his appetite, advise him to eat small, frequent meals. If the chemotherapy and adjunctive prednisone instead cause weight gain, he'll need dietary counseling.

• Instruct the patient to use a soft toothbrush and to avoid hot, spicy foods and commercial mouthwashes to prevent irritating the mouth ulcers that result from chemotherapy.

• Warn the patient to take care to prevent bleeding because his blood may not have enough platelets for proper clotting. Tell him to avoid aspirin and aspirin-containing drugs, and teach him how to recognize drugs that contain aspirin. Teach him the signs of abnormal bleeding (bruising, petechiae) and how to apply pressure and ice to the area to stop such bleeding. Urge him to report excessive bleeding or bruising to his doctor.

• Advise the patient to limit his activities and to plan rest periods during the day.

• Stress the importance of follow-up care, frequent blood tests, and taking all medications exactly as prescribed. Teach the patient the signs of recurrence (swollen lymph nodes in the neck, axillae, and groin; increased abdominal size or discomfort), and tell him to notify his doctor immediately if these signs occur.

• As appropriate, refer the patient and his family to the social service department, home health care agencies, hospices, and support groups such as the American Cancer Society.

Lithotripsy

A noninvasive procedure for removing obstructive renal calculi or gallstones, extracorporeal shock-wave lithotripsy (ESWL) uses high-energy shock waves to break up calculi and allow their normal passage. In this treatment, the patient is anesthetized. His affected kidney or the area containing the gallstone is positioned over an electric spark generator, which creates high-energy shock waves that shatter calculi without damaging surrounding tissue. Afterward, the patient is easily able to excrete the fine gravel-like remains of the calculi through the urinary tract or biliary ductal system.

ESWL may be performed as a preventive measure in a patient with potentially obstructive calculi or as an emergency treatment for an acute obstruction. Because ESWL is noninvasive, the procedure may be performed in the outpatient department and the patient can resume normal activities immediately after discharge. ESWL also minimizes many of the potentially serious complications associated with invasive methods of calculi removal, such as infection and hemorrhage.

ESWL isn't suitable for all patients, however. For instance, it may be contraindicated during pregnancy or in a patient with a pacemaker (because of potential electrical interference), with urinary or biliary tract obstruction distal to the calculi (which would prevent passage of fragments), with renal or gallbladder cancer, or with calculi that are fixed to the kidney, ureter, or gallbladder or located below the level of the iliac crest. Repeat treatments may be necessary for large or multiple calculi. (For information about another form of lithotripsy, see *Understanding percutaneous ultrasonic lithotripsy,* page 542.)

Procedure

Before undergoing ESWL, the patient receives a general or epidural anesthetic and has an I.V. line and indwelling urinary catheter inserted and electrocardiogram (ECG) electrodes attached. He's then placed in a semi-reclining position on the machine's hydraulic stretcher and positioned so that the shock-wave generator focuses directly on the calculi. Biplane fluoroscopy confirms proper positioning.

The generator is then activated to direct high-energy shock waves through the water at the calculi. To prevent disruption of the patient's cardiac rhythm, the shock waves are synchronized to the patient's R waves and fired during diastole. The number of waves fired depends on the size and composition of the stone; the patient may receive 500 to 2,000 shocks during a treatment.

After the shocks are delivered, the patient is removed from the tub and the ECG electrodes are removed.

Complications

Complications associated with ESWL include hemorrhage, hematoma formation, and obstruction from large fragments or collections of gravel.

Key nursing diagnoses and patient outcomes

Pain related to ESWL procedure. Based on this nursing diagnosis, you'll establish these patient outcomes. The patient will:

• express relief from pain following analgesic administration

• use relaxation techniques and diversional activities to minimize pain.

Fear related to inadequate knowledge or misunderstanding about shock-wave therapy. Based on this nursing diagnosis, you'll establish these patient outcomes. The patient will:

Understanding percutaneous ultrasonic lithotripsy

In this lithotripsy technique, an ultrasonic probe inserted through a nephrostomy tube into the renal pelvis generates ultrahigh-frequency sound waves to shatter calculi, while continuous suctioning removes the fragments. (See the illustration below.)

Percutaneous ultrasonic lithotripsy (PUL) may be used instead of ESWL, or it may be performed following ESWL to remove residual fragments. It's particularly useful for radiolucent calculi lodged in the kidney, which aren't treatable by ESWL.

Two stages

Some doctors prefer to perform PUL in two stages, with nephrostomy tube insertion on the 1st day followed by lithotripsy a day or two later, after intrarenal bleeding has subsided and the calculi can be better visualized. The day before scheduled treatment, the patient will have an I.V. pyelography or lower abdominal X-rays to locate the calculi.

Potential complications

Because PUL is an invasive procedure, it has many risks associated with surgical methods. Besides possibly causing hemorrhage and infection, it may lead to renal damage from nephrostomy tube insertion and ureteral obstruction from incomplete passage of calculi fragments.

Posttreatment care

After PUL, care measures include increased fluid intake, frequent nephrostomy tube irrigations, and straining of urine to capture passed calculi fragments and allow laboratory analysis of their composition. A day or two after treatment, the patient will have kidneys, ureters, and bladder X-ray or nephrostogram to check for retained fragments. If none are revealed, the doctor usually will remove the nephrostomy tube. Occasionally a patient will be discharged with the tube temporarily in place.

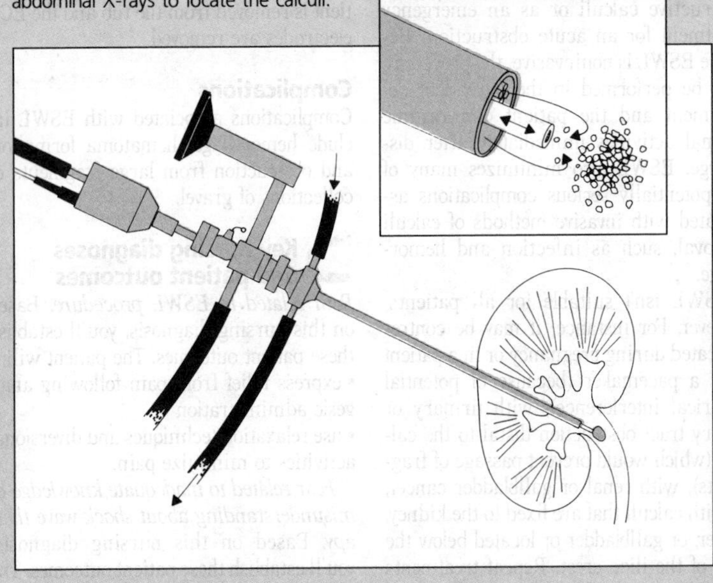

• verbalize his feelings of fear
• request information about ESWL from a knowledgeable source
• demonstrate fewer physical symptoms of fear.

Nursing interventions

When caring for a patient undergoing ESWL, your primary responsibilities will include instructing the patient and employing measures to ensure the passage of calculi fragments.

Before the procedure

• As necessary, review the doctor's explanation of ESWL with the patient and answer any questions. Explain who will perform the treatment and where, and tell him that it should take 30 minutes to 1 hour. Tell him that he'll receive a general or epidural anesthetic, depending on the doctor's preference, and that the treatment should be painless. However, if the patient will be receiving ESWL for gallstones, warn him that he may experience mild pain if his gallbladder undergoes spasms as it tries to expel the stone fragments. Tell the patient that he'll have an I.V. line and indwelling urinary catheter in place for a short time after ESWL.
• If possible, arrange for the patient to see the ESWL device before his first scheduled treatment. Explain its components and how they work.

After the procedure

• Check the patient's vital signs regularly. Notify the doctor of any abnormal findings.
• Maintain indwelling urinary catheter and I.V. line patency, and closely monitor intake and output. Strain all urine for calculi fragments, and send these to the laboratory for analysis. Note urine color and test pH. Remember that slight hematuria normally occurs for several days after ESWL. However, notify the doctor if you detect frank or persistent bleeding.
• Encourage ambulation as early as possible after treatment to aid passage of calculi fragments. For the same reason, increase fluid intake as ordered.
• To help remove any particles lodged in gravity-dependent kidney pockets, instruct the patient to lie face down with his head and shoulders over the edge of the bed for about 10 minutes. Have him perform this maneuver twice a day. To enhance its effectiveness, encourage fluids 30 to 45 minutes before starting.
• Assess for pain on the treated side, and administer analgesics, as ordered. Keep in mind that severe pain may indicate biliary or ureteral obstruction from new calculi; promptly report such findings to the doctor.

Home care instructions

• Instruct the patient to drink 3 to 4 qt (or liters) of fluid each day for about a month after treatment. Explain that this will aid passage of fragments and help prevent formation of new calculi.
• Teach the patient how to strain his urine for fragments. Tell him to strain all urine for the 1st week after treatment, to save all fragments in the container you've provided, and to bring the container with him on his first follow-up doctor's appointment.
• Discuss expected adverse effects of ESWL, including pain in the treated side as fragments pass, slight redness or bruising on the treated side, blood-tinged urine for several days after treatment (after removal of renal calculi), and mild GI upset. Reassure the patient that these effects are normal and are no cause for concern. However, tell him to report severe unremitting pain, persistent hematuria, inability to void, fever and chills, or recurrent nausea and vomiting.
• Encourage the patient to resume normal activities, including exercise and work, as soon as he feels able (unless the doctor instructs otherwise). Explain that physical activity will enhance the passage of calculi fragments.

• Stress the importance of complying with any special dietary or drug regimen designed to reduce the risk for new calculi formation.

Liver cancer

Having a high mortality, primary liver cancer accounts for roughly 2% of all cancers in North America and for 10% to 50% of cancers in Africa and parts of Asia. It's most prevalent in men, particularly those over age 60, and the incidence increases with age.

Most primary liver tumors (90%) originate in the parenchymal cells and are hepatomas (also called hepatocellular carcinomas or primary liver cell carcinomas). Some primary tumors originate in the intrahepatic bile ducts and are known as cholangiomas (also known as cholangiocarcinomas or cholangiocellular carcinomas). Rarer tumors include a mixed-cell type, Kupffer cell sarcoma, and hepatoblastoma, which occurs almost exclusively in children. Roughly 30% to 70% of patients with hepatomas also have cirrhosis, and a person with cirrhosis is about 40 times more likely to develop hepatomas than someone with a normal liver.

The liver is one of the most common sites of metastasis from other primary cancers, particularly melanoma and cancers of the colon, rectum, stomach, pancreas, esophagus, lung, or breast. In North America, metastatic liver cancer is about 20 times more common than primary liver cancer and, after cirrhosis, is the leading cause of fatal hepatic disease. Liver metastasis may occur as a solitary lesion, the first sign of recurrence after a remission.

No particular staging system exists for liver cancer. Although most hepatoblastomas are resectable, the prognosis is almost always poor. The disease is rapidly fatal – usually within 6 months – from GI hemorrhage, progressive cachexia, liver failure, or metastatic spread. When cirrhosis is present, the prognosis is especially grim, with death from liver failure usually occurring within 2 months of diagnosis.

Causes

The immediate cause is unknown. Liver cancer may result from environmental exposure to carcinogens, including the chemical compound aflatoxin (a mold that grows on rice and peanuts), thorium dioxide (a contrast medium used for liver radiography in the past), *Senecio* alkaloids and, possibly, androgens and oral estrogens. Another high-risk factor is exposure to the hepatitis B virus.

Whether cirrhosis is a premalignant state or whether alcohol or malnutrition predisposes the liver to hepatomas is unclear.

Complications

Progression of this disease may cause GI hemorrhage, progressive cachexia, and liver failure.

Assessment

The patient's history may show weight loss, resulting from anorexia, as well as weakness, fatigue, and fever. The patient also may complain of severe pain in the epigastrium or the right upper quadrant.

On inspection, you may note jaundice (including scleral icterus) and dependent edema. Peripheral edema may suggest decreased plasma albumin levels related to liver dysfunction and malnutrition. Auscultation may reveal a bruit, hum, or rubbing sound if the tumor involves a large part of the liver. Percussing the abdomen may uncover an increased span of liver dullness, indicating an enlarged liver. Dull sounds on percussion indicate ascites. Palpation may disclose a mass in the right upper quadrant and a tender, nodular liver.

Diagnostic tests

These findings support a diagnosis of liver cancer.

• *Liver biopsy,* by needle or open biopsy, reveals cancerous cells.
• *Liver function studies* are abnormal.
• *Alpha-fetoprotein* levels rise above 500 mcg/ml.
• *Chest X-rays* may rule out metastasis to the lungs.
• *Liver scan* may show filling defects.
• *Arteriography* may define large tumors.
• *Electrolyte studies* may indicate increased sodium retention (resulting in functional renal failure), hypoglycemia, hypercalcemia, or hypocholesterolemia.

Treatment

Because liver cancer may reach an advanced stage before diagnosis, few hepatic tumors are resectable. A resectable tumor must be solitary and not accompanied by cirrhosis, jaundice, or ascites. Resection is performed by lobectomy or partial hepatectomy.

Radiation therapy may be used alone or with chemotherapy. Chemotherapeutic drugs include fluorouracil, doxorubicin, methotrexate, cyclophosphamide, and vincristine. Combined therapy produces a better response rate than either therapy used alone.

Key nursing diagnoses and patient outcomes

Altered nutrition: Less than body requirements related to anorexia. Based on this nursing diagnosis, you'll establish these patient outcomes. The patient will:
• receive adequate nutritional intake daily, either orally or I.V.
• not develop signs or symptoms of malnutrition.

Anticipatory grieving related to threat of death. Based on this nursing diagnosis, you'll establish these patient outcomes. The patient will:
• verbalize his feelings about his diagnosis
• use appropriate coping behaviors to deal with the threat of death
• seek support from his family and friends.

Pain related to pressure from liver tumor on surrounding tissue. Based on this nursing diagnosis, you'll establish these patient outcomes. The patient will:
• express relief from pain after the administration of an analgesic
• use diversional activities to minimize pain.

Nursing interventions

• Give analgesics as ordered, and encourage the patient to identify care measures that promote comfort.
• As ordered, provide the patient with a special diet that restricts sodium, fluids, and protein and that prohibits alcohol.
• To increase venous return and prevent edema, elevate the patient's legs whenever possible.
• Keep the patient's fever down. Administer sponge baths and aspirin suppositories if the patient has no signs of GI bleeding. Avoid acetaminophen; the diseased liver can't metabolize it. If a high fever develops, the patient has an infection and needs antibiotics.
• Provide meticulous skin care. Turn the patient frequently, and keep his skin clean to prevent pressure ulcers. Apply lotion to prevent chafing, and administer an antipruritic for severe itching.
• As ordered, control ammonia accumulation with sorbitol (to induce osmotic diarrhea), neomycin (to reduce bacterial flora in the GI tract), lactulose (to control bacterial elaboration of ammonia), and sodium polystyrene sulfonate (to lower the potassium level).
• Prepare the patient for surgery, if indicated.
• If the patient has a transhepatic catheter in place to relieve obstructive jaundice, irrigate it frequently with the prescribed solution (0.9% sodium chloride or, sometimes, 5,000 units of heparin in 500 ml dextrose 5% in water).
• Throughout therapy, provide comprehensive supportive care and emotional assistance. Remember that throughout this in-

tractable illness, your primary concern is to keep the patient as comfortable as possible.
• At all times, listen to the concerns and fears of the patient and his family.

Monitoring
• Monitor the patient for fluid retention and ascites. Weigh the patient daily, and note intake and output accurately. If signs of ascites develop – peripheral edema, orthopnea, and dyspnea on exertion – measure and record the patient's abdominal girth daily.
• Monitor respiratory function. Note any shortness of breath or increase in respiratory rate. Bilateral pleural effusion (evident on chest X-ray) and metastasis to the lungs are common. Watch carefully for signs of hypoxemia from intrapulmonary arteriovenous shunting.
• Monitor the patient's temperature, and watch for signs and symptoms of infection.
• Watch for encephalopathy. Many patients develop end-stage symptoms of ammonia intoxication, including confusion, restlessness, irritability, agitation, delirium, asterixis, lethargy and, finally, coma. Monitor the patient's serum ammonia level, vital signs, and neurologic status.
• After surgery, watch for intraperitoneal bleeding and sepsis, which may precipitate coma. Monitor for renal failure by checking the patient's urine output, blood urea nitrogen, and serum creatinine levels hourly.

Patient teaching
• Explain the treatments to the patient and his family, including adverse reactions the patient may experience.
• Explain the importance of restricting sodium and protein intake and eliminating alcohol from the diet.
• Encourage the patient to learn and practice relaxation techniques to promote comfort and ease anxiety.
• If appropriate, direct the patient and his family to local support groups and services.

Lumpectomy

A lumpectomy is the removal of a malignant lump in the breast, leaving the breast itself intact. A lumpectomy with node dissection is the removal of the malignant lump along with nearby lymph nodes. Patients with early, small, well-defined lesions less than 5 cm in size and staged as 0, I, or II are candidates for lumpectomy. Unfortunately, fewer than 20% of breast cancer patients have this type of lesion. Following lumpectomy, most patients will undergo radiation therapy.

Lumpectomy has 5- and 10-year survival and local recurrence rates at least equivalent to those of the modified radical mastectomy. In addition, the psychological benefits of avoiding breast removal are significant, making this an especially appealing option for many women with breast cancer.

Procedure
After the patient has received anesthesia, the surgeon makes a small incision near the nipple. He then removes the tumor, a narrow margin of normal tissue surrounding the tumor and, possibly, nearby lymph nodes. The wound is closed and a small sterile dressing is applied.

Complications
Complications, although uncommon, include wound infection and delayed healing.

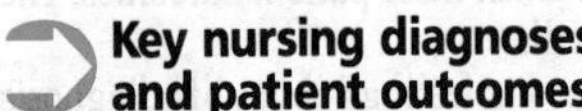

Key nursing diagnoses and patient outcomes
Anxiety related to potential change in breast appearance. Based on this nursing diagnosis, you'll establish these patient outcomes. The patient will:

• verbalize any feelings of anxiety
• use appropriate coping behaviors to deal with her anxiety
• show diminished physical signs of anxiety.

Knowledge deficit related to use of lumpectomy to treat breast cancer. Based on this nursing diagnosis, you'll establish these patient outcomes. The patient will:
• express a desire to learn the benefits and risks of lumpectomy for treating breast cancer
• obtain accurate information about lumpectomy
• make an educated decision regarding the potential use of lumpectomy in treating her breast cancer.

Nursing interventions

When caring for a patient undergoing lumpectomy, your primary responsibilities will include instructing the patient and providing general postoperative care.

Before surgery

• Always evaluate the patient's feelings about needing a lumpectomy for breast cancer, and determine her level of knowledge and expectations. Listen to her fears and concerns. Stay with her during periods of severe anxiety.
• Explain the surgical procedure to her, and inform her that she will have a dressing over the site and possibly a drain. If the patient is having the procedure done in the outpatient department, tell her that she can go home when she is fully recovered from the anesthesia.
• Check to be sure the consent form has been signed by the patient.

After surgery

• Inspect the dressing immediately upon return from the postanesthesia room and regularly thereafter. Report excessive bleeding promptly.
• Monitor vital signs. If a general anesthetic was given during surgery, monitor intake and output for at least 48 hours.
• Use strict aseptic technique when changing the dressing. Monitor the patient's temperature and white blood cell count closely.
• Administer an analgesic for pain as ordered, and perform comfort measures such as repositioning to promote relaxation and pain relief.
• Have the patient ambulate as soon as the anesthesia wears off.

Home care instructions

• Teach the patient how to care for the incision (and drain, if present) and change the dressing. Stress the importance of strict aseptic technique.
• Instruct the patient to wear a brassiere for support continuously for at least 1 week after surgery.
• Emphasize the importance of breast self-examination. Teach the patient how to do it, if necessary. Also review breast cancer warning signs with the patient. Women who have had breast cancer have a higher risk for recurrent cancer in the same breast as well as cancer in the other breast.
• Refer the patient and her family to hospital and community support personnel and services as indicated.

Lung cancer

The most common forms of lung cancer are squamous cell (epidermoid) carcinoma, small-cell (oat cell) carcinoma, adenocarcinoma, and large-cell (anaplastic) carcinoma. The most common site is the wall or epithelium of the bronchial tree.

For most patients, the prognosis is poor, depending on the cancer's extent when diagnosed and the cells' growth rate. Only about 13% of patients with lung cancer survive 5 years after diagnosis. Although the disease is largely preventable, it's the most common cause of cancer death in men. In women, lung cancer ranks with breast cancer as a leading cause of death.

Causes

Lung cancer's exact cause remains unclear. Risk factors include tobacco smoking, exposure to carcinogenic and industrial air pollutants (asbestos, arsenic, chromium, coal dust, iron oxides, nickel, radioactive dust, and uranium), and genetic predisposition.

Complications

Disease progression and metastasis cause various complications. When the primary tumor spreads to intrathoracic structures, complications may include tracheal obstruction; esophageal compression with dysphagia; phrenic nerve paralysis with hemidiaphragm elevation and dyspnea; sympathetic nerve paralysis with Horner's syndrome; eighth cervical and first thoracic nerve compression with ulnar and Pancoast's syndrome (shoulder pain radiating to the ulnar nerve pathways); lymphatic obstruction with pleural effusion; and hypoxemia. Other complications are anorexia and weight loss, sometimes leading to cachexia, digital clubbing, and hypertrophic osteoarthropathy. Endocrine syndromes may involve production of hormones and hormone precursors.

Assessment

Because early lung cancer may cause no symptoms, the disease may be advanced when it's diagnosed. While taking the patient's history, be sure to assess his exposure to carcinogens. If he's a smoker, determine pack years.

The patient's chief complaints may include coughing (induced by tumor stimulation of nerve endings), hemoptysis, dyspnea (from the tumor occluding air flow) and, sometimes, hoarseness (from tumor or tumor-bearing lymph nodes pressing on the laryngeal nerve).

On inspection, you may notice the patient become short of breath when he walks or exerts himself. You may also observe finger clubbing; edema of the face, neck, and upper torso; dilated chest and abdominal veins (superior vena cava syndrome); weight loss; and fatigue.

Palpation may reveal enlarged lymph nodes and an enlarged liver. Percussion findings may include dullness over the lung fields in a patient with pleural effusion.

Auscultation may disclose decreased breath sounds, wheezing, and pleural friction rub (with pleural effusion).

Diagnostic tests

- *Chest X-rays* usually show an advanced lesion and can detect a lesion up to 2 years before signs and symptoms appear. Findings may indicate tumor size and location.
- *Cytologic sputum analysis,* which is 75% reliable, requires a sputum specimen expectorated from the lungs and tracheobronchial tree, *not* from postnasal secretions or saliva.
- *Bronchoscopy* can identify the tumor site. Bronchoscopic washings provide material for cytologic and histologic study. The flexible fiber-optic bronchoscope increases test effectiveness.
- *Needle biopsy* of the lungs relies on biplanar fluoroscopic visual control to locate peripheral tumors before withdrawing a tissue specimen for analysis. The biopsy allows a firm diagnosis in 80% of patients.
- *Tissue biopsy* of metastatic sites (including supraclavicular and mediastinal nodes and pleura) helps to assess disease extent. Based on histologic findings, staging determines the disease's extent and prognosis and helps direct treatment. (See *Staging lung cancer.*)
- *Thoracentesis* allows chemical and cytologic examination of pleural fluid.

Additional studies include chest tomography, magnetic resonance imaging (MRI), bronchography, esophagography, and angiocardiography (contrast studies of bronchial tree, esophagus, and cardiovascular tissues). Tests that can detect metastasis include a

Staging lung cancer

The American Joint Committee on Cancer stages lung cancer using the tumor, node, metastasis (TNM) classification system.

Primary tumor

TX—primary tumor can't be assessed, or malignant tumor cells detected in sputum or bronchial washings but undetected by X-ray or bronchoscopy
T0—no evidence of primary tumor
Tis—carcinoma in situ
T1—tumor 3 cm or less in greatest dimension, surrounded by normal lung or visceral pleura; no bronchoscopic evidence of cancer closer to the center of the body than the lobar bronchus
T2—tumor larger than 3 cm; or one that involves the main bronchus and is 2 cm or more from the carina; or one that invades the visceral pleura; or one that's accompanied by atelectasis or obstructive pneumonitis that extends to the hilar region but doesn't involve the entire lung
T3—tumor of any size that extends into neighboring structures, such as the chest wall, diaphragm, or mediastinal pleura; or tumor in the main bronchus that doesn't involve but is less than 2 cm from the carina; or tumor that's accompanied by atelectasis or obstructive pneumonitis of the entire lung
T4—tumor of any size that invades the mediastinum, heart, great vessels, trachea, esophagus, vertebral body, or carina; or tumor with malignant pleural effusion

Regional lymph nodes

NX—regional lymph nodes can't be assessed
N0—no detectable metastasis to lymph nodes
N1—metastasis to the ipsilateral peribronchial or hilar lymph nodes or both
N2—metastasis to the ipsilateral mediastinal and the subcarinal lymph nodes or both
N3—metastasis to the contralateral mediastinal or hilar lymph nodes, the ipsilateral or the contralateral scalene, or the supraclavicular lymph nodes

Distant metastasis

MX—distant metastasis can't be assessed
M0—no evidence of distant metastasis
M1—distant metastasis

Staging categories

Lung cancer progresses from mild to severe as follows:
Occult carcinoma—TX, N0, M0
Stage 0—Tis, NO, MO
Stage I—T1, N0, M0; T2, N0, M0
Stage II—T1, N1, M0; T2, N1, M0
Stage IIIA—T1, N2, M0; T2, N2, M0; T3, N0, M0; T3, N1, M0; T3, N2, M0
Stage IIIB—any T, N3, M0; T4, any N, M0
Stage IV—any T, any N, M1

bone scan (abnormal findings may lead to a bone marrow biopsy, which is typically recommended in patients with small-cell carcinoma); a computed tomography scan or MRI of the brain; liver function studies; and gallium scans of the liver and spleen.

Treatment

Various combinations of surgery, radiation therapy, and chemotherapy improve the prognosis and prolong patient survival. Because lung cancer is usually advanced at diagnosis, most treatment is palliative.

Surgery is the primary treatment for Stage I, Stage II, or selected Stage III squamous cell carcinoma, adenocarcinoma, and large-cell carcinoma, unless the tumor is inoperable or other conditions (such as cardiac disease) rule out surgery. Surgery may involve partial lung removal (wedge resection, segmental resection, lobectomy, radical lobectomy) or total removal (pneumonectomy, radical pneumonectomy).

Preoperative radiation therapy may reduce tumor bulk to allow for surgical resection and may also improve response rates. Radiation therapy is ordinarily recommended for Stage I and Stage II lesions if surgery is contraindicated, and for Stage III disease confined to the involved hemithorax and the ipsilateral supraclavicular lymph nodes. Radiation therapy usually begins about 1 month after surgery (to allow the wound to heal). It's directed to the chest area most likely to develop metastasis.

Chemotherapy drug combinations of fluorouracil, vincristine, mitomycin, cisplatin, and vindesine induce a response rate ranging from 30% to 50% yet have minimal effect on long-term survival. Promising combinations of drugs for treating small-cell carcinomas include cyclophosphamide, doxorubicin, and vincristine; cyclophosphamide, doxorubicin, vincristine, and etoposide; and etoposide, cisplatin, cyclophosphamide, and doxorubicin.

Immunotherapy is investigational. Nonspecific regimens using bacille Calmette-Guérin vaccine or, possibly, *Corynebacterium parvum* offer the most promise.

In laser therapy, also largely investigational, a laser beam is directed through a bronchoscope to destroy local tumors.

Key nursing diagnoses and patient outcomes

Anticipatory grieving related to poor prognosis. Based on this nursing diagnosis, you'll establish these patient outcomes. The patient will:
- express his feelings about his diagnosis and the potential for death
- maintain control by making decisions about his care
- use appropriate behaviors to cope with the threat of death.

Fatigue related to hypoxia caused by impaired gas exchange. Based on this nursing diagnosis, you'll establish these patient outcomes. The patient will:
- explain the relationship between fatigue and his activity level
- employ measures to prevent and modify fatigue.

Impaired gas exchange related to pulmonary dysfunction. Based on this nursing diagnosis, you'll establish these patient outcomes. The patient will:
- express feelings of comfort in maintaining adequate air exchange
- perform his activities of daily living as tolerated
- maintain his respiratory rate within 5 breaths/minute of his baseline.

Nursing interventions

- Give comprehensive supportive care and provide patient teaching to minimize complications and speed the patient's recovery from surgery, radiation therapy, and chemotherapy.
- Urge the patient to voice his concerns, and schedule time to answer his questions. Be sure to explain procedures before performing them. This will help reduce the patient's anxiety.
- Prepare the patient for surgery, as indicated. (See the entry "Thoracotomy.")
- Ask the dietary department to provide soft, nonirritating, protein-rich foods. Encourage the patient to eat high-calorie between-meal snacks.
- Give antiemetics and antidiarrheals as needed with chemotherapy. Schedule patient care to help the patient conserve his energy.
- Impose reverse isolation if bone marrow suppression develops during chemotherapy.
- Provide meticulous skin care to minimize skin breakdown.

Monitoring

- Monitor the patient's respiratory status. Obtain arterial blood gases regularly, as ordered.

- Monitor the patient for adverse effects associated with surgery, chemotherapy, and radiation.
- Be alert for signs and symptoms of complications and metastasis.
- Evaluate the effectiveness of any medication administered, such as analgesics, antiemetics, and antidiarrheals.

Patient teaching

- Before surgery, supplement and reinforce what the doctor has told the patient about the disease and the operation.
- If the patient is receiving chemotherapy or radiation therapy, explain possible adverse effects of these treatments. Teach him ways to avoid complications such as infection. Also review reportable adverse reactions.
- Educate high-risk patients to reduce their chances of developing lung cancer or recurrent cancer.
- Refer smokers to local branches of the American Cancer Society or Smokenders. Provide information about group therapy, individual counseling, and hypnosis.
- Urge all heavy smokers over age 40 to have a chest X-ray annually and cytologic sputum analysis every 6 months. Also encourage patients who have recurring or chronic respiratory tract infections, chronic lung disease, or a nagging or changing cough to seek prompt medical evaluation.

Lupus erythematosus

A chronic inflammatory autoimmune disorder affecting the connective tissues, lupus erythematosus takes two forms: discoid lupus erythematosus (DLE) and systemic lupus erythematosus (SLE). DLE affects only the skin (see *Discoid lupus erythematosus,* page 552), whereas SLE affects multiple organs (including the skin) and can be fatal.

Researchers think that clinical signs and symptoms result from antibody-antigen trapping in specific organ capillaries. Like rheumatoid arthritis, SLE is characterized by recurrent seasonal remissions and exacerbations, especially during the spring and summer.

The annual incidence of SLE in urban populations varies from 15 to 50 per 100,000 persons. It strikes women 8 times more often than men (15 times more often during childbearing years). SLE occurs worldwide but is most prevalent among Asians and Blacks.

The prognosis improves with early detection and treatment but remains poor for patients who have cardiovascular, renal, or neurologic complications or severe bacterial infections. The disease is incurable.

Causes

The exact cause of SLE remains a mystery, but available evidence points to interrelated immune, environmental, hormonal, and genetic factors. Scientists think that autoimmunity is the primary cause. In autoimmunity, the body produces antibodies, such as antinuclear antibodies (ANAs), against its own cells. The formed antigen-antibody complexes then suppress the body's normal immunity and damage tissues. A significant feature in patients with SLE is their ability to produce antibodies against many different tissue components, such as red blood cells (RBCs), neutrophils, platelets, lymphocytes, or almost any organ or tissue in the body.

Certain predisposing factors may make a person susceptible to SLE. These include stress, streptococcal or viral infections, exposure to sunlight or ultraviolet light, immunization, pregnancy, and abnormal estrogen metabolism.

Complications

Concomitant infections, particularly urinary tract infections, and renal failure represent the leading causes of death for SLE patients.

Discoid lupus erythematosus

A form of lupus erythematosus marked by chronic skin eruptions, DLE can cause scarring and permanent disfigurement if untreated. About 5% of patients with DLE later develop SLE. An estimated 60% of patients with DLE are women in their late 20s or older. The disease seldom occurs in children. Its exact cause isn't known, although evidence suggests an autoimmune process.

Assessment

The patient with DLE has lesions that appear as raised, red, scaling plaques with follicular plugging and central atrophy. The raised edges and sunken centers give the lesions a coinlike appearance. Although these lesions can appear anywhere on the body, they usually erupt on the face, scalp, ears, neck, and arms or on any part of the body that is exposed to sunlight. Such lesions can resolve completely or may cause hypopigmentation or hyperpigmentation, atrophy, and scarring. Facial plaques sometimes assume the butterfly pattern characteristic of SLE. Hair becomes brittle and may fall out in patches.

Diagnostic tests

As a rule, the patient's history and the rash are enough to form the diagnosis. Positive findings in the LE cell test (in which polymorphonuclear leukocytes engulf cell nuclei to form so-called LE cells) occur in less than 10% of patients. Positive lesional skin biopsy results typically disclose immunoglobulins or complement components. SLE must be ruled out.

Treatment

Patients with DLE must avoid prolonged exposure to the sun, fluorescent lighting, and reflected sunlight. They should wear protective clothing, use sunscreen, avoid outdoor activity during peak sunlight periods (between 10 a.m. and 2 p.m.), and report any changes in the lesions.

As in SLE, drug treatment consists of topical, intralesional, and systemic medications.

Assessment

The onset of SLE, which may be acute or insidious, produces no characteristic clinical pattern. However, the patient may complain of fever, anorexia, weight loss, malaise, fatigue, abdominal pain, nausea, vomiting, diarrhea, constipation, rashes, and polyarthralgia. When taking the patient history, be sure to check the medication history.

SLE can involve every organ system. Women may report irregular menstruation or amenorrhea, particularly during flareups. In about 90% of patients, joint involvement resembles that of rheumatoid arthritis. Raynaud's phenomenon affects about 20% of patients. The patient may complain that sunlight (or ultraviolet light) provokes or aggravates skin eruptions. She may report chest pain (indicating pleuritis) and dyspnea (suggesting parenchymal infiltrates and pneumonitis).

Cardiopulmonary signs and symptoms occur in about 50% of patients. Watch for repeated arterial clotting to manifest itself in dyspnea, tachycardia, central cyanosis, and hypotension. These signs and symptoms may herald pulmonary emboli. Also be alert for altered level of consciousness, weakness of the extremities, and speech disturbances that point to cerebrovascular accident.

Seizure disorders and mental dysfunction may indicate neurologic damage. And some signs and symptoms signal added central nervous system (CNS) involvement.

They include emotional instability, psychosis, organic brain syndrome, headaches, irritability, and depression.

If the patient reports oliguria, be alert for possible renal failure. If she complains of urinary frequency, dysuria, and bladder spasms, watch for other signs of urinary tract infection.

During inspection, observe for skin lesions. Ordinarily, these eruptions appear as an erythematous rash in areas exposed to light. The classic butterfly rash over the nose and cheeks appears in less than 50% of patients. The rash may vary in severity from malar erythema to discoid lesions (plaque). Also watch for patchy alopecia, which is common.

Check the patient's vital signs, intake and output, and weight. Inspect the mucous membranes, noting any painless ulcers. Look at the patient's hands and feet. Vasculitis may develop, especially in the digits. Inspect the skin of the arms and legs for infarctive lesions, necrotic leg ulcers, and digital gangrene.

With palpation, you may detect lymph node enlargement (diffuse or local and nontender). During auscultation, note any signs of cardiopulmonary abnormalities, such as pericardial friction rub (signaling pericarditis). Also note tachycardia and other signs of myocarditis and endocarditis.

Diagnostic tests

Laboratory tests include a complete blood count with differential (which may show anemia and a reduced white blood cell [WBC] count); platelet count (which may be decreased); erythrocyte sedimentation rate (usually elevated); and serum electrophoresis (which may detect hypergammaglobulinemia).

Difficult to detect, CNS involvement may account for abnormal EEG results in about 70% of patients. But brain and magnetic resonance imaging scans may be normal in patients with SLE despite CNS disease. (For more information, see *Criteria for identifying SLE.*) Specific tests for SLE include the following studies.

- *ANA, anti-deoxyribonucleic acid (DNA),* and *lupus erythematosus (LE) cell tests* produce positive findings in most patients with active SLE, but they're only marginally useful in diagnosing the disease. The ANA test is sensitive but not specific for SLE, the anti-DNA test is specific but not sensitive, and the LE cell test is neither sensitive nor specific for SLE.
- *Urine studies* may detect RBCs, WBCs, urine casts and sediment, and significant protein loss (more than 3.5 g in 24 hours).
- *Blood studies* may demonstrate decreased serum complement (C3 and C4) levels, indicating active disease. Leukopenia, mild thrombocytopenia, and anemia also are seen during active disease.

Criteria for identifying SLE

Diagnosing SLE is far from easy because the disease so often mimics other disorders. Signs may be vague and may vary from patient to patient. For these reasons, the American Rheumatism Association has devised criteria for identifying SLE. Usually, four or more of the following signs must appear at some time in the disease course:

- discoid rash
- facial erythema (butterfly rash)
- hematologic abnormality (hemolytic anemia, leukopenia, lymphopenia, or thrombocytopenia)
- immune dysfunction (identified by positive LE cell, anti-DNA, or anti-Smith antibody tests; or false-positive test results for syphilis for more than 6 months)
- neurologic disorder
- nonerosive arthritis
- oral ulcers
- photosensitivity
- positive ANA test results
- renal disorder
- serositis.

• *Chest X-rays* may disclose pleurisy or lupus pneumonitis.
• *Electrocardiography* may show a conduction defect with cardiac involvement or pericarditis.
• *Renal biopsy* can show progression of SLE and the extent of renal involvement.

Treatment

The mainstay of SLE treatment is drug therapy. The patient with mild disease requires little or no medication. Nonsteroidal anti-inflammatory drugs, including aspirin, usually control arthritis and arthralgia symptoms. Skin lesions need topical medications and protection from exposure to the sun. Recommend that the patient use a sunscreen with a sun protection factor of at least 15. Topical corticosteroid creams, such as triamcinolone and hydrocortisone, may be administered for mild disease.

Fluorinated steroids may control acute or discoid lesions. And refractory skin lesions may respond to intralesional or systemic corticosteroids or antimalarials, such as hydroxychloroquine and chloroquine. Because hydroxychloroquine and chloroquine can cause retinal damage, such treatment requires ophthalmologic examination every 6 months. Dapsone helps many patients.

Corticosteroids remain the treatment of choice for systemic symptoms of SLE, for acute generalized exacerbations, and for serious disease-related injury to vital organ systems from pleuritis, pericarditis, nephritis related to SLE, vasculitis, and CNS involvement. With initial prednisone doses (equivalent to 60 mg or more), the patient's condition usually improves noticeably within 48 hours. With symptoms under control, the patient discontinues or slowly tapers prednisone use. (*Note:* Rising serum complement levels and decreasing anti-DNA titers indicate patient response.)

If the patient has glomerulonephritis, she'll need treatment with large doses of corticosteroids. Then, if renal failure occurs despite treatment, dialysis or kidney transplantation may be necessary.

In some patients, cytotoxic drugs such as azathioprine, cyclophosphamide, and methotrexate may delay or prevent renal deterioration. Antihypertensive drugs and dietary changes may also be effective. Additionally, warfarin is indicated for antiphospholipid antibodies, which can cause clotting in vascular structures.

Key nursing diagnoses and patient outcomes

Body image disturbance related to chronic skin eruptions. Based on this nursing diagnosis, you'll establish these patient outcomes. The patient will:
• acknowledge the change in her body image
• comply with the treatment regimen to minimize scarring and disfigurement
• express positive feelings about herself.

Impaired physical mobility related to chronic inflammation of connective tissues. Based on this nursing diagnosis, you'll establish these patient outcomes. The patient will:
• attain the highest degree of mobility possible
• not develop complications, such as contractures, venous stasis, thrombus formation, or skin breakdown.

Pain related to chronic inflammation of connective tissues. Based on this nursing diagnosis, you'll establish these patient outcomes. The patient will:
• express relief from pain following analgesic administration
• comply with the treatment regimen to minimize inflammatory response and thus reduce pain
• avoid activities that increase or precipitate pain.

Nursing interventions

• Provide a balanced diet. Foods high in protein, vitamins, and iron help maintain optimum nutrition and prevent anemia.

However, renal involvement may mandate a low-sodium, low-protein diet. Provide bland, cool foods if the patient has a sore mouth.
• Urge the patient to get plenty of rest. Schedule diagnostic tests and procedures to allow adequate rest.
• Explain all tests and procedures. Tell the patient that several blood samples are needed initially and periodically thereafter to monitor progress.
• Apply heat packs to relieve joint pain and stiffness. Encourage regular exercise to maintain full range of motion and to prevent contractures.
• Institute seizure precautions if you suspect CNS involvement.
• Warm and protect the patient's hands and feet if she has Raynaud's phenomenon.
• Arrange a physical therapy and occupational therapy consultation if musculoskeletal involvement compromises the patient's mobility.
• Support the patient's self-image. Offer female patients helpful tips. Suggest hypoallergenic cosmetics. As needed, refer her to a hairdresser who specializes in scalp disorders. Offer male patients similar advice, suggesting hypoallergenic hair care and shaving products.
• Offer the patient encouragement, emotional support, and thorough patient teaching.

Monitoring

• Continually assess for signs and symptoms of organ involvement. Specifically, monitor for hypertension, weight gain, and other signs of renal involvement.
• Assess for possible neurologic damage, signaled by personality changes, paranoid or psychotic behavior, depression, ptosis, and diplopia.
• Check urine, stools, and GI secretions for blood. Check the scalp for hair loss and the skin and mucous membranes for petechiae, bleeding, ulceration, pallor, and bruising.
• Watch for adverse reactions when administering medications, especially when administering high doses of corticosteroids or nonsteroidal anti-inflammatory drugs.
• Monitor the patient's response to therapy.
• Monitor the patient for signs and symptoms of infection. Take her temperature regularly.

Patient teaching

• Teach range-of-motion exercises and body alignment and postural techniques.
• Be sure the patient understands ways to avoid infection. Direct her to avoid crowds and people with known infections.
• Advise the patient to notify the doctor if fever, cough, or rash occurs or if chest, abdominal, muscle, or joint pain worsens.
• Instruct the photosensitive patient to wear protective clothing (hat, sunglasses, long-sleeved shirts or sweaters, and slacks) and to use a sunscreen when outdoors.
• Teach the patient to perform meticulous mouth care to relieve discomfort and prevent infection.
• Because SLE usually strikes women of childbearing age, questions associated with pregnancy commonly arise. The best evidence available indicates that a woman with SLE can have a safe, successful pregnancy if she sustains no serious renal or neurologic impairment. Advise her to seek additional medical care from a rheumatologist during her pregnancy. As indicated, explain that her doctors may order low-dose aspirin to reduce the risk of thrombosis during pregnancy.
• Warn the patient against trying unproven "miracle" drugs to relieve arthritis symptoms.
• Refer the patient to the Lupus Foundation of America and the Arthritis Foundation, as necessary.

Lyme disease

Named for the small Connecticut town in which it was first recognized in 1975, Lyme disease affects multiple body systems. It typically begins in summer or early fall with the classic skin lesion called erythema chronicum migrans. Weeks or months later, cardiac, neurologic, or joint abnormalities develop, possibly followed by arthritis. The incidence has risen in most states over the past 8 years.

Causes

Lyme disease is caused by the spirochete *Borrelia burgdorferi*. Carried by the minute tick *Ixodes dammini* (or another tick in the Ixodidae family), the disease occurs when a tick injects spirochete-laden saliva into the bloodstream or deposits fecal matter on the skin. After incubating for 3 to 32 days, the spirochetes migrate outward on the skin, causing a rash and disseminating to other skin sites or organs by the bloodstream or lymph system. The spirochetes' life cycle is incompletely understood; they may survive for years in the joints, or they may die after triggering an inflammatory response in the host.

Complications

Myocarditis, pericarditis, arrhythmias, heart block, meningitis, encephalitis, cranial or peripheral neuropathies, and arthritis are among the known complications of Lyme disease.

Assessment

Your assessment findings may be deceptive. Patient complaints vary in frequency and severity, probably because the illness typically occurs in stages.

The patient's history may reveal recent exposure to ticks—especially if he lives, works, or plays in wooded areas where Lyme disease is endemic. And he may report the onset of symptoms in warmer months. Typically reported symptoms include fatigue, malaise, and migratory myalgias and arthralgias. Nearly 10% of patients report cardiac symptoms, such as palpitations and mild dyspnea, especially in the early stage. Severe headache and stiff neck, suggestive of meningeal irritation, also may occur in the early stage when the rash erupts. At a later stage, the patient may report neurologic symptoms, such as memory loss.

Body temperature may rise to 104° F (40° C) in the early stage and be accompanied by chills. You may see erythema chronicum migrans, which begins as a red macule or papule at the tick bite site and may grow as large as 2″ (5 cm) in diameter. The patient may describe the lesion as hot and pruritic. Characteristic lesions (not seen in all patients) have bright red outer rims and white centers. They usually appear on the axillae, thighs, and groin. Within a few days, other lesions may erupt, as may a migratory, ringlike rash and conjunctivitis. In 3 to 4 weeks, the lesions fade to small red blotches, which persist for several more weeks.

Bell's palsy may be seen in the second stage and may occur alone. In the later stage, inspection may disclose signs and symptoms of intermittent arthritis: joint swelling, redness, and limited movement. Typically, the disease affects one or only a few joints, especially large ones, such as the knee.

Palpation of the pulse may detect tachycardia or irregular heartbeat. During the first or second stage, you may detect regional lymphadenopathy as well. The patient may complain of tenderness in the skin lesion site or the posterior cervical area. You'll note generalized lymphadenopathy less commonly.

If the patient has neurologic involvement, Kernig's and Brudzinski's signs usually aren't positive and neck stiffness usually occurs only with extreme flexion.

Diagnostic tests

Blood tests, including antibody titers to identify *B. burgdorferi,* are the most practical diagnostic tests. Or, the enzyme-linked immunosorbent assay (ELISA) may be ordered because of its greater sensitivity and specificity. However, serologic test results don't always confirm the diagnosis – especially in Lyme disease's early stages, before the body produces antibodies – or show seropositivity for *B. burgdorferi.* Also, the validity of test results depends on laboratory techniques and interpretation.

Mild anemia in addition to elevated erythrocyte sedimentation rate, white blood cell count, serum immunoglobulin M levels, and aspartate aminotransferase (formerly SGOT) levels support the diagnosis.

A lumbar puncture may be ordered if Lyme disease involves the central nervous system. Analysis of cerebrospinal fluid may detect antibodies to *B. burgdorferi.*

Treatment

A 10- to 20-day course of antibiotics is the treatment of choice. Adults typically receive tetracycline or doxycycline; penicillin and erythromycin are alternatives. Children usually receive oral penicillin. Administered early in the disease, these medications can minimize later complications. In later stages, high-dose penicillin (administered I.V.) or ceftriaxone (administered I.V. or I.M.) may produce good results.

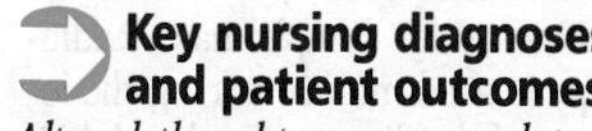

Key nursing diagnoses and patient outcomes

Altered thought processes related to neurologic dysfunction. Based on this nursing diagnosis, you'll establish these patient outcomes. The patient will:

- remain safe in his environment
- regain normal thought processes.

Fatigue related to infectious process. Based on this nursing diagnosis, you'll establish these nursing diagnoses. The patient will:

- express his understanding of measures to prevent or minimize fatigue
- incorporate measures necessary to modify fatigue into his daily routine
- regain his normal energy level.

Hyperthermia related to infectious process. Based on this nursing diagnosis, you'll establish these patient outcomes. The patient will:

- regain and maintain a normal temperature by taking antipyretic agents and by complying with treatment
- not develop any complications associated with hyperthermia, such as seizures and dehydration.

Nursing interventions

- Plan care to provide adequate rest.
- Ask the patient about possible drug allergies before administering antibiotics.
- Administer analgesics and antipyretics, as ordered.
- If the patient has arthritis, help him with range-of-motion and strengthening exercises, but avoid overexerting him.
- Protect the patient from sensory overload, and reorient him if needed. Also, encourage him to express his feelings and concerns about memory loss, if appropriate.

Monitoring

- Monitor the patient's vital signs, especially his temperature.
- Watch for signs and symptoms of complications, such as cardiovascular or neurologic dysfunction and arthritis.
- Monitor the effectiveness of administered medication.

Patient teaching

- Instruct the patient to take antibiotic medications as prescribed.
- Urge the patient to return for follow-up care and to report recurrent or new symptoms to the doctor.

HEALTH PROMOTION POINTERS

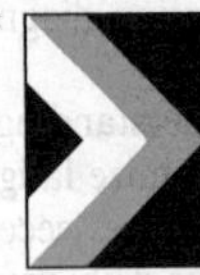

Preventing Lyme disease

To prevent Lyme disease, teach your patient to avoid tick exposure and how to remove attached ticks.

- Advise the patient, his family, and others to avoid tick-infested areas such as woods. If this is not possible, suggest they cover their skin with clothing, use insect repellents, and inspect exposed skin for attached ticks at least every 4 hours.
- If the patient comes in contact with a tick, advise him to use tweezers or forceps to pull the tick out, using firm traction. Caution him to carefully and firmly grasp the tick, taking care not to crush the insect or fail to remove the entire embedded body. Advise thorough hand washing after tick removal.

- Inform the patient, his family, and other caregivers about ways to prevent Lyme disease. (See *Preventing Lyme disease.*)

Lymphomas, malignant

Also called non-Hodgkin's lymphomas and lymphosarcomas, malignant lymphomas are a heterogeneous group of malignant diseases. They originate in lymph glands and other lymphoid tissue and are classified by different systems (see *Classifying malignant lymphomas*).

Causes

The cause of malignant lymphomas is unknown.

Complications

Malignant lymphomas can lead to hypercalcemia, hyperuricemia, lymphomatosis, meningitis, and anemia from bone marrow involvement. As tumors grow, they may produce liver, kidney, and lung problems. Central nervous system involvement can lead to increased intracranial pressure.

Assessment

Signs of malignant lymphomas may mimic those of Hodgkin's disease. Most patients' histories often reveal painless, swollen lymph glands. Swelling may appear and disappear over several months. As the lymphoma progresses, the patient may complain of fatigue, malaise, weight loss, and night sweats. Inspection may reveal enlarged tonsils and adenoids, and palpation may disclose rubbery nodes in the cervical and supraclavicular areas.

Diagnostic tests

Biopsies – of lymph nodes; of tonsils, bone marrow, liver, bowel, or skin; or, as needed, of tissue removed during exploratory laparotomy – differentiate a malignant lymphoma from Hodgkin's disease. Chest X-rays, lymphangiography, a computed tomography scan of the abdomen, excretory urography, and liver, bone, and spleen scans indicate disease progression.

A complete blood count may show anemia. The patient may have a normal or elevated uric acid level and an elevated serum calcium level, resulting from bone lesions.

The staging system for Hodgkin's disease also applies to malignant lymphomas.

Treatment

Radiation and chemotherapy serve as the main treatments for lymphomas. Radiation therapy is used mainly during the localized stage of the disease. Total nodal irradiation often effectively treats both nodular and diffuse lymphomas.

Chemotherapy is most effective with a combination of antineoplastic agents. Combinations – such as the cyclophosphamide, doxorubicin, vincristine (Oncovin), and prednisone protocol and the methotrexate, leucovorin, doxorubicin (Adria-

Classifying malignant lymphomas

Several classification and staging systems are being used to evaluate the extent of malignant lymphoma. Among the most common are the National Cancer Institute's (NCI) system (named the "working formulation for classification of non-Hodgkin's lymphomas for clinical usage"), the Rappaport histologic classification, and Lukes classification.

NCI working formulation	Rappaport histologic classification	Lukes classification
Low grade		
• Small lymphocytic	• Diffuse, well-differentiated, lymphocytic	• Small lymphocytic and plasmacytoid lymphocytic
• Follicular, predominantly small cleaved cell	• Nodular, poorly differentiated, lymphocytic	• Small cleaved follicular center cell, follicular only or follicular and diffuse
• Follicular mixed small and large cell	• Nodular, mixed lymphoma	• Small cleaved follicular center cell, follicular; large cleaved follicular center cell, follicular
Intermediate grade		
• Follicular, predominantly large cell	• Nodular, histiocytic lymphoma	• Large cleaved or noncleaved follicular center cell, or both, follicular
• Diffuse, small cleaved cell	• Diffuse, poorly differentiated lymphoma	• Small cleaved follicular center cell, diffuse
• Diffuse mixed, small and large cell	• Diffuse mixed, lymphocytic-histiocytic	• Small cleaved, large cleaved, or large noncleaved follicular center cell, diffuse
• Diffuse large cell, cleaved or noncleaved	• Diffuse, histiocytic lymphoma	• Large cleaved or noncleaved follicular center cell, diffuse
High grade		
• Diffuse large cell, immunoblastic	• Diffuse, histiocytic lymphoma	• Immunoblastic sarcoma, T-cell or B-cell type
• Small noncleaved cell	• Lymphoblastic, convoluted or nonconvoluted	• Convoluted T cell
• Large cell, lymphoblastic	• Undifferentiated, Burkitt's and non-Burkitt's diffuse undifferentiated lymphoma	• Small noncleaved follicular center cell
Miscellaneous		
• Composite • Mycosis fungoides • Histiocytic • Extramedullary plasmacytoma • Unclassifiable		

mycin), cyclophosphamide, vincristine (Oncovin), prednisone, and bleomycin protocol—can induce a prolonged remission and possibly a cure for diffuse lymphoma.

Because perforation commonly occurs in patients with gastric lymphomas, these patients usually undergo a debulking procedure before chemotherapy, such as a subtotal or total gastrectomy.

Key nursing diagnoses and patient outcomes

Altered nutrition: Less than body requirements related to chemotherapy or radiation therapy. Based on this nursing diagnosis, you'll establish these patient outcomes. The patient will:

- regain any lost weight and then maintain his weight within a normal range
- consume a nutritionally balanced diet each day
- not develop signs of malnutrition.

Fatigue related to anemia. Based on this nursing diagnosis, you'll establish these patient outcomes. The patient will:

- verbalize his understanding of measures to prevent or minimize fatigue
- incorporate the measures necessary to modify fatigue into his daily routine
- experience an increased energy level.

Risk for injury related to potential for hypercalcemia caused by bone involvement. Based on this nursing diagnosis, you'll establish these patient outcomes. The patient will:

- maintain a normal serum calcium level
- not exhibit signs of hypercalcemia.

Nursing interventions

- Administer pain medication, as ordered.
- Provide for rest periods if the patient tires easily.
- Offer the patient fluids such as orange juice or ginger ale to counteract nausea.
- Because this disease causes large numbers of tumors, provide the patient with plenty of fluids to help flush out the cells that are destroyed during treatment. This helps prevent tumor lysis syndrome.
- Provide a well-balanced, high-calorie, high-protein diet. Consult with the dietitian and plan small, frequent meals that include the patient's favorite foods. Schedule meals around the patient's treatment.
- If the patient can't tolerate oral feedings, administer I.V. fluids. If necessary, give antiemetics and sedatives, as ordered.
- Throughout therapy, listen to the patient's fears and concerns. Stay with him during periods of severe stress or anxiety. Encourage him to express his anger and concerns, and offer reassurance when appropriate.
- Involve the patient and his family in his care whenever possible.
- Prepare the patient for surgery, if indicated.

Monitoring

- Monitor the effectiveness of administered analgesics and other medications.
- Watch for complications of radiation and chemotherapy, such as nausea, vomiting, anorexia, hair loss, oral ulcers, and infection.
- Monitor the patient's complete blood count, uric acid level, and serum calcium level for abnormalities.
- Monitor the patient's nutritional and fluid intake. Weigh him daily.

Patient teaching

- Make sure the patient receives thorough explanations about all treatment.
- Instruct him to keep irradiated skin dry.
- Before surgery, explain preoperative and postoperative procedures thoroughly to the patient. Tell him that he may have a nasogastric tube or an indwelling urinary catheter inserted postoperatively.
- After chemotherapy and radiation therapy, advise the patient to avoid crowds and anyone who has an infection. Urge him to report any infection to his doctor.
- Stress the importance of a well-balanced, high-calorie, high-protein diet.
- Emphasize the importance of maintaining good oral hygiene during treatment to

prevent stomatitis. Instruct him to clean his teeth with a soft-bristled toothbrush and to avoid commercial mouthwashes.

• Teach relaxation and comfort measures, and encourage their use.

• If appropriate, refer the patient to the social service department, home health care agencies, hospices, and support groups such as the American Cancer Society.

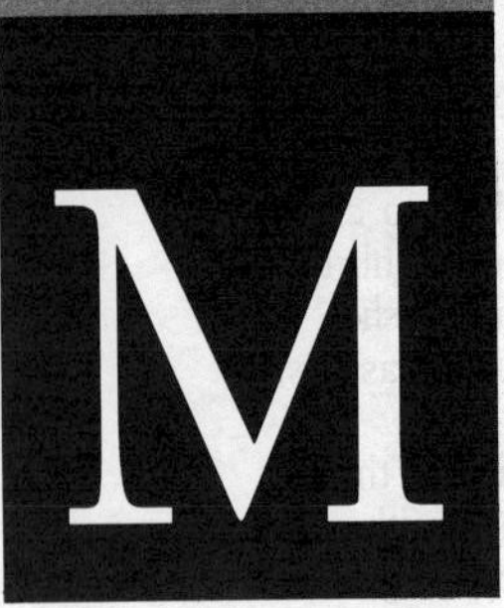

Magnesium imbalance

The second most abundant intracellular cation, magnesium functions chiefly to enhance neuromuscular integration. Changes in magnesium level affect neuromuscular irritability and contractility. Magnesium also stimulates parathyroid hormone (PTH) secretion, thus regulating intracellular fluid calcium levels.

Magnesium may also regulate skeletal muscle contraction through its influence on calcium utilization by depressing acetylcholine release at synaptic junctions. In addition, it activates many enzymes for proper carbohydrate and protein metabolism, aids in cell metabolism and the transport of sodium and potassium across cell membranes, and influences sodium, potassium, calcium, and protein levels.

Causes

Hypomagnesemia most commonly results from chronic alcoholism. The deficiency may also result from malabsorption syndromes, chronic diarrhea, prolonged nasogastric suction, or postoperative complications after bowel resection. It also may follow decreased intake or administration of parenteral fluids without magnesium salts; enteral or total parenteral nutrition without adequate magnesium content; increased renal excretion associated with prolonged diuretic therapy; and cisplatin, amphotericin, tobramycin, or gentamicin therapy. It may also follow excessive loss of magnesium, as in severe dehydration and diabetic acidosis; hyperaldosteronism and hypoparathyroidism; hyperparathyroidism and hypercalcemia; and excessive release of adrenocortical hormones.

Hypermagnesemia usually results from the kidneys' inability to excrete magnesium that was either absorbed from the intestines or infused. Common causes of hypermagnesemia include chronic renal insufficiency; overuse of magnesium-containing antacids, especially with renal insufficiency; severe dehydration; overdose of magnesium salts; and adrenal insufficiency.

Complications

Hypomagnesemia may result in transient hypoparathyroidism, interference with the peripheral action of PTH, seizures, and confusion that deteriorates to coma. Serious cardiac arrhythmias may also occur. Hypermagnesemia may cause complete heart block and respiratory paralysis.

Assessment

Generally, a patient with hypomagnesemia exhibits neuromuscular irritability and cardiac arrhythmias. A patient with hypermagnesemia may exhibit central nervous system and respiratory depression in addition to neuromuscular and cardiac effects. (See *Detecting magnesium imbalance.*)

Diagnostic tests

Serum magnesium levels determine imbalance. Values less than 1.5 mEq/liter or

Detecting magnesium imbalance

Both hypomagnesemia and hypermagnesemia may produce neuromuscular, central nervous system, cardiovascular, and GI effects.

System	Hypomagnesemia	Hypermagnesemia
Neuromuscular	• Hyperirritability, athetoid tetany • Leg and foot cramps • Chvostek's sign (facial muscle spasms induced by tapping branches of the facial nerve)	• Diminished deep tendon reflexes • Weakness, flaccid paralysis, respiratory muscle paralysis with high magnesium levels
Central nervous system	• Mood changes, confusion • Delusions, hallucinations • Seizures	• Drowsiness, confusion, diminished sensorium • Possible progression to coma
Cardiovascular	• Arrhythmias	• Bradycardia, weak pulse, hypotension, diffuse vasodilation • Heart block, cardiac arrest with high magnesium levels
GI	• Anorexia, nausea, vomiting	• Nausea, vomiting

1.8 mg/dl confirm hypomagnesemia; values more than 2.5 mEq/liter or 3.0 mg/dl indicate hypermagnesemia.

Low levels of other serum electrolytes (especially potassium and calcium) typically coexist with hypomagnesemia. In fact, unresponsiveness to correct treatment for hypokalemia strongly suggests hypomagnesemia. Similarly, elevated levels of other serum electrolytes are associated with hypermagnesemia.

Serum magnesium levels should be evaluated in combination with serum albumin levels because low albumin levels will decrease total magnesium while leaving the amount of free ionized magnesium unchanged.

Treatment

Therapy aims to identify and correct the underlying cause. Therapy for mild hypomagnesemia consists of dietary replacement and possibly daily oral magnesium supplements. For severe hypomagnesemia, it includes I.V. administration of magnesium sulfate (10 to 40 mEq/liter diluted in I.V. fluid). Magnesium intoxication is a possible adverse effect; its treatment requires calcium gluconate I.V.

Therapy for hypermagnesemia includes increased fluid intake and loop diuretics such as furosemide for the patient with impaired renal function; calcium gluconate (10%) I.V. (a magnesium antagonist) along with ventilatory support, for temporary relief of serious symptoms in an emergency, and peritoneal dialysis or hemodialysis if renal function fails or if excess magnesium can't be eliminated.

Key nursing diagnoses and patient outcomes

Decreased cardiac output related to arrhythmias. Based on this nursing diagnosis, you'll establish these patient outcomes. The patient will:

• maintain an adequate cardiac output, as evidenced by normal blood pressure and orientation to time, person, and place

• avoid signs and symptoms of cardiovascular collapse
• regain a normal heart rhythm.

Risk for injury related to neuromuscular irritability. Based on this nursing diagnosis, you'll establish these patient outcomes. The patient will:
• avoid complications associated with magnesium imbalance
• regain and maintain a normal serum magnesium level
• remain safe and injury free during times of magnesium imbalance.

Impaired gas exchange related to respiratory muscle paralysis. Based on this nursing diagnosis, you'll establish these patient outcomes. The patient will:
• maintain adequate ventilation with supportive care, such as mechanical ventilation
• avoid complications associated with impaired gas exchange
• regain normal respiratory function when his serum magnesium level returns to normal.

Nursing interventions

For hypomagnesemia:
• Provide a diet high in magnesium, and administer magnesium supplements, as ordered.
• With severe hypomagnesemia, initiate seizure precautions and take other measures to ensure patient safety if he's confused.
• Infuse magnesium supplements slowly, using an I.V. controller. Have calcium gluconate I.V. available for administration if the patient develops hypermagnesemia from overcorrection.
• Refer the alcoholic patient to a support group.

For hypermagnesemia:
• Provide sufficient fluids to ensure adequate hydration and maintain renal function.
• Administer diuretics and calcium gluconate (10%), as ordered.
• Prepare the patient for peritoneal dialysis or hemodialysis, as indicated. (See the entries "Peritoneal dialysis" and "Hemodialysis.")

Monitoring

For hypomagnesemia:
• Watch for and report signs of hypomagnesemia in patients at risk.
• Monitor serum electrolyte levels (including magnesium, calcium, and potassium) daily for mild deficits and every 6 to 12 hours during replacement therapy. Assess for signs and symptoms of electrolyte imbalances.
• Before giving food or medications, assess for dysphagia by testing the patient's ability to swallow water.
• Closely observe the patient who's receiving digitalis glycosides because hypomagnesemia predisposes him to digitalis toxicity.
• Monitor the electrocardiogram for arrhythmias, especially bradycardia and heart block.
• Assess the patient's vital signs during I.V. replacement therapy. Watch for decreased respirations and pulse rate.

For hypermagnesemia:
• Watch for signs of the disorder in patients at risk.
• Frequently assess the patient's level of consciousness, muscle activity, and vital signs, noting hypotension and shallow respirations.
• Monitor serum magnesium levels. Respiratory paralysis may occur when the serum magnesium level measures 10 to 15 mEq/liter. Report abnormal serum electrolyte levels immediately.
• Keep accurate intake and output records.
• Carefully monitor the patient who's receiving digitalis glycosides and calcium gluconate simultaneously. Calcium excess enhances digitalis glycosides' action, predisposing the patient to digitalis toxicity.

Patient teaching

For hypomagnesemia:

- Advise the patient to eat foods high in magnesium, such as seed grains, nuts, and legumes. Inform him that fresh meat, fish, and fresh fruits usually contain small amounts of magnesium.
- Warn a patient receiving parenteral magnesium that he may experience flushing and warmth secondary to peripheral vasodilation.
- Advise the patient to avoid laxative or diuretic abuse; this practice may result in loss of magnesium.

For hypermagnesemia:

- Advise a patient with renal failure to check with his doctor before taking any nonprescription medication.
- Caution the patient not to abuse laxatives and antacids containing magnesium, particularly if he's elderly or has compromised renal function.

Mallory-Weiss syndrome

Characterized by mild to massive and usually painless bleeding, Mallory-Weiss syndrome results from a tear in the mucosa or submucosa of the cardia or lower esophagus. Such a tear, usually singular and longitudinal, results from prolonged or forceful vomiting.

Sixty percent of these tears involve the cardia; 15%, the terminal esophagus; and 25%, the region across the esophagogastric junction. Mallory-Weiss syndrome is most common in men over age 40, especially alcoholics.

Causes

Forceful or prolonged vomiting is the direct cause of Mallory-Weiss syndrome. The tear in the gastric mucosa probably occurs when the upper esophageal sphincter fails to relax during vomiting. This lack of sphincter coordination seems more common after excessive intake of alcohol. Other factors or conditions that may increase intra-abdominal pressure and predispose a person to esophageal tearing include coughing, straining during defecation, trauma, seizures, childbirth, hiatal hernia, esophagitis, gastritis, and atrophic gastric mucosa.

Complications

Hypovolemia may develop if bleeding is excessive. Rarely, massive bleeding – usually from a tear on the gastric side near the cardia – quickly leads to fatal shock.

Assessment

Typically, the history will reveal a recent bout of forceful vomiting, followed by vomiting of bright red blood. The patient may describe this bleeding as mild to massive and may complain of accompanying epigastric or back pain. He also may report passing large amounts of blood rectally a few hours to several days after normal vomiting. Be alert for a history of hiatal hernia or alcoholism.

Diagnostic tests

- *Fiberoptic endoscopy* of esophageal tears confirms Mallory-Weiss syndrome. In most patients, lesions appear as recently produced, erythematous, longitudinal cracks in the mucosa. In older tears, lesions appear as raised, white streaks surrounded by erythema.
- *Angiography* (selective celiac arteriography) can determine the bleeding site but not the cause. This procedure may be used when endoscopy isn't available.
- *Serum hematocrit* helps quantify blood loss.

Treatment

Because GI bleeding usually stops spontaneously, treatment often consists of supportive measures and careful observation. However, treatment must be geared to the severity of bleeding. In some patients, blood transfusion is necessary. If severe

bleeding continues, other treatments may include:
• angiography, with infusion of a vasoconstrictor (vasopressin) into the superior mesenteric artery or direct infusion into a vessel that leads to the bleeding artery
• endoscopy with electrocoagulation or heater probe for hemostasis
• transcatheter embolization or thrombus formation with an autologous blood clot or other hemostatic material (insertion of artificial material, such as shredded absorbable gelatin sponge or, less often, the patient's own clotted blood through a catheter into the bleeding vessel to aid thrombus formation)
• surgery to suture each laceration (rare).

Key nursing diagnoses and patient outcomes

Altered nutrition: Less than body requirements related to inability to eat during acute bleeding episodes. Based on this nursing diagnosis, you'll establish these patient outcomes. The patient will:
• receive adequate nutritional supplementation during bleeding episodes
• avoid signs and symptoms of malnutrition
• resume a normal intake after treatment for the esophageal tear.

Anxiety related to bleeding caused by the esophageal tear. Based on this nursing diagnosis, you'll establish these patient outcomes. The patient will:
• express his feelings of anxiety
• develop effective coping mechanisms
• avoid severe signs of anxiety when a bleeding episode occurs.

Risk for fluid volume deficit related to potential for hemorrhage. Based on this nursing diagnosis, you'll establish these patient outcomes. The patient will:
• maintain stable vital signs and remain oriented to time, person, and place
• maintain an adequate fluid volume
• avoid hemorrhage.

Nursing interventions

• Provide support for the patient, particularly if bleeding has frightened him.
• Keep the patient warm during bleeding episodes.
• Insert a large-bore (14G to 18G) I.V. line, and start a temporary infusion of 0.9% sodium chloride solution, as ordered, in case transfusion is necessary.
• Draw blood for coagulation studies (prothrombin time, partial thromboplastin time, and platelet count), as well as typing and crossmatching. As ordered, keep units of crossmatched blood on hand. Transfuse blood if ordered.
• Avoid giving the patient medications that may cause nausea or vomiting.
• If surgery is necessary, prepare the patient for the scheduled operation.

Monitoring

• Regularly assess the patient's vital signs, urine output, and general clinical status.
• Monitor the patient's hemoglobin and hematocrit levels and red blood cell count.

Patient teaching

• Explain the disorder and its treatment.
• Advise the patient to avoid alcohol, aspirin, and other substances irritating to the GI tract.
• Encourage an alcoholic patient to join a support group, such as Alcoholics Anonymous, or refer him for counseling.

Mammoplasty

During mammoplasty, a surgical procedure to reshape the breast, the breast may be reduced, augmented, or reconstructed.

Breast reduction mammoplasty reduces breast size by removing excess breast skin and underlying tissue and reshaping the contour of large breasts. The surgeon also repositions the nipple and areola. Breast reduction usually is performed to relieve physical discomfort related to large breast size, including backache, shoulder ache, and irritation and fungal infection under the breast. However, it may be done simply because a woman is self-conscious about the size of her breasts. Although the procedure is permanent, breast size can increase with weight gain, use of birth control pills, and pregnancy. Breast reduction also may be performed on the unaffected breast in a patient who has had a mastectomy followed by breast reconstruction mammoplasty. In this case, the goal is to make the size of the unaffected breast closer to that of the reconstructed breast.

Breast augmentation mammoplasty may be performed to augment or enlarge breast size and shape. It usually is done because a woman is self-conscious about her small breasts.

Breast reconstruction mammoplasty is done to reconstruct the breast after surgery for cancer. Besides restoring a more normal breast shape, the surgery may help relieve emotional distress caused by mastectomy, improve the patient's self-image, and restore her sexual identity.

Mammoplasty is usually performed after the breasts are fully developed. It is not recommended for women who want to breast-feed. Breast reconstruction is contraindicated when metastasis is possible, if healing is impaired, or if the patient has unrealistic expectations about the procedure.

Procedure

The location of the incision varies, depending on the type of procedure and the surgeon's preference. For breast reduction, the surgeon may make an incision around the edge of the nipple or in the crease below the breast, following the breast's natural contour. He also may make a vertical, keyhole-shaped incision around the areola to allow repositioning of the nipple. He then removes excess tissue, fat, and skin from the sides of the breast and around the areola. Next, he moves the nipple, areola, and underlying tissue to a new, higher location on the breast. If the breasts are extremely large, he may completely detach the nipple and areola and then relocate them after removing the excess tissue. He then brings the skin flaps together to reform the breast.

In breast augmentation mammoplasty, the surgeon makes an incision under the breast just large enough to insert an implant. After inserting the implant, he closes the incision and applies a dressing.

In breast reconstruction mammoplasty, the surgeon may take one of three approaches. He may place an implant matching the size of the other breast under the muscle of the mastectomy site, creating a breast mound. Or, he may place a tissue expander under the muscle of the mastectomy site and gradually expand the area with 0.9% sodium chloride solution. This stretches the overlying skin and creates a pocket. The surgeon may remove the tissue expander and insert a permanent implant or the tissue expander may remain in place once the correct breast size has been achieved by saline injection. A third alternative involves autogenous procedures in which a flap of skin, fat, and muscle is transferred from a donor site to the mastectomy site. The flap contains an appropriate amount of fat to match the other breast and resembles breast tissue in appearance. To establish a blood supply, the surgeon reanastomoses vessels from the operative area to those of the flap when possible. Regardless of the procedure used, if the patient's own nipple is not available, the surgeon will construct a nipple using similar tissue, such as from the other nipple, the labia, or the thigh. After the nipple is attached, a dressing is applied or a surgical bra may be fitted.

Complications

Breast reduction causes scarring on the breast. Also, breast and nipple sensitivity may be reduced for up to 6 months. Other potential complications include hematoma formation and tissue ischemia in the nipple or areola.

Complications of breast augmentation vary with the type of implant. Recent studies show that silicone implants may leak or even burst, causing silicone to migrate into surrounding breast tissue. This may result in pain and tissue hardening.

Key nursing diagnoses and patient outcomes

Anxiety related to anticipated appearance of the breast after mammoplasty. Based on this nursing diagnosis, you'll establish these patient outcomes. The patient will:
• express her feelings of anxiety regarding mammoplasty
• discuss her concerns and fears with the surgeon before surgery, then express an understanding of the anticipated results
• exhibit no physical signs of anxiety.

Altered peripheral tissue perfusion related to tissue transferred for breast reconstruction. Based on this nursing diagnosis, you'll establish these patient outcomes. The patient will:
• maintain adequate perfusion in the transferred tissue, as evidenced by normal color, appearance, and temperature
• avoid complications, such as infection at the incision site, that could alter tissue perfusion.

Sensory/perceptual alterations (tactile) related to decreased sensation of the breast and nipple. Based on this nursing diagnosis, you'll establish these patient outcomes. The patient will:
• use safety measures to prevent injury to her breast and nipple
• regain normal sensation in the breast and nipple.

Nursing interventions

When caring for a patient undergoing mammoplasty, your primary responsibilities include instructing the patient and monitoring for postoperative complications.

Before surgery

• Explain the procedure to the patient and answer any questions, to reduce her anxiety.
• Inform the patient that blood transfusions may be necessary during surgery, and suggest that she give blood in advance for autotransfusion.
• Verify that the patient has signed a consent form.

After surgery

• Inspect the dressing for drainage. When changing dressings, assess the incision and flap (if present) for signs of infection, such as redness, drainage, and odor. Assess transplanted tissue used in breast reconstruction for poor perfusion, as shown by blanching, duskiness, and decreased capillary refill. Notify the doctor if you detect excessive bleeding, infection, or decreased perfusion.
• Avoid pressure on flap or suture lines by positioning the patient on the nonoperative side.
• Administer analgesics, as ordered, to relieve pain.
• Encourage the patient to ambulate and to move her arms and legs.
• Monitor the patient's vital signs closely.

Home care instructions

• Teach the patient the importance of taking analgesics to avoid impaired arm movement.
• Inform the patient that the surgical dressings will be removed after 1 week. Instruct her to wear a soft bra for several weeks, keeping it on even at night. Also tell her the sutures will be removed 2 to 3 weeks after surgery.
• Reassure the patient that swelling and skin discoloration of the breast are normal and will subside in several days. Also tell her that scars may remain visible for up to 1 year but will eventually fade.
• Instruct the patient to avoid excessive movement and overhead lifting for 3 to 4 weeks or as advised by the doctor. Inform

her that she may return to work 2 weeks after surgery.

Mastectomy

A mastectomy is performed primarily to remove malignant breast tissue and any regional lymphatic metastases. It may be combined with radiation therapy and chemotherapy. Until recently, radical mastectomy was the treatment of choice for breast cancer. Now, several different types of mastectomy can be performed, depending on the size of the tumor and the presence of any metastases. (See *Types of mastectomy.*)

Procedure

In a total mastectomy, the surgeon removes the entire breast without dissecting the lymph nodes. He may apply a skin graft if necessary.

If the surgeon is performing a modified radical mastectomy, he may use one of several techniques to remove the entire breast. He also resects all axillary lymph nodes, while leaving the pectoralis major intact. He may or may not remove the pectoralis minor. If the patient has small lesions and no metastases, the surgeon may perform breast reconstruction immediately or a few days later.

In a radical mastectomy, the surgeon removes the entire breast, axillary lymph nodes, underlying pectoral muscles, and adjacent tissues. He covers the skin flaps and exposed tissue with moist packs for protection and, before closure, irrigates the chest wall and axilla.

In an extended radical mastectomy, the surgeon removes the breast, underlying pectoral muscles, axillary contents, and upper internal mammary (mediastinal) lymph node chain.

After closing the mastectomy site, the surgeon may make a stab wound and insert a drain or catheter. The drain or catheter removes blood that may collect under the skin flaps, where it could prevent healing and lead to infection. Less commonly, he may use large pressure dressings instead.

If a graft was needed to close the wound, he'll probably place a pressure dressing over the donor site.

Types of mastectomy

If a tumor is confined to breast tissue and no lymph node involvement is detected, a lumpectomy or *total (simple) mastectomy* may be performed. A total mastectomy may also be used palliatively for advanced, ulcerative cancer and as a treatment for extensive benign disease.

A *modified radical mastectomy,* the standard surgery for Stage I and II lesions, removes small, localized tumors. It has replaced radical mastectomy as the most widely used surgical procedure for treating breast cancer. Besides causing less disfigurement than a radical mastectomy, it reduces postoperative arm edema and shoulder problems.

A *radical mastectomy* controls the spread of larger, metastatic lesions. Later, breast reconstruction may be performed using a portion of the latissimus dorsi. Rarely, an *extended radical mastectomy* may be used to treat cancer in the medial quadrant of the breast or in subareolar tissue. This procedure is done to prevent possible metastasis to the internal mammary lymph nodes.

Complications

After any type of mastectomy, infection and delayed healing are possible. However, the major complication of radical mastectomy and axillary dissection is lymphedema, which may occur soon after surgery and persist for years. Dissection of the lymph nodes draining the axilla may interfere with lymphatic drainage of the arm on the affected side.

Key nursing diagnoses and patient outcomes

Body image disturbance related to loss of a breast. Based on this nursing diagnosis, you'll establish these patient outcomes. The patient will:
• express recognition of the change in her body image
• demonstrate control over her situation by participating in care decisions after the mastectomy
• express positive feelings about herself.

Risk for infection related to lymph fluid stasis caused by lymphedema secondary to mastectomy with axillary lymph node dissection. Based on this nursing diagnosis, you'll establish these patient outcomes. The patient will:
• take precautions to prevent lymphedema
• maintain a normal temperature and white blood cell count
• avoid signs and symptoms of infection.

Impaired physical mobility related to surgical incision on the affected side, loss of muscle tissue with radical and extended radical mastectomy, and potential lymphedema. Based on this nursing diagnosis, you'll establish these patient outcomes. The patient will:
• correctly perform prescribed postoperative exercises
• take safety precautions to prevent injuring her affected arm, such as avoiding blood pressure measurement on or blood withdrawal from the affected arm
• regain movement of the affected arm.

Nursing interventions

When caring for a patient undergoing a mastectomy, your primary responsibilities include instruction and monitoring for postoperative complications.

Before surgery

• Mastectomy may be more threatening to a woman's self-image than any other type of surgery. Be sure to explore the patient's feelings about it. Typically, she'll be afraid and anxious. She may have many questions but may feel too confused or upset to ask them. Be a supportive, caring listener, and help her express her concerns. Discuss her sexuality and her relationship with her sex partner to identify possible conflicts about the surgery and the degree of support she can expect from her partner afterward.
• Review the surgeon's explanation of the procedure. Also prepare the patient for her postoperative care. Explain that a drain or catheter and suction may be used to drain the incision and that the arm on her affected side will be elevated. She'll have to sit up and turn in bed by pushing up with her unaffected arm (but not pulling). Tell her she'll begin arm and shoulder exercises shortly after surgery. Demonstrate the exercises and have her repeat them.
• Provide other information, such as about the types of breast prostheses available. However, most women will need to concentrate on dealing with the upcoming surgery and the immediate recovery period. Consequently, defer discussion of rehabilitation until after surgery.
• Take arm measurements on both sides to obtain baseline data. If the patient will have a radical mastectomy, explain that the skin on the anterior surface of one thigh may be shaved and prepared in case she needs a graft.
• Verify that the patient has signed a consent form.

After surgery

• When the patient returns to the unit, elevate her arm on a pillow to enhance circulation and prevent edema. Periodically check the suction tubing to ensure proper function, and observe the drainage site for erythema, induration, and drainage. Using aseptic technique, measure and record drainage every 8 hours. Keep in mind that drainage should change from sanguineous to serosanguineous fluid. After 2 to 3 days, you may need to milk the drain periodically to prevent clots from occluding the tubing.

• As ordered, teach the patient arm exercises to prevent muscle shortening and contracture of the shoulder joint and to promote lymph drainage. The surgeon will determine the optimal time for initiating these exercises, based on the degree of healing, the presence of a drainage tube, and the tension placed on skin flaps and sutures with movement. You can usually initiate arm flexion and extension on the first postoperative day and then add exercises each day, depending on the patient's needs and the procedure performed.
• Plan an exercise program with the patient. Such exercises may include climbing the wall with her hands, arm swinging, and rope pulling.
• To prevent lymphedema, make sure no blood pressure readings, injections, or venipunctures are performed on the affected arm. Place a sign bearing this message at the head of the patient's bed.
• Because mastectomy causes emotional distress, teach the patient to conserve her energy and to recognize early signs of fatigue. Gently encourage her to look at the operative site by describing its appearance and allowing her to express her feelings. Be sure to be present when she looks at the wound for the first time.
• Arrange for a volunteer who's had a mastectomy to talk with the patient. Contact the American Cancer Society's rehabilitation program, Reach to Recovery.
• After 2 to 3 days, initiate a fitting for a temporary breast pad. Soft and lightweight, the pad may be inserted into a bra without stays or underwires.

If appropriate, explain breast reconstruction.

Home care instructions

• Inform the patient that preventing lymphedema is critical. Explain that swelling may follow even minor trauma to the arm on her affected side. Tell her to promptly wash cuts and scrapes on the affected side and to contact the doctor immediately if erythema, edema, or induration occurs.
• Advise the patient to use the affected arm as much as possible and to avoid keeping it in a dependent position for a prolonged period.
• Reinforce the importance of performing range-of-motion exercises daily. Instruct the patient to do them with both arms to maintain symmetry and prevent additional deformities.
• Emphasize the importance of not allowing blood pressure readings, injections, or venipunctures on the affected arm.
• Remind the patient that her energy level will wax and wane. Instruct her to be alert for signs of fatigue and to rest frequently during the day for the first few weeks after discharge.
• Stress the importance of monthly self-examination of the unaffected breast and the mastectomy site. Demonstrate the correct examination technique, and have the patient repeat it.
• Explain the importance of keeping scheduled postoperative appointments.
• If necessary, provide information regarding a permanent prosthesis, which can be fitted 3 to 4 weeks after surgery. Prostheses are available in a wide range of styles, skin tones, and weights from lingerie shops, medical supply stores, and department stores.
• Reassure the patient that she can wear the same type of clothing she wore before her surgery.

Mastitis

Parenchymatous inflammation of the mammary glands, or mastitis, occurs postpartum in about 1% of lactating women, mainly in primiparas who are breast-feeding. It occurs occasionally in nonlactating women and rarely in men. The prognosis is good.

Causes

Mastitis develops when a pathogen that typically originates in the nursing infant's nose or pharynx invades breast tissue through a fissured or cracked nipple and disrupts normal lactation. The most common pathogen is *Staphylococcus aureus;* less frequently, it's *S. epidermidis* or beta-hemolytic streptococci. Rarely, mastitis may result from disseminated tuberculosis or the mumps virus.

Predisposing factors include a fissure or abrasion of the nipple, blocked milk ducts, and an incomplete let-down reflex, usually due to emotional trauma. Blocked milk ducts can result from a tight bra or prolonged intervals between breast-feedings.

Complications

An untreated breast infection can lead to abscess.

Assessment

Usually the patient reports a fever of 101° F (38.3° C) or higher, malaise, and flulike symptoms that develop 2 to 4 weeks postpartum (although these findings may develop at any time during lactation). Inspection and palpation typically uncover such classic signs as redness, swelling, warmth, hardness, tenderness, nipple cracks or fissures, and enlarged axillary lymph nodes.

Diagnostic tests

Cultures of expressed milk confirm generalized mastitis; cultures of breast skin surface confirm localized mastitis. Such cultures also determine appropriate antibiotic treatment.

Treatment

Antibiotic therapy, the primary treatment, usually consists of penicillin G to combat staphylococci; erythromycin or kanamycin is used for penicillin-resistant strains. Cephalosporin or dicloxacillin are also used. Symptoms usually subside in 2 to 3 days, but antibiotic therapy should continue for 10 days.

Other appropriate measures include analgesics for pain and, rarely, incision and drainage of a breast abscess.

Key nursing diagnoses and patient outcomes

Risk for impaired skin integrity related to potential development or exacerbation of cracks or fissures. Based on this nursing diagnosis, you'll establish these patient outcomes. The patient will:

- avoid cracks and fissures or, if these are present, avoid exacerbation of the condition
- regain normal tissue integrity.

Ineffective breast-feeding related to inflammation of breast tissue. Based on this nursing diagnosis, you'll establish these patient outcomes. The patient will:

- maintain her ability to lactate
- resume effective breast-feeding after mastitis resolves.

Pain related to inflammation of breast tissue. Based on this nursing diagnosis, you'll establish these patient outcomes. The patient will:

- express relief of pain after analgesic administration
- use nonpharmacologic measures to reduce and alleviate pain
- become pain free.

Nursing interventions

- Give analgesics as needed. Provide comfort measures, such as warm soaks.
- Use meticulous hand-washing technique and provide good skin care.

Monitoring

- Regularly measure the patient's temperature and assess the effectiveness of antipyretic agents.
- Monitor the patient's response to administered analgesics and comfort measures.
- Inspect the patient's breasts daily for signs of impaired skin integrity, such as cracks or fissures.

Patient teaching

- Advise the patient to take antibiotics as ordered. Stress the need to take the entire prescribed amount even if symptoms improve in the meantime.

• Reassure the patient that breast-feeding during mastitis won't harm her infant because the infant is the source of the infection.
• If only one breast is affected, instruct the patient to offer the infant this breast first to promote complete emptying and prevent clogged ducts. However, if an open abscess develops, she must stop breast-feeding with this breast and use a breast pump until the abscess heals. She should continue to breast-feed on the unaffected side.
• Suggest applying a warm, wet towel to the affected breast or taking a warm shower to relax and improve her ability to breast-feed.

To prevent mastitis:
• Stress the need to completely empty the breasts because stasis of milk causes infection.
• Teach the patient to alternate nursing positions to facilitate complete breast emptying and rotate pressure areas on the nipples.
• Show the patient how to position the infant properly on the breast to prevent cracked nipples. The entire areola of the nipple should be in the infant's mouth.
• Advise the patient to expose sore nipples to the air as often as possible.
• Teach her proper hand-washing technique and personal hygiene.
• Stress the importance of getting plenty of rest, drinking sufficient fluids, and maintaining a balanced diet to enhance her ability to breast-feed.

Medullary sponge kidney

In this disorder, the collecting ducts in the renal pyramids dilate and cavities, clefts, and cysts form in the medulla. Medullary sponge kidney may affect only a single pyramid in one kidney or all pyramids in both kidneys. Although an affected kidney may be of normal size, it's usually somewhat enlarged and spongy.

Because this disorder typically is asymptomatic and benign, it's commonly overlooked until the patient reaches adulthood. Although found in both sexes and in all age-groups, it's usually diagnosed in adolescents and in adults ages 30 to 50. It occurs in about 1 in every 5,000 persons. The prognosis is good.

Medullary sponge kidney is unrelated to medullary cystic disease, a hereditary disorder. These conditions are similar only in the presence and location of the cysts.

Causes

Medullary sponge kidney may be transmitted as an autosomal dominant trait, but this remains unproven. Most nephrologists consider it a congenital abnormality.

Complications

Occurring in 30% to 60% of patients, complications include formation of calcium oxalate calculi, which lodge in the dilated cystic collecting ducts or pass through a ureter, and infection from dilation of the ducts. Hypertension and renal failure seldom occur, except in patients with severe infection or nephrolithiasis. Secondary impairment of renal function from obstruction and infection occurs in about 10% of patients.

Assessment

Clinical features usually appear only as a result of complications and seldom occur before young adulthood. The patient may complain of severe colic, hematuria, burning on urination, urgency, and frequency – all signs and symptoms of a lower urinary tract infection (UTI). He also may report signs and symptoms of pyelonephritis – sudden onset of chills, fever, dull flank pain, and costovertebral angle tenderness.

Diagnostic tests

Excretory urography, usually the key to diagnosis, typically reveals a characteristic flowerlike appearance of the pyramidal cavities when they fill with contrast medium. It also may show renal calculi.

Urinalysis is normal unless complications develop, such as an increased white blood cell count and casts with infection or an increased red blood cell count with hematuria. It may show hypercalciuria or a slight reduction in concentrating ability.

Diagnosis must distinguish medullary sponge kidney from renal tuberculosis, renal tubular acidosis, and papillary necrosis. If infection is suspected, calculi should be evaluated.

Treatment

Treatment focuses on preventing or treating complications caused by calculi and infection. Specific measures include increasing fluid intake and monitoring renal function and urine output. If new symptoms develop, the patient needs immediate evaluation.

Because medullary sponge kidney is benign, surgery seldom is necessary, except to remove calculi during acute obstruction. Only serious, uncontrollable infection or hemorrhage necessitates nephrectomy.

Key nursing diagnoses and patient outcomes

Altered urinary elimination related to renal complications. Based on this nursing diagnosis, you'll establish these patient outcomes. The patient will:

- avoid signs and symptoms of severe renal impairment, such as oliguria and anuria
- regain a normal urinary elimination pattern.

Risk for infection related to dilation of collecting ducts in the renal pyramids. Based on this nursing diagnosis, you'll establish these patient outcomes. The patient will:

- maintain a normal temperature and white blood cell count
- avoid signs or symptoms of UTI or pyelonephritis
- remain free of infection.

Pain related to renal calculi. Based on this nursing diagnosis, you'll establish these patient outcomes. The patient will:

- express relief of pain after analgesic administration
- become pain free after calculi are removed.

Nursing interventions

- Limit the patient's dietary calcium intake to prevent calculus formation.
- When the patient is hospitalized for calculi, strain all urine and give analgesics to relieve pain.
- Before diagnostic tests that use a contrast medium, ask about previous allergic reaction to shellfish, iodine, or contrast medium. If the patient has had such a reaction, the doctor may cancel the test, do a limited study without a contrast medium, or pretreat the patient with antihistamines or steroids.
- If infection occurs, administer the prescribed antibiotic either I.V. or by mouth.
- Provide at least 2,000 ml of fluids daily by mouth (or parenterally if the patient has difficulty swallowing).

Monitoring

- Observe the patient for signs and symptoms of renal complications, such as calculi, infection, and renal impairment.
- Monitor the patient's response to therapy.

Patient teaching

- Explain the disorder to the patient and his family. Stress that the condition is benign and the prognosis is good, but warn them to watch for and report any signs of calculus passage or UTI.
- Explain all tests, and demonstrate how to collect a clean-catch urine specimen for culture and sensitivity tests.
- To prevent UTI, instruct the patient to bathe often and use proper toilet hygiene.

Melanoma, malignant

A neoplasm that arises from melanocytes, malignant melanoma is potentially the most lethal of the skin cancers. It accounts for 3% of all cancers and its incidence is rapidly increasing. Melanoma is slightly more common in women than in men and is unusual in children. Peak incidence occurs between ages 50 and 70, although the incidence in younger age-groups is increasing.

Melanoma spreads through the lymphatic and vascular systems and metastasizes to the regional lymph nodes, skin, liver, lungs, and central nervous system. Its course is unpredictable, however, and recurrence and metastases may not appear for more than 5 years after resection of the primary lesion. The prognosis varies with the tumor thickness. In most patients, superficial lesions are curable, whereas deeper lesions tend to metastasize.

Common sites for melanoma are the head and neck in men, the legs in women, and the backs of people exposed to excessive sunlight. Up to 70% of malignant melanomas arise from a preexisting nevus.

There are four types of melanomas.

- *Superficial spreading melanoma,* the most common type (accounting for 50% to 70% of cases), usually develops between ages 40 and 50.
- *Nodular melanoma* usually develops between ages 40 and 50 (accounting for 12% to 30% of cases). It grows vertically, invades the dermis, and metastasizes early.
- *Acral-lentiginous melanoma* is the most common melanoma among Hispanics, Asians, and Blacks. It occurs on palms and soles and in sublingual locations.
- *Lentigo maligna melanoma* is relatively rare (accounting for 4% to 10% of cases). This is the most benign, the slowest growing, and the least aggressive of the four types. It most commonly occurs in areas heavily exposed to the sun. It arises from a lentigo maligna on an exposed skin surface and usually occurs between ages 60 and 70.

Causes

Several factors may influence the development of melanoma.

- *Excessive exposure to sunlight.* Melanoma occurs most commonly in sunny, warm areas and often develops on body parts that are exposed to the sun.
- *Skin type.* Most people who develop melanoma have blond or red hair, fair skin, and blue eyes; are prone to sunburn; and are of Celtic or Scandinavian ancestry. Melanoma is rare among Blacks; when it does develop, it usually arises in lightly pigmented areas (the palms, plantar surface of the feet, or mucous membranes).
- *Genetic factors.* Familial atypical multiple mole melanoma (FAMMM) syndrome is characterized by multiple dysplastic nevi; it carries an extremely high lifetime risk of melanoma.
- *Family history.* Melanoma occurs slightly more often within families.
- *Past history of melanoma.* A person who has had one melanoma is at greater risk for developing a second.

Complications

This cancer has a strong tendency to metastasize, and complications result from disease progression to the lungs, liver, or brain.

Assessment

A sore that doesn't heal, a persistent lump or swelling, and changes in preexisting skin markings, such as moles, birthmarks, scars, freckles, or warts, may be part of the patient history. Suspect melanoma when any preexisting skin lesion or nevus enlarges, changes color, becomes inflamed or sore, itches, ulcerates, bleeds, changes texture, or shows signs of surrounding pigment regression.

In superficial spreading melanoma, inspection may reveal lesions on the ankles or the inside surfaces of the knees. These lesions may appear red, white, or blue over a brown or black background. They may have an irregular, notched margin. Palpation may reveal small, elevated tumor nodules that may ulcerate and bleed. These tumors may grow horizontally for years, but when vertical growth occurs, the prognosis worsens.

In nodular melanoma, inspection may reveal a uniformly discolored nodule. It may appear grayish and resemble a blackberry. Occasionally, this melanoma is flesh-colored, with flecks of pigment around its base, which may be inflamed. Palpation may disclose polypoidal nodules that resemble the surface of a blackberry.

In acral-lentiginous melanoma, inspection may show pigmented lesions on the palms and soles. The color may resemble a mosaic of rich browns, tans, and black. Inspection of the nail beds may reveal a streak in the nail associated with an irregular tan or brown stain that diffuses from the nail bed.

In lentigo maligna melanoma, the patient history may reveal a long-standing lesion that has now ulcerated. Inspection may disclose a large lesion (3 to 6 cm) that appears as a freckle of tan, brown, black, whitish, or slate color on the face, back of the hand, or under the fingernails. There may be irregular scattered black nodules on the surface. Palpation may reveal a flat nodule with smaller nodules scattered over the surface.

Diagnostic tests

• *Excisional biopsy* and *full-depth punch biopsy* with histologic examination can distinguish malignant melanoma from a benign nevus, seborrheic keratosis, or pigmented basal cell epithelioma and can also determine tumor thickness and stage of the disease. (See *Staging malignant melanoma.*)

• *Baseline laboratory studies* may include complete blood count with differential, erythrocyte sedimentation rate, platelet count, and liver function studies, in addition to urinalysis.

Depending on the depth of tumor invasion and any metastatic spread, baseline diagnostic studies may also include such tests as chest X-rays, computed tomography (CT) scans of the chest and abdomen, and a gallium scan. Signs of bone metastasis may require a bone scan; central nervous system metastasis, a CT scan of the brain. Magnetic resonance imaging may be used to assess metastasis.

Treatment

A patient with malignant melanoma always requires surgical resection to remove the tumor. A 1-cm margin is recommended for thin melanomas (less than 1 mm thick) and a 2- to 3-cm margin for intermediate and thick melanomas (greater than 1 mm thick). The extent of resection depends upon the size and location of the primary lesion. Closure of a wide resection may necessitate a skin graft. Plastic surgery techniques can provide excellent cosmetic repair. Surgical treatment may, in addition, include regional lymphadenectomy.

Treatment with interferon alpha-2b has recently been approved as adjuvant treatment for high-risk melanoma (T4 or N1). Induction interferon is given I.V. for 1 month followed by subcutaneous interferon three times a week for a total of 48 weeks. Occasionally, isolated limb perfusion with chemotherapy is used to prevent recurrence and control metastasis.

Chemotherapy is useful only in metastatic disease. Dacarbazine and the nitrosoureas have generated some response. Similarly, radiation therapy is usually reserved for metastatic disease. It doesn't prolong survival but may reduce tumor size and relieve pain.

Regardless of treatment, melanomas require close long-term follow-up care to detect metastases and recurrences. Statistics show that about 13% of recurrences develop more than 5 years after primary surgery.

Staging malignant melanoma

Several systems exist for staging malignant melanoma, including the tumor, node, metastasis (TNM) system and Clark's system, which classifies tumor progression according to skin layer penetration.

Primary tumor

TX—primary tumor can't be assessed
T0—no evidence of primary tumor
Tis—melanoma in situ (atypical melanotic hyperplasia, severe melanotic dysplasia), not an invasive lesion (Clark's Level I)
T1—tumor 0.75 mm in thickness or less invades the papillary dermis (Clark's Level II)
T2—tumor between 0.75 and 1.5 mm thick, or tumor invades the interface between the papillary and reticular dermis (Clark's Level III), or both
T3—tumor between 1.5 and 4 mm thick, or tumor invades the reticular dermis (Clark's Level IV), or both
T3a—tumor between 1.5 and 3 mm thick
T3b—tumor between 3 and 4 mm thick
T4—tumor more than 4 mm thick, or tumor invades subcutaneous tissue (Clark's Level V), or tumor has one or more satellites within 2 cm of the primary tumor
T4a—tumor more than 4 mm thick, or invades subcutaneous tissue, or both
T4b—one or more satellites exist within 2 cm of the primary tumor

Regional lymph nodes

NX—regional lymph nodes can't be assessed
N0—no evidence of regional lymph node involvement
N1—metastasis 3 cm or less in greatest dimension in any regional lymph node
N2—metastasis greater than 3 cm in greatest dimension in any regional lymph node, or in-transit metastasis, or both

Distant metastasis

MX—distant metastasis can't be assessed
M0—no evidence of distant metastasis
M1—distant metastasis
M1a—metastasis in skin, subcutaneous tissue, or lymph nodes beyond the regional nodes
M1b—visceral metastasis

Staging categories

Malignant melanoma progresses from mild to severe as follows:
Stage I—T1, N0, M0; T2, N0, M0
Stage II—T3, N0, M0
Stage III—T4, N0, M0; any T, N1, M0; any T, N2, M0
Stage IV—any T, any N, M1

Clark's levels

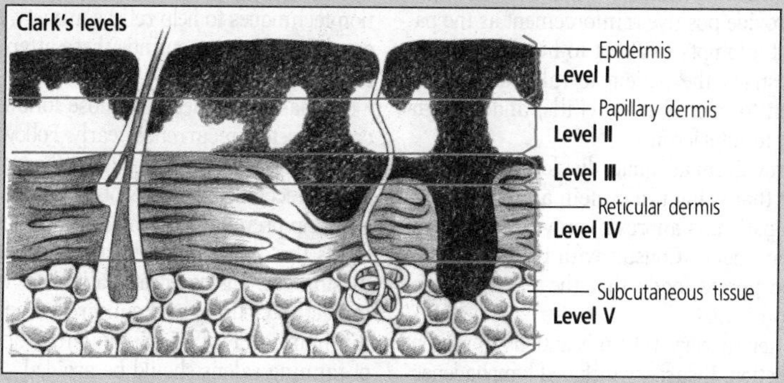

Key nursing diagnoses and patient outcomes

Anxiety related to potential for metastasis. Based on this nursing diagnosis, you'll establish these patient outcomes. The patient will:
- express his feelings of anxiety
- demonstrate effective coping strategies
- cope with his diagnosis and the requirements of follow-up care without exhibiting severe signs of anxiety.

Body image disturbance related to skin changes associated with melanoma and surgery. Based on this nursing diagnosis, you'll establish these patient outcomes. The patient will:
- express recognition of his changed body image
- express positive feelings about himself.

Impaired skin integrity related to skin cancer. Based on this nursing diagnosis, you'll establish these patient outcomes. The patient will:
- regain normal skin integrity
- inspect his skin daily for changes and seek medical attention if changes occur
- maintain a skin care routine to prevent or minimize the risk of melanoma recurrence.

Nursing interventions

- Listen to the patient's fears and concerns. Stay with him during episodes of stress and anxiety. Include the patient and family in care decisions.
- Provide positive reinforcement as the patient attempts to adapt to his disease.
- Instruct the patient to take acetaminophen to control fever, chills, and myalgia due to interferon.
- Provide an adequate diet for the patient—one that is high in protein and calories. If the patient is anorexic, provide small, frequent meals. Consult with the dietitian to incorporate foods that the patient enjoys into his diet.
- After surgery, take precautions to prevent infection. If surgery included lymphadenectomy, apply a compression stocking and instruct the patient to keep the extremity elevated to minimize lymphedema.

In advanced metastatic disease:
- Control and prevent pain with regularly scheduled administration of analgesics.
- If the patient has a poor prognosis, identify the needs of patient, family, and friends and provide appropriate support and care.

Monitoring

- Watch for complications associated with interferon, such as fever, chills, malaise, and fatigue.
- After surgery, check dressings often for excessive drainage, foul odor, redness, and swelling.
- Monitor the patient's response to analgesic administration.

Patient teaching

- Make sure the patient understands the procedures and treatments associated with his diagnosis. Review the doctor's explanation of treatment alternatives. Honestly answer any questions the patient or his family may have about surgery, interferon, chemotherapy, and radiation therapy.
- Tell the patient what to expect before and after surgery, what the wound will look like, and what type of dressing he'll have. Warn him that the donor site for a skin graft may be as painful, if not more so, than the tumor excision site.
- Teach the patient and his family relaxation techniques to help relieve anxiety, and encourage him to continue these after discharge.
- Emphasize the need for close follow-up care to detect recurrences early. Follow up needs to continue for years. Teach the patient how to recognize the signs of recurrence.
- To help prevent recurrence of melanoma, stress the detrimental effects of exposure to sunlight. Instruct the patient to wear protective clothing and sunscreens with a minimum SPF of 15. Sunburning or use of tanning salons should be avoided.

• When appropriate, refer the patient and his family to community support services, such as a local chapter of the American Cancer Society or a hospice.

Meningitis

In this disorder, the brain and the spinal cord meninges become inflamed. Such inflammation may involve all three meningeal membranes – the dura mater, the arachnoid membrane, and the pia mater.

For most patients, meningitis follows onset of respiratory symptoms. In about 50% of patients, it develops over a period of 1 to 7 days; in just under 20% of patients, it occurs 1 to 3 weeks after respiratory symptoms appear. Unheralded by respiratory symptoms, meningitis has a sudden onset in about 25% of patients, who become seriously ill within 24 hours.

The prognosis is good and complications are rare, especially if the disease is recognized early and the infecting organism responds to antibiotics. However, mortality in untreated meningitis is 70% to 100%. The prognosis is poorer for infants and elderly people.

Causes

Meningitis can be caused by various bacteria, viruses, protozoa, or fungi. It most commonly results from bacterial infection, usually caused by *Neisseria meningitidis, Hemophilus influenzae, Streptococcus pneumoniae,* and *Escherichia coli.* In some patients, no causative organism can be found.

In most patients, the infection that causes meningitis is secondary to another bacterial infection, such as bacteremia (especially from pneumonia, empyema, osteomyelitis, and endocarditis), sinusitis, otitis media, encephalitis, myelitis, and brain abscess. Meningitis may also follow skull fracture, a penetrating head wound, lumbar puncture, or ventricular shunting procedures.

When meningitis is caused by a virus, it's known as aseptic viral meningitis. (See *What you should know about aseptic viral meningitis,* page 580.)

Infants, children, and elderly people have the highest risk of developing meningitis. In addition to age, other risk factors include malnourishment, immunosuppression (as from radiation therapy, chemotherapy, or long-term steroid therapy), and central nervous system trauma.

Complications

Depending on the cause and severity of the illness, potential complications of meningitis include visual impairment, optic neuritis, cranial nerve palsies, deafness, personality change, headache, paresis or paralysis, endocarditis, coma, vasculitis, and cerebral infarction.

Other complications, seen primarily in children, include unilateral or bilateral sensory hearing loss, epilepsy, mental retardation, hydrocephalus, and subdural effusions.

Assessment

Signs and symptoms of infection and increased intracranial pressure (ICP) are the cardinal signs of meningitis.

The patient's history may detail headache, stiff neck and back, malaise, photophobia, chills and, in some patients, vomiting, twitching, and seizures. The patient or a family member may also report altered level of consciousness (LOC), such as confusion and delirium. Vital signs may reveal fever. (Vomiting and fever occur more often in children than in adults.) In addition, the history for an infant may list fretfulness and refusal to eat.

In pneumococcal meningitis, the patient's history may uncover a recent lung, ear, or sinus infection or endocarditis. It may also reveal the presence of other conditions, such as alcoholism, sickle cell dis-

What you should know about aseptic viral meningitis

A benign syndrome, aseptic viral meningitis is characterized by headache, fever, vomiting, and meningeal symptoms. It results from some form of viral infection, such as from an enterovirus (most common), arbovirus, herpes simplex virus, mumps virus, or lymphocytic choriomeningitis virus.

Assessment

The history of a patient with aseptic viral meningitis usually shows that the disease began suddenly with a fever up to 104° F (40° C), alterations in LOC (drowsiness, confusion, stupor), and neck or spinal stiffness, that is slight at first. The patient experiences such stiffness when bending forward. The history also may reveal a recent illness.

Other signs and symptoms may include headache, nausea, vomiting, abdominal pain, poorly defined chest pain, and sore throat.

The patient history and your knowledge of seasonal epidemics are essential in differentiating among the many forms of aseptic viral meningitis. Negative bacteriologic cultures and CSF analysis showing pleocytosis and increased protein suggest the diagnosis. Isolation of the virus from CSF confirms it.

Supportive treatment

Management of aseptic meningitis includes bed rest, maintenance of fluid and electrolyte balance, analgesics for pain, and exercises to combat residual weakness. Isolation isn't necessary. Careful handling of excretions and good hand-washing technique prevent the spread of the disease.

ease, basal skull fracture, recent splenectomy, or organ transplant.

In *H. influenzae* meningitis, patient history may reveal recent respiratory tract or ear infection.

Physical findings vary, depending on the severity of the meningitis. You may note opisthotonos (a spasm in which the back and extremities arch backward so that the body rests on the head and heels), a sign of meningeal irritation. In meningococcal meningitis, you may also see a petechial, purpuric, or ecchymotic rash on the lower part of the body.

Neurologic examination may uncover other indications of meningeal irritation, including positive Brudzinski's and Kernig's signs and exaggerated and symmetrical deep tendon reflexes. Neurologic examination may also reveal altered LOC, ranging from confusion or delirium to deep stupor or coma.

Vision testing may demonstrate diplopia and other visual problems. Ophthalmoscopic examination may show papilledema (another sign of increased ICP), although this is rare.

Diagnostic tests

- *Lumbar puncture* shows typical cerebrospinal fluid (CSF) findings associated with meningitis (elevated CSF pressure, cloudy or milky white CSF, high protein level, positive Gram stain and culture that usually identifies the infecting organism [unless it's a virus] and depressed CSF glucose concentration).
- *Chest X-rays* are especially important because they may reveal pneumonitis or lung abscess, tubercular lesions, or granulomas secondary to fungal infection. *Sinus* and *skull films* may help identify the presence of cranial osteomyelitis, paranasal sinusitis, or skull fracture.
- *White blood cell count* usually indicates leukocytosis, and *serum electrolyte* levels often are abnormal.

• *Computed tomography scan* can rule out cerebral hematoma, hemorrhage, or tumor.

Treatment

Medical management of meningitis includes appropriate antibiotic therapy and vigorous supportive care.

Usually, I.V. antibiotics are given for at least 2 weeks, followed by oral antibiotics. Such antibiotics include penicillin G, ampicillin, or nafcillin. However, if the patient is allergic to penicillin, anti-infective therapy includes tetracycline, chloramphenicol, or kanamycin. Other drugs include a digitalis glycoside (such as digoxin) to control arrhythmias, mannitol to decrease cerebral edema, an anticonvulsant (usually given I.V.) or a sedative to reduce restlessness, and aspirin or acetaminophen to relieve headache and fever.

Supportive measures consist of bed rest, hypothermia, and fluid therapy to prevent dehydration. Isolation is necessary if nasal cultures are positive. Treatment includes appropriate therapy for any coexisting conditions, such as endocarditis or pneumonia.

To prevent meningitis, prophylactic antibiotics are sometimes used after ventricular shunting procedures, skull fracture, or penetrating head wounds, but this use is controversial.

Key nursing diagnoses and patient outcomes

Risk for injury related to increased ICP. Based on this nursing diagnosis, you'll establish these patient outcomes. The patient will:

• avoid permanent neurologic deficits caused by increased ICP
• regain and maintain normal ICP.

Hyperthermia related to infection caused by the organism responsible for meningitis. Based on this nursing diagnosis, you'll establish these patient outcomes. The patient will:

• exhibit a reduced temperature after antipyretic measures
• avoid complications associated with hyperthermia, such as dehydration and seizures
• regain and maintain a temperature within the normal range.

Pain related to meningeal irritation. Based on this nursing diagnosis, you'll establish these patient outcomes. The patient will:

• express relief of pain after analgesic administration
• become pain free.

Nursing interventions

• Maintain droplet precautions for 24 hours after the start of antibiotic therapy. Discharges from the nose and the mouth are considered infectious. Follow strict aseptic technique when treating patients with head wounds or skull fractures.
• Administer prescribed medications.
• Administer oxygen as required to maintain partial pressure of oxygen at desired levels. If necessary, maintain the patient on mechanical ventilation and care for his endotracheal tube or tracheostomy.
• Maintain adequate fluid intake to avoid dehydration, but avoid fluid overload because of the danger of cerebral edema.
• Position the patient carefully to prevent joint stiffness and neck pain. Turn him often, according to a planned positioning schedule. Assist with range-of-motion exercises.
• Maintain adequate nutrition. You may need to provide small, frequent meals or to supplement these meals with nasogastric tube or parenteral feedings.
• To prevent constipation and minimize the risk of increased ICP from straining during defecation, give a mild laxative or stool softener, as ordered. (See *Nursing care in meningitis,* pages 582 and 583.)
• Provide mouth care regularly.
• Ensure the patient's comfort, and maintain a quiet environment. Darkening the room may decrease photophobia. Relieve

NURSING PRIORITY

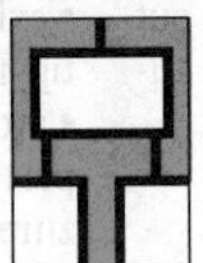

Nursing care in meningitis

History of headache, stiff neck and back, malaise, photophobia, chills, vomiting (possible), twitching and seizures, altered level of consciousness (possible), and contributing factors

Physical findings, including fever, opisthotonos, rash (petechial, purpuric, or ecchymotic), positive Brudzinski's and Kernig's signs, exaggerated and symmetrical deep tendon reflexes, possible change in mental status (ranging from confusion to coma), visual abnormalities, and possible papilledema

Results of diagnostic tests, including lumbar puncture, X-rays (chest, sinus, skull), white blood cell count, serum electrolyte levels, and computed tomography scan

Risk for injury related to increased intracranial pressure (ICP)

- Assess neurologic status and vital signs frequently.
- Be alert for signs and symptoms of increased ICP.

Maintain calm environment; avoid exciting patient.

Implement measures to avoid increasing ICP, such as preventing constipation and restricting fluids, as prescribed.

Does patient show signs and symptoms of increased ICP?

YES

Notify doctor immediately.

Expect to administer an osmotic diuretic or corticosteroids or both to reduce ICP.

Increase frequency of neurologic assessment.

Prepare for possible insertion of ICP monitoring device for more precise measurement.

Expect to transfer patient to intensive care unit.

NO

Continue supportive care.

Patient does not experience injury related to increased ICP as evidenced by:
- regaining and maintaining normal ICP
- presence of normal neurologic function.

KEY

- Assessment
- Nursing diagnoses
- Interventions
- Evaluation

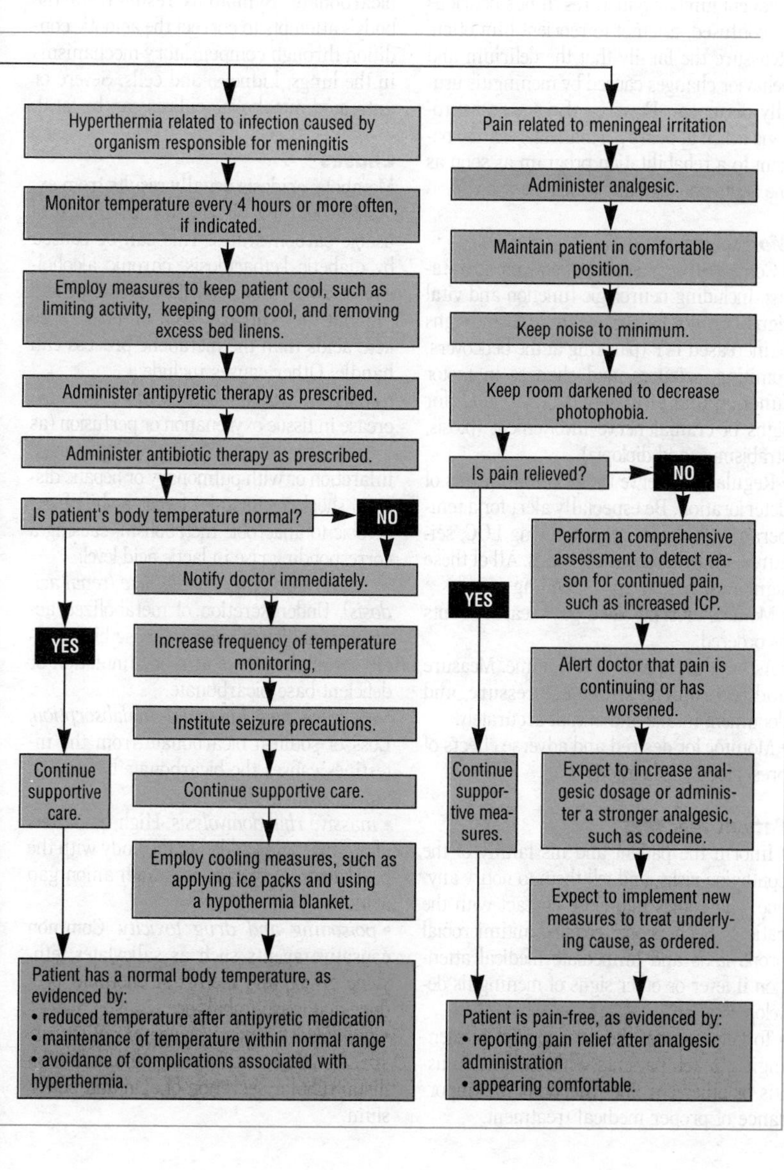
Hyperthermia related to infection caused by organism responsible for meningitis
Monitor temperature every 4 hours or more often, if indicated.
Employ measures to keep patient cool, such as limiting activity, keeping room cool, and removing excess bed linens.
Administer antipyretic therapy as prescribed.
Administer antibiotic therapy as prescribed.
Is patient's body temperature normal?
NO
Notify doctor immediately.
YES
Increase frequency of temperature monitoring,
Institute seizure precautions.
Continue supportive care.
Continue supportive care.
Employ cooling measures, such as applying ice packs and using a hypothermia blanket.
Patient has a normal body temperature, as evidenced by:
• reduced temperature after antipyretic medication
• maintenance of temperature within normal range
• avoidance of complications associated with hyperthermia.
Pain related to meningeal irritation
Administer analgesic.
Maintain patient in comfortable position.
Keep noise to minimum.
Keep room darkened to decrease photophobia.
Is pain relieved?
NO
Perform a comprehensive assessment to detect reason for continued pain, such as increased ICP.
YES
Alert doctor that pain is continuing or has worsened.
Continue supportive measures.
Expect to increase analgesic dosage or administer a stronger analgesic, such as codeine.
Expect to implement new measures to treat underlying cause, as ordered.
Patient is pain-free, as evidenced by:
• reporting pain relief after analgesic administration
• appearing comfortable.

headache with a nonnarcotic analgesic, such as aspirin or acetaminophen, as ordered. (Narcotics interfere with accurate neurologic assessment.)
• Provide reassurance and support. The patient may be frightened by his illness and frequent lumbar punctures. If he's delirious or confused, attempt to reorient him often. Reassure the family that the delirium and behavior changes caused by meningitis usually disappear. However, if a severe neurologic deficit appears permanent, refer the patient to a rehabilitation program as soon as the acute phase of this illness has passed.

Monitoring

• Continually assess the patient's clinical status, including neurologic function and vital signs. Monitor for changes in LOC and signs of increased ICP (plucking at the bedcovers, vomiting, seizures, and changes in motor function and vital signs). Also watch for signs of cranial nerve involvement (ptosis, strabismus, and diplopia).
• Regularly observe the patient for signs of deterioration. Be especially alert for a temperature increase, deteriorating LOC, seizures, and altered respirations. All of these signs may herald an impending crisis.
• Monitor arterial blood gas measurements as ordered.
• Assess the patient's fluid volume. Measure and record central venous pressure, and document intake and output accurately.
• Monitor for desired and adverse effects of prescribed medications.

Patient teaching

• Inform the patient and his family of the contagion risks, and tell them to notify anyone who comes into close contact with the patient. Such people require antimicrobial prophylaxis and immediate medical attention if fever or other signs of meningitis develop.
• To help prevent the development of meningitis, teach patients with chronic sinusitis or other chronic infections the importance of proper medical treatment.

Metabolic acidosis

Produced by an underlying disorder, metabolic acidosis is a physiologic state of excess acid accumulation and deficient base bicarbonate. Symptoms result from the body's attempts to correct the acidotic condition through compensatory mechanisms in the lungs, kidneys, and cells. Severe or untreated metabolic acidosis can be fatal.

Causes

Metabolic acidosis usually results from excessive burning of fats in the absence of usable carbohydrates. This can be caused by diabetic ketoacidosis, chronic alcoholism, malnutrition, or a low-carbohydrate, high-fat diet – all of which produce more keto acids than the metabolic process can handle. Other causes include:
• *anaerobic carbohydrate metabolism.* A decrease in tissue oxygenation or perfusion (as occurs with pump failure after myocardial infarction or with pulmonary or hepatic disease, shock, or anemia) forces a shift from aerobic to anaerobic metabolism, causing a corresponding rise in lactic acid level.
• *renal insufficiency and failure (renal acidosis).* Underexcretion of metabolized acids or inability to conserve base bicarbonate results in excess acid accumulation or deficient base bicarbonate.
• *diarrhea and intestinal malabsorption.* Loss of sodium bicarbonate from the intestines causes the bicarbonate buffer system to shift to the acidic side.
• *massive rhabdomyolysis.* High quantities of organic acids added to the body with the breakdown of cells causes high anion gap acidosis.
• *poisoning and drug toxicity.* Common causative agents such as salicylates, ethylene glycol, and methyl alcohol may produce acid-base imbalance.
• *hypoaldosteronism or use of potassium-sparing diuretics.* These conditions inhibit distal tubular secretion of acid and potassium.

Complications

If untreated, metabolic acidosis may lead to coma, arrhythmias, and cardiac arrest.

Assessment

The history of a patient with metabolic acidosis may point to the presence of risk factors, including associated disorders or the use of medications that contain alcohol or aspirin. Information about the patient's urine output, fluid intake, and dietary habits (including any recent fasting) may help to establish the underlying cause and severity of metabolic acidosis.

The patient's history (obtained from a family member, if necessary) also may reveal central nervous system (CNS) symptoms, such as changes in level of consciousness (LOC) that range from lethargy, drowsiness, and confusion to stupor and coma.

Inspection findings may include Kussmaul's respirations (as the lungs attempt to compensate by "blowing off" carbon dioxide). Underlying diabetes mellitus may cause a fruity breath odor from catabolism of fats and excretion of accumulated acetone through the lungs.

Palpation may reveal cold and clammy skin. As acidosis grows more severe, the skin feels warm and dry, indicating ensuing shock. Auscultation may detect hypotension and arrhythmias. Neuromuscular assessment may reveal diminished muscle tone and deep tendon reflexes.

Diagnostic tests

For critical laboratory test values, see *Key abnormal test values in metabolic acidosis.* Other characteristic laboratory findings are:

- *Urine pH* is 4.5 in the absence of renal disease.
- *Serum potassium levels* are usually elevated, as hydrogen ions move into the cells and potassium moves out of the cells to maintain electroneutrality.
- *Blood glucose levels* rise in diabetes.
- *Serum ketone body levels* increase in diabetes mellitus.
- *Plasma lactic acid levels* are elevated in lactic acidosis.

CHECKLIST

Key abnormal test values in metabolic acidosis

If your patient has metabolic acidosis, expect the following test values.

- ☐ pH below 7.35.
- ☐ Decreased PCO_2, representing compensation for acidosis.
- ☐ Bicarbonate level below 24 mEq/liter in acute metabolic acidosis.
- ☐ Anion gap value above 14 mEq/liter from increased acid production or renal insufficiency.

Also, check the patient's respiratory function. (See *Using arterial blood gas values to assess metabolic acid-base imbalance.*)

Treatment

For acute metabolic acidosis, treatment may include I.V. administration of sodium bicarbonate (when arterial pH is less than 7.2) to neutralize blood acidity. For chronic metabolic acidosis, oral bicarbonate may be given. Other measures include careful evaluation and correction of electrolyte imbalances and, correction of the underlying cause. For example, diabetic ketoacidosis requires insulin administration and fluid replacement.

Mechanical ventilation may be required to ensure adequate respiratory compensation.

Key nursing diagnoses and patient outcomes

Altered thought processes related to neurologic dysfunction. Based on this nursing diagnosis, you'll establish these patient outcomes. The patient will:

- remain safe and free from injury
- exhibit orientation to time, person, and place.

NURSING PRIORITY

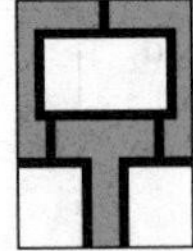

Using ABGs to assess metabolic acid base imbalances

To help determine if a patient is experiencing a metabolic acid-base imbalance, follow the decision tree steps below to interpret the patients ABGs.

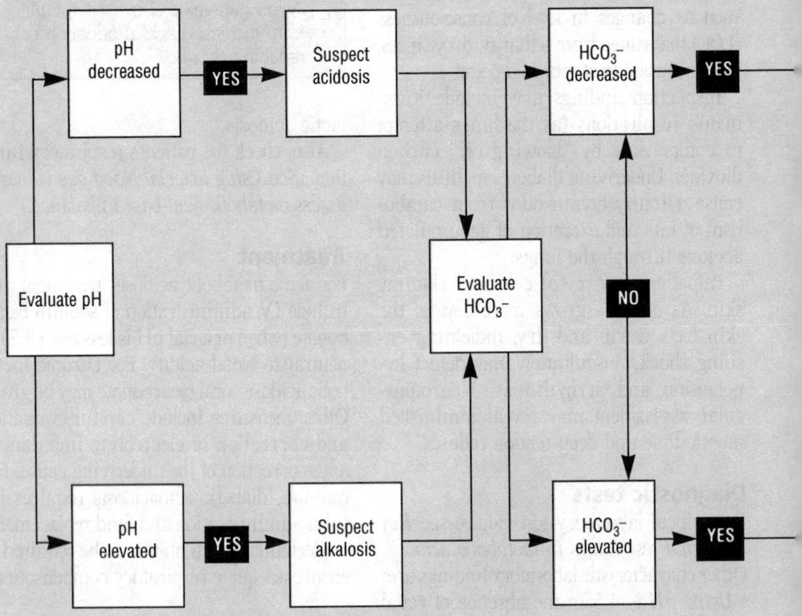

Evaluate pH

pH decreased → YES → Suspect acidosis → Evaluate HCO_3^-

pH elevated → YES → Suspect alkalosis → Evaluate HCO_3^-

Evaluate HCO_3^- → HCO_3^- decreased → YES

Evaluate HCO_3^- → HCO_3^- elevated → YES

HCO_3^- decreased ↔ NO ↔ HCO_3^- elevated

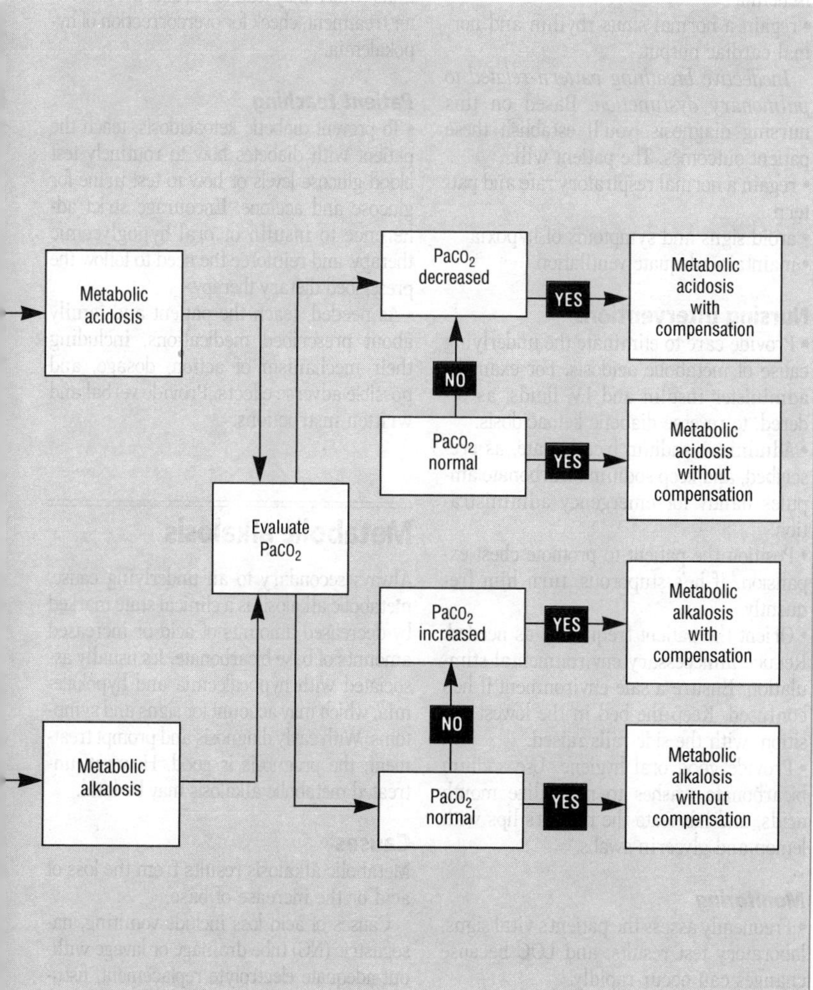
Metabolic acidosis
Metabolic alkalosis
Evaluate $PaCO_2$
$PaCO_2$ decreased
NO
$PaCO_2$ normal
$PaCO_2$ increased
NO
$PaCO_2$ normal
YES
YES
YES
YES
Metabolic acidosis with compensation
Metabolic acidosis without compensation
Metabolic alkalosis with compensation
Metabolic alkalosis without compensation

Decreased cardiac output related to arrhythmias. Based on this nursing diagnosis, you'll establish these patient outcomes. The patient will:
- remain hemodynamically stable
- avoid manifestations of profoundly decreased cardiac output, such as shock or ischemia
- regain a normal sinus rhythm and normal cardiac output.

Ineffective breathing pattern related to pulmonary dysfunction. Based on this nursing diagnosis, you'll establish these patient outcomes. The patient will:
- regain a normal respiratory rate and pattern
- avoid signs and symptoms of hypoxia
- maintain adequate ventilation.

Nursing interventions
- Provide care to eliminate the underlying cause of metabolic acidosis. For example, administer insulin and I.V. fluids, as ordered, to reverse diabetic ketoacidosis.
- Administer sodium bicarbonate, as prescribed, and keep sodium bicarbonate ampules handy for emergency administration.
- Position the patient to promote chest expansion. If he's stuporous, turn him frequently.
- Orient the patient frequently, as needed. Reduce unnecessary environmental stimulation. Ensure a safe environment if he's confused. Keep the bed in the lowest position, with the side rails raised.
- Provide good oral hygiene. Use sodium bicarbonate washes to neutralize mouth acids, and lubricate the patient's lips with lemon and glycerin swabs.

Monitoring
- Frequently assess the patient's vital signs, laboratory test results, and LOC because changes can occur rapidly.
- Monitor the patient's respiratory function. Check his arterial blood gas values frequently.
- If the patient has diabetic acidosis, watch for secondary changes caused by hypovolemia, such as decreasing blood pressure.
- Record the patient's intake and output accurately to monitor renal function. Watch for signs of excessive serum potassium, such as weakness, flaccid paralysis, and arrhythmias (which may lead to cardiac arrest). After treatment, check for overcorrection of hypokalemia.

Patient teaching
- To prevent diabetic ketoacidosis, teach the patient with diabetes how to routinely test blood glucose levels or how to test urine for glucose and acetone. Encourage strict adherence to insulin or oral hypoglycemic therapy, and reinforce the need to follow the prescribed dietary therapy.
- As needed, teach the patient and family about prescribed medications, including their mechanism of action, dosage, and possible adverse effects. Provide verbal and written instructions.

Metabolic alkalosis

Always secondary to an underlying cause, metabolic alkalosis is a clinical state marked by decreased amounts of acid or increased amounts of base bicarbonate. It's usually associated with hypocalcemia and hypokalemia, which may account for signs and symptoms. With early diagnosis and prompt treatment, the prognosis is good. However, untreated metabolic alkalosis may be fatal.

Causes
Metabolic alkalosis results from the loss of acid or the increase of base.

Causes of acid loss include vomiting, nasogastric (NG) tube drainage or lavage without adequate electrolyte replacement, fistulas, and the use of steroids and certain diuretics (furosemide, thiazides, and ethacrynic acid). Hyperadrenocorticism is another cause of severe acid loss. Cushing's disease, primary hyperaldosteronism, and Bartter's syndrome, for example, all lead to retention of sodium and chloride and urinary loss of potassium and hydrogen.

Excessive retention of base can result from excessive intake of bicarbonate of soda or other antacids (usually for treatment of gastritis or peptic ulcer), excessive intake of absorbable alkali (as in milk-alkali syndrome, often seen in patients with peptic ulcers), administration of excessive amounts of I.V. fluids with high concentrations of bicarbonate or lactate, massive blood transfusions, or respiratory insufficiency.

Complications

Untreated metabolic alkalosis may result in coma, atrioventricular arrhythmias, and death.

Assessment

The patient's history (obtained from a family member, if necessary) may disclose such risk factors as excessive ingestion of alkali antacids. The history may include extracellular fluid (ECF) volume depletion, which is frequently associated with conditions leading to metabolic alkalosis (for example, vomiting or NG tube suctioning). The patient or a family member may report irritability, belligerence, and paresthesia.

Inspection may reveal the presence of tetany if serum calcium levels are borderline or low. The rate and depth of the patient's respirations may be decreased as a compensatory mechanism; however, this mechanism is limited because of the development of hypoxemia, which stimulates ventilation.

Assessment of the patient's level of consciousness (LOC) may find apathy, confusion, seizures, stupor, or coma if alkalosis is severe. Neuromuscular assessment may discover hyperactive reflexes and muscle weakness if serum potassium is markedly low. Auscultation may detect cardiac arrhythmias occurring with hypokalemia.

Diagnostic tests

• *Arterial blood gas analysis* may reveal a blood pH over 7.45 and a bicarbonate level over 29 mEq/liter in metabolic alkalosis. A partial pressure of carbon dioxide over 45 mm Hg indicates attempts at respiratory compensation.
• *Serum electrolyte studies* usually show low potassium, calcium, and chloride levels in metabolic alkalosis.
• *Electrocardiogram (ECG)* findings disclose a low T wave merging with a P wave and atrial or sinus tachycardia.

Treatment

Correcting the underlying cause of metabolic alkalosis is the goal of treatment. Mild metabolic alkalosis generally requires no treatment. Rarely, therapy for severe alkalosis includes cautious I.V. administration of ammonium chloride to release hydrogen chloride and restore concentration of ECF and chloride levels. Potassium chloride and 0.9% sodium chloride solution (except with heart failure) are usually sufficient to replace losses from gastric drainage.

Electrolyte replacement with potassium chloride and discontinuation of diuretics correct metabolic alkalosis resulting from potent diuretic therapy.

Oral or I.V. acetazolamide, which enhances renal bicarbonate excretion, may be prescribed to correct metabolic alkalosis without rapid volume expansion. Because acetazolamide also enhances potassium excretion, potassium administration before giving this drug may be necessary.

Key nursing diagnoses and patient outcomes

Altered thought processes related to neurologic dysfunction. Based on this nursing diagnosis, you'll establish these patient outcomes. The patient will:
• remain safe and protected from injury
• become oriented to time, person, and place with effective treatment.

Decreased cardiac output related to atrioventricular arrhythmias. Based on this

nursing diagnosis, you'll establish these patient outcomes. The patient will:
- maintain hemodynamic stability
- avoid manifestations of profoundly decreased cardiac output, such as shock and tissue ischemia
- demonstrate correction of arrhythmia and improved cardiac output with treatment.

Risk for injury related to tetany. Based on this nursing diagnosis, you'll establish these patient outcomes. The patient will:
- maintain a normal calcium level
- avoid signs and symptoms of tetany.

Nursing interventions

- When administering I.V. solutions containing potassium salts, dilute potassium with the prescribed I.V. solution and use an I.V. infusion pump. Infuse ammonium chloride 0.9% I.V. no faster than 1 liter over 4 hours; faster administration may cause hemolysis of red blood cells. Avoid administering excessive amounts of these solutions because this could cause overcorrection leading to metabolic acidosis. Don't give ammonium chloride to a patient who has signs of hepatic or renal disease.
- Observe seizure precautions, and provide a safe environment for the patient with altered thought processes. Orient the patient as needed.
- Irrigate the patient's NG tube with 0.9% sodium chloride solution instead of plain water to prevent loss of gastric electrolytes.

Monitoring

- Monitor I.V. fluid concentrations of bicarbonate or lactate. Observe the infusion rate of I.V. solutions containing potassium salts to prevent damage to blood vessels. Monitor I.V. solutions containing ammonium chloride to prevent hemolysis of red blood cells. Watch for signs of phlebitis.
- Assess the patient's laboratory values, including pH, serum bicarbonate, serum potassium, and serum calcium levels. Notify the doctor if you detect significant changes or if the patient responds poorly to treatment.
- Observe the ECG for arrhythmias.
- Watch closely for signs of muscle weakness, tetany, or decreased activity.
- Check the patient's vital signs frequently, and record intake and output to evaluate respiratory, fluid, and electrolyte status. Keep in mind that the respiratory rate usually slows in an effort to compensate for alkalosis. Tachycardia may indicate electrolyte imbalance, especially hypokalemia.
- Assess the patient's LOC frequently.

Patient teaching

- To prevent metabolic alkalosis, warn the patient not to overuse alkaline agents.
- If the patient has an ulcer, teach him how to recognize signs of milk-alkali syndrome, including a distaste for milk, anorexia, weakness, and lethargy.
- If potassium-wasting diuretics or potassium chloride supplements are prescribed, make sure the patient understands the medication regimen, including the purpose, dosage, and possible adverse effects.

Mitral insufficiency

Also known as mitral regurgitation, mitral insufficiency occurs when a damaged mitral valve allows blood from the left ventricle to flow back into the left atrium during systole. As a result, the atrium enlarges to accommodate the backflow. The left ventricle also dilates to accommodate the increased volume of blood from the atrium and to compensate for diminishing cardiac output.

Mitral insufficiency tends to be progressive. As left ventricular dilation continues to lead to left atrial and ventricular enlargement, the insufficiency increases further.

Causes

Damage to the mitral valve can result from rheumatic fever, hypertrophic cardiomyopathy, mitral valve prolapse, myocardial infarction, severe left ventricular failure, or ruptured chordae tendineae.

In older patients, mitral insufficiency may occur because the mitral annulus has become calcified. The cause is unknown, but it may be linked to a degenerative process. Mitral insufficiency is sometimes associated with congenital anomalies, such as transposition of the great arteries.

Complications

Ventricular hypertrophy and increased end-diastolic pressure result in increased pulmonary artery pressure, eventually leading to left and right ventricular failure with pulmonary edema and cardiovascular collapse.

Assessment

Depending on the disorder's severity, the patient may either be asymptomatic or may complain of orthopnea, exertional dyspnea, fatigue, weakness, weight loss, chest pain, and palpitations.

Inspection may reveal jugular vein distention with an abnormally prominent *a* wave. You may also note peripheral edema.

Auscultation may detect a soft S_1 that may be buried in the systolic murmur. A grade 3 to 6 holosystolic murmur, most characteristic of mitral insufficiency, is best heard at the apex. You'll also hear a split S_2 and a low-pitched S_3. The S_3 may be followed by a short, rumbling diastolic murmur. An S_4 may be evident in patients with a recent onset of severe mitral insufficiency and who are in normal sinus rhythm.

Auscultation of the lungs may reveal crackles if the patient has pulmonary edema.

Palpation of the chest may disclose a regular pulse rate with a sharp upstroke. You can probably palpate a systolic thrill at the apex. In patients with marked pulmonary hypertension, you may be able to palpate a right ventricular tap and the shock of the pulmonary valve closing. When the left atrium is markedly enlarged, it may be palpable along the sternal border late during ventricular systole. It resembles a right ventricular lift. Abdominal palpation may reveal hepatomegaly if the patient has right ventricular failure.

Diagnostic tests

- *Cardiac catheterization* detects mitral insufficiency, with increased left ventricular end-diastolic volume and pressure, increased atrial and pulmonary capillary wedge pressures, and decreased cardiac output.
- *Chest X-rays* demonstrate left atrial and ventricular enlargement, pulmonary venous congestion, and calcification of the mitral leaflets in long-standing mitral insufficiency and stenosis.
- *Echocardiography* reveals abnormal motion of the valve leaflets, left atrial enlargement, and a hyperdynamic left ventricle.
- *Electrocardiography (ECG)* may show left atrial and ventricular hypertrophy, sinus tachycardia, and atrial fibrillation.

Treatment

The nature and severity of associated symptoms determine treatment in valvular heart disease. The patient may need to restrict activities to avoid extreme fatigue and dyspnea.

Heart failure requires digoxin, diuretics, a sodium-restricted diet and, in acute cases, oxygen. Other appropriate measures include anticoagulant therapy to prevent thrombus formation around diseased or replaced valves and prophylactic antibiotics before and after surgery or dental care.

If the patient has severe signs and symptoms that can't be managed medically, he may need open-heart surgery, with cardiopulmonary bypass for valve replacement.

Valvuloplasty may be used in elderly patients with end-stage disease who cannot tolerate general anesthesia.

Key nursing diagnoses and patient outcomes

Activity intolerance related to fatigue and dyspnea. Based on this nursing diagnosis, you'll establish these patient outcomes. The patient will:
- state the activities that increase fatigue or dyspnea, then avoid them or request assistance to perform them
- perform self-care activities as tolerated.

Decreased cardiac output related to the disease process. Based on this nursing diagnosis, you'll establish these patient outcomes. The patient will:
- remain hemodynamically stable
- avoid manifestations of profoundly decreased cardiac output, such as shock and tissue ischemia
- comply with the prescribed treatment regimen to enhance cardiac output.

Fluid volume excess related to pulmonary edema. Based on this nursing diagnosis, you'll establish these patient outcomes. The patient will:
- respond to treatment measures to alleviate excess fluid, as evidenced by a normal respiratory rate and pattern and a fluid output that exceeds intake
- take measures to prevent or minimize pulmonary edema, such as adhering to dietary and activity restrictions
- regain and maintain normal pulmonary function.

Nursing interventions

- Provide periods of rest alternating with activity to prevent excessive fatigue.
- To reduce anxiety, allow the patient to express his concerns about the effects of activity restrictions on his responsibilities and routines. Assure him that the restrictions are temporary.
- Keep the patient on a low-sodium diet; consult with the dietitian to ensure that the patient receives as many favorite foods as possible during the restriction.
- Provide oxygen to prevent tissue hypoxia, as needed and ordered.
- Prepare the patient for valve replacement or valvuloplasty, as indicated.
- Before giving penicillin, ask the patient if he's ever had a hypersensitivity reaction to it. Even if he hasn't, warn that such a reaction is possible. Administer antibiotics on time to maintain consistent drug levels in the blood.

Monitoring

- Observe the patient for signs and symptoms of left ventricular failure, pulmonary edema, and adverse reactions to drug therapy.
- Monitor vital signs, arterial blood gas values, intake and output, daily weights, blood chemistry studies, chest X-rays, and ECG.

Patient teaching

- Teach the patient about diet restrictions, medications, signs and symptoms that should be reported, and the importance of consistent follow-up care.
- Explain all tests and treatments.
- If valve replacement or valvuloplasty is scheduled, teach the patient and family about the surgery or procedure and what care to expect afterwards.
- Make sure the patient and his family understand the need to comply with prolonged antibiotic therapy and follow-up care and the need for additional antibiotics during dental surgery.
- Instruct the patient and his family to watch for and report early signs of heart failure, such as dyspnea and a hacking, nonproductive cough.

Mitral stenosis

In this disorder, valve leaflets become diffusely thickened by fibrosis and calcification. The mitral commissures fuse, the chordae tendineae fuse and shorten, the valvular cusps become rigid, and the apex of the valve becomes narrowed, obstructing blood flow from the left atrium to the left ventricle.

As a result of these changes, left atrial volume and pressure rise and the atrial chamber dilates. The increased resistance to blood flow causes pulmonary hypertension, right ventricular hypertrophy and, eventually, right ventricular failure. What's more, inadequate filling of the left ventricle reduces cardiac output.

Two-thirds of all patients with mitral stenosis are female.

Causes

Mitral stenosis most commonly results from rheumatic fever. It may also be associated with congenital anomalies.

Complications

Pulmonary hypertension caused by mitral stenosis can rupture pulmonary-bronchial venous connections, which results in hemorrhage. Pulmonary hypertension also increases transudation of fluid from pulmonary capillaries, which can cause fibrosis in the alveoli and pulmonary capillaries. This action reduces vital capacity, total lung capacity, maximal breathing capacity, and oxygen uptake per unit of ventilation.

Thrombi may form in the left atrium and–if they embolize–travel to the brain, kidneys, spleen, and extremities, possibly causing infarction. Embolization occurs most commonly in patients with arrhythmias.

Assessment

In mild mitral stenosis, the patient may have no symptoms. In moderate to severe mitral stenosis, you may find a history of dyspnea on exertion, paroxysmal nocturnal dyspnea, orthopnea, weakness, fatigue, and palpitations. Hemoptysis suggests rupture of pulmonary-bronchial venous connections. Inspection, palpation, and auscultation may reveal characteristic findings in mitral stenosis. (See *Physical findings in mitral stenosis.*)

Physical findings in mitral stenosis

With mitral stenosis, *inspection* may reveal peripheral and facial cyanosis, particularly in severe cases. The patient's face may appear pinched and blue, and she may have a malar rash. You may note jugular vein distention and ascites in the patient with severe pulmonary hypertension or associated tricuspid stenosis.

Palpation may reveal peripheral edema, hepatomegaly, and a diastolic thrill at the cardiac apex.

Auscultation may detect a loud S_1 or opening snap and a diastolic murmur at the apex, along the left sternal border or at the base of the heart. In a patient with pulmonary hypertension, the S_2 may be accentuated and the two components of the S_2 are closely split. You may hear a pulmonary systolic ejection click in a patient with severe pulmonary hypertension. Crackles also may be audible.

Diagnostic tests

- *Cardiac catheterization* shows a diastolic pressure gradient across the valve. It also shows elevated left atrial and pulmonary capillary wedge pressures (greater than 15 mm Hg) with severe pulmonary hypertension and pulmonary arterial pressures. It detects elevated right ventricular pressure, decreased cardiac output, and abnormal contraction of the left ventricle. However, this test may not be indicated in patients who have isolated mitral stenosis with mild symptoms.
- *Chest X-rays* show left atrial and ventricular enlargement (in severe mitral stenosis), straightening of the left border of the cardiac silhouette, enlarged pulmonary arteries, dilation of the upper lobe pul-

monary veins, and mitral valve calcification.

- *Echocardiography* discloses thickened mitral valve leaflets and left atrial enlargement.
- *Electrocardiography (ECG)* reveals cardiac hypertrophy, atrial fibrillation, right ventricular hypertrophy, and right axis deviation.

Treatment

In valvular heart disease, treatment depends on the nature and severity of associated symptoms. In asymptomatic mitral stenosis in a young patient, penicillin is an important prophylactic.

If the patient is symptomatic, treatment varies. Heart failure requires bed rest, digoxin, diuretics, a sodium-restricted diet and, in acute cases, oxygen. Small doses of beta blockers may also be used to slow ventricular rate when digitalis glycosides fail to control atrial fibrillation or flutter.

If hemoptysis develops, the patient requires bed rest, salt restriction, and diuretics to decrease pulmonary venous pressure. Embolization mandates anticoagulants along with symptomatic treatments.

If the patient has severe signs and symptoms that can't be managed medically, she may need open-heart surgery, with cardiopulmonary bypass for commissurotomy or valve replacement.

Percutaneous balloon valvuloplasty may be used in young patients who have no calcification or subvalvular deformity, in symptomatic pregnant women, and in elderly patients with end-stage disease who couldn't withstand general anesthesia. This procedure is performed in the cardiac catheterization laboratory.

Key nursing diagnoses and patient outcomes

Activity intolerance related to fatigue, dyspnea, or palpitations. Based on this nursing diagnosis, you'll establish these patient outcomes. The patient will:

- state the activities that increase fatigue, dyspnea, and palpitations, then avoid them or request assistance to perform them
- perform self-care activities as tolerated.

Decreased cardiac output related to the disease process. Based on this nursing diagnosis, you'll establish these patient outcomes. The patient will:

- remain hemodynamically stable
- avoid manifestations of profoundly decreased cardiac output, such as shock and tissue ischemia
- regain a normal cardiac output after valve replacement or percutaneous balloon valvuloplasty.

Impaired gas exchange related to pulmonary hypertension. Based on this nursing diagnosis, you'll establish these patient outcomes. The patient will:

- maintain adequate tissue oxygenation
- express ease in maintaining air exchange
- avoid further pulmonary dysfunction caused by pulmonary hypertension.

Nursing interventions

- Before giving penicillin, ask the patient if she's ever had a hypersensitivity reaction to it. Even if she never has, warn her that such a reaction is possible.
- If the patient needs bed rest, stress its importance. Assist with bathing as necessary. Provide a bedside commode because using a commode puts less stress on the heart than using a bedpan. Offer diversional, physically undemanding activities.
- To reduce anxiety, allow the patient to express concerns over being unable to meet her responsibilities because of activity restrictions. Give reassurance that activity limitations are temporary.
- Place the patient in an upright position to relieve dyspnea, if needed. Administer oxygen to prevent tissue hypoxia, as needed.
- Prepare the patient for valve replacement or percutaneous balloon valvuloplasty, as indicated. (See the entries "Heart valve replacement" and "Valvuloplasty, balloon.")
- Keep the patient on a low-sodium diet. Provide as many favorite foods as possible.

Monitoring

- Watch closely for signs of pulmonary dysfunction caused by pulmonary hypertension, tissue ischemia caused by emboli, and adverse reactions to drug therapy.
- Assess the patient's vital signs, arterial blood gas values, intake and output, daily weights, blood chemistry studies, chest X-rays, and ECG.

Patient teaching

- Explain all tests and treatments to the patient.
- Advise the patient to plan for periodic rest in her daily routine to prevent undue fatigue.
- Teach the patient about diet restrictions, medications, symptoms that should be reported, and the importance of consistent follow-up care.
- If the patient is scheduled for a valve replacement or percutaneous balloon valvuloplasty, explain the surgery or procedure to the patient and family and tell them what to expect afterward.

Mononucleosis

An acute infectious disease, mononucleosis causes fever, sore throat, and cervical lymphadenopathy, the hallmarks of the disease. It also causes hepatic dysfunction, increased lymphocytes and monocytes, and development and persistence of heterophil antibodies. The disease primarily affects young adults and children although, in children, it's usually so mild that it's often overlooked.

The disease is fairly prevalent in the United States, Canada, and Europe, and both sexes are affected equally. Incidence varies seasonally among college students but not among the general population.

The prognosis is excellent, and major complications are uncommon.

Causes

Infectious mononucleosis is caused by the Epstein-Barr virus (EBV), a member of the herpes group. Apparently, the reservoir of EBV is limited to humans.

The disease probably spreads by the oropharyngeal route. About 80% of patients carry EBV in the throat during the acute stage and for an indefinite time afterward. It also can be transmitted by blood transfusion and has been reported in cardiac surgery patients as the "postpump perfusion" syndrome. The disease is probably contagious from before symptoms develop until the fever subsides and oropharyngeal lesions disappear.

Complications

Although major complications are rare, mononucleosis may cause splenic rupture, aseptic meningitis, encephalitis, hemolytic anemia, pericarditis, and Guillain-Barré syndrome.

Assessment

The patient's history may reveal contact with a person who has infectious mononucleosis.

After an incubation period of about 30 to 50 days in adults, the patient may experience prodromal symptoms. He usually reports headache, malaise, profound fatigue, anorexia, myalgia and, possibly, abdominal discomfort. After 3 to 5 days he develops a sore throat, which he may describe as the worst he's ever had, and dysphagia related to adenopathy. He'll usually have a fever, typically with a late afternoon or evening peak of 101° to 102° F (38.3° to 38.9° C).

Your inspection commonly reveals exudative tonsillitis, pharyngitis and, sometimes, palatal petechiae, periorbital edema, maculopapular rash that resembles rubella, and jaundice.

On palpation, you'll probably note that nodes are mildly tender. You'll usually find cervical adenopathy with slight tenderness, but the patient also may have inguinal and axillary adenopathy. You may detect splenomegaly and, less commonly, hepatomegaly.

Auscultation of the chest usually is normal.

Diagnostic tests

The following abnormal laboratory test results confirm infectious mononucleosis.

- An increase in white blood cell (WBC) count of 10,000 to 20,000/mm³ during the 2nd and 3rd weeks of illness. Lymphocytes and monocytes account for 50% to 70% of the total WBC count; 10% of the lymphocytes are atypical.
- A fourfold rise in heterophil antibodies (agglutinins for sheep red blood cells) in serum drawn during the acute phase and at 3- to 4-week intervals.
- Antibodies to EBV and cellular antigens shown on indirect immunofluorescence. Such testing usually is more definitive than heterophil antibodies but may not be necessary because the vast majority of patients are heterophil-positive.
- Abnormal liver function studies.

Treatment

Infectious mononucleosis isn't easily prevented, and it's resistant to standard antimicrobial treatment. Thus, therapy is essentially supportive, including relief of symptoms, bed rest during the acute febrile period, and aspirin or another salicylate for headache and sore throat.

If severe throat inflammation causes airway obstruction, steroids can relieve swelling and prevent a tracheotomy. Splenic rupture, marked by sudden abdominal pain, requires splenectomy. About 20% of patients with infectious mononucleosis also have streptococcal pharyngotonsillitis and should receive antibiotic therapy for at least 10 days.

Key nursing diagnoses and patient outcomes

Fatigue related to the infection process. Based on this nursing diagnosis, you'll establish these patient outcomes. The patient will:

- avoid activities that increase fatigue
- obtain adequate rest to minimize fatigue
- regain his normal energy level.

Hyperthermia related to the infectious process. Based on this nursing diagnosis, you'll establish these patient outcomes. The patient will:

- exhibit a decrease in temperature after antipyretic measures
- avoid complications associated with hyperthermia, such as seizures and shock
- regain and maintain a normal temperature.

Pain related to throat inflammation and swelling. Based on this nursing diagnosis, you'll establish these patient outcomes. The patient will:

- express relief from discomfort after analgesic administration
- use diversional activities to minimize pain
- exhibit resolution of throat discomfort after treatment.

Nursing interventions

- Administer medications to treat symptoms, as needed.
- Provide warm saline gargles for symptomatic relief of sore throat.
- Provide adequate fluids and nutrition.
- Plan care to provide frequent rest periods.

Monitoring

- Check the patient's temperature regularly.
- Monitor the patient's response to analgesics, antipyretics, and other supportive care measures.
- Monitor the patient for complications.

Patient teaching

- Explain that convalescence may take several weeks, usually until the patient's WBC count returns to normal.
- Stress the need for bed rest during the acute illness. Warn the patient to avoid ex-

cessive activity, which could lead to splenic rupture.

- If the patient is a student, tell him that he can continue less demanding school assignments and see his friends but that he should avoid long, difficult projects until after recovery.
- To minimize throat discomfort, encourage the patient to drink milk shakes, fruit juices, and broths and to eat cool, bland foods. Advise using warm saline gargles, analgesics, and antipyretics as needed.

Multiple myeloma

Also called malignant plasmacytoma, plasma cell myeloma, and myelomatosis, multiple myeloma is a disseminated neoplasm of marrow plasma cells. The disease infiltrates bone to produce osteolytic lesions throughout the skeleton (flat bones, vertebrae, skull, pelvis, and ribs). With disease progression, bone marrow replacement with tumor, renal failure, and vertebral compression fractures are common occurrences.

Multiple myeloma strikes about 14,400 persons yearly – predominantly in persons over age 60. The median survival time is 2½ to 3 years, and men are affected slightly more often than women.

Although myeloma can improve with therapy and some long-term survivors are seen, it is generally considered an incurable disease.

Causes

Although the cause of multiple myeloma isn't known, genetic factors and occupational exposure to radiation have been linked to the disease.

Complications

Multiple myeloma can cause infections (such as pneumonia), pyelonephritis (caused by tubular damage from large amounts of Bence Jones protein, hypercalcemia, and hyperuricemia), renal calculi, renal failure, hematologic imbalance, fractures, hypercalcemia, hyperuricemia, and dehydration.

Patients may also develop a predisposition toward bleeding because of impaired platelet function and thrombocytopenia. This bleeding usually occurs in the GI tract or the nose.

Assessment

The patient may have a history of pathologic fractures. He usually complains of severe, constant back pain, which may increase with exercise. The patient may also report symptoms similar to those of arthritis, such as aches, joint swelling, and tenderness, probably from vertebral compression. Other complaints that may be reported include numbness, prickling, and tingling of the extremities (peripheral paresthesia).

Inspection may reveal that the patient has pain on movement or weight bearing, especially in the thoracic and lumbar vertebrae.

As the disease advances, the patient will become progressively weaker because of vertebral compression, anemia, and weight loss. As the nerves associated with respiratory function are affected, he may develop pneumonia as well as noticeable thoracic deformities and a reduction in body height of 5″ (13 cm) or more as vertebral collapse occurs.

Diagnostic tests

- *Complete blood count* shows moderate or severe anemia. The differential may show 40% to 50% lymphocytes but seldom more than 3% plasma cells. Rouleau formation, often the first clue, is seen on differential smear and results from elevation of the erythrocyte sedimentation rate.
- *Urine studies* may show proteinuria, Bence Jones protein, and hypercalciuria.

Understanding Bence Jones protein

The hallmark of multiple myeloma, this protein – a light chain of gamma globulin – was named for Henry Bence Jones, an English doctor. In 1848, he noticed that patients with a certain bone disease excreted a unique protein – unique in that it coagulated at 113° to 131° F (45° to 55° C), then redissolved when heated to boiling.

It remained for Otto Kahler, an Austrian, to demonstrate in 1889 that Bence Jones protein was related to myeloma. Bence Jones protein isn't found in the urine of all multiple myeloma patients, but it's almost never found in patients without this disease.

Absence of Bence Jones protein doesn't rule out multiple myeloma, but its presence almost invariably confirms the disease. (See *Understanding Bence Jones protein.*)

- *Bone marrow aspiration* detects myelomatous cells (abnormal number of immature plasma cells) – 10% to 95% instead of the normal 3% to 5%.
- *Serum electrophoresis* shows an elevated globulin spike that is electrophoretically and immunologically abnormal.
- *X-rays* during the early stages may reveal only diffuse osteoporosis. Eventually, they show multiple, sharply circumscribed osteolytic (punched out) lesions, particularly on the skull, pelvis, and spine – the characteristic lesions of multiple myeloma.
- *Excretory urography* can assess renal involvement. To avoid precipitation of Bence Jones protein, iothalamate or diatrizoate is used instead of the usual contrast medium.

Treatment

Long-term treatment of multiple myeloma consists mainly of chemotherapy to suppress plasma cell growth and control pain. Combinations of melphalan and prednisone or of vincristine, BCNU, melphalan, cyclophosphamide, and prednisone (VBMCP) are used. Adjuvant local irradiation reduces acute lesions and relieves the pain of collapsed vertebrae.

Other treatment usually includes administration of analgesics for pain. If the patient develops vertebral compression, he may require a laminectomy; if he has renal complications, he may need dialysis. Maintenance therapy with interferon may prolong the plateau phase once the initial chemotherapy is complete.

Because the patient may have bone demineralization and may lose large amounts of calcium into blood and urine, he's a prime candidate for renal calculi, nephrocalcinosis and, eventually, renal failure from hypercalcemia. Hydration, diuretics, corticosteroids, and pamidronate are given to decrease serum calcium levels. Plasmapheresis removes the M protein from the blood and returns the cells to the patient, although this effect is only temporary.

Key nursing diagnoses and patient outcomes

Anxiety related to the fear of death. Based on this nursing diagnosis, you'll establish these patient outcomes. The patient will:
- express his feelings about his diagnosis and prognosis
- use available support systems to help cope with his anxiety
- exhibit a reduction in anxiety after participating in decisions about his care
- exhibit fewer physical symptoms of anxiety.

Risk for infection related to bone disease. Based on this nursing diagnosis, you'll establish these patient outcomes. The patient will:
- maintain a normal temperature
- avoid signs and symptoms of infection.

Pain related to bone tissue destruction. Based on this nursing diagnosis, you'll establish these patient outcomes. The patient will:

• express relief of pain after analgesic administration
• avoid performing activities that cause or worsen pain or seek assistance when performing them
• use nonpharmacologic measures, such as guided imagery and relaxation techniques, to help cope with pain.

Nursing interventions

• Encourage the patient to drink 3,000 to 4,000 ml of fluids daily, particularly before excretory urography.
• Administer prescribed analgesics for pain as necessary. Provide comfort measures, such as repositioning and relaxation techniques.
• Prepare the patient for laminectomy, if indicated.
• The patient with multiple myeloma is particularly vulnerable to pathologic fractures. Never allow him to walk unaccompanied, and make sure he uses a walker or other supportive aid to prevent falls. Reassure him if he's fearful, and allow him to move at his own pace.
• If the patient is bedridden, change his position every 2 hours or position him as ordered; maintain alignment; and logroll him when turning. Provide passive range-of-motion and deep-breathing exercises; promote active exercises when he can tolerate them.
• Throughout therapy, listen to the patient's fears and concerns. Offer reassurance when appropriate, and stay with him if he experiences periods of severe stress and anxiety.
• Encourage the patient to identify actions and measures that promote comfort and relaxation. Try to perform these measures, and encourage the patient and his family to do so, too.
• Involve the patient and his family in decisions about his care whenever possible.
• Help relieve the patient's and his family's anxiety by answering their questions.

Monitoring

• Monitor the patient's fluid intake and output, which shouldn't fall below 1,500 ml/day.
• Assess the effectiveness of analgesics and nonpharmacologic measures used to alleviate or minimize pain.
• During chemotherapy, watch for complications such as fever and malaise; these may signal the onset of infection. Also observe for signs of other problems, such as severe anemia and fractures.
• If the patient is receiving melphalan, a phenylalanine derivative of nitrogen mustard that depresses bone marrow, obtain a platelet and white blood cell count before each treatment. If he's receiving prednisone, watch closely for signs of infection, which this drug masks.
• Monitor the patient for hemorrhage, motor and sensory deficits, and loss of bowel or bladder function.
• Observe the patient for signs and symptoms of infection.

Patient teaching

• Reinforce the doctor's explanation of the disease, diagnostic tests, treatment options, and prognosis. Make sure the patient understands what to expect from the treatment and diagnostic tests (including painful procedures, such as bone marrow aspiration and biopsy). Tell him to notify the doctor if the adverse effects of treatment persist.
• Prepare the patient for the effects of surgery.
• Explain the procedures the patient will undergo, such as insertion of an I.V. line and an indwelling urinary catheter.
• Emphasize the importance of deep breathing and changing position every 2 hours after surgery.
• Tell the patient to dress appropriately because multiple myeloma may make him particularly sensitive to cold.
• Caution the patient to avoid crowds and people with known infections because che-

motherapy and the disease itself impair the body's natural resistance to infection.
• If appropriate, direct the patient and his family to community resources – such as a local chapter of the American Cancer Society – for support.

Multiple sclerosis

This chronic disease is characterized by exacerbations and remissions caused by progressive demyelination of the white matter of the brain and spinal cord. Sporadic patches of demyelination in various parts of the long conduction pathways of the central nervous system cause widespread and varied neurologic dysfunction.

Multiple sclerosis (MS) is a major cause of chronic disability in young adults ages 20 to 40. The prognosis varies. MS may progress rapidly, disabling the patient by early adulthood or causing death within months of onset. However, about 70% of patients lead active, productive lives with prolonged remissions.

The incidence of MS is highest in women and among people in higher socioeconomic groups as well as those living in northern climates and in urban areas. A family history of MS also increases the risk.

Causes

The exact cause of MS is unknown, but theories suggest a slow-acting viral infection, an autoimmune response of the nervous system, or an allergic response to an infectious agent. Other possible causes include trauma, anoxia, toxins, nutritional deficiencies, vascular lesions, and anorexia, all of which may contribute to destruction of axons and the myelin sheath.

Emotional stress, overwork, fatigue, pregnancy, and acute respiratory tract infections all have been known to precede the onset of this illness. Genetic factors may also be involved.

Complications

In MS, complications include injuries from falls, urinary tract infections (UTIs), constipation, joint contractures, pressure ulcers, rectal distention, and pneumonia.

Assessment

Clinical findings in MS correspond to the extent and site of myelin destruction, the extent of remyelination, and the adequacy of subsequent restored synaptic transmission. Symptoms may be transient or may last for hours or weeks. They may vary from day to day, with no predictable pattern, and be bizarre and difficult for the patient to describe.

The patient history commonly reveals initial visual problems and sensory impairment, such as numbness and tingling sensations (paresthesia).

After the initial episode, signs and symptoms may vary widely. Patient history may reveal blurred vision or diplopia; urinary problems, such as incontinence, frequency, urgency, and UTIs; emotional lability, such as mood swings, irritability, euphoria, and depression; and possibly dysphagia.

As the patient speaks, you may notice scanning or poorly articulated speech. Neurologic examination and muscle function testing may discover muscle weakness of the involved area, such as an arm or leg, and spasticity, hyperreflexia, intention tremor, gait ataxia, and paralysis that ranges from monoplegia to quadriplegia. Visual examination may reveal nystagmus, scotoma, optic neuritis, or ophthalmoplegia.

Diagnostic tests

Because diagnosis is difficult, some patients may undergo years of periodic testing and close observation. These tests are helpful in diagnosing the disease.
• *EEG* shows abnormalities in one-third of patients.
• *Cerebrospinal fluid analysis* reveals elevated immunoglobulin G (IgG) levels but normal total protein levels. Such elevated

IgG levels are significant only when serum gamma globulin levels are normal, and they reflect hyperactivity of the immune system due to chronic demyelination. The white blood cell count may be slightly increased.

• *Evoked potential studies* demonstrate slowed conduction of nerve impulses in 80% of MS patients.

• *Computed tomography scan* may disclose lesions within the brain's white matter.

• *Magnetic resonance imaging* is the most sensitive method of detecting MS lesions. More than 90% of patients with MS show multifocal white matter lesions when this test is performed. It is also used to evaluate disease progression.

Other tests, such as *neuropsychological tests,* may help rule out other disorders.

Treatment

The aim of treatment is to shorten exacerbations and, if possible, relieve neurologic deficits, so the patient can resume a normal life-style.

Because MS is thought to have allergic and inflammatory causes, corticotropin, prednisone, or dexamethasone is used to reduce the associated edema of the myelin sheath during exacerbations. Corticotropin and corticosteroids seem to relieve symptoms and hasten remission but don't prevent future exacerbations.

Other useful drugs include chlordiazepoxide to mitigate mood swings, baclofen or dantrolene to relieve spasticity, and bethanechol or oxybutynin to relieve urine retention and minimize urinary frequency and urgency.

During acute exacerbations, supportive measures include bed rest, comfort measures (such as massages), prevention of fatigue and pressure ulcers, bowel and bladder training (if necessary), treatment of bladder infections with antibiotics, physical therapy, and counseling.

Key nursing diagnoses and patient outcomes

Altered urinary elimination related to urinary incontinence. Based on this nursing diagnosis, you'll establish these patient outcomes. The patient will:

• regain bladder control with bladder training

• avoid complications associated with urinary incontinence, such as infection and skin breakdown.

Impaired physical mobility related to neurologic dysfunction. Based on this nursing diagnosis, you'll establish these patient outcomes. The patient will:

• maintain muscle strength and joint range of motion

• avoid complications associated with impaired mobility, such as contractures, venous stasis, thrombus formation, and skin breakdown

• achieve the highest level of mobility possible with effective treatment of MS.

Sensory/perceptual alterations (visual, tactile, kinesthetic) related to neurologic deficits. Based on this nursing diagnosis, you'll establish these patient outcomes. The patient will:

• compensate for visual, tactile, and kinesthetic loss by using adaptive devices

• express feelings of safety, comfort, and security

• regain at least part of lost sensory/perceptual functioning during remission.

Nursing interventions

• Provide emotional and psychological support for the patient and the family, and answer their questions honestly. Stay with them during crisis periods. Encourage the patient by suggesting ways to help her cope with her disease.

• Assist with physical therapy. Increase patient comfort with massages and relaxing baths. Make sure the water isn't too hot because it may temporarily intensify otherwise subtle symptoms. Assist with active, resistive, and stretching exercises to maintain muscle tone and joint mobility, decrease spasticity, improve coordination, and boost morale. Provide rest periods between exercises because fatigue may contribute to exacerbations.

• Administer medications, as ordered.
• Promote emotional stability. Help the patient establish a daily routine to maintain optimal functioning. Her activity level is regulated by her tolerance level. Encourage regular rest periods, as well as daily physical exercise.
• Keep the bedpan or urinal readily accessible because the need to void is immediate.
• Encourage adequate fluid intake and regular urination. Institute bowel and bladder training as indicated. Eventually, the patient may require urinary drainage by self-catheterization or, in men, condom catheter.

Monitoring

• Watch for adverse reactions to administered medications. For instance, dantrolene may cause muscle weakness and decreased muscle tone.
• Monitor bowel and bladder function during hospitalization.
• Assess the patient's neurologic status for deficits.
• Monitor the patient for exacerbations and remissions of MS.

Patient teaching

• Educate the patient and her family about this chronic disease. Emphasize the need to avoid stress, infections, and fatigue and to maintain independence by developing new ways of performing daily activities.
• Emphasize the importance of exercise. Tell the patient that walking exercise may improve her gait. If her motor dysfunction causes coordination or balance problems, teach her to walk with a wide base of support. If she has trouble with position sense, tell her to watch her feet while walking. If she's still in danger of falling, a walker or a wheelchair may be required.
• Stress the importance of taking rest periods, preferably lying down.
• Teach the importance of eating a nutritious, well-balanced diet that contains sufficient roughage to prevent constipation.
• Teach the patient about bowel and bladder training if necessary. Also, teach her how to use suppositories to establish a regular bowel elimination schedule.
• Inform the patient that exacerbations are unpredictable, necessitating physical and emotional adjustments in life-style.
• Refer the patient to the social service department, when appropriate, and to a local chapter of the National Multiple Sclerosis Society.

Muscular dystrophy

Actually a group of hereditary disorders, muscular dystrophy is characterized by progressive symmetrical wasting of skeletal muscles but no neural or sensory defects. Four main types of muscular dystrophy occur: Duchenne's (pseudohypertrophic) muscular dystrophy, which accounts for 50% of all cases; Becker's (benign pseudohypertrophic) muscular dystrophy; facioscapulohumeral (Landouzy-Dejerine) dystrophy; and limb-girdle (Erb's) dystrophy.

Depending on the type, the disorder may affect vital organs and lead to severe disability or even death. Early in the disease, muscle fibers necrotize and regenerate in various states. Over time, regeneration slows and degeneration dominates. Fat and connective tissue replace muscle fibers, causing weakness.

Duchenne's and Becker's muscular dystrophies affect males almost exclusively; the incidence of Duchenne's in males is 13 to 33 per 100,000, and of Becker's, about 1 to 3 per 100,000. The remaining two types affect both sexes about equally.

The prognosis varies. Duchenne's muscular dystrophy typically begins during early childhood and causes death within 10 to 15 years. Patients with Becker's muscular dystrophy usually live into their

40s. Facioscapulohumeral and limb-girdle dystrophies usually don't shorten life expectancy.

Causes

Muscular dystrophy is caused by various genetic mechanisms. The basic defect can be mapped genetically to band Xp 21. Duchenne's and Becker's muscular dystrophies are X-linked recessive, and facioscapulohumeral dystrophy is autosomal dominant. Limb-girdle dystrophy may be inherited in several ways but usually is autosomal recessive.

Exactly how these inherited defects cause progressive muscle weakness isn't known. They may create an abnormality in the intracellular metabolism of muscle cells. The abnormality may be related to an enzyme deficiency or dysfunction or to an inability to synthesize, absorb, or metabolize an unknown substance vital to muscle function.

Complications

Duchenne's and Becker's muscular dystrophies lead to crippling disability and contractures. Progressive skeletal deformity and thoracic muscle weakness inhibit pulmonary function, increasing the risk of pneumonia and other respiratory infections. These diseases can also lead to such cardiac problems as arrhythmias and hypertrophy; sudden heart failure may cause death. Most patients with Duchenne's or Becker's muscular dystrophy die from respiratory complications.

Complications from other types of dystrophy vary with the site and severity of muscle involvement.

Assessment

The patient's family history may point to evidence of genetic transmission. If another family member has muscular dystrophy, its clinical characteristics can indicate the type of dystrophy the patient has and how he may be affected.

The patient may complain of progressive muscle weakness. The onset and characteristics of the increasing weakness vary with the type of dystrophy involved.

Duchenne's muscular dystrophy begins insidiously. Onset typically occurs when the child is between ages 3 and 5. Weakness begins in the pelvic muscles and interferes with the child's ability to run, climb, and walk. The disease progresses rapidly; by age 12, the child usually can't walk.

Signs and symptoms of Becker's muscular dystrophy resemble those of Duchenne's, but they progress more slowly. They start after age 5, but the patient can still walk well beyond age 15 – sometimes into his 40s.

Facioscapulohumeral dystrophy – a slowly progressive and relatively benign form of muscular dystrophy – typically begins before the child reaches age 10. However, symptoms may develop during adolescence. Early symptoms include weakness of eye, face, and shoulder muscles. The patient may complain that he's unable to raise his arms over his head or close his eyes completely. The patient or the patient's parents may notice other early signs, including an inability to pucker the lips or whistle, abnormal facial movements, and the absence of facial movements when laughing or crying. Pelvic muscles weaken as the disease progresses.

Limb-girdle dystrophy follows a similarly slow course and commonly causes only slight disability. Onset usually occurs when the child is between ages 6 and 10 but may occur in early adulthood. Muscle weakness first appears in the upper arm and pelvic muscles.

Inspection reveals the effects of muscle weakness and eventually muscle wasting. Findings vary according to the type of dystrophy. Early in Duchenne's and Becker's muscular dystrophies, you may notice that the patient has a wide stance and a waddling gait. He may also display Gowers' sign when rising from a sitting or supine position.

During the initial stage, you may notice muscle hypertrophy. As the disease progresses, however, most muscles atrophy.

The calves remain enlarged because of fat infiltration into the muscle. As abdominal and paravertebral muscles weaken, you may observe posture changes. The patient develops lordosis and a protuberant abdomen. Weakened thoracic muscles may cause scapular "winging" or flaring when the patient raises his arms. Bone outlines become prominent as surrounding muscles atrophy. In later stages, you may note contractures as well as pulmonary signs such as tachypnea and shortness of breath.

A patient with facioscapulohumeral dystrophy may develop a pendulous lower lip, and the nasolabial fold may disappear. Diffuse facial flattening leads to a masklike expression. The scapulae develop a winglike appearance, and the patient can't raise his arms above his head.

With limb-girdle dystrophy, you may note winging of the scapulae, lordosis with abdominal protrusion, a waddling gait, poor balance, and an inability to raise the arms.

Diagnostic tests

Several tests help confirm the diagnosis.

- *Muscle biopsy* shows fat and connective tissue deposits and confirms the diagnosis. It also shows degeneration and necrosis of muscle fibers and, in Duchenne's and Becker's dystrophies, a deficiency of the muscle protein dystrophin.
- *Electromyography* typically demonstrates short, weak bursts of electrical activity in affected muscles.
- *Urine creatinine, serum creatine phosphokinase (CPK), lactate dehydrogenase, alanine aminotransferase (formerly SGPT)* and *aspartate aminotransferase (formerly SGOT) levels* are elevated. CPK levels rise before muscle weakness becomes severe, providing an early indicator of Duchenne's and Becker's muscular dystrophies. These diagnostic tests are also useful for genetic screening because unaffected carriers also show elevated enzyme levels.
- *Amniocentesis* can't detect muscular dystrophy definitively, but because it reveals the sex of the fetus, it may be recommended for pregnant patients known to carry the gene for Duchenne's or Becker's muscular dystrophy.
- *Genetic testing* can detect the gene defect that leads to muscular dystrophy in some families.

Treatment

Currently, no treatment can stop the progressive muscle impairment. However, orthopedic appliances, exercise, physical therapy, and surgery to correct contractures can help preserve the patient's mobility and independence.

Key nursing diagnoses and patient outcomes

Activity intolerance related to weakness. Based on this nursing diagnosis, you'll establish these patient outcomes. The patient will:

- express an understanding of the need to maintain his activity level
- avoid risk factors that may increase his activity intolerance, such as obesity
- perform self-care activities as tolerated.

Impaired physical mobility related to skeletal muscle wasting. Based on this nursing diagnosis, you'll establish these patient outcomes. The patient will:

- avoid complications associated with impaired physical mobility, such as skin breakdown, venous stasis, and thrombus formation
- seek assistance to carry out his mobility regimen
- achieve the highest mobility level possible.

Ineffective breathing pattern related to thoracic muscle weakness. Based on this nursing diagnosis, you'll establish these patient outcomes. The patient will:

- achieve maximum lung expansion with adequate ventilation
- avoid pulmonary complications, such as pneumonia and atelectasis
- exhibit normal arterial blood gas values.

Nursing interventions

- If a patient with Duchenne's or Becker's muscular dystrophy develops respiratory involvement, encourage coughing and deep-breathing exercises.
- Help the patient to preserve joint mobility and prevent muscle atrophy by encouraging and assisting with active and passive range-of-motion exercises.
- The patient may need splints, braces, grab bars, and overhead slings. For comfort and to prevent footdrop, use a footboard or high-topped shoes and a foot cradle.
- Because inactivity may cause constipation, encourage adequate fluid intake, increase dietary bulk, and obtain an order for a stool softener. Because the patient is prone to obesity from reduced physical activity, provide him with a low-calorie, high-protein, high-fiber diet.
- Allow the patient plenty of time to perform even simple physical tasks.

Monitoring

- Regularly assess the patient's respiratory status for signs of pulmonary complications.
- Monitor the patient's self-care abilities.
- Observe the patient for complications associated with immobility, such as skin breakdown, contractures, and venous stasis.

Patient teaching

- Encourage communication between the family members and the patient to help them handle emotional strain and cope with changes in body image.
- Encourage the patient and his family to express their concerns. Listen to them and answer their questions.
- Help a child with Duchenne's muscular dystrophy maintain peer relationships and realize his intellectual potential by encouraging his parents to keep him in a regular school as long as possible.
- Teach the patient and his parents ways to maintain the patient's mobility and independence for as long as possible.
- Inform the patient and his parents about possible complications and the steps they can take to prevent them.
- Explain the possibility of respiratory tract infections, what signs to watch for, and what to do if the patient develops such an infection. Urge the patient and his parents to report signs of infection to the doctor at once.
- When the patient becomes confined to a wheelchair, help him and his family to see the chair as a way to preserve his independence. Have an occupational therapist teach the patient about his wheelchair and other supportive devices that can help him with activities of daily living.
- Help the patient and his family plan a low-calorie, high-protein, high-fiber diet to prevent obesity caused by reduced physical activity.
- Advise the patient to avoid long periods of bed rest and inactivity; if necessary, he should limit television viewing and other sedentary activities.
- If desired, refer adult patients for sexual counseling.
- Refer the patient for appropriate physical therapy, vocational rehabilitation, social services, and financial assistance. Suggest the Muscular Dystrophy Association as a source of information and support.
- Refer family members who carry the muscular dystrophy trait to genetic counseling so they understand the risk of transmitting this disorder.

Myasthenia gravis

This disorder produces sporadic but progressive weakness and abnormal fatigability of striated (skeletal) muscles. Muscle weakness is exacerbated by exercise and repeated movement but improved by anticholinesterase drugs. Usually, myasthenia gravis affects muscles innervated by the cranial nerves (face, lips, tongue, neck, and throat), but it can affect any muscle group. It commonly accompanies immune and thyroid disorders. In fact, 15% of myasthenic patients have thymomas. When the disease involves the respiratory system, it may be life-threatening.

Myasthenia gravis follows an unpredictable course of recurring exacerbations and periodic remissions. No cure is known. However, drug treatment has improved the prognosis and allows patients to lead relatively normal lives except during exacerbations.

Myasthenia gravis affects 2 to 20 persons per 100,000. It occurs at any age, but incidence is highest in women ages 18 to 25 and in men ages 50 to 60. About three times as many women as men develop this disease.

About 20% of infants born to myasthenic mothers have transient (or occasionally persistent) myasthenia. Spontaneous remissions occur in about 25% of patients.

Causes

Myasthenia gravis is thought to be an autoimmune disorder. For an unknown reason, the patient's blood cells and thymus gland produce antibodies that block, destroy, or weaken the neuroreceptors that transmit nerve impulses, causing a failure in transmission of nerve impulses at the neuromuscular junction.

Complications

In myasthenia gravis, complications include respiratory distress, pneumonia, and chewing and swallowing difficulties that may lead to choking and food aspiration.

Assessment

Depending on the muscles involved and the severity of the disease, assessment findings may vary. Muscle weakness is progressive, and eventually some muscles may lose function entirely.

Expect the patient to complain of extreme muscle weakness and fatigue. The muscles most often initially involved are those innervated by the cranial nerves; thus, the patient often mentions ptosis and diplopia (the most common sign and symptom). She may also report that chewing and swallowing are difficult, that her jaw hangs open (especially when she's tired), and that her head bobs. She may also say that she must tilt her head back to see properly. Some patients (about 15%) report weakness of arm or hand muscles; rarely, a patient may report leg weakness.

The patient usually notes that symptoms are milder on awakening and worsen as the day progresses and that short rest periods temporarily restore muscle function. On questioning, she may report that symptoms become more intense during menses and after emotional stress, prolonged exposure to sunlight or cold, or infections.

On inspection, the patient may have a sleepy, masklike expression (caused by involvement of the facial muscles) and a drooping jaw (especially if she's tired). Inspection may also confirm ptosis. Auscultation may reveal hypoventilation if the respiratory muscles are involved.

Respiratory muscle involvement may lead to decreased tidal volume, making breathing difficult; this may predispose the patient to pneumonia and other respiratory tract infections. Progressive weakness of the diaphragm and the intercostal muscles may eventually lead to severe respiratory distress and myasthenic crisis. (See *What to do in myasthenic crisis.*)

Diagnostic tests

- A positive *Tensilon test* confirms a diagnosis of myasthenia gravis. This test shows temporarily improved muscle function after an I.V. injection of edrophonium (or occasionally neostigmine). In myasthenic patients, muscle function improves within 30 to 60 seconds and lasts up to 30 minutes. However, long-standing ocular muscle dysfunction often fails to respond to such testing. The Tensilon test can also differentiate a myasthenic crisis from a cholinergic crisis, which is caused by acetylcholine overactivity at the neuromuscular

LIFE-THREATENING COMPLICATIONS

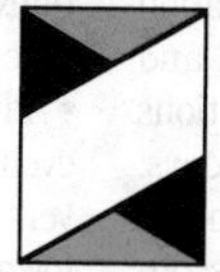

What to do in myasthenic crisis

Myasthenic crisis is an acute exacerbation of the muscular weakness that occurs in myasthenia gravis. It can be triggered by infection, surgery, emotional stress, an overdose or insufficiency of anticholinesterase medication, a drug interaction, alcohol intake, pregnancy, or seasonal or temperature changes.

Signs and symptoms

Typical signs and symptoms of myasthenic crisis include respiratory distress that progresses to periods of apnea, extreme fatigue, increased muscular weakness, dysphagia, dysarthria, and fever. The patient may be anxious, restless, irritable, and unable to move the jaws or to raise one or both eyelids.

If myasthenic crisis results from anticholinesterase toxicity, you may assess anorexia, nausea, vomiting, abdominal cramps, diarrhea, excessive salivation, sweating, lacrimation, blurred vision, vertigo, muscle cramps, spasms, general weakness, dysarthria, and respiratory distress.

Emergency interventions

- Notify the doctor immediately.
- Maintain a patent airway.
- Be prepared to administer oxygen therapy with assisted or controlled mechanical ventilation.
- Expect to withdraw anticholinergic drugs if the crisis is caused by toxicity; or, you may be asked to administer anticholinergic drugs to help identify the type of crisis.
- Administer supportive care as needed. For example, the patient may require parenteral fluids, antibiotics, nasogastric tube feedings, and insertion of an indwelling urinary catheter.
- Prepare the patient for transfer to the intensive care unit, where she'll remain until the crisis subsides.

junction, possibly caused by anticholinesterase overdose.

- *Electromyography* measures the electrical potential of muscle cells and helps differentiate nerve disorders from muscle disorders.
- *Nerve conduction studies* measure the speed at which electrical impulses travel along a nerve and also help distinguish nerve disorders from muscle disorders.
- *Chest X-rays* or *computed tomography scan* may identify a thymoma.

Treatment

Measures to relieve symptoms may include anticholinesterase drugs, such as neostigmine and pyridostigmine. These drugs counteract fatigue and muscle weakness and allow about 80% of normal muscle function. However, they become less effective as the disease worsens. Corticosteroids may also help to relieve symptoms.

Some patients may undergo plasmapheresis if medications prove ineffective. This procedure will remove acetylcholine-receptor antibodies and temporarily lessen the severity of symptoms.

Patients with thymomas require thymectomy, which leads to remission in adult-onset myasthenia in about 40% of patients if done within 2 years of diagnosis.

Acute exacerbations that cause severe respiratory distress may signal the onset of myasthenic crisis and necessitate emergency treatment. Tracheotomy, ventilation with a positive-pressure ventilator, and vigorous suctioning to remove secretions usually bring improvement in a few days. Because anticholinesterase drugs aren't effective in myasthenic crisis, they're discontinued until respiratory function begins to improve. Such a crisis requires immediate hospitalization and vigorous respiratory support.

Key nursing diagnoses and patient outcomes

Impaired gas exchange related to respiratory dysfunction. Based on this nursing diagnosis, you'll establish these patient outcomes. The patient will:
- maintain adequate gas exchange with mechanical assistance during myasthenic crisis
- perform bronchial hygiene correctly to keep his airways clear
- regain normal gas exchange after myasthenic crisis, as evidenced by normal arterial blood gas values and normal respiratory function.

Impaired physical mobility related to muscle weakness. Based on this nursing diagnosis, you'll establish these patient outcomes. The patient will:
- maintain normal joint range of motion
- avoid complications associated with impaired mobility, such as contractures, venous stasis, thrombus formation, and skin breakdown
- achieve the highest level of mobility possible.

Impaired swallowing related to muscle weakness. Based on this nursing diagnosis, you'll establish these patient outcomes. The patient will:
- exhibit correct eating or feeding techniques to maximize his ability to swallow
- maintain an adequate nutritional intake
- avoid aspiration pneumonia.

Nursing interventions

- Provide psychological support. Listen to the patient's concerns, and answer questions honestly. Encourage her to participate in her own care.
- Administer medications on time and at evenly spaced intervals, as ordered, to prevent relapses. Be prepared to give atropine for anticholinesterase overdose or toxicity.
- Plan exercise, meals, patient care, and activities to make the most of energy peaks. For example, administer the patient's medication 20 to 30 minutes before meals to facilitate chewing or swallowing.
- When swallowing is difficult, give soft, semisolid foods (applesauce, mashed potatoes) instead of liquids to lessen the risk of choking.
- After a severe exacerbation, try to increase social activity as soon as possible.
- If surgery is scheduled, prepare the patient according to hospital policy.

Monitoring

- Establish an accurate neurologic and respiratory baseline. Thereafter, regularly monitor the patient's tidal volume, vital capacity, and inspiratory force.
- Stay alert for signs of impending myasthenic crisis (increased muscle weakness, respiratory distress, and difficulty talking or chewing). The patient may need a ventilator and frequent suctioning to remove accumulated secretions.

Patient teaching

- Help the patient plan daily activities to coincide with energy peaks.
- Stress the need for frequent rest periods throughout the day. Emphasize that periodic remissions, exacerbations, and day-to-day fluctuations are common.
- Teach the patient to recognize adverse effects of anticholinesterase drugs (headaches, weakness, sweating, abdominal cramps, nausea, vomiting, diarrhea, excessive salivation, and bronchospasm) and corticosteroids (decreased or blurred vision; increased thirst; frequent urination; rectal bleeding, burning, or itching; restlessness; depression).

• Warn the patient to avoid strenuous exercise, stress, infection, and needless exposure to the sun or cold weather. All of these things may worsen signs and symptoms. Wearing an eye patch or glasses with one frosted lens may help the patient with diplopia.
• Teach the patient who has swallowing difficulties to eat semisolid foods and to avoid alcohol because it increases weakness. Tell her that eating warm (not hot) foods can help ease swallowing.
• If surgery is scheduled, provide preoperative teaching. Explain to the patient that before surgery, her chest will be cleaned and shaved and she'll receive a general anesthetic. Tell her that, depending on where the surgeon makes the incision, she may awaken from surgery with a chest tube or a drain in place. Also tell her that she may require intubation and mechanical ventilation after surgery and that she'll have antimyasthenic drugs administered I.V. or I.M. until she's well enough to take them orally. Explain that these medications will be progressively withdrawn so that the doctor can assess her muscle strength after surgery.
• For information and an opportunity to meet patients with myasthenia gravis who lead productive lives, refer the patient to the Myasthenia Gravis Foundation.

Myocardial infarction

Myocardial infarction (MI) results from reduced blood flow through one of the coronary arteries, which causes myocardial ischemia and necrosis. The infarction site depends on the vessels involved. For instance, occlusion of the circumflex coronary artery causes a lateral wall infarction; occlusion of the left anterior coronary artery causes an anterior wall infarction. True posterior and inferior wall infarctions result from occlusion of the right coronary artery or one of its branches. Right ventricular infarctions can also result from right coronary artery occlusion, can accompany inferior infarctions, and may cause right ventricular failure. In transmural (Q wave) MI, tissue damage extends through all myocardial layers; in subendocardial (non–Q wave) MI, usually only the innermost layer is damaged.

Men are more susceptible to MI than premenopausal women, although incidence is rising among women who smoke and take oral contraceptives. The incidence in postmenopausal women is similar to that in men.

In North America and western Europe, MI is one of the most common causes of death, which usually results from cardiac damage or complications. Mortality is about 25%. However, more than 50% of sudden deaths occur within 1 hour after onset of signs and symptoms, before the patient reaches the hospital. Of those who recover, up to 10% die within the first year.

Causes

MI results from occlusion of one of the coronary arteries. Such occlusion can stem from atherosclerosis, thrombosis, platelet aggregration, or coronary artery stenosis or spasm. Predisposing factors include:
• aging
• diabetes mellitus
• elevated serum triglyceride, low-density lipoprotein, and cholesterol levels and decreased serum high-density lipoprotein levels
• excessive intake of saturated fats, carbohydrates, or salt
• hypertension
• obesity
• family history of coronary artery disease
• sedentary life-style
• smoking
• stress or a type A personality (aggressive, competitive attitude, addiction to work, chronic impatience).

In addition, use of drugs such as amphetamines or cocaine can cause an MI.

Assessing and managing complications of MI

Complication	Assessment	Treatment
Arrhythmias	• ECG shows premature ventricular contractions, ventricular tachycardia, or ventricular fibrillation; in inferior wall MI, bradycardia and junctional rhythms or atrioventricular (AV) block; in anterior wall MI, tachycardia or heart block.	• Antiarrhythmics, atropine, cardioversion, defibrillation, and pacemaker
Heart failure	• In left ventricular failure, chest X-rays show venous congestion and cardiomegaly. • Catheterization shows increases in pulmonary artery systolic and diastolic pressures, pulmonary capillary wedge pressure (PCWP), central venous pressure, and systemic vascular resistance (SVR).	• Diuretics, vasodilators, inotropics, and cardiac glycosides
Cardiogenic shock	• Catheterization shows decreased cardiac output, increased pulmonary artery systolic and diastolic pressures, decreased cardiac index, increased SVR, and increased PCWP. • Signs are hypotension, tachycardia, decreased level of consciousness, decreased urine output, neck vein distention, S_3 and S_4, and cool, pale skin.	• I.V. fluids, vasodilators, cardiotonics, cardiac glycosides, intra-aortic balloon pump (IABP), vasopressors, and beta-adrenergic stimulants
Mitral insufficiency	• Auscultation reveals apical holosystolic murmur. • Dyspnea is prominent. • Catheterization shows increased pulmonary artery pressure (PAP) and PCWP. • Echocardiogram shows valve dysfunction.	• Nitroglycerin, nitroprusside, IABP, and surgical replacement of the mitral valve and possible concomitant myocardial revascularization with significant coronary artery disease
Ventricular septal rupture	• In left-to-right shunt, auscultation reveals a harsh holosystolic murmur and thrill. • Catheterization shows increased PAP and PCWP. • Increased oxygen saturation of right ventricle and pulmonary artery confirms the diagnosis.	• Surgical correction (may be postponed, but more patients have surgery immediately or up to 7 days after septal rupture), IABP, nitroglycerin, nitroprusside, low-dose inotropics (dopamine), and cardiac pacing when high-grade AV blocks occur

Assessing and managing complications of MI *(continued)*

Complication	Assessment	Treatment
Pericarditis or Dressler's syndrome	• Auscultation reveals a pericardial friction rub. • Chest pain is relieved in sitting position. • Sharp pain unlike previously experienced anginal pain.	• Anti-inflammatory agents, such as aspirin or other nonsteroidal anti-inflammatory drugs or corticosteroids
Ventricular aneurysm	• Chest X-rays may show cardiomegaly. • ECG may show arrhythmias and persistent ST-segment elevation. • Left ventriculography shows altered or paradoxical left ventricular motion.	• Cardioversion, defibrillation (if ventricular tachycardia or fibrillation occurs), antiarrhythmics, vasodilators, anticoagulants, cardiac glycosides, diuretics and, possibly, surgery
Cerebral or pulmonary embolism	• Dyspnea and chest pain or neurologic changes occur. • Nuclear scan shows ventilation-perfusion mismatch in pulmonary embolism. • Angiography shows arterial blockage.	• Oxygen and heparin • Cardiopulmonary resuscitation (CPR), epinephrine, or cardiac pacing
Ventricular rupture	• Cardiac tamponade occurs. • Arrhythmias, such as ventricular tachycardia and ventricular fibrillation, or sudden death results.	• Resuscitation for advanced cardiac life support protocol • Possible emergency surgical repair if CPR is successful

Complications

Cardiac complications of acute MI include arrhythmias, cardiogenic shock, heart failure causing pulmonary edema, and pericarditis. Other complications include rupture of the atrial or ventricular septum, ventricular wall, or valves; ventricular aneurysms; mural thrombi causing cerebral or pulmonary emboli; and extensions of the original infarction. Dressler's syndrome (post-MI pericarditis) can occur days to weeks after an MI and cause residual pain, malaise, and fever. (See *Assessing and managing complications of MI.*)

Typically, elderly patients are more prone to complications and death. Psychological problems can also occur, either from the patient's fear of another MI or from an organic brain disorder caused by tissue hypoxia. Occasionally, a patient may have a personality change.

Assessment

Typically, the patient reports the cardinal symptom of MI – persistent, crushing substernal pain that may radiate to the left arm, jaw, neck, and shoulder blades. He commonly describes the pain as heavy, squeezing, or crushing, and it may persist for 12 or more hours. However, in some patients – particularly elderly patients or those with diabetes – pain may not occur; in others, it may be mild and may be confused with indigestion.

CHECKLIST

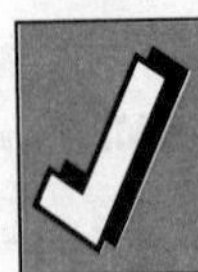

Key abnormal diagnostic findings in MI

To help diagnose an MI, the patient will undergo a 12-lead ECG as well as serum laboratory analysis. Expect the following results.

- ☐ Serial 12-lead ECG revealing serial ST-segment depression in subendocardial MI and ST-segment elevation and Q waves (representing scarring and necrosis) in transmural MI. However, be aware that during the first few hours after an MI, the ECG may be normal or inconclusive.
- ☐ Total serum creatine phosphokinase (CPK) level above 175 U/L for men and above 140 U/L for women. (*Note:* Different measurement methods give different ranges. Check the normal range used by the laboratory at your health care facility.)
- ☐ CPK-MB isoenzyme level that starts to rise within 4 hours of an acute MI, peaks in 12 to 48 hours, and usually returns to normal in 24 to 48 hours. Persistent elevations or increasing levels indicate ongoing myocardial damage.
- ☐ LDH_1-LDH_2 isoenzyme ratio above 1.

Patients with coronary artery disease may report increasing anginal frequency, severity, or duration (especially when not precipitated by exertion, a heavy meal, or cold and wind). The patient may also report a feeling of impending doom, fatigue, nausea, vomiting, and shortness of breath. Sudden death, however, may be the first and only indication of MI.

Inspection may reveal an extremely anxious and restless patient with dyspnea and diaphoresis. If right ventricular failure is present, you may note jugular venous distention. Within the first hour after an anterior MI, about 25% of patients exhibit sympathetic nervous system hyperactivity, such as tachycardia and hypertension. Up to 50% of patients with an inferior MI exhibit parasympathetic nervous system hyperactivity, such as bradycardia and hypotension.

In patients who develop ventricular dysfunction, auscultation may disclose an S_4, an S_3, paradoxical splitting of S_2, and decreased heart sounds. A systolic murmur of mitral insufficiency may be heard with papillary muscle dysfunction secondary to infarction. A pericardial friction rub may also be heard, especially in patients who have a transmural MI or have developed pericarditis.

Fever is unusual at the onset of an MI. However, a low-grade fever may develop during the next few days.

Diagnostic tests

For critical diagnostic test results, see *Key abnormal diagnostic findings in MI.* Other characteristic diagnostic results include the following:

- *Echocardiography* shows ventricular wall dyskinesia with a transmural MI and helps evaluate the ejection fraction.
- *Scans,* using I.V. technetium Tc99m can identify acutely damaged muscle by picking up accumulations of radioactive nucleotide, which appears as a "hot spot" on the film. Myocardial perfusion imaging with thallium-201 reveals a "cold spot" in most patients during the first few hours after a transmural MI.

Treatment

The goals of treatment are to relieve chest pain, to stabilize heart rhythm, and to reduce cardiac work load. Treatment includes revascularization to preserve myocardial tissue. Arrhythmias, the most common problem during the first 48 hours after MI, may require antiarrhythmics, possibly a pacemaker and, rarely, cardioversion.

Drug therapy usually includes:

- lidocaine for ventricular arrhythmias; if lidocaine is ineffective, procainamide, quinidine sulfate, bretylium, or disopyramide
- atropine I.V. or a temporary pacemaker for heart block or bradycardia
- nitroglycerin (sublingual, topical, transdermal, or I.V.); calcium channel blockers, such as nifedipine, verapamil, and diltiazem (sublingual, oral, or I.V.); or isosorbide dinitrate (sublingual, oral, or I.V.) to relieve pain by redistributing blood to ischemic area of the myocardium, increasing cardiac output, and reducing myocardial work load
- morphine I.V., the drug of choice for pain and sedation, and possibly meperidine or hydromorphone
- drugs that increase contractility or blood pressure
- inotropic drugs, such as dobutamine and amrinone, to treat reduced myocardial contractility
- beta-adrenergic blockers, such as propranolol and timolol, after acute MI to help prevent reinfarction.

Other therapies may be used.

- Oxygen is usually administered (by face mask or nasal cannula) at a modest flow rate for 24 to 48 hours; a lower concentration is necessary if the patient has chronic obstructive pulmonary disease.
- Bed rest with bedside commode is enforced to decrease cardiac work load.
- Pulmonary artery catheterization may be performed to detect left or right ventricular failure and to monitor response to treatment, but it's not routinely done.
- Intra-aortic balloon pump may be used for cardiogenic shock.
- Revascularization therapy can be used if the patient is less than age 70 and doesn't have a history of cerebrovascular accident, bleeding, GI ulcers, marked hypertension, recent surgery, or chest pain lasting longer than 6 hours. Thrombolytic therapy must be started up to 12 hours after infarction, using intracoronary or systemic streptokinase (I.V.) or tissue plasminogen activator. The best response occurs when treatment begins within the first hour after onset of symptoms.
- Cardiac catheterization, percutaneous transluminal coronary angioplasty (PTCA), and coronary artery bypass grafting may also be performed.

Key nursing diagnoses and patient outcomes

Altered cardiac tissue perfusion related to narrowing or closure of one or more coronary arteries. Based on this nursing diagnosis, you'll establish these patient outcomes. The patient will:

- seek emergency intervention immediately to minimize myocardial damage.
- exhibit no arrhythmias on electrocardiogram (ECG)
- regain adequate cardiac tissue perfusion.

Risk for injury related to complications of MI. Based on this nursing diagnosis, you'll establish these patient outcomes. The patient will:

- seek immediate medical treatment if complications arise
- avoid permanent deficits caused by complications of MI.

Pain related to myocardial tissue ischemia. Based on this nursing diagnosis, you'll establish these patient outcomes. The patient will:

- express relief of chest discomfort after treatment
- avoid new episodes of chest pain and exhibit no ischemic changes on ECG
- comply with the prescribed treatment regimen to prevent further tissue ischemia.

Nursing interventions

- Administer analgesics, as ordered. Avoid giving I.M. injections because absorption from muscles is unpredictable and I.V. administration provides more rapid symptomatic relief.
- Organize patient care and activities to allow periods of uninterrupted rest.

EXPERT GERIATRIC CARE

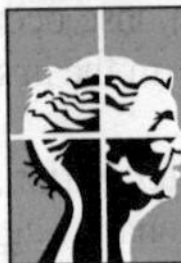

Monitoring signs and symptoms of MI in the elderly

The diagnosis of MI may be delayed or even missed because the elderly patient doesn't exhibit the typical signs and symptoms associated with an MI. These atypical signs and symptoms include low body temperature, decreased blood pressure, vague complaints of discomfort, mild perspiration, stroke-like symptoms, dizziness, and changes in sensorium. Pain is often absent. The elderly patient also is more likely to suffer a silent MI. Therefore, thorough assessment and evaluation of the patient's complaints are essential.

- Provide a clear-liquid diet until nausea subsides. A low-cholesterol, low-sodium diet without caffeine may be ordered.
- Provide a stool softener to prevent straining during defecation. Allow the patient to use a bedside commode, and provide as much privacy as possible.
- Assist with range-of-motion exercises. If the patient is immobilized, turn him often and use antiembolism stockings.
- Provide emotional support, and help reduce stress and anxiety; administer tranquilizers as needed.
- Prepare the patient for PTCA and thrombolytic therapy, as indicated. (See the entries "Angioplasty, percutaneous transluminal coronary" and "Thrombolytic therapy.")

Monitoring

- On admission to the intensive care unit (ICU), monitor and record the patient's ECG, blood pressure, temperature, and heart and breath sounds.
- Assess and record the patient's severity, location, type, and duration of pain.
- Check his blood pressure after giving nitroglycerin, especially the first dose.
- Frequently monitor ECG rhythm strips to detect heart rate changes and arrhythmias. (See *Monitoring signs and symptoms of MI in the elderly.*)
- During episodes of chest pain, monitor the ECG and blood pressure and pulmonary artery catheter measurements (if applicable) to determine changes.
- Watch for crackles, cough, tachypnea, and edema, which may indicate impending left ventricular failure. Carefully monitor daily weight, intake and output, respiratory rate, serum enzyme levels, ECG waveforms, and blood pressure. Auscultate for adventitious breath sounds periodically. Also auscultate for S_3 or S_4 gallops.

Patient teaching

- Explain procedures and answer questions for both the patient and his family. Explain the ICU environment and routine.
- Thoroughly explain medication and treatment regimen. Inform the patient of the drug's adverse effects and advise him to watch for and report signs of toxicity (for example, anorexia, nausea, vomiting, mental depression, vertigo, blurred vision, and yellow vision, if the patient is receiving a digitalis glycoside).
- Review dietary restrictions with the patient. If he must follow a low-sodium or low-fat and low-cholesterol diet, provide a list of foods to avoid. Ask the dietitian to speak to the patient and his family.
- Encourage the patient to participate in a cardiac rehabilitation exercise program.
- Advise the patient to resume sexual activity progressively. He may need to take nitroglycerin before sexual intercourse to prevent chest pain from the increased activity.
- Advise the patient about appropriate responses to new or recurrent symptoms.
- Advise the patient to report typical or atypical chest pain. Post-MI syndrome may develop, producing chest pain that

must be differentiated from recurrent MI, pulmonary infarction, and heart failure.
• Stress the need to stop smoking. If necessary, refer the patient to a support group.

Myocarditis

A focal or diffuse inflammation of the myocardium, myocarditis typically is uncomplicated and self-limiting. It may be acute or chronic and can occur at any age. In many patients, myocarditis fails to produce specific cardiovascular symptoms or electrocardiogram (ECG) abnormalities. Recovery usually is spontaneous and without residual defects.

Occasionally, myocarditis may become serious and induce myofibril degeneration, right and left ventricular failure with cardiomegaly, and arrhythmias.

Causes

Myocarditis may result from any of the following:
• viruses – the most common causes in the United States and western Europe – including coxsackievirus A and B; possibly, those that cause poliomyelitis, influenza, rubeola, and rubella; human immunodeficiency virus; adenoviruses; and echoviruses
• bacteria, including those that cause diphtheria, tuberculosis, typhoid fever, tetanus, and Lyme disease, and staphylococcal, pneumococcal, and gonococcal bacteria
• hypersensitive immune reactions, such as acute rheumatic fever and postcardiotomy syndrome
• radiation therapy, especially large doses to the chest during treatment of lung or breast cancer
• chemical poisoning, such as in chronic alcoholism
• parasitic infections, especially toxoplasmosis and South American trypanosomiasis (Chagas' disease) in infants and immunosuppressed adults
• helminthic infections, such as trichinosis.

Complications

Occasionally, myocarditis is complicated by left ventricular failure. Rarely, it leads to cardiomyopathy. Sometimes myocarditis recurs or produces chronic valvulitis (when it results from rheumatic fever), cardiomyopathy, arrhythmias, or thromboembolism.

Assessment

The patient history commonly reveals a recent upper respiratory tract infection with fever, viral pharyngitis, or tonsillitis. The patient may complain of nonspecific symptoms, such as fatigue, dyspnea, palpitations, persistent tachycardia, and persistent fever, all of which reflect the accompanying systemic infection. Occasionally, the patient may complain of a mild, continuous pressure or soreness in the chest. This pain, however, is unlike the recurring, stress-related pain of angina pectoris.

Auscultation commonly reveals S_3 and S_4 gallops, a muffled S_1, possibly a murmur of mitral regurgitation (from papillary muscle dysfunction) and, if the patient has pericarditis, a pericardial friction rub. If the patient also has left ventricular failure, you may notice neck vein distention, dyspnea, and resting or exertional tachycardia disproportionate to the degree of fever.

Diagnostic tests

Endomyocardial biopsy confirms a myocarditis diagnosis. These test results can support the diagnosis:
• *Cardiac enzyme levels,* including creatine-kinase (CK), CK-MB, serum aspartate aminotransferase (formerly SGOT), and lactate dehydrogenase, are elevated.
• *White blood cell count* and *erythrocyte sedimentation rate* are elevated.
• *Antibody titers* are elevated, such as antistreptolysin-O titer in rheumatic fever.

• *Electrocardiography* typically shows diffuse ST-segment and T-wave abnormalities as in pericarditis, conduction defects (prolonged PR interval), and other ventricular and supraventricular ectopic arrhythmias.
• *Cultures* of stool, throat, pharyngeal washings, or other body fluids may identify the causative bacteria or virus.

Treatment

For most patients, treatment includes anti-infectives for the underlying causative infection, modified bed rest to decrease the heart's work load, and careful management of complications. Left ventricular failure requires activity restriction to minimize myocardial oxygen consumption; supplemental oxygen therapy; sodium restriction; diuretics to decrease fluid retention; and digitalis glycosides to increase myocardial contractility. However, digitalis glycosides must be administered carefully because some patients with myocarditis may show a paradoxical sensitivity even to small doses.

Arrhythmias necessitate prompt but cautious administration of antiarrhythmics, such as quinidine or procainamide, to depress myocardial contractility. Thromboembolism requires anticoagulant therapy.

Treatment with corticosteroids or other immunosuppressants is controversial and therefore limited to combating life-threatening complications, such as intractable heart failure.

Key nursing diagnoses and patient outcomes

Activity intolerance related to fatigue, dyspnea, and palpitations. Based on this nursing diagnosis, you'll establish these patient outcomes. The patient will:
• maintain bed rest as prescribed
• seek assistance when performing activities of daily living
• regain his normal activity level.

Hyperthermia related to the inflammatory process. Based on this nursing diagnosis, you'll establish these patient outcomes. The patient will:
• regain a normal temperature after administration of antipyretic agents
• avoid complications associated with hyperthermia, such as dehydration and seizures
• maintain a normal temperature without using antipyretic agents after myocarditis resolves.

Decreased cardiac output related to reduced myocardial contractility caused by inflammation. Based on this nursing diagnosis, you'll establish these patient outcomes. The patient will:
• remain hemodynamically stable, as evidenced by normal vital signs, alertness, and orientation to time, person, and place
• avoid complications associated with decreased cardiac output, such as left ventricular failure and tissue ischemia
• regain and maintain a normal cardiac output.

Nursing interventions

• Stress the importance of bed rest. Assist the patient with bathing if necessary. Provide a bedside commode because this method puts less stress on the heart than using a bedpan. Offer diversional activities that are physically undemanding.
• To reduce anxiety, allow the patient to express his concerns about the effects of activity restrictions on his responsibilities and routines. Reassure him that the restrictions are temporary.
• Administer oxygen as needed.
• Administer parenteral anti-infectives, as ordered.

Monitoring

• Assess the patient's cardiovascular status frequently, watching for signs of left ventricular failure (dyspnea, hypotension, and tachycardia). Observe for changes in cardiac rhythm or conduction.
• Monitor arterial blood gas values regularly to ensure adequate oxygenation.

• Observe for signs of digitalis toxicity (anorexia, nausea, vomiting, blurred vision, and arrhythmias) and for complicating factors that may potentiate toxicity, such as electrolyte imbalance and hypoxia.

Patient teaching

• Teach the patient about anti-infective drugs. Stress the importance of taking the drug and restricting his activities for as long as the doctor orders.

• If the patient will be taking a digitalis glycoside at home, teach him to check his pulse for 1 full minute before taking the dose. Direct him to withhold the dose and notify the doctor if his heart rate falls below the predetermined rate (usually 60 beats/minute).

• During recovery, recommend that the patient resume normal activities slowly and avoid competitive sports.

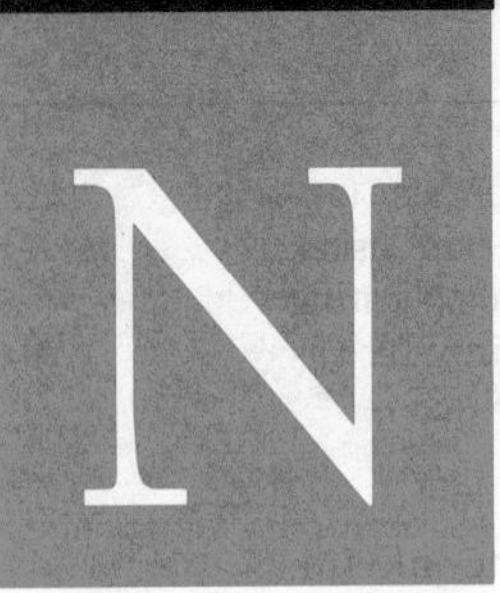

Necrotizing fasciitis

Necrotizing fasciitis, or streptococcal gangrene, is commonly referred to as the "flesh-eating disease" because it involves an infection of the skin. This disorder mimics gas gangrene and is more common in elderly patients with arteriosclerotic vascular disease or diabetes. (For more information, see *Differentiating necrotizing fasciitis from gas gangrene.*)

Causes

The cause of necrotizing fasciitis is the organism *Streptococcus pyogenes;* the disease is spread by direct contact. Several predisposing factors have been identified, including surgery, wounds, and skin ulcers.

Complications

As the disorder progresses, there is extensive necrotic sloughing. If left untreated, bacteremia, metastatic abscesses, and death may result. If the lower extremities are involved, thrombophlebitis also can occur.

Assessment

Typically, within 72 hours of onset, the patient shows red-streaked, painful skin lesions with dusky red surrounding tissue. Bullae with yellow or reddish black fluid develop and rupture. Other findings include fever, tachycardia, lethargy, prostration, disorientation, hypotension, jaundice, hypovolemia, and severe pain followed by anesthesia (due to nerve destruction).

Diagnostic tests

Culture and Gram stain usually show *S. pyogenes* in early bullous lesions and frequently in blood.

Treatment

Immediate, wide, deep surgery of all necrotic tissues is performed. In addition, high-dose I.V. penicillin therapy is administered.

Because the infection is transmitted through direct contact, good preoperative skin preparation and aseptic surgical and suturing technique are crucial in preventing the transmission of infection.

Key nursing diagnoses and patient outcomes

Risk for infection related to impaired skin integrity. Based on this nursing diagnosis, you'll establish these patient outcomes. The patient will:
• exhibit a temperature within normal limits
• remain free of any further signs and symptoms of infection.

Impaired skin integrity related to subcutaneous skin infection. Based on this nursing diagnosis, you'll establish these patient outcomes. The patient will:
• exhibit signs of improved wound status and healing
• take precautions to prevent recurrent skin infections
• comply and participate in prescribed course of therapy.

Pain related to infectious process. Based

Differentiating necrotizing fasciitis from gas gangrene

Necrotizing fasciitis often mimics gas gangrene. Because both are serious skin infections that can lead to death if left untreated, you must be able to distinguish between them.

	Necrotizing fasciitis	Gas gangrene
Cause	*Streptococcal pyogenes* (gram-positive cocci)	*Clostridium perfringens* (gram-positive bacilli)
Transmission	• Spread by direct contact	• Spread by direct contact during trauma or surgery
Predisposing factors	• Recent surgery • Wounds • Skin ulcers • Elderly with arteriosclerotic vascular disease or diabetes	• Deep wounds with tissue necrosis • Compromized arterial circulation after trauma or surgery
Assessment findings	• Red-streaked, painful lesions within 72 hours of onset • Surrounding tissue is dusky red • Development of bullae with yellow or reddish black fluid, possibly rupture • Fever • Tachycardia • Lethargy • Prostration • Disorientation • Severe pain followed by anesthesia	• History of recent surgery, traumatic injury, septic abortion or delivery • Sudden complaints of severe pain at wound site • Normal body temperature followed by moderate rise (usually not above 101° F [38.3° C]) • Hypotension • Tachycardia • Tachypnea • Localized swelling and discoloration (dusky brown or reddish) • Bullae and necrosis within 36 hours of onset • Rupturing skin over wound with darkened or black necrotic muscle • Foul smelling, watery, or frothy discharge • Subcutaneous emphysema (hallmark)
Complications	• Extensive necrotic sloughing • Thrombophlebitis (if lower extremities involved) • Bacteremia • Metastatic abscesses • Death	• Renal failure • Hypotension • Shock • Hemolytic anemia • Tissue death and amputation • Death

on this nursing diagnosis, you'll establish these patient outcomes. The patient will:
• verbalize relief of pain
• express feelings of increasing comfort as the infection diminishes.

Nursing interventions

• Institute standard and contact precautions to minimize risk of transmission.
• Practice thorough hand washing before and after any contact with the patient. Encourage the patient to do the same.
• Obtain cultures as ordered.
• Administer I.V. therapy, as ordered, to maintain fluid and electrolyte balance. Encourage fluid intake, as tolerated.
• Administer antibiotics, as ordered, to treat the infection.
• Keep the patient as comfortable as possible. Administer analgesics, as ordered, to decrease pain and antipyretics to reduce fever.
• Use sterile technique when performing dressing changes or care to open lesions.
• Allow for frequent rest periods alternating with activity, as tolerated by the patient.
• Provide frequent, small, high-protein, high-calorie meals to promote wound healing.
• Prepare the patient for an extensive surgical procedure and the possibility of a large wound after surgery.
• Offer emotional support and guidance to the patient and family. Explain all treatments and procedures openly and honestly.

Monitoring

• Monitor vital signs, noting any changes, especially in pulse and blood pressure, which may be early signs of bacteremia. Monitor temperature.
• Assess intake and output frequently, noting any decreased urine output.
• Observe the affected sites. Note color, temperature, and presence of edema. Assess any drainage for quantity, color, and odor.
• Evaluate the patient's degree of comfort and the effectiveness of analgesics.
• Monitor culture and sensitivity results.

Patient teaching

• Reinforce the importance of completing the full course of antibiotic therapy as prescribed.
• Teach the patient and family about the signs and symptoms of infection and the need to notify the doctor if they occur.
• Instruct the patient and family on how to assess for signs of healing.
• Discuss any wound care procedures. Explain the procedure to the patient and family, and have them demonstrate the procedure in return. Anticipate the need for home care services to assist with wound care.

Nephrectomy

The surgical removal of a kidney, nephrectomy is the treatment of choice for renal cell carcinoma. The procedure also is used to harvest a healthy kidney for transplantation. And when conservative treatments fail, nephrectomy may be used to treat renal trauma, infection, hypertension, hydronephrosis, and inoperable renal calculi.

Nephrectomy may be unilateral or bilateral. Unilateral nephrectomy, the more commonly performed procedure, usually doesn't interfere with renal function as long as one healthy kidney remains. However, bilateral nephrectomy (removal of both kidneys) requires lifelong dialysis or transplantation to support renal function.

Four major types of nephrectomy are performed: partial nephrectomy, involving resection of only a portion of the kidney; simple nephrectomy, removal of the entire kidney; radical nephrectomy, resection of the entire kidney and the surrounding fat tissue; and nephroureterectomy, removal of the entire kidney, the perinephric fat, and the entire ureter. Except for variations in the extent of tissue resection, the surgical approach is basically the same.

Procedure

To perform a unilateral nephrectomy, the surgeon makes a flank incision to expose the kidney. (Alternatively, he may make a thoracicoabdominal or transthoracic incision if extensive renovascular repair or radical excision of the kidney and surrounding structures is necessary, or if the patient has respiratory or cardiac dysfunction.) He then mobilizes the kidney, frees it of fat and adhesions, releases the lower pole, and locates the ureter and frees its upper third. He orders the ureter double-clamped, then cuts between the clamps and ligates both ends. Next, he frees and double-clamps the vascular pedicle. The renal artery is clamped first, followed by clamping of the renal vein. The kidney is then removed distal to the clamps. After resecting surrounding perinephric fat and the ureter, if necessary, he inserts a flank catheter and Penrose drain and sutures the wound closed.

Complications

Nephrectomy can cause serious complications. The most common are infection, hemorrhage, atelectasis, pneumonia, deep vein thrombosis, and pulmonary embolism.

Key nursing diagnoses and patient outcomes

Anxiety related to possible renal dysfunction secondary to nephrectomy. Based on this nursing diagnosis, you'll establish these patient outcomes. The patient will:
- state the source of his anxiety
- express his feelings of anxiety
- communicate his understanding of how renal function is managed postoperatively.

Pain related to the flank incision used during nephrectomy. Based on this nursing diagnosis, you'll establish these patient outcomes. The patient will:
- express feelings of comfort after analgesic administration
- exhibit ease in breathing and maintain adequate ventilation with pain management
- become pain free once the incision heals completely.

Risk for fluid volume deficit related to hemorrhage caused by nephrectomy. Based on this nursing diagnosis, you'll establish these patient outcomes. The patient will:
- maintain hemodynamic stability postoperatively, as evidenced by stable vital signs, alertness, and orientation to time, person, and place
- avoid excessive bleeding at the incisional site.

Nursing interventions

When caring for a person undergoing nephrectomy, your primary responsibilities include instruction and monitoring for postoperative complications.

Before surgery

- As with any organ excision, the patient will have many concerns and questions. He'll probably want to know how the surgery will affect his kidney function. If he's having unilateral nephrectomy, reassure him that one healthy kidney is all he'll need for adequate function. If he's scheduled for bilateral nephrectomy or removal of his only kidney, prepare him for radical changes in his life-style, most notably the need for regular dialysis. If appropriate, discuss the possibility of a future kidney transplant to restore normal function.
- Describe postoperative measures. Tell the patient that he'll return from surgery with an indwelling urinary catheter in place to allow precise measurement of urine output and a nasogastric (NG) tube in place to prevent abdominal pain, distention, and vomiting. Explain that he won't receive food or fluids by mouth after surgery until bowel sounds have returned but that he'll receive I.V. fluids to maintain hydration.

He'll also have a dressing and possibly a drain at the incision site. Prepare him for frequent dressing changes.
• Stress the need for postoperative deep breathing and coughing to prevent pulmonary complications. Demonstrate these exercises, and have him practice them before surgery.
• Ensure that the patient or a responsible family member has signed a consent form.

After surgery

• Provide routine I.V. line, NG tube, and indwelling urinary catheter care. Carefully monitor the rate, volume, and type of I.V. fluids. Keep in mind that mistakes in fluid therapy can be particularly devastating for a patient with only one kidney. Measure and record urine output, and notify the doctor if it falls below 50 ml/hour. Assess for signs of electrolyte imbalance and fluid overload.
• Check the patient's dressing and drain every 4 hours for the first 24 to 48 hours, then once every shift to assess the amount and nature of drainage. Maintain drain patency.
• Unless otherwise ordered, the doctor will perform the first dressing change after surgery. Thereafter, you will change the dressing whenever it becomes wet or once a day, using sterile technique and taking care not to dislodge the drain. During dressing changes, assess the suture line for swelling, redness, and purulent drainage.
• Maintain food and fluid restrictions, as ordered. Periodically auscultate for bowel sounds. When they return and the patient is able to pass flatus (usually by the 4th day after surgery), notify the doctor and prepare to resume oral feedings. When oral intake is permitted, encourage fluids – up to 3,000 ml/day.
• Encourage coughing, deep breathing, incentive spirometry, and position changes. Regularly assess the patient's respiratory status. Be alert for signs of pulmonary embolism, especially 5 to 10 days after surgery. Watch for dyspnea, tachypnea, pleuritic chest pain, and hemoptysis. If these develop, immediately notify the doctor, raise the head of the patient's bed at least 30 degrees, and administer oxygen.
• To reduce the risk of deep vein thrombosis, encourage early and regular ambulation and apply antiembolism stockings, as ordered. Assess for signs and symptoms of deep vein thrombosis.
• Monitor for signs of hemorrhage and shock. Keep in mind that the risk of hemorrhage is greatest 8 to 12 days after surgery, owing to tissue sloughing.

Home care instructions

• Teach the patient how to monitor intake and output at home, and explain how this helps assess renal function. Instruct him to call the doctor immediately if he detects a significant decrease in urine output, a reliable sign of renal failure.
• Tell the patient to notify the doctor if he experiences fever, chills, hematuria, or flank pain. Explain that these signs and symptoms may indicate urinary tract infection, a potentially serious complication.
• If the patient has undergone nephrectomy to treat renal cell carcinoma, convey the importance of reporting any weight loss, bone pain, altered mental status, and paresthesia in the extremities – possible signs of tumor metastasis.
• Emphasize the importance of following the doctor's guidelines on fluid intake and dietary restrictions.
• Inform the patient that he may experience incisional pain and fatigue for several weeks after discharge; reassure him that these are normal postoperative effects. Encourage him to refrain from strenuous exercise, heavy lifting, and sexual activity until his doctor grants permission.
• Stress the need for regular follow-up examinations to evaluate kidney function and to assess for possible complications.
• Provide information about medical identification bracelets for patients who now have a solitary kidney.

Nephrotic syndrome

Although not a disease in itself, nephrotic syndrome is characterized by marked proteinuria, hypoalbuminemia, hyperlipidemia, and edema. It results from a glomerular defect that affects the vessels' permeability and indicates renal damage. The prognosis is highly variable, depending on the underlying cause, but age plays no part in progression or prognosis. Some forms of nephrotic syndrome may eventually progress to end-stage renal failure.

Causes

About 75% of nephrotic syndrome cases result from primary (idiopathic) glomerulonephritis. There are several causes of nephrotic syndrome.

- *Lipid nephrosis (nil lesions)* exhibits a normal glomeruli by light microscopy. Some tubules may contain increased lipid deposits.
- *Membranous glomerulonephritis* is the most common lesion in adult idiopathic nephrotic syndrome. It's characterized by the appearance of immune complexes, seen as dense deposits, within the glomerular basement membrane and by the uniform thickening of the basement membrane. It eventually progresses to renal failure.
- *Focal glomerulosclerosis* can develop spontaneously at any age, can occur after kidney transplantation, or can result from heroin injection. Up to 20% of adults with nephrotic syndrome develop this condition. Lesions initially affect some of the deeper glomeruli, causing hyaline sclerosis. Involvement of the superficial glomeruli occurs later. These lesions usually cause slowly progressive deterioration in renal function, although remissions may occur in children.
- *Membranoproliferative glomerulonephritis* causes slowly progressive lesions to develop in the subendothelial region of the basement membrane. This disorder may follow infection, particularly streptococcal infection, and occurs primarily in children and young adults.

Other causes of nephrotic syndrome are metabolic diseases such as diabetes mellitus; collagen-vascular disorders such as systemic lupus erythematosus; circulatory diseases, such as congestive heart failure, sickle cell anemia, and renal vein thrombosis; nephrotoxins, such as mercury and gold; infections, such as tuberculosis and enteritis; allergic reactions; pregnancy; hereditary nephritis; and certain neoplastic diseases such as multiple myeloma.

All of these diseases increase glomerular protein permeability, which leads to increased urinary excretion of protein (especially albumin) and subsequent hypoalbuminemia.

Complications

Major complications include malnutrition, infection, coagulation disorders, hypovolemia, thromboembolic vascular occlusion (especially in the lungs and legs), and accelerated atherosclerosis. Hypochromic anemia can develop from excessive urinary excretion of transferrin. Acute renal failure may occur and may progress to end-stage renal disease.

Assessment

The patient may complain of lethargy and depression. Your assessment may reveal two problems: periorbital edema, which occurs primarily in the morning, and mild to severe dependent edema of the ankles or sacrum. (See *Evaluating edema.*) You may note orthostatic hypotension, ascites, swollen external genitalia, signs of pleural effusion, anorexia, and pallor.

Diagnostic tests

Consistent, heavy proteinuria (levels over 3.5 mg/dl for 24 hours) strongly suggests nephrotic syndrome. Examination of urine also reveals an increased number of hyaline, granular, and waxy, fatty casts as well as oval fat bodies.

Serum values that support the diagnosis include increased levels of cholesterol, phospholipids (especially low-density and

Evaluating edema

To assess pitting edema, press firmly for 5 to 10 seconds over a bony surface, such as the subcutaneous part of the tibia, fibula, sacrum, or sternum. Then remove your finger and note how long the depression remains. Document your observation on a scale from +1 (barely detectable depression) to +4 (persistent pit as deep as 1" [2.5 cm]).

In severe edema, tissue swells so much that fluid can't be displaced, making pitting impossible. The surface feels rock-hard, and subcutaneous tissue becomes fibrotic. Brawny edema eventually may develop.

+1 pitting edema

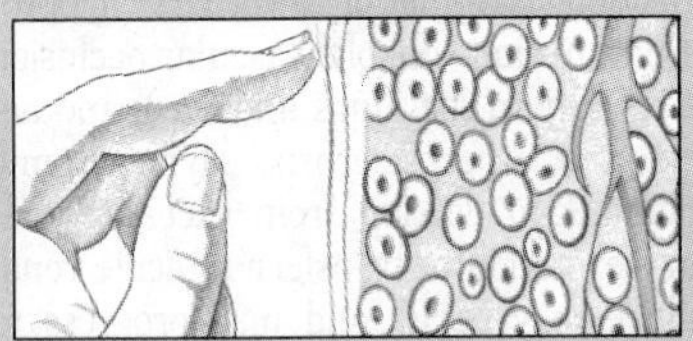

+4 pitting edema

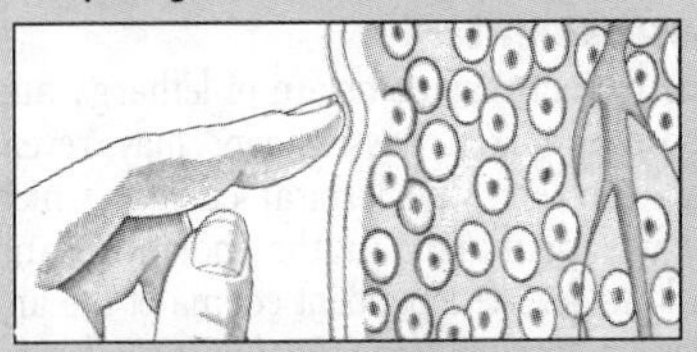

Brawny edema

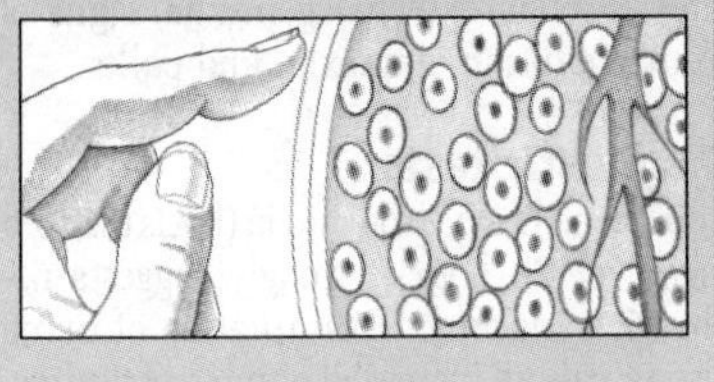

very-low-density lipoproteins), and triglycerides, as well as decreased albumin levels.

Histologic identification of the lesion necessitates a renal biopsy.

Treatment

Effective treatment requires correction of the underlying cause, if possible. Supportive treatment consists of a nutritious diet of 0.6 g of protein/kg of body weight, with restricted sodium intake, diuretics for edema, and antibiotics for infection.

Some patients respond to an 8-week course of a corticosteroid, such as prednisone, followed by maintenance therapy. Others respond better to a combination of prednisone and azathioprine or cyclophosphamide. Treatment for hyperlipidemia frequently is unsuccessful.

Key nursing diagnoses and patient outcomes

Altered nutrition: Less than body requirements related to loss of protein in urine. Based on this nursing diagnosis, you'll establish these patient outcomes. The patient will:

- consume a nutritionally balanced diet
- avoid signs and symptoms of malnutrition

Fluid volume excess related to edema. Based on this nursing diagnosis, you'll establish these patient outcomes. The patient will:

- comply with sodium restrictions and diuretic therapy to minimize edema
- avoid complications associated with edema, such as skin breakdown and impaired mobility
- regain a normal fluid balance.

Risk for infection related to nephrotic syndrome. Based on this nursing diagnosis, you'll establish these patient outcomes. The patient will:

- maintain a normal temperature and white blood cell count
- maintain a urine output that is clear, odorless, and free from white blood cells
- avoid infection.

Nursing interventions

- Administer medications, such as diuretics, antibiotics, and corticosteroids, as ordered.

- Ask the dietitian to plan a low-sodium diet with moderate amounts of protein.
- Provide meticulous skin care to combat the edema that usually occurs with nephrotic syndrome. Use a reduced-pressure mattress or padding to help prevent pressure ulcers.
- To avoid thrombophlebitis, encourage activity and exercise and provide antiembolism stockings, as ordered.
- Offer the patient and his family reassurance and support, especially during the acute phase, when edema is severe and the patient's body image changes.

Monitoring

- Frequently check the patient's urine for protein, indicated by a frothy appearance.
- Monitor and document the location and character of edema.
- Measure blood pressure while the patient is both supine and standing. Immediately report any drop in systolic or diastolic pressure that exceeds 20 mm Hg.
- After a renal biopsy, watch for bleeding and signs of shock.
- Monitor intake and output, and weigh the patient each morning after he voids and before he eats. Make sure he's wearing the same kind of clothing each time you weigh him.
- Monitor plasma albumin and transferrin concentrations to evaluate the patient's overall nutritional status.
- Assess the patient's response to prescribed medications, including both desired and adverse reactions.

Patient teaching

- If the patient is taking immunosuppressants, teach him and his family to report even mild signs of infection. If he's undergoing long-term corticosteroid therapy, teach him and his family to report muscle weakness and mental changes.

To prevent GI complications, suggest to the patient that he take steroids with an antacid or with cimetidine or ranitidine. Explain that adverse effects of steroids will subside when therapy stops, but warn the patient not to discontinue the drug abruptly or without a doctor's consent.
- Stress the importance of adhering to the special diet.
- If the doctor prescribes antiembolism stockings for home use, show the patient how to safely apply and remove them.

Neurogenic bladder

All types of bladder dysfunction caused by an interruption of normal bladder innervation by the nervous system are referred to as neurogenic bladder. (Other names for this disorder include neuromuscular dysfunction of the lower urinary tract, neurologic bladder dysfunction, and neuropathic bladder.) Neurogenic bladder can be hyperreflexic (hypertonic, spastic, or automatic) or flaccid (hypotonic, atonic, or autonomous).

An upper motor neuron lesion (at or above the second to fourth sacral vertebrae) causes spastic neurogenic bladder, with spontaneous contractions of detrusor muscles, increased intravesical voiding pressure, bladder wall hypertrophy with trabeculation, and urinary sphincter spasms. A lower motor neuron lesion (below the second to fourth sacral vertebrae) causes flaccid neurogenic bladder, with decreased intravesical pressure, increased bladder capacity and residual urine retention, and poor detrusor contraction.

Causes

At one time, neurogenic bladder was thought to result primarily from spinal cord injury; now it appears to stem from a host of underlying conditions, including:

- *cerebral disorders,* such as cerebrovascular accident, brain tumor (meningioma and glioma), Parkinson's disease, multiple sclerosis, and dementia
- *spinal cord disease or trauma,* such as spinal stenosis (causing cord compression)

Assessing neurogenic bladder

In neurogenic bladder, a spinal cord lesion at the upper thoracic (cervical) level may cause hyperactive autonomic reflexes (autonomic dysreflexia) when the bladder is distended. Assessment also may reveal severe hypertension, bradycardia, vasodilation (blotchy skin) above the level of the lesion, piloerection, and profuse sweating. The patient may complain of a headache.

With *hyperreflexic neurogenic bladder,* the patient may have involuntary or frequent scanty urination without a feeling of bladder fullness and, possibly, spontaneous spasms of the arms and legs. Anal sphincter tone may be increased. Tactile stimulation of the abdomen, thighs, or genitalia may trigger voiding and spontaneous contractions of the arms and legs.

With *flaccid neurogenic bladder,* the patient may have overflow incontinence and diminished anal sphincter tone. Palpation and percussion reveal a greatly distended bladder but without the accompanying feeling of bladder fullness because of sensory impairment.

or arachnoiditis (causing adhesions between the membranes covering the cord), cervical spondylosis, spinal cord tumors, spina bifida, myelopathies from hereditary or nutritional deficiencies and, rarely, tabes dorsalis

- *disorders of peripheral innervation,* including autonomic neuropathies resulting from endocrine disturbances, such as diabetes mellitus (most common)
- *metabolic disturbances,* such as hypothyroidism, porphyria, or uremia (infrequent)
- *acute infectious diseases,* such as Guillain-Barré syndrome and transverse myelitis
- *heavy metal toxicity*
- *chronic alcoholism*
- *collagen diseases,* such as systemic lupus erythematosus
- *vascular diseases,* such as atherosclerosis
- *distant effects of certain cancers,* such as primary oat cell carcinoma of the lung
- *herpes zoster*
- *sacral agenesis.*

Complications

Conditions that can complicate neurogenic bladder include incontinence, residual urine retention, urinary tract infection (UTI), calculus formation, hydronephrosis, and renal failure.

Assessment

The patient's history includes a condition or disorder that can cause neurogenic bladder. The patient may have some degree of incontinence and will experience changes in initiation or interruption of micturition or an inability to completely empty the bladder. He also may have a history of frequent UTIs. Other assessment findings may be present. (See *Assessing neurogenic bladder.*)

Diagnostic tests

These tests will help assess bladder function.

- *Voiding cystourethrography* evaluates bladder neck function, vesicoureteral reflux, and continence.
- *Urodynamic studies* help evaluate how urine is stored in the bladder, how well the bladder empties, and the rate of movement of urine out of the bladder during voiding. These studies consist of four components:
  - *urine flow study (uroflow)* shows diminished or impaired urine flow
  - *cystometry* evaluates bladder nerve supply, detrusor muscle tone, and intravesical pressures during bladder filling and contraction
  - *urethral pressure profile* determines urethral function with respect to length of the urethra and outlet pressure resistance
  - *sphincter electromyelography* correlates the neuromuscular function of the exter-

nal sphincter with bladder muscle function during bladder filling and contraction; this evaluates how well the bladder and urinary sphincter muscles work together.

• *Retrograde urethrography* reveals strictures and diverticula. This test may not be done routinely.

Treatment

The goals of treatment are to maintain the integrity of the upper urinary tract; control infection; and prevent urinary incontinence through evacuation of the bladder, drug therapy, surgery or, less often, nerve blocks and electrical stimulation.

Techniques for bladder evacuation include Credé's maneuver, Valsalva's maneuver, and intermittent self-catheterization. Credé's maneuver – application of manual pressure over the lower abdomen – promotes complete bladder emptying and is used only if reflux isn't evident. After instruction, most patients can perform this maneuver themselves. Even when performed properly, this method isn't always successful and doesn't always eliminate the need for catheterization. Tapping over the bladder also can initiate voiding, but it has the same shortcomings as Credé's maneuver.

The patient can perform Valsalva's maneuver himself by sitting on the toilet and forcefully exhaling (while keeping his mouth closed). This helps the bladder release urine and promotes complete emptying.

Intermittent self-catheterization – more effective than either Credé's maneuver or Valsalva's maneuver – is a major advance in treatment because it completely empties the bladder without the risks of an indwelling urinary catheter. A male can perform this procedure more easily, a female can learn self-catheterization with the help of a mirror. Intermittent self-catheterization, along with a bladder retraining program, is especially useful in patients with flaccid neurogenic bladder. Anticholinergics and alpha-adrenergic stimulators can help the patient with hyperreflexic neurogenic bladder until intermittent self-catheterization is performed.

Treatment with drugs is not effective in promoting bladder emptying. Drugs such as oxybutinin, hycosamine, imipramine, or propantheline may facilitate urine storage.

When conservative treatment fails, surgery may correct the structural impairment through transurethral resection of the bladder neck, urethral dilatation, external sphincterotomy, or urinary diversion procedures. Implantation of an artificial urinary sphincter may be necessary if permanent incontinence occurs after surgery.

Key nursing diagnoses and patient outcomes

Risk for infection related to urinary stasis. Based on this nursing diagnosis, you'll establish these patient outcomes. The patient will:

• maintain a temperature and white blood cell count within the normal range

• avoid complications associated with UTI, such as sepsis and dehydration

• demonstrate normal urinalysis results and produce odorless urine with a normal appearance.

Urge incontinence related to neurologic dysfunction. Based on this nursing diagnosis, you'll establish these patient outcomes. The patient will:

• comply with conservative measures and drug therapy prescribed to control incontinence

• avoid complications caused by incontinence, such as skin breakdown and UTI

• achieve bladder control with effective management of neurogenic bladder.

Urinary retention related to neurogenic bladder caused by a lower motor neuron lesion. Based on this nursing diagnosis, you'll establish these patient outcomes. The patient will:

• demonstrate complete bladder emptying through such methods as self-catheterization, Credé's or Valsalva's maneuver, and bladder retraining
• avoid UTIs caused by urine retention.

Nursing interventions

• Nursing care for patients with neurogenic bladder varies, depending on the underlying cause and the method of treatment.
• Use strict aseptic technique during insertion of an indwelling urinary catheter (a temporary measure to drain the incontinent patient's bladder). Don't interrupt the closed drainage system for any reason. Obtain urine specimens with a syringe and small-bore needle inserted through the aspirating port of the catheter itself (below the junction of the balloon instillation site). Irrigate in the same manner, if ordered.
• Clean the catheter insertion site with soap and water at least twice a day. Don't allow the catheter to become encrusted. Keep the drainage bag below the tubing and below the level of the bladder. Clamp the tubing or empty the bag before transferring the patient to a wheelchair or stretcher, to prevent accidental urine reflux if the drainage container doesn't have an antireflux valve. If the urine output is considerable, empty the bag more frequently than once every 8 hours because bacteria can multiply in standing urine and migrate up the catheter and into the bladder.
• For those patients who are on an intermittent self-catheterization program, adjust the frequency of catheterization until a volume of 300 to 500 ml is obtained each time (usually four times daily). Catheterization can be stopped when the amount of postvoiding residual urine is consistently less than 100 ml.
• Try to keep the patient as mobile as possible, or perform passive range-of-motion exercises if necessary.
• Neurogenic bladder can produce emotional turmoil. Recommend a support group at a local rehabilitation center or hospital.

Monitoring

• Monitor the patient's urine output. Palpate and percuss his bladder at regular intervals to check for urine retention. Measure postvoid residuals, as needed.
• Watch for signs of UTI (fever, cloudy or foul-smelling urine) and other complications, such as incontinence, renal calculi, and renal failure.
• Monitor the effectiveness of administered medications and procedures, and remain alert for adverse reactions.
• Watch for adverse skin problems, such as dermatitis, fungal infections, and skin breakdown.

Patient teaching

• Explain all diagnostic tests clearly so that the patient understands the procedure, the time involved, and the possible results. Assure him that the lengthy diagnostic process is necessary to identify the most effective treatment plan. After the treatment plan is chosen, explain it to him in detail.
• Encourage the patient to drink plenty of fluids to prevent calculus formation and infection from urinary stasis.
• Before discharge, teach the patient and his family evacuation techniques as necessary (for example, Credé's maneuver or intermittent self-catheterization). Also teach him how to care for the catheter, if appropriate.
• Discuss sexual activities. The incontinent patient will feel embarrassed and worried about sexual function, so provide emotional support.
• Demonstrate good hand-washing technique, and encourage meticulous cleaning of the drainage site.
• Teach the patient the signs of UTI, and warn him to report them immediately.

Neuropathic arthropathy

Most common in men over age 40, neuropathic arthropathy (also called Charcot's arthropathy) is a progressively degenerative disease of peripheral and axial joints that results from impaired sensory innervation. Trauma or disease results in loss of sensation in the joint, which damages the supporting ligaments. Eventually, the affected joint disintegrates.

The specific joints affected vary. Diabetes mellitus usually attacks joints and bones of the feet. Tabes dorsalis affects large, weight-bearing joints, such as the knee, hip, ankle, or lumbar and dorsal vertebrae. Syringomyelia involves the shoulder, elbow, or cervical intervertebral joint. Neuropathic arthropathy caused by intra-articular corticosteroid injections may develop in the hip or knee joint.

Causes

In adults, the most common cause of neuropathic arthropathy is diabetes mellitus. Other causes include syringomyelia (which progresses to neuropathic arthropathy in about one of four patients), myelopathy of pernicious anemia, spinal cord trauma, paraplegia, hereditary sensory radicular neuropathy, and Charcot-Marie-Tooth disease. Rarely, tabes dorsalis, amyloidosis, peripheral nerve injury, leprosy, or alcoholism causes neuropathic arthropathy.

Frequent intra-articular injection of corticosteroids has also been linked to neuropathic arthropathy. The analgesic effect of the corticosteroids may mask symptoms and allow continuous damaging stress to accelerate joint destruction.

Complications

Neuropathic arthropathy can lead to joint subluxation or dislocation, pathologic fractures, infection, pseudogout, or neurovascular compression.

Assessment

The patient's history may reveal an insidious onset, underlying neurologic disease, previous pathologic fractures, trauma and swelling in the affected area, and progressively worsening symptoms. Even with marked swelling over the joints, the patient may report no pain.

Inspection and other physical assessment techniques disclose extreme joint swelling, increased joint range of motion, joint deformity and instability, dislocation or subluxation, and loss of muscle tone around the joint. Palpation may detect warmth or tenderness over the involved joints. In rare cases, loose objects and abnormal calcifications in the joint may be felt.

Diagnostic tests

- *X-rays* confirm the diagnosis and allow evaluation of damage. Early in the disease, soft-tissue swelling or effusion may be the only overt effect. Later, X-rays may display articular fracture, subluxation, and cartilaginous erosion; periosteal new bone formation; and excessive growth of marginal loose bodies (osteophytosis). Bone resorption also may be evident.
- *Vertebral examination* shows narrowed disk spaces, vertebral deterioration, and osteophyte formation, leading to ankylosis and deforming kyphoscoliosis.
- *Synovial biopsy* detects bony fragments and bits of calcified cartilage.
- *Neuromuscular tests* may reveal motor and sensory deficits and diminished deep tendon reflexes.

Treatment

Pain relief – the immediate treatment goal – may be achieved with analgesics, nonsteroidal anti-inflammatory drugs, and joint immobilization (crutches, splints, braces, and weight-bearing restrictions). Although surgical correction, such as joint fusion or amputation, may be necessary in severe disease, surgery has a high failure rate because of nonunion, infection, or dislocation.

Key nursing diagnoses and patient outcomes

Body image disturbance related to deforming kyphoscoliosis. Based on this nursing diagnosis, you'll establish these patient outcomes. The patient will:
- state that he recognizes the change in his body image
- express his feelings about his altered body image
- express positive feelings about himself.

Risk for impaired skin integrity related to skin fragility from joint swelling. Based on this nursing diagnosis, you'll establish these patient outcomes. The patient will:
- comply with treatment to reduce joint swelling
- use precautions to minimize or prevent skin breakdown in the swollen area
- maintain skin integrity in the area.

Impaired physical mobility related to joint degeneration. Based on this nursing diagnosis, you'll establish these patient outcomes. The patient will:
- avoid complications associated with impaired physical mobility, such as skin breakdown and venous stasis
- achieve the highest level of mobility possible
- use prescribed assistive devices correctly.

Nursing interventions

- Assist the patient to overcome anxiety and fear by expressing his feelings and concerns about his disorder. Listen, offering support and encouragement when appropriate. Include the patient and his family in all phases of his care. Answer questions as honestly as you can.
- Encourage the patient to perform as much self-care as his immobility and pain allow. Recognize that he may need extra time to perform activities at his own pace.
- Maintain neutral joint alignment. Apply splints and restrict weight bearing, as ordered.
- Administer prescribed analgesics for pain.

Monitoring

- Assess the patient's pain pattern, and monitor his response to analgesics.
- Monitor the patient's sensory perception, range of motion, alignment, and joint swelling, and evaluate the status of the underlying disease.
- Assess skin regularly for breakdown.

Patient teaching

- Teach the patient joint protection techniques. Advise him to avoid physical stress that could cause pathologic fractures and to take safety precautions to avoid falls. Tell him to remove throw rugs and clutter from passageways.
- Instruct the patient to report severe joint pain, swelling, or instability. Suggest applying warm compresses to relieve local pain and tenderness.
- Teach the patient how to use crutches or other orthopedic devices. Stress the importance of proper fitting and regular professional readjustment of such devices. Forewarn him that impaired sensation might allow these aids to cause tissue damage without causing discomfort.
- Explain treatments, tests, and procedures.
- Review prescribed medications and possible adverse reactions. Tell the patient to notify his doctor of adverse reactions.
- Urge the patient to continue with regular treatment of the underlying disease.
- Refer the patient to an occupational therapist or a home health nurse to help him cope with activities of daily living.

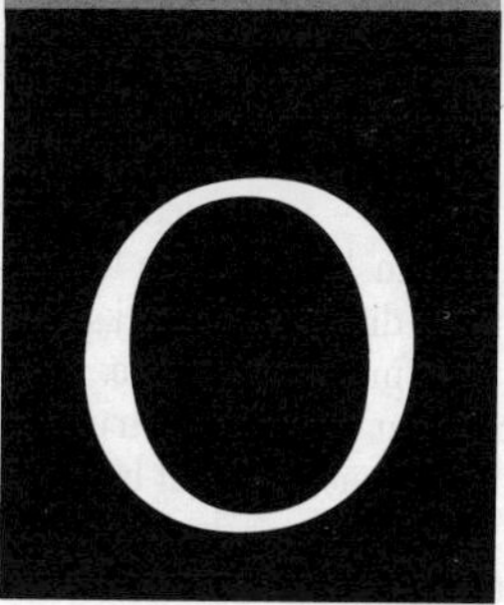

Oophorectomy and salpingectomy

Oophorectomy is the surgical removal of one (unilateral) or both (bilateral) ovaries. Salpingectomy is the surgical removal of one or both fallopian tubes. When done together, the procedures may be referred to as a salpingo-oophorectomy.

Oophorectomy is performed to treat ovarian cysts, ovarian cancer, or an estrogen-dependent tumor. Bilateral oophorectomy may be done during a hysterectomy if disease has spread to the ovaries.

Salpingectomy may be performed to treat salpingitis (infection of the fallopian tubes), severe pelvic inflammatory disease, endometriosis, or ectopic pregnancy. In some cases, it's done to achieve contraception.

Procedure

With the patient under general anesthesia, the surgeon makes a transverse or vertical incision through the abdominal wall. After locating the internal reproductive organs, he excises one or both ovaries, one or both fallopian tubes, or both the ovaries and fallopian tubes. When doing this procedure in conjunction with a hysterectomy, the surgeon also removes the uterus. The abdominal incision is then closed with sutures or staples, and a sterile dressing is applied.

Complications

Complications are rare, but may include hemorrhage, infection, atelectasis, and pulmonary embolism. The patient may experience a change in self-concept as well as physical changes related to loss of estrogen. However, these changes usually don't arise for several days or weeks after surgery unless a bilateral oophorectomy was performed.

Key nursing diagnoses and patient outcomes

Altered protection related to loss of ability to produce estrogen. Based on this nursing diagnosis, you'll establish these patient outcomes. The patient will:

- express an understanding of the need for estrogen replacement therapy
- comply with prescribed estrogen therapy
- avoid signs and symptoms of estrogen deficiency.

Anticipatory grieving related to loss of fertility caused by bilateral salpingo-oophorectomy. Based on this nursing diagnosis, you'll establish these patient outcomes. The patient will:

- express her feelings about loss of fertility
- use healthy coping mechanisms to deal with loss of fertility.

Nursing interventions

When caring for a patient undergoing an oophorectomy or a salpingectomy, your primary responsibilities include instruction and monitoring for postoperative complications.

Before surgery

- Careful preoperative teaching can help prevent or minimize self-concept disturbances. If both ovaries will be removed, encourage the patient to discuss her feelings about the loss of her reproductive ability.
- Insert an indwelling urinary catheter and connect it to gravity drainage to prevent accidental perforation of the urinary bladder during surgery. Tell the patient the catheter will remain in place for 24 hours after surgery.
- Make sure the patient has signed a consent form.

After surgery

- Monitor the patient's vital signs closely. Report any sudden or radical change from preoperative baseline findings.
- Inspect dressings frequently for signs of drainage. Report excessive bleeding to the surgeon promptly.
- Encourage the patient to cough and deep-breathe every hour. Help her splint the incision with a pillow during these measures.
- Assist the patient out of bed as soon as anesthesia wears off, and encourage her to ambulate to help prevent phlebitis and atelectasis.
- Administer I.V. therapy to ensure adequate hydration and prevent hypotension until the patient is able to tolerate oral intake.
- Monitor the patient for pain, and administer analgesics as needed and prescribed.
- Administer estrogen replacement drugs, as prescribed.
- Administer calcium supplements, as prescribed.

Home care instructions

- Teach the patient the importance of taking prescribed medication as directed. Make sure she understands why estrogen and calcium replacement is given as well as the risks and benefits of this therapy.
- Teach the patient the importance of having a follow-up pelvic examination in 6 to 8 weeks to ensure that her healing is adequate.
- Instruct the patient to report any abnormal bleeding, pain, fever, or voiding problems to the doctor immediately.

Orchiopexy

This surgical procedure secures a testis in the scrotum. It's indicated for the patient with cryptorchidism (undescended testis) or testicular torsion. Orchiopexy is performed when other treatments, such as hormonal therapy with human chorionic gonadotropin, fail to make the testis descend. When successful, this surgery reduces the risk of sterility, testicular cancer, and testicular trauma from abnormal positioning. It also precludes harmful psychological effects caused by poor sexual image.

In testicular torsion, which can affect males of all ages, orchiopexy is indicated when the testis remains viable. However, if the testis can't be saved, an orchiectomy (removal of the testis) may be performed.

Procedure

With the patient under general anesthesia, the surgeon makes the incision. If the patient has testicular torsion, the surgeon makes an incision in the scrotal skin and attempts to untwist and stabilize the spermatic cord. He may also remove a hydrocele, if present. However, if he's unable to save the testis, he performs an orchiectomy.

If the patient has an undescended testis, the surgeon makes an incision in the inguinal area or lower abdomen to expose the testis and makes a small incision in the scrotal skin to open the scrotum. He then frees the testis and lowers it into the scrotal sac, where he secures it in place with sutures. If bilateral cryptorchidism is present, he repeats this procedure for the other testis.

Complications

Although uncommon, complications of orchiopexy may include hemorrhage and dysuria.

Key nursing diagnoses and patient outcomes

Altered sexuality patterns related to the need to abstain temporarily from sexual activity. Based on this nursing diagnosis, you'll establish these patient outcomes. The patient will:

- verbalize his understanding of the need to restrict sexual activity following surgery
- comply with sexual activity restrictions for the prescribed period
- resume normal sexual activity when permitted.

Fear related to the effect of orchiopexy on sexuality. Based on this nursing diagnosis, you'll establish these patient outcomes. The patient will:

- express his feelings of fear
- express an understanding of how orchiopexy affects sexuality
- exhibit no physical signs or symptoms of fear.

Pain related to the surgical incision. Based on this nursing diagnosis, you'll establish these patient outcomes. The patient will:

- express relief of pain after analgesic administration
- use cold therapy to help reduce pain
- become pain free.

Self-esteem disturbance related to the effects of surgery on sexuality. Based on this nursing diagnosis, you'll establish these patient outcomes. The patient will:

- verbalize positive feelings about himself
- demonstrate knowledge of the effects of surgery on sexuality
- demonstrate positive behaviors about himself.

Nursing interventions

When caring for a patient undergoing orchiopexy, your primary responsibilities are instructing and reassuring the patient and monitoring for postoperative complications.

Before surgery

- If the patient has testicular torsion, briefly explain the surgery. Tell him that the surgeon will untwist and permanently stabilize the spermatic cord. If this isn't possible, he'll remove the twisted appendage.
- If the patient has an undescended testis, review the doctor's explanation of the surgery, using terms the patient can understand. If appropriate, use simple diagrams or anatomically detailed models to enhance your explanation.
- Reassure the postpubescent patient that surgery shouldn't impair his sexual performance and reproductive function. In fact, it may enhance them by correcting a potential source of problems and improving the appearance of his sexual organs. Also reassure the patient that recovery should be rapid and that he'll be able to resume most normal activities within a week.

After surgery

- Monitor the patient's vital signs, looking for evidence of hemorrhage or infection. Check the incision site and dressing frequently for redness, inflammation, and bleeding. Change the dressing frequently.
- Carefully monitor and record the patient's intake and output. Watch for urine retention or dysuria, which may result from postsurgical edema or the effects of the anesthetic.
- Take measures to promote patient comfort, such as applying an ice pack or a scrotal support. Administer analgesics, as ordered.

Home care instructions

- Instruct the patient to promptly report increased scrotal pain or swelling or other changes in the testis. Explain that these symptoms may indicate infection or ischemia and require immediate medical attention.

- Advise the patient to resume normal activities gradually starting about 1 week after surgery but to avoid heavy lifting and other strenuous activities until the doctor advises otherwise.
- Encourage the patient to wear a scrotal support to enhance comfort and control edema.
- Advise the patient to refrain from sexual activity for 6 weeks after surgery or for the duration recommended by the doctor.
- Teach the patient how to perform testicular self-examination. Advise him to examine both testes regularly and to report any lumps or unusual findings. For as-yet-unclear reasons, the patient with cryptorchidism has an increased risk for testicular cancer.

Osteoarthritis

The most common form of arthritis, osteoarthritis causes deterioration of the joint cartilage and formation of reactive new bone at the margins and subchondral areas of the joints. This chronic degeneration results from a breakdown of chondrocytes, most often in the hips and knees.

Osteoarthritis occurs equally in both sexes. More than half of people over age 30 have some features of primary osteoarthritis. And nearly all people over age 60 have radiographic evidence of the disorder, although fewer than half experience symptoms.

Depending on the site and severity of joint involvement, disability can range from minor limitation of the fingers to near immobility in persons with hip or knee disease. Progression rates vary; joints may remain stable for years in the early stage of deterioration.

Causes

Primary osteoarthritis may be related to aging, although researchers don't understand why. This form of the disease seems to lack any predisposing factors. In some patients, however, it may be hereditary.

Secondary osteoarthritis usually follows an identifiable event – most commonly a traumatic injury or congenital abnormality, such as hip dysplasia. Endocrine disorders (such as diabetes mellitus), metabolic disorders (such as chondrocalcinosis), and other types of arthritis also can lead to secondary osteoarthritis.

Complications

Osteoarthritis may cause flexion contractures, subluxation and deformity, ankylosis, bony cysts, gross bony overgrowth, central cord syndrome (with cervical spine osteoarthritis), nerve root compression, and cauda equina syndrome.

Assessment

The patient usually complains of gradually increasing signs and symptoms. He may report a predisposing event, such as a traumatic injury. Most commonly, the patient has a deep, aching joint pain, particularly after he exercises or bears weight on the affected joint. Rest may relieve the pain.

Additional complaints include stiffness in the morning and after exercise, aching during changes in weather, a "grating" feeling when the joint moves, contractures, and limited movement. These symptoms tend to be worse in patients with poor posture, obesity, or occupational stress.

Inspection may reveal joint swelling, muscle atrophy, deformity of the involved areas, and gait abnormalities (when arthritis affects the hips or knees). Osteoarthritis of the interphalangeal joints produces hard nodes on the distal and proximal joints. Painless at first, these nodes eventually become red, swollen, and tender. The fingers may become numb and lose their dexterity. (See *Signs of osteoarthritis.*)

Palpation may reveal joint tenderness and warmth without redness, grating with movement, joint instability, muscle spasms, and limited movement.

Diagnostic tests

- *X-rays* of the affected joint may help confirm the diagnosis; however, findings may be normal in the early stages. X-ray studies may require many views and typically show a narrowing of the joint space or margin, cystlike bony deposits in the joint space and margins, sclerosis of the subchondral space, joint deformity caused by degeneration or articular damage, bony growths at weight-bearing areas, and joint fusion in patients with erosive, inflammatory osteoarthritis.
- *Synovial fluid analysis* can rule out inflammatory arthritis.
- *Radionuclide bone scan* can also rule out inflammatory arthritis by showing normal uptake of the radionuclide.
- *Arthroscopy* identifies soft-tissue swelling by showing internal joint structures.
- *Magnetic resonance imaging* produces clear cross-sectional images of the affected joint and adjacent bones. Scan results also show disease progression.
- *Neuromuscular tests* may disclose reduced muscle strength (reduced grip strength, for example).

Treatment

To relieve pain, improve mobility, and minimize disability, treatment includes medications, rest, physical therapy, assistive mobility devices and, possibly, surgery.

Medications include aspirin and other salicylates and such nonsteroidal anti-inflammatory drugs as piroxicam, tolmetin, naproxen, indomethacin, fenoprofen, ibuprofen, and diclofenac. In some patients, intra-articular injections of corticosteroids may be necessary. Such injections, given every 4 to 6 months, may delay nodal development in the hands.

Adequate rest is essential and should be balanced with activity. Physical therapy includes massage, moist heat, paraffin dips for the hands, supervised exercise to decrease muscle spasms and atrophy, and protective techniques for preventing undue joint stress. Some patients may reduce stress and increase stability by using crutches, braces, a cane, a walker, a cervical collar, or traction. Weight reduction may help an obese patient.

In some instances, a patient with severe disability or uncontrollable pain may undergo surgery, including:

- *arthroplasty (partial or total)*–replacement of deteriorated part of joint with prosthetic appliance
- *arthrodesis*–surgical fusion of bones, used primarily in the spine (laminectomy)

Signs of osteoarthritis

Heberden's nodes appear on the dorsolateral aspect of the distal interphalangeal joints. Usually hard and painless, these bony and cartilaginous enlargements typically occur in middle-aged and elderly osteoarthritis patients. Bouchard's nodes, similar to Heberden's nodes but less common, appear on the proximal interphalangeal joints.

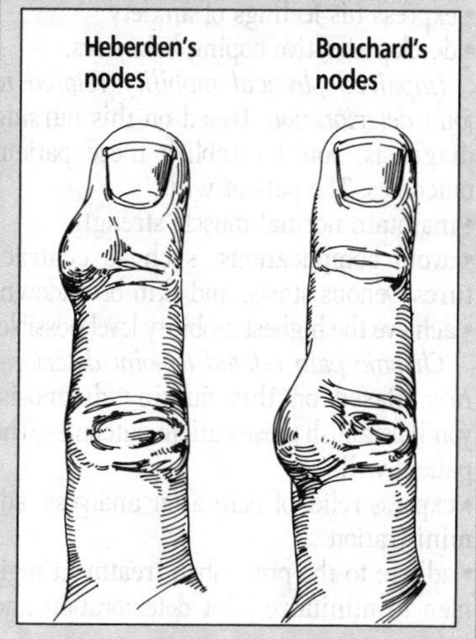

- *osteoplasty*–scraping and lavage of deteriorated bone from the joint
- *osteotomy*–excision or cutting of a wedge of bone (usually in the lower leg) to change alignment and relieve stress.

Key nursing diagnoses and patient outcomes

Anxiety related to the potential crippling effects of osteoarthritis. Based on this nursing diagnosis, you'll establish these patient outcomes. The patient will:

- express his feelings of anxiety
- develop effective coping behaviors.

Impaired physical mobility related to joint deterioration. Based on this nursing diagnosis, you'll establish these patient outcomes. The patient will:

- maintain normal muscle strength
- avoid complications, such as contractures, venous stasis, and skin breakdown
- achieve the highest mobility level possible.

Chronic pain related to joint deterioration. Based on this nursing diagnosis, you'll establish these patient outcomes. The patient will:

- express relief of pain after analgesic administration
- adhere to the prescribed treatment regimen to minimize joint deterioration and pain.

Nursing interventions

- Administer anti-inflammatory medication and other drugs, as ordered.
- Provide emotional support and reassurance to help the patient cope with limited mobility. Give him opportunities to voice his feelings about immobility and nodular joints. Include him and his family in all phases of his care. Answer questions as honestly as you can.
- Encourage the patient to perform as much self-care as his immobility and pain allow. Provide him with adequate time to perform activities at his own pace.
- To help promote sleep, adjust pain medications to allow for maximum rest. Provide the patient with sleep aids such as a pillow, bath, or back rub.
- Help the patient identify techniques and activities that promote rest and relaxation. Encourage him to perform them.
- For joints in the hand, provide hot soaks and paraffin dips to relieve pain, as ordered.
- For lumbosacral spinal joints, provide a firm mattress (or bed board) to decrease morning pain.
- For cervical spinal joints, adjust the patient's cervical collar to avoid constriction.
- For the hip, use moist heat pads to relieve pain. Administer antispasmodic drugs, as ordered.
- For the knee, assist with prescribed range-of-motion (ROM) exercises twice daily to maintain muscle tone. Also help perform progressive resistance exercises to increase the patient's muscle strength.
- Provide elastic supports or braces if needed.
- Check crutches, cane, braces, or walker for proper fit. A patient with unilateral joint involvement should use an orthopedic appliance (such as a cane or walker) on the unaffected side.

Monitoring

- Assess the patient's pain pattern. Give analgesics as needed and prescribed, and monitor his response.
- Monitor for desired and adverse effects of anti-inflammatory medications.
- Watch for skin irritation caused by prolonged use of assistive devices such as a cervical collar or braces.

Patient teaching

- Instruct the patient to plan for adequate rest during the day, after exertion, and at night. Encourage him to learn and use energy conservation methods, such as pacing activities, simplifying work procedures, and protecting joints.
- Instruct him to take medications exactly as prescribed. Tell him which adverse reactions to report immediately.

- Advise against overexertion. Tell him that he should take care to stand and walk correctly, to minimize weight-bearing activities, and to be especially careful when stooping or picking up objects.
- Tell the patient to wear well-fitting support shoes and to repair worn heels.
- Tell him to have safety devices installed at home, such as grab bars in the bathroom.
- Teach him to do ROM exercises, performing them as gently as possible.
- Advise maintaining proper body weight to minimize strain on joints.
- Teach the patient how to use crutches or other orthopedic devices properly. Stress the importance of proper fitting and regular professional readjustment of such devices. Warn that impaired sensation might allow tissue damage from these aids without discomfort.
- Recommend using cushions when sitting. Also suggest using an elevated toilet seat. Both reduce stress when rising from a seated position.
- Positively reinforce the patient's efforts to adapt. Point out improving or stabilizing physical functioning.
- As necessary, refer the patient to an occupational therapist or a home health nurse to help him cope with activities of daily living.

Osteomyelitis

A pyogenic bone infection, osteomyelitis may be chronic or acute. The disease commonly results from combined traumatic injury – usually minor but severe enough to cause a hematoma – and acute infection originating elsewhere in the body. Although osteomyelitis usually remains a local infection, it can spread through the bone to the marrow, cortex, and periosteum.

Typically a blood-borne disease, acute osteomyelitis most often affects rapidly growing children, particularly boys. The rarer chronic osteomyelitis is characterized by multiple draining sinus tracts and metastatic lesions. The incidence of both types of osteomyelitis is declining, except in drug abusers.

In children, the most common disease sites include the lower end of the femur and the upper end of the tibia, humerus, and radius. In adults, the disease commonly localizes in the pelvis and vertebrae and usually results from contamination related to surgery or trauma.

The prognosis for a patient with acute osteomyelitis is good if he receives prompt treatment. The prognosis for a patient with chronic osteomyelitis (more prevalent in adults) is poor.

Causes

Infection causes osteomyelitis. Bacterial pyogens are the most common agents, but the disease also may result from fungi or viruses. The most common pyogenic organism in osteomyelitis is *Staphylococcus aureus*; others include *Streptococcus pyogenes, Pseudomonas aeruginosa, Escherichia coli,* and *Proteus vulgaris.*

Typically, these organisms find a culture site in a recent hematoma or a weakened area, such as a site of local infection (as in furunculosis). From there, they spread directly to bone. As the organisms grow and produce pus within the bone, pressure builds within the rigid medullary cavity and forces the pus through the haversian canals. A subperiosteal abscess forms, depriving the bone of its blood supply and eventually causing necrosis.

In turn, necrosis stimulates the periosteum to create new bone (involucrum). The old, dead bone (sequestrum) detaches and works its way out through an abscess or the sinuses. By the time the body processes sequestrum, osteomyelitis is chronic.

Complications

Osteomyelitis may lead to chronic infection, skeletal deformities, joint deformities,

Detecting osteomyelitis

Suspect osteomyelitis if your patient complains of a sudden, severe pain in a bone—especially if he has chills, nausea, and malaise and if his history reveals a previous injury, surgery, or primary infection. He may describe the pain as unrelieved by rest and worse with motion.

The patient's vital signs may show tachycardia and a fever. Inspection may reveal swelling and restricted movement over the infection site. The patient may refuse to use the affected area. Palpation may detect tenderness and warmth over the infection site.

disturbed bone growth (in children), differing leg lengths, and impaired mobility.

Assessment

Usually, chronic and acute osteomyelitis have similar clinical features. (See *Detecting osteomyelitis.*) However, chronic infection can persist intermittently for years, flaring up spontaneously after minor trauma. Sometimes, the only sign of chronic infection is persistent pus drainage from an old pocket in a sinus tract.

Diagnostic tests

- *White blood cell (WBC) count* shows leukocytosis if the patient has osteomyelitis.
- *Erythrocyte sedimentation rate* rises in osteomyelitis.
- *Blood culture* can identify the pathogen.
- *X-rays* may show bone involvement only after the disease has been active for some time, usually 2 to 3 weeks.
- *Bone scans* can detect early infection.

Diagnosis must rule out poliomyelitis, rheumatic fever, myositis, and bone fractures.

Treatment

To decrease internal bone pressure and prevent infarction, treatment for acute osteomyelitis begins even before confirming the diagnosis. After drawing samples for blood culture, you'll typically administer high doses of I.V. antibiotics (usually a penicillinase-resistant agent, such as nafcillin or oxacillin). The infected site may be drained surgically to relieve pressure and remove sequestrum. Usually the infected bone is immobilized with a cast or traction or by complete bed rest. The patient receives analgesics and I.V. fluids as needed.

If an abscess forms, treatment includes incision and drainage, followed by a culture of the drainage. Anti-infective therapy may include systemic antibiotics; intracavitary instillation of antibiotics through closed-system continuous irrigation with low intermittent suction; limited irrigation with a blood drainage system equipped with suction (such as a Hemovac); or local application of packed, wet, antibiotic-soaked dressings.

Some patients may receive hyperbaric oxygen therapy to increase the activity of naturally occurring WBCs. Additional measures include using free tissue transfers and local muscle flaps to fill in dead space and increase blood supply.

Chronic osteomyelitis also may require surgery: sequestrectomy to remove dead bone and saucerization to promote drainage and decrease pressure. The typical patient reports great pain and requires prolonged hospitalization. Unrelieved chronic osteomyelitis in an arm or a leg may require amputation.

Key nursing diagnoses and patient outcomes

Activity intolerance related to the inflammatory process. Based on this nursing diagnosis, you'll establish these patient outcomes. The patient will:

- seek assistance when performing activities
- comply with prescribed activity restrictions to minimize tissue damage

• regain his normal activity level.

Impaired physical mobility related to bone necrosis. Based on this nursing diagnosis, you'll establish these patient outcomes. The patient will:
• maintain normal muscle strength and joint range of motion
• avoid complications, such as contractures, venous stasis, and skin breakdown
• regain normal physical mobility.

Impaired tissue integrity related to bone necrosis and inflammation. Based on this nursing diagnosis, you'll establish these patient outcomes. The patient will:
• express relief of pain with prescribed therapy
• avoid permanent deficits in tissue integrity.

Nursing interventions

• Focus care on controlling infection, protecting the bone from injury, and providing support.
• Encourage the patient to verbalize his concerns about his disorder. Offer support and encouragement. Answer questions as honestly as you can.
• Encourage the patient to perform as much self-care as his condition allows. Allow him adequate time to perform these activities at his own pace.
• Help the patient identify care techniques and activities that promote rest and relaxation, and encourage him to perform them.
• Use strict aseptic technique when changing dressings and irrigating wounds.
• If the patient has a cast, check circulation and drainage in the affected limb. If a wet spot appears on the cast, circle it with a marking pen and note the time of its appearance (on the cast). Be aware of how much drainage to expect. Keep in mind that one drop of blood can cause a 3″ (7.6-cm) stain on the cast. Check the circled spot at least every 4 hours. Assess and report increasing drainage as appropriate. Monitor vital signs to help detect excessive blood loss.
• If the patient is in skeletal traction for compound fractures, cover the pin insertion points with small, dry dressings. Tell the patient not to touch the skin around the pins and wires. Make sure that there is adequate drainage of pin sites.
• Provide a diet high in protein and vitamin C to promote healing.
• Support the affected limb with firm pillows. Keep it level with the body; don't let it sag.
• Provide thorough skin care. Turn the patient gently every 2 hours.
• Provide complete cast care. Support the cast with firm pillows, and petal the edges with pieces of adhesive tape or moleskin to smooth rough edges.
• Protect the patient from mishaps, such as jerky movements and falls, which may threaten bone integrity.
• Administer prescribed analgesics for pain.

Monitoring

• Assess vital signs, observe wound appearance, and note any new pain (which may indicate secondary infection) daily.
• Carefully monitor drainage and suctioning equipment. Keep containers nearby that are filled with the irrigant being instilled. Monitor the amount of solution instilled and drained.
• Watch for signs of pressure ulcer formation.
• Look for sudden malpositioning of the affected limb, which may indicate fracture.
• Assess the patient's pain pattern and response to administered analgesics.

Patient teaching

• Explain all test and treatment procedures.
• Review prescribed medications. Discuss possible adverse reactions to drug administration, and instruct the patient to report them to the doctor.
• Tell him to report sudden pain, unusual bone sensations and noises (crepitus), or deformity immediately.

• Before surgery, explain all preoperative and postoperative procedures to the patient and his family.
• Teach the patient techniques for promoting rest and relaxation. Encourage him to perform them.
• Before discharge, teach the patient how to protect and clean the wound site and, most important, how to recognize signs of recurring infection (elevated temperature, redness, localized heat, and swelling).
• Urge the patient to schedule follow-up examinations and to seek treatment for possible sources of recurrent infection – blisters, boils, sties, and impetigo.
• As necessary, refer the patient to an occupational therapist or a home health nurse to help him manage the activities of daily living.

Osteoporosis

In this metabolic bone disorder, the rate of bone resorption accelerates and the rate of bone formation slows. As a result, bone mass decreases. Bones affected by this disease lose calcium and phosphate and become porous, brittle, and abnormally vulnerable to fracture. Osteoporosis may be primary or secondary to an underlying disease.

Primary osteoporosis can be classified as idiopathic, type I, or type II. Idiopathic osteoporosis affects children and adults. Type I (postmenopausal) osteoporosis usually affects women ages 51 to 75. Related to the loss of estrogen's protective effect on bone, type I osteoporosis results in trabecular bone loss and some cortical bone loss. Vertebral and wrist fractures are common. Type II (or senile) osteoporosis occurs most commonly between ages 70 and 85. Trabecular and cortical bone loss and consequent fractures of the proximal humerus, proximal tibia, femoral neck, and pelvis characterize type II osteoporosis.

Causes

The cause of primary osteoporosis is unknown. However, clinicians suspect these contributing factors:
• mild but prolonged negative calcium balance resulting from inadequate dietary intake
• declining gonadal adrenal function
• faulty protein metabolism caused by estrogen deficiency
• a sedentary life-style.

Secondary osteoporosis may result from prolonged therapy with steroids or heparin, bone immobilization or disuse (as occurs with hemiplegia), alcoholism, malnutrition, rheumatoid arthritis, liver disease, malabsorption, scurvy, lactose intolerance, hyperthyroidism, osteogenesis imperfecta, and Sudeck's atrophy (localized in hands and feet, with recurring attacks).

Complications

Bone fractures are the major complication of osteoporosis. They occur most commonly in the vertebrae, the femoral neck, and the distal radius.

Assessment

The history may typically disclose a postmenopausal patient or one with a condition known to cause secondary osteoporosis. The patient (usually an elderly woman) may report that she bent down to lift something, heard a snapping sound, and felt a sudden pain in her lower back. Or, she may say that the pain developed slowly over several years. If the patient has vertebral collapse, she may describe a backache and pain radiating around the trunk. Any movement or jarring aggravates the pain.

Inspection may reveal that the patient has a humped back and a markedly aged appearance. She may report a loss of height. Palpation may reveal muscle spasm. The patient may also have decreased spinal movement, with flexion more limited than extension.

Diagnostic tests

Differential diagnosis must exclude other causes of rarefying bone disease, especially those that affect the spine, such as metastatic carcinoma and advanced multiple myeloma.

- *X-ray studies* show characteristic degeneration in the lower thoracolumbar vertebrae. The vertebral bodies may appear flatter and denser than usual. Loss of bone mineral appears in later disease.
- *Serum calcium, phosphorus,* and *alkaline phosphatase levels* remain within normal limits.
- *Parathyroid hormone levels* may be elevated.
- *Transiliac bone biopsy* allows direct examination of osteoporotic changes in bone cells.
- *Computed tomography scan* allows accurate assessment of spinal bone loss.
- *Bone scans* that use a radionuclide agent display injured or diseased areas as darker portions.

Treatment

To control bone loss, prevent additional fractures, and control pain, treatment focuses on a physical therapy program of gentle exercise and activity and drug therapy to slow disease progress. Other treatment measures include supportive devices and possibly surgery.

Estrogen may be prescribed within 3 years after menopause to decrease the rate of bone resorption. Sodium fluoride may be given to stimulate bone formation. Calcium and vitamin D supplements may help to support normal bone metabolism. Calcitonin may be used to reduce bone resorption and slow the decline in bone mass.

Etidronate is the first agent that has proved to restore lost bone. Studies show that using etidronate for 2 weeks every 4 months increases bone mass.

Weakened vertebrae should be supported, usually with a back brace. Surgery (open reduction and internal fixation) can correct pathologic fractures of the femur. Colles' fracture requires reduction and immobilization (with a cast) for 4 to 10 weeks.

Key nursing diagnoses and patient outcomes

Risk for injury related to potential for fractures. Based on this nursing diagnosis, you'll establish these patient outcomes. The patient will:

- incorporate safety precautions into her daily life
- avoid fracture.

Impaired physical mobility related to decreased spinal flexion. Based on this nursing diagnosis, you'll establish these patient outcomes. The patient will:

- maintain normal muscle mass and joint range of motion
- seek assistance with activities of daily living
- achieve the highest level of physical mobility possible.

Chronic pain related to stress on a bone with decreased bone mass. Based on this nursing diagnosis, you'll establish these patient outcomes. The patient will:

- express relief of pain after analgesic administration
- avoid activities that precipitate or increase pain
- perform diversional activities to decrease the perception of pain.

Nursing interventions

- Design your care plan to consider the patient's fragility. Focus on careful positioning, ambulation, and prescribed exercises.
- Administer analgesics and heat to relieve pain, as ordered.
- Provide emotional support and reassurance to help the patient cope with limited mobility. Give her opportunities to voice her feelings. If possible, arrange for her to interact with others who have similar problems.

• Include the patient and her family in all phases of care. Answer questions as honestly as you can.
• Encourage the patient to perform as much self-care as her immobility and pain allow. Allow her adequate time to perform these activities at her own pace.
• Provide the patient with activities that involve mild exercise; help her to walk several times daily. As appropriate, perform passive range-of-motion exercises or encourage her to perform active exercises. Make sure she attends scheduled physical therapy sessions.
• Impose safety precautions. Keep side rails up on the patient's bed. Move the patient gently and carefully at all times. Discuss with ancillary hospital personnel how easily an osteoporotic patient's bones can fracture.
• Provide a balanced diet rich in nutrients that support skeletal metabolism: vitamin D, calcium, and protein.

Monitoring

• Check the patient's skin daily for redness, warmth, and new pain sites, which may indicate new fractures.
• Monitor the patient's pain level, and assess her response to analgesics, heat therapy, and diversional activities.
• Evaluate the patient's dietary intake of vitamin D, calcium, and protein.

Patient teaching

• Explain all treatments, tests, and procedures. For example, if the patient is undergoing surgery, explain all preoperative and postoperative procedures and treatments to the patient and her family.
• Make sure the patient and her family clearly understand the prescribed drug regimen. Tell them how to recognize significant adverse reactions. Instruct them to report them immediately.
• Teach the patient who's taking estrogen to perform breast self-examination. Tell her to perform this examination at least once a month and to report any lumps immediately. Emphasize the need for regular gynecologic examinations. Also instruct her to report abnormal vaginal bleeding promptly.
• If the patient takes a calcium supplement, encourage liberal fluid intake to help maintain adequate urine output and thereby avoid renal calculi, hypercalcemia, and hypercalciuria.
• Tell the patient to report any new pain sites immediately, especially after trauma.
• Advise the patient to sleep on a firm mattress and to avoid excessive bed rest.
• Teach the patient how to use a back brace properly, if appropriate.
• Thoroughly explain osteoporosis to the patient and her family. If they don't understand the disease process, they may feel needless guilt, thinking that they could have acted to prevent bone fractures.
• Demonstrate proper body mechanics. Show the patient how to stoop before lifting anything and how to avoid twisting movements and prolonged bending.
• Encourage the patient to install safety devices, such as grab bars and railings, at home.
• Advise the patient to eat a diet rich in calcium. Give her a list of calcium-rich foods. Explain that type II osteoporosis may be prevented by adequate dietary calcium intake and regular exercise. Hormonal and fluoride treatments also may help prevent osteoporosis.
• Explain that secondary osteoporosis may be prevented by effective treatment of underlying disease, early mobilization after surgery or trauma, decreased alcohol consumption, careful observation for signs of malabsorption, and prompt treatment of hyperthyroidism.
• Reinforce the patient's efforts to adapt, and show her how her condition is improving or stabilizing. As necessary, refer her to an occupational therapist or a home health nurse to help her cope with activities of daily living.

Ovarian cancer

After cancers of the lung, breast, and colon, primary ovarian cancer ranks as the most common cause of cancer death among American women. In women with previously treated breast cancer, metastatic ovarian cancer is more common than cancer of any other organ.

The highest incidence of ovarian cancer occurs in postmenopausal women between the ages of 55 and 59. However, the disease may occur during childhood or even pregnancy.

The prognosis varies with the histologic type and stage of the disease, but it's often poor because ovarian tumors are difficult to diagnose and progress rapidly. Although about 40% of women with ovarian cancer survive for 5 years, no major improvement in the overall survival rate has been made in the past 30 years.

Causes

Environmental and life-style factors seem to play a role in ovarian cancer. Women who live in industrialized nations are at greater risk, as are those whose diet is high in saturated fat. Other risk factors include infertility problems or nulliparity, celibacy, exposure to asbestos and talc, a history of breast or uterine cancer, and a family history of ovarian cancer.

Primary epithelial tumors arise in the müllerian epithelium; germ cell tumors, in the ovum itself; and sex cord tumors, in the ovarian stroma. Ovarian tumors rapidly spread intraperitoneally by local extension or surface seeding and, occasionally, through the lymphatics and the bloodstream. In most cases, extraperitoneal spread is through the diaphragm into the chest cavity, which may cause pleural effusions. Other metastasis is rare.

Three main types of ovarian cancer exist.

- *Primary epithelial tumors* account for 90% of all ovarian cancers and include serous cystadenocarcinoma, mucinous cystadenocarcinoma, and endometrioid and mesonephric malignant tumors.
- *Germ cell tumors* include endodermal sinus malignant tumors, embryonal carcinoma (a rare ovarian cancer that appears in children), immature teratomas, and dysgerminoma.
- *Sex cord (stromal) tumors* include granulosa cell tumors (which produce estrogen and may have feminizing effects), thecomas, and the rare arrhenoblastomas (which produce androgen and have virilizing effects).

Complications

Fluid and electrolyte imbalance, leg edema, ascites, and intestinal obstruction, causing nausea, malnutrition, and hunger, are common complications of progressive disease. Profound cachexia and recurrent malignant effusions, such as pleural effusions, may also occur.

Assessment

Because of ovarian cancer's lack of obvious signs, it's seldom diagnosed early. Usually, the cancer has metastasized before a diagnosis is made. Signs and symptoms vary with the tumor's size and the extent of metastasis.

In later stages, the history may disclose urinary frequency, constipation, pelvic discomfort, distention, and weight loss. The patient may complain of pain, possibly associated with tumor rupture, torsion, or infection. In a young patient, the pain may mimic that of appendicitis.

Inspection reveals a patient who is alert but gaunt. It often discloses a grossly distended abdomen accompanied by ascites – typically the sign that prompts the patient to seek treatment.

Palpation of the abdominal organs and peritoneum may disclose masses. On palpation, an ovarian tumor may vary from a rocky hardness to a rubbery or cyst-like quality. Postmenopausal women who have palpable, premenopausal-size ovaries require further evaluation for an ovarian tumor.

Staging ovarian cancer

The International Federation of Gynecology and Obstetrics has established this staging system, which is based on findings at clinical examination, surgical exploration, or both. Histology is taken into consideration, as is cytology in effusions. Ideally, biopsies should be obtained from any suspicious areas outside the pelvis.

Stage I
Growth limited to the ovaries.

Stage IA
Growth limited to one ovary; no ascites. No tumor on the external surface; capsule intact.

Stage IB
Growth limited to both ovaries; no ascites. No tumor on the external surfaces; capsules intact.

Stage IC
Tumor either Stage IA or IB but with tumor on surface of one or both ovaries; or with capsule ruptured; or with ascites present containing malignant cells or with positive peritoneal washings.

Stage II
Growth involving one or both ovaries with pelvic extension.

Stage IIA
Extension or metastasis, or both, to the uterus or tubes (or both).

Stage IIB
Extension to other pelvic tissues.

Stage IIC
Tumor either Stage IIA or IIB but with tumor on surface of one or both ovaries; or with capsule (or capsules) ruptured; or with ascites present containing malignant cells or with positive peritoneal washings.

Stage III
Tumor involving one or both ovaries with peritoneal implants outside the pelvis or positive retroperitoneal or inguinal nodes. Superficial liver metastasis equals Stage III.

Tumor limited to the true pelvis but with histologically proven malignant extension to small bowel or omentum.

Stage IIIA
Tumor grossly limited to the true pelvis with negative nodes but with histologically confirmed microscopic seeding of abdominal peritoneal surfaces.

Stage IIIB
Tumor of one or both ovaries with histologically confirmed implants of abdominal peritoneal surfaces, none exceeding 2 cm in greatest dimension. Nodes are negative.

Stage IIIC
Abdominal implants greater than 2 cm in greatest dimension or positive retroperitoneal or inguinal nodes or both.

Stage IV
Growth involving one or both ovaries with distant metastasis. If pleural effusion is present, there must be positive cytology to suggest Stage IV.

Parenchymal liver metastasis equals Stage IV.

Diagnostic tests

There are many tests ordered to help assess the patient's condition, including a complete blood count, blood chemistries, and electrocardiography (see *Staging ovarian cancer*).

• *Exploratory laparotomy,* including lymph node evaluation and tumor resection, is required for accurate diagnosis and staging.
• *Abdominal ultrasonography, computed tomography scan,* or *X-rays* delineate tumor size.
• *Excretory urography* provides information on renal function and possible urinary tract obstruction.
• *Chest X-rays* can help identify distant metastasis and pleural effusions.
• *Barium enema* (especially in patients with GI symptoms) may reveal obstruction and tumor size.
• *Lymphangiography* can show lymph node involvement.
• *Mammography* can rule out primary breast cancer.
• *Liver function studies* or a *liver scan* can help identify metastasis with ascites.
• *Aspiration of ascitic fluid* can reveal atypical cells.
• *Laboratory tumor marker studies,* such as ovarian carcinoma antigen, carcinoembryonic antigen, and human chorionic gonadotropin, are also evaluated.

Treatment

Depending on the cancer stage and the patient's age, treatment requires varying combinations of surgery, chemotherapy and, possibly, radiation therapy.

Occasionally, in girls or young women with a unilateral encapsulated tumor who wish to maintain fertility, the following conservative approach may be appropriate:
• resection of the involved ovary
• biopsies of the omentum and the uninvolved ovary
• biopsies of the pelvic and periaortic lymph nodes
• peritoneal washings for cytologic examination of pelvic fluid
• careful follow-up, including periodic X-rays, to rule out metastasis.

However, ovarian cancer usually requires more aggressive treatment, including total abdominal hysterectomy and bilateral salpingo-oophorectomy with tumor resection, omentectomy, appendectomy, lymph node palpation with probable lymphadenectomy, tissue biopsies, and peritoneal washings. Complete tumor resection is impossible if the tumor has matted around other organs or if it involves organs that can't be resected. Bilateral salpingo-oophorectomy in a prepubertal girl requires hormonal replacement therapy, starting at puberty, to induce the development of secondary sex characteristics.

Chemotherapy after surgery extends survival time in most patients but is largely palliative in advanced disease, although prolonged remissions are achieved in some patients. Primary chemotherapeutic regimens include cisplatinum or taxol. A newer chemotherapy drug, topotecan, has recently been approved for the treatment of adenocarcinoma of the ovary. Topotecan is used after patients don't respond to the more traditional chemotherapy agents. Intraperitoneal administration of cisplatin is under investigation, but the technique hasn't slowed disease progression or prolonged survival.

Radiation therapy isn't commonly used because ovarian tumors are normally not radio-sensitive. Radioisotopes have been used as adjuvant therapy but cause small-bowel obstructions and stenosis.

Under investigation, immunotherapy consists of I.V. injection of *Corynebacterium parvum* or bacille Calmette-Guérin vaccine, lymphokine-activated killer cells, and interleukin-2.

Key nursing diagnoses and patient outcomes

Altered nutrition: Less than body requirements related to malnutrition. Based on this nursing diagnosis, you'll establish these patient outcomes. The patient will:
• regain any lost weight, then maintain weight within a normal range
• eat a well-balanced diet high in calories and protein
• take supplements as needed to gain weight and alleviate malnutrition.

Anticipatory grieving related to the threat of death. Based on this nursing di-

agnosis, you'll establish these patient outcomes. The patient will:
- express her feelings about her diagnosis and prognosis
- use healthy coping mechanisms to deal with grief
- demonstrate control over her situation by participating in decisions about her care.

Fluid volume excess related to ascites. Based on this nursing diagnosis, you'll establish these patient outcomes. The patient will:
- comply with prescribed sodium and fluid restrictions to minimize fluid retention
- ambulate and carry out activities of daily living safely and comfortably
- describe the signs and symptoms of worsening fluid retention and seek medical treatment if they occur.

Nursing interventions

- If the patient has pain, make her as comfortable as possible. Administer prescribed analgesics as necessary, provide distractions, and have the patient perform relaxation techniques.
- Listen to the patient's concerns and fears. Answer her questions honestly. Provide support for the patient and her family. If the patient is a young woman who must undergo surgery and lose her childbearing ability, help her and her family overcome feelings of despair. If the patient is a child, find out whether her parents have told her she has cancer and respond to her questions accordingly.
- Provide supportive care for the adverse effects of therapy. If the patient is undergoing intraperitoneal chemotherapy, help alleviate her discomfort by infusing the fluid at a slower rate and repositioning her in an attempt to distribute the fluid evenly.
- If the patient develops flulike symptoms with immunotherapy, give acetaminophen for fever. Keep her covered with blankets, and provide warm liquids to relieve chills. Administer meperidine for rigors, as ordered. Administer an antiemetic as needed.
- If the patient has effusions and must undergo paracentesis and thoracentesis, assist with the procedure as necessary. Help her find a comfortable position during the procedure, then help her maintain it, using pillows. After the procedure, encourage her to drink fluids.
- For the malnourished patient, administer supplementary enteral or parenteral nutrition, as ordered. If her GI tract is intact, offer her frequent, small meals. If her GI tract is obstructed, discuss the possibility of a gastrostomy or jejunostomy tube with the doctor and the patient.
- Prepare the patient for surgery, as indicated. (See the entry "Oophorectomy and salpingectomy.")

Monitoring

- Monitor the patient for adverse effects of therapy.
- If the patient is receiving immunotherapy, watch for flulike symptoms that may last 12 to 24 hours after drug administration.
- Monitor the patient's fluid status, and measure intake and output. If she has ascites, measure her abdominal girth daily.
- Assess the patient's response to therapy and comfort measures.
- Monitor the patient's nutritional status and weigh her daily.

Patient teaching

- Teach the patient relaxation techniques and other measures that may help ease her discomfort.
- Stress the importance of preventing infection, emphasizing good hand-washing technique.
- Explain measures that may help maintain adequate nutrition, such as eating small, frequent meals.
- If the patient will undergo drug therapy or radiation therapy, explain the adverse effects that she can expect and suggest ways to alleviate and prevent them.
- Before surgery, thoroughly explain all preoperative tests, the expected course of

treatment, and surgical and postoperative procedures. In premenopausal women, explain that bilateral oophorectomy induces early menopause. Such patients may experience hot flashes, headaches, palpitations, insomnia, depression, and excessive perspiration.

• As appropriate, refer the patient and her family to the social service department, home health care agencies, hospices, and support groups such as the American Cancer Society.

Ovarian cysts

Usually nonneoplastic, ovarian cysts are sacs on an ovary. These cysts contain fluid or semisolid material. Although they are usually small and produce no symptoms, they require thorough investigation as possible sites of malignant change. Common ovarian cysts include follicular cysts and lutein cysts (granulosa-lutein, corpus luteum, and theca-lutein cysts). Ovarian cysts can develop anytime between puberty and menopause, including during pregnancy. Granulosa-lutein cysts occur infrequently, usually during early pregnancy. The prognosis for nonneoplastic cysts is excellent.

Causes

Follicular cysts are usually small and arise from follicles that overdistend instead of going through the atretic stage of the menstrual cycle. They appear semitransparent and are filled with a watery fluid visible through their thin walls. When such cysts persist into menopause, they secrete excessive amounts of estrogen in response to the hypersecretion of follicle-stimulating hormone and luteinizing hormone that normally occurs during menopause.

Granulosa-lutein cysts, which occur within the corpus luteum, are functional, nonneoplastic enlargements of the ovaries caused by excessive accumulation of blood during menstruation. Theca-lutein cysts are commonly bilateral and filled with clear, straw-colored fluid; they're often associated with hydatidiform mole, choriocarcinoma, or hormone therapy (with human chorionic gonadotropin [HCG] or clomiphene citrate). They may also be associated with multiple gestation, diabetes, and Rh sensitization.

Polycystic ovarian disease is part of Stein-Leventhal syndrome and stems from endocrine abnormalities.

Complications

Possible complications include amenorrhea, oligomenorrhea, secondary dysmenorrhea, and infertility. Torsion of the ovary and fallopian tube may result in rupture of the cyst with resulting peritonitis or intraperitoneal hemorrhage, shock, and death.

Assessment

Small ovarian cysts (such as follicular cysts) usually don't produce symptoms unless torsion or rupture occurs. The patient may report mild pelvic discomfort, low back pain, dyspareunia, or abnormal uterine bleeding secondary to a disturbed ovulatory pattern. Inspection may reveal signs of an acute abdomen similar to signs of appendicitis (abdominal tenderness, distention, and rigidity).

Granulosa-lutein cysts that appear early in pregnancy may grow as large as 2″ to 2½″ (5 to 6.5 cm) in diameter and produce unilateral pelvic discomfort. If rupture occurs, massive intraperitoneal hemorrhage may result. A nonpregnant patient may report delayed menses, followed by prolonged or irregular bleeding.

Palpation may detect enlarged ovaries caused by lack of ovulation. It may also reveal large follicular cysts. Theca-lutein cysts, however, usually aren't palpable.

Diagnostic tests

Visualization of the ovary through ultrasonography, laparoscopy, or surgery (often for another condition) confirms ovarian cysts. The following tests provide additional diagnostic information.

- *HCG titers* that are extremely elevated strongly suggest theca-lutein cysts.
- *Urine 17-ketosteroid concentrations* that are slightly elevated accompany polycystic ovarian disease.
- *Basal body temperature graphs* and *endometrial biopsy* results indicate anovulation.

Direct visualization must rule out paraovarian cysts of the broad ligament, salpingitis, endometriosis, and neoplastic cysts.

Treatment

Follicular cysts generally don't require treatment because they tend to disappear spontaneously by reabsorption or silent rupture within 60 days. Follicular cysts are usually observed for one menstrual cycle; if they persist, oral contraceptives are used to accelerate involution.

Treatment for granulosa-lutein cysts that occur during pregnancy is based on the patient's symptoms because these cysts diminish during the third trimester and rarely require surgery. Theca-lutein cysts disappear spontaneously after elimination of the hydatidiform mole, destruction of choriocarcinoma, or discontinuation of HCG or clomiphene citrate therapy.

Treatment for polycystic ovarian disease may include drugs such as hydrocortisone or clomiphene citrate to induce ovulation or, if drug therapy fails to induce ovulation, surgical wedge resection of one-third to one-half of the ovary.

Indications for surgical intervention (cystectomy) for both diagnosis and treatment include the following: a cyst that remains after one menstrual period, a cystic mass that is larger than 3″ (8 cm) or that persists longer than 8 weeks, a solid mass, or an adnexal mass after menopause.

Key nursing diagnoses and patient outcomes

Altered role performance related to infertility. Based on this nursing diagnosis, you'll establish these patient outcomes. The patient will:

- express her feelings about her inability to conceive a child
- conceive a child, if desired, through treatment of the ovarian cyst.

Anxiety related to the presence of an ovarian cyst. Based on this nursing diagnosis, you'll establish these patient outcomes. The patient will:

- identify and express her feelings of anxiety
- cope with her anxiety by participating in decisions about her care
- exhibit no physical symptoms of anxiety.

Pain related to pressure caused by the ovarian cyst. Based on this nursing diagnosis, you'll establish these patient outcomes. The patient will:

- express relief of pain after analgesic administration or nonpharmacologic measures such as heat therapy and diversion
- express an understanding of the need to seek immediate care if sudden acute abdominal pain develops
- become pain free after removal of the ovarian cyst.

Nursing interventions

- Administer hydrocortisone or clomiphene, as ordered.
- Administer mild analgesics and provide nonpharmacologic measures such as heat therapy for pain control.
- Prepare the patient for surgery, as ordered and appropriate. Administer sedatives, as ordered, to ensure adequate preoperative rest.
- After surgery, encourage frequent movement in bed and early ambulation.
- Encourage the patient to discuss her feelings. Provide emotional support, and help her develop effective coping strategies.

Monitoring

- Before surgery, watch for signs of cyst rupture, such as increasing abdominal pain, distention, and rigidity. Monitor the patient's vital signs to detect fever, tachy-

pnea, or hypotension, a possible sign of peritonitis or intraperitoneal hemorrhage.
• Assess the patient's response to drug therapy, and stay alert for adverse drug reactions.
• Monitor the patient's menstrual cycle and flow for abnormalities.

Patient teaching
• Carefully explain the nature of the particular cyst, the type of discomfort the patient may experience, and how long the condition may last.
• Before discharge, advise the patient to increase her at-home activity gradually—preferably over 4 to 6 weeks. Tell her to abstain from intercourse, tampon use, and douching during this time.

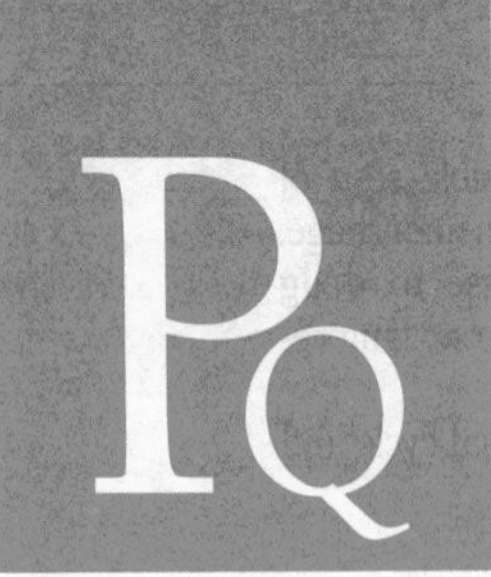

Pacemaker insertion

Pacemakers are battery-operated generators that emit timed electrical signals, triggering contraction of the heart muscle and controlling the heart rate. Whether temporary or permanent, they're used when the heart's natural pacemaker fails to work properly.

Temporary pacemakers may be used in emergency situations – for example, when drug therapy fails to correct dangerous bradycardia or heart block, when the patient's condition doesn't permit implantation of a permanent pacemaker, or during open-heart surgery. They're also used before a permanent pacemaker is implanted, to observe pacing's effects on cardiac function so that an optimum rate can be selected.

Permanent pacemakers are used when the heart's natural pacemaker is irreversibly disrupted. Indications include symptomatic bradycardia, advanced symptomatic atrioventricular (AV) block, sick sinus syndrome, sinus arrest, sinoatrial block, Stokes-Adams syndrome, tachyarrhythmias, and ectopic rhythms caused by antiarrhythmic drugs. Permanent pacemaker implantation is a common procedure.

The doctor's choice of a pacemaker depends on the patient's underlying cardiac condition and electrocardiogram (ECG) findings. More than 300 types of pacemakers exist, and many of them are programmable to perform varied functions. They're categorized according to their capabilities. (See *Reviewing pacemaker codes.*)

Procedure

Insertion or application of a temporary pacemaker varies, depending on the device. (See *Types of temporary pacemakers,* page 653.)

Although a permanent pacemaker can be implanted through a thoracotomy (which requires a general anesthetic), most are implanted using the transvenous endocardial approach. In this method, done under a local anesthetic, the patient is sedated and his chest or abdomen is prepared. Then, the surgeon makes a 3″ to 4″ (7.5- to 10-cm) incision in the selected site, inserts the electrode catheter through a vein, and uses fluoroscopy to guide it into the heart chamber appropriate for the type of pacemaker. After inserting the leads, he uses a pacing system analyzer to set the pulse generator to the proper stimulating and sensing thresholds, attaches the pulse generator to the leads, and then implants it into a pocket of muscle in the patient's chest or abdominal wall. He uses nonabsorbable sutures to tie the connection, leaving extra lengths of leads coiled under the pulse generator to decrease tension on the leads and to simplify subsequent replacement of the pulse generator, if necessary. He then closes the incision and applies a tight occlusive dressing.

Reviewing pacemaker codes

A three-letter coding system developed by the Intersociety Commission for Heart Disease provides a simple description of a pacemaker's capabilities. The first letter signifies the heart chamber being paced: **A** (atrium), **V** (ventricle), or **D** (dual, or both chambers). The second letter identifies the heart chamber that the pacemaker senses: **A, V, D,** or **O** (none). The third letter indicates how the pacemaker responds to the sensed event: **T** (triggered by event), **I** (inhibited by event), **D** (triggered and inhibited by event), **O** (not applicable), or **R** (reverse—pacemaker *slows* the heartbeat).

Pacemaker code and indications	Advantages	Disadvantages
AAI, AAT • Sick sinus syndrome with intact AV conduction	• Simplest system with sequential AV depolarization • Requires single lead • Easily understood function	• Won't pace ventricle if AV block develops • Inhibits atrial impulses by sensing QRS complexes
VVI, VVT • Atrial flutter or fibrillation, or multifocal atrial tachycardia with slow ventricular response • Infrequent bradycardia • Insufficient hemodynamic response to AV sequential pacing • Recurrent pacemaker-mediated tachycardia (PMT)	• Requires single lead • Relatively simple to operate	• Doesn't change rate in response to increased metabolic demands • Doesn't preserve AV synchrony • May cause retrograde AV conduction and echo beats • May cause pacemaker syndrome
VDD • Impaired AV conduction with normal sinus node function	• Maintains AV synchrony and rate responsiveness to increased metabolic demands when atrial rate stays within tracking limits	• Requires two leads • Doesn't pace atrium • May cause PMT • Lacks AV synchrony and rate responsiveness during atrial bradycardia
DVI • Atrial bradycardia • PMT in VDD and DDD modes	• Maintains AV synchrony during atrial bradycardia • Permits AV rate control to decrease myocardial oxygen demands during angina • Lack of atrial sensing may prevent PMT	• Requires two leads • Doesn't maintain AV synchrony unless pacemaker's programmed rate exceeds spontaneous atrial rate • Doesn't respond to increased metabolic demands • Lack of atrial sensing may cause competitive rhythms
DDD • Atrial bradycardia • Normal sinus node function with abnormal AV conduction	• Maintains AV synchrony • Most closely mimics normal cardiac physiology	• Requires two leads • May cause PMT • Paced rate doesn't increase to meet metabolic demands in sinus node dysfunction unless programmed to do so

Complications

Early complications include serous or bloody drainage from the insertion site, swelling, ecchymosis, incisional pain, and impaired mobility; less common complications include venous thrombosis, embolism, infection, pneumothorax, pectoral or diaphragmatic muscle stimulation from the pacemaker, arrhythmias, cardiac tamponade, heart failure, and abnormal pacemaker operation with lead dislodgment. Late complications (up to several years) include failure to capture, failure to sense, firing loss, and pacemaker rejection.

Key nursing diagnoses and patient outcomes

Anxiety related to lack of understanding of pacemaker unit function. Based on this nursing diagnosis, you'll establish these patient outcomes. The patient will:

- express fears and concerns related to pacemaker
- cope with anxiety by obtaining information about pacemaker function from appropriate sources
- communicate an understanding of pacemaker procedure and function.

Risk for injury related to potential for pacemaker malfunction. Based on this nursing diagnosis, you'll establish these patient outcomes. The patient will:

- identify reportable signs and symptoms of pacemaker malfunction, such as hiccups, confusion, and slurred speech
- have pacemaker function checked regularly
- maintain hemodynamic stability with a properly functioning pacemaker.

Impaired physical mobility related to pacemaker incision temporarily affecting shoulder and arm movement on operative side. Based on this nursing diagnosis, you'll establish these patient outcomes. The patient will:

- perform range-of-motion (ROM) exercises as prescribed postoperatively
- regain and maintain normal physical mobility on affected side.

Nursing interventions

When preparing for pacemaker insertion or managing a patient afterward, expect to implement these nursing interventions.

Before the procedure

- If pacing is done in an emergency, briefly explain the procedure to the patient if possible.
- If the patient is scheduled for permanent implantation, ensure that he and his family understand the doctor's explanation of the need for an artificial pacemaker, the potential complications, and the alternatives. Also be sure they understand pacemaker terminology. (See *Understanding pacemaker vocabulary,* page 654.)
- Before permanent implantation, obtain baseline vital signs and record a 12-lead ECG or rhythm strip. Evaluate radial and dorsalis pedis pulses and assess the patient's mental status.
- Restrict food and fluids for 12 hours before the procedure.
- Explain to the patient that he may receive a sedative before the procedure and will probably have his upper chest or abdomen shaved and scrubbed with an antiseptic solution. Inform him that when he arrives in the operating room, his hands may be restrained so that they don't inadvertently touch the sterile area and his chest or abdomen will be draped with sterile towels.
- Unless he's scheduled to undergo a thoracotomy, explain that he'll receive a local, rather than a general, anesthetic. Tell him that he'll be in the operating room for about an hour.
- Check that the patient or a responsible family member has signed a consent form.

After the procedure

- After pacemaker insertion, provide continuous ECG monitoring. Chart the type of insertion, lead system, pacemaker mode, and pacing guidelines. Take vital signs every 30 minutes until the patient stabilizes, and watch the ECG for signs of pacemaker problems.

Types of temporary pacemakers

Temporary pacemakers come in four types: transcutaneous, transvenous, transthoracic, and epicardial. They're used to pace the heart after cardiac surgery, during cardiopulmonary resuscitation, and when sinus arrest, symptomatic sinus bradycardia, or complete heart block occurs. Temporary pacing may also correct tachyarrhythmias that fail to respond to drug therapy.

Transcutaneous pacemaker

Completely noninvasive and easily applied, this pacemaker proves especially useful in an emergency. To perform pacing with this device, the doctor places electrodes on the skin directly over the heart and connects them to a pulse generator.

Transvenous pacemaker

This device, a balloon-tipped pacing catheter, is inserted via the subclavian or jugular vein into the right ventricle. The procedure can be done at the bedside or in the cardiac catheterization laboratory. Transvenous pacemakers offer better control of the heartbeat than either transcutaneous or transthoracic pacemakers, but electrode insertion takes longer, thus limiting its usefulness in emergencies.

Transthoracic pacemaker

Transthoracic pacing involves needle insertion of leads into the heart. Used in emergencies, it rarely stimulates the heart and commonly causes complications.

Epicardial pacemaker

Implanted during open-heart surgery, the epicardial pacemaker permits rapid treatment of postoperative complications. During surgery, the doctor attaches the leads to the heart and runs them out through the chest incision. Afterward, they're coiled on the patient's chest, insulated, and covered with a dressing. If pacing is needed, the leads are simply uncovered and attached to a pulse generator. When pacing is no longer needed, the leads can be removed under a local anesthetic.

- Be on guard for signs of a perforated ventricle, with resultant cardiac tamponade. Ominous signs include persistent hiccups, distant heart sounds, pulsus paradoxus, hypotension accompanied by narrow pulse pressure, increased venous pressure, bulging neck veins, cyanosis, decreased urine output, restlessness, and complaints of fullness in the chest. Report any of these signs immediately and prepare the patient for emergency surgery.
- If your patient's condition worsens dramatically and he requires defibrillation, follow these guidelines to avoid damaging the pacemaker. Place the paddles at least 4" (10 cm) from the pulse generator, and avoid anterior-posterior paddle placement. Have a backup temporary pacemaker available. If your patient has an external pacemaker, turn it off. Keep the current under 200 joules if possible.
- Assess the area around the incision for swelling, tenderness, and hematoma, but don't remove the occlusive dressing for the first 24 hours without a doctor's order. When you do remove it, check the wound for drainage, redness, and unusual warmth or tenderness.
- After the first 24 hours, begin passive ROM exercises for the affected arm, if ordered. Progress to active ROM in 2 weeks.

Home care instructions

- Tell the patient to take his pulse every day before getting out of bed. Instruct him to record his heart rate, along with the date and time, to help his doctor determine

Understanding pacemaker vocabulary

"The firing loss seems to be caused by undersensing. The threshold needs to be increased to be sure the heartbeat is captured." A patient who overhears comments such as these may find them confusing or even frightening. Like any specialized field, cardiac pacing has its own jargon, which can seem overwhelming if you don't know what's being said. To help you convert this jargon into plain English, here's a quick primer.

Artifact
The spike recorded on the ECG depicting the electrical energy discharged from the pulse generator

Capture
Contraction of the heart muscle in response to discharge from the pulse generator

Electrode
The thin, electrically conductive wire that's enclosed within the lead wire of the system; comes in direct contact with the heart and sends signals to the pulse generator

Failure to pace
Absence of an artifact on the ECG when the pacemaker, according to program, should be firing

Failure to sense
A condition in which the pulse generator doesn't respond at all to the heart's signals

Firing loss
Combined failure to sense and capture, caused by mechanical failure of the unit

Lead
The wire and electrode unit, which delivers the electrical energy from the pulse generator to the heart and receives the sensing information; can be unipolar (single terminal) or bipolar (double terminal)

Noncapture (failure to capture)
The failure of the heart to respond to a correctly synchronized pacing stimulus

Oversensing
A condition in which the pulse generator responds too readily to signals for impulse generation

Pulse generator
The device that includes the power source and circuitry for transmitting pacing signals as well as for sensing the heart's intrinsic activity

Sensing
The ability to recognize the electrical signal that stimulates (or inhibits) the discharge of electrical energy by the pulse generator

Threshold
The amount of electrical energy necessary to consistently cause depolarization

Undersensing
A condition in which the pulse generator occasionally fails to respond to the heart's signals

whether the pacemaker requires adjustment.

• Stress the importance of calling the doctor immediately if his pulse rate drops below the minimal pacemaker setting or if it exceeds 100 beats/minute. Also have him report difficulty breathing, dizziness, fainting, or swollen hands or feet. Similarly, have him report redness, warmth, pain, drainage, or swelling at the insertion site.

• Warn the patient to avoid placing excessive pressure over the insertion site, moving suddenly or jerkily, or extending his arms over his head for 8 weeks after discharge.
• Tell the patient that he's free to follow his normal routines, including sexual activity, and that he may bathe and shower normally. Urge him to follow dietary and exercise instructions.
• Remind the patient to carry his pacemaker identification at all times and to show his card to airline clerks when he travels; the pacemaker will set off metal detectors but won't be harmed.
• Explain the special precautions that he'll have to take to prevent disruption of the pacemaker by electrical or electronic devices. For example, he should avoid placing electric hair clippers or shavers directly over the pacemaker, maintain a distance of at least 3′ (1 m) from microwave ovens, and avoid close contact with electric motors and gasoline engines. He should also keep away from automobile antitheft devices and high-voltage electrical lines. Advise him to tell any doctor that he has an implanted pacemaker before undergoing certain diagnostic tests, such as magnetic resonance imaging.
• Mention that the doctor may provide instructions for testing the pacemaker by using a transistor radio or the telephone.
• Stress the importance of follow-up care. Doctor visits are usually scheduled 2 to 4 weeks after implantation and then periodically thereafter, according to the patient's needs.

Paget's disease

Also known as osteitis deformans, this slowly progressive metabolic bone disease is characterized by an initial phase of excessive bone resorption (osteoclastic phase), followed by a reactive phase of excessive abnormal bone formation (osteoblastic phase). The new bone structure, which is chaotic, fragile, and weak, causes painful deformities of the external contour and the internal structures.

Paget's disease usually affects one or several skeletal areas (most commonly the spine, pelvis, femur, and skull). Occasionally, the patient will have widely distributed skeletal deformity. In about 5% of patients, the involved bone will undergo malignant changes.

The disease can be fatal, particularly when associated with congestive heart failure (widespread disease creates a continuous need for high cardiac output), bone sarcoma, or giant-cell tumors.

Paget's disease occurs worldwide but only rarely in Asia, the Middle East, Africa, and Scandinavia. In the United States, it affects about 2.5 million people over age 40, primarily men.

Causes

Although the disease's exact cause isn't known, one theory suggests that a slow or dormant viral infection (possibly mumps) causes a dormant skeletal infection, which surfaces many years later as Paget's disease.

Complications

Involved sites may fracture easily after only minor trauma. These fractures heal slowly and usually incompletely. Vertebral collapse or vascular changes that affect the spinal cord could lead to paraplegia. Bony impingement on the cranial nerves may cause blindness and hearing loss with tinnitus and vertigo.

Other complications include osteoarthritis, sarcoma, hypertension, renal calculi, hypercalcemia, gout, congestive heart failure, and a waddling gait (from softened pelvic bones).

Assessment

Clinical effects vary. The patient with early disease may be asymptomatic. As the disease progresses, he may report severe, persistent pain. If abnormal bone impinges on the spinal cord or sensory nerve root, he may complain of impaired mobility and pain increasing with weight bearing.

If the patient's head is involved, inspection may reveal characteristic cranial enlargement over the frontal and occipital areas. The patient may comment that his hat size has increased, and he may have headaches. Other deformities include kyphosis (spinal curvature caused by compression fractures of affected vertebrae) accompanied by a barrel-shaped chest and asymmetrical bowing of the tibia and femur, which typically reduces height. Palpation may detect warmth and tenderness over affected sites.

Diagnostic tests

- *X-ray studies* performed before overt symptoms develop show bone expansion and increased bone density.
- *Bone scans* (more sensitive than X-rays) clearly show early pagetic lesions (the radioisotope concentrates in areas of active disease).
- *Bone biopsy* may show bone tissue that has a characteristic mosaic pattern.
- *Red blood cell count* indicates anemia.
- *Serum alkaline phosphatase level*—an index of osteoblastic activity and bone formation—is elevated.
- *A 24-hour urinalysis* demonstrates elevated hydroxyproline levels. Hydroxyproline, an amino acid excreted by the kidneys, provides an index of osteoblastic hyperactivity.

Treatment

If the patient is asymptomatic, treatment isn't needed. The patient with symptoms requires drug therapy.

The hormone calcitonin may be given subcutaneously or I.M. Although the patient will require long-term maintenance therapy with calcitonin, noticeable improvement occurs after the first few weeks of treatment. The patient also may receive oral etidronate to retard bone resorption (and relieve bone lesions) and to reduce serum alkaline phosphatase and urinary hydroxyproline excretion. Etidronate produces improvement after 1 to 3 months.

Plicamycin (a cytotoxic antibiotic used to decrease serum calcium, urinary hydroxyproline, and serum alkaline phosphatase levels) produces remission of symptoms within 2 weeks and biochemically detectable improvement in 1 to 2 months. However, plicamycin may destroy platelets or compromise renal function; it's usually given only to patients who have severe disease, who require rapid relief, or who don't respond to other treatment.

Self-administration of calcitonin and etidronate helps patients with Paget's disease lead nearly normal lives. Even so, these patients may need surgery to reduce or prevent pathologic fractures, correct secondary deformities, and relieve neurologic impairment. To decrease the risk of excessive bleeding caused by hypervascular bone, drug therapy with calcitonin and etidronate or plicamycin must precede surgery. Joint replacement is difficult because methyl methacrylate (a gluelike bonding material) doesn't set properly on bone affected by Paget's disease. Other treatments vary according to symptoms. Aspirin, indomethacin, or ibuprofen typically controls pain.

Key nursing diagnoses and patient outcomes

Risk for injury related to bone fractures. Based on this nursing diagnosis, you'll establish these patient outcomes. The patient will:

- incorporate safety precautions into every-day life to prevent bone fractures
- comply with therapy to stabilize bone metabolism
- not develop fractures.

Impaired physical mobility related to bone deformities. Based on this nursing diagnosis, you'll establish these patient outcomes. The patient will:

• maintain muscle strength and joint range of motion
• show no evidence of complications related to impaired physical mobility, such as contractures, venous stasis, or skin breakdown
• attain the highest degree of mobility possible within the confines of the disease.

Pain related to bone reformation. Based on this nursing diagnosis, you'll establish these patient outcomes. The patient will:
• express feelings of comfort after analgesic administration
• avoid or minimize activity that precipitates or increases pain.

Nursing interventions

• Administer prescribed medications, including analgesics, as ordered.
• If bed rest confines the patient for prolonged periods, prevent pressure ulcers with meticulous skin care. Reposition the patient frequently, and use a flotation mattress. Provide high-topped sneakers or a footboard to manage footdrop.
• Prepare the patient for surgery if appropriate.

Monitoring

• Monitor intake and output. Encourage adequate fluid intake to minimize renal calculi formation.
• Assess the patient's pain level daily to evaluate the effectiveness of analgesic therapy. Watch for new areas of pain or newly restricted movements – which may indicate new fracture sites – and sensory or motor disturbances, such as difficulty in hearing, seeing, or walking.
• Monitor serum calcium and alkaline phosphatase levels.

Patient teaching

• Help the patient adjust to the life-style changes imposed by Paget's disease. Teach him to pace activities and, if necessary, to use assistive devices.
• Encourage the patient to follow a recommended exercise program. Urge him to avoid both immobility and excessive activity.
• Suggest a firm mattress or a bed board to minimize spinal deformities.
• To prevent falls at home, urge the patient to remove throw rugs and other small obstacles from the floor.
• Emphasize the importance of regular checkups, including examination of the eyes and ears, to assess for complications.
• Explain all medications to the patient. Instruct him to use analgesics cautiously.
• Demonstrate how to inject calcitonin properly and how to rotate injection sites. Caution the patient that adverse reactions may occur (including nausea, vomiting, local inflammation at the injection site, facial flushing, itchy hands, and fever). Reassure him that these reactions are usually mild and occur infrequently.
• Tell the patient receiving etidronate to take this medication with fruit juice 2 hours before or after meals (milk or other calcium-rich fluids impair absorption), to divide the daily dosage to minimize adverse reactions, and to watch for and report stomach cramps, diarrhea, fractures, and new or increasing bone pain.
• Instruct the patient receiving plicamycin to watch for signs of infection, easy bruising, bleeding, and temperature elevation. Urge him to schedule and report for regular follow-up laboratory tests.
• Refer the patient and his family to community support resources, such as a home health care agency and a local chapter of the Paget's Disease Foundation.

Pancreatectomy

In pancreatectomy, various resections, drainage procedures, and anastomoses may be used to treat pancreatic diseases in which more conservative techniques have failed. It's indicated for palliative treatment of pancreatic cancer as well as chronic pancreatitis, which often stems from prolonged alcohol abuse. It's also used to treat islet cell tumors (insulinomas).

The type of procedure used depends on the patient's condition, the extent of the disease and its metastasis, and the amount of endocrine and exocrine function the pancreas retains. Often, the procedure is determined only after surgical exploration of the abdomen.

Procedure

After the patient is anesthetized, the surgeon makes an abdominal incision. He selects the procedure based on evaluation of the pancreas, liver, gallbladder, and common bile duct. If the disease is localized, he may resect a portion of the pancreas and the surrounding organs. If the surgeon detects either metastatic disease in the liver or lymph nodes or tumor invasion of the aorta or superior mesenteric artery, he may decide to bypass the obstruction to lessen the patient's pain.

Complications

Major complications of pancreatectomy include hemorrhage (during and after surgery), fistulas, abscesses (common with distal pancreatectomy), common bile duct obstruction, and pseudocysts. Subtotal resection sometimes causes insulin dependence, whereas total pancreatectomy always causes permanent and complete insulin dependence.

Key nursing diagnoses and patient outcomes

Altered nutrition: Less than body requirements related to malabsorption of nutrients caused by loss of digestive enzymes. Based on this nursing diagnosis, you'll establish these patient outcomes. The patient will:

- receive an adequate nutritional intake with enteral feedings (or total parenteral nutrition when enteral feedings can't be given)
- show no signs of intolerance to enteral feedings, such as nausea and vomiting
- have an adequate intake and output
- not exhibit signs and symptoms of malnutrition.

Risk for injury related to potential coagulation abnormalities. Based on this nursing diagnosis, you'll establish these patient outcomes. The patient will:

- exhibit normal coagulation studies
- show no signs of bleeding from his incision site
- maintain hemodynamic stability, as evidenced by stable vital signs, output that equals intake, and normal mental status.

Ineffective breathing pattern related to guarded respirations caused by abdominal incision. Based on this nursing diagnosis, you'll establish these patient outcomes. The patient will:

- maintain adequate ventilation and stable respiratory status
- comply with measures to prevent respiratory complications, such as turning, coughing, and deep breathing every 2 to 4 hours and using an incentive spirometer correctly
- not exhibit respiratory complications, such as pneumonia or atelectasis.

Nursing interventions

When preparing for or managing a patient with a pancreatectomy, expect to implement these nursing interventions.

Before surgery

- Explain to the patient that the specific procedure will be selected by the surgeon during abdominal exploration. (See *Understanding types of pancreatectomy,* pages 660 and 661.) Provide emotional support, and encourage the patient to express his feelings.
- Give analgesics, as ordered.
- Arrange for necessary diagnostic studies, as ordered, to help the surgeon determine the existing endocrine and exocrine structure of the pancreas and any anatomic anomalies.

• For the patient with chronic pancreatitis or cancer, provide enteral or parenteral nutrition before surgery. As ordered, give low-fat, high-calorie feedings to combat the malnutrition and steatorrhea that result from malabsorption.
• Give meticulous skin care to prevent tissue breakdown that could complicate postoperative healing.
• If the patient is hyperglycemic, give oral hypoglycemic agents or insulin, as ordered, and monitor blood and urine glucose levels.
• Monitor the patient who has a recent history of alcohol abuse for withdrawal symptoms: agitation, tachycardia, tremors, anorexia, and hypertension. Remember that delirium tremens may occur 72 to 96 hours after the patient's last drink and that surgery should be delayed until after this period.
• If the patient smokes (many patients with pancreatic cancer are heavy smokers), advise him to stop smoking before surgery. Evaluate his pulmonary status to provide baseline information.
• Instruct the patient in deep-breathing and coughing techniques. Tell him to turn in bed, perform deep-breathing exercises, and cough every 2 hours for 24 to 72 hours after surgery. If incentive spirometry is indicated, instruct him as appropriate.
• Assess the patient for jaundice and increased hematoma formation – signs of liver dysfunction, which commonly accompanies pancreatic disease. As ordered, arrange for liver function and coagulation studies before surgery. If the patient has a prolonged prothrombin time, expect to give vitamin K to prevent postoperative hemorrhage.
• Because resection of the transverse colon may be necessary, the doctor may order mechanical and antibiotic bowel preparation as well as prophylactic systemic antibiotics (started 6 hours before surgery and continuing for 72 hours after surgery). Carry out these measures as directed, and expect to assist with nasogastric (NG) tube and indwelling urinary catheter insertion.
• Make sure that the patient or a responsible family member has signed a consent form.

After surgery

• The patient may be admitted to the intensive care unit after surgery. Monitor his vital signs closely, and administer plasma expanders as ordered. Use central, arterial, or pulmonary catheter readings to evaluate hemodynamic status; correlate these readings with urine output and wound drainage. If central venous pressure and urine output drop, give fluids to avoid hypovolemic shock.
• Evaluate NG tube drainage, which should be green tinged as bile drains from the stomach.
• If the patient has a T tube in his common bile duct, evaluate this drainage, too. Normal bile drainage is 600 to 800 ml daily, decreasing as more bile goes to the intestine. Notify the doctor if bile drainage doesn't decrease, as this may indicate a biliary obstruction leading to possibly fatal peritonitis.
• Assess drainage tubes for drainage and inspect sites for frank bleeding, which may signal hemorrhage. If a pancreatic drain is in place, prevent skin breakdown from highly excoriating pancreatic enzymes by changing dressings frequently or by using a wound pouching system to contain the drainage.
• Monitor the patient's fluid and electrolyte balance closely, evaluate arterial blood gases, and provide I.V. fluid replacements, as ordered. Keep in mind that constant gastric drainage can cause metabolic alkalosis, signaled by apathy, irritability, dehydration, and slow, shallow breathing. Report these signs to the doctor, and expect to administer isotonic fluids. Alternatively, loss of bile and pancreatic secretions can lead to metabolic acidosis, signaled by elevated blood pressure, rapid pulse and respirations, and arrhythmias.

Understanding types of pancreatectomy

Surgery and indications	Procedure	
Pancreaticojejunostomy • Chronic pancreatitis with extensive pathology • Multiple strictures • Palpable ductal dilation • Pancreatic ascites	• Pancreatic duct, if large enough, is connected to the jejunum, bypassing obstruction; pancreatic tissue is preserved	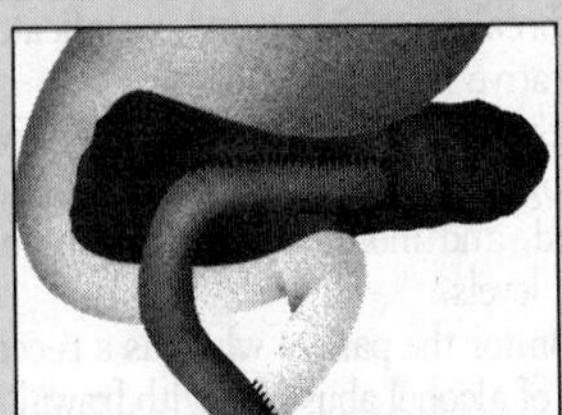
Distal pancreatectomy (subtotal) • Islet cell tumors (insulinomas) confined to tail of pancreas	• Removes the neck, body, and tail of the pancreas plus the spleen and splenic vessels; pancreatic duct may be drained into stomach or jejunum; leaves the head and uncinate process of the pancreas to the left of the mesenteric vessels	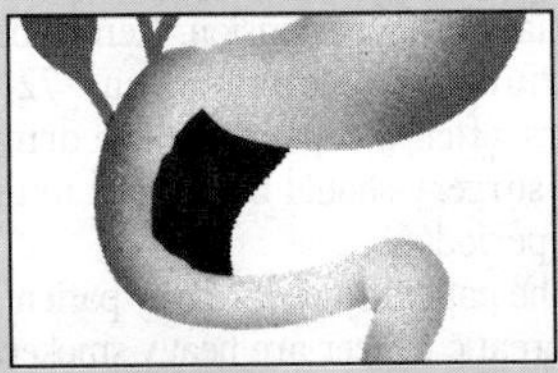
Distal pancreatectomy (95%) • Acute pancreatitis • Chronic pancreatitis with extensive pathology and diffuse calcification • Multiple strictures or obstructions • Intrahepatic cyst formation • Failure of other procedures, such as surgical repair of biliary or pancreatic ducts or the sphincter of Oddi	• Removes the neck, body, and tail of the pancreas as well as a major portion of the head and uncinate process and the entire spleen; leaves only a rim of pancreatic tissue, containing the blood supply to the duodenum and common bile duct; also includes vagotomy and gastrojejunostomy	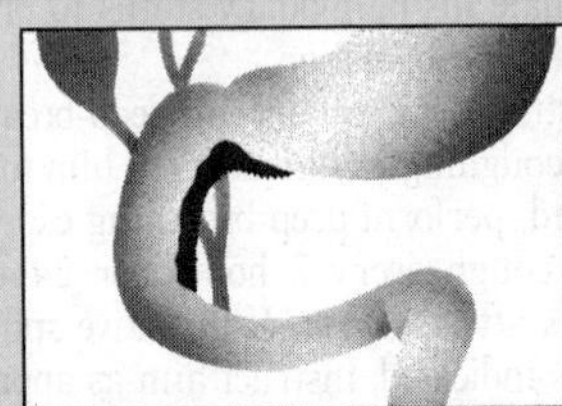
Total pancreatectomy • Chronic pancreatitis with marked pancreatic destruction • Multiple intraductal obstructions • Failure of more conservative measures, such as medication and diet, to control severe pain • Pancreatic cancer	• Removes the pancreas and spleen completely, leaving the hepatic duct anastomosed to the jejunum; also includes hemigastrectomy and vagotomy or 75% gastrectomy and duodenectomy	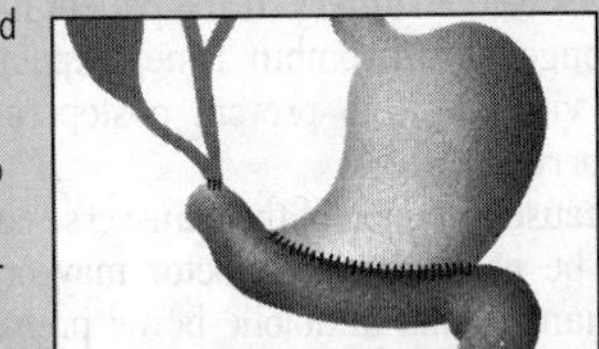

Understanding types of pancreatectomy *(continued)*

Surgery and indications	Procedure	
Fortner regional pancreatectomy • Pancreatic cancer	• Removes the portal vein, entire pancreas, spleen, transverse colon, gallbladder, and common bile duct	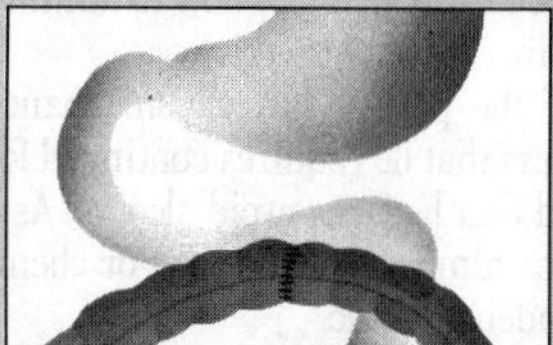
Radical pancreaticoduodenectomy (Whipple procedure) • Cancer confined to head of pancreas	• Removes the head of the pancreas along with the duodenum, pylorus, distal half of the stomach, gallbladder, and lower end of the common bile duct	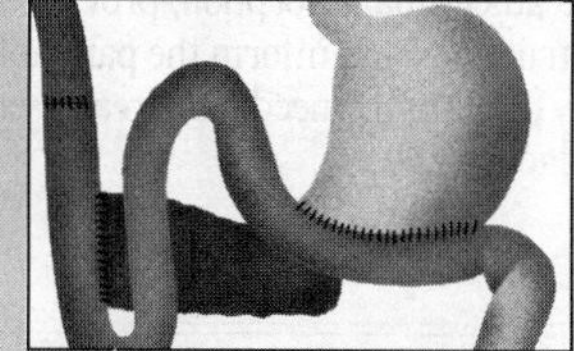
Partial pancreaticoduodenectomy (Modified Whipple procedure) • Cancer confined to head of pancreas	• Preserves the pylorus and stomach by anastomosing the pancreatic remnant to the antrum of the stomach (pancreaticogastrostomy)	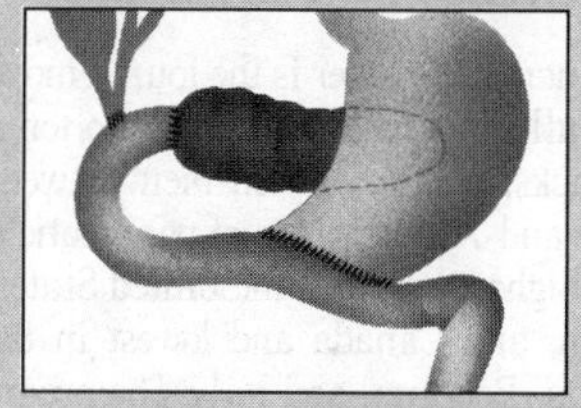

Report these signs to the doctor, and give I.V. bicarbonate as ordered.

• Have I.V. calcium ready because serum amylase levels commonly rise after pancreatic surgery and amylase can bind to calcium. Evaluate serum calcium levels periodically.

• Check blood glucose levels periodically for possible fluctuations. Give insulin, if ordered.

• Monitor the patient's respiratory status, being alert for shallow breathing, decreased respiratory rate, and respiratory distress. Administer oxygen, if necessary and ordered. Reinforce deep-breathing techniques, and encourage the patient to cough.

• Be alert for absent bowel sounds, severe abdominal pain, vomiting, or fever – evidence of such complications as fistula development and paralytic ileus. Also, check the patient's wound for redness, pain, edema, unusual odor, or suture line separation. Report any of these findings to the doctor.

• If no complications develop, expect the patient's GI function to return in 24 to 48 hours. Remove his NG tube as ordered, and start him on fluids.

Home care instructions

• Teach the patient how to care for his wound, including careful cleaning and

dressing each day. Tell him to report any signs of wound infection promptly.
- As appropriate, teach the patient how to test his urine for ketones or how to monitor his blood glucose levels. If he had a total pancreatectomy, provide routine diabetic teaching and show him or a responsible family member how to administer insulin.
- If the patient has chronic pancreatitis, stress that he requires continued follow-up and that he *must* avoid alcohol. As needed, refer him to an outpatient or chemical dependency clinic.
- Because pancreatic exocrine insufficiency leads to malabsorption, provide dietary instructions and inform the patient that he may eventually need pancreatic enzyme replacement.

Pancreatic cancer

Pancreatic cancer is the fourth most lethal of all cancers. It occurs most often among blacks, particularly in men between ages 35 and 70. Incidence of pancreatic cancer is highest in Israel, the United States, Sweden, and Canada and lowest in Switzerland, Belgium, and Italy. The prognosis is poor: most patients die within a year of diagnosis.

Causes

Evidence suggests that pancreatic cancer is linked to inhalation or absorption of carcinogens that are then excreted by the pancreas. Examples of such carcinogens include:
- cigarette smoke (pancreatic cancer is three to four times more common among smokers)
- excessive fat and protein (a diet high in fat and protein induces chronic hyperplasia of the pancreas, with increased turnover of cells)
- food additives
- industrial chemicals, such as beta-naphthalene, benzidine, and urea.

Other possible predisposing factors include chronic pancreatitis, diabetes mellitus, and chronic alcohol abuse.

Tumors of the pancreas are almost always adenocarcinomas. They arise most frequently (67% of the time) in the head of the pancreas. Tumors in this location commonly obstruct the ampulla of Vater and common bile duct and metastasize directly to the duodenum. Adhesions anchor the tumor to the spine, stomach, and intestines.

Less frequently, tumors arise in the body and tail of the pancreas. When this happens, large nodular masses become fixed to retropancreatic tissues and the spine. The spleen, left kidney, suprarenal gland, and diaphragm are directly invaded, and the celiac plexus becomes involved, resulting in splenic vein thrombosis and spleen infarction. Among the rarest of pancreatic tumors are islet cell tumors. (See *Islet cell tumors.*)

In pancreatic cancer, two main tissue types form fibrotic nodes. Cylinder cells arise in ducts and degenerate into cysts, and large, fatty, granular cells arise in parenchyma.

Complications

Related to the progression of the disease, complications may include malabsorption of nutrients, insulin-dependent diabetes, liver and GI problems, and mental status changes.

Assessment

A patient who seeks treatment early in the disease usually reports a dull, intermittent epigastric pain. Later, he may report continuous pain that radiates to the right upper quadrant or dorsolumbar area. He may describe it as colicky, dull, or vague and unrelated to posture or activity. Or, he may state that meals seem to aggravate the epigastric pain. He also may report anorexia, nausea, vomiting, and a rapid, profound weight loss.

Inspection may reveal jaundice. On palpation, you may note a palpable, well-defined, large mass in the subumbilical or left hypochondrial region – an indication that the tail of the pancreas is involved. The mass may adhere to the large vessels or the vertebral column and may produce a pulsation. If the tumor has involved or compressed the splenic artery, auscultation of the left hypochondrium may reveal an abdominal bruit.

Diagnostic tests

Several tests may be ordered to help diagnose the disease and determine its extent. (See *Staging pancreatic cancer,* page 664.)

Percutaneous fine-needle aspiration biopsy of the pancreas may detect tumor cells, and laparotomy with a biopsy allows a definitive diagnosis. However, a biopsy may miss relatively small or deep-seated cancerous tissue or create a pancreatic fistula. Retroperitoneal insufflation, cholangiography, scintigraphy and, particularly, barium swallow (to locate the neoplasm and detect changes in the duodenum or stomach relating to cancer of the head of the pancreas) also can be performed to detect the disease.

Ultrasonography helps identify a mass, but not its histology. A computed tomography scan shows greater detail of the mass than ultrasonography. A magnetic resonance imaging scan discloses the tumor's location and size in great detail.

Angiography reveals the tumor's vascular supply. Endoscopic retrograde cholangiopancreatography allows visualization, instillation of contrast medium, and specimen biopsy.

A secretin test reveals the absence of pancreatic enzymes and suggests pancreatic duct obstruction and tumors of the body and tail.

Other laboratory tests that support the diagnosis include:

- serum bilirubin (increased)
- serum amylase-lipase (occasionally increased)
- prothrombin time (prolonged)
- aspartate aminotransferase (formerly SGOT) and alanine aminotransferase (formerly SGPT) (elevated enzyme levels when liver cell necrosis is present)
- alkaline phosphatase (markedly elevated, with biliary obstruction)

Islet cell tumors

Relatively uncommon, islet cell tumors (insulinomas) may be benign or malignant. They produce symptoms in three stages, and despite treatment, the prognosis is unfavorable.

Stage 1: Slight hypoglycemia
Fatigue, restlessness, malaise, and excessive weight gain result from slight hypoglycemia.

Stage 2: Compensatory secretion of epinephrine
This stage is characterized by pallor, clamminess, perspiration, palpitations, finger tremors, hunger, decreased temperature, and increased pulse rate and blood pressure.

Stage 3: Severe hypoglycemia
Ataxia, clouded sensorium, diplopia, and episodes of violence and hysteria are the effects of severe hypoglycemia.

Therapy and prognosis
Treatment consists of enucleation of tumor (if benign) and chemotherapy with streptozocin and fluorouracil and resection to include pancreatic tissue (if malignant). Most islet cell tumors metastasize to the liver only. Some metastasize to the bone, brain, and lungs. Death results from hypoglycemic reactions and widespread metastasis.

Staging pancreatic cancer

Using the tumor, node, metastasis (TNM) system, the American Joint Committee on Cancer has established the following stages for pancreatic cancer.

Primary tumor

TX—primary tumor can't be assessed
T0—no evidence of primary tumor
T1—tumor limited to the pancreas
T1a—tumor 2 cm or less in greatest dimension
T1b—tumor more than 2 cm in greatest dimension
T2—tumor penetrates the duodenum, common bile duct, or peripancreatic tissues
T3—tumor penetrates the stomach, spleen, colon, or adjacent large vessels

Regional lymph nodes

NX—regional lymph nodes can't be assessed
N0—no evidence of regional lymph node metastasis
N1—regional lymph node metastasis

Distant metastasis

MX—distant metastasis can't be assessed
M0—no known distant metastasis
M1—distant metastasis

Staging categories

Pancreatic cancer progresses from mild to severe as follows:
Stage I—T1, N0, M0; T2, N0, M0
Stage II—T3, N0, M0
Stage III—any T, N1, M0
Stage IV—any T, any N, M1

- plasma insulin immunoassay (shows measurable serum insulin in the presence of islet cell tumors)
- hemoglobin and hematocrit (may show mild anemia)
- fasting blood glucose (may indicate hypoglycemia or hyperglycemia)
- stool studies (may show occult blood if ulceration in the GI tract or ampulla of Vater has occurred)
- specific tumor markers for pancreatic cancer, including carcinoembryonic antigen, pancreatic oncofetal antigen, alphafetoprotein, and serum immunoreactive elastatase I (all levels elevated in the presence of cancer).

Treatment

Because pancreatic cancer may metastasize widely before it's diagnosed, treatment seldom succeeds in curing the disease. Treatment consists of surgery and, possibly, chemotherapy and radiation therapy.

Some surgical procedures help increase the survival rate slightly.

- Total pancreatectomy may increase survival time by resecting a localized tumor or by controlling postoperative gastric ulceration.
- Cholecystojejunostomy, choledochoduodenostomy, and choledochojejunostomy have partially replaced radical resection. These procedures bypass the obstructing common bile duct extensions, easing jaundice and pruritus.
- If radical resection isn't indicated and duodenal obstruction is expected to develop later, a gastrojejunostomy is performed.

Whipple's procedure, or radical pancreaticoduodenectomy, can obtain wide lymphatic clearance—except with tumors located near the portal vein, superior mesenteric vein and artery, and celiac axis. Recent studies have demonstrated a reduction in mortality and morbidity with this procedure, and improvement in the 5-year survival rate for patients.

Although pancreatic cancer usually responds poorly to chemotherapy, recent studies using combinations of fluorouracil, streptomycin, mitomycin, and doxorubicin show a trend toward longer survival time.

Radiation therapy usually doesn't increase long-term survival, although it may prolong survival time by 6 to 11 months when used as an adjunct to fluorouracil chemotherapy. It also can ease the pain associated with nonresectable tumors.

Medications used in pancreatic cancer include:

- antibiotics to prevent infection and relieve symptoms
- anticholinergics, particularly propantheline, to decrease GI tract spasm and motility and reduce pain and secretions
- antacids and H_2–receptor antagonists to suppress peptic activity, thus reducing stress-induced damage to gastric mucosa
- diuretics to mobilize extracellular fluid from ascites
- insulin to provide an adequate exogenous insulin supply after pancreatic resection
- opioid analgesics to relieve pain (used only after other analgesics fail because morphine, meperidine, and codeine can lead to biliary tract spasm and increase common bile duct pressure)
- pancreatic enzymes to assist with digestion of proteins, carbohydrates, and fats when pancreatic juices are insufficient because of surgery or obstruction.

Key nursing diagnoses and patient outcomes

Altered nutrition: Less than body requirements related to adverse GI signs and symptoms. Based on this nursing diagnosis, you'll establish these patient outcomes. The patient will:

- obtain relief from GI signs and symptoms with therapy
- be able to ingest a nutritionally balanced diet daily
- regain and maintain weight within normal limits.

Anticipatory grieving related to poor prognosis. Based on this nursing diagnosis, you'll establish these patient outcomes. The patient will:

- acknowledge feelings about his diagnosis and prognosis
- seek support from family, friends, and support groups
- use healthy coping mechanisms to deal with the threat of death.

Pain related to pancreatic dysfunction. Based on this nursing diagnosis, you'll establish these patient outcomes. The patient will:

- express feelings of comfort following analgesic administration
- use diversional activities to help minimize pain.

Nursing interventions

- If weight loss occurs, replace nutrients by mouth or through an I.V. line or nasogastric (NG) tube. If the patient gains weight from ascites, impose dietary restrictions, such as a low-sodium diet, as ordered.
- Maintain a 2,500-calorie diet by serving small, frequent meals. Consult the dietitian to ensure proper nutrition, and make mealtimes as pleasant as possible. Administer an oral pancreatic enzyme at mealtimes, if needed. As ordered, give an antacid and H_2-receptor antagonists to prevent stress ulcers.
- To prevent constipation, administer laxatives, stool softeners, and cathartics, as ordered. Also, modify the patient's diet and increase his fluid intake. To increase GI motility, position him properly during and after meals and assist him with walking.
- Prepare the patient for surgery, as indicated. (See the entry "Pancreatectomy.")
- Before surgery, make sure the patient is medically stable – particularly regarding nutrition. This may take 4 to 5 days. If he can't tolerate oral feedings, provide total parenteral nutrition and I.V. fat emulsions to correct deficiencies and maintain a positive nitrogen balance.

- Administer blood transfusions (to combat anemia), vitamin K (to overcome prothrombin deficiency), antibiotics (to prevent postoperative complications), and gastric lavage (to maintain gastric decompression), as ordered.
- If the patient is receiving chemotherapy, symptomatically treat its toxic effects.
- Ensure adequate rest and sleep (with a sedative, if necessary). Assist with range-of-motion (ROM) and isometric exercises, as appropriate.
- Administer analgesics for pain and antibiotics and antipyretics for fever, as ordered.
- Give the patient glucose or an antidiabetic agent (such as tolbutamide), as ordered.
- Provide scrupulous skin care to prevent pruritus and necrosis, and keep the patient's skin clean and dry. If he develops overwhelming pruritus, you can prevent excoriation by clipping his nails and having him wear light cotton gloves.
- To control active bleeding, promote gastric vasoconstriction with medication and with cool saline or water lavage through an NG tube or a duodenal tube. Replace any lost fluids.
- Ease discomfort from pyloric obstruction with an NG tube.
- To prevent thrombosis, apply antiembolism stockings and assist with ROM exercises. If thrombosis occurs, elevate the patient's legs and apply moist heat to the thrombus site. Give an anticoagulant, as ordered, to prevent further clot formation and pulmonary embolus.
- Throughout therapy, answer any questions the patient has and tell him what to expect from surgery and other therapies. Listen to his fears and concerns, and stay with him during periods of severe stress and anxiety.
- Encourage the patient to identify actions and care measures that will promote his comfort and relaxation. Try to perform these measures, and encourage the patient and his family to do so, too.
- Whenever possible, include the patient and his family in care decisions.

Monitoring

- Monitor the patient's pain level and response to administered analgesics. Monitor his response to drug therapy, assessing him frequently for adverse reactions.
- Assess the patient's fluid balance, abdominal girth, metabolic state, and weight daily.
- Watch for signs of hypoglycemia or hyperglycemia. Monitor the patient's blood glucose, urine glucose, and acetone levels and his response to treatment.
- Watch for signs of upper GI bleeding. Test stools and emesis for blood, and maintain a flow sheet of frequent hemoglobin and hematocrit determinations.
- Monitor and document the patient's degree of jaundice daily.

Patient teaching

- Describe expected postoperative procedures and the adverse effects of radiation therapy and chemotherapy.
- If appropriate, provide information on diabetes.
- Help the patient and his family cope with the impending reality of death.
- Refer the patient to resource and support services, such as the social service department, local home health care agencies, hospices, and the American Cancer Society.
- Encourage the patient to follow as normal a routine as possible. Explain that leading a near-normal life will help foster feelings of independence and control.

Pancreatitis

Inflammation of the pancreas, or pancreatitis, occurs in acute and chronic forms and may stem from edema, necrosis, or hemorrhage. In men, the disorder is commonly associated with alcoholism, trauma, or peptic ulcer; in women, with biliary tract disease. The prognosis is good when pancreatitis follows biliary tract disease but poor when it follows alcoholism. Mortality reaches 60% when pancreatitis is associated with necrosis or hemorrhage.

Causes

The most common causes of pancreatitis are biliary tract disease and alcoholism, but the disorder can also result from abnormal organ structure, metabolic or endocrine disorders (such as hyperlipidemia or hyperparathyroidism), pancreatic cysts or tumors, penetrating peptic ulcers, or trauma (blunt or iatrogenic). This disorder also can develop after the use of certain drugs, such as glucocorticoids, sulfonamides, thiazides, and oral contraceptives.

Pancreatitis may be a complication of renal failure, kidney transplantation, open-heart surgery, and endoscopic retrograde cholangiopancreatography (ERCP). Predisposing factors include heredity and, in some patients, emotional or neurogenic factors.

Acute pancreatitis involves autodigestion: the enzymes normally excreted by the pancreas digest pancreatic tissue. Chronic pancreatitis is progressive destruction and calcification of pancreatic tissue.

Complications

If pancreatitis damages the islets of Langerhans, diabetes mellitus may occur. Fulminant pancreatitis (which occurs late in chronic pancreatitis) causes massive hemorrhage and total destruction of the pancreas, resulting in diabetic acidosis, shock, or coma. Respiratory complications include adult respiratory distress syndrome, atelectasis, pleural effusion, and pneumonia. Proximity of the inflamed pancreas to the bowel may cause paralytic ileus. Other complications include GI bleeding, pancreatic abscess, pseudocysts and, rarely, cancer.

Assessment

Commonly, the patient describes intense epigastric pain centered close to the umbilicus and radiating to the back, between the 10th thoracic and 6th lumbar vertebrae. He typically reports that this pain is aggravated by eating fatty foods, consuming alcohol, or lying in a recumbent position. He may also complain of weight loss, with nausea and vomiting.

Investigation may uncover predisposing factors, such as alcoholism, biliary tract disease, or pancreatic disease. Other medical problems, such as peptic ulcer disease or hyperlipidemia, may be discovered.

Assessment of vital signs may reveal decreased blood pressure, tachycardia, and fever. These signs, if present, indicate respiratory complications. Other signs of respiratory complications are dyspnea or orthopnea. Observe the patient for changes in behavior and sensorium; these signs may be related to alcohol withdrawal or may indicate hypoxia or impending shock.

Abdominal inspection may disclose generalized jaundice, Cullen's sign (bluish periumbilical discoloration), and Turner's sign (bluish flank discoloration). Inspection of stools may reveal steatorrhea, a sign of chronic pancreatitis.

During abdominal palpation, you may note tenderness, rigidity, and guarding. If you hear a dull sound while percussing, suspect pancreatic ascites. If bowel sounds are absent or decreased on abdominal auscultation, suspect paralytic ileus.

Diagnostic tests

For key abnormal laboratory test values, see *Critical test values in pancreatitis,* page 668.

- *Supportive laboratory studies* include elevated white blood cell count and serum bilirubin level. In many patients, hypocalcemia occurs and appears to be associated with the severity of the disease. Blood and urine glucose tests may reveal transient glucosuria and hyperglycemia. In chronic pancreatitis, significant laboratory findings include elevations in serum alkaline phosphatase, amylase, and bilirubin levels. Serum glucose levels may be

CHECKLIST

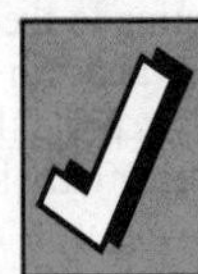

Critical test values in pancreatitis

The following findings confirm acute pancreatitis.

- ☐ Serum amylase levels above 180 Somogyi units/dl (130 U/L). This is the diagnostic hallmark that confirms acute pancreatitis. Characteristically, serum amylase reaches peak levels in 24 hours after onset of pancreatitis, then returns to normal within 48 to 72 hours despite continued symptoms.
- ☐ Urinary amylase level above 80 amylase units/hour (17 U/h). Because urine amylase is reported in various units of measurement, values differ among laboratories. Check your hospital's normal range for urine amylase. Urine amylase levels remain elevated longer than serum amylase levels.
- ☐ Serum lipase level above 80 U/L. Serum lipase levels along with urine amylase levels remain elevated longer than serum amylase levels.

transiently elevated. Stools contain elevated lipid and trypsin levels.
• *Abdominal and chest X-rays* differentiate pancreatitis from other diseases that cause similar symptoms and detect pleural effusions.
• *Computed tomography scan* and *ultrasonography* reveal an increased pancreatic diameter; these tests also identify pancreatic cysts and pseudocysts.
• *ERCP* shows the anatomy of the pancreas; identifies ductal system abnormalities, such as calcification or strictures; and differentiates pancreatitis from other disorders, such as pancreatic cancer.

Treatment

The goals are to maintain circulation and fluid volume, relieve pain, and decrease pancreatic secretions. Emergency treatment for shock (the most common cause of death in early stage pancreatitis) consists of vigorous I.V. replacement of electrolytes and proteins. Metabolic acidosis secondary to hypovolemia and impaired cellular perfusion requires vigorous fluid volume replacement. Blood transfusions may be needed if shock occurs. Food and fluids are withheld to allow the pancreas to rest and to reduce pancreatic enzyme secretion.

In acute pancreatitis, nasogastric (NG) tube suctioning is usually required to decrease gastric distention and suppress pancreatic secretions. Prescribed medications may include:
• meperidine to relieve abdominal pain (this drug causes less spasm at the ampulla of Vater than opiates, such as morphine)
• antacids to neutralize gastric secretions
• histamine$_2$-receptor antagonists, such as cimetidine or ranitidine, and proton pump inhibitors, such as omeprazole, to decrease hydrochloric acid production
• antibiotics, such as clindamycin or gentamicin, to treat bacterial infections
• anticholinergics to reduce vagal stimulation, decrease GI motility, and inhibit pancreatic enzyme secretion
• insulin to correct hyperglycemia, if present.

Once the crisis begins to resolve, oral low-fat, low-protein feedings are gradually implemented. Alcohol and caffeine are eliminated from the diet. If the crisis occurred during treatment with glucocorticoids, oral contraceptives, or thiazide diuretics, these drugs are discontinued.

Surgery usually isn't indicated in acute pancreatitis. However, if complications such as pancreatic abscess or pseudocyst occur, surgical drainage may be necessary. If biliary tract obstruction causes acute pancreatitis, a laparotomy may be required.

For chronic pancreatitis, treatment depends on the cause. Nonsurgical measures are appropriate if the patient isn't a suitable candidate for surgery or if he refuses this treatment. Measures to prevent and relieve abdominal pain are similar to those used in acute pancreatitis. Meperidine usually is the drug of choice; however, pentazocine also effectively relieves pain. Treatments for diabetes mellitus may include dietary modification, insulin replacement, or antidiabetic agents. Malabsorption and steatorrhea are treated with pancreatic enzyme replacement.

Surgical intervention relieves abdominal pain, restores pancreatic drainage, and reduces the frequency of acute pancreatic attacks. Surgical drainage is required for an abscess or pseudocyst. If biliary tract disease is the underlying cause, cholecystectomy or choledochotomy is performed. A sphincterotomy is indicated to enlarge a pancreatic sphincter that has become fibrotic. To relieve obstruction and allow drainage of pancreatic secretions, pancreaticojejunostomy (anastomosis of the jejunum with the opened pancreatic duct) may be required.

Key nursing diagnoses and patient outcomes

Altered nutrition: Less than body requirements related to malabsorption caused by pancreatic enzyme deficiency. Based on this nursing diagnosis, you'll establish these patient outcomes. The patient will:
- comply with pancreatic enzyme replacement therapy
- not exhibit signs and symptoms of malnutrition
- regain and maintain normal weight.

Altered protection related to loss of ability to control blood glucose levels naturally, caused by alpha- and beta-cell damage. Based on this nursing diagnosis, you'll establish these patient outcomes. The patient will:
- communicate his understanding of early signs and symptoms of hypoglycemia and hyperglycemia
- comply with the prescribed treatment to control blood glucose levels
- regain and maintain normal serum blood glucose and not have ketones in urine.

Pain related to inflammatory process. Based on this nursing diagnosis, you'll establish these patient outcomes. The patient will:
- express feelings of comfort following analgesic administration
- avoid eating foods or engaging in activities that precipitate or increase pain
- not develop chronic pain.

Nursing interventions

- Administer meperidine or other analgesics, as ordered, and document the drugs' effectiveness.
- Maintain the NG tube for drainage or suctioning.
- In case of hypocalcemia, keep airway and suction apparatus handy and pad the side rails of the bed.
- Restrict the patient to bed rest, and provide a quiet and restful environment.
- Place the patient in a comfortable position that also allows maximal chest expansion, such as Fowler's position.
- Keep water and other beverages at the bedside, and encourage the patient to drink plenty of fluids.
- Provide I.V. fluids and parenteral nutrition, as ordered. As soon as the patient can tolerate it, provide a diet high in carbohydrates, low in proteins, and low in fat.
- Prepare the patient for surgery, as indicated. (See the entries "Cholecystectomy" and "Pancreatectomy.")
- If the patient has chronic pancreatitis, allow him to express feelings of anger, depression, and sadness related to his condition and help him to cope with these feelings. Encourage him to use appropriate physical outlets to express his emo-

tions, such as pounding a punching bag or throwing pillows.
- Counsel the patient to contact a self-help group, such as Alcoholics Anonymous, if needed.

Monitoring
- Assess the patient's level of pain. Evaluate his response to administered analgesics, and monitor for adverse reactions.
- Assess pulmonary status at least every 4 hours to detect early signs of respiratory complications.
- Monitor fluid and electrolyte balance, and report any abnormalities. Maintain an accurate record of intake and output. Weigh the patient daily and record his weight.
- Evaluate the patient's present nutritional status and metabolic requirements.
- Monitor serum glucose levels, and administer insulin as ordered.
- Don't confuse thirst due to hyperglycemia (indicated by serum glucose levels up to 350 mg/dl and glucose and acetone in the urine) with dry mouth due to NG intubation and anticholinergics.
- Watch for signs of calcium deficiency: tetany, cramps, carpopedal spasm, and seizures.

Patient teaching
- Emphasize the importance of avoiding factors that precipitate acute pancreatitis, especially alcohol.
- Refer the patient and his family to the dietitian. Stress the need for a diet high in carbohydrates and low in protein and fats. Caution the patient to avoid caffeinated beverages and irritating foods.
- Point out the need to comply with pancreatic enzyme replacement therapy. Instruct the patient to take the enzymes with meals or snacks to help digest food and to promote fat and protein absorption. Advise him to watch for and report any of the following signs and symptoms: fatty, frothy, foul-smelling stools; abdominal distention; cramping; and skin excoriation.
- If the patient has chronic pain, teach a family member how to give I.M. injections as ordered.

Parathyroidectomy

Parathyroidectomy, the surgical removal of one or more of the four parathyroid glands, treats primary hyperparathyroidism. In this disorder, the parathyroids secrete excessive amounts of parathyroid hormone (PTH), causing high serum calcium and low serum phosphorus levels.

The number of glands removed depends on the underlying cause of excessive PTH secretion. For example, if the patient has a single adenoma, excision of the affected gland corrects the problem. If more than one gland is enlarged, subtotal parathyroidectomy (removal of the three largest glands and part of the fourth gland) can correct hyperparathyroidism. The remaining glandular segment decreases the risk of postoperative hypoparathyroidism and resulting hypocalcemia since it resumes normal function.

Total parathyroidectomy is necessary when glandular hyperplasia results from cancer. In this case, the patient will require lifelong treatment for hypoparathyroidism. The doctor may also perform subtotal thyroidectomy along with parathyroidectomy if he's unable to locate the abnormal tissue or adenoma and suspects an intrathyroid lesion.

Serum calcium levels typically decrease within 24 to 48 hours after surgery and become normal within 4 to 5 days.

Procedure
After the patient is anesthetized, the doctor makes a cervical neck incision and exposes the thyroid gland. He then locates the four parathyroids (usually within ¾" [2 cm] above or below the point where the recurrent laryngeal nerve and the inferior

thyroid artery cross) and identifies and tags them.

If he can't find one of them, he'll do a cervical thymectomy and thyroid lobectomy on the side where the gland is missing and send a sample for an immediate frozen section. If the missing gland is not found in the removed tissue, the doctor may stop the procedure and order localization studies before a second surgery. Or, he may continue surgery by opening the sternum and exploring the mediastinum for the missing gland.

Once he has found all four glands, he examines them for hyperplasia and removes the affected ones. The surgeon tags the remaining glands or any of the gland that isn't removed (remnant). Before he sutures the incision, he inserts a Penrose drain or a closed wound drainage device. (See *What happens in parathyroidectomy,* page 672.) The surgeon should document the number and location of glands identified and removed so postoperative treatment can be planned for the patient's specific needs.

Complications

Complications seldom occur but may include hemorrhage, damage to the recurrent laryngeal nerve, and hypoparathyroidism.

Key nursing diagnoses and patient outcomes

Altered protection related to potential for hypocalcemia caused by transient parathyroidism. Based on this nursing diagnosis, you'll establish these patient outcomes. The patient will:

- maintain a normal serum calcium level postoperatively
- not demonstrate signs and symptoms of hypocalcemia.

Risk for trauma related to potential for damage to recurrent laryngeal nerve. Based on this nursing diagnosis, you'll establish these patient outcomes. The patient will:

- acknowledge that damage to the recurrent laryngeal nerve is a potential complication of parathyroidectomy
- be able to speak postoperatively.

Impaired swallowing related to swelling and pain caused by neck incision. Based on this nursing diagnosis, you'll establish these patient outcomes. The patient will:

- maintain a patent airway
- achieve adequate nutritional intake
- show no evidence of aspiration pneumonia.

Nursing interventions

When preparing for or managing a patient with a parathyroidectomy, expect to implement these nursing interventions.

Before surgery

- Tell the patient that this surgery will remove diseased parathyroid tissue. Explain all aspects of care, surgery, and treatment.
- Show the patient how to support his neck and perform coughing and deep-breathing exercises postoperatively. Warn him that talking and swallowing will be painful for the first few days after surgery.
- As ordered, take measures to bring the patient's calcium levels to near normal before surgery. For example, maintain calcium restrictions and provide plenty of fluids to dilute excess calcium. Also give medications such as diuretics, mithramycin (an antihypercalcemic agent), and inorganic phosphates, as ordered, to lower calcium levels.
- Be sure that the patient or a responsible family member has signed a consent form.

After surgery

- Keep the patient in high Fowler's position after surgery to promote venous return from the head and neck and to decrease oozing into the incision. As soon as he begins to awaken from anesthesia, check for laryngeal nerve damage by asking him to speak.
- Check the patient's dressing, and palpate the *back* of his neck, where drainage tends to flow. Expect about 50 ml of drainage in the first 24 hours; if you find no drainage,

What happens in parathyroidectomy

The surgeon makes a transverse cervical incision and explores the exposed area to identify the parathyroid gland (or glands). The superior glands prove easier to locate than the inferior glands. (In this illustration, the surgeon has located the left inferior parathyroid gland.) Before removing the gland, he will take a tissue sample for biopsy to ensure correct gland identification.

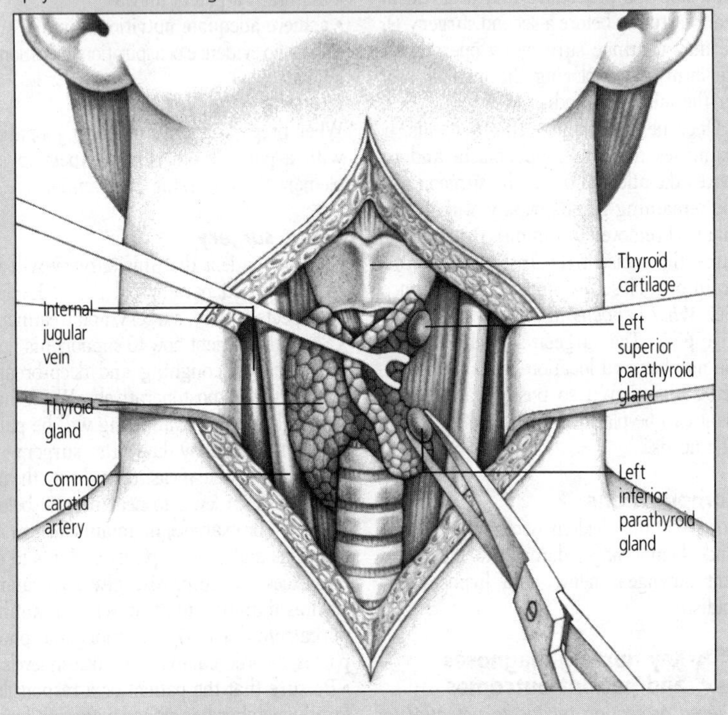

check for drain kinking or the need to reestablish suction. Expect only scant drainage after 24 hours.

• Keep a tracheotomy tray at the patient's bedside for the first 24 hours after surgery, and assess the patient frequently for signs of respiratory distress, such as dyspnea and cyanosis. Upper airway obstruction may result from tracheal collapse, mucus accumulation in the trachea, laryngeal edema, or vocal cord paralysis.

• Expect the patient to complain of a sore neck (from hyperextension during surgery), a sore throat (from manipulation), and hoarseness and swallowing difficulty (from anesthesia and intubation). Give mild analgesics, as ordered.

• Because transient hypoparathyroidism with resulting hypocalcemia can occur 1 to 4 days after surgery, watch closely for signs of increased neuromuscular excitability. Check for positive Chvostek's and Trousseau's signs, and tell the patient to report numbness and tingling of his fingers and toes or around his mouth (early signs of hypocalcemia) as well as muscle cramps. Keep I.V. calcium on hand in case tetany occurs.

Home care instructions

• Tell the patient to keep his incision site clean and dry, and explain that it will need to be checked in follow-up appointments. Also tell him that he'll need periodic serum calcium determinations to help evaluate the surgery's outcome.
• Advise him not to take any nonprescription drugs without consulting his doctor. In particular, tell him to avoid magnesium-containing laxatives and antacids, mineral oil, and vitamins A and D.
• If the patient has had a total parathyroidectomy, instruct him to follow a high-calcium, low-phosphorus diet, as ordered, and to take his calcium medications. If he'll be receiving dihydrotachysterol and calciferol, tell him not to take vitamins without consulting his doctor. Tell him to call his doctor if he develops signs of hypercalcemia, such as excessive thirst, headache, vertigo, tinnitus, and anorexia.

Parkinson's disease

Named for the English doctor who first accurately described the disease in 1817, Parkinson's disease is a slowly progressive movement disorder that characteristically produces progressive muscle rigidity, akinesia, and involuntary tremors. The disorder is not fatal but death may result from aspiration pneumonia or some other infection.

Also called parkinsonism, paralysis agitans, or shaking palsy, Parkinson's disease is one of the most common crippling diseases in the United States. It affects men more often than women and usually occurs in middle age or later. This disease strikes 1 in every 100 persons over age 60. Because of increased longevity, this amounts to roughly 60,000 new cases diagnosed annually in the United States alone.

Causes

The cause of Parkinson's disease is unknown in most cases. However, studies of the extrapyramidal brain nuclei (corpus striatum, globus pallidus, substantia nigra) have established that in this disease, a dopamine deficiency prevents affected brain cells from performing their normal inhibitory function within the central nervous system.

Some cases of Parkinson's disease are caused by exposure to toxins (such as manganese dust and carbon monoxide), which destroy cells in the substantia nigra.

Complications

Common complications associated with Parkinson's disease include injury from falls, food aspiration because of impaired voluntary movements, urinary tract infections, and skin breakdown, as the patient becomes less mobile.

Assessment

The patient history notes the cardinal symptoms of Parkinson's disease, which include muscle rigidity, akinesia, and an insidious tremor known as unilateral pill-roll tremor, which begins in the fingers. Although the patient often can't pinpoint exactly when tremors began, he typically reports that they increase during stress or anxiety and decrease with purposeful movement and sleep. He may also report dysphagia.

The patient may complain that he becomes fatigued when he tries to perform activities of daily living and that he experiences muscle cramps of the legs, neck, and trunk. He may also mention oily skin, increased perspiration, insomnia, and mood changes. You may note dysarthria and find that the patient speaks in a high-pitched monotone.

Inspection may reveal drooling, a mask-like facial expression, and difficulty walking. The patient's gait often lacks normal parallel motion and may be retropulsive or propulsive. In addition, the patient may demonstrate a loss of posture control when he walks. Typically, the patient who loses posture control walks with the body bent forward. These signs result from akinesia.

You may note other results of akinesia: oculogyric crisis (eyes fixed upward, with involuntary tonic movements) or blepharospasm (eyelids closed). You may also discover that the patient takes a long time to initiate movement to perform a purposeful action.

In addition to gait changes, musculoskeletal and neurologic assessment may point to muscle rigidity that results in resistance to passive muscle stretching. Such rigidity may be uniform (lead-pipe rigidity) or jerky (cogwheel rigidity). The patient may also pivot with difficulty and lose his balance easily.

As you assess this patient, keep in mind that Parkinson's disease itself doesn't impair the intellect but that a coexisting disorder, such as arteriosclerosis, may.

Diagnostic tests

Although urinalysis may reveal decreased dopamine levels, laboratory test results usually have little value in identifying Parkinson's disease.

Computed tomography scan or magnetic resonance imaging may be performed to rule out other disorders, such as intracranial tumors.

Treatment

No cure exists for Parkinson's disease, so treatment aims to relieve symptoms and keep the patient functional as long as possible. Treatment consists of drugs, physical therapy and, in severe disease unresponsive to drugs, stereotaxic neurosurgery.

Drug therapy usually includes levodopa, a dopamine replacement that is most effective for the first few years after it's initiated. The drug is given in increasing doses until signs and symptoms are relieved or adverse reactions appear. Because adverse reactions can be serious, levodopa is frequently given in combination with carbidopa (a dopa-decarboxylase inhibitor) to halt peripheral dopamine synthesis. The patient may receive bromocriptine as an additive to reduce the levodopa dose. When levodopa proves ineffective or too toxic, alternative drug therapy includes anticholinergics (such as trihexyphenidyl or benztropine) and antihistamines (such as diphenhydramine).

Antihistamines may help decrease tremors because of their central anticholinergic and sedative effects. Anticholinergics may be used to control tremors and rigidity. They may also be used in combination with levodopa.

Amantadine, an antiviral agent, is used early in treatment to reduce rigidity, tremors, and akinesia.

When drug therapy fails, stereotaxic neurosurgery sometimes offers an effective alternative. In this procedure, electrical coagulation, freezing, radioactivity, or ultrasound destroys the ventrolateral nucleus of the thalamus to prevent involuntary movement. Such neurosurgery is most effective in comparatively young, otherwise healthy people with unilateral tremor or muscle rigidity. Like drug therapy, neurosurgery is a palliative measure that can only relieve symptoms.

Physical therapy complements drug treatment and neurosurgery to maintain the patient's normal muscle tone and function. Appropriate physical therapy includes both active and passive range-of-motion exercises, routine daily activities, walking, and baths and massage to help relax muscles.

Tricyclic antidepressants may be given to decrease the depression that often accompanies the disease.

Key nursing diagnoses and patient outcomes

Chronic low self-esteem related to involuntary movement and drooling. Based on this nursing diagnosis, you'll establish these patient outcomes. The patient will:
- acknowledge feelings of low self-esteem
- seek help in raising self-esteem
- demonstrate an increase in self-esteem.

Impaired home maintenance management related to self-care deficits caused by neuromuscular dysfunction. Based on this nursing diagnosis, you'll establish these patient outcomes. The patient will:
- describe changes needed to promote maximum health and safety at home
- seek and get help from family, friends, and agencies to meet personal needs
- be able to remain at home at optimal level of health within the disease limitations.

Impaired physical mobility related to involuntary movement. Based on this nursing diagnosis, you'll establish these patient outcomes. The patient will:
- maintain functional mobility without injury
- use appropriate safety precautions.

Nursing interventions

- Provide emotional and psychological support to the patient and his family. Encourage him to participate in care decisions and to perform as much of his own care as possible.
- Encourage independence. Provide assistive devices as appropriate.
- To help the patient who has severe tremors gain partial control of his body, have him sit on a chair and use its arms to steady himself.
- Provide rest periods between activities.
- Work with the physical therapist to develop a program of daily exercises to increase muscle strength, decrease muscle rigidity, prevent contractures, and improve coordination.
- Provide frequent warm baths and massage to help relax muscles and relieve muscle cramps.
- Protect the patient from injury and assist as necessary.

EXPERT GERIATRIC CARE

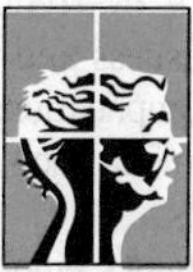

The elderly patient and parkinsonism

Because of age-related changes affecting pharmacodynamics and pharmacokinetics, the elderly patient receiving antiparkinsonian drugs is at risk for developing adverse reactions.

Monitor drug treatment so dosage can be adjusted to minimize these reactions. Watch for adverse psychiatric responses, such as anxiety and confusion, or for cardiac reactions, such as orthostatic hypotension and pulse irregularities. Be especially alert for eyelid twitching, an early sign of toxicity.

Although intellectual functioning isn't affected, speech problems and the patient's physical appearance may cause others to question his mental ability. He may become extremely frustrated and feel degraded and may react with irritability or depression. Support the patient and his family and help them understand and cope with the disease.

- Help the patient overcome problems related to eating and elimination. Offer supplementary feedings or small, frequent meals to increase caloric intake. Help establish a regular bowel elimination routine.
- To decrease the possibility of aspiration, have the patient sit in an upright position when eating. Remember that these patients are often silent aspirators.
- Provide the patient with a semisolid diet, which is easier to swallow than a diet consisting of solids and liquids.

Monitoring

- Monitor drug treatment and report any adverse reactions. (See *The elderly patient and parkinsonism.*)
- If the patient has surgery, be alert for signs of hemorrhage and increased intra-

cranial pressure by frequently checking level of consciousness and vital signs.
• Monitor for complications caused by involuntary movement, such as aspiration or injury from falls.
• Assess the patient's emotional health for signs of ineffective coping and low self-esteem.
• Evaluate the patient's nutritional intake, and weigh him regularly.

Patient teaching

• Teach the patient and his family about the disease, its progressive stages, and the treatments that may help the patient. Explain the actions of prescribed medications and their possible adverse effects.
• If appropriate, show the family how to prevent pressure ulcers and contractures by proper positioning.
• Explain household safety measures, such as installing or using side rails in halls and stairs and removing throw rugs from frequently traveled floors to prevent patient injury.
• Explain the importance of daily bathing to the patient who has oily skin and increased perspiration.
• To make dressing easier, teach the patient to wear clothing fitted with zippers or Velcro fasteners rather than buttons.
• To improve communication, instruct the patient to make a conscious effort to speak, to speak slowly, to take a few deep breaths before he begins to speak, and to think about what he wants to say before he begins to speak.
• If appropriate, advise the patient how to eat. Tell him to place food on the tongue, close the lips, chew first on one side and then the other, then lift the tongue up and back and make a conscious effort to swallow. Because these patients eat slowly, allow them plenty of time to eat.
• Refer the patient and his family to the National Parkinson Foundation, the American Parkinson Disease Association, or the United Parkinson Foundation for more information.

Pelvic inflammatory disease

An umbrella term, pelvic inflammatory disease (PID) refers to any acute, subacute, recurrent, or chronic infection of the oviducts and ovaries, with adjacent tissue involvement. It includes inflammation of the cervix (cervicitis), uterus (endometritis), fallopian tubes (salpingitis), and ovaries (oophoritis), which can extend to the connective tissue lying between the broad ligaments (parametritis). (See *Features and test findings in PID.*)

About 60% of cases result from overgrowth of one or more of the common bacterial species found in the cervical mucus. Early diagnosis and treatment helps prevent damage to the reproductive system, as does well-planned nursing care. Untreated PID may be fatal.

Causes

PID can result from infection with aerobic or anaerobic organisms. The organisms *Neisseria gonorrhoeae* and *Chlamydia trachomatis* are the most common causes because they most readily penetrate the bacteriostatic barrier of cervical mucus.

Common bacteria found in cervical mucus include staphylococci, streptococci, diphtheroids, chlamydiae, and coliforms, including *Pseudomonas* and *Escherichia coli.* Uterine infection can result from any one or several of these organisms or may follow the multiplication of normally nonpathogenic bacteria in an altered endometrial environment. Bacterial multiplication is most common during parturition because the endometrium is atrophic, quiescent, and not stimulated by estrogen.

Risk factors include:
• any sexually transmitted infection
• multiple sex partners
• conditions or procedures, such as conization or cauterization of the cervix, that

Features and test findings in PID

Clinical features	Diagnostic findings
Salpingo-oophoritis • *Acute:* sudden onset of lower abdominal and pelvic pain, usually following menses; increased vaginal discharge; fever; malaise; lower abdominal pressure and tenderness; tachycardia; pelvic peritonitis • *Chronic:* recurring acute episodes	• Blood studies show leukocytosis or a normal white blood cell (WBC) count. • X-rays may show ileus. • Pelvic examination reveals extreme tenderness. • Smear of cervical or periurethral gland exudate shows gram-negative intracellular diplococci.
Cervicitis • *Acute:* purulent, foul-smelling vaginal discharge; vulvovaginitis, with itching or burning; red, edematous cervix; pelvic discomfort; sexual dysfunction; metrorrhagia; infertility; spontaneous abortion • *Chronic:* cervical dystocia; laceration or eversion of the cervix; ulcerative vesicular lesion (when cervicitis results from herpes simplex virus 2)	• Cultures for *N. gonorrhoeae* are positive in more than 90% of patients. • Cytologic smears may reveal severe inflammation. • If cervicitis isn't complicated by salpingitis, WBC count is normal or slightly elevated and erythrocyte sedimentation rate (ESR) is elevated. • In *acute cervicitis,* cervical palpation reveals tenderness. • In *chronic cervicitis,* causative organisms are usually staphylococcus or streptococcus.
Endometritis (generally postpartum or postabortion) • *Acute:* mucopurulent or purulent vaginal discharge oozing from the cervix; edematous, hyperemic endometrium, possibly leading to ulceration and necrosis (with virulent organisms); lower abdominal pain and tenderness; fever; rebound pain; abdominal muscle spasm; thrombophlebitis of uterine and pelvic vessels (in severe forms) • *Chronic:* recurring acute episodes (increasingly common because of widespread use of intrauterine devices)	• In severe infection, palpation may reveal a boggy uterus. • Uterine and blood samples are positive for causative organism, usually staphylococcus. • WBC count and ESR are elevated.

alter or destroy cervical mucus, allowing bacteria to ascend into the uterine cavity
- any procedure that risks transfer of contaminated cervical mucus into the endometrial cavity by an instrument (such as a biopsy curet, an intrauterine device, or an irrigation catheter) or by tubal insufflation or abortion
- infection during or after pregnancy
- infectious foci within the body, such as drainage from a chronically infected fallopian tube, a pelvic abscess, a ruptured appendix, or diverticulitis of the sigmoid colon.

Complications

Possible complications of PID may include potentially fatal septicemia from a ruptured pelvic abscess, pulmonary emboli, infertility, and shock.

Assessment

The patient with PID may complain of profuse, purulent vaginal discharge, sometimes accompanied by low-grade fever and malaise (particularly if gonorrhea is the cause). She may also describe lower abdominal pain and vaginal bleeding. Vaginal examination may reveal pain during movement of the cervix or palpation of the adnexa.

Diagnostic tests

• *Complete blood count and erythrocyte sedimentation rate* help to identify the existence of an infection.
• *Pregnancy test* rules out ectopic pregnancy.
• *Gram stain* of secretions from the endocervix or cul-de-sac determines the causative agent.
• *Culture and sensitivity testing* aids selection of the appropriate antibiotic. Urethral and rectal secretions may also be cultured.
• *Ultrasonography, computed tomography scan,* and *magnetic resonance imaging* may help to identify and locate an adnexal or uterine mass.
• *Culdocentesis* obtains peritoneal fluid or pus for culture and sensitivity testing.

Treatment

To prevent progression of PID, antibiotic therapy begins immediately after culture specimens are obtained. Infection may become chronic if treated inadequately.

The preferred antibiotic therapy for PID includes I.V. doxycycline and cefoxitin for 4 to 6 days (alternative therapy includes clindamycin and gentamicin), followed by oral doxycycline for another 10 to 14 days. Outpatient therapy may consist of cefoxitin I.M., procaine penicillin G I.M., oral amoxicillin, or oral ampicillin (each with probenecid), followed by oral doxycycline for 10 to 14 days. The patient may also require therapy for syphilis.

Supplemental treatment of PID may include bed rest, analgesics, and I.V. fluids as needed.

Development of a pelvic abscess necessitates adequate drainage. A ruptured pelvic abscess is a life-threatening condition. If this complication develops, the patient may need a total abdominal hysterectomy, with bilateral salpingo-oophorectomy.

Key nursing diagnoses and patient outcomes

Altered sexuality patterns related to infection of the reproductive system. Based on this nursing diagnosis, you'll establish these patient outcomes. The patient will:
• abstain from sexual activity until the infection is eradicated
• identify and avoid sexual risk factors that increase the chance of reinfection
• resume normal sexual activity when the infection is cured.

Risk for injury related to inflammation of reproductive structures. Based on this nursing diagnosis, you'll establish these patient outcomes. The patient will:
• comply with the prescribed therapy to minimize the risk of permanent damage
• demonstrate normal reproductive function following PID.

Pain related to inflammation caused by PID. Based on this nursing diagnosis, you'll establish these patient outcomes. The patient will:
• express feelings of comfort following analgesic administration
• use diversional activities to minimize pain perception
• become pain free when PID is eradicated.

Nursing interventions

• After establishing that the patient has no drug allergies, administer antibiotics and analgesics, as ordered.
• Provide frequent perineal care if vaginal drainage occurs.

• Use meticulous hand-washing technique; follow wound and skin precautions if necessary.
• Encourage the patient to discuss her feelings, offer her emotional support, and help her develop effective coping strategies.

Monitoring

• Monitor vital signs for fever and fluid intake and output for signs of dehydration. Watch for abdominal rigidity and distention, possible signs of developing peritonitis.
• Monitor the patient's level of pain and the effectiveness of analgesics.
• Assess the patient for adverse reactions to administered medications and other complications.

Patient teaching

• To prevent recurrence, encourage compliance with treatment and explain the disease and its severity.
• Stress the need for the patient's sexual partner to be examined and, if necessary, treated for infection.
• Discuss the use of condoms to prevent the spread of sexually transmitted diseases.
• Because PID may cause dyspareunia, advise the patient to consult with her doctor about sexual activity.
• To prevent infection after minor gynecologic procedures such as dilatation and curettage, tell the patient to immediately report any fever, increased vaginal discharge, or pain. After such procedures, instruct her to avoid douching or intercourse for at least 7 days.

Peptic ulcers

Occurring as circumscribed lesions in the mucosal membrane, peptic ulcers can develop in the lower esophagus, stomach, duodenum, or jejunum. The major forms are duodenal ulcer and gastric ulcer; both are chronic conditions resulting from contact of the mucosa with gastric juice (especially hydrochloric acid and pepsin).

Duodenal ulcers, which account for about 80% of peptic ulcers, affect the proximal part of the small intestine. These ulcers follow a chronic course characterized by remissions and exacerbations; 5% to 10% of patients develop complications that necessitate surgery. They occur most commonly in men between ages 20 and 50.

Gastric ulcers, which affect the stomach mucosa, are most common in middle-aged and elderly men, especially among the poor and undernourished, and in chronic users of aspirin or alcohol.

Causes

The relationship of gastric acid to ulcer disease remains strong. In gastric ulcers, the stomach mucosa is less resistant to acid. In duodenal ulcers, there is increased acid production. Recent findings indicate that a bacterial infection with *Helicobacter pylori* is a leading factor of peptic ulcer disease. Two other leading causes of peptic ulcer include the use of nonsteroidal anti-inflammatory drugs (NSAIDs) and pathological hypersecretory states such as Zollinger-Ellison syndrome. (See *Causes of peptic ulcer,* page 680.)

Complications

Erosion of the mucosa can cause GI hemorrhage, which can progress to hypovolemic shock, perforation, and obstruction. Obstruction may cause the stomach to distend with food and fluid and result in abdominal or intestinal infarction.

Penetration (the ulcer crater extends beyond the duodenal walls into attached structures, such as the pancreas, biliary tract, liver, or gastrohepatic omentum) occurs fairly frequently in duodenal ulcer.

Assessment

Typically, the patient describes periods of exacerbation and remission of his symptoms, with remissions lasting longer than exacerbations. The patient's history may

Causes of peptic ulcer

Although more research is needed to unveil the exact mechanisms of ulcer formation, several causative factors are known.

- *Helicobacter* pylori. How *H. pylori* produces the ulcer isn't clear. Acid seems to be mainly a contributor to the consequences of the bacterial infection rather than the dominant cause.
- *Drug therapy.* Salicylates and other NSAIDs, reserpine, or caffeine may erode the mucosal lining. NSAIDs may cause a gastric ulcer by inhibiting prostaglandins (the fatty acids)—particularly the E-series prostaglandins. These substances, present in large quantities in the gastric mucosa, inhibit injury by stimulating secretion of gastric mucus and gastric and duodenal mucosal bicarbonate (a neutralizing agent). They also promote gastric mucosal blood flow, maintain the integrity of the gastric mucosal barrier, and help renew the epithelium after a mucosal injury.
- *Certain illnesses.* Pancreatitis, hepatic disease, Crohn's disease, preexisting gastritis, and Zollinger-Ellison syndrome are associated with ulcer development. In Zollinger-Ellison syndrome, for example, gastrinomas (commonly found in the pancreas) stimulate gastric acid secretion. This large volume of acid eventually erodes the gastric mucosa and contributes to ulcer formation.
- *Blood type.* For unknown reasons, gastric ulcers commonly strike people with type A blood. Duodenal ulcers tend to afflict people with type O blood, perhaps because these people don't secrete blood group antigens (mucopolysaccharides, which may serve to protect the mucosa) in their saliva and other body fluids.
- *Genetic factors.* Duodenal ulcers are about three times more common in first-degree relatives of duodenal ulcer patients than in the general population.
- *Exposure to irritants.* Like certain other drugs, alcohol inhibits prostaglandin secretion, triggering a mechanism much like the one caused by NSAIDs. Cigarette smoking also appears to encourage ulcer formation by inhibiting pancreatic secretion of bicarbonate. It also may accelerate the emptying of gastric acid into the duodenum and promote mucosal breakdown.
- *Trauma.* Critical illness, shock, or severe tissue injury from extensive burns or from intracranial surgery may lead to a stress ulcer.
- *Normal aging.* The pyloric sphincter may wear down in the course of aging, which permits the reflux of bile into the stomach. This appears to be a common contributor to the development of gastric ulcers in elderly persons.

reveal possible causes or predisposing factors, such as smoking, use of aspirin or other medications, or associated disorders.

The patient with a gastric ulcer may report a recent loss of weight or appetite. He may not feel like eating or report that he has developed an aversion to food because eating causes discomfort. He may have pain in the left epigastrium, which he describes as heartburn or indigestion. His discomfort may be accompanied by a feeling of fullness or distention. Usually, the onset of pain signals the start of an attack.

The patient's history will help distinguish between a gastric or a duodenal ulcer. Ask the patient whether his pain worsens after eating or is relieved by it. In the patient with a gastric ulcer, eating often triggers or aggravates pain. Conversely, food often relieves the pain of a duodenal ulcer. Also ask whether the patient has experienced pain that disrupts his sleep. The patient with a duodenal ulcer typically reports night awakenings because of pain; the patient with a gastric ulcer does not.

The patient with a duodenal ulcer may have epigastric pain that he describes as sharp, gnawing, or burning. Alternatively, he may describe the pain as boring or aching and poorly defined. Or, he may liken it to a sensation of hunger, abdominal pressure, or fullness. Typically, pain occurs 90 minutes to 3 hours after eating. Because eating often reduces the pain of a duodenal ulcer, the patient may report a recent weight gain. Vomiting and other digestive disturbances are rare in these patients.

If the patient is anemic from blood loss, you may notice pallor on inspection. Palpation in the midline and midway between the umbilicus and the xiphoid process may reveal epigastric tenderness. Hyperactive bowel sounds may be heard upon auscultation.

Diagnostic tests

• *Upper GI endoscopy* or *esophagogastroduodenoscopy* confirms the presence of an ulcer and permits biopsy and cytologic studies to rule out *H. pylori* or cancer. Endoscopy is the major diagnostic test for peptic ulcers.
• *Barium swallow* or *upper GI and small-bowel series* may reveal the presence of the ulcer. This is the initial test performed on a patient whose symptoms are not severe.
• *Upper GI tract X-rays* reveal abnormalities in the mucosa.
• *Laboratory analysis* may detect occult blood in stools.
• *Serologic testing* may disclose clinical signs of infection, such as an elevated white blood cell count. Serology can also detect antibodies to *H. pylori.*
• *Gastric secretory studies* show hyperchlorhydria.
• *Carbon 13 (^{13}C) urea breath test* results reflect activity of *H. pylori.* (*H. pylori* contains the enzyme urease, which breaks down orally administered urea containing the radioisotope ^{13}C before it's absorbed systemically. Low levels of ^{13}C in exhaled breath point to *H. pylori* infection.) This test is expected to be available in the United States shortly.

Treatment

Medical management is essentially symptomatic, emphasizing drug therapy, physical rest, dietary changes, and stress reduction. For patients with severe symptoms or complications, surgery may be required.

Drug therapy aims to eradicate *H. pylori,* reduce gastric secretions, protect the mucosa from further damage, and relieve pain. Medications may include:
• bismuth and two other antimicrobial agents, usually tetracycline or amoxicillin and metronidazole
• antacids to reduce gastric acidity
• histamine$_2$-receptor antagonists, such as cimetidine or ranitidine, or a proton pump inhibitor such as omeprazole to reduce gastric secretion for short-term therapy (up to 8 weeks)
• coating agents, such as sucralfate, for duodenal ulcers; sucralfate forms complexes with proteins at the base of an ulcer, making a protective coat that prevents further digestive action of acid and pepsin
• anticholinergics, such as propantheline, to inhibit the vagus nerve effect on the parietal cells and to reduce gastrin production and excessive gastric activity in duodenal ulcers. (These drugs are usually contraindicated in gastric ulcers because they prolong gastric emptying and can aggravate the ulcer.)

Standard therapy also includes rest and decreased activity to help reduce gastric secretions. Diet therapy may consist of eating six small meals daily (or small hourly meals) rather than three regular meals. Usually, diet therapy involves the elimination of foods that cause distress, including nicotine, caffeine, and alcohol. Some doctors allow small amounts of alcohol with meals.

If GI bleeding occurs, emergency treatment begins with passage of a nasogastric tube to allow for cool saline or water lavage, possibly containing norepinephrine. Gastroscopy allows visualization of the bleeding site and coagulation by laser or cautery to control bleeding. This therapy allows surgery to be postponed until the patient's condition stabilizes.

Surgery is indicated for perforation, unresponsiveness to conservative treatment, suspected cancer, and other complications. The type of surgery chosen for peptic ulcers depends on the location and the extent of the disorder. Choices include bilateral vagotomy, pyloroplasty, and gastrectomy. (See the entry "Gastric surgery.")

Key nursing diagnoses and patient outcomes

Altered nutrition: Less than body requirements related to adverse GI effects. Based on this nursing diagnosis, you'll establish these patient outcomes. The patient will:
- regain and maintain weight
- consume and tolerate a well-balanced diet daily
- not exhibit signs and symptoms of nutritional deficiencies.

Knowledge deficit related to peptic ulcer. Based on this nursing diagnosis, you'll establish these patient outcomes. The patient will:
- express a desire to learn about peptic ulcer disease and his treatment regimen
- obtain information about peptic ulcer disease and treatment from appropriate sources
- communicate an understanding of peptic ulcer disease and his prescribed treatment.

Risk for fluid volume deficit related to bleeding. Based on this nursing diagnosis, you'll establish these patient outcomes. The patient will:
- maintain hemodynamic stability, as evidenced by normal vital signs, orientation to time, person, and place, and equal intake and output
- show no evidence of GI bleeding; stools will be negative for occult blood
- maintain normal fluid volume balance.

Nursing interventions

- Support the patient emotionally and offer reassurance.
- Administer prescribed medications.
- Provide six small meals a day or small hourly meals, as ordered. Advise the patient to eat slowly, chew thoroughly, and have small snacks between meals. Strive for a relaxed and comfortable atmosphere during meals.
- Schedule care so that the patient gets plenty of rest.
- Prepare the patient for surgery, as indicated.

Monitoring

- Monitor the effectiveness of administered medications, and also watch for adverse reactions.
- Assess the patient's nutritional status and the effectiveness of measures used to maintain it. Weigh him regularly.
- Continuously monitor the patient for complications: hemorrhage (sudden onset of weakness, fainting, chills, dizziness, thirst, the desire to defecate, and passage of loose, tarry, or even red stools); perforation (acute onset of epigastric pain, followed by lessening of the pain and the onset of a rigid abdomen, tachycardia, fever, or rebound tenderness); obstruction (feeling of fullness or heaviness, copious vomiting of undigested food after meals); and penetration (pain radiating to the back, night distress). If any of the above occurs, notify the doctor immediately.

Patient teaching

- Teach the patient about peptic ulcer disease, and help him to recognize its signs and symptoms. Explain scheduled diagnostic tests and prescribed therapies. Review symptoms associated with complications, and urge him to notify the doctor if any of these occur. Emphasize the importance of complying with treatment even after his symptoms disappear.

• Review the proper use of prescribed medications, discussing the desired actions and possible adverse effects of each drug.
• Instruct the patient to take antacids 1 hour after meals. If he has cardiac disease or follows a sodium-restricted diet, advise him to take low-sodium antacids. Caution him that antacids may cause changes in bowel habits (diarrhea with magnesium-containing antacids, constipation with aluminum-containing antacids) or affect absorption of other medications (advise him not to take them simultaneously).
• Warn the patient to avoid aspirin-containing drugs, reserpine, ibuprofen, indomethacin, and phenylbutazone because they irritate the gastric mucosa. Also, warn against excessive intake of coffee and alcoholic beverages during exacerbations.
• Tell the patient to avoid nonprescription medications that contain corticosteroids, aspirin, or other nonsteroidal anti-inflammatory drugs, such as ibuprofen. Explain that these drugs inhibit mucus secretion and leave the GI tract vulnerable to injury from gastric acid. Advise him to use alternative analgesics, such as acetaminophen. Caution him to avoid systemic antacids, such as sodium bicarbonate, because they can cause an acid-base imbalance.
• If steroid medication is essential, advise the patient to take it with an antacid.
• Encourage the patient to make appropriate life-style changes.
• If the patient smokes, urge him to stop because smoking stimulates gastric acid secretion. Refer him to a smoking-cessation program.
• Teach the patient to avoid foods that cause pain, such as those that contain caffeine, if possible.

Pericardiocentesis

Typically performed at bedside in a critical care unit, pericardiocentesis involves the needle aspiration of excess fluid from the pericardial sac. It may be the treatment of choice for life-threatening cardiac tamponade (except when fluid accumulates rapidly, in which case immediate surgery is usually preferred).

Pericardiocentesis may also be used to aspirate fluid in subacute conditions, such as viral or bacterial infections and pericarditis. What's more, it provides a sample for laboratory analysis to confirm diagnosis and identify the cause of pericardial effusion.

Procedure

After starting continuous electrocardiogram (ECG) monitoring and administering a local anesthetic at the puncture site, the doctor inserts the aspiration needle in one of three areas. He'll probably choose the xiphocostal approach, with needle insertion in the angle between the left costal margin and the xiphoid process, to avoid needle contact with the pleura and the coronary vessels and thus decrease the risk of damage to these structures.

As an alternative, he may use the parasternal approach, inserting the needle into the fifth or sixth intercostal space next to the left side of the sternum, where the pericardium normally isn't covered by lung tissue; however, this method poses a risk of puncture of the left anterior descending coronary artery or the internal mammary artery.

He may opt for a third method, the apical approach, in which he inserts the needle at the cardiac apex; however, because this method poses the greatest risk of complications, such as pneumothorax, he needs to proceed cautiously.

After inserting the needle tip, the doctor slowly advances it into the pericardial sac to a depth of 1" to 2" (2.5 to 5 cm) or until he can aspirate fluid. He then clamps a hemostat to the needle at the chest wall to prevent needle movement.

The doctor aspirates pericardial fluid slowly. If he finds large amounts of fluid, he may place an indwelling catheter into the pericardial sac to allow continuous slow drainage. After the doctor has removed the fluid, he withdraws the needle and places a dressing over the puncture site.

Complications

Pericardiocentesis carries some risk of potentially fatal complications, such as inadvertent puncture of internal organs (particularly the heart, lung, stomach, or liver) or laceration of the myocardium or of a coronary artery. Therefore, keep emergency equipment readily available during the procedure.

Key nursing diagnoses and patient outcomes

Fear related to a lack of understanding about pericardiocentesis. Based on this nursing diagnosis, you'll establish these patient outcomes. The patient will:
- express fears and concerns about pericardiocentesis and ask questions
- obtain information from appropriate sources and communicate an understanding of the procedure
- exhibit relaxed body posture.

Risk for injury related to complications associated with pericardiocentesis. Based on this nursing diagnosis, you'll establish these patient outcomes. The patient will:
- maintain hemodynamic stability throughout the procedure
- not develop signs and symptoms of complications.

Nursing interventions

When preparing a patient for pericardiocentesis or managing him afterwards, expect to implement these nursing interventions.

Before the procedure

- Help the patient comply by clearly explaining the procedure. Briefly discuss possible complications, such as arrhythmias and organ or artery puncture, but reassure him that such complications occur rarely. Tell him he'll have an I.V. line inserted to provide access for medications, if needed.
- Make sure the patient (or a family member, if appropriate) has signed a consent form.
- Place the patient in a supine position in his bed, with his upper torso raised 60 degrees and his arms supported by pillows. Shave the needle insertion site on his chest if necessary, and clean the area with an antiseptic solution. Then apply 12-lead ECG electrodes. If ordered, assist the doctor in attaching the pericardial needle to the precordial lead (V) of the ECG and also to a three-way stopcock.

During the procedure

- During pericardiocentesis, closely monitor the patient's blood pressure and central venous pressure. Check the ECG pattern continuously for premature ventricular contractions and elevated ST segments, which may indicate that the needle has touched the ventricle; for elevated PR segments, which may indicate that the needle has touched the atrium; and for large, erratic QRS complexes, which may indicate that the needle has penetrated the heart. Also watch for signs of organ puncture, such as hypotension, decreased breath sounds, chest pain, dyspnea, hematoma, and tachycardia.
- Note and record the volume and character of any aspirated fluid. Blood that has accumulated slowly in the patient's pericardial sac usually doesn't clot after it has been aspirated; blood from a sudden hemorrhage, however, will clot.

After the procedure

- After pericardiocentesis, check vital signs at least hourly and maintain continuous ECG monitoring. Expect the patient's blood pressure to rise as tamponade is relieved. Be alert for the development of recurring tamponade; watch for decreased blood pressure, narrowing pulse pressure, increased central venous pressure, tachycardia, muffled heart sounds, tachypnea, pleural friction rub, distended neck veins, anxiety, and chest pain. Notify the doctor of these signs; he may need to repeat pericardiocentesis or surgically drain the pericardium in the operating room.

Home care instructions

• Urge the patient to keep follow-up medical appointments.

Pericarditis

The pericardium is the fibroserous sac that envelops, supports, and protects the heart. Inflammation of this sac is called pericarditis.

This condition occurs in acute and chronic forms. The acute form can be fibrinous or effusive, with serous, purulent, or hemorrhagic exudate. The chronic form (called constrictive pericarditis) is characterized by dense, fibrous pericardial thickening.

The prognosis depends on the underlying cause but typically is good in acute pericarditis unless constriction occurs.

Causes

Common causes of this disorder include:

• bacterial, fungal, or viral infection (infectious pericarditis)
• neoplasms (primary or metastatic from lungs, breasts, or other organs)
• high-dose radiation to the chest
• uremia
• hypersensitivity or autoimmune disease, such as acute rheumatic fever (the most common cause of pericarditis in children), systemic lupus erythematosus, and rheumatoid arthritis
• drugs such as hydralazine or procainamide
• idiopathic factors (most common in acute pericarditis)
• postcardiac injury, such as myocardial infarction (which later causes an autoimmune reaction known as Dressler's syndrome in the pericardium); other types of postcardiac injury include trauma and surgery that leave the pericardium intact but allow blood to leak into the pericardial cavity.

Less common causes of pericarditis include aortic aneurysm with pericardial leakage as well as myxedema with cholesterol deposits in the pericardium.

Complications

Pericardial effusion is the major complication of acute pericarditis. If fluid accumulates rapidly, cardiac tamponade may occur, resulting in shock, cardiovascular collapse, and eventually death.

Assessment

The patient's history may include an event or disease that can cause pericarditis, such as chest trauma, myocardial infarction, or recent bacterial infection.

The patient with acute pericarditis typically complains of sharp, sudden pain, usually starting over the sternum and radiating to the neck, shoulders, back, and arms. The pain is usually pleuritic, increasing with deep inspiration and decreasing when the patient sits up and leans forward. This decrease occurs because leaning forward pulls the heart away from the diaphragmatic pleurae of the lungs. The patient may complain of dyspnea.

Pericarditis can mimic the pain of myocardial infarction. However, the patient may have no pain if he has slowly developing tuberculous pericarditis or postirradiation, neoplastic, or uremic pericarditis.

Auscultation almost always reveals a pericardial friction rub, which is a grating sound heard as the heart moves. You can hear it best during forced expiration, while the patient leans forward or is on his hands and knees in bed. The rub may have up to three components that correspond to atrial systole, ventricular systole, and the rapid-filling phase of ventricular diastole.

Occasionally, the friction rub is heard only briefly or not at all. If acute pericarditis has caused very large pericardial effusions, heart sounds may be distant.

Palpation may reveal a diminished or an absent apical impulse.

Constrictive pericarditis causes the membrane to calcify and become rigid. It also causes a gradual increase in systemic venous pressure and symptoms similar to those of chronic right ventricular failure (fluid retention, ascites, hepatomegaly).

Tachycardia, an ill-defined substernal chest pain, and a feeling of fullness in the chest may indicate pericardial effusion.

Pallor, clammy skin, hypotension, pulsus paradoxus (drop in systolic blood pressure of 15 mm Hg or greater during slow inspiration), neck vein distention, and dyspnea indicate cardiac tamponade.

Diagnostic tests

Laboratory results reflect inflammation and may identify the disorder's cause. They include the following:

- normal or elevated white blood cell count, especially in infectious pericarditis
- elevated erythrocyte sedimentation rate
- slightly elevated serum creatine phosphokinase-MB levels with associated myocarditis
- culture of pericardial fluid obtained by open surgical drainage or pericardiocentesis (which sometimes identifies the causative organism in bacterial or fungal pericarditis).

Other pertinent laboratory data include blood urea nitrogen levels to check for uremia, antistreptolysin-O titers to detect rheumatic fever, and a purified protein derivative skin test to check for tuberculosis.

Electrocardiography shows characteristic changes in acute pericarditis. They include elevated ST segments in the standard limb leads and most precordial leads without the significant changes in QRS morphology that occur with myocardial infarction. They also include atrial ectopic rhythms, such as atrial fibrillation. And, in pericardial effusion, they include diminished QRS voltage.

Echocardiography diagnoses pericardial effusion when it shows an echo-free space between the ventricular wall and the pericardium.

Treatment

Appropriate treatment aims to relieve symptoms, manage underlying systemic disease, and prevent or treat pericardial effusion and cardiac tamponade.

In idiopathic pericarditis, postmyocardial infarction pericarditis, and postthoracotomy pericarditis, treatment consists of bed rest as long as fever and pain persist and the administration of nonsteroidal drugs, such as aspirin and indomethacin, to relieve pain and reduce inflammation. If symptoms continue, the doctor may prescribe corticosteroids. Although they provide rapid and effective relief, corticosteroids must be used cautiously because the disorder may recur when drug therapy stops.

When infectious pericarditis results from disease of the left pleural space, mediastinal abscesses, or septicemia, the patient will require antibiotics, surgical drainage, or both. If cardiac tamponade develops, the doctor may perform emergency pericardiocentesis and may inject antibiotics directly into the pericardial sac.

Recurrent pericarditis may require partial pericardectomy, which creates a window that allows fluid to drain into the pleural space. In constrictive pericarditis, total pericardectomy may be necessary to permit the heart to fill and contract adequately. Treatment must also include management of rheumatic fever, uremia, tuberculosis, and other underlying disorders.

Key nursing diagnoses and patient outcomes

Decreased cardiac output related to thickening of the pericardial membrane or

pericardial effusion constricting the movement of the heart. Based on this nursing diagnosis, you'll establish these patient outcomes. The patient will:
• maintain hemodynamic stability, as reflected by stable vital signs
• show no evidence of impaired tissue perfusion, such as pain or changes in mental status or organ function
• maintain adequate cardiac output to perform activities of daily living.

Diversional activity deficit related to bed rest. Based on this nursing diagnosis, you'll establish these patient outcomes. The patient will:
• participate in activities that require little energy expenditure, such as watching television, listening to music or tapes, and reading
• report acceptance of his time while on bed rest.

Pain related to inflammation of the pericardial sac. Based on this nursing diagnosis, you'll establish these patient outcomes. The patient will:
• express feelings of comfort following analgesic administration
• become pain free as inflammation subsides.

Nursing interventions

• Stress the importance of bed rest. Assist the patient with bathing, if necessary. Provide a bedside commode because this method puts less stress on the heart than using a bedpan. Offer diversional activities that are physically undemanding.
• Place the patient in an upright position to relieve dyspnea and chest pain.
• Provide analgesics to relieve pain and oxygen to prevent tissue hypoxia.
• Before giving antibiotics, obtain a patient history of allergies. Administer antibiotics on time to maintain consistent drug levels in the blood.
• To reduce the risk of infiltration or inflammation at the I.V. venipuncture site, rotate venous access sites.
• Because cardiac tamponade requires immediate treatment, keep a pericardiocentesis set handy whenever you suspect pericardial effusion.
• To reduce anxiety, allow the patient to express his concerns about the effects of activity restrictions on his responsibilities and routines. Reassure him that the restrictions are temporary.
• Prepare the patient for pericardiocentesis, as indicated.
• Provide appropriate postoperative care, similar to that given after cardiothoracic surgery.

Monitoring

• Assess the patient's cardiovascular status frequently, watching for signs of cardiac tamponade.
• Observe for signs of infiltration or inflammation at the venipuncture site, a possible complication of long-term I.V. administration.
• Monitor the patient's pain level and the effectiveness of analgesics.

Patient teaching

• Explain all tests and treatments to the patient.
• If surgery will be necessary, teach the patient how to perform deep-breathing and coughing exercises before he undergoes the procedure.
• Tell the patient to resume his daily activities slowly and to schedule rest periods into his daily routine for a while.

Peritoneal dialysis

Like hemodialysis, peritoneal dialysis removes toxins from the blood of a patient with acute or chronic renal failure who doesn't respond to other treatments. But unlike hemodialysis, it uses the patient's peritoneal membrane as a semipermeable dialyzing membrane. In this technique, a hypertonic dialyzing solution is instilled through a catheter inserted into the peritoneal cavity. (See *Catheters for peritoneal dialysis,* pages 690 and 691.) Then, by diffusion, excessive concentrations of electrolytes and uremic toxins in the blood move across the peritoneal membrane and into the dialysis solution. Next, by osmosis, excessive water in the blood does the same. After an appropriate dwelling time, the dialysis solution is drained, taking toxins and wastes with it.

Peritoneal dialysis may be performed manually, by an automatic or semiautomatic cycler machine, or as continuous ambulatory peritoneal dialysis (CAPD). In manual dialysis, the nurse, the patient, or a family member instills dialyzing solution through the catheter into the peritoneal cavity, allows it to dwell for a specified time, and then drains it from the peritoneal cavity. Typically, this process is repeated for 4 to 8 hours at a time, five or six times a week.

The cycler machine requires sterile setup and connection technique, and then it automatically completes dialysis.

CAPD is performed by the patient himself. He fills a special plastic bag with dialyzing solution and then instills the solution through a catheter into his peritoneal cavity. While the solution remains in the peritoneal cavity, the patient can roll up the empty bag, place it under his clothing, and go about his normal activities. After 4 to 8 hours of dwelling time, he drains the spent solution into the bag, removes and discards the full bag, and attaches a new bag and instills a new batch of dialyzing solution. He repeats the process to ensure continuous dialysis 24 hours a day, 7 days a week. As its name implies, CAPD allows the patient to be out of bed and active during dialysis and thus only minimally disrupts his life-style.

Some patients use CAPD in combination with an automatic cycler, in a treatment called continuous-cycling peritoneal dialysis (CCPD). In CCPD, the cycler performs dialysis at night while the patient sleeps and the patient performs CAPD in the daytime.

Peritoneal dialysis has several advantages over hemodialysis – it's simpler, less costly, and less stressful. What's more, it's nearly as effective as hemodialysis while posing fewer risks.

Procedure

To begin dialysis, open the clamps on the infusion lines and infuse the prescribed amount of dialyzing solution over a period of 5 to 10 minutes. When the bottle is empty, immediately close the clamps to prevent air from entering the tubing.

Allow the solution to dwell in the peritoneal cavity for the prescribed length of time (usually between 10 minutes and 4 hours) so that excess water, electrolytes, and accumulated wastes can move from the blood through the peritoneal membrane and into the solution. At the completion of the prescribed dwelling time, open the outflow clamps and allow the solution to drain from the peritoneal cavity into the collection bag.

Repeat the infusion-dwell-drainage cycle, using new solution each time, until you've instilled the prescribed amount of solution and completed the prescribed number of cycles. When dialysis is completed, put on sterile gloves and clamp the catheter with a small, sterile plastic clamp. Disconnect the inflow line from the catheter, taking care not to dislodge or pull on the catheter, and place a sterile protective cap over the catheter's distal end. Apply povidone-iodine or antibiotic ointment to the catheter insertion site with a sterile gauze sponge, then place two split-drain sponges around the site and secure them with tape.

Complications

Peritoneal dialysis can cause severe complications. The most serious one, peritonitis, results from bacteria entering the peritoneal cavity through the catheter or the insertion site. Other complications include catheter obstruction from clots, lodgment against the abdominal wall, or kinking; hypotension; and hypovolemia from excessive plasma fluid removal.

Key nursing diagnoses and patient outcomes

Risk for infection related to catheter insertion into the peritoneum. Based on this nursing diagnosis, you'll establish these patient outcomes. The patient will:
• identify and use infection control measures while performing the procedure and caring for the catheter insertion site
• identify and report signs and symptoms of infection, such as redness, swelling, and discomfort around the catheter insertion site
• remain free from infection, as evidenced by a normal temperature and a white blood cell count within normal range.

Knowledge deficit related to unfamiliarity with peritoneal dialysis. Based on this nursing diagnosis, you'll establish these patient outcomes. The patient will:
• identify and express the need to learn about peritoneal dialysis
• obtain information about peritoneal dialysis from appropriate sources
• communicate an understanding of the procedure and the importance of compliance and life-style changes required.

Risk for fluid volume deficit related to excessive fluid removal during peritoneal dialysis. Based on this nursing diagnosis, you'll establish these patient outcomes. The patient will:
• have normal vital signs
• show no signs and symptoms of dehydration and hypovolemic shock during or after peritoneal dialysis.

Nursing interventions

When preparing a patient for peritoneal dialysis or managing his care during and after the procedure, expect to implement these nursing interventions.

Before the procedure

• For the first-time peritoneal dialysis patient, explain the purpose of the treatment and what he can expect during and after the procedure. Tell him that first the doctor will insert a catheter into his abdomen to allow instillation of dialyzing solution; explain the appropriate insertion procedure.
• Before catheter insertion, take and record the patient's baseline vital signs and weight. (Be sure to check blood pressure in both the supine and standing positions.) Ask him to urinate to reduce the risk of bladder perforation and increase comfort during catheter insertion. If he can't urinate, perform straight catheterization, as ordered, to drain the bladder.
• While the patient is undergoing peritoneal catheter insertion, warm the dialysate to body temperature in a warmer, heating pad, or water bath. The dialysate may be a 1.5%, 2.5%, or 4.25% dextrose solution, usually with heparin added to prevent clotting in the catheter. The dialysate should be clear and colorless. Add any prescribed medication at this time.
• Next, put on a surgical mask and prepare the dialysis administration set. Place the drainage bag below the patient to facilitate gravity drainage, and connect the outflow tubing to it. Then, connect the dialysis infusion lines to the bags or bottles of dialyzing solution and hang the containers on an I.V. pole at the patient's bedside. Maintain sterile technique during solution and equipment preparation to avoid introducing pathogens into the patient's peritoneal cavity during treatment.
• When the equipment and solution are ready, place the patient in a supine position, have him put on a surgical mask, and tell him to relax. Prime the tubing with solution, keeping the clamps closed, and connect one infusion line to the abdominal catheter.
• To test the catheter's patency, open the clamp on the infusion line and rapidly instill 500 ml of dialyzing solution into the patient's

Catheters for peritoneal dialysis

The first step in any type of peritoneal dialysis is insertion of a catheter to allow instillation of dialyzing fluid. The surgeon may insert one of three different catheters, as described below.

Tenckhoff catheter

To implant a Tenckhoff catheter, the surgeon inserts the first 6¾" (17 cm) of the catheter into the patient's abdomen. The next 2¾" (7-cm) segment, which has a Dacron cuff at each end, is imbedded subcutaneously. Within a few days after insertion, the patient's tissues grow around these Dacron cuffs, forming a tight barrier against bacterial infiltration. The remaining 3⅞" (10 cm) of the catheter extends outside of the abdomen and is equipped with a metal adapter at the tip to allow connection to dialyzer tubing.

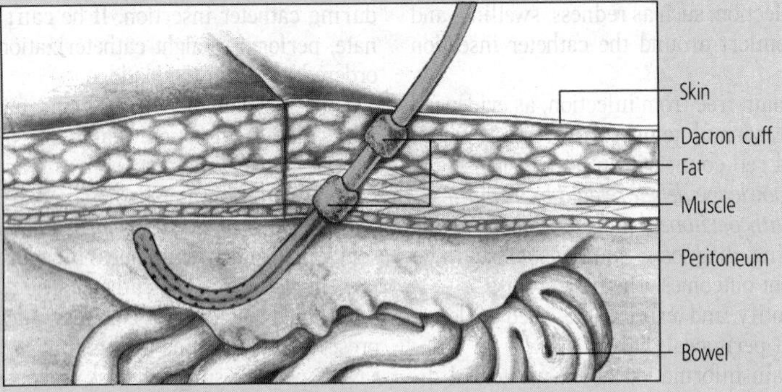

Flanged-collar catheter

To insert this kind of catheter, the surgeon positions its flanged collar just below the dermis so that the device extends through the abdominal wall. He keeps the distal end of the cuff from extending into the peritoneum, where it could cause adhesions.

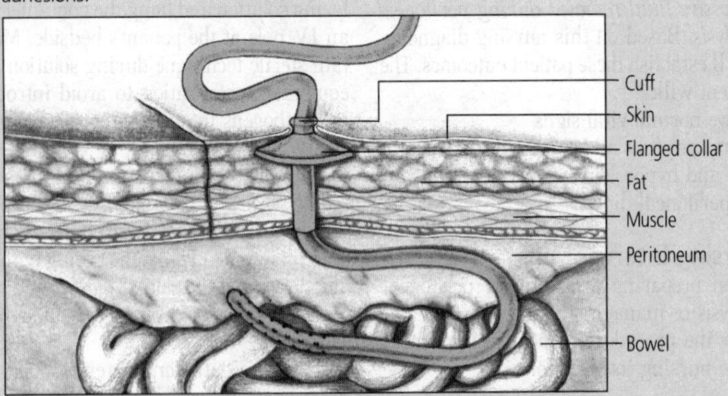

Catheters for peritoneal dialysis *(continued)*

Column-disk peritoneal catheter (CDPC)

To insert a CDPC, the surgeon rolls up the flexible disk section of the implant, inserts it into the peritoneal cavity, and retracts it against the abdominal wall. The implant's first cuff rests just outside the peritoneal membrane, whereas the second cuff rests just beneath the skin. Because the CDPC doesn't float freely in the peritoneal cavity, it keeps inflowing dialyzing solution from being directed at sensitive organs; this increases patient comfort during dialysis.

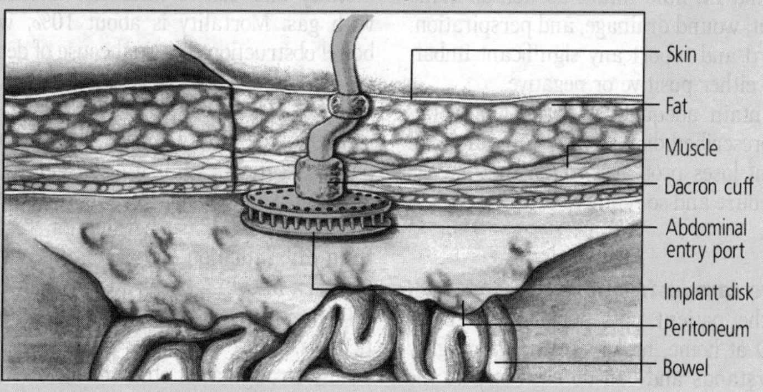

peritoneal cavity. Immediately unclamp the outflow line and let fluid drain into the collection bag; outflow should be brisk. Once you've established catheter patency, you're ready to start dialysis.

During the procedure

- During dialysis, monitor the patient's vital signs every 10 minutes until they stabilize, then every 2 to 4 hours or as ordered. Report any abrupt or significant changes.
- Watch closely for developing complications. Peritonitis may be manifested by fever, persistent abdominal pain and cramping, slow or cloudy dialysis drainage, swelling and tenderness around the catheter, and an increased white blood cell count. If you detect these signs and symptoms, notify the doctor and send a dialysate specimen to the laboratory for smear and culture.
- Observe the outflow drainage for blood. Keep in mind that drainage is commonly blood tinged after catheter placement but should clear after a few fluid exchanges. Notify the doctor of bright-red or persistent bleeding.
- Watch for respiratory distress, which may indicate fluid overload or leakage of dialyzing solution into the pleural space. If it's severe, drain the patient's peritoneal cavity and call the doctor.
- Periodically check the outflow tubing for clots or kinks that may be obstructing drainage. If you cannot clear an obstruction, notify the doctor.
- Have the patient change position frequently. Provide passive range-of-motion exercises, and encourage deep breathing and coughing. This will improve patient comfort, reduce the risk of skin breakdown and respiratory problems, and enhance dialysate drainage.

After the procedure

• Periodically check the patient's weight, and report any gain. Using aseptic technique, change the catheter dressing every 24 hours or whenever it becomes wet or soiled.
• To help prevent fluid imbalance, calculate the patient's fluid balance at the end of each dialysis session or after every 8-hour period in a longer session. Include both oral and I.V. fluid intake as well as urine output, wound drainage, and perspiration. Record and report any significant imbalance, either positive or negative.
• Maintain adequate nutrition, following any prescribed diet. Keep in mind that the patient loses protein through the dialysis procedure and so requires protein replacement.

Home care instructions

• If the patient will perform CAPD or CCPD at home, make sure he thoroughly understands and can do each step of the procedure. Normally, he'll go through a 2-week training program before beginning treatment on his own.
• Instruct the patient to wear a medical identification bracelet or carry a card identifying him as a dialysis patient. Also tell him to keep the phone number of the dialysis center on hand at all times in case of an emergency.
• Tell the patient to watch for and report signs of infection and fluid imbalance. Make sure he knows how to take his vital signs to provide a record of response to treatment.
• Stress the importance of follow-up appointments with the doctor and dialysis team to evaluate the success of treatment and detect any problems.
• If possible, introduce the patient to other patients on peritoneal dialysis, to help him develop a support system. Arrange for periodic visits by a home care nurse to assess his adjustment to CAPD or CCPD.

Peritonitis

An acute or chronic disorder, peritonitis is an inflammation of the peritoneum, the membrane that lines the abdominal cavity and covers the visceral organs. Such inflammation may extend throughout the peritoneum or be localized as an abscess. Peritonitis commonly decreases intestinal motility and causes intestinal distention with gas. Mortality is about 10%, with bowel obstruction the usual cause of death.

Causes

Although the GI tract normally contains bacteria, the peritoneum is sterile. In peritonitis, bacteria invade the peritoneum. Generally, such infection results from inflammation and perforation of the GI tract, allowing bacterial invasion. Usually, this is a result of appendicitis, diverticulitis, peptic ulcer, ulcerative colitis, volvulus, strangulated obstruction, abdominal neoplasm, or abdominal trauma. Peritonitis can also result from chemical inflammation after rupture of a fallopian tube, ovarian cyst, or the bladder; perforation of a gastric ulcer; or released pancreatic enzymes.

In both bacterial and chemical inflammation, fluid containing protein and electrolytes accumulates in the peritoneal cavity and makes the transparent peritoneum opaque, red, inflamed, and edematous. Because the peritoneal cavity is so resistant to contamination, such infection is often localized as an abscess instead of disseminated as a generalized infection.

Complications

Peritonitis can lead to abscess formation, septicemia, respiratory compromise, bowel obstruction, and shock.

Assessment

The patient's symptoms depend on whether the disorder is assessed early or late in its course. In the early phase, he may report vague, generalized abdominal pain. If peritonitis is localized, he may describe pain over a specific area (usually over the site of inflammation); if peritonitis is generalized, he may complain of diffuse pain over the abdomen.

As the disorder progresses, the patient typically reports increasingly severe and unremitting abdominal pain. Pain often increases with movement and respirations. Occasionally, pain may be referred to the shoulder or the thoracic area. Other signs and symptoms include abdominal distention, anorexia, nausea, vomiting, and an inability to pass feces and flatus.

Assessment of vital signs may reveal fever, tachycardia (a response to the fever), and hypotension. On inspection, the patient usually appears acutely distressed. He may lie very still in bed, often with his knees flexed to try to alleviate abdominal pain. He tends to breathe shallowly and move as little as possible to minimize pain. If he loses excessive fluid, electrolytes, and proteins into the abdominal cavity, you may observe excessive sweating, cold skin, pallor, abdominal distention, and such signs of dehydration as dry mucous membranes.

Early in peritonitis, auscultation usually discloses bowel sounds; as the inflammation progresses, these sounds tend to disappear. Abdominal rigidity is usually felt on palpation. If peritonitis spreads throughout the abdomen, palpation may disclose general tenderness; if peritonitis stays in a specific area, you may detect local tenderness. Rebound tenderness may also be present.

Diagnostic tests

- *White blood cell count* shows leukocytosis (commonly more than 20,000/mm³).
- *Abdominal X-rays* demonstrate edematous and gaseous distention of the small and large bowel. With perforation of a visceral organ, the X-ray shows air in the abdominal cavity.
- *Chest X-ray* may reveal elevation of the diaphragm.
- *Paracentesis* discloses the nature of the exudate and permits bacterial culture so appropriate antibiotic therapy can be instituted.
- *Urinalysis* may reveal a urinary tract problem as the primary source of infection.
- *Arterial blood gases* may show metabolic acidosis with respiratory compensation.
- *Computed tomography scan* of the abdomen may reveal abscess formation.

Treatment

To prevent peritonitis, early treatment of GI inflammatory conditions and preoperative and postoperative antibiotic therapy are important. After peritonitis develops, emergency treatment must combat infection, restore intestinal motility, and replace fluids and electrolytes.

Antibiotic therapy depends on the infecting organism but usually includes administration of cefoxitin with an aminoglycoside, or penicillin G and clindamycin with an aminoglycoside. To decrease peristalsis and prevent perforation, the patient should receive nothing by mouth; instead, he requires supportive fluids and electrolytes parenterally.

Supplementary treatment includes administration of an analgesic, such as meperidine; nasogastric (NG) intubation to decompress the bowel; and possible use of a rectal tube to facilitate the passage of flatus.

Surgery, which is necessary as soon as the patient's condition is stable enough to tolerate it, aims to control the source of the peritonitis. For example, an appendectomy may be performed for a ruptured appendix or a colon resection for a ruptured colon.

Peritoneal lavage also may be performed to remove the infected contents of the peritoneum and to prevent recurrent infection. Peritoneal lavage may be carried out laparoscopically.

Key nursing diagnoses and patient outcomes

Altered GI tissue perfusion related to inflammatory process. Based on this nursing diagnosis, you'll establish these patient outcomes. The patient will:
• develop increased GI tissue perfusion as inflammation subsides with treatment
• regain and maintain normal GI function with treatment.

Risk for fluid volume deficit related to excessive fluid loss into abdomen. Based on this nursing diagnosis, you'll establish these patient outcomes. The patient will:
• maintain hemodynamic stability, as exhibited by normal vital signs
• not have signs and symptoms of ascites, dehydration, and hypovolemic shock
• maintain normal vascular fluid volume balance.

Pain related to inflammatory process. Based on this nursing diagnosis, you'll establish these patient outcomes. The patient will:
• express feelings of comfort after analgesic administration
• comply with antibiotic therapy to alleviate inflammation and pain.

Nursing interventions

• Provide psychological support, and offer encouragement when appropriate.
• Administer prescribed medications, such as analgesics and antibiotics, as ordered.
• Maintain parenteral fluid and electrolyte administration, as ordered.
• Maintain bed rest, and place the patient in semi-Fowler's position to help him breathe deeply with less pain and thus prevent pulmonary complications.
• Counteract mouth and nose dryness due to fever, dehydration, and NG intubation with regular hygiene and lubrication.
• Prepare the patient for surgery, as indicated.
• If necessary, refer the patient to the hospital's social service department or a home health care agency that can help him obtain needed services during convalescence.

Monitoring

• Monitor the patient for the desired effects of medications and possible adverse reactions to them.
• Assess fluid volume by checking skin turgor, mucous membranes, urine output, weight, vital signs, amount of NG tube drainage, and amount of I.V. infusion. Record intake and output, including NG tube drainage.
• Monitor the patient for surgical complications if appropriate.

Patient teaching

• Teach the patient about peritonitis, what caused his problem, and necessary treatments.
• Provide preoperative teaching. Review postoperative care procedures.
• Discuss the proper use of prescribed medications, reviewing their correct administration, desired effects, and possible adverse effects.

Pernicious anemia

Also known as Addison's anemia, pernicious anemia is a megaloblastic anemia characterized by decreased gastric production of hydrochloric acid and deficiency of intrinsic factor, a substance normally secreted by the parietal cells of the gastric mucosa that is essential for vitamin B_{12} absorption. The resulting deficiency of vitamin B_{12} causes serious neurologic, psychological, gastric, and intestinal abnormalities. Increasingly fragile cell membranes induce widespread destruction of red blood cells (RBCs), resulting in low hemoglobin levels.

In the United States, pernicious anemia is most common in New England and the Great Lakes region. It's rare in children, Blacks, and Asians. Onset typically is between ages 50 and 60; incidence rises with increasing age.

Causes

Familial incidence of pernicious anemia suggests a genetic predisposition. This disorder is significantly more common in patients with immunologically related diseases, such as thyroiditis, myxedema, and Graves' disease.

These facts seem to support a widely held theory that an inherited autoimmune response causes gastric mucosal atrophy and consequently decreases hydrochloric acid and intrinsic factor production. Intrinsic factor deficiency impairs vitamin B_{12} absorption. The resultant vitamin B_{12} deficiency inhibits the growth of all cells, particularly RBCs, leading to insufficient and deformed RBCs with poor oxygen-carrying capacity.

Pernicious anemia also impairs myelin formation. Initially, it affects the peripheral nerves, but gradually it extends to the spinal cord, causing neurologic dysfunction.

Secondary pernicious anemia can result from partial removal of the stomach, which limits the amount of productive mucosa.

Complications

Patients treated with vitamin B_{12} injections have few permanent complications. Those who go untreated may experience permanent neurologic disability (including paralysis) and psychotic behavior; they also may lose sphincter control of bowel and bladder, and some eventually may die of the disorder. Although the reason is unclear, the incidence of peptic ulcer disease is four to five times greater in patients with pernicious anemia than in the general population.

Assessment

Although pernicious anemia usually has an insidious onset, the patient's history may reveal this characteristic triad of symptoms: weakness, a beefy red sore tongue, and numbness and tingling in the extremities. The patient may also complain of nausea, vomiting, anorexia, weight loss, flatulence, diarrhea, and constipation.

On inspection, the tongue appears beefy red and smooth. Slightly jaundiced sclera and pale to bright-yellow skin may be present with hemolysis-induced hyperbilirubinemia.

The pulse rate is rapid, and auscultation may reveal a systolic murmur. Percussion or palpation may reveal an enlarged liver and spleen.

When neurologic involvement occurs, the patient may complain of weakness in the extremities; peripheral numbness and paresthesia; disturbed position sense; lack of coordination; impaired fine finger movement; light-headedness; headache; altered vision (diplopia, blurred vision), taste, and hearing (tinnitus); loss of bowel and bladder control; and, in males, impotence.

You may observe that the patient is irritable, depressed, delirious, and ataxic and has poor memory. You also may note positive Babinski's and Romberg's signs and optic muscle atrophy. Although some of these symptoms are temporary, irreversible central nervous system changes may have occurred before treatment is initiated.

Complaints of weakness, fatigue, and light-headedness stem from the impaired oxygen-carrying capacity of the blood owing to lowered hemoglobin levels. Compensatory increased cardiac output may cause palpitations, dyspnea, orthopnea, tachycardia, premature beats and, eventually, congestive heart failure.

Diagnostic tests

The Schilling test is the definitive test for pernicious anemia. (See *Understanding the Schilling test,* page 696.) Results of blood, bone marrow, and gastric analyses also help establish the diagnosis. Laboratory screening must rule out other ane-

> **Understanding the Schilling test**
>
> In the Schilling test—the definitive test for pernicious anemia—the patient receives a small (0.5- to 2-mcg) oral dose of radioactive vitamin B_{12} after fasting for 12 hours. A larger (1-mg) dose of nonradioactive vitamin B_{12} is given I.M. 2 hours later, as a parenteral flush. Then, the radioactivity of a 24-hour urine specimen is measured.
>
> Normally, vitamin B_{12} is absorbed, and excess amounts—about 7%—are excreted in the urine within 24 hours. But in pernicious anemia, the vitamin remains unabsorbed, with less than 3% excreted in the stool. When the Schilling test is repeated with intrinsic factor added, the test shows normal excretion of vitamin B_{12}.

mias with similar symptoms, such as folic acid deficiency anemia, because treatment differs. Diagnosis must also rule out vitamin B_{12} deficiency, resulting from malabsorption due to GI disorders, gastric surgery, radiation therapy, or drug therapy.

Blood study results that suggest pernicious anemia include:

- *hemoglobin levels* are decreased (4 to 5 g/dl) and *RBC count* is decreased
- *mean corpuscular volume* is increased (under 120 mm³); because larger-than-normal RBCs each contain increased amounts of hemoglobin, *mean corpuscular hemoglobin concentration* is also increased
- *white blood cell* and *platelet counts* may possibly be decreased; platelets may be large and malformed
- *serum vitamin B_{12} levels* are less than 0.1 mcg/ml
- *serum lactate dehydrogenase levels* are elevated.

Bone marrow studies reveal erythroid hyperplasia (crowded red bone marrow) with increased numbers of megaloblasts but few normally developing RBCs. Gastric analysis shows absence of free hydrochloric acid after histamine or pentagastrin injection.

Treatment

Early I.M. vitamin B_{12} replacement can reverse pernicious anemia and may prevent permanent neurologic damage. An initial high dose of parenteral vitamin B_{12} causes rapid RBC regeneration. Within 2 weeks, hemoglobin should rise to normal and the patient's condition should markedly improve. Because rapid cell regeneration increases the patient's iron requirements, concomitant iron replacement is necessary to prevent iron deficiency anemia. After the patient's condition improves, vitamin B_{12} doses can be decreased to maintenance levels and given monthly. Because such injections must be continued for life, patients should learn self-administration.

If anemia causes extreme fatigue, the patient may require bed rest until hemoglobin rises. If he is critically ill, with severe anemia and cardiopulmonary distress, he may need blood transfusions, digitalis glycosides, a diuretic, and a low-sodium diet for congestive heart failure. Most important is the replacement of vitamin B_{12} to control the condition that led to this failure. Antibiotics help combat accompanying infections, and topical anesthetics may relieve mouth pain.

Key nursing diagnoses and patient outcomes

Activity intolerance related to fatigue and weakness. Based on this nursing diagnosis, you'll establish these patient outcomes. The patient will:

- identify controllable factors that cause fatigue and weakness
- demonstrate skill in conserving energy while performing daily activities to tolerance level

• regain and maintain his normal activity level with effective treatment.

Altered nutrition: Less than body requirements related to vitamin B_{12} deficiency and adverse GI effects. Based on this nursing diagnosis, you'll establish these patient outcomes. The patient will:
• regain and maintain his weight within the normal range
• comply with vitamin B_{12} replacement therapy
• report alleviation of adverse GI effects with effective treatment.

Risk for injury related to falls and hand injuries associated with neurologic changes. Based on this nursing diagnosis, you'll establish these patient outcomes. The patient will:
• incorporate safety precautions into his activities of daily living
• seek and obtain assistance with activities as needed
• remain free of injury.

Nursing interventions

• If the patient has severe anemia, plan activities, rest periods, and necessary diagnostic tests to conserve his energy.
• To ensure accurate Schilling test results, make sure that all urine over a 24-hour period is collected and that the specimens remain uncontaminated by bacteria.
• Administer vitamin B_{12} as prescribed.
• Provide a well-balanced diet, including foods high in vitamin B_{12} (meat, liver, fish, eggs, and milk). Offer between-meal snacks, and encourage the family to bring favorite foods from home.
• Because a sore mouth and tongue make eating painful, ask the dietitian to avoid giving the patient irritating foods. If these symptoms make talking difficult, supply a pad and pencil or some other aid to facilitate nonverbal communication; explain this problem to the family. Provide diluted mouthwash or, with severe conditions, swab the patient's mouth with tap water or warm saline solution. Oral anesthetics diluted in 0.9% sodium chloride solution also may be used.
• If the patient is incontinent, establish a regular bowel and bladder routine. After the patient is discharged, a visiting nurse should follow up on this schedule and make adjustments as needed.
• Institute safety precautions to prevent falls.

Monitoring

• Monitor the patient's pulse rate often; tachycardia means the patient's activities are too strenuous.
• Check for signs and symptoms of decreased perfusion to vital organs, such as dyspnea, chest pain, and dizziness, and for signs and symptoms of neuropathy, such as peripheral tingling.
• If neurologic damage causes behavioral problems, assess mental and neurologic status often. If necessary, give tranquilizers, as ordered; if needed, apply a soft restraint at night.
• Monitor the patient's compliance with vitamin B_{12} replacement therapy.

Patient teaching

• Warn the patient to guard against infections, and tell him to report signs of infection promptly, especially pulmonary and urinary tract infections. The patient's weakened condition may increase his susceptibility to infection.
• Caution the patient with a sensory deficit to avoid exposure of his extremities to extreme heat or cold.
• If neurologic involvement is present, advise the patient to avoid clothing with small buttons and activities of daily living that require fine motor skills.
• Teach family members to observe for confusion or irritability and to report these findings to the doctor.
• Stress that vitamin B_{12} replacement isn't a permanent cure and that these injections *must* be continued for life, even after symptoms subside.

• If possible, teach the patient or his caregiver proper injection techniques.
• To prevent pernicious anemia, emphasize the importance of vitamin B_{12} supplements for patients who have had extensive gastric resections or who follow strict vegetarian diets.

Pheochromocytoma

A rare disease, pheochromocytoma (also known as chromaffin tumor) is characterized by paroxysmal or sustained hypertension due to oversecretion of the catecholamines epinephrine and norepinephrine. By some estimates, about 0.5% of newly diagnosed patients with hypertension have pheochromocytoma. Although this tumor is usually benign, it may be malignant in a few patients.

Pheochromocytoma affects all races and both sexes and is diagnosed most commonly between ages 30 and 40. It can also occur during childhood (in children with a history of hypertension). Although this disorder is potentially fatal, the prognosis is generally favorable with the appropriate treatment.

Causes

Pheochromocytoma stems from a chromaffin cell tumor of the adrenal medulla or sympathetic ganglia, occurring more commonly in the right adrenal gland than in the left. Extra-adrenal pheochromocytomas may be located in the abdomen, thorax, urinary bladder, neck, and in association with the 9th and 10th cranial nerves.

Epinephrine overproduction occurs only with adrenal pheochromocytoma, but norepinephrine overproduction can occur with either adrenal or extra-adrenal pheochromocytoma. In about 5% of patients, pheochromocytoma is inherited as an autosomal dominant trait.

Complications

Pheochromocytoma produces the same complications as those of severe, persistent hypertension: cerebrovascular accident (CVA), retinopathy, heart disease, and irreversible kidney damage. Often, the disorder is diagnosed during pregnancy when uterine pressure on the tumor induces more frequent attacks of hypertensive crisis. Such attacks can prove fatal for both mother and fetus as a result of CVA, acute pulmonary edema, cardiac arrhythmias, or hypoxia. In such patients, the risk of spontaneous abortion is high, but most fetal deaths occur during labor or immediately after birth. Cholelithiasis is often associated with this disorder.

Patients with pheochromocytoma have an increased risk of serious complications and death during invasive diagnostic testing and surgery. After adrenalectomy, severe hypotension resulting in circulatory collapse and shock may occur.

Assessment

The cardinal sign of pheochromocytoma is persistent or paroxysmal hypertension. The patient's history may reveal unpredictable episodes of hypertensive crisis, paroxysmal symptoms suggestive of seizure disorder or anxiety attacks, hypertension that responds poorly to conventional treatment and, in some cases, hypotension or shock resulting from surgery or diagnostic procedures.

The patient may detail attacks that include headache, palpitations, visual blurring, nausea, vomiting, severe diaphoresis, feelings of impending doom, and precordial or abdominal pain. The attacks may be precipitated by any activity or condition that displaces the abdominal contents, such as heavy lifting, exercise, bladder distention, or pregnancy. Severe attacks may be triggered by the administration of opiates, histamine, glucagon, and corticotropin although, sometimes, no precipitating event is found.

The patient may also report mild to moderate weight loss caused by increased metabolism. In addition, she may have symptoms related to orthostatic hypotension: dizziness, light-headedness, or faintness when rising to an upright position.

Inspection may find tachypnea, pallor, or flushing accompanied by profuse sweating. Tremor and seizures may also occur.

Palpation may reveal moist, cool hands and feet or generalized warmth and flushing. Tachycardia is usually present. The tumor itself is rarely palpable, but when it is, palpation of the surrounding area may induce a typical acute attack and help confirm the diagnosis.

Auscultation of blood pressure reveals hypertension, the most common manifestation. Although hypertension is sustained in most patients, some lability is usually noted. During an attack, blood pressure may rise to dangerously high levels.

Diagnostic tests

Diagnosis is usually based on the following tests and test findings.

- Increased urinary excretion of total free catecholamine and its metabolites, vanillylmandelic acid (VMA) and metanephrine confirms pheochromocytoma.
- Labile blood pressure necessitates urine collection during a hypertensive episode and comparison of this specimen to a baseline specimen. Direct assay of total plasma catecholamines may show levels 10 to 50 times higher than normal.
- Adrenal computed tomography (CT) scan or magnetic resonance imaging is usually successful in identifying the intra-adrenal lesions. CT scanning, chest X-rays, or abdominal aortography may identify extra-adrenal pheochromocytomas.
- Glucagon test may be indicated when a patient has infrequent episodes. The glucagon injection of 1 mg I.V. induces a paroxysm in more than 90% of patients with this disorder. Phentolamine should be available to terminate the induced reaction. The test is not indicated for patients with a history of angina, visual changes, or other severe symptoms during a spontaneous attack.

Treatment

Surgical removal of the tumor is the treatment of choice.

If marked hypotension occurs postoperatively, the patient may require I.V. fluids, plasma volume expanders, vasopressors and, possibly, transfusions. However, persistent hypertension in the immediate postoperative period is more common.

If surgery isn't feasible, alpha- and beta-adrenergic blocking agents – such as phenoxybenzamine and prazosin, respectively – are beneficial in controlling catecholamine effects and preventing attacks. Patients with inoperable malignant tumors have benefited symptomatically from treatment with alpha-methylmetatyrosine. The use of combination chemotherapeutic agents has been effective in controlling soft tissue lesions in some patients. ^{131}I-meta-iodobenzylguanidine has also been used for treating malignant pheochromocytomas with a certain degree of success.

Management of acute attacks or hypertensive crisis requires administration of phentolamine (by I.V. push or drip) or nitroprusside to bring the blood pressure level back to normal.

Key nursing diagnoses and patient outcomes

Altered renal tissue perfusion related to adverse effects of hypertension on renal vascular system. Based on this nursing diagnosis, you'll establish these patient outcomes. The patient will:

- maintain adequate renal function
- have normal renal function studies.

Anxiety related to potential seriousness and associated complications of pheochromocytoma. Based on this nursing diagnosis, you'll establish these patient outcomes. The patient will:

- identify and express her feelings about the diagnosis
- perform activities that help lower anxiety
- demonstrate positive coping methods.

Risk for injury related to potential for hypertensive crisis. Based on this nursing diagnosis, you'll establish these patient outcomes. The patient will:
- identify early signs and symptoms of hypertensive crisis and seek medical treatment immediately if they develop
- avoid factors known to precipitate a hypertensive crisis
- remain free from injury.

Nursing interventions

- To ensure the reliability of urine catecholamine measurements, keep the patient at rest and make sure she avoids foods high in vanillin (such as coffee, nuts, chocolate, and bananas) for 2 days before urine collection of VMA. Also, be aware that some drugs – such as guaifenesin and salicylates – may interfere with the accurate determination of VMA. When possible, avoid administering these medications before the test. Collect the urine in a special receptacle, containing hydrochloric acid, that's been prepared by the laboratory. Keep the urine specimen refrigerated during and after the test. Don't schedule the test if the patient has recently been exposed to radiographic contrast medium.
- Administer analgesics for headache. Provide comfort measures: decrease environmental stimuli, apply ice packs, and avoid abrupt jarring motions.
- Consult a dietitian to plan a high-protein diet that has adequate calories.
- Encourage the patient to verbalize her feelings and fears to help decrease anxiety. Help her identify her strengths and use them to develop coping strategies.
- Prepare the patient for adrenalectomy, as indicated. (See the entry "Adrenalectomy.")

Monitoring

- Monitor blood pressure; transient hypertensive attacks are possible. Tell the patient to report headaches, palpitations, nervousness, or other symptoms of an acute attack. If hypertensive crisis develops, monitor blood pressure and heart rate every 2 to 5 minutes until blood pressure stabilizes at an acceptable level.
- Monitor serum glucose levels, and observe for weight loss from hypermetabolism.
- Assess peripheral circulation, neurologic status, and renal and cardiac function for signs of adequate perfusion.

Patient teaching

- Provide honest and clear explanations of all procedures to allay the patient's fears.
- Teach the patient methods that help prevent paroxysmal attacks – for example, relaxation techniques to reduce anxiety, adequate fluids and fiber to avoid constipation, and adequate rest to avoid fatigue.
- Prepare the patient for adrenalectomy by explaining what to expect preoperatively and postoperatively.
- Encourage the patient to wear medical identification and to carry her medication with her at all times.

Phosphorus imbalance

The primary intracellular anion, phosphorus is critical for normal cellular functioning. It's mainly found in inorganic combination with calcium in teeth and bones.

Phosphorus has a variety of important functions, such as formation of energy-storing substances (adenosine triphosphate) and support to bones and teeth. It also plays a role in utilization of B vitamins, acid-base homeostasis, nerve and muscle activity, cell division, and metabolism of carbohydrates, proteins, and fats.

Renal tubular reabsorption of phosphate is inversely regulated by calcium levels – an increase in phosphorus causes a decrease in calcium. An imbalance causes hypophosphatemia or hyperphosphatemia.

The incidence of hypophosphatemia varies with the underlying cause. Hyperphosphatemia is most common in children, who tend to consume more phosphorus-rich foods and beverages than adults, and in children and adults with renal insufficiency.

Causes

Hypophosphatemia may result from respiratory, urinary, or dietary problems; hyperphosphatemia from renal, thyroid, or dietary problems. For more information about why phosphorus imbalance occurs, see *Causes of phosphorus imbalance.*

Complications

Possible complications of hypophosphatemia include heart failure, shock, and arrhythmias. Also, rhabdomyolysis (destruction of striated muscle), seizures, and coma may occur. Hypophosphatemia also may increase susceptibility to infection.

Hyperphosphatemia may result in soft-tissue calcifications and complications resulting from hypocalcemia.

Assessment

A patient with chronic hypophosphatemia may have a history of anorexia, memory loss, muscle and bone pain, and fractures. With acute hypophosphatemia, the patient may complain of chest pain, muscle pain, apprehension, and paresthesia.

On inspection, you may detect a tremor and weakness in the patient's speaking voice and hand grasp. Depending on the severity of hypophosphatemia, you may note confusion, seizures, and coma. You also may detect bruises and bleeding due to platelet dysfunction.

A patient with hyperphosphatemia usually remains asymptomatic unless his condition results in hypocalcemia; in that case, his chief complaint may be tetany. The patient may describe tingling sensations in the fingertips and around the mouth. He also may complain of muscle cramps.

If the patient has soft-tissue calcifications, inspection may reveal oliguria, conjunctivitis, and papular eruptions. Auscultation may reveal an irregular heart rate.

Causes of phosphorus imbalance

Most commonly, hypophosphatemia stems from respiratory alkalosis. (Prolonged, intense hyperventilation can cause severe hypophosphatemia.) Also, increased urinary excretion associated with such conditions as hyperparathyroidism, aldosteronism, renal tubular defects, and administration of mineralocorticoids, glucocorticoids, or diuretics may lead to hypophosphatemia.

Other important causes include the use of total parenteral nutrition with inadequate phosphate content, diabetic ketoacidosis, chronic alcoholism, alcohol withdrawal, and during forced nutrition of undernourished patients, which may lead to severe hypophosphatemia.

Rarely, mild hypophosphatemia results from decreased dietary intake. When combined with overuse of phosphate-binding antacids, hypophosphatemia may become severe. Decreased absorption due to such conditions as vitamin D deficiency, malabsorption syndromes, or diarrhea may also cause this condition.

Hyperphosphatemia most commonly results from renal failure with decreased renal phosphorus excretion. It also may stem from overuse of laxatives with phosphates or phosphate enemas, excessive administration of phosphate supplements, and vitamin D excess with increased GI absorption.

Hyperthyroidism may be associated with hyperphosphatemia. Conditions that result in cellular destruction, such as malignant tumors (especially when treated with chemotherapy), cause phosphorus to shift out of the cell and accumulate in extracellular fluid. Respiratory acidosis may also cause such a shift.

Diagnostic tests

- *Serum phosphorus values* less than 1.7 mEq/liter or 2.5 mg/dl confirm hypophosphatemia; results that are more than 2.6 mEq/liter or 4.5 mg/dl confirm hyperphosphatemia.
- *Urine phosphorus values* above 1.3 g/24 hours support hypophosphatemia; values under 0.9 g/24 hours support hyperphosphatemia.
- *Serum calcium values* less than 9 mg/dl support the diagnosis of hyperphosphatemia.

Treatment

The goal of treatment is to correct the underlying cause of phosphorus imbalance. In the meantime, management of hypophosphatemia consists of phosphorus replacement, with a high phosphorus diet and oral administration of phosphate salt tablets or capsules. Severe hypophosphatemia requires I.V. infusion of potassium phosphate. I.V. supplements are also required when the GI tract can't be used to administer supplements.

Hyperphosphatemia is commonly treated with aluminum, magnesium, or calcium gels or antacids, which bind with phosphorus in the intestine and increase its elimination. Reduced phosphorus intake may be used in conjunction with these phosphorus-binding antacids. Severe hyperphosphatemia may require peritoneal dialysis or hemodialysis to lower the serum phosphorus level.

Key nursing diagnoses and patient outcomes

Pain related to bone, chest, or muscle discomfort caused by hypophosphatemia. Based on this nursing diagnosis, you'll establish these patient outcomes. The patient will:

- express feelings of comfort following administration of an analgesic
- regain and maintain a normal phosphorus level and thus be pain free.

Risk for injury related to hypocalcemia caused by hyperphosphatemia. Based on this nursing diagnosis, you'll establish these patient outcomes. The patient will:

- identify early signs and symptoms of tetany and seek medical attention immediately if they occur
- regain and maintain a normal serum calcium level
- remain safe from injury until his phosphorus level returns to normal.

Knowledge deficit related to phosphorus imbalance. Based on this nursing diagnosis, you'll establish these patient outcomes. The patient will:

- identify and express the need to learn about the cause of his phosphorus imbalance and the prescribed treatment for it
- obtain information about his condition and prescribed treatment from appropriate sources
- communicate an understanding of his condition and treatment.

Nursing interventions

For hypophosphatemia:

- Administer I.V. potassium phosphate slowly to prevent overcorrection leading to hyperphosphatemia. Administer the infusion at a rate no greater than 10 mEq/hour. If phosphate salt tablets cause nausea, use capsules instead.
- Administer medication for bone pain, as ordered. Assist the patient with ambulation and activities of daily living.
- Observe safety precautions. Keep the patient's bed in its lowest position, with the wheels locked and all four side rails raised. If seizures are possible, pad the side rails and keep an artificial airway at the patient's bedside.
- Orient the patient as needed.

For hyperphosphatemia:

- Obtain a dietary consultation if the condition results from chronic renal insufficiency.
- Administer medications as prescribed.
- If hyperphosphatemia is severe, prepare the patient for hemodialysis or peritoneal

dialysis. (See the entries "Hemodialysis" and "Peritoneal dialysis.")

Monitoring

For hypophosphatemia:

- Carefully monitor serum electrolyte, calcium, magnesium, and phosphorus levels. Report any changes immediately. Monitor patients at risk for phosphorus imbalance.
- Assess the patient's renal function, and be alert for signs of hypocalcemia (such as tetany) when giving phosphate supplements.
- Monitor and record the patient's fluid intake and output accurately.
- Observe for signs of infiltration at the I.V. site when administering potassium phosphate, which can cause tissue sloughing and necrosis.
- Monitor the rate and depth of respirations. Report signs of hypoxia, such as confusion and cyanosis.
- Frequently assess the patient's level of consciousness and neurologic status.

For hyperphosphatemia:

- Carefully monitor serum electrolyte, calcium, magnesium, and phosphorus levels. Report any changes immediately. Monitor patients at risk for phosphorus imbalance.
- Watch for signs of hypocalcemia, such as muscle twitching and tetany, which often accompany hyperphosphatemia.
- Monitor the patient's intake and output. If urine output falls below 25 ml/hour or 600 ml/day, notify the doctor immediately; decreased output can seriously affect renal clearance of excess serum phosphorus.

Patient teaching

For hypophosphatemia:

- To prevent recurrence, advise the patient to follow a high-phosphorus diet.
- Provide verbal and written instructions for the patient taking prescribed oral phosphate supplements.
- Encourage the patient on oral phosphate preparations to take the medication every 4 hours while awake and gradually increase the dose over 1 to 2 weeks to decrease adverse effects.

For hyperphosphatemia:

- Make sure the patient and family understand the medication regimen, including dosage and possible adverse effects of prescribed phosphate binders.
- Encourage the patient to avoid foods with high phosphorus content. Review foods with low phosphorus content such as vegetables.
- Stress the importance of avoiding nonprescription preparations containing phosphorus or phosphate, such as laxatives and enemas.

Pilonidal disease

In this disorder, a lesion called a coccygeal or pilonidal cyst develops in the sacral area. The cyst – which usually contains hair – becomes infected and commonly produces an abscess, a draining sinus, or a fistula. Generally, a pilonidal cyst produces no symptoms until it becomes infected. The incidence is highest among hirsute, white men ages 18 to 30.

Causes

Pilonidal disease may develop congenitally from a tendency to hirsutism, or it may be acquired from stretching or irritation of the sacrococcygeal area (intergluteal fold) from prolonged rough exercise (such as horseback riding), heat, excessive perspiration, or constricting clothing.

Complications

Pain and discomfort associated with pilonidal disease can cause psychosocial complications for the patient, such as impaired social interaction and difficulty performing work-related activities. This is most likely if his life-style or occupation requires vigorous activity that irritates the cyst, causing increased pain.

Assessment

Investigation of the patient history may turn up one or more predisposing factors for pilonidal disease. Typically, the patient complains of localized pain, tenderness, swelling, and heat over the affected area. He may also describe continuous or intermittent purulent drainage. If the infection is severe enough, signs and symptoms include chills, fever, headache, and malaise.

On inspection, you may detect a series of openings along the midline, with thin, brown, foul-smelling drainage or a protruding tuft of hair. Palpation of the area may produce purulent drainage, if the drainage is not already continuous.

Diagnostic tests

Cultures of discharge from the infected cyst may show staphylococci or skin bacteria; the discharge doesn't usually contain bowel bacteria.

Treatment

Conservative measures consist of incision and drainage of abscesses, regular extraction of protruding hairs, and sitz baths (four to six times daily). However, persistent infections may result in abscess formation and require surgical excision of the infected area.

After excision of a pilonidal abscess, the patient requires regular follow-up care to monitor wound healing. The surgeon may periodically palpate the wound during healing with a cotton-tipped applicator, curette excess granulation tissue, and extract loose hairs to promote wound healing from the inside out and to prevent dead cells from collecting in the wound. Complete healing may take several months.

Key nursing diagnoses and patient outcomes

Risk for infection related to tendency to hirsutism or repeated stretching or irritation of the sacrococcygeal area. Based on this nursing diagnosis, you'll establish these patient outcomes. The patient will:

- identify and avoid activities that increase the risk of recurrent infection
- maintain a normal temperature and white blood cell count
- not develop signs and symptoms of a recurrent infection.

Impaired social interaction related to pain and discomfort. Based on this nursing diagnosis, you'll establish these patient outcomes. The patient will:

- interact with family or significant other and with staff members
- recover from negative feelings associated with social isolation
- achieve the expected state of wellness.

Pain related to inflammatory process. Based on this nursing diagnosis, you'll establish these patient outcomes. The patient will:

- state and carry out appropriate interventions for pain relief
- express feelings of comfort following analgesic administration.

Nursing interventions

- Administer analgesics and antibiotics, as prescribed.
- Provide sitz baths four to six times daily.
- Prepare the patient for incision and drainage of a pilonidal abscess, as indicated. (See the entry "Incision and drainage.")
- After surgery, change the patient's dressing as directed, using sterile technique to avoid infection. Provide stool softeners, as ordered, and record the time of the first bowel movement. When the patient's condition is stable, resume a normal diet. Encourage the patient to walk within 24 hours.

Monitoring

- Monitor the effectiveness of administered analgesics and sitz baths in relieving pain.
- Assess the patient for adverse reactions to administered analgesics and antibiotics.
- Monitor the patient for recurrent infection in the sacral area.

• After surgery, monitor vital signs often until the patient is stable; check compression dressings for signs of excessive bleeding, such as large amounts of blood on the perianal dressing.

Patient teaching

• Teach the patient about pilonidal disease, and explain his treatment plan. Reassure him that the disorder usually resolves completely with proper treatment.
• Before surgery, reinforce the doctor's explanation of the procedure and answer the patient's questions.
• After surgery or incision and drainage, instruct the patient to wear a gauze sponge over the site once the dressing has been removed. Explain that this protective covering will provide ventilation and prevent friction from clothing from irritating the wound. Recommend the continued use of sitz baths, followed by air-drying instead of towel drying.
• Review the proper use of prescribed medications, usually analgesics and antibiotics. Teach the patient about the desired action of each drug and any adverse reactions that he should report to his doctor.

Pituitary tumors

Originating most often in the anterior pituitary (adenohypophysis), pituitary tumors constitute 10% to 15% of intracranial neoplasms. They occur in adults of both sexes, usually between ages 30 and 50.

The most common tumor tissue types include chromophobe adenoma (90%), basophil adenoma, and eosinophil adenoma. As pituitary adenomas grow, they replace normal glandular tissue and enlarge the sella turcica, which houses the pituitary gland. The prognosis is fair to good, depending on the extent to which the tumor spreads beyond the sella turcica.

Causes

The exact cause is unknown, but a predisposition to a pituitary tumor may be inherited through an autosomal dominant trait. A pituitary tumor isn't malignant in the strict sense; however, its invasive growth categorizes it as a neoplastic condition.

Chromophobe adenoma may be associated with production of corticotropin, melanocyte-stimulating hormone, growth hormone, and prolactin; basophil adenoma, with excess corticotropin production and consequently Cushing's syndrome; and eosinophil adenoma, with excessive growth hormone.

Complications

The loss of pituitary hormone action results in endocrine abnormalities throughout the body if lost hormones are not replaced. Tumor compression of the hypothalamus may result in diabetes insipidus.

Assessment

The patient's history may reveal complaints related to neurologic and endocrine abnormalities. Typically, the patient complains of a frontal headache and visual disturbances (blurred vision progressing to field cuts and eventually blindness). The patient's family may describe personality changes or dementia. The patient may also report amenorrhea, decreased libido, impotence, lethargy, weakness, increased fatigability, sensitivity to cold, constipation (from decreased production of corticotropin and thyroid-stimulating hormone), and seizures.

Inspection may reveal rhinorrhea, a sign that the tumor has eroded the base of the skull. History and inspection may reveal cranial nerve (III, IV, VI) involvement from lateral extension of the tumor. With cranial nerve involvement, the patient typically reports diplopia and dizziness. You may observe head tilting to compensate for diplopia, conjugate deviation of gaze, nystagmus, eyelid ptosis, and limited eye movements.

Inspection may also disclose skin changes that indicate endocrine involvement. Examples include a waxy appearance, fewer wrinkles (which the patient may report during the history), and pubic and axillary hair loss.

Inspection of the eyes may reveal strabismus.

Diagnostic tests

- *Skull X-rays with tomography* may show an enlarged sella turcica or erosion of its floor. If growth hormone secretion predominates, X-ray findings show enlarged paranasal sinuses and mandible, thickened cranial bones, and separated teeth.
- *Carotid angiography* may identify displacement of the anterior cerebral and internal carotid arteries from tumor enlargement. This study can also rule out an intracerebral aneurysm.
- *Computed tomography scan* may confirm an adenoma and accurately depict its size.
- *Cerebrospinal fluid (CSF) analysis* may disclose increased protein levels.
- *Endocrine function tests* may or may not contribute helpful information. In many cases, results are ambiguous and inconclusive.
- *Magnetic resonance imaging scan* differentiates healthy, benign, and malignant tissues and blood vessels.

Treatment

Surgical options include transfrontal removal of large tumors impinging on the optic apparatus and transsphenoidal resection of smaller tumors confined to the pituitary fossa. Radiation therapy is the primary treatment for small, nonsecretory tumors confined to the sella turcica or for patients considered poor surgical risks. Otherwise, radiation is an adjunct to surgery, especially when only part of the tumor can be removed.

Postoperative measures include replacement therapy with corticosteroids or thyroid or sex hormones, correction of electrolyte imbalances and, as necessary, insulin therapy. Other drug therapy may include bromocriptine, an ergot derivative that shrinks prolactin-secreting and growth hormone–secreting tumors. Cyproheptadine, an antiserotonin drug, can reduce increased corticosteroid levels in Cushing's syndrome.

Cryohypophysectomy (freezing the area with a probe inserted transsphenoidally) is an alternative to surgical resection.

Key nursing diagnoses and patient outcomes

Fatigue related to decreased production of corticotropin and thyroid-stimulating hormone. Based on this nursing diagnosis, you'll establish these patient outcomes. The patient will:

- communicate an understanding of the relationship between fatigue, the disease process, and his activity level
- incorporate into his daily activities measures that reduce fatigue
- express a feeling of increased energy with effective treatment.

Sensory/perceptual alterations (visual) related to neurologic dysfunction. Based on this nursing diagnosis, you'll establish these patient outcomes. The patient will:

- compensate for visual changes by using adaptive devices and appropriate resources
- express feelings of safety, comfort, and security
- regain normal visual functioning with effective treatment.

Sexual dysfunction related to hormonal imbalance. Based on this nursing diagnosis, you'll establish these patient outcomes. The patient will:

- acknowledge that his sexual function has changed
- communicate an understanding of the reason for sexual dysfunction
- reestablish his previous level of sexual activity with effective treatment.

Nursing interventions

- Establish a supportive, trusting relationship with the patient and family to help them cope with the diagnosis, treatment, and potential long-term consequences of this disease.
- Maintain a safe, clutter-free environment for the visually impaired or acromegalic patient. Reassure him that treatment will probably restore his eyesight.
- Provide for periods of rest to avoid undue fatigue.
- Administer analgesics, as ordered, to relieve headache.
- Prepare the patient for a craniotomy or a supratentorial or transsphenoidal hypophysectomy, as indicated. (See the entries "Craniotomy" and "Hypophysectomy.")

Monitoring

- Use the patient's comprehensive health history and physical assessment data as the baseline for later comparison.
- Monitor the patient for signs and symptoms of hormonal imbalance.
- Assess the patient for excessive urine output, suggestive of diabetes insipidus.
- Monitor the patient for visual disturbances, and assess him for neurologic dysfunction.

Patient teaching

- Provide necessary preoperative instruction, taking care that the patient understands the information and recognizes possible postoperative problems.
- Instruct the patient to immediately report a persistent postnasal drip or constant swallowing – signs of CSF drainage, not necessarily nasal drainage.
- Encourage the patient to wear a medical identification bracelet that identifies his hormonal condition and its proper treatment.
- Make sure the patient understands the need for lifelong health evaluations and possibly hormone replacement.

Platelet function disorders

These hemorrhagic disorders resemble thrombocytopenia but stem from platelet dysfunction rather than platelet deficiency. They characteristically cause defects in platelet adhesion or procoagulation activity (ability to bind coagulation factors to their surface to form a stable fibrin clot). Such disorders may also create defects in platelet aggregation and thromboxane A_2 and may produce abnormalities by preventing the release of adenosine diphosphate (defective platelet release reaction). The prognosis varies widely.

Causes

Platelet function disorders may be inherited (autosomal recessive) or acquired. Inherited disorders cause the bone marrow to produce platelets that are ineffective in the clotting mechanism. Acquired disorders result from the effects of drugs such as aspirin and carbenicillin; from systemic diseases such as uremia; and from other hematologic disorders.

Complications

Hemorrhage is the most serious complication of platelet function disorders.

Assessment

The patient history discloses the sudden occurrence of excessive bruising and both nasal and gingival bleeding. It may also reveal the use of drugs (especially aspirin) that might be the cause of the problem or a family history of bleeding disorders that cause platelet dysfunction.

Skin inspection reveals petechiae and purpura. External hemorrhage may also be present. The patient's vital signs are usually normal. However, with hemorrhage, the patient's pulse and respiratory rates will rise and his blood pressure will decrease.

Another serious sign – internal hemorrhage into the muscles and visceral or-

Understanding plasmapheresis

In plasmapheresis, blood drawn from a patient's vein (usually in the antecubital fossa or via a large-bore double lumen central venous [CV] access device) flows to a cell separator. Here it is divided into plasma and formed elements (red cells, white cells, and platelets) by centrifugation or by microporous membrane filtration.

The plasma is then collected in a container for disposal, and the formed elements are mixed with a plasma replacement fluid (proteins, fluid, and electrolytes) and returned to the patient through another vein or a CV access device.

In another method of plasmapheresis, the plasma is separated, filtered to remove the disease mediator, then returned to the patient. In both methods, the extracorporeal circuit contains 150 to 400 ml of blood during plasma exchange, which means that the patient must be able to tolerate decreased blood volume.

The procedure can be performed at the bedside or in a special unit and requires a specially trained technician or nurse to operate the cell separator, another to monitor and maintain the patient, and a specialized doctor to be in the facility.

Candidates for plasmapheresis

This procedure may benefit patients with immune-related disorders, such as multiple myeloma, rapidly progressive glomerulonephritis, systemic lupus erythematosus, and rheumatoid arthritis. It may also benefit patients with a neuromuscular disorder, such as myasthenia gravis. It is commonly combined with steroid immunosuppressant therapy to suppress pathologic immune responses, thereby preventing further organ or system destruction.

gans – may not be immediately obvious. Occasionally, this disorder is first identified by excessive bleeding during surgery.

Diagnostic tests

Prolonged bleeding time in a patient with both a normal platelet count and normal clotting factors suggests this diagnosis. Determination of the defective mechanism requires a blood film and a platelet function test to measure platelet release reaction and aggregation. Depending on the type of platelet dysfunction, some or all test results may be abnormal.

Other typical laboratory findings include poor clot retraction; decreased prothrombin conversion; and normal prothrombin, activated partial thromboplastin, and thrombin times. Baseline testing includes a complete blood count and differential and appropriate tests to determine hemorrhage sites.

Treatment

Platelet replacement is the only satisfactory treatment for inherited platelet dysfunction. However, platelets may need to be human leukocyte antigen (HLA)-matched to ensure that the body doesn't reject them.

Acquired platelet function disorders respond to adequate treatment of the underlying disease or discontinuation of damaging drug therapy.

Plasmapheresis effectively controls bleeding caused by a plasma element that's inhibiting platelet function. During this procedure, one or more units of whole blood are removed from the patient, the plasma is removed from the whole blood, and the remaining packed red blood cells are reinfused. (See *Understanding plasmapheresis.*)

Key nursing diagnoses and patient outcomes

Altered protection related to bleeding tendencies. Based on this nursing diagnosis, you'll establish these patient outcomes. The patient will:

- demonstrate the use of protective measures to minimize or prevent bruising and bleeding
- comply with the prescribed treatment regimen
- maintain a safe environment.

Knowledge deficit related to platelet function disorders. Based on this nursing diagnosis, you'll establish these patient outcomes. The patient will:

- identify and express the need to learn about platelet function disorders
- seek and obtain information about his condition from appropriate sources
- communicate an understanding of his condition and the prescribed treatment.

Risk for fluid volume deficit related to hemorrhage. Based on this nursing diagnosis, you'll establish these patient outcomes. The patient will:

- maintain hemodynamic stability, as exhibited by stable vital signs and equal intake and output
- show no signs and symptoms of hemorrhage during bleeding episodes
- maintain fluid volume balance during bleeding episodes.

Nursing interventions

- Provide emotional support as necessary. Listen to the patient's fears and concerns. Reassure him when possible. If the patient is distressed by the appearance of the ecchymoses and petechiae, reassure him that they will heal as the disease resolves.
- Protect all areas of ecchymoses and petechiae from further injury to avoid further discomfort for the patient.
- Alert other care team members to the patient's hemorrhagic potential, especially before he undergoes diagnostic tests that may cause trauma and bleeding.
- Keep the bed's side rails raised, and pad them if possible. Avoid invasive procedures, such as venipuncture and urinary catheterization, if possible. When venipuncture is unavoidable, exert pressure on the puncture site for at least 20 minutes or until the bleeding stops.
- During active bleeding, maintain the patient on strict bed rest if necessary, with the head of the bed elevated to prevent gravity-related pressure increases possibly leading to intracranial bleeding.
- When administering platelet concentrate, remember that platelets are extremely fragile; infuse them quickly, using the administration set recommended by the blood bank.
- Administer HLA-typed platelets, as ordered, to prevent febrile reaction. If the patient has a history of minor reactions, he may benefit from acetaminophen and diphenhydramine before the transfusion.
- Prepare the patient for plasmapheresis, as indicated.

Monitoring

- Watch for bleeding (petechiae, ecchymoses, surgical or GI bleeding, menorrhagia, and bleeding from the skin, nose, gums, or an injury site). Identify the amount of bleeding or size of the ecchymoses at least every 24 hours. Test stools, urine, and vomitus for blood.
- Monitor the patient's platelet count daily.
- During platelet transfusion, monitor for febrile reaction (flushing, chills, fever, headache, tachycardia, hypertension). Such reactions are common, and a fever will destroy the blood products.
- Perform a platelet count 1 to 2 hours after the platelet transfusion to evaluate the patient's response.
- Observe the patient undergoing plasmapheresis for hypovolemia, hypotension, tachycardia, vasoconstriction, and other signs of volume depletion.

Patient teaching

- Teach the patient about the disease, its signs and symptoms, and treatment.
- If platelet dysfunction is inherited, help the patient and his family understand and accept the disorder. Teach them how to manage potential bleeding episodes. Warn them that petechiae, ecchymoses, and bleeding from the nose, gums, and GI tract signal abnormal bleeding and should be reported immediately. Be sure that the patient knows the significance of tarry stools and coffee-ground vomitus.
- Teach the patient to avoid unnecessary trauma. Advise him to tell his dentist that he has this condition before undergoing oral surgery. Also, stress the need for good oral hygiene, using a soft toothbrush. Tell him to use an electric razor to avoid skin injury.
- Advise the patient to avoid coughing or straining during defecation; both can lead to increased intracranial pressure, possibly causing cerebral hemorrhage in the patient with thrombocytopenia. Provide a stool softener, if necessary, because constipation and passage of hard stools are likely to tear the rectal mucosa and cause bleeding.
- Teach the patient to monitor his condition by examining his skin for ecchymoses and petechiae. Teach him how to test his stools for occult blood.
- Tell the patient with a known coagulopathy to avoid aspirin, aspirin compounds, and other agents that impair coagulation. Teach him how to recognize aspirin compounds and nonsteroidal anti-inflammatory drugs listed on the labels of over-the-counter remedies.
- Advise the patient to carry medical identification to alert others that he is a potential bleeder.

Pleural effusion and empyema

Normally, the pleural space contains a small amount of extracellular fluid that lubricates the pleural surfaces. But if fluid builds up from either increased production or inadequate removal, pleural effusion results. An accumulation of pus and necrotic tissue in the pleural space results in empyema, a type of pleural effusion. Blood (hemothorax) and chyle (chylothorax) may also collect in this space.

The incidence of pleural effusion increases with congestive heart failure (the most common cause), parapneumonia, cancer, and pulmonary embolism.

Causes

Pleural effusion may be transudative or exudative. For more information see *What causes pleural effusion?*

Empyema usually stems from an infection in the pleural space. The infection may be idiopathic or may be related to pneumonitis, cancer, perforation, penetrating chest trauma, or esophageal rupture.

Complications

Large pleural effusions may result in atelectasis, infection, and hypoxemia.

Assessment

The patient's history characteristically shows underlying pulmonary disease. If he has a large amount of effusion, he'll typically complain of dyspnea. If he has pleurisy, he may report pleuritic chest pain. If he has empyema, he may also complain of a general feeling of malaise.

Inspection may indicate that the trachea has deviated away from the affected side. With empyema, the patient may also have a fever.

On palpation, you may note decreased tactile fremitus with a large amount of effusion. Percussion may disclose dullness over the effused area that doesn't change with respiration.

When you auscultate the chest, you may hear diminished or absent breath sounds over the effusion and a pleural friction rub during both inspiration and expiration. (This pleural friction rub is transitory, however, and disappears as fluid accumulates in the pleural space.) You'll also hear bronchial breath sounds, sometimes with the patient's pronunciation of the letter E sounding like the letter A.

Diagnostic tests

Thoracentesis allows analysis of aspirated fluid and may show the following.

- Transudative effusion usually has a specific gravity below 1.015 and contains less than 3 g/dl of protein.
- Exudative effusion has a ratio of protein in the fluid to serum of more than or equal to 0.5, pleural fluid lactate dehydrogenase (LDH) of greater than or equal to 200 IU, and a ratio of LDH in pleural fluid to LDH in serum of more than or equal to 0.6.
- Aspirated fluid in empyema contains acute inflammatory white blood cells and microorganisms and shows leukocytosis.
- Fluid in empyema and rheumatoid arthritis – which can be the cause of an exudative pleural effusion – shows an extremely decreased pleural fluid glucose level.
- Pleural effusion that results from esophageal rupture or pancreatitis usually has fluid amylase levels higher than serum levels.

Aspirated fluid may also be tested for lupus erythematosus cells, antinuclear antibodies, and neoplastic cells. Plus, it may be analyzed for color and consistency; acid-fast bacillus, fungal, and bacterial cultures; and triglycerides (in chylothorax).

Other diagnostic tests may also be ordered. A negative tuberculin skin test helps rule out tuberculosis as a cause. If thoracentesis doesn't provide a definitive diagnosis in exudative pleural effusion, a pleural biopsy can help confirm tuberculosis or cancer.

What causes pleural effusion?

Transudative and exudative pleural effusions result from varying disorders and conditions.

Transudative pleural effusion

An ultrafiltrate of plasma containing a low concentration of protein, a transudative pleural effusion may result from congestive heart failure, hepatic disease with ascites, peritoneal dialysis, hypoalbuminemia, and disorders that increase intravascular volume.

The effusion stems from an imbalance of osmotic and hydrostatic pressures. Normally, the balance of these pressures in parietal pleural capillaries causes fluid to move into the pleural space; balanced pressure in visceral pleural capillaries promotes reabsorption of this fluid. But when excessive hydrostatic pressure or decreased osmotic pressure causes excessive fluid to pass across intact capillaries, a transudative pleural effusion results.

Exudative pleural effusions

This type of pleural effusion can result from tuberculosis, subphrenic abscess, pancreatitis, bacterial or fungal pneumonitis or empyema, cancer, parapneumonia, pulmonary embolism (with or without infarction), collagen disease (lupus erythematosus and rheumatoid arthritis), myxedema, intra-abdominal abscess, esophageal perforation, and chest trauma.

Such an effusion occurs when capillary permeability increases, with or without changes in hydrostatic and colloid osmotic pressures, allowing protein-rich fluid to leak into the pleural space.

Treatment

Depending on the amount of fluid present, symptomatic effusion may require thoracentesis to remove fluid or careful monitoring of the patient's own reabsorption of the fluid. Chemical pleurodesis – the instillation of a sclerosing agent such as tetracycline, bleomycin, or nitrogen mustard through the chest tube to create adhesions between the two pleura – may prevent recurrent effusions.

The patient with empyema needs one or more chest tubes inserted after thoracentesis. These tubes allow purulent material to drain. He may also need decortication (surgical removal of the thick coating over the lung) or rib resection to allow open drainage and lung expansion. He'll also require parenteral antibiotics and, if he has hypoxia, oxygen administration.

Hemothorax requires drainage to prevent fibrothorax formation.

Key nursing diagnoses and patient outcomes

Risk for infection related to introduction of foreign object (thoracentesis needle, chest tube, or both) into chest cavity. Based on this nursing diagnosis, you'll establish these patient outcomes. The patient will:

- maintain a normal temperature and white blood cell count
- not develop empyema; if empyema is already present, it won't become worse following invasive treatment.

Impaired gas exchange related to ineffective breathing pattern. Based on this nursing diagnosis, you'll establish these patient outcomes. The patient will:

- maintain adequate ventilation with treatment
- not have signs and symptoms of hypoxia
- regain and maintain normal arterial blood gas values.

Ineffective breathing pattern related to compromised lung expansion. Based on this nursing diagnosis, you'll establish these patient outcomes. The patient will:

- report the ability to breathe comfortably with effective treatment
- perform activities of daily living without dyspnea
- regain his normal breathing pattern when the condition is eradicated.

Nursing interventions

- Prepare the patient for thoracentesis, as indicated. (See the entry "Thoracentesis.")
- Reassure the patient throughout the procedure.
- Prepare the patient for chest tube insertion, as indicated. (See the entry "Chest drainage.")
- Provide meticulous chest tube care, and use aseptic technique for changing dressings around the tube insertion site in the patient with empyema.
- Follow your hospital's policy for milking the tube. Keep petroleum gauze at the bedside in case of chest tube dislodgment.
- Don't clamp the chest tube; doing so may cause tension pneumothorax.
- If the patient has open drainage through a rib resection or intercostal tube, use secretion precautions. The patient will usually need weeks of such drainage to obliterate the space, so make home health nurse referrals if he'll be discharged with the tube in place.
- Administer oxygen and, in empyema, antibiotics, as ordered. Record the patient's response to these care measures.
- Use an incentive spirometer to promote deep breathing, and encourage the patient to perform deep-breathing exercises to promote lung expansion.
- Throughout therapy, listen to the patient's fears and concerns and remain with him during periods of extreme stress and anxiety. Encourage him to identify care measures and actions that will make him comfortable and relaxed. Then, try to perform these measures and encourage the patient to do so, too.

Monitoring

• After thoracentesis, watch for respiratory distress and signs of pneumothorax (sudden onset of dyspnea and cyanosis).

• Ensure chest tube patency by watching for bubbles in the underwater-seal chamber. Record the amount, color, and consistency of any tube drainage.

• Monitor the patient's respiratory status frequently. Obtain arterial blood gas analysis if signs and symptoms of hypoxia develop.

• Monitor the patient for adverse reactions to administered medications.

Patient teaching

• Explain all tests and procedures to the patient, including thoracentesis, and answer any questions he may have.

• Before thoracentesis, tell the patient to expect a stinging sensation from the local anesthetic and a feeling of pressure when the needle is inserted. Instruct him to tell you immediately if he feels uncomfortable or has trouble breathing during the procedure.

• If the patient developed pleural effusion because of pneumonia or influenza, tell him to seek medical attention promptly whenever he gets a chest cold.

• Teach the patient the signs and symptoms of respiratory distress. If any of these develops, tell him to notify his doctor.

• Fully explain the medication regimen, including adverse effects. Emphasize the importance of completing the prescribed drug regimen.

• If the patient smokes, urge him to stop.

Pleurisy

Also called pleuritis, pleurisy is an inflammation of the visceral and parietal pleurae that line the inside of the thoracic cage and envelop the lungs. The disorder causes the pleurae to become swollen and congested, hampering pleural fluid transport and increasing friction between the pleural surfaces.

Causes

Pleurisy can result from pneumonia, tuberculosis, viruses, systemic lupus erythematosus, rheumatoid arthritis, uremia, Dressler's syndrome, cancer, pulmonary infarction, and chest trauma.

Complications

Extensively inflamed pleural membranes may result in permanent adhesions that can restrict lung expansion. The inflammation can also stimulate excessive production and hinder reabsorption of pleural fluid, leading to pleural effusion.

Assessment

The patient may report a sudden, sharp, stabbing pain that worsens on inspiration, the result of inflammation or irritation of sensory nerve endings in the parietal pleura that rub against one another during respiration. He may tell you that the pain is so severe it limits his movement on the affected side during breathing. He may also have dyspnea. Other symptoms vary, depending on the underlying pathologic process.

When you auscultate the chest, you may hear a characteristic pleural friction rub – a coarse, creaky sound heard during late inspiration and early expiration – directly over the area of pleural inflammation. Palpation over the affected area may reveal coarse vibration.

Diagnostic tests

Although diagnosis generally rests on the patient's history and your respiratory assessment, diagnostic tests help rule out other causes and pinpoint the underlying disorder. Electrocardiography rules out coronary artery disease as the source of the patient's pain, and chest X-rays can identify pneumonia.

Treatment

Symptomatic treatment includes anti-inflammatory agents, analgesics, and bed rest. Severe pain may require blocking two or three intercostal nerves. Pleurisy with pleural effusion calls for thoracentesis as both a diagnostic and a therapeutic measure.

Key nursing diagnoses and patient outcomes

Activity intolerance related to pain and dyspnea. Based on this nursing diagnosis, you'll establish these patient outcomes. The patient will:

- maintain muscle strength and joint range of motion
- demonstrate skill in performing activities of daily living without increasing pain and dyspnea
- resume his normal activity level when pleurisy is cured.

Ineffective breathing pattern related to pain. Based on this nursing diagnosis, you'll establish these patient outcomes. The patient will:

- report the ability to breathe comfortably without depressing respirations with prescribed pain management
- have normal arterial blood gas levels
- show no signs and symptoms of hypoxia.

Pain related to inflammatory process. Based on this nursing diagnosis, you'll establish these patient outcomes. The patient will:

- express feelings of comfort following analgesic administration
- comply with the prescribed therapy to eradicate pleurisy and thus pain
- become pain free when pleurisy is cured.

Nursing interventions

- Administer antitussives and pain medication, but don't overmedicate the patient. Pain relief allows for maximum chest expansion.
- Encourage the patient to take deep breaths and to cough. To minimize pain, apply firm pressure at the site of the pain while the patient coughs.
- Position the patient in high Fowler's position to help lung expansion. Lying on his affected side may aid in splinting.
- Plan your care to allow the patient as much uninterrupted rest as possible.
- Pain may impair the patient's mobility, so help him perform active and passive range-of-motion exercises to prevent contractures and promote muscle strength.
- Prepare the patient for thoracentesis, as indicated. Reassure him during the procedure. (See the entry "Thoracentesis.")
- Throughout therapy, listen to the patient's fears and concerns and answer any questions.
- Whenever possible, include the patient in care decisions and include the family in various phases of the patient's care.

Monitoring

- Assess the patient's respiratory status at least every 4 hours to detect early signs of compromise. Also monitor for such complications as fever, increased dyspnea, and changes in breath sounds.
- Monitor the patient for pain at least every 3 hours and for the effectiveness of administered analgesics after each dose.
- After thoracentesis, watch for respiratory distress and signs of pneumothorax (sudden onset of dyspnea and cyanosis).

Patient teaching

- Explain all procedures, including thoracentesis, to the patient and his family.
- If the patient about to be discharged receives a prescription for a narcotic analgesic for pain, warn him about the dangers of overuse. Explain that the drug depresses coughing and respiration and decreases alertness. Also, teach him about the drug's other possible adverse effects and tell him to call his doctor if such effects occur.
- Teach the patient how to splint and perform deep-breathing exercises.

• Emphasize the need for regular rest periods.
• Teach the patient the signs and symptoms of possible complications, such as increased shortness of breath, fever, increasing fatigue, or any change in the quality or quantity of secretions. Tell him to call his doctor if such signs or symptoms occur.
• Reassure the patient that the pain should subside after several days.

Pneumocystis carinii pneumonia

Because of its association with human immunodeficiency virus (HIV) infection, *Pneumocystis carinii* pneumonia (PCP), an opportunistic infection, has increased in incidence since the 1980s. Before PCP prophylaxis, this disease was the first clue, in about 60% of patients, that an HIV infection was present.

PCP occurs in up to 90% of HIV-infected patients in the United States during their lifetime. It is the leading cause of death in these patients. PCP also is associated with other conditions involving immunosuppression, including organ transplantation, leukemia, and lymphoma.

Causes

P. carinii, the cause of PCP, usually is classified as a protozoan, although some investigators consider it more closely related to fungi. The organism exists as a saprophyte in the lungs of humans and various animals. Part of the normal flora in most healthy people, *P. carinii* becomes an aggressive pathogen in the immunocompromised patient. Impaired cell-mediated (T-cell) immunity is thought to be more important than impaired humoral (B-cell) immunity in predisposing the patient to PCP, but the immune defects involved are poorly understood.

The organism invades the lungs bilaterally and multiplies extracellularly. As the infestation grows, alveoli fill with organisms and exudate, impairing gas exchange. The alveoli hypertrophy and thicken progressively, eventually leading to extensive consolidation.

The primary transmission route seems to be air, although the organism is already resident in most people. The incubation period probably lasts for 4 to 8 weeks.

Complications

PCP can progress to pulmonic insufficiency and possibly death. Disseminated infection doesn't occur.

Assessment

The patient typically has a history of an immunocompromising condition or procedure, such as HIV infection, leukemia, lymphoma, or organ transplantation.

PCP begins insidiously with increasing shortness of breath and a nonproductive cough. Anorexia, generalized fatigue, and weight loss may be reported. Although the patient may have hypoxemia and hypercapnea, he may not exhibit significant clinical symptoms. Throughout the illness, he may report a low-grade, intermittent fever.

Inspection may reveal tachypnea, dyspnea, and accessory muscle use when the patient breathes. With acute illness, he may appear cyanotic.

Late in the disease, when consolidation develops, chest percussion discloses dullness. Auscultation findings include crackles (in about one-third of patients) and decreased breath sounds (in patients with advanced pneumonia).

Diagnostic tests

Histologic studies can confirm *P. carinii.* In many patients with HIV, initial examination of a first-morning sputum specimen (induced by inhaling an ultrasonically dispersed 0.9% sodium chloride mist) may be sufficient. This technique usually is ineffective in patients without HIV.

In all patients, fiber-optic bronchoscopy remains the most commonly used diagnostic tool to confirm PCP. Invasive procedures, such as transbronchial biopsy and open lung biopsy, are less commonly used.

In addition, chest X-ray may show slowly progressing, fluffy infiltrates and occasional nodular lesions or a spontaneous pneumothorax. These findings must be differentiated from findings in other types of pneumonia or in adult respiratory distress syndrome.

A gallium scan may show increased uptake over the lungs even when the chest X-ray appears relatively normal.

In PCP, arterial blood gas studies detect hypoxia and an increased A-a gradient.

Treatment

PCP may respond to drug therapy with co-trimoxazole or pentamidine isethionate. Because of immune system impairment, many patients with HIV experience severe adverse reactions to drug therapy. These reactions include bone marrow suppression, thrush, fever, hepatotoxicity, and anaphylaxis. Nausea, vomiting, and rashes are common. To treat the latter effects, the doctor may prescribe diphenhydramine.

Leucovorin may reduce bone marrow suppression and may be used prophylactically in patients with HIV infection.

Pentamidine may be administered I.V. or in aerosol form. I.V. pentamidine is associated with severe toxic effects, whereas the inhaled form usually is well tolerated. However, inhaled pentamidine may not effectively reach the lung apices.

Supportive measures, such as oxygen therapy, mechanical ventilation, adequate nutrition, and fluid balance, are important adjunctive therapies. Oral morphine sulfate solution may reduce respiratory rate and anxiety, enhancing oxygenation.

Key nursing diagnoses and patient outcomes

Altered nutrition: Less than body requirements related to adverse GI effects. Based on this nursing diagnosis, you'll establish these patient outcomes. The patient will:
- regain and maintain weight within the normal range
- eat a nutritionally balanced diet daily
- show no evidence of malnutrition.

Hyperthermia related to inflammatory process. Based on this nursing diagnosis, you'll establish these patient outcomes. The patient will:
- regain a normal temperature with antipyretic administration
- not develop dehydration or other complications of hyperthermia.

Impaired gas exchange related to inflammatory process in lung tissue. Based on this nursing diagnosis, you'll establish these patient outcomes. The patient will:
- maintain adequate ventilation
- regain and maintain normal arterial blood gas levels with treatment
- perform activities of daily living without experiencing dyspnea.

Nursing interventions

- Implement standard precautions.
- Encourage ambulation, deep-breathing exercises, and incentive spirometry to facilitate effective gas exchange.
- Administer antipyretics, as ordered, to relieve fever.
- Give antimicrobial drugs, as ordered. Never give pentamidine I.M. because it can cause pain and sterile abscesses. Administer the I.V. drug form slowly over 60 minutes to reduce the risk of hypotension.
- Administer oxygen therapy as ordered.
- Replace fluids as ordered.
- Supply nutritional supplements as needed. Encourage the patient to eat a high-calorie, protein-rich diet. Offer small, frequent meals if the patient cannot tolerate large amounts of food.

• Give emotional support, and help the patient identify and use meaningful support systems.

Monitoring

• Frequently assess the patient's respiratory status, and monitor arterial blood gas levels.
• Monitor intake and output and daily weight to evaluate fluid balance.
• Assess for adverse effects of antimicrobial drugs. If the patient is receiving co-trimoxazole, watch for nausea, vomiting, rash, bone marrow suppression, thrush, fever, hepatotoxicity, and anaphylaxis. If he's receiving pentamidine, watch for cardiac arrhythmias, hypotension, dizziness, azotemia, hypocalcemia, and hepatic disturbances.
• Check the patient's temperature regularly to determine the effectiveness of antipyretic medications.
• Monitor the patient's nutritional intake daily. Weigh him twice a week.

Patient teaching

• Instruct the patient about the medication regimen, especially about its adverse effects.
• Teach the patient energy conservation techniques.
• If the patient requires oxygen therapy at home, explain that an oxygen concentrator may be most effective.

Pneumonia

An acute infection of the lung parenchyma that often impairs gas exchange, pneumonia can be classified in several ways. Based on microbiological etiology, it may be viral, bacterial, fungal, protozoal, mycobacterial, mycoplasmal, or rickettsial in origin.

Based on location, pneumonia may be classified as bronchopneumonia, lobular pneumonia, or lobar pneumonia. Bronchopneumonia involves distal airways and alveoli; lobular pneumonia, part of a lobe; and lobar pneumonia, an entire lobe.

Finally, the infection can be classified as one of three types – primary, secondary, or aspiration pneumonia. Primary pneumonia results directly from inhalation or aspiration of a pathogen, such as bacteria or a virus; it includes pneumococcal and viral pneumonia. Secondary pneumonia may follow initial lung damage from a noxious chemical or other insult (superinfection) or may result from hematogenous spread of bacteria from a distant area. Aspiration pneumonia results from inhalation of foreign matter, such as vomitus or food particles, into the bronchi. (See *Understanding types of pneumonia*, pages 718 to 720.)

Pneumonia occurs in both sexes and at all ages. More than 3 million cases of pneumonia occur annually in the United States. The infection carries a good prognosis for patients with normal lungs and adequate immune systems. In debilitated patients, however, bacterial pneumonia ranks as the leading cause of death. Pneumonia is also the leading cause of death from infectious disease in the United States.

Causes

In bacterial pneumonia, which can occur in any part of the lungs, an infection initially triggers alveolar inflammation and edema. Capillaries become engorged with blood, causing stasis. As the alveolocapillary membrane breaks down, alveoli fill with blood and exudate, resulting in atelectasis. In severe bacterial infections, the lungs assume a heavy, liverlike appearance, as in adult respiratory distress syndrome (ARDS).

Viral infection, which typically causes diffuse pneumonia, first attacks bronchiolar epithelial cells, causing interstitial inflammation and desquamation. It then spreads to the alveoli, which fill with blood and fluid. In advanced infection, a hyaline

(Text continues on page 721.)

Understanding types of pneumonia

Characteristics	Diagnostic tests	Treatment
Viral pneumonias		
Influenza • Prognosis poor, even with treatment • 50% mortality from cardiopulmonary collapse • Signs and symptoms include cough (initially nonproductive; later, purulent sputum), marked cyanosis, dyspnea, high fever, chills, substernal pain and discomfort, moist crackles, frontal headache, myalgia	• *Chest X-ray:* diffuse bilateral bronchopneumonia radiating from hilus • *WBC count:* normal to slightly elevated • *Sputum smears:* no specific organisms	• Supportive treatment for respiratory failure includes endotracheal intubation and ventilator assistance; for fever, hypothermia blanket or antipyretics; for influenza A, amantadine.
Adenovirus • Insidious onset • Generally affects young adults • Good prognosis; usually clears with no residual effects • Signs and symptoms include sore throat, fever, cough, chills, malaise, small amounts of mucoid sputum, retrosternal chest pain, anorexia, rhinitis, adenopathy, scattered crackles, and rhonchi	• *Chest X-ray:* patchy distribution of pneumonia, more severe than indicated by physical examination • *WBC count:* normal to slightly elevated	• Treatment aims to relieve symptoms.
Respiratory syncytial virus • Most prevalent in infants and children • Complete recovery in 1 to 3 weeks • Signs and symptoms include listlessness, irritability, tachypnea with retraction of intercostal muscles, slight sputum production, fine moist crackles, fever, severe malaise, and possibly cough or croup	• *Chest X-ray:* patchy bilateral consolidation • *WBC count:* normal to slightly elevated	• Supportive treatment includes humidified air, oxygen, and antimicrobials (often given until viral cause is confirmed).
Measles (rubeola) • Signs and symptoms include fever, dyspnea, cough, small amounts of sputum, coryza, rash, and cervical adenopathy	• *Chest X-ray:* reticular infiltrates, sometimes with hilar lymph node enlargement • *Lung tissue specimen:* characteristic giant cells	• Supportive treatment includes bed rest, adequate hydration, antimicrobials and, if necessary, assisted ventilation.

Understanding types of pneumonia *(continued)*

Characteristics	Diagnostic tests	Treatment
Viral pneumonias *(continued)*		
Chicken pox (varicella) • Uncommon in children, but present in 30% of adults with varicella • Signs and symptoms include characteristic rash, cough, dyspnea, cyanosis, tachypnea, pleuritic chest pain, and hemoptysis and rhonchi 1 to 6 days after onset of rash	• *Chest X-ray:* more extensive pneumonia than indicated by physical examination, and bilateral, patchy, diffuse, nodular infiltrates • *Sputum analysis:* predominant mononuclear cells and characteristic intranuclear inclusion bodies	• Supportive treatment includes adequate hydration and, in critically ill patients, oxygen therapy.
Cytomegalovirus • Difficult to distinguish from other nonbacterial pneumonias • In adults with healthy lung tissue, resembles mononucleosis and is generally benign; in neonates, occurs as devastating multisystemic infection; in immunocompromised hosts, varies from clinically inapparent to fatal infection • Signs and symptoms include fever, cough, shaking chills, dyspnea, cyanosis, weakness, and diffuse crackles	• *Chest X-ray:* in early stages, variable patchy infiltrates; later, bilateral, nodular, and more predominant in lower lobes • *Percutaneous aspiration of lung tissue, transbronchial biopsy, or open lung biopsy:* typical intranuclear and cytoplasmic inclusions on microscopic examination (the virus can be cultured from lung tissue)	• Supportive treatment includes adequate hydration and nutrition, oxygen therapy, and bed rest.
Bacterial pneumonias		
Streptococcus • Caused by *Streptococcus pneumoniae* • Signs and symptoms include sudden onset of a single, shaking chill, and sustained temperature of 102° to 104° F (38.9° to 40° C); often preceded by upper respiratory tract infection	• *Chest X-ray:* areas of consolidation, often lobar • *WBC count:* elevated • *Sputum culture:* possibly gram-positive *S. pneumoniae*	• Antimicrobial therapy consists of penicillin G or, if the patient is allergic to penicillin, erythromycin; therapy begins after obtaining culture specimen but without waiting for results and continues for 7 to 10 days.

(continued)

Understanding types of pneumonia *(continued)*

Characteristics	Diagnostic tests	Treatment
Bacterial pneumonias *(continued)*		
Klebsiella • More likely in patients with chronic alcoholism, pulmonary disease, and diabetes • Signs and symptoms include fever and recurrent chills; cough producing rusty, bloody, viscous sputum (currant jelly); cyanosis of lips and nail beds from hypoxemia; shallow, grunting respirations	• *Chest X-ray:* typically, but not always, consolidation in the upper lobe that causes bulging of fissures • *WBC count:* elevated • *Sputum culture and Gram stain:* possibly gram-negative cocci *Klebsiella*	• Antimicrobial therapy consists of an aminoglycoside and, in serious infections, a cephalosporin.
Staphylococcus • Commonly occurs in patients with viral illness, such as influenza or measles, and in those with cystic fibrosis • Signs and symptoms include a temperature of 102° to 104° F, recurrent shaking chills, bloody sputum, dyspnea, tachypnea, and hypoxemia	• *Chest X-ray:* multiple abscesses and infiltrates; frequently empyema • *WBC count:* elevated • *Sputum culture and Gram stain:* possibly gram-positive staphylococci	• Antimicrobial therapy consists of nafcillin or oxacillin for 14 days if staphylococci are penicillinase-producing. • A chest tube drains empyema.
Aspiration pneumonia		
• Results from vomiting and aspiration of gastric or oropharyngeal contents into trachea and lungs • Noncardiogenic pulmonary edema possible with damage to respiratory epithelium from contact with gastric acid • Subacute pneumonia possible with cavity formation • Lung abscess possible if foreign body present • Signs and symptoms include crackles, dyspnea, cyanosis, hypotension, and tachycardia	• *Chest X-ray:* location of areas of infiltrates (suggests diagnosis)	• Antimicrobial therapy consists of penicillin G or clindamycin. • Supportive therapy includes oxygen therapy, suctioning, coughing, deep breathing, adequate hydration, and I.V. corticosteroids.

membrane may form. As with bacterial infection, severe viral infection may clinically resemble ARDS.

In aspiration pneumonia, aspiration of gastric juices or hydrocarbons triggers similar inflammatory changes and also inactivates surfactant over a large area. Decreased surfactant leads to alveolar collapse. Acidic gastric juices may directly damage the airways and alveoli. Particles in the aspirated gastric juices may obstruct the airways and reduce airflow, which in turn leads to secondary bacterial pneumonia.

Certain predisposing factors increase the risk of pneumonia. For bacterial and viral pneumonia, these include chronic illness and debilitation, cancer (particularly lung cancer), abdominal and thoracic surgery, atelectasis, common colds or other viral respiratory infections, chronic respiratory disease (chronic obstructive pulmonary disease, asthma, bronchiectasis, cystic fibrosis), influenza, smoking, malnutrition, alcoholism, sickle cell disease, tracheostomy, exposure to noxious gases, aspiration, and immunosuppressant therapy.

Aspiration pneumonia is more likely to occur in elderly or debilitated patients, those receiving nasogastric tube feedings, and those with an impaired gag reflex, poor oral hygiene, or a decreased level of consciousness.

Complications

Without proper treatment, pneumonia can lead to such life-threatening complications as septic shock, hypoxemia, and respiratory failure. The infection can also spread within the patient's lungs, causing empyema or lung abscess. Or, it may spread by way of the bloodstream or by cross-contamination to other parts of the body, causing bacteremia, endocarditis, pericarditis, or meningitis.

Assessment

In bacterial pneumonia, the patient may report pleuritic chest pain, a cough, excessive sputum production, and chills.

On assessment, you may note that the patient has a fever. During inspection, you may observe that the patient is shaking and coughs up sputum. Creamy yellow sputum suggests staphylococcal pneumonia; green sputum denotes pneumonia caused by *Pseudomonas* organisms; and sputum that looks like currant jelly indicates pneumonia caused by *Klebsiella*. (Clear sputum means that the patient doesn't have an infective process.)

In advanced cases of all types of pneumonia, you'll hear dullness when you percuss. Auscultation may disclose crackles, wheezing, or rhonchi over the affected lung area as well as decreased breath sounds and decreased vocal fremitus.

Diagnostic tests

- *Chest X-rays* disclose infiltrates, confirming the diagnosis.
- *Sputum specimen* for Gram stain and culture and sensitivity tests shows acute inflammatory cells.
- *White blood cell (WBC) count* indicates leukocytosis in bacterial pneumonia and a normal or low count in viral or mycoplasmal pneumonia.
- *Blood cultures* reflect bacteremia and help determine the causative organism.
- *Arterial blood gas (ABG) levels* vary, depending on the severity of pneumonia and the underlying lung state.
- *Bronchoscopy* or *transtracheal aspiration* allows the collection of material for culture. *Pleural fluid culture* may also be obtained.
- *Pulse oximetry* may show a reduced arterial oxygen saturation level.

Treatment

The patient needs antimicrobial therapy based on the causative agent. Therapy should be reevaluated early in the course of treatment.

EXPERT GERIATRIC CARE

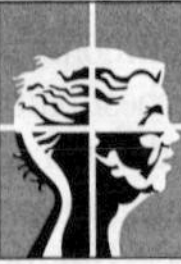

The elderly patient and pneumonia

If an elderly patient with pneumonia requires oxygen, administer it cautiously. High oxygen levels can depress the respiratory stimulus in the brain, reducing respiration and promoting carbon dioxide retention. Elderly patients have a diminished cough and gag reflex, weaker respiratory muscles, and a reduced maximum breathing capacity. Because sedatives, cough suppressants, and narcotics suppress respiratory drive and the cough and gag reflex, their use is often contraindicated in these patients.

Supportive measures include humidified oxygen therapy for hypoxia, bronchodilator therapy, antitussives, mechanical ventilation for respiratory failure, a high-calorie diet and adequate fluid intake, bed rest, and an analgesic to relieve pleuritic chest pain. A patient with severe pneumonia who's on mechanical ventilation may require positive end-expiratory pressure or pressure support ventilation to maintain adequate oxygenation.

Key nursing diagnoses and patient outcomes

Risk for infection related to potential for sepsis, lung abscess, and other complications. Based on this nursing diagnosis, you'll establish these patient outcomes. The patient will:

- remain free from signs and symptoms of a second infection or cardiac dysfunction
- comply with the prescribed treatment.

Impaired gas exchange related to acute infection of the lung parenchyma. Based on this nursing diagnosis, you'll establish these patient outcomes. The patient will:

- maintain his respiratory rate within 5 breaths of baseline
- regain and maintain normal blood gas levels
- express feelings of comfort in maintaining air exchange with treatment.

Ineffective airway clearance related to thick sputum production. Based on this nursing diagnosis, you'll establish these patient outcomes. The patient will:

- use measures to lessen sputum thickness
- cough and expectorate sputum effectively
- maintain a patent airway.

Nursing interventions

- Maintain a patent airway and adequate oxygenation. Administer supplemental oxygen if the patient's partial pressure of oxygen in arterial blood falls below 55 to 60 mm Hg. If the patient has an underlying chronic lung disease, administer oxygen cautiously. (See *The elderly patient and pneumonia.*)
- In severe pneumonia that requires endotracheal intubation or a tracheostomy with or without mechanical ventilation, provide thorough respiratory care and suction often, using sterile technique, to remove secretions.
- Obtain sputum specimens as needed. Use suction if the patient can't produce a specimen. Encourage incentive spirometry.
- Give antibiotics, analgesics, I.V. fluids, and electrolyte replacement, as ordered.
- Provide a high-calorie, high-protein diet of soft foods. Supplement oral feedings with enteral or parenteral nutrition, if needed.
- To prevent aspiration during NG tube feedings, elevate the patient's head, check the tube position, and administer the feeding slowly. Don't give large volumes at one time because this could cause vomiting.

If the patient has an endotracheal tube, inflate the tube cuff before feeding. Keep his head elevated for at least ½ hour after feeding.

- To control the spread of infection, dispose of secretions properly.
- Provide a quiet, calm environment, with frequent rest periods.
- Listen to the patient's fears and concerns, and remain with him during periods of severe stress and anxiety. Encourage him to identify actions and care measures that promote comfort and relaxation.

Monitoring

- Monitor the patient's ABG levels, especially if he's hypoxic.
- Assess the patient's respiratory status. Auscultate for breath sounds at least every 4 hours.
- Monitor fluid intake and output.
- Monitor nutritional intake.
- Evaluate the effectiveness of administered medications, and check the patient for adverse reactions.
- Periodically evaluate the patient's ability to perform bronchial hygiene.

Patient teaching

- Explain all procedures (especially intubation and suctioning) to the patient and his family.
- Emphasize the importance of adequate rest to promote full recovery and prevent a relapse. Explain that the doctor will advise the patient when he can resume full activity and return to work.
- Review the patient's medication. Stress the need to take the entire course of medication to prevent a relapse.
- Teach the patient procedures and therapies for clearing lung secretions, such as deep-breathing and coughing exercises as well as home oxygen therapy. Explain deep breathing and pursed-lip breathing.
- Urge the patient to drink 2 to 3 qt (or liters) of fluid a day to maintain adequate hydration and keep mucus secretions thin for easier removal.
- Teach the patient and his family about chest physiotherapy. Explain that postural drainage, percussion, and vibration help to mobilize and remove mucus from the patient's lungs.
- Urge all bedridden and postoperative patients to perform deep-breathing and coughing exercises frequently. Position such patients properly to promote full aeration and drainage of secretions.
- Advise patients to avoid using antibiotics indiscriminately for minor infections. Doing so could result in upper airway colonization with antibiotic-resistant bacteria. If pneumonia develops, the organisms that produce the pneumonia may require treatment with more toxic antibiotics.
- Encourage the high-risk patient to ask his doctor about an annual influenza vaccination and the pneumococcal pneumonia vaccination.
- Urge the patient to avoid irritants that stimulate secretions, such as cigarette smoke, dust, and significant environmental pollution. If necessary, refer him to community programs or agencies that can help him stop smoking.
- Discuss ways to avoid spreading the infection to others. Remind the patient to sneeze and cough into tissues and to dispose of the tissues in a waxed or plastic bag. Advise him to wash his hands thoroughly after handling contaminated tissues.

Pneumothorax

An accumulation of air or gas between the parietal and visceral pleurae characterizes pneumothorax. The amount of air or gas trapped in the intrapleural space determines the degree of lung collapse. The most common types of pneumothorax are open, closed, and tension. Many factors contribute to pneumothorax.

Causes

Open pneumothorax – also called an open or sucking chest wound – results when atmospheric air (positive pressure) flows directly into the pleural cavity (negative pressure). As the air pressure in the pleural cavity becomes positive, the lung collapses on the affected side, resulting in substantially decreased total lung capacity, vital capacity, and lung compliance. The resulting ventilation-perfusion imbalances lead to hypoxia. Types of open pneumothorax include penetrating pneumothorax and traumatic pneumothorax.

Closed pneumothorax occurs when air enters the pleural space from within the lung, causing increased pleural pressure and preventing lung expansion during normal inspiration. Closed pneumothorax may be called traumatic pneumothorax when blunt chest trauma causes lung tissue to rupture, which results in air leakage.

Spontaneous pneumothorax, another type of closed pneumothorax, is more common in men than in women. It's common in older patients with chronic pulmonary disease, but it may occur in healthy, tall, young adults. Both types of closed pneumothorax can result in a collapsed lung with hypoxia and decreased total lung capacity, vital capacity, and lung compliance. The total amount of lung collapse can range from 5% to 95%.

In tension pneumothorax, air in the pleural space is under higher pressure than air in adjacent lung and vascular structures. The air cannot escape, and the accumulating pressure causes the lung to collapse. As air continues to accumulate and intrapleural pressures rise, the mediastinum shifts away from the affected side and decreases venous return. This forces the heart, trachea, esophagus, and great vessels to the unaffected side, compressing the heart and the contralateral lung. Without immediate treatment, this emergency can rapidly become fatal.

Complications

Extensive pneumothorax can lead to fatal pulmonary and circulatory impairment.

Assessment

The patient history reveals sudden, sharp, pleuritic pain. The patient may report that chest movement, breathing, and coughing exacerbate the pain. He may also report shortness of breath.

Inspection typically reveals asymmetrical chest wall movement with overexpansion and rigidity on the affected side. The patient may appear cyanotic. In tension pneumothorax, he may have distended neck veins and pallor and may exhibit anxiety. (Test results may confirm increased central venous pressure.)

Palpation may reveal crackling beneath the skin, indicating subcutaneous emphysema (air in tissues) and decreased vocal fremitus. In tension pneumothorax, palpation may disclose tracheal deviation away from the affected side and a weak and rapid pulse. Percussion may demonstrate hyperresonance on the affected side, and auscultation may disclose decreased or absent breath sounds over the collapsed lung. The patient may be hypotensive with tension pneumothorax. Spontaneous pneumothorax that releases only a small amount of air into the pleural space may cause no signs and symptoms.

Diagnostic tests

- *Chest X-rays* reveal air in the pleural space and, possibly, a mediastinal shift, which confirms the diagnosis.
- *Arterial blood gas studies* may show hypoxemia, possibly accompanied by respiratory acidosis and hypercapnia. Arterial oxygen saturation levels may fall initially but typically return to normal within 24 hours.

Treatment

Typically, treatment is conservative for spontaneous pneumothorax with no signs of increased pleural pressure (indicating tension pneumothorax), with lung collapse less than 30%, and with no dyspnea or other indications of physiologic compromise. Such treatment consists of bed rest, careful monitoring (blood pressure and pulse and respiratory rates), oxygen administration and, possibly, aspiration of air with a large-bore needle attached to a syringe.

If more than 30% of the lung collapses, treatment to reexpand the lung includes placing a thoracostomy tube in the second or third intercostal space in the midclavicular line. The thoracostomy tube then connects to an underwater seal or to low-pressure suction.

Recurring spontaneous pneumothorax requires thoracotomy and pleurectomy. These procedures prevent recurrence by causing the lung to adhere to the parietal pleura. Traumatic and tension pneumothorax require chest tube drainage; traumatic pneumothorax may also require surgical repair. Analgesics may be prescribed.

Key nursing diagnoses and patient outcomes

Altered tissue perfusion related to decreased oxygen availability in blood. Based on this nursing diagnosis, you'll establish these patient outcomes. The patient will:

- restrict his activities to reduce tissue oxygen need until pneumothorax is resolved
- not exhibit signs and symptoms of tissue hypoxia.

Impaired gas exchange related to air trapped in pleural space impeding lung expansion. Based on this nursing diagnosis, you'll establish these patient outcomes. The patient will:

- regain and maintain adequate ventilation with prompt treatment
- regain and maintain normal arterial blood gas levels
- show resolution of pneumothorax on chest X-ray with treatment.

Pain related to air pressure change in pleural cavity. Based on this nursing diagnosis, you'll establish these patient outcomes. The patient will:

- express feelings of chest comfort following analgesic administration
- sit upright to increase comfort
- become pain free with resolution of pneumothorax.

Nursing interventions

- Listen to the patient's fears and concerns. Offer reassurance as appropriate. Include the patient and his family in care-related decisions whenever possible.
- Keep the patient as comfortable as possible, and administer analgesics as necessary. The patient with pneumothorax usually feels most comfortable sitting upright.
- Prepare the patient for chest tube insertion. (See the entry "Chest drainage.")
- Prepare the patient for thoracotomy, as indicated. (See the entry "Thoracotomy.")

Monitoring

- Assess the patient's respiratory status. Monitor arterial blood gas levels regularly, as ordered. (See *Nursing care in pneumothorax,* pages 726 and 727.)
- Watch for complications, signaled by pallor, gasping respirations, and sudden chest pain. Carefully monitor vital signs at least every hour for indications of shock, increasing respiratory distress, or mediastinal shift. Listen for breath sounds over both lungs.
- Watch for signs of tension pneumothorax (especially if the patient has chest tubes inserted). These include falling blood pressure and rising pulse and respiratory rates, which could be fatal without prompt treatment.
- Assess the effectiveness of administered analgesics, and monitor the patient for adverse reactions.

Patient teaching

- Reassure the patient. Explain what pneumothorax is, what causes it, and all diagnostic tests and procedures. If the patient is having surgery or chest tubes inserted, explain why he needs these procedures. Reassure him that the chest tubes will make him more comfortable.

NURSING PRIORITY

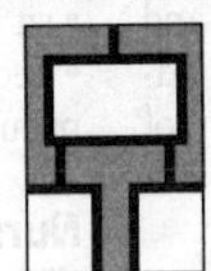

Nursing care in pneumothorax

Presence of sudden, sharp pleuretic pain; shortness of breath; pain with chest movement, breathing, or coughing; contributing factors

Physical findings, including asymmetrical chest wall movement with overexpansion and rigidity on the affected side, skin color changes, distended neck veins (tension pneumothorax), crackling beneath skin on touch, decreased vocal fremitus, tracheal deviation away from affected side (tension pneumothorax), hyperresonance on affected side, decreased or absent breath sounds on affected side, rapid, weak pulse and hypotension (tension pneumothorax)

Results of chest X-ray, arterial blood gas (ABG) analysis

Altered cerebral, cardiopulmonary, and renal tissue perfusion related to decreased oxygen availability in blood

Institute bed rest immediately to reduce oxygen requirements.

Attend to patient's physical needs to resolve pneumothorax.

Monitor brain, heart, and kidney function closely.

Is tissue perfusion adequate?

YES

Continue supportive care.

NO

Expect to implement measures to combat shock.

Monitor vital signs more frequently.

Prepare to transfer patient to intensive care unit.

Patient exhibits adequate cerebral, cardiopulmonary, and renal tissue perfusion by:
- regaining and maintaining normal vital signs
- exhibiting normal ECG pattern and mental status
- maintaining urine output greater than 30 ml/hr.

KEY
- Assessment
- Nursing diagnoses
- Interventions
- Evaluation

Impaired gas exchange related to air trapped in pleural space impeding lung expansion

Administer oxygen (O_2) therapy.

- Monitor respiratory function, including breath sounds.
- Monitor ABG values and O_2 saturation levels.
- Check mental status frequently.

Is gas exchange adequate?

YES

Continue O_2 therapy as prescribed.

NO

Expect to insert chest tubes.

Provide supportive care for chest tubes.

Continue monitoring respiratory function closely.

Patient exhibits adequate gas exchange by:
- having normal ABG and O_2 saturation values
- being alert and oriented to time, person and place
- reporting breathing comfort.

Pain related to air pressure change in pleural cavity

Administer analgesic.

Maintain patient in upright sitting position.

Monitor analgesic effectiveness.

Is pain relieved?

YES

Continue prescribed analgesic therapy.

NO

Expect to increase analgesic dosage or administer a stronger analgesic.

Monitor analgesic effectiveness.

Patient will be pain-free as exhibited by:
- reporting pain relief
- appearing comfortable.

• Encourage the patient to perform deep-breathing exercises every hour when awake.
• Discuss the potential for recurrent spontaneous pneumothorax, and review its signs and symptoms. Emphasize the need for immediate medical intervention if these should occur.

Poliomyelitis

Also called polio and infantile paralysis, poliomyelitis is an acute communicable disease caused by the poliovirus. It ranges in severity from inapparent infection to fatal paralytic illness.

First recognized in 1840, the disease became epidemic in Norway and Sweden in 1905. Outbreaks reached pandemic proportions in Europe, North America, Australia, and New Zealand during the first half of this century. Incidence peaked during the 1940s and early 1950s and led to the development of the Salk vaccine. (See *Polio protection*.)

Minor polio outbreaks still occasionally occur among nonimmunized groups; one such outbreak occurred among the Amish of Pennsylvania in 1979. Otherwise, only 5 to 10 cases (associated with the use of oral poliovirus vaccine) are reported in the United States annually.

Polio strikes most often during the summer and fall. Once mainly confined to infants and children, it's now more common in people over age 15. Among children, it most often paralyzes boys; girls and adults are at greater risk for infection but not for paralysis.

The prognosis largely depends on the site affected. If the central nervous system (CNS) is spared, the prognosis is excellent. However, CNS infection can cause paralysis and death. The mortality for all types of polio is 5% to 10%.

Causes

The poliovirus (an enterovirus) has three antigenically distinct serotypes – types 1, 2, and 3 – that cause polio. These polioviruses are found worldwide and are transmitted from person to person by direct contact with infected oropharyngeal secretions or feces. The incubation period ranges from 5 to 35 days (7 to 14 days is average).

The virus usually enters the body through the alimentary tract, multiplies in the oropharynx and lower intestinal tract, and then spreads to regional lymph nodes and blood. Factors that increase the probability of paralysis include pregnancy, old age, unusual physical exertion at or just before the clinical onset of poliomyelitis, and localized trauma, such as a recent tonsillectomy, tooth extraction, or inoculation.

Most major cases in the United States are related to the oral poliovirus vaccine (OPV) and occur in children under age 4. Infection occurs 7 to 21 days after administration of OPV and usually is associated with the first dose of the vaccine. OPV-related cases also occur in young adults, who show symptoms 20 to 29 days after vaccine administration.

Complications

Possible complications include respiratory failure, pulmonary edema, pulmonary embolism, hypertension, urinary tract infection, urolithiasis, atelectasis, pneumonia, myocarditis, cor pulmonale, soft-tissue and skeletal deformities, and paralytic ileus.

In polio survivors, latent poliomyelitis can lead to muscle spasticity and weakness 10 to 15 years after the initial infection. Delayed poliomyelitis also can affect respiratory muscles, leading to hypoxemia.

Assessment

Today, most cases of polio are so minor that the patient doesn't even visit the doctor. Inapparent, or subclinical, poliomyelitis (about 95% of all cases) has no symp-

Polio protection

Dr. Jonas Salk's poliomyelitis vaccine, which became available in 1955, has been one of the miracle drugs of modern medicine. The vaccine contains dead (formalin-inactivated) polioviruses that stimulate production of circulating antibodies in the human body. It has effectively eliminated the once-feared disease.

The vaccine of choice

However, even miracle drugs can be improved. Today, the Sabin vaccine, which can be taken orally and is more than 90% effective, is the vaccine of choice in preventing poliomyelitis. This vaccine is available in trivalent and monovalent forms. Both forms contain live but weakened viruses. The trivalent form is the vaccine of choice because it contains all three poliovirus serotypes in one solution. The monovalent form contains one viral type and is useful only when the particular serotype is known.

All infants should be immunized with the Sabin vaccine, and pregnant women may be vaccinated without risk.

Sabin vaccine risks

Because of the small risk of contracting polio from the vaccine, it's contraindicated in patients with immunodeficiency diseases, leukemia, or lymphoma and in those receiving corticosteroids, antimetabolites, other immunosuppressants, or radiation therapy. These patients usually are immunized with the Salk vaccine, instead.

When possible, immunodeficient patients should avoid contact with family members who've received the Sabin vaccine for at least 2 weeks after vaccination. The Sabin vaccine is no longer routinely advised for adults unless they're apt to be exposed to the disease or plan to travel to endemic areas.

toms. Abortive poliomyelitis (4% to 8% of all cases) is over in about 72 hours, with the patient experiencing only a slight fever, malaise, headache, sore throat, and vomiting.

The third type, major poliomyelitis, is most likely to be reported. It involves the CNS and takes two forms: nonparalytic and paralytic. In children, the course often is biphasic, with the onset of major illness occurring after recovery from the minor illness stage.

The most perilous paralytic form, bulbar paralytic poliomyelitis, occurs when the virus affects the medulla of the brain. This type usually weakens the muscles supplied by the cranial nerves (particularly the 9th and 10th).

A patient with nonparalytic poliomyelitis complains of moderate fever, headache, vomiting, lethargy, irritability, and pains in the neck, back, arms, legs, and abdomen.

Paralytic poliomyelitis usually develops within 5 to 7 days after the onset of fever. The patient complains of symptoms similar to those of nonparalytic poliomyelitis and then develops weakness and paralysis. The patient also may report related signs and symptoms, such as paresthesia, urine retention, constipation, and abdominal distention.

The patient with bulbar paralytic poliomyelitis may complain of facial weakness, dysphasia, difficulty in chewing, inability to swallow or expel saliva, regurgitation of food through the nasal passages, and dyspnea.

Your examination of the patient with nonparalytic poliomyelitis may reveal muscle tenderness and spasms in the extensors of the neck and back and sometimes in the hamstring and other muscles. (These spasms may be observed during maximum range-of-motion exercises.) This type of polio usually lasts about 1 week, with meningeal irritation persisting for about 2 weeks.

Examination of the patient with paralytic poliomyelitis may show asymmetrical weakness and flaccid paralysis of various muscles. He'll display Hoyne's sign – his head will fall back when he's supine and his shoulders are elevated. He also won't be able to raise his legs a full 90 degrees. The extent of paralysis depends on the level of the spinal cord lesions, which may be cervical, thoracic, or lumbar.

In both nonparalytic and paralytic polio, you may observe resistance to neck flexion – the patient will extend his arms behind him for support ("tripod") when he sits up.

Diagnostic tests

Isolation of the poliovirus from throat washings early in the disease and from stools throughout the disease confirms the diagnosis. If the patient has a CNS infection, cerebrospinal fluid cultures may aid diagnosis. Coxsackie virus and echovirus infections must be ruled out. Convalescent serum antibody titers four times greater than acute titers support a diagnosis of poliomyelitis.

Treatment

Poliomyelitis calls for supportive treatment, including analgesics to ease headache, back pain, and leg spasms. Morphine is contraindicated because of the danger of additional respiratory depression. Moist heat applications also may reduce muscle spasm and pain.

Bed rest is necessary until extreme discomfort subsides. It also helps prevent increased paralysis. Patients with paralytic polio may be bedridden for a long time and then require long-term rehabilitation using physical therapy, braces, and corrective shoes. Orthopedic surgery also may be necessary.

Bladder involvement may require catheterization, and respiratory muscle involvement may require mechanical ventilation. Postural drainage and suction may be sufficient to manage pooling of secretions in patients with nonparalytic polio.

Key nursing diagnoses and patient outcomes

Risk for disuse syndrome related to potential for prolonged inactivity. Based on this nursing diagnosis, you'll establish these patient outcomes. The patient will:
- maintain normal body function during the period of inactivity
- not have signs and symptoms of inactivity-related complications, such as pneumonia, constipation, or renal calculi.

Impaired physical mobility related to neurologic dysfunction. Based on this nursing diagnosis, you'll establish these patient outcomes. The patient will:
- maintain muscle strength and tone as well as joint range of motion
- achieve the highest level of mobility possible within the confines of the disease
- use available resources to help maintain this level of functioning.

Ineffective breathing pattern related to respiratory muscle weakness or paralysis. Based on this nursing diagnosis, you'll establish these patient outcomes. The patient will:
- maintain adequate ventilation with treatment, which may include mechanical ventilation
- not have signs and symptoms of hypoxia, such as restlessness, confusion, and cyanosis
- report feeling comfortable with his breathing pattern.

Nursing interventions

- Maintain a patent airway, and keep a tracheotomy tray at the patient's bedside. A tracheotomy commonly is performed at

the first sign of respiratory distress, and the patient is placed on a ventilator.
- Don't demand any vigorous muscle activity. Encourage a return to mild activity as soon as possible.
- Prevent fecal impaction by giving enough fluids (1.5 to 2 qt [or liters] per day for adults) to ensure an adequate daily urine output of low specific gravity.
- Provide tube feedings when needed.
- To prevent pressure ulcers, provide good skin care, reposition the patient often, and keep the bed linens dry.
- Have the patient wear high-top sneakers or use a footboard to prevent footdrop. To alleviate discomfort, use foam rubber pads and sandbags or light splints, as ordered.
- To control the spread of infection, wash your hands thoroughly after contact with the patient or any of his secretions and excretions.
- Provide emotional support to the patient and his family.
- When caring for a paralyzed patient, help set up an interdisciplinary rehabilitation program with physical and occupational therapists and doctors. A psychiatrist also may help the patient and family accept the patient's physical disabilities.
- Report all polio cases to local public health authorities.

Monitoring

- Carefully observe the patient for signs of paralysis and other neurologic damage, which can occur rapidly. Watch for respiratory weakness and difficulty swallowing. Perform a brief neurologic assessment at least once a day.
- Frequently check blood pressure, especially if the patient has bulbar poliomyelitis. This form of the disease can cause hypertension or shock.
- Monitor the bedridden patient's food intake to make sure he's receiving an adequate, well-balanced diet.
- Assess bladder distention. Muscle paralysis may cause bladder weakness or transient bladder paralysis with urine retention.
- Monitor the patient for complications associated with inactivity: constipation that can lead to fecal impaction, skin breakdown, renal calculi, and pneumonia.

Patient teaching

- Inform the ambulatory patient about the need for careful hand washing.
- Warn any hospital worker who hasn't been vaccinated against polio to avoid contact with the patient.
- Instruct the patient or caregivers about measures needed to manage symptoms and prevent complications.
- Help the patient establish a support system of family, friends, or health care workers to assist him at home.
- Encourage parents to have children vaccinated against polio. Reassure them that the risk of vaccine-related disease is small.

Polycystic kidney disease

This inherited disorder is characterized by multiple, bilateral, grapelike clusters of fluid-filled cysts that enlarge the kidneys, compressing and eventually replacing functioning renal tissue. The disease affects males and females equally. It has an insidious onset but usually becomes obvious between ages 30 and 50; rarely, it may not cause symptoms until the patient is in his 70s. Renal deterioration gradually occurs, and the disease progresses relentlessly to fatal uremia.

The prognosis is extremely variable. Progression may be slow, even after symptoms of renal insufficiency appear. Once uremic symptoms develop, polycystic kidney disease usually is fatal within 4 years unless the patient receives dialysis.

Causes

Polycystic kidney disease is genetically transmitted as an autosomal dominant trait.

Complications

This disease may cause recurrent hematuria, life-threatening retroperitoneal bleeding from cyst rupture, proteinuria, and colicky abdominal pain from the ureteral passage of clots or calculi. In most cases, progressive compression of kidney structures by the enlarging mass produces renal failure about 10 years after symptoms appear.

Assessment

The patient with polycystic kidney disease commonly is asymptomatic while in his 30s and 40s, but he may report polyuria, urinary tract infections (UTIs), and other nonspecific symptoms. Your assessment may show hypertension.

Later assessment reveals overt symptoms caused by the enlarging kidney mass, such as lumbar pain, widening girth, and a swollen or tender abdomen. The patient states that abdominal pain usually is worsened by exertion and relieved by lying down. In advanced stages, palpation easily reveals grossly enlarged kidneys.

Diagnostic tests

In a patient with polycystic disease, these laboratory test results are typical.

- *Excretory* or *retrograde urography* reveals enlarged kidneys, with elongation of the pelvis, flattening of the calyces, and indentations caused by cysts.
- *Ultrasonography, tomography,* and *radioisotopic scans* show kidney enlargement and cysts; *tomography, computed tomography,* and *magnetic resonance imaging* show multiple areas of cystic damage.
- *Urinalysis* and *creatinine clearance tests*–nonspecific tests that evaluate renal function–indicate abnormalities.

Diagnosis must rule out renal tumors.

Treatment

Polycystic kidney disease can't be cured. The primary goal of treatment is to preserve renal parenchyma and prevent pyelonephritis. Progressive renal failure requires treatment similar to that for other types of renal disease, including dialysis or, rarely, kidney transplantation.

When polycystic kidney disease is discovered in the asymptomatic stage, careful monitoring is required, including urine cultures and creatinine clearance tests every 6 months. When urine culture detects infection, the patient needs prompt and vigorous antibiotic treatment, even if he has no symptoms.

As renal impairment progresses, selected patients may undergo dialysis, transplantation, or both. Cystic abscess or retroperitoneal bleeding may necessitate surgical drainage; intractable pain (an uncommon symptom) also may require surgery. Nephrectomy usually isn't recommended because this disease occurs bilaterally and the infection could recur in the remaining kidney.

Key nursing diagnoses and patient outcomes

Altered urinary elimination related to progressive renal failure. Based on this nursing diagnosis, you'll establish these patient outcomes. The patient will:

- maintain fluid balance with or without dialysis or transplantation
- demonstrate skill in managing urinary elimination problems caused by renal failure.

Risk for infection related to predisposition to UTI. Based on this nursing diagnosis, you'll establish these patient outcomes. The patient will:

- maintain a normal temperature and white blood cell count
- maintain a normal urine color and odor
- not show signs and symptoms of UTI, such as dysuria and hematuria.

Pain related to enlarging kidney mass. Based on this nursing diagnosis, you'll es-

tablish these patient outcomes. The patient will:

- express feelings of comfort following analgesic administration
- avoid or seek help with activities that precipitate or heighten pain.

Nursing interventions

- Provide supportive care to minimize any associated symptoms.
- Encourage the patient to rest, and help with activities of daily living when the patient has abdominal pain. Offer analgesics as needed.
- Acquaint yourself with all aspects of end-stage renal disease, including dialysis and transplantation, so that you can provide appropriate care and patient teaching as the disease progresses.
- Administer antibiotics, as ordered, for UTI. Provide adequate hydration during antibiotic therapy.
- Observe universal precautions when handling all blood and body fluids.
- Prepare the patient for peritoneal dialysis or hemodialysis, as indicated. (See the entries "Peritoneal dialysis" and "Hemodialysis.")
- Allow the patient to verbalize his fears and concerns about this progressive disorder.

Monitoring

- Monitor the patient's renal function regularly, as ordered. Measure his intake and output.
- Carefully evaluate the patient's life-style and physical and mental state. Determine how rapidly the disease is progressing. Use this information to plan individualized patient care.
- Screen urine for blood, cloudiness, and calculi or granules. Report any of these findings immediately.
- Before beginning excretory urography and other procedures that use an iodine-based contrast medium, ask the patient if he's ever had an allergic reaction to iodine or shellfish. Even if he says no, watch for a possible allergic reaction after the procedures.
- Monitor the patient for complications associated with polycystic kidney disease.

Patient teaching

- Discuss the patient's prognosis honestly, including such possible treatments as dialysis or transplantation; answer any questions.
- Explain all diagnostic procedures to the patient and his family. Review any treatments, such as dialysis.
- Discuss prescribed medications and their possible adverse effects. Stress the need to take medications exactly as prescribed even if symptoms are minimal or absent.
- Discuss possible screening and genetic counseling for other family members.

Polycythemia, secondary

Also called reactive polycythemia, secondary polycythemia is characterized by excessive production of circulating red blood cells (RBCs) due to hypoxia, tumor, or disease. It occurs in about 2 out of every 100,000 people who live at or near sea level; incidence is greater among people who live at high altitudes.

Causes

Secondary polycythemia may result from increased production of erythropoietin. This hormone, which is possibly produced and secreted in the kidneys, stimulates bone marrow production of RBCs. This increased production may be an appropriate (compensatory) physiologic response to hypoxemia, which may result from:

- chronic obstructive pulmonary disease
- hemoglobin abnormalities (such as carboxyhemoglobinemia, which occurs in heavy smokers)
- congestive heart failure (causing a decreased ventilation-perfusion ratio)
- right-to-left shunting of blood in the heart (as in transposition of the great vessels)

CHECKLIST

Key abnormal test values in secondary polycythemia

The following are critical laboratory values in secondary polycythemia.

- ☐ Erythrocyte count more than 6.2 million/μL in adult males and more than 5.4 million/μL in adult females
- ☐ Hematocrit higher than 54% for adult males and higher than 47% for adult females
- ☐ Hemoglobin levels above 18 g/dl for adult males and above 16 g/dl for adult females
- ☐ Mean corpuscular volume greater than 99 μ³/red cell
- ☐ Mean corpuscular hemoglobin more than 32 pg/red cell

• central or peripheral alveolar hypoventilation (as in barbiturate intoxication or Pickwickian syndrome)
• low oxygen content of air at high altitudes.

Increased production of erythropoietin may also be an inappropriate (pathologic) response to renal disease (such as renovascular impairment, renal cysts, and hydronephrosis), to central nervous system disease (such as encephalitis and parkinsonism), to neoplasms (such as renal tumors, uterine myomas, and cerebellar hemangiomas), and to endocrine disorders (such as Cushing's syndrome and pheochromocytomas). Rarely, secondary polycythemia results from a recessive genetic trait.

Complications

A patient with secondary polycythemia has an increased risk of hemorrhage due to problems with platelet quality, especially during surgery. Thromboemboli secondary to hemoconcentration may occur spontaneously; after prolonged immobility, as may occur with arthritic conditions or decreased mobility; or after surgery.

Assessment

The patient's history usually reveals shortness of breath (associated with emphysema). Inspection reveals a ruddy cyanosis of the skin and possibly clubbing of the fingers (in underlying cardiac or pulmonary disease). Hypoxemia is found without hepatosplenomegaly or hypertension, which constitutes a major difference between primary (vera) and secondary polycythemia.

Secondary polycythemia that isn't caused by hypoxemia is usually an incidental finding during treatment for an underlying disease.

Diagnostic tests

For critical laboratory test values, see *Key abnormal test values in secondary polycythemia.* Other characteristic results include:
• elevated urinary erythropoietin levels
• increased blood histamine levels
• decreased or normal arterial oxygen saturation.

Bone marrow biopsies reveal hyperplasia confined to the erythroid series. Unlike polycythemia vera, secondary polycythemia isn't associated with leukocytosis or thrombocytosis.

Treatment

The goal of treatment is correction of the underlying disease or environmental condition. When altitude is a contributing factor in severe secondary polycythemia, relocation may be advisable. If secondary polycythemia has produced hazardous hyperviscosity or if the patient doesn't respond to treatment for the primary disease, reduction of blood volume by phlebotomy or pheresis may be effective.

Emergency phlebotomy is indicated for prevention of impending vascular occlusion and before emergency surgery. In the latter case, removal of excess RBCs and reinfusion of the patient's plasma is usually advisable.

Key nursing diagnoses and patient outcomes

Activity intolerance related to hypoxemia. Based on this nursing diagnosis, you'll establish these patient outcomes. The patient will:
- identify controllable factors that cause fatigue
- demonstrate skill in conserving energy while carrying out daily activities to tolerance level
- communicate an understanding of the relationship between activity intolerance and secondary polycythemia.

Risk for fluid volume deficit related to potential for hemorrhage. Based on this nursing diagnosis, you'll establish these patient outcomes. The patient will:
- maintain hemodynamic stability, as exhibited by stable vital signs
- produce adequate urine volume to match fluid intake
- not show signs of excessive bleeding.

Risk for injury related to hyperviscosity. Based on this nursing diagnosis, you'll establish these patient outcomes. The patient will:
- maintain a tolerable activity level to prevent venous stasis
- show no signs or symptoms of tissue hypoxia as a result of thrombi or emboli
- comply with the prescribed treatment regimen.

Nursing interventions

- Encourage the patient to express any concerns about the disease, its treatments, and the effect that it may have on his life. Answer questions and provide emotional support. If possible, stay with the patient during periods of severe stress and anxiety.
- During phlebotomy, make sure the patient is lying down comfortably to prevent vertigo and syncope.
- After phlebotomy, have the patient sit up for about 5 minutes before allowing him to walk; this prevents vasovagal stimulation and orthostatic hypotension. Also, administer 24 oz (710 ml) of juice or water to replenish fluid volume.
- Support the patient's efforts to perform activities.
- Keep the patient as active as possible to decrease the risk of thrombosis due to increased blood viscosity. Provide rest periods between activities, as needed; the well-rested patient may be more active. If bed rest is necessary, incorporate a program of active and passive range-of-motion exercises into the patient's daily routine.
- Reduce caloric and sodium intake to counteract the tendency to hypertension. Provide meals that meet these requirements.
- Administer ordered medications, such as analgesics for headaches, as appropriate. Administer oxygen as ordered to maintain adequate tissue perfusion.

Monitoring

- Monitor the patient's blood studies for signs of improvement with therapy.
- Before phlebotomy or pheresis, check the patient's blood pressure while he's lying down. Also note pulse and respiratory rates. Stay alert for tachycardia, clamminess, and complaints of vertigo. If these reactions occur, the procedure should be stopped.
- Immediately after phlebotomy, check the patient's blood pressure and pulse rate while he's lying down.
- Monitor the patient for complications associated with secondary polycythemia.

Patient teaching

- Teach the patient and his family about the underlying disorder. Help them understand its relation to polycythemia, and describe measures to control both. Explain the disease process, its signs and symptoms, prescribed treatments, and any complications that may occur.

- Emphasize the importance of regular blood studies (every 2 to 3 months), even after the disease is controlled.
- Help the patient overcome potential noncompliance with a low-sodium, reduced-calorie diet. Suggest using herbs and spices to add flavor and removing fat and skin from meat before cooking. Refer the patient to the dietitian for additional teaching, if necessary.
- Instruct the patient to use an electric razor and to maintain a clutter-free environment to minimize falls and contusions.
- Caution the patient to avoid high altitudes, which may exacerbate polycythemia.
- Explain that alternating periods of rest and activity will reduce the body's demand for oxygen and prevent fatigue.
- Describe the advantages of following a cardiovascular fitness program (affirmed by the doctor), and encourage the patient to participate. If appropriate, suggest walking at a pace of at least 4 mph for 20 to 30 minutes four times per week.
- Refer the patient to the social service department and local home health care agencies, as appropriate.

Polycythemia, spurious

Characterized by increased hematocrit and normal or decreased red blood cell (RBC) total mass, spurious polycythemia results from decreasing plasma volume and subsequent hemoconcentration. This disease is also known as relative polycythemia, stress erythrocytosis, stress polycythemia, benign polycythemia, Gaisböck's syndrome, and pseudopolycythemia.

Causes

Possible causes of spurious polycythemia include the following.

- *Dehydration.* Conditions that promote severe fluid loss decrease plasma levels and lead to hemoconcentration. Such conditions include persistent vomiting or diarrhea, burns, adrenocortical insufficiency, aggressive diuretic therapy, decreased fluid intake, diabetic ketoacidosis, and renal disease.
- *Hemoconcentration due to stress.* Nervous stress leads to hemoconcentration by some unknown mechanism, possibly by temporarily decreasing circulating plasma volume or by vascular redistribution of erythrocytes.
- *High-normal RBC mass and low-normal plasma volume.* In many patients, an increased hematocrit merely reflects a normally high RBC mass and low plasma volume.

Other factors that may be associated with spurious polycythemia include hypertension, thromboembolic disease, pregnancy, elevated serum cholesterol and uric acid levels, and familial tendency.

Complications

Spurious polycythemia can be complicated by hypercholesterolemia, hyperlipidemia, and hyperuricemia. Thromboembolic complications may result if the condition goes untreated.

Assessment

The patient with spurious polycythemia usually has no specific signs or symptoms but may have vague complaints, such as headache, dizziness, and fatigue. Less commonly, the patient may report diaphoresis, dyspnea, and claudication. The patient's history may reveal existing cardiac or pulmonary disease.

Inspection typically reveals a patient with a ruddy appearance and a short neck. Palpation usually discloses associated hepatosplenomegaly. Auscultation may detect slight hypertension and hypoventilation when the patient is recumbent.

Diagnostic tests

Spurious polycythemia is distinguishable from polycythemia vera by its characteristic normal or decreased RBC mass, elevated hematocrit, and the absence of leukocytosis.

The results of other commonly performed laboratory tests include:
- elevated hemoglobin levels and hematocrit
- elevated RBC count
- normal arterial oxygen saturation and bone marrow studies
- normal or decreased plasma volume.

Treatment

The principal goals of treatment are to correct dehydration and to prevent life-threatening thromboembolism. Rehydration with appropriate fluids and electrolytes is the primary therapy for spurious polycythemia secondary to dehydration. Therapy must also include appropriate measures to prevent continuing fluid loss.

Key nursing diagnoses and patient outcomes

Fatigue related to decreased RBC mass. Based on this nursing diagnosis, you'll establish these patient outcomes. The patient will:
- identify measures to prevent or modify fatigue
- demonstrate skill in performing activities of daily living with minimal fatigue
- report increased energy with treatment.

Fluid volume deficit related to dehydration. Based on this nursing diagnosis, you'll establish these patient outcomes. The patient will:
- regain normal fluid volume balance
- take precautions to prevent a recurrence of dehydration.

Risk for injury related to potential for thromboembolism. Based on this nursing diagnosis, you'll establish these patient outcomes. The patient will:
- maintain a tolerable activity level to prevent venous stasis
- not have signs and symptoms of tissue ischemia as a result of thrombi or emboli formation
- comply with the prescribed treatment.

Nursing interventions

- Focus your care on rehydration, a cardiovascular diet and exercise regimen, and patient teaching about the condition and related stress factors.
- Encourage the patient to discuss his concerns about the disease, its treatments, and the effect it may have on his life. Answer questions appropriately, and provide emotional support.
- Keep the patient active and ambulatory to prevent thrombosis. If he complains of fatigue, alternate periods of rest and activity.
- To prevent thromboemboli in predisposed patients, initiate a cardiovascular exercise program coupled with a reduced dietary cholesterol plan. (Studies show that hypertension and hypercholesterolemia can be reduced by the combination of regular exercise and a diet low in fat and cholesterol.) Antilipemics, such as cholestyramine or gemfibrozil, may be added to the treatment plan when exercise and dietary control are unsuccessful.
- If the patient hypoventilates when recumbent, elevate the head of the bed.

Monitoring

- Assess the patient's hematologic status regularly.
- During rehydration, monitor intake and output to maintain fluid balance. Also monitor laboratory studies to maintain electrolyte balance.
- Auscultate the patient's breath sounds every 4 hours.
- Monitor the patient for complications of spurious polycythemia.

Patient teaching

- Thoroughly explain the disease, including its diagnosis and treatment. The hard-driving person who is predisposed to spurious polycythemia is likely to be more inquisitive and anxious than the average patient. Answer his questions honestly, and reassure him that he can effectively control symptoms by complying with the prescribed treatment.

- Emphasize the need for follow-up examinations every 3 to 4 months after leaving the hospital.
- Caution the patient to follow a doctor-prescribed exercise program and diet. Results should be checked during follow-up examinations.
- When appropriate, suggest counseling about the patient's work habits and lack of relaxation. If the patient is a smoker, emphasize the importance of stopping. Then, refer him to an antismoking program if necessary.
- Teach the patient to recognize and report signs and symptoms of increasing polycythemia and thromboembolism.
- Instruct the patient to use an electric razor and to maintain a clutter-free environment to minimize falls and contusions.
- Refer the patient to the social service department and local home health care agencies, as appropriate.

Polycythemia vera

A chronic, myeloproliferative disorder, polycythemia vera is characterized by increased red blood cell (RBC) mass, leukocytosis, thrombocytosis, and increased hemoglobin concentration, with normal or decreased plasma volume. It usually occurs between ages 40 and 60, most commonly among men of Jewish ancestry; it seldom affects children or blacks and doesn't appear to be familial.

The onset of polycythemia is gradual, and the disease runs a chronic but slowly progressive course. The prognosis depends on age at diagnosis, treatment used, and complications. Mortality is high if polycythemia is untreated or is associated with leukemia or myeloid metaplasia. (Polycythemia vera is also known as primary polycythemia, erythremia, polycythemia rubra vera, splenomegalic polycythemia, and Vaquez's disease.)

Causes

In polycythemia vera, uncontrolled and rapid cellular reproduction and maturation cause proliferation or hyperplasia of all bone marrow cells (panmyelosis). The cause of such uncontrolled cellular activity is unknown, but it is probably the result of a multipotential stem cell defect.

Complications

Hyperviscosity may lead to thrombosis of small vessels, with ruddy cyanosis of the nose and clubbing (stunting) of the digits. Further thromboembolic involvement can lead to splenomegaly, renal calculus formation, and abdominal organ thrombosis.

Paradoxically, hemorrhage is a complication of polycythemia vera. It may be due to defective platelet function or to hyperviscosity and the local effects from excess RBCs exerting pressure on distended venous and capillary walls.

Cerebrovascular accident (CVA) may also complicate the disease. As well, incidence of peptic ulcer disease is four to five times greater in patients with polycythemia vera than in the general population.

Assessment

In its early stages, polycythemia vera may produce no signs or symptoms. However, as altered circulation (secondary to increased RBC mass) produces hypervolemia and hyperviscosity, the patient may report a vague feeling of fullness in the head, rushing in the ears, tinnitus, headache, dizziness, vertigo, epistaxis, night sweats, epigastric and joint pain, and visual alterations such as scotomas, double vision, and blurred vision. He may also report a decrease in urine output, possibly due to increased uric acid production.

Late in the disease, the patient may report pruritus (which worsens after bathing and may be disabling), a sense of abdominal fullness, and pain such as pleuritic chest pain or left upper quadrant pain. (See *Clinical features of polycythemia vera,* page 740.)

Diagnostic tests

Laboratory studies confirm polycythemia vera by showing increased RBC mass and normal arterial oxygen saturation in association with splenomegaly or two of the following:

- platelet count above 400,000/mm³ (thrombocytosis)
- white blood cell (WBC) count above 10,000/mm³ in adults (leukocytosis)
- elevated leukocyte alkaline phosphatase level
- elevated serum vitamin B_{12} levels or increased B_{12}–binding capacity.

Another common finding is increased uric acid production, leading to hyperuricemia and hyperuricuria. Other laboratory results include increased blood histamine, decreased serum iron concentration, and decreased or absent urinary erythropoietin. Bone marrow biopsy reveals panmyelosis.

Treatment

Phlebotomy, the primary treatment, can be performed repeatedly and can reduce RBC mass promptly. It's best used for patients with mild disease or for young patients. The frequency of phlebotomy and the amount of blood removed each time depend on the patient's condition. Typically, 350 to 500 ml of blood can be removed every other day until the patient's hematocrit is reduced to the low-normal range. After repeated phlebotomies, the patient will develop iron deficiency, which stabilizes RBC production and reduces the need for phlebotomy. However, phlebotomy doesn't reduce the WBC or platelet count and won't control the hyperuricemia associated with marrow cell proliferation.

Myelosuppressant therapy may be used for patients with severe symptoms, such as extreme thrombocytosis, a rapidly enlarging spleen, and hypermetabolism. It's also used for elderly patients who have difficulty tolerating the phlebotomy procedure. Radioactive phosphorus (^{32}P) or chemotherapeutic agents, such as melphalan, busulfan, and chlorambucil, can satisfactorily control the disease in most cases. However, these agents may cause leukemia and should be reserved for older patients and those with serious problems not controlled by phlebotomy. Patients of any age who have had previous thrombotic problems should be considered for myelosuppressant therapy.

Pheresis technology allows removal of RBCs, WBCs, and platelets individually or collectively (and provides these cellular components for blood banks). Pheresis also permits the return of plasma to the patient, thereby diluting the blood and reducing hypovolemic symptoms.

As appropriate, additional treatments include administration of cyproheptadine (12 to 16 mg/day) and allopurinol (300 mg/day) to reduce serum uric acid levels. Treatment usually improves symptomatic splenomegaly; rarely, splenectomy may be performed.

Key nursing diagnoses and patient outcomes

Altered nutrition: Less than body requirements related to adverse GI effects. Based on this nursing diagnosis, you'll establish these patient outcomes. The patient will:

- regain and maintain his weight within the normal range
- be able to tolerate an oral intake and consume a nutritionally balanced diet daily
- show no signs and symptoms of malnutrition.

Altered cardiovascular tissue perfusion related to hyperviscosity and hypervolemia. Based on this nursing diagnosis, you'll establish these patient outcomes. The patient will:

Clinical features of polycythemia vera

Signs and symptoms	Causes
Eye and ear • Visual disturbances (blurring, diplopia, scotoma, engorged veins of fundus and retina) and congestion of conjunctiva, retina, and retinal veins	• Hypervolemia and hyperviscosity • Engorgement of capillary beds
Nose and mouth • Epistaxis or gingival bleeding • Oral mucous membrane congestion	• Hypervolemia and hyperviscosity • Engorgement of capillary beds
Central nervous system • Headache or fullness in the head, lethargy, weakness, fatigue, syncope, dizziness, vertigo, tinnitus, paresthesia of digits, and impaired mentation	• Hypervolemia and hyperviscosity
Cardiovascular system • Hypertension • Intermittent claudication, thrombosis and emboli, angina, thrombophlebitis • Hemorrhage	• Hypervolemia and hyperviscosity • Hypervolemia, thrombocytosis, and vascular disease • Engorgement of capillary beds
Skin • Pruritus (especially after hot bath) • Urticaria • Ruddy cyanosis • Night sweats • Ecchymosis	• Basophilia (secondary histamine release) • Altered histamine metabolism • Hypervolemia and hyperviscosity due to congested vessels, increased oxyhemoglobin, and reduced hemoglobin levels • Hypermetabolism • Hemorrhage
GI system • Epigastric distress • Early abdominal fullness • Peptic ulcer pain • Hepatosplenomegaly • Weight loss	• Hypervolemia and hyperviscosity • Hepatosplenomegaly • Gastric thrombosis and hemorrhage • Congestion, extramedullary hemopoiesis, and myeloid metaplasia • Hypermetabolism
Respiratory system • Dyspnea	• Hypervolemia and hyperviscosity
Musculoskeletal system • Joint pain	• Increased urate production secondary to nucleoprotein turnover

- comply with the prescribed treatment to decrease blood viscosity and volume
- not show ischemic changes suggestive of angina or intermittent claudication
- regain and maintain normal tissue perfusion.

Sensory/perceptual alteration (visual) related to increased RBC mass. Based on

this nursing diagnosis, you'll establish these patient outcomes. The patient will:
• remain safe in his environment
• use safety precautions when ambulating and performing activities of daily living
• regain normal visual functioning.

Nursing interventions

• Encourage the patient to express any concerns about the disease, its treatment, and the effect that it may have on his life. Answer questions appropriately, and provide emotional support. If possible, stay with the patient during periods of acute stress and anxiety.
• Keep the patient active and ambulatory to prevent thrombosis. If bed rest is necessary, incorporate a program of both active and passive range-of-motion exercises into the patient's daily routine.
• To compensate for increased uric acid production, give the patient additional fluids, administer allopurinol (as ordered), and alkalinize the urine to prevent uric acid calculus formation.
• If the patient has symptomatic splenomegaly, suggest or provide small, frequent meals, followed by a rest period, to prevent nausea and vomiting.
• If the patient has pruritus, give medications (as ordered) and provide distractions to help him cope.
• During phlebotomy, make sure the patient is lying down comfortably, to prevent vertigo and syncope. After the phlebotomy, have the patient sit up for about 5 minutes before allowing him to walk; this prevents vasovagal attack and orthostatic hypotension. Also, administer 24 oz (710 ml) of juice or water to replenish fluid volume.
• If leukopenia develops during myelosuppressant chemotherapy in a hospitalized patient, follow hospital guidelines for reverse isolation, as ordered.
• If nausea and vomiting occur with myelosuppressant chemotherapy, begin antiemetic therapy and adjust the patient's diet.
• Make sure you have a blood sample for complete blood count (CBC) and platelet count before beginning treatment with ^{32}P. (*Note:* The health care professional who administers ^{32}P should take radiation precautions to prevent contamination.) Have the patient lie down during I.V. administration (to facilitate the procedure and prevent extravasation) and for 15 to 20 minutes afterward.

Monitoring

• Watch for complications, such as hypervolemia, thrombocytosis, and signs of an impending CVA (decreased sensation, numbness, transitory paralysis, fleeting blindness, headache, and epistaxis).
• Regularly examine the patient for bleeding.
• Monitor and report acute abdominal pain immediately; it may signal splenic infarction, renal calculus formation, or abdominal organ thrombosis.
• Before phlebotomy, check the patient's blood pressure and pulse and respiratory rates. Stay alert for tachycardia, clamminess, and complaints of vertigo. If these effects occur, the procedure should be stopped. Then, immediately after phlebotomy, check the patient's blood pressure and pulse rate.
• Monitor CBC and platelet count before and during myelosuppressant therapy. Watch for and report all adverse reactions that occur after administration of an alkylating agent.

Patient teaching

• Determine what the patient knows about the disease, especially if he has been diagnosed for some time. As necessary, reinforce the doctor's explanation of the disease process, signs and symptoms, and prescribed treatment.
• Tell the patient to remain as active as possible to help maintain his self-esteem.
• Instruct the patient to use an electric razor to prevent accidental cuts and to keep

his environment free of clutter to minimize falls and contusions.
• If the patient develops thrombocytopenia, tell him which are the most common bleeding sites (such as the nose, gingiva, and skin), so he can check for bleeding. Advise him to report any abnormal bleeding promptly.
• Advise the patient to avoid high altitudes, which may exacerbate polycythemia.
• If the patient requires phlebotomy, describe the procedure and explain that it will relieve distressing symptoms. Tell the patient to watch for and report any symptoms of iron deficiency (pallor, weight loss, asthenia, glossitis).
• If the patient requires myelosuppressant therapy, tell him about possible adverse reactions (nausea, vomiting, and susceptibility to infection) that may follow administration of an alkylating agent. As appropriate, mention that alopecia may follow the use of busulfan, cyclophosphamide, and uracil mustard and that sterile hemorrhagic cystitis may follow the use of cyclophosphamide (forcing fluids can prevent this adverse reaction).
• If an outpatient develops leukopenia, reinforce instructions about preventing infection. Warn the patient that his resistance to infection is low; advise him to avoid crowds, and make sure he knows the symptoms of infection.
• If the patient requires treatment with ^{32}P, explain the procedure. Tell him that he may require repeated phlebotomies until ^{32}P takes effect.
• Refer the patient to the social service department and local home health care agencies, as appropriate.

Porphyrias

An umbrella term, porphyrias are metabolic disorders that affect the biosynthesis of heme (a component of hemoglobin) and cause excessive production and excretion of porphyrins or their precursors. Porphyrins, which are present in all protoplasm, play a role in energy storage and use. The classification of porphyrias depends on the site of excessive porphyrin production: They may be erythropoietic (erythroid cells in bone marrow), hepatic (in the liver), or erythrohepatic (in bone marrow and in the liver).

Causes

Porphyrias are inherited as autosomal dominant traits, except for Günther's disease (an autosomal recessive trait) and toxic-acquired porphyria (usually a result of lead ingestion or lead exposure). Enzymatic defects occurring in the heme synthetic pathway cause porphyrias.

Complications

Hepatic porphyrias may result in neurologic and hepatic dysfunction. Acute intermittent porphyria may result in flaccid paralysis, respiratory paralysis, and death. Erythropoietic porphyrias may cause hemolytic anemia.

Assessment

Clinical findings vary widely, depending on the clinical variant of porphyria. (See *Types of porphyria.*)

A patient with hepatic porphyria may complain of mild or severe abdominal pain, possibly accompanied by nausea, vomiting, and constipation. Many patients with porphyrias also report photosensitivity. The patient history may help pinpoint precipitating factors, such as the use of certain medications, hormonal changes during the menstrual and premenstrual cycles, infection, and malnutrition.

Neurologic examination may reveal paresthesia, hypoesthesia, neuritic pain, psychosis, and seizures.

Depending on the type of porphyria, inspection findings may include skin lesions (possibly associated with erythema, altered pigmentation, and edema in areas exposed to light); changes in urine color;

Types of porphyria

Type	Clinical findings	Treatment
Erythropoietic porphyria *Günther's disease* • Usual onset before age 5 • Extremely rare	• Red urine (earliest, most characteristic sign); severe cutaneous photosensitivity, leading to vesicular or bullous eruptions on exposed areas and eventual scarring and ulceration • Hypertrichosis • Brown- or red-stained teeth • Splenomegaly, hemolytic anemia	• Beta carotene for photosensitivity, anti-inflammatory ointments, prednisone to reverse anemia • Packed RBCs inhibit erythropoiesis and excreted porphyrins • Hemin for recurrent attacks • Splenectomy for hemolytic anemia • Topical dihydroxyacetone and Lawson sunscreen filter • Cholestyramine and charcoal reduce porphyrin reabsorption
Erythrohepatic porphyria *Protoporphyria* • Usually affects children • More common in males	• Photosensitive dermatitis • Hemolytic anemia • Chronic hepatic disease	• Avoidance of causative factors • Beta carotene to reduce photosensitivity
Toxic-acquired porphyria • Usually affects children • Significant mortality	• GI symptoms; neuromuscular weakness; behavioral changes; seizures; coma	• Chlorpromazine I.V. for GI symptoms • Avoidance of lead exposure
Hepatic porphyria *Acute intermittent porphyria* • Most common form • More prevalent in females, usually between ages 15 and 40	• Colicky abdominal pain with fever, general malaise, and hypertension • Peripheral neuritis, behavior changes, possibly leading to frank psychosis • Respiratory paralysis possible	• Chlorpromazine I.V. for psychic abnormalities; meperidine for pain • Avoidance of precipitating medications, infections, alcohol, and fasting • Hemin for recurrent attacks • High carbohydrate diet; I.V. glucose
Variegate porphyria • Onset: ages 30 to 50 • Occurs almost exclusively among South African whites • Affects males and females equally	• Skin lesions, fragile skin • Hypertrichosis of face and temples; hyperpigmentation • Abdominal pain in acute attack; behavioral changes	• High-carbohydrate diet • Avoidance of sunlight, or wearing of protective clothing and use of sunscreen • Hemin for recurrent attacks
Porphyria cutanea tarda • Most common in men ages 40 to 60; highest incidence in South Africans	• Facial pigmentation • Red-brown urine • Photosensitivity dermatitis • Hypertrichosis	• Avoidance of alcohol, estrogen, sun exposure, and iron • Phlebotomy at 2-week intervals to lower serum iron level
Hereditary coproporphyria • Rare • Affects males and females equally	• Asymptomatic or mild neurologic, abdominal, or psychiatric symptoms	• High-carbohydrate diet • Avoidance of barbiturates • Hemin for recurrent attacks

and neurologic signs, such as wristdrop and footdrop. If hemolytic anemia occurs, expect to find splenomegaly on palpation.

In a patient with acute intermittent porphyria, auscultation may reveal wheezing and dyspnea, compounded by the patient's anxiety. During an acute attack, fever may occur.

Diagnostic tests

- In acute intermittent porphyria, the Watson-Schwartz test may be positive for porphobilinogen in the urine; the ion exchange chromatography test may identify aminolevulinic acid in the urine.
- In variegate porphyria, protoporphyrin and coproporphyrin may be positive in the stools. With hereditary coproporphyria, large amounts of coproporphyrin appear in the stools and, to a lesser extent, in the urine.
- Porphyria cutanea tarda results in increased excretion of uroporphyrins; the amount of fecal porphyrins varies.
- With Günther's disease, porphyrins are found in the urine, especially uroporphyrin I.
- With erythropoietic protoporphyria, fluorescent microscopy is used to confirm the diagnosis by detecting excess protoporphyrin in the red blood cells.
- A urine lead level of 0.2 mg/liter helps confirm toxic-acquired porphyria.

Other laboratory values may include increased serum iron levels in porphyria cutanea tarda; leukocytosis and elevated bilirubin and alkaline phosphatase levels in acute intermittent porphyria.

Treatment

Depending on the type of porphyria, treatment may include the administration of beta carotene to reduce photosensitivity, chlorpromazine I.V. to treat mild abdominal discomfort, meperidine to treat severe pain, levulose I.V. to increase carbohydrate intake, and hemin to suppress hepatic aminolevulinic acid and porphobilinogen. Splenectomy may be performed to treat hemolytic anemia. Patients with photosensitivity are advised to avoid direct sunlight or to use sunscreen.

Key nursing diagnoses and patient outcomes

Altered protection related to photosensitivity. Based on this nursing diagnosis, you'll establish these patient outcomes. The patient will:

- incorporate sun precautions into his daily routine
- show no evidence of skin lesions caused by sun exposure.

Risk for injury related to neurologic dysfunction. Based on this nursing diagnosis, you'll establish these patient outcomes. The patient will:

- remain safe in his environment
- incorporate safety precautions into his daily routine
- not suffer injury because of neurologic dysfunction.

Impaired gas exchange related to respiratory muscle weakness caused by acute intermittent porphyria. Based on this nursing diagnosis, you'll establish these patient outcomes. The patient will:

- regain and maintain adequate ventilation
- regain and maintain normal arterial blood gas levels
- show no signs and symptoms of hypoxia.

Nursing interventions

- Before administering medications to the patient, make certain the drugs don't precipitate an acute attack. (See *Drugs that aggravate porphyria.*)
- Administer hemin by a large arm vein or central venous catheter, as ordered. Overdosage may result in renal shutdown.
- Provide emotional support, and encourage the patient to verbalize his concerns about his condition.
- Prepare the patient with hemolytic anemia for splenectomy, if indicated. (See the entry "Splenectomy.")

In acute intermittent porphyria:

• Provide active and passive range-of-motion exercises every 8 hours. Position the patient's body in proper alignment, using splinting as necessary.
• Take safety precautions, as indicated. Use padded side rails, and keep an oral airway at the bedside if seizure activity is possible.
• If the patient is experiencing an acute attack, administer comfort measures, including mouth care, skin care, and massage every 2 hours, with positioning and pulmonary hygiene. Administer analgesics, as ordered.

Monitoring

• During acute intermittent porphyria, assess respiratory status every 2 hours; respiratory depression or paralysis requires mechanical ventilation. Observe for signs and symptoms of decreased GI motility, resulting in distention, ileus, vomiting, and constipation.
• Monitor the patient for photosensitivity reactions, such as the appearance of skin lesions after sun exposure.
• Monitor the patient's pain level and response to meperidine, if appropriate.

Patient teaching

• Warn the patient against excessive sun exposure.
• Stress the importance of wearing a medical identification bracelet or necklace.
• If the patient has toxic-acquired porphyria, discuss sources of lead and refer him to resources that can identify such sources in the home.
• Warn the patient to avoid precipitating factors, including crash dieting; fasting; and the use of specific drugs, such as alcohol, estrogens, and barbiturates. Teach stress-management techniques because emotional stress may also precipitate an acute attack. Discuss measures to help prevent infection, another precipitating factor.

NURSING ALERT

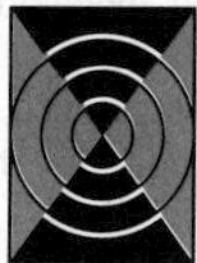

Drugs that aggravate porphyria

Make sure the patient with porphyria doesn't receive any of the following drugs, which are known to precipitate signs and symptoms of porphyria:

• alcohol
• barbiturates
• carbamazepine
• carisoprodol
• chloramphenicol
• chlordiazepoxide
• danazol
• diazepam
• ergot alkaloids
• estrogens
• glutethimide
• griseofulvin
• imipramine
• meprobamate
• methsuximide
• methyldopa
• methylprylon
• pentazocine
• phenytoin
• progesterones
• sulfonamides
• tolbutamide.

• Encourage a high-carbohydrate diet to provide sufficient calories without taxing the liver to break down proteins.

Potassium imbalance

A cation that's the dominant cellular electrolyte, potassium facilitates contraction of both skeletal and smooth muscles, including myocardial contraction. It figures prominently in nerve impulse conduction, acid-base balance, enzyme action, and cell membrane function. Because serum potassium level has such a narrow range (3.5 to 5 mEq/liter), a slight deviation in either direction can produce profound consequences.

Causes

Hypokalemia rarely results from a dietary deficiency because many foods contain po-

tassium. Instead, potassium loss results from:
• excessive GI losses, such as from vomiting, gastric suction, diarrhea, villous adenoma, or laxative abuse
• chronic renal disease, with tubular potassium wasting
• certain drugs, especially potassium-wasting diuretics, steroids, and certain sodium-containing antibiotics (carbenicillin)
• alkalosis or insulin effect, which causes potassium shifting into cells without true depletion of total body potassium
• prolonged potassium-free I.V. therapy
• hyperglycemia, causing osmotic diuresis and glycosuria
• Cushing's syndrome, primary hyperaldosteronism, excessive ingestion of licorice, and severe serum magnesium deficiency.

Hyperkalemia usually results from reduced excretion by the kidneys. This may be due to acute or severe chronic renal failure, oliguria due to shock or severe dehydration, or the use of potassium-sparing diuretics (such as triamterene) by patients with renal disease. Inadequate potassium excretion may also be due to hypoaldosteronism or Addison's disease.

Hyperkalemia may also result from failure to excrete excessive amounts of potassium infused I.V. or administered orally. Another cause is massive release of intracellular potassium, such as can occur with burns, crushing injuries, severe infection, or acidosis.

Complications

Potassium imbalances may result in muscle weakness and flaccid paralysis and may also lead to cardiac arrest. (See *ECG changes in potassium imbalance.*)

Assessment

The patient's history and physical examination may reveal cardiovascular irregularities manifested by dizziness, postural hypotension, and arrhythmias.

GI complaints may include nausea and vomiting, anorexia, abdominal distention, constipation, paralytic ileus, and decreased peristalsis (with hypokalemia) or nausea, diarrhea, and abdominal cramps (with hyperkalemia).

The patient may also experience neuromuscular symptoms, such as weakness and hyporeflexia (with hypokalemia); skeletal muscle weakness, numbness, and tingling (with hyperkalemia); and flaccid paralysis or respiratory paralysis (with both imbalances).

Diagnostic tests

Serum potassium levels definitively diagnose a potassium abnormality. In hypokalemia, potassium levels are less than 3.5 mEq/liter. In hyperkalemia, levels are more than 5 mEq/liter.

Additional tests may be necessary to determine the cause of the imbalance.

Treatment

Hypokalemia treatment should involve increased dietary intake of potassium or oral supplements with potassium salts. Potassium chloride is the preferred choice. Edematous patients with diuretic-induced hypokalemia should receive a potassium-sparing diuretic, such as spironolactone.

Patients with GI potassium loss or severe potassium depletion require I.V. potassium replacement therapy. If hypocalcemia is also present, treatment should include calcium replacement. (See *Guidelines for I.V. potassium administration,* page 748.)

For hyperkalemia, treatment consists of withholding potassium and administering a cation exchange resin orally or by enema. Sodium polystyrene sulfonate (Kayexalate) with 70% sorbitol produces exchange of sodium ions for potassium ions in the intestine.

In an emergency, rapid infusion of 10% calcium gluconate decreases myocardial irritability and temporarily prevents cardiac arrest but doesn't correct serum po-

ECG changes in potassium imbalance

Hypokalemia and hyperkalemia can induce cardiac arrhythmias. The solid-line waveforms below represent normal sinus rhythms and the dotted waveforms show ECG changes caused by hypokalemia and hyperkalemia.

Hypokalemia

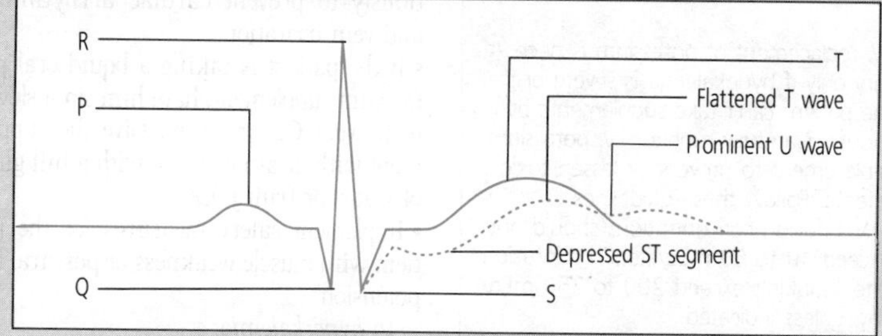

Hyperkalemia

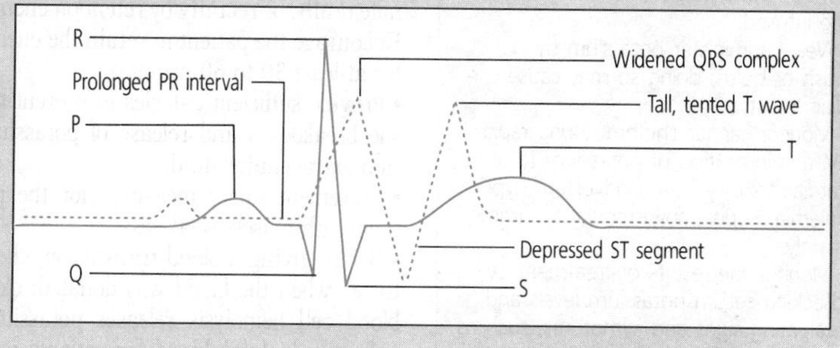

tassium excess; this therapy is contraindicated in patients receiving digitalis glycosides.

Also as an emergency measure, sodium bicarbonate I.V. increases pH and causes potassium to shift back into the cells. Insulin and 10% to 50% glucose I.V. also move potassium back into cells. Infusions should be followed by dextrose 5% in water because infusion of 10% to 15% glucose will stimulate secretion of endogenous insulin. Hemodialysis or peritoneal dialysis also aids in removal of excess potassium; however, these are slow techniques.

Key nursing diagnoses and patient outcomes

Activity intolerance related to neuromuscular dysfunction. Based on this nursing diagnosis, you'll establish these patient outcomes. The patient will:

- seek and obtain assistance with activities of daily living
- regain normal neuromuscular function with restoration of a normal serum potassium level.

Altered nutrition: Less than body requirements related to adverse GI effects. Based on this nursing diagnosis, you'll establish these patient outcomes. The patient will:

NURSING ALERT

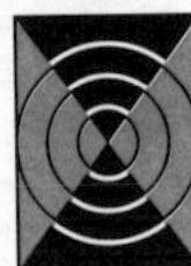

Guidelines for I.V. potassium administration

I.V. replacement of potassium is necessary only if hypokalemia is severe or if the patient can't take supplements by mouth. Carefully monitor I.V. potassium replacement to prevent or lessen toxic effects. Follow these guidelines.

- I.V. infusion concentrations should not exceed 40 to 60 mEq/liter. The infusion rate shouldn't exceed 200 to 250 mEq/day, unless indicated.
- Use volumetric devices whenever concentrations of more than 40 mEq/liter are infused.
- *Never* administer potassium by I.V. push or bolus; doing so may cause cardiac arrest.
- Monitor cardiac rhythm during rapid I.V. administration of potassium to avoid cardiac toxicity from inadvertent hyperkalemia. Report any irregularities immediately.
- Monitor the results of treatment by checking serum potassium levels and evaluating signs and symptoms, such as muscle weakness or paralysis.
- Monitor the I.V. site for signs and symptoms of infiltration, phlebitis, or tissue necrosis.

- maintain a normal weight
- tolerate oral food intake
- obtain relief from adverse GI effects with restoration of a normal serum potassium level.

Decreased cardiac output related to arrhythmias. Based on this nursing diagnosis, you'll establish these patient outcomes. The patient will:

- regain and maintain normal cardiac output, as exhibited by stable vital signs
- regain a normal electrocardiogram (ECG) pattern with alleviation of potassium imbalance.

Nursing interventions

In hypokalemia:

- Because of the risk of potassium toxicity, administer I.V. potassium slowly and cautiously to prevent cardiac arrhythmias and vein irritation.
- If the patient is taking a liquid oral potassium supplement, have him sip it slowly to prevent GI irritation. Give the supplement with or after meals, with a full glass of water or fruit juice.
- Implement safety measures for the patient with muscle weakness or postural hypotension.

In hyperkalemia:

- Administer sodium polystyrene sulfonate orally, or rectally by retention enema. Encourage the patient to retain the enema for at least 30 to 60 minutes.
- Provide sufficient calories to prevent tissue breakdown and release of potassium into extracellular fluid.
- Implement safety measures for the patient with muscle weakness.
- Before giving a blood transfusion, check to see when the blood was donated; older blood cell hemolysis releases potassium. Infuse only *fresh* blood for patients with average to high serum potassium levels.

Monitoring

In hypokalemia:

- Frequently monitor serum potassium and other electrolyte levels during potassium replacement therapy to avoid overcorrection leading to hyperkalemia.
- Assess intake and output carefully. Remember, the kidneys excrete 80% to 90% of ingested potassium. Never give supplementary potassium to a patient whose urine output is below 600 ml/day. Also, measure GI loss from suctioning or vomiting.
- Assess for abdominal distention, decreased bowel sounds, and constipation.

• Carefully monitor patients receiving digitalis glycosides because hypokalemia enhances their action. Assess for signs of digitalis toxicity (anorexia, nausea, vomiting, blurred vision, and arrhythmias).
• Monitor cardiac rhythm, and report any irregularities immediately.

In hyperkalemia:

• As in hypokalemia, frequently monitor serum potassium and other electrolyte levels and carefully record intake and output.
• Watch for signs of hypokalemia with prolonged use of sodium polystyrene sulfonate.
• Assess for clinical effects of hypoglycemia (muscle weakness, syncope, hunger, diaphoresis) with repeated insulin and glucose treatment.
• Monitor for and report cardiac arrhythmias.
• Assess GI functioning for abdominal distention, intestinal cramping, and diarrhea.
• Watch for signs of hyperkalemia in predisposed patients, especially those with poor urine output or those receiving potassium supplements by mouth or I.V.

Patient teaching

• To prevent hypokalemia, instruct patients (especially those taking diuretics) to include potassium-rich foods in their diets. Such foods include oranges, bananas, tomatoes, milk, dried fruits, apricots, peanuts, and dark-green, leafy vegetables.
• To prevent hyperkalemia, tell patients who use salt substitutes containing potassium to discontinue them if urine output decreases.
• Emphasize the importance of taking potassium supplements as prescribed, particularly if the patient is also taking digitalis glycosides or diuretics. If appropriate, teach the patient to recognize and report signs of digitalis toxicity, such as pulse irregularities. Demonstrate the proper technique for assessing the patient's pulse.
• Make sure the patient can recognize signs of hypokalemia and hyperkalemia, including weakness and pulse irregularities. Tell him to report such signs to the doctor.

Pressure ulcers

Localized areas of cellular necrosis, pressure ulcers occur most often in the skin and subcutaneous tissue over bony prominences, particularly the sacrum, ischial tuberosities, greater trochanter, heels, malleoli, and elbows. These ulcers – also called decubitus ulcers, pressure sores, or bedsores – may be superficial, caused by local skin irritation (with subsequent surface maceration), or deep, originating in underlying tissue. Deep lesions often go undetected until they penetrate the skin; by then, they've usually caused subcutaneous damage.

Causes

Pressure, particularly over bony prominences, interrupts normal circulatory function and causes most pressure ulcers. The intensity and duration of such pressure govern the severity of the ulcer; pressure exerted over an area for a moderate period (1 to 2 hours) produces tissue ischemia and increased capillary pressure, leading to edema and multiple small-vessel thromboses. An inflammatory reaction gives way to ulceration and necrosis of ischemic cells. In turn, necrotic tissue predisposes the body to bacterial invasion and infection.

Shearing force, the force applied when tissue layers move over one another, can also cause ulcerations. This force stretches the skin, compressing local circulation. As an example, if the head of the patient's bed is raised, gravity tends to pull the patient downward and forward, creating a shearing force. The friction of the patient's skin against the bed, such as occurs when a patient slides himself up in bed rather than lifting his hips, compounds the problem.

Moisture, whether from perspiration or incontinence, can also cause pressure ulcers. Such moisture softens skin layers and provides an environment for bacterial growth, leading to skin breakdown.

Other factors that can predispose a patient to pressure ulcers and also delay healing include poor nutrition, diabetes mellitus, paralysis, cardiovascular disorders, and aging. Added risks include obesity, insufficient weight, edema, anemia, poor hygiene, and exposure to chemicals.

Complications

Bacterial invasion and secondary infection, possibly leading to bacteremia and septicemia, are common complications of pressure ulcers. If the ulcer is large, a continuous loss of serum may deplete the body of its normal circulating fluids and essential proteins. In severe cases, ulcers may extend through subcutaneous fat layers, fibrous tissue, and muscle until reaching the bone.

Assessment

The patient with a pressure ulcer will have a history of one or more predisposing factors. Inspection of an early, superficial lesion notes shiny, erythematous changes over the compressed area, caused by localized vasodilation when pressure is relieved. If the superficial erythema has progressed, you'll see small blisters or erosions and ultimately necrosis and ulceration.

In underlying damage from pressure between deep tissue and bone, you'll note an inflamed skin surface area. Bacteria in a compressed site cause inflammation and, eventually, infection, which leads to further necrosis. You may detect a foul-smelling, purulent discharge seeping from a lesion that has penetrated the skin from beneath. A black eschar may develop around and over the lesion because infected, necrotic tissue prevents healthy granulation of scar tissue. (See *Stages of pressure ulcers.*)

Diagnostic tests

Wound culture and sensitivity testing of the ulcer exudate identify infecting organisms. Serum protein and serum albumin studies may be ordered to determine severe hypoproteinemia.

Treatment

Prevention is most important in pressure ulcers, by such means as movement and exercise to improve circulation and adequate nutrition to maintain skin health. When pressure ulcers do develop, successful management involves relieving pressure on the affected area, keeping the area clean and dry, and promoting healing. To relieve pressure, devices such as pads, mattresses, and special beds may be used. Bear in mind that turning and repositioning are still necessary. (See *Pressure-relief devices,* page 752.) In addition, a diet high in protein, iron, and vitamin C will help promote healing.

Other treatments depend on the ulcer stage. Stage 1 treatment aims to increase tissue pliability, stimulate local circulation, promote healing, and prevent skin breakdown. Specific measures include the use of lubricants (such as Lubriderm), clear plastic dressings (Op-Site), gelatin-type wafers (DuoDerm), vasodilator sprays (Proderm), and whirlpool baths.

For Stage 2 ulcers, additional treatments include cleaning the ulcer with 0.9% sodium chloride solution or water and hydrogen peroxide. This removes ulcer debris and helps prevent further skin damage and infection.

Therapy for Stage 3 or 4 ulcers aims to treat existing infection, prevent further infection, and remove necrotic tissue. Specific measures include cleaning the ulcer with saline, hydrogen peroxide, or other ordered solutions and applying granular and absorbent dressings. These dressings promote wound drainage and absorb any exudate. In addition, enzymatic ointments (such as Elase or Travase) break down dead tissue, whereas healing ointments

Stages of pressure ulcers

To protect the patient from pressure ulcer complications, learn to recognize the four stages of ulcer formation.

Stage 1
In this stage, the skin stays red for 5 minutes after removal of pressure and may develop an abrasion of the epidermis. (A black person's skin may look purple.) The skin also feels warm and firm. The sore is usually reversible if you remove pressure.

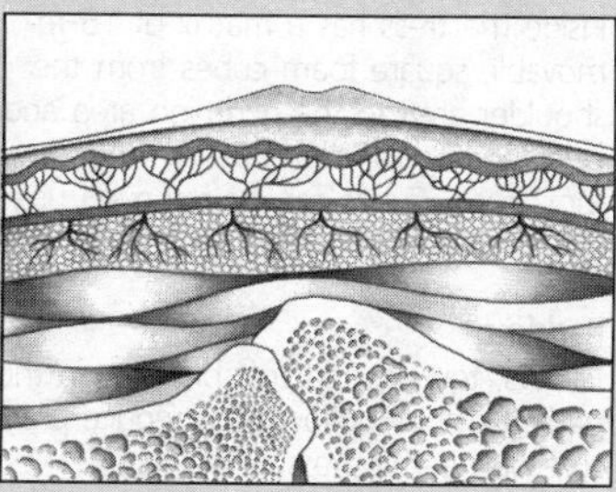

Stage 2
Breaks appear in the skin, and discoloration may occur. Penetrating to the subcutaneous fat layer, the sore is painful and visibly swollen. If pressure is removed, the sore may heal within 1 to 2 weeks.

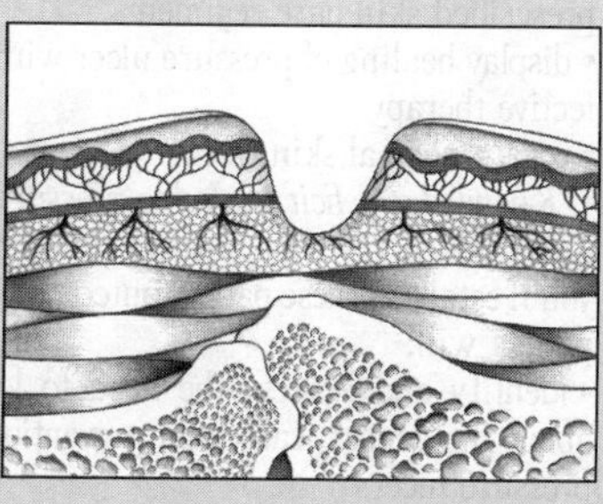

Stage 3
A hole develops that oozes foul-smelling yellow or green fluid. Extending into the muscle, the ulcer may develop a black leathery crust or eschar at its edges and eventually at the center. The ulcer isn't painful, but healing may take months.

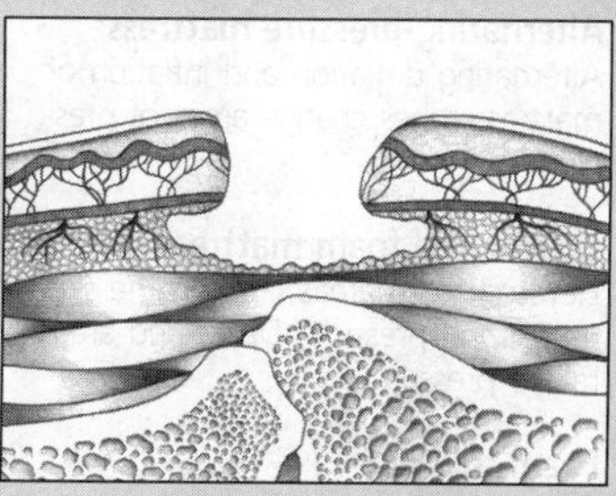

Stage 4
The ulcer destroys tissue from the skin to the bone and becomes necrotic. Findings include foul drainage and deep tunnels that extend from the ulcer. Months or even a year may elapse before the ulcer heals.

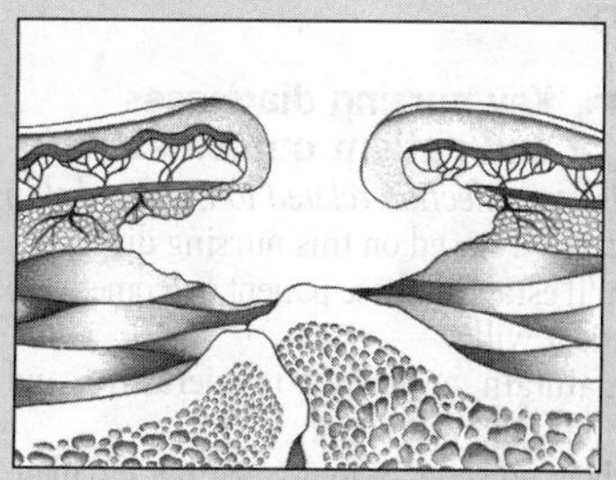

clean deep or infected ulcers and stimulate new cell growth.

Debridement of necrotic tissue may be necessary to allow healing. One method is to apply open wet dressings and allow them to dry on the ulcer. Removal of the dressings mechanically debrides exudate and necrotic tissue. On occasion, the ulcer may require debridement using surgical, mechanical, or chemical techniques. In se-

Pressure-relief devices

Numerous special pads, mattresses, and beds are available to help relieve pressure for the patient who is confined to one position for long periods and in danger of developing pressure ulcers. Examples of devices available follow.

Gel flotation pads
These wide pads disperse pressure over a wide surface area.

Alternating-pressure mattress
Alternating deflation and inflation of mattress tubes change areas of pressure.

Convoluted foam mattress or pads
Elevated foam areas cushion the skin, minimizing pressure. Depressed areas relieve pressure.

Foam rubber
Cut to just the right size and shape, foam rubber cushions individual areas on the patient.

Clinitron bed
This bed contains beads that move under airflow to support the patient, thus eliminating shearing force and friction.

Stryker or Foster frame or CircOlectric bed
These devices ease turning of immobile patients to relieve pressure.

Comfortex DeCube mattress
Inside mattress has a matrix of 15 removable square foam cubes from the shoulder area to the midthigh area and two rectangular cubes at the head and foot areas. Cubes can be removed under areas of pressure.

Padding
Pillows, towels, and soft blankets in the patient's body hollows can reduce pressure on nearby pressure points.

Foot cradle
This device lifts the bedclothes to relieve pressure over the patient's feet.

vere cases, skin grafting may be necessary.

Key nursing diagnoses and patient outcomes

Risk for infection related to impaired skin integrity. Based on this nursing diagnosis, you'll establish these patient outcomes. The patient will:
• maintain a normal temperature and white blood cell count
• show no signs of foul-smelling, purulent drainage at the ulcer site
• remain free of infection.

Impaired skin integrity related to decreased blood flow. Based on this nursing diagnosis, you'll establish these patient outcomes. The patient will:
• demonstrate skill in carrying out the prescribed skin care regimen
• display healing of pressure ulcer with effective therapy
• regain normal skin integrity.

Knowledge deficit related to pressure ulcers. Based on this nursing diagnosis, you'll establish these patient outcomes. The patient will:
• identify and express the need to learn about the causes, care, and prevention of pressure ulcers
• seek and obtain information about pressure ulcers from appropriate sources
• communicate an understanding of the care required for the existing pressure ulcer and of measures to prevent further ulcers.

Nursing interventions

- Reposition the bedridden patient at least every 2 hours around the clock. Minimize the effects of shearing force by using a footboard and not raising the head of the bed more than 60 degrees. Keep the patient's knees slightly flexed for short periods.
- Perform passive range-of-motion (ROM) exercises, or encourage the patient to do active exercises if possible.
- To prevent pressure ulcers in an immobilized patient, use pressure-relief aids on his bed.
- Give the patient meticulous skin care. Keep his skin clean and dry without using harsh soaps. Gently massaging the skin around the affected area (not on it) promotes healing. Rub moisturizing lotions into the skin thoroughly to prevent maceration of the skin surface. Change bed linens frequently for a diaphoretic or incontinent patient.
- If the patient is incontinent, offer him a bedpan or commode frequently. Use only a single layer of padding for urine and fecal incontinence because excessive padding increases perspiration, which leads to maceration. Excessive padding also may wrinkle, irritating the skin.
- Clean open lesions with a 0.9% sodium chloride solution. If possible, expose the lesions to air and sunlight to promote healing. Dressings, if needed, should be porous and lightly taped to healthy skin.
- Encourage adequate food and fluid intake to maintain body weight and promote healing. Consult the dietitian to provide a diet that promotes granulation of new tissue. Encourage the debilitated patient to eat frequent, small meals that include protein- and calorie-rich supplements. Assist the weakened patient with meals.

Monitoring

- During each shift, check the bedridden patient's skin for changes in color, turgor, temperature, and sensation. Examine an existing ulcer for any change in size or degree of damage.
- Monitor the patient for infection at the ulcer site.
- Because anemia and elevated blood glucose levels may lead to skin breakdown, monitor hemoglobin and blood glucose levels and hematocrit.

Patient teaching

- Explain the function of pressure-relief aids and topical agents, and demonstrate their proper use.
- Teach the patient and his family position-changing techniques and active and passive ROM exercises.
- Stress good hygiene. Teach the patient to avoid skin-damaging agents, such as harsh soaps, alcohol-based products, tincture of benzoin, and hexachlorophene.
- As indicated, explain debridement procedures and prepare the patient for skin graft surgery.
- Teach the patient and his family to recognize and record signs of healing. Explain that treatment typically varies according to the stage of healing.
- Encourage the patient to eat a well-balanced diet and consume an adequate amount of fluids, explaining their importance for skin health. Point out dietary sources rich in vitamin C, which aids wound healing, promotes iron absorption, and helps in collagen formation.

Proctitis

An inflammation of the rectal mucosa, proctitis has a good prognosis unless massive bleeding occurs.

Causes

Proctitis may develop secondary to rectal gonorrhea, candidiasis, syphilis, or nonspecific sexually transmitted infections. The most common causative pathogens are

Neisseria gonorrhoeae, chlamydiae, and herpesvirus.

Other causes include chronic constipation, habitual laxative use, emotional upset, radiation therapy, endocrine dysfunction, rectal surgery, rectal medications, allergies, vasomotor disturbance that interferes with normal muscle control, and food poisoning.

Complications

Proctitis can lead to ulcerations, crypt abscesses, bleeding, fissures, and fistulas. Submucosal inflammation with fibrosis may occur, leading to stricture.

Assessment

The patient typically complains of these key symptoms: constipation, a feeling of rectal fullness, and cramps in the left abdomen. The history may also reveal tenesmus producing a few bloody or mucoid stools.

Diagnostic tests

- *Sigmoidoscopy* in acute proctitis shows edematous, bright red or pink rectal mucosa that is shiny, thick, friable, and possibly ulcerated. In chronic proctitis, sigmoidoscopy shows thickened mucosa, loss of vascular pattern, and stricture of the rectal lumen.
- *Biopsy* is performed to rule out cancer.
- *Bacteriologic and viral analyses* detect the cause.

Treatment

Therapy aims to remove the underlying cause of proctitis, such as fecal impaction or laxative abuse. Anti-infective medications are given for infection. Corticosteroids (in enema or suppository form) may reduce inflammation, as may sulfasalazine, mesalamine, or similar agents. Tranquilizers may relieve emotional stress.

Key nursing diagnoses and patient outcomes

Impaired tissue integrity related to fissure or fistula formation. Based on this nursing diagnosis, you'll establish these patient outcomes. The patient will:

- comply with the prescribed treatment to facilitate healing
- regain normal rectal tissue integrity
- not develop chronic proctitis.

Pain related to inflammation of rectal tissue. Based on this nursing diagnosis, you'll establish these patient outcomes. The patient will:

- express feelings of comfort with treatment
- become pain free when rectal infection is cured.

Nursing interventions

- Offer emotional support and reassurance during rectal examinations and treatment.
- Administer anti-infective medications, sulfasalazine, and tranquilizers, as ordered. Provide soothing enemas, steroid foam, or steroid suppositories, as ordered, to relieve pain.

Monitoring

- Evaluate the patient's response to administered medications, and observe for adverse drug reactions.
- Monitor the patient for complications.

Patient teaching

- Explain proctitis and its treatment to help the patient understand the disorder and prevent its recurrence.
- Instruct the patient to watch for and report anal bleeding and other persistent signs and symptoms.
- Review prescribed medications.
- Teach the patient how to administer steroid enemas, foam, or suppositories as needed.
- If constipation adds to symptoms, teach about fluid intake, a high-fiber diet, and stool softeners.

Prostatectomy

Radical prostatectomy is a treatment option for early stages of prostate cancer. Total or partial prostatectomy is also an option for men with significantly obstructive benign prostatic hyperplasia (BPH), and it's performed to remove diseased or obstructive tissue and restore urine flow through the urethra. Depending on the disease, one of four approaches is used. Transurethral resection of the prostate (TURP), the most common approach, involves insertion of a resectoscope into the urethra. Open surgical approaches include suprapubic, retropubic, and perineal prostatectomy. (See *Comparing types of prostatectomy,* pages 756 and 757, for indications, advantages, and drawbacks of each approach.)

Procedure

In TURP, the patient is placed in a lithotomy position and anesthetized. The surgeon then introduces a resectoscope into the urethra and advances it to the prostate. After instilling a clear irrigating solution and visualizing the obstruction, he uses the resectoscope's cutting loop to resect prostatic tissue and restore the urethral opening.

In suprapubic prostatectomy, the patient is given a general anesthetic and placed in a supine position. The surgeon begins by making a horizontal incision just above the pubic symphysis. After instilling fluid into the bladder to distend it, he makes a small incision in the bladder wall to expose the prostate. He then shells the obstructing prostatic tissue out of its bed with his finger. After clearing the obstruction and ligating all bleeding points, he usually inserts a suprapubic drainage tube and a Penrose drain.

In retropubic prostatectomy, the patient is anesthetized and placed in a supine position. The surgeon makes a horizontal suprapubic incision and approaches the prostate from between the bladder and the pubic arch. He then makes another incision in the prostatic capsule and removes the obstructing tissue. After controlling any bleeding, he usually inserts a suprapubic tube and a Penrose drain. This allows for pelvic lymph node dissection, which is necessary to stage prostate cancer.

In perineal prostatectomy, the patient is anesthetized and placed in an exaggerated lithotomy position in which the knees are drawn up against the chest and the buttocks are slightly elevated. The surgeon makes an inverted U-shaped incision in the perineum, then removes the entire prostate and the seminal vesicles. He anastomoses the urethra to the bladder and closes the incision, leaving a Penrose drain in place. This approach is safer in patients who are obese or who have had previous lower abdominal or pelvic surgery.

Complications

Hemorrhage, infection, urine retention, impotence, and incontinence may be complications of prostatectomy.

Key nursing diagnoses and patient outcomes

Body image disturbance related to incontinence. Based on this nursing diagnosis, you'll establish these patient outcomes. The patient will:

- communicate an understanding of the relationship between incontinence and prostatectomy
- demonstrate skill in temporarily managing incontinence
- express positive feelings about himself.

Risk for infection related to drains and catheters left in place. Based on this nursing diagnosis, you'll establish these patient outcomes. The patient will:

- maintain a normal temperature and white blood cell count
- identify and carry out interventions to prevent or minimize the risk of infection
- remain free from signs and symptoms of infection.

(Text continues on page 758.)

Comparing types of prostatectomy

Procedure and indications	Advantages and disadvantages
Perineal prostatectomy • Prostate cancer • BPH, if the prostate is too large for transurethral resection and the patient is no longer sexually active	• Allows direct visualization of gland • Permits drainage by gravity • Low mortality and decreased incidence of shock • High incidence of impotence and incontinence • Risk of damage to rectum and external sphincter • Restricted operative field
Retropubic prostatectomy • BPH, if the prostate is too large for transurethral resection • Prostate cancer, when total removal of gland is necessary	• Allows direct visualization of gland • Avoids bladder incision • Short convalescence period • Patient may remain potent • Can't be used to treat associated bladder pathology • Increased risk of hemorrhage from prostate venous plexus
Suprapubic prostatectomy • BPH, if the prostate is too large for transurethral resection • Bladder lesions	• Allows exploration of wide area, such as into lymph nodes • Simple procedure • Requires bladder incision • Hemorrhage control difficult • Urine leakage common around suprapubic tube • Prolonged and uncomfortable recovery
TURP • BPH • Moderately enlarged prostate • Prostate cancer, as a palliative measure to remove obstruction	• Safer and less painful and invasive than other prostate procedures • Doesn't require surgical incision • Short hospital stay • Little risk of impotence • Urethral stricture and delayed bleeding may occur • Not a curative surgery for prostate cancer • Results in retrograde ejaculation

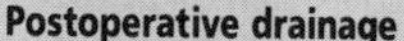

Postoperative drainage

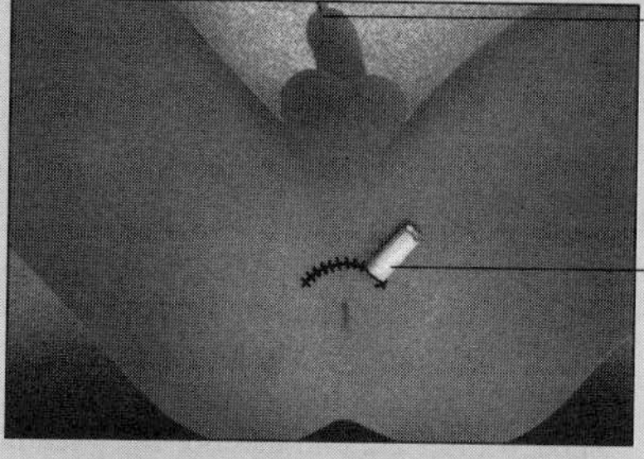

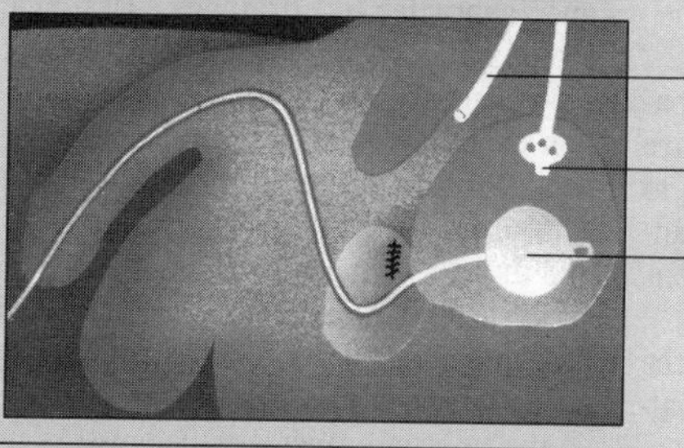

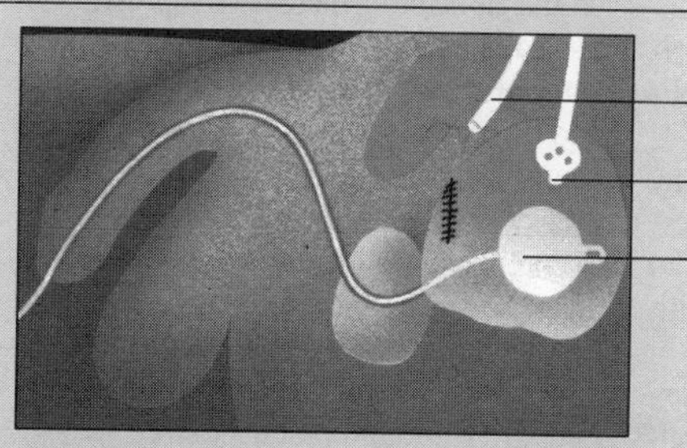

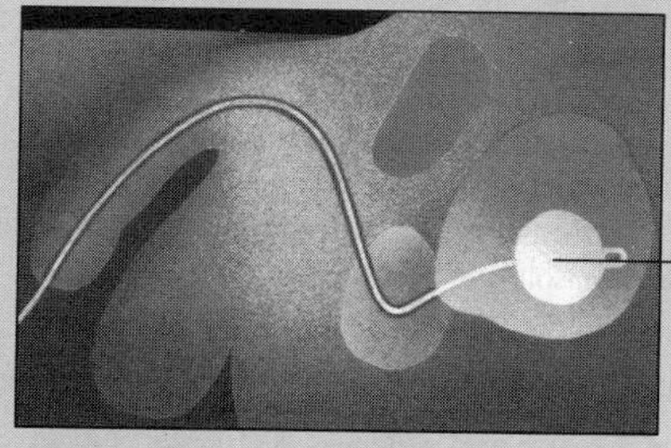

Sexual dysfunction related to impotence. Based on this nursing diagnosis, you'll establish these patient outcomes. The patient will:

- communicate an understanding of the relationship between impotence and prostatectomy
- identify treatment options to restore erectile ability or alternative sexual practices that are satisfying and acceptable to him and his partner.

Nursing interventions

In caring for a patient undergoing prostatectomy, your main responsibilities will be patient teaching and monitoring for postoperative complications.

Before surgery

- Review the planned surgery. Ask the patient what he knows about the procedure and its aftermath, and encourage him to ask questions. Provide straightforward answers to help clear up any misconceptions he may have.
- Offer emotional support. Encourage the patient to express his fears, and help to allay them by emphasizing the positive aspects of the surgery, such as improved urination and prevention of further complications.
- Because some types of prostatectomy can result in impotence, it may be necessary to arrange for sexual counseling to help the patient and his partner cope with this often devastating loss.
- If the patient is scheduled for TURP, explain that this procedure often causes retrograde ejaculation but otherwise doesn't impair sexual function.
- Before surgery, administer a cleansing enema. Explain to the patient that he may have a catheter in place for several days to several weeks to ensure proper urine drainage and healing.
- Be sure that the patient or a responsible family member has signed a consent form.

After surgery

- Monitor the patient's vital signs closely, looking for indications of possible hemorrhage and shock. Frequently check the incision site (if present) for signs of infection, and change dressings as necessary. Also watch for and report signs of epididymitis: fever, chills, groin pain, and a tender, swollen epididymis.
- Record the amount and nature of urine drainage. Maintain indwelling urinary catheter patency through intermittent or continuous irrigation, as ordered. Watch for catheter blockage from kinking or clot formation, and correct as necessary.
- Maintain the patency of the suprapubic tube, if inserted, and monitor the amount and character of drainage. Drainage should be amber or slightly blood tinged; report any abnormalities. Keep the collection container below the patient's bladder level to promote drainage, and keep the skin around the tube insertion site clean and dry.
- Expect and report frank bleeding the first day after surgery. If bleeding is venous, the doctor may increase the traction on the catheter or increase the pressure in the catheter's balloon end. If bleeding is arterial (bright red, with numerous clots and increased viscosity), it may need to be controlled surgically.
- As ordered, administer antispasmodics to control painful bladder spasms and analgesics to relieve incisional pain. Offer sitz baths to reduce perineal discomfort. Never administer medication rectally in a patient after a total prostatectomy.
- Watch for signs of dilutional hyponatremia: altered mental status, muscle twitching, and seizures. If these occur, raise the bed's side rails to prevent injury; notify the doctor; draw blood for serum sodium determination; and prepare hypertonic saline solution for possible I.V. infusion.
- Offer emotional support to the patient with a perineal prostatectomy because this procedure usually causes impotence. Try to arrange for psychological and sex-

ual counseling during the recovery period.

Home care instructions

- Tell the patient to drink ten 8-oz glasses of water a day, to urinate at least every 2 hours, and to notify the doctor promptly if he has trouble urinating.
- Explain that after catheter removal, transient urinary frequency and dribbling may occur. Reassure the patient that he'll gradually regain control over urination. Teach him Kegel exercises to tighten the perineum and speed the return of sphincter control. Suggest that he avoid caffeine-containing beverages, which cause mild diuresis.
- Reassure the patient that slightly blood-tinged urine normally occurs for the first few weeks after surgery. But tell him to report bright-red urine or persistent hematuria.
- Tell the patient to immediately report any signs of infection, such as fever, chills, and flank pain.
- Warn the patient not to have sexual relations, lift anything heavier than 10 lb (4.5 kg), perform strenuous exercise (short walks are usually permitted), take long car trips, or drive a car until the doctor gives permission. Explain that performing these activities too soon after surgery can cause bleeding.
- Tell the patient to take his prescribed medications as ordered. Suggest sitz baths for perineal discomfort.
- Urge the patient to keep all follow-up appointments and to have a yearly prostate examination (unless he's had a total prostatectomy). Tell men who've had radical prostatectomies to have a prostate-specific antigen test every year or as ordered.

Prostatic cancer

The most common neoplasm in men over age 50, prostatic cancer is a leading cause of male cancer death. Adenocarcinoma is the most common form; only seldom does prostatic cancer occur as a sarcoma. About 85% of prostatic cancers originate in the posterior prostate gland, with the rest growing near the urethra. Malignant prostatic tumors seldom result from the benign hyperplastic enlargement that commonly develops around the prostatic urethra in older men.

Slow-growing prostatic cancer seldom produces signs and symptoms until it's well advanced. Typically, when primary prostatic lesions spread beyond the prostate gland, they invade the prostatic capsule and then spread along the ejaculatory ducts in the space between the seminal vesicles or perivesicular fascia. When prostatic cancer is treated in its localized form, the 5-year survival rate is 70%; after metastasis, it's under 35%. Death usually results from widespread bone metastases. Prostatic cancer accounts for about 22% of all cancers, with highest incidence among Blacks and lowest among Asians. It appears unaffected by socioeconomic status or fertility.

Causes

The primary risk factor for prostatic cancer is age (the cancer seldom develops in men under age 40). Endocrine factors also have a role. It is known that androgens are necessary for tumor growth.

Complications

Progressive disease can lead to spinal cord compression, deep vein thrombosis, and pulmonary emboli.

Assessment

The patient's history may reveal urinary problems, such as dysuria, frequency, complete urine retention, back or hip pain, and hematuria. When the patient reports these signs and symptoms, the disease is likely to be advanced. What's more, back or hip pain may signal bone metastasis.

Staging prostatic cancer

Developed by the American Joint Committee on Cancer, descriptive categories, known as the tumor, node, metastasis (TNM) cancer staging system, interpret prostatic cancer's progress.

Primary tumor
TX—primary tumor can't be assessed
T0—no evidence of primary tumor
T1—tumor an incidental histologic finding
T1a—three or fewer microscopic foci of cancer
T1b—more than three microscopic foci of cancer
T2—tumor limited to the prostate gland
T2a—tumor less than 1.5 cm in greatest dimension, with normal tissue on at least three sides
T2b—tumor larger than 1.5 cm in greatest dimension or present in more than one lobe
T3—unfixed tumor extends into the prostatic apex or into or beyond the prostatic capsule, bladder neck, or seminal vesicle
T4—tumor fixed or invades adjacent structures not listed in T3

Regional lymph nodes
NX—regional lymph nodes can't be assessed
N0—no evidence of regional lymph node metastasis
N1—metastasis in a single lymph node, 2 cm or less in greatest dimension
N2—metastasis in a single lymph node, between 2 and 5 cm in greatest dimension, or metastasis to several lymph nodes, none more than 5 cm in greatest dimension
N3—metastasis in a lymph node, more than 5 cm in greatest dimension

Distant metastasis
MX—distant metastasis can't be assessed
M0—no known distant metastasis
M1—distant metastasis

Staging categories
Prostatic cancer progresses from mild to severe as follows:
Stage 0 or Stage I—T1a, N0, M0; T2a, N0, M0
Stage II—T1b, N0, M0; T2b, N0, M0
Stage III—T3, N0, M0
Stage IV—T4, N0, M0; any T, N1, M0; any T, N2, M0; any T, N3, M0; any T, any N, M1

The patient usually has no signs or symptoms in early disease.

Inspection may reveal edema of the scrotum or leg in advanced disease. During rectal examination, prostatic palpation may detect a nonraised, firm, nodular mass with a sharp edge (in early disease) or a hard lump (in advanced disease).

Diagnostic tests

• *Digital rectal examination (DRE),* recommended yearly by the American Cancer Society for men over age 50, is the standard screening test.

• *Blood tests* may show elevated levels of prostate-specific antigen (PSA). Although most men with metastasized prostatic cancer will have an elevated PSA level, the finding also occurs with other prostatic disease. PSA levels are recommended yearly for men over age 50.

• *Transrectal prostatic ultrasonography* may be used for patients with abnormal DRE and PSA test findings.

• *Bone scan* and *excretory urography* may determine the disease's extent. (See *Staging prostatic cancer.*)

• *Magnetic resonance imaging* and *computed tomography scans* can help define the tumor's extent.

Treatment

Therapy varies by cancer stage and may include radiation, prostatectomy, orchiectomy (removal of the testes) to reduce androgen production, and hormonal therapy. Radical prostatectomy is usually effective for localized lesions without metastasis. A transurethral resection of the prostate may be performed to relieve an obstruction in metastatic disease.

Radiation therapy may cure locally invasive lesions in early disease and may relieve bone pain from metastatic skeletal involvement. It also may be used prophylactically for patients with tumors in regional lymph nodes. Alternatively, brachytherapy or implantation of radioactive seeds or pellets into the prostate may be recommended because it permits increased radiation to reach the prostate but minimizes the surrounding tissues' exposure to radiation.

Hormonal therapy is used for advanced or metastatic prostate cancer. Because prostate cancer cells depend on testosterone for growth, drugs that block its production result in a temporary remission of the cancer. The most commonly used drugs are luteinizing hormone-releasing hormone (LHRH) agonists: goserelin acetate and leuprolide acetate. Both drugs block testosterone production by the testes and are given as injections monthly or every 3 months. Oral flutamide is given daily to block the 10% of circulating testosterone that is produced by the adrenal glands.

Key nursing diagnoses and patient outcomes

Altered urinary elimination related to functional changes in lower urinary system. Based on this nursing diagnosis, you'll establish these patient outcomes. The patient will:

• express feelings of increased comfort when urinating
• avoid complications or have minimal ones
• regain a normal urinary elimination pattern with removal of prostatic cancer.

Anxiety related to diagnosis. Based on this nursing diagnosis, you'll establish these patient outcomes. The patient will:

• identify and express his feelings of anxiety
• identify and perform activities that decrease anxiety
• cope with the diagnosis without showing signs of severe anxiety.

Pain related to metastasis of prostatic cancer to bone. Based on this nursing diagnosis, you'll establish these patient outcomes. The patient will:

• express feelings of comfort after analgesic administration
• identify and carry out appropriate interventions for pain relief
• become pain free with eradication of prostatic cancer.

Nursing interventions

• Encourage the patient to express his fears and concerns, including those about changes in his sexual identity. Offer reassurance when possible.
• Administer ordered analgesics and provide comfort measures to reduce pain. Encourage the patient to identify care measures that promote his comfort and relaxation.
• Prepare the patient for orchiectomy or prostatectomy, as indicated. (See the entries "Orchiopexy" and "Prostatectomy.")
• Encourage the patient undergoing radiation to drink at least eight 8-oz glasses of fluid daily. Administer analgesics and antispasmodics to decrease his discomfort.
• Provide supportive care for adverse reactions to hormonal therapy or chemotherapy.

Monitoring

• Evaluate the patient's pain level and the effectiveness of administered analgesics.
• Monitor the patient's urinary system for dysfunction. Measure intake and output.
• Watch for the common adverse effects of radiation to the prostate: proctitis, diarrhea, bladder spasms, and urinary fre-

quency. Internal radiation of the prostate almost always results in cystitis in the first 2 to 3 weeks of therapy.

• Watch for adverse reactions (hot flashes, decreased libido, and gynecomastia) in a patient receiving hormonal therapy with LHRH agonists. During the first 2 to 4 weeks of therapy, symptoms of bone pain may increase due to "the flare phenomenon" – the hormonal therapy initially causes an increase in testosterone production. Administer increased amounts of analgesics during this period, as needed.

Patient teaching

• Prepare the patient for his particular type of surgery.
• If appropriate, discuss the adverse effects of pelvic radiation therapy, such as diarrhea, urinary frequency, nocturia, bladder spasms, rectal irritation, and tenesmus.
• Encourage him to maintain as normal a life-style as possible during recovery.
• When appropriate, refer the patient to the social service department, local home health care agencies, hospices, and prostate cancer support organizations.

Prostatitis

An inflammation of the prostate gland, prostatitis occurs in several forms. Acute prostatitis most often results from gram-negative bacteria and is easily recognized and treated. Chronic prostatitis, which affects up to 35% of men over age 50 and is the most common cause of recurrent urinary tract infection (UTI) in men, is harder to recognize. Other classifications include granulomatous prostatitis (also called tuberculous prostatitis), nonbacterial prostatitis, and prostatodynia (painful prostate).

Causes

About 80% of bacterial prostatitis cases result from infection by *Escherichia coli.* The rest result from infection by *Klebsiella, Enterobacter, Proteus, Pseudomonas, Serratia, Streptococcus, Staphylococcus,* and diphtheroids, which are contaminants from the anterior urethra's normal flora.

Infection probably spreads to the prostate gland by the hematogenous route or from ascending urethral infection, invasion of rectal bacteria by way of the lymphatic vessels, or reflux of infected bladder urine into prostate ducts. Less commonly, infection may result from urethral procedures performed with instruments, such as cystoscopy and catheterization.

Chronic prostatitis usually results from bacterial invasion from the urethra. Granulomatous prostatitis occurs secondary to a miliary spread of *Mycobacterium tuberculosis.* Nonbacterial prostatitis is probably caused by *Mycoplasma, Ureaplasma, Chlamydia, Trichomonas vaginalis,* or some viruses. The cause of prostatodynia is unknown.

Complications

UTI is the most common complication of prostatitis. An untreated infection can progress to prostatic abscess, acute urine retention from prostatic edema, pyelonephritis, and epididymitis.

Assessment

The patient with acute prostatitis may report sudden fever, chills, low-back pain, myalgia, perineal fullness, arthralgia, frequent urination, urinary urgency, dysuria, and nocturia. Some degree of urinary obstruction also may occur, and the urine may appear cloudy. The bladder may feel distended when palpated. When palpated rectally, the prostate is markedly tender and boggy or soft.

Clinical features of chronic bacterial prostatitis vary. Although some patients are asymptomatic, this condition usually elicits the same urinary symptoms as the acute form but to a lesser degree. Other possible signs and symptoms include hemospermia, persistent urethral discharge, and painful ejaculation that's responsible for some sexual dysfunction. The prostate is usually normal.

Digital examination in granulomatous prostatitis may reveal a stony, hard induration of the prostate (mimicking cancer or a calculus). This finding may suggest prostatitis if the patient has a history of pulmonary or GI tuberculosis or has been receiving intravesical therapy for superficial bladder cancer.

With nonbacterial prostatitis, the patient usually complains of dysuria, mild perineal or low-back pain, and frequent nocturia. With prostatodynia, he may complain of perineal, low-back, or pelvic pain.

Diagnostic tests

Although a urine culture often can identify the causative infectious organism, and characteristic rectal examination findings suggest prostatitis (especially in the acute phase), firm diagnosis depends on comparison of bacterial growth in specimens obtained by the Meares and Stamey technique.

This test requires four specimens: one collected when the patient starts voiding (voided bladder one [VB1]); another midstream (VB2); another after the patient stops voiding and the doctor massages the prostate to produce secretions (expressed prostate secretions [EPS]); and a final voided specimen (VB3). A significant increase in colony count of the prostatic specimens (EPS and VB3) confirms prostatitis.

In granulomatous prostatitis, demonstration of *M. tuberculosis* in the urine or a tissue biopsy from the prostate confirms the diagnosis.

In nonbacterial prostatitis, smears of prostatic secretions reveal inflammatory cells but often no causative organism. In prostatodynia, urine cultures are negative and no inflammatory cells are present in smears of prostatic secretions. Urodynamic evaluation may reveal detrusor hyperreflexia and pelvic floor myalgia from chronic spasms.

Rectal examination frequently reveals a tender, painful, warm, and swollen prostate. White blood cell count is elevated in bacterial prostatitis.

Treatment

Systemic antibiotic therapy, guided by sensitivity studies, is the treatment of choice for acute prostatitis. Aminoglycosides, in combination with penicillins or cephalosporins, may be most effective for severe cases. Urine retention may be managed with a suprapubic cystostomy. Urethral catheterization is to be avoided.

In chronic prostatitis, antibiotics are prescribed only if the patient has severe symptoms and a positive culture. Quinolones, trimethoprim, and trimethoprim combined with sulfa are widely used, and treatment for 6 weeks is often necessary. Prolonged therapy may be necessary to control symptoms and prevent bacteriuria. Oral antispasmodics may be used to relieve urinary frequency and urgency.

Treatment for granulomatous prostatitis consists of antitubercular drug combinations. Minocycline, doxycycline, or erythromycin is used for nonbacterial prostatitis for 4 weeks, but antibiotic therapy isn't repeated if symptoms don't subside.

Supportive therapy includes bed rest, adequate hydration, and administration of analgesics, antipyretics, and stool softeners as necessary. If symptoms are present in chronic prostatitis, treatment may consist of sitz baths and regular sexual intercourse or ejaculation to promote drainage of prostatic secretions. Regular prostatic massage for several weeks or months is most effective. Anticholinergics and analgesics may help relieve the symptoms of nonbacterial prostatitis. Alpha-adrenergic blocking agents and muscle relaxants may be used for prostatodynia.

Key nursing diagnoses and patient outcomes

Altered urinary elimination related to involvement of lower urinary tract in inflammatory process. Based on this nursing diagnosis, you'll establish these patient outcomes. The patient will:
- express feelings of increased comfort when voiding
- be able to void
- regain and maintain a normal urinary elimination pattern with eradication of prostatitis.

Risk for infection related to potential for UTI. Based on this nursing diagnosis, you'll establish these patient outcomes. The patient will:
- have urine with a clear appearance and a normal odor
- have a normal urinalysis and urine culture
- not show signs and symptoms of UTI.

Pain related to prostatic inflammation. Based on this nursing diagnosis, you'll establish these patient outcomes. The patient will:
- express feelings of comfort following analgesic administration
- comply with the prescribed therapy to treat prostatitis and thus reduce pain.

Nursing interventions

- Administer analgesics for pain, as ordered.
- Ensure bed rest and adequate hydration.
- Provide stool softeners and administer sitz baths, as ordered. Avoid rectal examination because it may precipitate bleeding.
- As necessary, prepare to assist with suprapubic needle aspiration of the bladder or a suprapubic cystostomy.

Monitoring

- Monitor the patient's vital signs.
- Assess the patient's response to therapy, and monitor him for adverse reactions to administered medications.
- Monitor the patient for infection, especially UTI. Assess his urinary elimination pattern, and measure intake and output.

Patient teaching

- Familiarize the patient with any prescribed drugs and their possible adverse effects. Tell him to take oral antibiotics and other drugs exactly as ordered and to complete the prescribed drug regimens. Also, review the indications for using gentle laxatives.
- Tell the patient to immediately report adverse drug reactions, such as rash, nausea, vomiting, fever, chills, and GI irritation.
- Instruct the patient to drink at least eight 8-oz glasses of water a day (about 2 qt or liters).
- If the patient has chronic prostatitis, recommend that he remain sexually active and ejaculate regularly to promote drainage of prostatic secretions. Advise the patient to use a condom during sexual intercourse when he's having a bout of prostatitis.
- Urge the patient to seek medical care immediately if he can't void, if he passes bloody urine, or if he develops a fever.

Pseudomembranous enterocolitis

An acute inflammation and necrosis of the small and large intestines, pseudomembranous enterocolitis usually affects the mucosa but may extend into the submucosa and, rarely, other layers. This rare condition, marked by severe diarrhea, can be fatal in 1 to 7 days from severe dehydration and from toxicity, peritonitis, or perforation.

Causes

What triggers the acute inflammation and necrosis characteristic of this disorder is unknown; however, *Clostridium difficile* may produce a toxin that plays a role in its development. The disease typically occurs in patients who are undergoing treatment with broad-spectrum antibiotics or who have received such therapy within the past 4 weeks. Nearly all broad-spectrum antibiotics, especially clindamycin, ampicillin, and the cephalosporins, have been linked with its onset. Possible exceptions are vancomycin and aminoglycosides.

Pseudomembranous enterocolitis may also occur postoperatively in debilitated patients undergoing abdominal surgery. Whatever the cause, the necrosed mucosa is replaced by a pseudomembrane filled with staphylococci, leukocytes, mucus, fibrin, and inflammatory cells.

Complications

Severe dehydration, electrolyte imbalance, hypotension, shock, colonic perforation, and peritonitis are among the potentially fatal complications associated with this disorder.

Assessment

The patient's history usually reveals current or recent antibiotic treatment. Typically, the patient reports the sudden onset of copious, watery or, rarely, bloody diarrhea; abdominal pain; and fever. Palpation may reveal abdominal tenderness.

Careful consideration of the patient history is essential because the abrupt onset of enterocolitis and the emergency situation it creates may make diagnosis difficult.

Diagnostic tests

A rectal biopsy through sigmoidoscopy confirms pseudomembranous enterocolitis. Stool cultures can identify *C. difficile.*

Treatment

If the patient is receiving broad-spectrum antibiotic treatment, the first priority is immediate discontinuation of the offending drug. Usually, the patient is then treated with oral metronidazole or oral vancomycin. Metronidazole generally is used first; if it's ineffective, vancomycin is given. Anion exchange resins such as cholestyramine, which bind the toxin produced by *C. difficile,* may be ordered for patients with mild pseudomembranous enterocolitis. However, patient response to this treatment has proved inferior to that with oral vancomycin or metronidazole.

Supportive treatments maintain fluid and electrolyte balance and combat hypotension and shock with vasopressors, such as dopamine and norepinephrine.

Key nursing diagnoses and patient outcomes

Diarrhea related to inflammation of the intestines. Based on this nursing diagnosis, you'll establish these patient outcomes. The patient will:
- control diarrhea with treatment
- not develop complications of diarrhea, such as skin breakdown and fluid and electrolyte imbalance
- regain and maintain a normal elimination pattern.

Risk for fluid volume deficit related to loss of fluids from diarrhea. Based on this nursing diagnosis, you'll establish these patient outcomes. The patient will:
- restore and maintain fluid and electrolyte balance
- not have signs and symptoms of dehydration.

Pain related to inflammation of the intestines. Based on this nursing diagnosis, you'll establish these patient outcomes. The patient will:
- express increased feelings of comfort with therapy
- use nonpharmacologic measures to alleviate or minimize abdominal pain

• become pain free when pseudomembranous enterocolitis is cured.

Nursing interventions

• If ordered, administer I.V. therapy to restore and maintain fluid and electrolyte balance.
• Administer medications as ordered.
• Keep the patient as comfortable as possible. Administer analgesics to decrease abdominal pain and antipyretics to control high fever. Teach the patient how to perform relaxation techniques, such as distraction or guided imagery, to help him cope with abdominal pain.
• Keep a bedpan within the patient's reach to help prevent embarrassing accidents.

Monitoring

• Monitor vital signs, skin color, and level of consciousness. Immediately report signs of shock.
• Record fluid intake and output, including fluid lost in stools. Watch for indications of dehydration (poor skin turgor, sunken eyes, and decreased urine output).
• Check serum electrolyte levels daily, and watch for clinical signs of hypokalemia (especially malaise) and a weak, rapid, irregular pulse.
• Monitor the patient for the desired effects of administered medications and for adverse reactions.

Patient teaching

• Teach the patient about the disorder and its possible causes; discuss signs and symptoms, ordered diagnostic tests, and treatments.
• Review prescribed medications, explaining their desired effects, potential adverse effects, and proper administration.
• Point out that because pseudomembranous enterocolitis recurs in about 20% of cases, the patient must immediately report symptoms of recurrence. Reassure him that a second course of therapy resolves the disorder.
• If the disorder was antibiotic-related, instruct the patient to caution doctors who might prescribe similar medications in the future.

Pseudomonas infections

A genus of small, gram-negative bacilli, *Pseudomonas* primarily produces nosocomial infections, superinfections of various parts of the body, and a rare disease called melioidosis. The most common infections associated with *Pseudomonas* include skin infections (such as burns and pressure ulcers), urinary tract infections (UTIs), diarrheal illnesses, bronchitis, pneumonia, bronchiectasis, meningitis, corneal ulcers, mastoiditis, otitis externa, and otitis media. These bacilli are especially associated with bacteremia, endocarditis, and osteomyelitis in drug addicts.

In local *Pseudomonas* infections, treatment usually is successful and complications are rare. However, in patients with poor resistance to infection – for example, premature infants, elderly people, and persons with debilitating disease, burns, or wounds – septicemic *Pseudomonas* infections are considered serious. In some patients they may even cause death. (See *Melioidosis*.)

Causes

The most common species of *Pseudomonas* is *P. aeruginosa*. Other pathogenic species include *P. maltophilia, P. cepacia, P. fluorescens, P. testosteroni, P. acidovorans, P. alcaligenes, P. stutzeri, P. putrefaciens,* and *P. putida*.

These organisms frequently are found in hospital liquids that have been allowed to stand for a long time, such as benzalkonium chloride, hexachlorophene soap, saline solution, water in flower vases, and fluids in incubators, humidifiers, and respiratory therapy equipment. Outside the hospital, *Pseudomonas* skin infections have been associated with the use of contaminated whirlpools, hot tubs, spas, and swimming pools.

In elderly patients, *Pseudomonas* infection usually enters through the genitourinary (GU) tract.

Complications

Septic shock—the most serious complication of *Pseudomonas* infections—can cause death in people who are severely immunocompromised or resistant to antibiotics. *Pseudomonas* produces severe mucopurulent pneumonia, which may be necrotizing.

Assessment

The immunocompromised hospital patient is the most vulnerable to *Pseudomonas.* Signs and symptoms vary with the infection site. In respiratory infection, the patient may complain of dyspnea, a cough producing purulent sputum, and chills. In UTI, he may report urinary urgency and frequency, dysuria, nocturia, low-back pain, and malaise. In otitis externa, he may describe a painful or itching ear that is draining.

Although the patient's body temperature may be normal in some local infections, it will be elevated in severe infection, such as bacteremia associated with *Pseudomonas.*

Inspection findings also vary. For example, in a respiratory infection you may note cyanosis, apprehension, dyspnea and, possibly, mental confusion. In otitis externa, you may observe a tender, swollen external auditory canal filled with drainage. The drainage has a sickly sweet odor and consists of a greenish blue pus that forms a crust on wounds.

Abscesses may be palpable and tender on the skin surface. In *Pseudomonas* pneumonia, percussion discloses dullness over areas of mucopurulent drainage consolidation and auscultation of the lungs may reveal crackles in areas of drainage collection.

Melioidosis

Wound penetration, inhalation, or ingestion of the gram-negative bacterium *Pseudomonas pseudomallei* causes melioidosis. Once confined to Southeast Asia, Central America, South America, Madagascar, and Guam, incidence in the United States is rising because of the recent influx of Southeast Asian immigrants.

Two forms: Chronic and acute

Melioidosis occurs in two forms: chronic melioidosis, which causes osteomyelitis and lung abscesses; and acute melioidosis (rare), which causes pneumonia, bacteremia, and prostration. Acute melioidosis commonly is fatal. Most infections are chronic, however, and produce clinical symptoms only with accompanying malnutrition, major surgery, or severe burns.

Diagnostic measures consist of isolation of *P. pseudomallei* in a culture of exudate, blood, or sputum; serology tests (complement fixation, passive hemagglutination); and chest X-ray, with findings that resemble tuberculosis.

Treatment includes oral tetracycline as well as co-trimoxazole, abscess drainage and, in severe cases, chloramphenicol until X-rays show resolution of the primary abscesses.

The prognosis is good because most patients experience mild infections and acquire permanent immunity. The aggressive use of antibiotics and sulfonamides has improved the prognosis in acute melioidosis.

Diagnostic tests

Diagnosis relies on isolation of the *Pseudomonas* organism in blood, cerebrospinal fluid, urine, exudate, or sputum culture.

Treatment

In the debilitated or otherwise vulnerable patient with clinical evidence of *Pseudomonas* infection, treatment should begin immediately, without waiting for laboratory test results. Antibiotic treatment includes aminoglycosides, such as gentamicin or amikacin, combined with a *Pseudomonas*-sensitive penicillin, such as ceftazidime or imipenem–cilastatin. Such combination therapy is necessary because *Pseudomonas* quickly becomes resistant to penicillin derivatives alone.

In UTI, carbenicillin indanyl sodium can be used alone if the organism is susceptible and the infection doesn't have systemic effects; the drug is excreted in urine and builds up high urine levels that prevent resistance.

Local *Pseudomonas* infection or septicemia secondary to wound infection requires 1% acetic acid irrigations, topical applications of colistimethate sodium and polymyxin B, and debridement or drainage of the infected wound.

Key nursing diagnoses and patient outcomes

Impaired skin integrity related to skin infections. Based on this nursing diagnosis, you'll establish these patient outcomes. The patient will:
- demonstrate skill in carrying out his skin care regimen
- exhibit improved or healed lesions or wounds
- take precautions to prevent recurrent skin infections.

Ineffective airway clearance related to presence of tracheobronchial secretions caused by respiratory infections. Based on this nursing diagnosis, you'll establish these patient outcomes. The patient will:
- cough and expectorate sputum effectively
- demonstrate skill in performing bronchial hygiene
- maintain a patent airway.

Pain related to inflammation. Based on this nursing diagnosis, you'll establish these patient outcomes. The patient will:
- describe and carry out appropriate interventions for pain relief
- express feelings of comfort and relief from pain as *Pseudomonas* infection is eradicated.

Nursing interventions

- For respiratory infections, maintain a patent airway by suctioning secretions whenever necessary and provide adequate oxygenation. Perform chest physiotherapy and postural drainage as needed.
- Administer ordered analgesics as needed.
- Protect immunocompromised patients from exposure to this infection. Attention to hand washing and aseptic techniques prevents further spread.
- Use strict sterile technique when changing dressings that involve infected wounds. Clean the wounds with a bactericidal solution and apply local antibiotic ointment, if ordered.
- To prevent *Pseudomonas* infection, maintain proper endotracheal and tracheostomy suctioning technique; use strict sterile technique when caring for I.V. lines, catheters, and other tubes; properly dispose of suction bottle contents; label and date solution bottles and change them frequently, according to policy. Change water for fresh flowers daily. Avoid using humidifiers in the patient's room.

Monitoring

- Observe and record the character of wound exudate and sputum.
- Before administering antibiotics, ask the patient about a history of allergies, especially to penicillin.
- Assess the effectiveness of the prescribed drug treatment, and watch for adverse reactions.
- Monitor the patient's hearing and renal function (urine output, specific gravity, urinalysis, and blood urea nitrogen and serum creatinine levels) during treatment with aminoglycosides.
- Monitor the body system infected by *Pseudomonas* for dysfunction.

• Monitor the patient for septic shock, exhibited by a high fever, hypotension, tachycardia, tachypnea, and confusion.

Patient teaching

• Reinforce the importance of completing the course of antibiotic therapy as prescribed.
• Teach the immunocompromised patient to avoid having sources of stagnant or contaminated water at home. Advise him to change the water for fresh flowers daily and, if a humidifier is essential, to change its water daily. Whirlpools and swimming pools must be scrupulously clean.
• Educate the patient who wears contact lenses, especially extended-wear soft lenses, to care for them properly and to report any associated eye trauma or other symptoms.
• Tell the patient to avoid drinking water when traveling to endemic areas.

Pulmonary edema

Marked by an accumulation of fluid in extravascular spaces of the lung, pulmonary edema is a common complication of cardiac disorders. The disorder may occur as a chronic condition, or it may develop quickly and rapidly become fatal.

Causes

Pulmonary edema usually results from left ventricular failure caused by arteriosclerotic, cardiomyopathic, hypertensive, or valvular heart disease. The disorder stems from either of two mechanisms: increased pulmonary capillary hydrostatic pressure or decreased colloid osmotic pressure. Normally, the two pressures are in balance. When this balance changes, pulmonary edema results.

If pulmonary capillary hydrostatic pressure increases, the compromised left ventricle requires increased filling pressures to maintain adequate output; these pressures are transmitted to the left atrium, pulmonary veins, and pulmonary capillary bed. This forces fluids and solutes from the intravascular compartment into the interstitium of the lungs. As the interstitium overloads with fluid, fluid floods the peripheral alveoli and impairs gas exchange.

If colloid osmotic pressure decreases, the natural pulling force that contains intravascular fluids is lost – nothing opposes the hydrostatic force. Thus, fluid flows freely into the interstitium and alveoli, resulting in pulmonary edema.

Other factors that may predispose the patient to pulmonary edema include:
• barbiturate or opiate poisoning
• congestive heart failure
• infusion of excessive volumes of I.V. fluids or an overly rapid infusion
• impaired pulmonary lymphatic drainage (from Hodgkin's disease or obliterative lymphangitis after radiation)
• inhalation of irritating gases
• mitral stenosis and left atrial myxoma (which impair left atrial emptying)
• pneumonia
• pulmonary veno-occlusive disease.

Complications

Acute pulmonary edema may progress to respiratory and metabolic acidosis, with subsequent cardiac or respiratory arrest.

Assessment

The history may include a predisposing factor for pulmonary edema. The patient typically complains of a persistent cough. He may report getting a cold and being dyspneic on exertion. He may experience paroxysmal nocturnal dyspnea and orthopnea.

On inspection, you may note restlessness and anxiety. With severe pulmonary edema, the patient's breathing may be visibly labored and rapid. His cough may sound intense and produce frothy, bloody sputum. In advanced stages, the patient's level of consciousness decreases.

NURSING ALERT

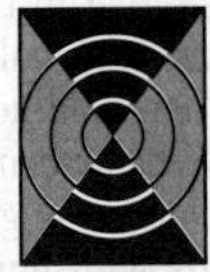

Detecting danger signs of pulmonary edema

If you detect inspiratory crackles, dry cough, or dyspnea, notify the doctor immediately. Chest X-ray results may not be available until 24 hours after you've assessed the patient. Don't wait for X-ray findings if you suspect pulmonary edema.

Typical palpation findings include neck vein distention. In acute pulmonary edema, the skin feels sweaty, cold, and clammy. Auscultation may reveal crepitant crackles and a diastolic (S_3) gallop. In severe pulmonary edema, you may hear wheezing as the alveoli and bronchioles fill with fluid. The crackles become more diffuse. (See *Detecting danger signs of pulmonary edema.*)

Additional findings include worsening tachycardia, falling blood pressure, thready pulse, and decreased cardiac output. In advanced pulmonary edema, breath sounds diminish.

Diagnostic tests

Clinical features of pulmonary edema permit a working diagnosis. Diagnostic tests provide the following information.

- *Arterial blood gas (ABG) analysis* usually shows hypoxia with variable partial pressure of carbon dioxide in arterial blood, depending on the patient's degree of fatigue. ABG results may also identify metabolic acidosis.
- *Chest X-rays* show diffuse haziness of the lung fields and, usually, cardiomegaly and pleural effusion.
- *Pulse oximetry* may reveal decreasing arterial oxygen saturation levels.
- *Pulmonary artery catheterization* identifies left ventricular failure (indicated by elevated pulmonary artery wedge pressures). These findings help to rule out adult respiratory distress syndrome, in which wedge pressure usually remains normal.
- *Electrocardiography* may disclose evidence of previous or current myocardial infarction.

Treatment

Treatment aims to reduce extravascular fluid, to improve gas exchange and myocardial function and, if possible, to correct underlying disease. High concentrations of oxygen can be administered by nasal cannula or mask. (Typically, the patient with pulmonary edema doesn't tolerate a mask.) If the patient's arterial oxygen levels remain too low, assisted ventilation can improve oxygen delivery to the tissues and usually improves his acid-base balance. A bronchodilator, such as aminophylline, may decrease bronchospasm and enhance myocardial contractility. Diuretics, such as furosemide, ethacrynic acid, and bumetanide, increase urination, which helps to mobilize extravascular fluid.

Treatment of myocardial dysfunction includes positive inotropic agents, such as digitalis glycosides, dobutamine, and milrinone lactate, to enhance contractility. Pressor agents may be given to enhance contractility and to promote vasoconstriction in peripheral vessels.

Antiarrhythmics may also be given, particularly in arrhythmias related to decreased cardiac output. Sometimes, arterial vasodilators, such as nitroprusside or nitroglycerin, can decrease peripheral vascular resistance, preload, and afterload.

Morphine may reduce anxiety and dyspnea and dilate the systemic venous bed, promoting blood flow from pulmonary circulation to the periphery.

Other treatments include rotating tourniquets and phlebotomy (both reduce preload). Phlebotomy will also remove hemoglobin, which may worsen the patient's hypoxemia.

Key nursing diagnoses and patient outcomes

Anxiety related to inability to breathe comfortably. Based on this nursing diagnosis, you'll establish these patient outcomes. The patient will:
• express feelings of anxiety
• perform stress-reduction techniques to decrease anxiety
• cope with pulmonary edema without demonstrating severe signs of anxiety.

Fluid volume excess related to fluid accumulation in lungs. Based on this nursing diagnosis, you'll establish these patient outcomes. The patient will:
• eliminate excess fluid safely with treatment
• not develop complications, such as respiratory and metabolic acidosis
• regain and maintain a normal fluid balance.

Impaired gas exchange related to fluid accumulation in lungs. Based on this nursing diagnosis, you'll establish these patient outcomes. The patient will:
• not demonstrate severe signs and symptoms of tissue hypoxia
• regain and maintain normal ABG levels
• regain normal gas exchange with alleviation of pulmonary edema.

Nursing interventions

• Help the patient relax to promote oxygenation, control bronchospasm, and enhance myocardial contractility.
• Reassure the patient, who will be frightened by his inability to breathe normally. Provide emotional support to his family as well.
• Place him in high Fowler's position to enhance lung expansion.
• Administer oxygen as ordered.
• Administer nitroprusside in dextrose 5% in water by I.V. drip. During administration, protect the solution from light by wrapping the bottle or bag with aluminum foil. Discard the unused solution after 24 hours.
• Carefully record the time morphine is given and the amount administered.

Monitoring

• Assess the patient's condition frequently, and document his responses to treatment. Monitor ABG and pulse oximetry values, oral and I.V. fluid intake, urine output and, in the patient with a pulmonary artery catheter, pulmonary end-diastolic and capillary wedge pressures. Check the cardiac monitor often. Report changes immediately. (See *Nursing care in acute pulmonary edema,* pages 772 and 773.)
• Watch for complications of treatment, such as electrolyte depletion. Also watch for complications of oxygen therapy and mechanical ventilation.
• Monitor vital signs every 15 to 30 minutes while administering nitroprusside or nitroglycerin. Watch for arrhythmias in patients receiving digitalis glycosides and for marked respiratory depression in those receiving morphine.

Patient teaching

• Urge the patient to comply with the prescribed medication regimen to avoid future episodes of pulmonary edema.
• Explain all procedures to the patient and his family.
• Emphasize reporting early signs of fluid overload.
• Explain the reasons for sodium restrictions. List high-sodium foods and drugs.
• Review all prescribed medications with the patient. If he takes digoxin, show him how to monitor his own pulse rate and warn him to report signs of toxicity. Encourage consumption of potassium-rich foods to lower the risk of toxicity and cardiac arrhythmias. If he takes a vasodilator, teach him the signs of hypotension and emphasize the need to avoid alcohol.
• Discuss ways to conserve physical energy.

(Text continues on page 774.)

NURSING PRIORITY

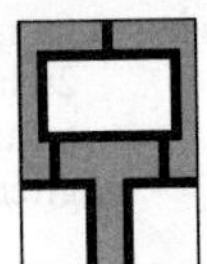

Nursing care in acute pulmonary edema

Presence of predisposing factors, such as cardiovascular disease; persistent cough; dyspnea on exertion; possible paroxysmal nocturnal dyspnea or orthopnea

Physical findings, including restlessness; anxiety; labored, rapid respirations; frothy, bloody sputum; decreased level of consciousness; neck vein distention; cold, clammy skin; crepitant crackles and wheezes; diastolic (S3) gallop; tachycardia; hypotension; thready pulse

Results of chest X-ray, arterial blood gas (ABG) analysis, pulse oximetry, pulmonary artery catheterization, electrocardiogram

Anxiety related to inability to breathe normally as a result of fluid accumulation

Thoroughly attend to patient's physical needs.

Maintain awareness and sensitivity to patient's emotional state.

Encourage patient to verbalize feelings of anxiety.

Is anxiety decreased or abated?

YES → Continue supportive care.

NO → Stay at patient's bedside as much as possible.

Listen attentively.

Give clear, concise explanations of care and procedures.

Continue to attend to physical needs.

Is anxiety decreased or abated now?

YES → Continue supportive care.

NO → Encourage a calm family member or friend (if available) also to remain at patient's bedside as much as possible.

Obtain an order for morphine and administer as needed.

Patient will experience decreased anxiety by:
- expressing that anxiety has decreased
- using available support systems
- demonstrating abated physical signs of anxiety.

KEY
- Assessment
- Nursing diagnoses
- Interventions
- Evaluation

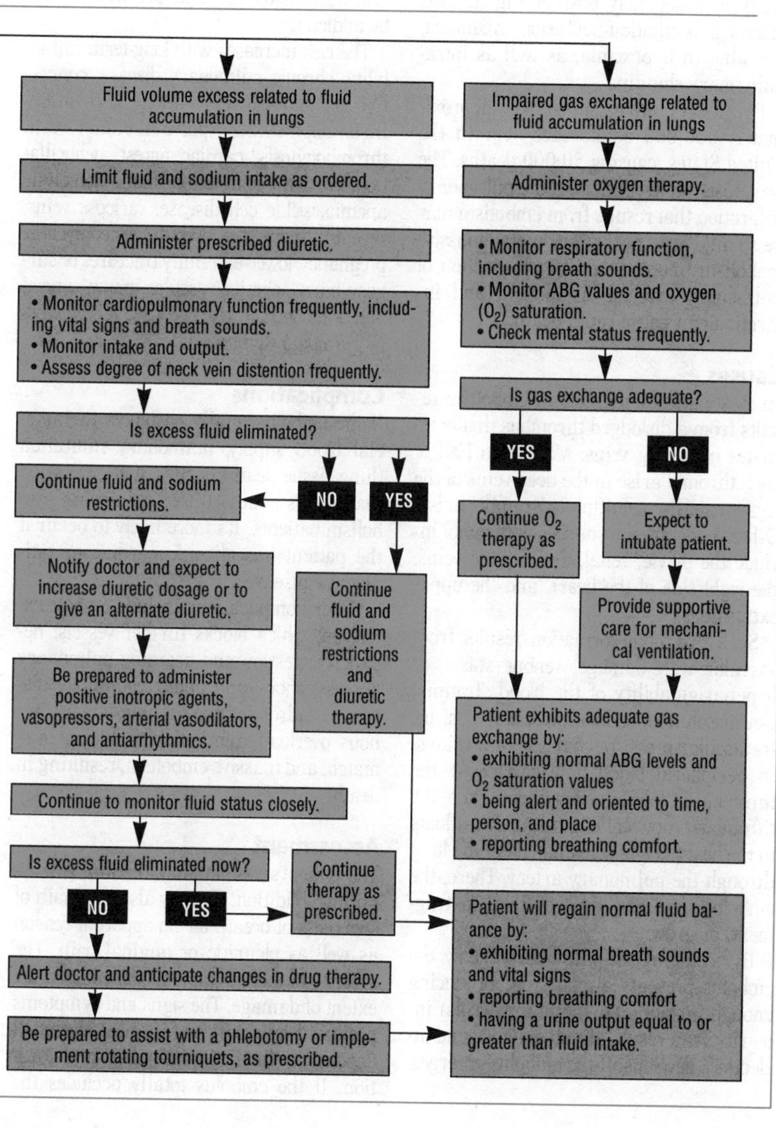
Fluid volume excess related to fluid accumulation in lungs
Limit fluid and sodium intake as ordered.
Administer prescribed diuretic.
• Monitor cardiopulmonary function frequently, including vital signs and breath sounds.
• Monitor intake and output.
• Assess degree of neck vein distention frequently.
Is excess fluid eliminated?
NO
YES
Continue fluid and sodium restrictions.
Notify doctor and expect to increase diuretic dosage or to give an alternate diuretic.
Be prepared to administer positive inotropic agents, vasopressors, arterial vasodilators, and antiarrhythmics.
Continue fluid and sodium restrictions and diuretic therapy.
Continue to monitor fluid status closely.
Is excess fluid eliminated now?
NO
YES
Continue therapy as prescribed.
Alert doctor and anticipate changes in drug therapy.
Be prepared to assist with a phlebotomy or implement rotating tourniquets, as prescribed.
Impaired gas exchange related to fluid accumulation in lungs
Administer oxygen therapy.
• Monitor respiratory function, including breath sounds.
• Monitor ABG values and oxygen (O_2) saturation.
• Check mental status frequently.
Is gas exchange adequate?
YES
NO
Continue O_2 therapy as prescribed.
Expect to intubate patient.
Provide supportive care for mechanical ventilation.
Patient exhibits adequate gas exchange by:
• exhibiting normal ABG levels and O_2 saturation values
• being alert and oriented to time, person, and place
• reporting breathing comfort.
Patient will regain normal fluid balance by:
• exhibiting normal breath sounds and vital signs
• reporting breathing comfort
• having a urine output equal to or greater than fluid intake.

Pulmonary embolism

An obstruction of the pulmonary arterial bed, pulmonary embolism occurs when a mass – such as a dislodged thrombus – lodges in a pulmonary artery branch, partially or completely obstructing it. This causes a ventilation-perfusion mismatch, resulting in hypoxemia, as well as intrapulmonary shunting.

Pulmonary embolism strikes approximately 500,000 adults each year in the United States, causing 50,000 deaths. The prognosis varies. Although the pulmonary infarction that results from embolism may be so mild as to be asymptomatic, massive embolism (more than 50% obstruction of pulmonary arterial circulation) and infarction can cause rapid death.

Causes

In most patients, pulmonary embolism results from a dislodged thrombus that originates in the leg veins. More than half of such thrombi arise in the deep veins of the legs; usually, multiple thrombi arise. Other, less common sources of thrombi include the pelvic, renal, and hepatic veins, the right side of the heart, and the upper extremities.

Such thrombus formation results from vascular wall damage, venous stasis, or hypercoagulability of the blood. Trauma, clot dissolution, sudden muscle spasm, intravascular pressure changes, or a change in peripheral blood flow can cause the thrombus to loosen or fragment. Then, the thrombus – now called an embolus – floats to the heart's right side and enters the lung through the pulmonary artery. There, the embolus may dissolve, continue to fragment, or grow.

By occluding the pulmonary artery, the embolus prevents alveoli from producing enough surfactant to maintain alveolar integrity. As a result, alveoli collapse and atelectasis develops. If the embolus enlarges, it may clog most or all pulmonary vessels and cause death.

Rarely, pulmonary embolism results from other types of emboli, including bone, air, fat, amniotic fluid, tumor cells, or a foreign object such as a needle, catheter part, or talc (from drugs intended for oral administration that are injected I.V. by addicts).

The risk increases with long-term immobility, chronic pulmonary disease, congestive heart failure or atrial fibrillation, thrombophlebitis, polycythemia vera, thrombocytosis, cardiac arrest, defibrillation, cardioversion, autoimmune hemolytic anemia, sickle cell disease, varicose veins, recent surgery, age over 40, osteomyelitis, pregnancy, lower-extremity fractures or surgery, burns, obesity, vascular injury, cancer, and oral contraceptive use. (See *Risk factors in pulmonary embolism.*)

Complications

If the embolus totally obstructs the arterial blood supply, pulmonary infarction (lung tissue death) occurs, a complication that affects about 10% of pulmonary embolism patients. It's more likely to occur if the patient has chronic cardiac or pulmonary disease.

Other complications include emboli extension, which blocks further vessels; hepatic congestion and necrosis; pulmonary abscess; shock and adult respiratory distress syndrome; massive atelectasis; venous overload; ventilation-perfusion mismatch; and massive embolism, resulting in death.

Assessment

The patient's history may reveal a predisposing condition. He may also complain of shortness of breath for no apparent reason as well as pleuritic or anginal pain. The severity of these symptoms depends on the extent of damage. The signs and symptoms produced by small or fragmented emboli depend on their size, number, and location. If the embolus totally occludes the main pulmonary artery, the patient will have severe signs and symptoms.

When you begin your assessment, you may find that the patient is tachycardic. He may also have a low-grade fever. If circulatory collapse has occurred, he'll have a weak, rapid pulse rate and hypotension.

On inspection, you may note a productive cough, possibly producing blood-tinged sputum. Less commonly, you may observe chest splinting, massive hemoptysis, leg edema and, with a large embolus, cyanosis, syncope, and distended neck veins. If you observe restlessness – a sign of hypoxia – the patient may have circulatory collapse.

Palpation may reveal a warm, tender area in the extremities, a possible area of thrombosis. On auscultation, you may hear transient pleural friction rub and crackles at the embolus site. You may also note an S_3 and S_4 gallop, with increased intensity of the pulmonic component of S_2.

In pleural infarction, the patient's history may include heart disease and left ventricular failure. He may complain of sudden, sharp pleuritic chest pain accompanied by progressive dyspnea. On inspection, you may note that the patient has a fever and is coughing up blood-tinged sputum. Auscultation may reveal a pleural friction rub.

Diagnostic tests

- *Lung perfusion scan (lung scintiscan)* can show a pulmonary embolus.
- *Ventilation scan,* usually performed with a lung perfusion scan, confirms the diagnosis.
- *Pulmonary angiography* may show a pulmonary vessel filling defect or an abrupt vessel ending, both of which indicate pulmonary embolism. Although the most definitive test, it's only used if the diagnosis can't be confirmed any other way and anticoagulant therapy would put the patient at significant risk.
- *Electrocardiography (ECG)* helps distinguish pulmonary embolism from myocar-

Risk factors in pulmonary embolism

Many disorders and treatments heighten the risk of pulmonary embolism. At particular risk are surgical patients. For example, the anesthetic used during surgery can injure lung vessels, and surgery itself or prolonged bed rest can promote venous stasis, which compounds the risk.

Predisposing disorders
- Lung disorders, especially chronic types
- Cardiac disorders
- Infection
- Diabetes mellitus
- History of thromboembolism, thrombophlebitis, or vascular insufficiency
- Sickle cell disease
- Autoimmune hemolytic anemia
- Polycythemia
- Osteomyelitis
- Long-bone fracture
- Manipulation or disconnection of central lines

Venous stasis
- Prolonged bed rest or immobilization
- Obesity
- Age over 40
- Burns
- Recent childbirth
- Orthopedic casts

Venous injury
- Surgery, particularly of the legs, pelvis, abdomen, or thorax
- Leg or pelvic fractures or injuries
- I.V. drug abuse
- I.V. therapy

Increased blood coagulability
- Cancer
- Use of high-estrogen oral contraceptives

dial infarction. If the patient has an extensive embolism, the ECG shows right axis deviation; right bundle-branch block; tall, peaked P waves; depressed ST segments; T-wave inversions (a sign of right ventricular heart strain); and supraventricular tachyarrhythmias.

- *Chest X-ray* helps rule out other pulmonary diseases, although it's inconclusive in the 1 to 2 hours after embolism. It may also show areas of atelectasis, an elevated diaphragm, pleural effusion, a prominent pulmonary artery and, occasionally, the characteristic wedge-shaped infiltrate that suggests pulmonary infarction.
- *Arterial blood gas (ABG) analysis* sometimes reveals decreased partial pressure of oxygen in arterial blood and partial pressure of carbon dioxide in arterial blood levels from tachypnea.
- *Thoracentesis* may rule out empyema, a sign of pneumonia, if the patient has pleural effusion.
- *Magnetic resonance imaging* can identify blood flow changes that point to an embolus or identify the embolus itself.

Treatment

The goal of treatment is to maintain adequate cardiovascular and pulmonary function until the obstruction resolves and to prevent any recurrence. (Most emboli resolve within 10 to 14 days.)

Treatment for an embolism caused by a thrombus generally consists of oxygen therapy, as needed, and anticoagulation with heparin to inhibit new thrombus formation. The patient on heparin therapy needs daily coagulation studies (partial thromboplastin time [PTT]). The patient may also receive warfarin for 3 to 6 months, depending on his risk factors. This patient's prothrombin time (PT) will be monitored daily and then biweekly.

If the patient has a massive pulmonary embolism and shock, he may need fibrinolytic therapy with urokinase, streptokinase, or alteplase. Initially, these thrombolytic agents dissolve clots within 12 to 24 hours. Seven days later, these drugs lyse clots to the same degree as heparin therapy alone.

If the embolus causes hypotension, the patient may need a vasopressor. A septic embolus requires antibiotic therapy, not anticoagulants, and evaluation for the infection's source (most likely endocarditis).

If the patient can't take anticoagulants or develops recurrent emboli during anticoagulant therapy, he'll need surgery. Surgery consists of vena caval ligation, plication, or insertion of a device (umbrella filter) to filter blood returning to the heart and lungs. Angiographic demonstration of pulmonary embolism should take place before surgery.

To prevent postoperative venous thromboembolism, the patient may require rotating tourniquets applied to his legs. Or, he can receive a combination of heparin and dihydroergotamine, which is more effective than heparin alone.

If the patient has a fat embolus, he'll need oxygen therapy. He may also need mechanical ventilation, corticosteroids and, if pulmonary edema arises, diuretics.

Key nursing diagnoses and patient outcomes

Altered cardiopulmonary perfusion related to obstruction of pulmonary artery. Based on this nursing diagnosis, you'll establish these patient outcomes. The patient will:

- regain and maintain cardiopulmonary tissue perfusion and cellular oxygenation
- not show signs and symptoms of pulmonary infarction or emboli extension
- eliminate risk factors when possible, to prevent recurrence.

Anxiety related to situational crisis. Based on this nursing diagnosis, you'll establish these patient outcomes. The patient will:

- express feelings of anxiety
- cope with his condition without showing signs of severe anxiety.

Impaired gas exchange related to collapsed alveoli. Based on this nursing diagnosis, you'll establish these patient outcomes. The patient will:
• regain and maintain adequate ventilation
• regain and maintain normal ABG levels
• not show signs and symptoms of severe hypoxia.

Nursing interventions

• As ordered, give oxygen by nasal cannula or mask. If breathing is severely compromised, provide endotracheal intubation with assisted ventilation, as ordered.
• Administer heparin, as ordered, by I.V. push or by continuous drip. Don't administer I.M. injections.
• If the patient has pleuritic chest pain, administer the ordered analgesic.
• After the patient's condition stabilizes, encourage him to move about and assist him with isometric and range-of-motion exercises. *Never* vigorously massage his legs; doing so could cause thrombi to dislodge.
• If the patient needs surgery, make sure he ambulates as soon as possible afterward to prevent venous stasis.
• Provide the patient with adequate nutrition and fluids to promote healing.
• If needed, provide incentive spirometry to help the patient with deep breathing. Provide tissues and a bag for easy disposal of tissues.
• Offer the patient diversional activities to promote relaxation and relieve restlessness.

Monitoring

• Monitor the patient's respiratory status closely. If he has worsening dyspnea, check his ABG levels.
• Monitor coagulation studies daily. Effective heparin therapy raises PTT to about 2 to 2½ times normal. During heparin therapy, watch closely for epistaxis, petechiae, and other signs of abnormal bleeding. Also check the patient's stools for occult blood.
• Watch for possible anticoagulant treatment complications, including gastric bleeding, cerebrovascular accident, and hemorrhage.
• Check the patient's temperature and the color of his feet to detect venous stasis.

Patient teaching

• Explain all procedures and treatments to the patient and his family.
• Teach the patient and his family the signs and symptoms of thrombophlebitis and pulmonary embolism.
• Teach the patient on anticoagulant therapy the signs of bleeding he should watch for (bloody stools, blood in urine, large bruises).
• Tell the patient he can help prevent bleeding by shaving with an electric razor and by brushing his teeth with a soft toothbrush.
• Make sure the patient understands the importance of taking his medication exactly as ordered. Tell him not to take any other medications, especially aspirin, without asking the doctor.
• Instruct the patient taking warfarin not to significantly vary the amount of vitamin K he takes in daily. Doing so could interfere with anticoagulation stabilization.
• Stress the importance of follow-up laboratory tests, such as PT, to monitor anticoagulant therapy.
• Tell the patient that he must inform all his health care providers – including dentists – that he's receiving anticoagulant therapy.
• To prevent pulmonary emboli in a high-risk patient, encourage him to walk and exercise his legs and to wear support or antiembolism stockings. Also, tell him not to cross or massage his legs.

Pulmonary hypertension

In both the rare primary form and the more common secondary form, pulmonary hypertension is indicated by a resting systolic pulmonary artery pressure (PAP) above 30 mm Hg and a mean PAP above 18 mm Hg.

Primary or idiopathic pulmonary hypertension is characterized by increased PAP and increased pulmonary vascular resistance, both without an obvious cause. This form is most common in women between ages 20 and 40 and is usually fatal within 3 to 4 years; mortality is highest in pregnant women.

Secondary pulmonary hypertension results from existing cardiac or pulmonary disease or both. The prognosis in secondary pulmonary hypertension depends on the severity of the underlying disorder.

Causes

Although the cause of primary pulmonary hypertension remains unknown, the tendency for the disease to occur within families points to a hereditary defect. It also occurs more commonly in those with collagen disease and is thought to result from altered immune mechanisms. In primary pulmonary hypertension, the intimal lining of the pulmonary arteries thickens for no apparent reason. This narrows the artery and impairs distensibility, increasing vascular resistance.

Secondary pulmonary hypertension results from hypoxemia. (See *Causes of secondary pulmonary hypertension.*)

Complications

Pulmonary hypertension may ultimately lead to cor pulmonale, cardiac failure, and cardiac arrest.

Assessment

The patient with primary pulmonary hypertension may have no signs or symptoms until lung damage becomes severe. (In fact, the disorder may not be diagnosed until an autopsy.)

Usually, a patient with pulmonary hypertension complains of increasing dyspnea on exertion, weakness, syncope, and fatigue. He may also have difficulty breathing, feel short of breath, and report that breathing causes pain. Such signs may result from left ventricular failure.

Inspection may show signs of right ventricular failure, including ascites and neck vein distention. The patient may appear restless and agitated and have a decreased level of consciousness (LOC). He may even be confused and have memory loss. You may observe decreased diaphragmatic excursion and respiration, and the point of maximal impulse may be displaced beyond the midclavicular line.

On palpation, you may also note signs of right ventricular failure, such as peripheral edema. The patient typically has an easily palpable right ventricular lift and a reduced carotid pulse. He may also have a palpable and tender liver as well as tachycardia.

Auscultation findings are specific to the underlying disorder but may include a systolic ejection murmur, a widely split S_2, and S_3 and S_4. You may also hear decreased breath sounds and loud tubular sounds. The patient may have decreased blood pressure.

Diagnostic tests

- *Arterial blood gas (ABG) studies* reveal hypoxemia (decreased partial pressure of oxygen in arterial blood).
- *Electrocardiography,* in right ventricular hypertrophy, shows right axis deviation and tall or peaked P waves in inferior leads.
- *Cardiac catheterization* discloses increased PAP, with a systolic pressure above 30 mm Hg. It may also show an increased pulmonary capillary wedge pressure (PCWP) if the underlying cause is left atrial myxoma, mitral stenosis, or left ven-

tricular failure; otherwise, PCWP is normal.

- *Pulmonary angiography* detects filling defects in pulmonary vasculature, such as those that develop with pulmonary emboli.
- *Pulmonary function tests* may show decreased flow rates and increased residual volume in underlying obstructive disease; in underlying restrictive disease, they may show reduced total lung capacity.
- *Radionuclide imaging* allows assessment of right and left ventricular functioning.
- *Open lung biopsy* may determine the type of disorder.
- *Echocardiography* allows the assessment of ventricular wall motion and possible valvular dysfunction. It can also demonstrate right ventricular enlargement, abnormal septal configuration consistent with right ventricular pressure overload, and a reduction in left ventricular cavity size.
- *Perfusion lung scan* may produce normal or abnormal results, with multiple patchy and diffuse filling defects that don't suggest pulmonary thromboembolism.

Treatment

Oxygen therapy decreases hypoxemia and resulting pulmonary vascular resistance. For patients with right ventricular failure, treatment also includes fluid restriction, digitalis glycosides to increase cardiac output, and diuretics to decrease intravascular volume and extravascular fluid accumulation. Vasodilators and calcium channel blockers can reduce myocardial work load and oxygen consumption. Bronchodilators and beta-adrenergic agents may also be prescribed.

For a patient with secondary pulmonary hypertension, treatment must also aim to correct the underlying cause. If that's not possible and the disease progresses, the patient may need a heart-lung transplant.

Key nursing diagnoses and patient outcomes

Activity intolerance related to dyspnea, fatigue, and pain. Based on this nursing di-

Causes of secondary pulmonary hypertension

Secondary pulmonary hypertension can stem from any of the following:

- *Alveolar hypoventilation.* This can result from diseases that cause alveolar destruction, such as chronic obstructive pulmonary disease (the most common cause in the United States), sarcoidosis, diffuse interstitial pneumonia, malignant metastases, and scleroderma. Or, it can stem from obesity or kyphoscoliosis, which don't damage lung tissue but prevent the chest wall from expanding sufficiently to let air into the alveoli.

  Either way, the decreased ventilation that results increases pulmonary vascular resistance. Hypoxemia resulting from this ventilation-perfusion mismatch also causes vasoconstriction, further increasing vascular resistance. The result is pulmonary hypertension.
- *Vascular obstruction.* Such obstruction can arise from pulmonary embolism or vasculitis. It can also result from disorders that cause obstructions of small or large pulmonary veins, such as left atrial myxoma, idiopathic veno-occlusive disease, fibrosing mediastinitis, and mediastinal neoplasm.
- *Primary cardiac disease.* Such disease may be congenital or acquired. Congenital defects that cause left-to-right shunting include patent ductus arteriosus and an atrial or a ventricular septal defect. This shunting into the pulmonary artery reroutes blood through the lungs twice, causing pulmonary hypertension.

  Acquired cardiac diseases, such as rheumatic valvular disease and mitral stenosis, result in left ventricular failure that diminishes the flow of oxygenated blood from the lungs. This increases pulmonary vascular resistance and right ventricular pressure.

agnosis, you'll establish these patient outcomes. The patient will:

- express an understanding of the need to increase his activity level gradually and stagger activities
- demonstrate skill in conserving energy while carrying out daily activities to tolerance level
- seek help with activities that precipitate or worsen signs and symptoms of pulmonary hypertension.

Altered cerebral tissue perfusion related to hypoxemia. Based on this nursing diagnosis, you'll establish these patient outcomes. The patient will:

- comply with oxygen therapy
- regain and maintain normal cerebral function, as exhibited by being oriented to time, person, and place
- not develop permanent neurologic deficits from altered cerebral tissue perfusion.

Impaired gas exchange related to alveolar hypoventilation. Based on this nursing diagnosis, you'll establish these patient outcomes. The patient will:

- regain and maintain adequate ventilation
- regain and maintain normal ABG levels
- not show signs and symptoms of severe hypoxia.

Nursing interventions

- Administer oxygen therapy as ordered.
- Make sure the patient alternates periods of rest and activity to reduce his body's oxygen demand and prevent fatigue.
- Arrange for diversional activities. The type of activity–whether active or passive–depends on the patient's physical condition.
- Before discharge, help the patient adjust to the limitations imposed by this disorder.
- Listen to the patient's fears and concerns, and remain with him during periods of extreme stress and anxiety. Answer any questions he may have as best you can. Encourage him to identify care measures and activities that will make him comfortable and relaxed. Then, try to perform these measures and encourage the patient to do so, too.
- Include the patient in care decisions, and include the patient's family in all phases of his care.

Monitoring

- Observe the patient's response to oxygen therapy. Report any signs of increasing dyspnea so the doctor can adjust treatment accordingly.
- Monitor ABG levels for acidosis and hypoxemia. Report any change in the patient's LOC immediately.
- When caring for a patient with right ventricular failure, especially one receiving diuretics, record weight daily and measure intake and output carefully. Check for increasing neck vein distention, which may signal fluid overload.
- Monitor the patient's vital signs, especially his blood pressure and heart rate. If hypotension or tachycardia develops, notify the doctor. If the patient has a pulmonary artery catheter, monitor his PAP and PCWP as ordered and report any changes.

Patient teaching

- Teach the patient what signs and symptoms to report to his doctor (increasing shortness of breath, swelling, increasing weight gain, increasing fatigue).
- Fully explain the medication regimen.
- If the patient smokes, encourage him to stop and give him the names of programs to help him stop smoking.
- If necessary, go over diet restrictions the patient should follow to maintain a low-sodium diet.
- Teach the patient taking a potassium-wasting diuretic which foods are high in potassium.
- Warn the patient not to overexert himself, and suggest frequent rest periods between activities.
- If the patient needs special equipment for home use, such as oxygen equipment, refer him to the social service department.

Pulmonic insufficiency

In this disorder, blood ejected into the pulmonary artery during systole flows back into the right ventricle during diastole, causing fluid overload in the ventricle, ventricular hypertrophy, and eventual right ventricular failure.

Causes

Pulmonic insufficiency may be congenital or may result from pulmonary hypertension. The most common acquired cause is dilation of the pulmonary valve ring from severe pulmonary hypertension.

Rarely, pulmonic insufficiency may result from prolonged use of a pressure monitoring catheter in the pulmonary artery.

Complications

If the patient has pulmonary hypertension, right ventricular failure may develop.

Assessment

The patient may complain of dyspnea on exertion, fatigue, chest pain, and syncope. Peripheral edema may cause him discomfort.

A patient with severe insufficiency that has progressed to right ventricular failure may appear jaundiced, with severe peripheral edema and ascites. He may also appear malnourished.

Auscultation may reveal a high-pitched, decrescendo, diastolic blowing murmur along the left sternal border (Graham Steell's murmur). This murmur may be difficult to distinguish from the murmur of aortic insufficiency.

Palpation may disclose hepatomegaly when the patient has right ventricular failure.

Diagnostic tests

- *Cardiac catheterization* shows pulmonary regurgitation, increased right ventricular pressure, and associated cardiac defects.
- *Chest X-rays* show right ventricular and pulmonary arterial enlargement.
- *Echocardiography* visualizes the pulmonary valve abnormality.
- *Electrocardiography* findings may be normal in mild cases or reveal right ventricular hypertrophy.

Treatment

In pulmonic insufficiency, treatment is based on the patient's symptoms. A low-sodium diet and diuretics help to reduce hepatic congestion before surgery. Valvulotomy or valve replacement may be required in severe cases.

Key nursing diagnoses and patient outcomes

Fatigue related to cardiac circulation disturbance. Based on this nursing diagnosis, you'll establish these patient outcomes. The patient will:

- communicate an understanding of the relationship between fatigue, pulmonary insufficiency, and activity level
- take measures to decrease fatigue during his daily activities
- perform activities of daily living to his level of tolerance.

Fluid volume excess related to right ventricular failure. Based on this nursing diagnosis, you'll establish these patient outcomes. The patient will:

- tolerate a restricted sodium intake with no physical or emotional discomfort
- show reduced fluid retention with effective therapy
- identify signs and symptoms that require medical treatment.

Ineffective breathing pattern related to dyspnea. Based on this nursing diagnosis, you'll establish these patient outcomes. The patient will:

- maintain adequate ventilation
- identify activities that precipitate or worsen dyspnea
- show no signs and symptoms of hypoxia.

Nursing interventions

- Alternate periods of activity and rest to prevent extreme fatigue and dyspnea.
- Keep the patient's legs elevated while he sits in a chair to improve venous return to the heart.
- Elevate the head of the bed to improve ventilation.
- Keep the patient on a low-sodium diet. Consult with a dietitian to ensure that the patient receives foods that he likes while adhering to the diet restrictions.
- To reduce anxiety, allow the patient to express his concerns about the effects of limited activity on his responsibilities and routines. Help him explore methods of coping.
- Prepare patient for surgery, as indicated. (See the entry "Heart valve replacement.")

Monitoring

- Assess the patient's cardiopulmonary function regularly, observing for signs of heart failure and pulmonary edema.
- Watch for adverse drug reactions.
- Check the patient for fluid retention, and weigh him regularly.
- Monitor the patient's compliance with restricted sodium intake and medication therapy.

Patient teaching

- Teach the patient about diet restrictions, medications, symptoms that should be reported, and the importance of consistent follow-up care.
- Tell the patient to elevate his legs whenever he sits.

Pulmonic stenosis

In this disorder, obstructed right ventricular outflow causes right ventricular hypertrophy as the right ventricle attempts to overcome resistance to the narrow valvular opening.

A congenital defect, pulmonic stenosis is associated with other congenital heart defects, such as tetralogy of Fallot. It's rare among elderly people.

Causes

Pulmonic stenosis results from congenital stenosis of the pulmonary valve cusp or (infrequently) from rheumatic heart disease. In cases of I.V. drug abuse, the valve can be damaged by vegetation or foreign substances (such as cotton from a cotton swab) caught on leaflets.

Complications

Right ventricular failure is the ultimate result of untreated pulmonic stenosis.

Assessment

The patient with mild stenosis may be asymptomatic. A patient with moderate to severe stenosis may complain of dyspnea on exertion, fatigue, chest pain, and syncope. Accompanying peripheral edema may cause him discomfort.

Inspection may reveal a prominent *a* wave in the jugular venous pulse. If severe stenosis has progressed to right ventricular failure, the patient may appear jaundiced, with severe peripheral edema and ascites. He may also appear malnourished.

Auscultation may reveal S_4, a thrill at the upper left sternal border, a harsh systolic ejection murmur, and a holosystolic decrescendo murmur of tricuspid insufficiency, particularly if the patient has heart failure.

Palpation may detect hepatomegaly when the patient has right ventricular failure, presystolic pulsations of the liver, and a right parasternal lift.

Diagnostic tests

- *Chest X-rays* usually show normal heart size and normal lung vascularity, although the pulmonary arteries may be evident. With severe obstruction and right ventricular failure, the right atrium and ventricle typically appear enlarged.

• *Echocardiography* visualizes the pulmonary valve abnormality.
• *Electrocardiography* results may be normal in mild cases, or they may show right axis deviation and right ventricular hypertrophy. High-amplitude P waves in leads II and V_1 indicate right atrial enlargement.

Treatment

A low-sodium diet and diuretics help reduce hepatic congestion before surgery. Additionally, cardiac catheter balloon valvuloplasty is usually effective even with moderate to severe obstruction.

Key nursing diagnoses and patient outcomes

Activity intolerance related to fatigue and dyspnea. Based on this nursing diagnosis, you'll establish these patient outcomes. The patient will:
• identify activities that precipitate or increase fatigue and dyspnea
• use available resources for assistance with activities of daily living
• perform activities of daily living to his tolerance level.

Decreased cardiac output related to restricted blood flow through the pulmonary valve. Based on this nursing diagnosis, you'll establish these patient outcomes. The patient will:
• maintain hemodynamic stability, as evidenced by stable vital signs and adequate output
• maintain adequate tissue perfusion
• not develop complications related to decreased cardiac output, such as ischemia and shock.

Fluid volume excess related to edema caused by pulmonic stenosis. Based on this nursing diagnosis, you'll establish these patient outcomes. The patient will:
• adhere to restricted sodium intake and diuretic therapy
• have decreased edema with therapy
• identify signs and symptoms that require medical attention.

Nursing interventions

• Alternate periods of activity and rest to prevent extreme fatigue and dyspnea.
• Keep the patient's legs elevated while he sits in a chair to improve venous return to the heart.
• Elevate the head of the bed to improve ventilation.
• Keep the patient on a low-sodium diet. Consult with a dietitian to ensure that the patient receives foods that he likes while adhering to the diet restrictions.
• To reduce anxiety, allow the patient to express his concerns about the effects of activity restrictions on his responsibilities and routines.
• After cardiac catheterization, apply firm pressure to the catheter insertion site, usually in the groin. If the site bleeds, remove the pressure dressing and manually apply firm pressure to the site.
• Notify the doctor of any changes in peripheral pulses distal to the insertion site, swelling or hematoma formation at the insertion site, changes in cardiac rhythm and vital signs, and complaints of chest pain.

Monitoring

• Monitor the patient's cardiopulmonary function, checking for signs of heart failure and pulmonary edema.
• Watch for adverse drug reactions.
• After cardiac catheterization, monitor the site for signs of bleeding according to hospital policy.
• Monitor the patient's compliance with dietary restrictions and his medication regimen.

Patient teaching

• Teach the patient about diet restrictions, medications, signs and symptoms that should be reported, and the importance of consistent follow-up care.
• Tell the patient to elevate his legs whenever he sits.
• Discuss the importance of adequate rest and spacing activities to prevent fatigue.

Pyelonephritis, acute

Acute pyelonephritis is one of the most common renal diseases. In this disorder, sudden inflammation is caused by bacterial invasion. It occurs mainly in the interstitial tissue and the renal pelvis and occasionally in the renal tubules. It may affect one or both kidneys. With treatment and continued follow-up care, the prognosis is good and extensive permanent damage is rare.

Pyelonephritis occurs more often in women than in men, probably because the shorter urethra and the proximity of the urinary meatus to the vagina and rectum allow bacteria to reach the bladder more easily. Women also lack the antibacterial prostatic secretions that men produce.

Typically, the infection spreads from the bladder to the ureters and then to the kidneys, commonly through vesicoureteral reflux. Vesicoureteral reflux may result from congenital weakness at the junction of the ureter and the bladder. Bacteria refluxed to intrarenal tissues may create colonies of infection within 24 to 48 hours.

Causes

Acute pyelonephritis results from bacterial infection of the kidneys. Infecting bacteria usually are normal intestinal and fecal flora that grow readily in urine. The most common causative organism is *Escherichia coli,* but *Proteus, Pseudomonas, Staphylococcus aureus,* and *Streptococcus faecalis* (enterococcus) also may cause such infections.

Infection also may result from procedures that involve the use of instruments (such as catheterization, cystoscopy, and urologic surgery) or from a hematogenic infection (such as septicemia and endocarditis).

Pyelonephritis may result from an inability to empty the bladder (for example, in patients with neurogenic bladder), from urinary stasis, or from urinary obstruction caused by tumors, strictures, or benign prostatic hyperplasia. Incidence increases with age and is higher in the following groups.

- *Sexually active women.* Intercourse increases the risk of bacterial contamination.
- *Pregnant women.* About 5% of pregnant women develop asymptomatic bacteriuria; if untreated, about 40% of these women develop pyelonephritis.
- *People with obstructive diseases.* Resulting hydronephrosis increases the risk of urinary tract infection (UTI), which can lead to pyelonephritis.
- *People with neurogenic bladder.* Seen in diabetes, spinal cord injury, multiple sclerosis, and tabes dorsalis, neurogenic bladder causes incomplete emptying and urinary stasis. Frequent catheterization increases the risk of introducing bacteria. Glycosuria may support bacterial growth in urine.
- *People with other renal diseases.* Compromised renal function increases susceptibility to acute pyelonephritis.

Complications

Associated complications include secondary arteriosclerosis, calculus formation, further renal damage, renal or perinephric abscesses with possible metastasis to other organs, septic shock, and chronic pyelonephritis. (See *Chronic pyelonephritis.*)

Assessment

A patient with acute pyelonephritis commonly looks quite ill. She usually complains of pain over one or both kidneys, urinary urgency and frequency, burning during urination, dysuria, nocturia, and hematuria (usually microscopic but possibly gross). Palpating the flank area may increase pain. Urine may appear cloudy and have an ammonia-like or fishy odor. Other common symptoms include a temperature of 102° F (38.9° C) or higher, shaking chills, anorexia, and general fatigue.

The patient usually reports that symptoms developed rapidly over a few hours or a few days. Although these symptoms may disappear within days, even without treatment, residual bacterial infection is likely and may cause recurrence of symptoms.

Diagnostic tests

Diagnosis requires a urinalysis and culture and sensitivity testing. Typical findings include the following.

- *Pyuria* (pus in urine). Urine sediment reveals leukocytes singly, in clumps, and in casts and possibly a few red blood cells.
- *Significant bacteriuria.* Urine culture reveals more than 100,000 organisms/mm^3 of urine.
- *Low specific gravity and osmolality.* These findings result from a temporarily decreased ability to concentrate urine.
- *Slightly alkaline urine pH.*
- *Proteinuria, glycosuria, and ketonuria.* These conditions occur less frequently.

Blood tests and X-rays also help in the evaluation of acute pyelonephritis. A complete blood count shows an elevated white blood cell count (up to 40,000/mm^3) and an elevated neutrophil count. The erythrocyte sedimentation rate also is elevated.

Kidney-ureter-bladder radiography may reveal calculi, tumors, or cysts in the kidneys and the urinary tract. Excretory urography may show asymmetrical kidneys.

Treatment

Appropriate treatment centers on antibiotic therapy appropriate to the specific infecting organism after identification by urine culture and sensitivity studies. For example, enterococcus requires treatment with ampicillin, penicillin G, or vancomycin. *Staphylococcus* requires penicillin G or, if the bacterium is resistant, a semisynthetic penicillin, such as nafcillin, or a cephalosporin. *Escherichia coli* may be treated with sulfisoxazole, nalidixic acid, or nitrofurantoin; *Proteus,* with ampicillin, sulfisoxazole, nalidixic acid, or a cephalosporin; and *Pseudomonas,* with gentamicin, tobramycin, or carbenicillin.

When the infecting organism can't be identified, therapy usually consists of a broad-spectrum antibiotic, such as ampicillin or cephalexin. Antibiotics must be prescribed cautiously for elderly patients because of the combined effects of aging and pyelonephritis on renal function. Antibiotics also are used with caution in pregnant patients. In these patients, urinary analgesics, such as phenazopyridine, can help relieve pain.

Chronic pyelonephritis

A persistent kidney inflammation, chronic pyelonephritis can scar the kidneys and lead to chronic renal failure. Its etiology may be bacterial, metastatic, or urogenous. This disease most frequently occurs in patients who are predisposed to recurrent acute pyelonephritis—for instance, those with urinary obstructions or vesicoureteral reflux.

Assessment and diagnosis

Patients with chronic pyelonephritis may have a childhood history of unexplained fevers or bed-wetting. Clinical signs and symptoms include flank pain, anemia, low urine specific gravity, proteinuria, leukocytes in urine, and hypertension (especially in late stages). Uremia seldom develops unless structural abnormalities exist in the excretory system. Intermittent bacteriuria may occur.

When no bacteria are found in the urine, diagnosis depends on excretory urography (the patient's renal pelvis may appear small and flattened) and renal biopsy.

Treatment

Effective treatment of chronic pyelonephritis requires control of hypertension, elimination of the obstruction (when possible), and long-term antimicrobial therapy.

Symptoms may disappear after several days of antibiotic therapy. Although urine usually becomes sterile within 48 to 72 hours, the course of such therapy ranges from 10 to 14 days. Follow-up treatment includes reculturing urine 1 week after drug therapy stops and then periodically for the next year to detect residual or recurring infection. A patient with an uncomplicated infection usually responds well to therapy and doesn't suffer reinfection.

If infection results from obstruction or vesicoureteral reflux, antibiotics may be less effective and surgery may be necessary to relieve the obstruction or correct the anomaly. A patient at high risk for recurring urinary tract and kidney infections – for example, a patient with a long-term indwelling urinary catheter or on maintenance antibiotic therapy – requires lengthy follow-up care.

Key nursing diagnoses and patient outcomes

Altered urinary elimination related to bladder inflammation. Based on this nursing diagnosis, you'll establish these patient outcomes. The patient will:
- maintain adequate urine output
- not develop complications related to altered urine elimination, such as urine retention or fluid retention
- regain and maintain a normal urinary elimination pattern with eradication of pyelonephritis.

Hyperthermia related to inflammatory process. Based on this nursing diagnosis, you'll establish these patient outcomes. The patient will:
- reestablish a normal body temperature with antipyretic and antibiotic therapy
- show no signs and symptoms of complications associated with hyperthermia, such as seizures and dehydration.

Pain in the back and pain related to dysuria. Based on this nursing diagnosis, you'll establish these patient outcomes. The patient will:
- state and carry out appropriate interventions for pain relief
- express feelings of comfort and relief from pain with eradication of pyelonephritis.

Nursing interventions

- Administer antipyretics for fever.
- Force fluids to achieve a urine output of more than 2,000 ml/day. This helps empty the bladder of contaminated urine and is the best way to prevent calculus formation. Don't encourage intake of more than 2 to 3 qt (or liters) because this may decrease the effectiveness of the antibiotics.
- Provide an acid-ash diet to prevent calculus formation.
- Observe strict sterile technique during catheter insertion and care.
- Be sure to refrigerate or culture a urine specimen within 30 minutes of collection to prevent overgrowth of bacteria.

Monitoring

- Assess the patient's temperature regularly to determine his response to administered antipyretics.
- Check the patient's voiding pattern and urine characteristics for evidence of improvement or complications. Measure his intake and output.

Patient teaching

- Instruct a female patient to avoid bacterial contamination by wiping the perineum from front to back after bowel movements.
- Teach proper technique for collecting a clean-catch urine specimen.
- Stress the need to complete the prescribed antibiotic regimen even after symptoms subside. Encourage long-term follow-up care for a high-risk patient.
- Advise routine checkups for a patient with a history of UTIs. Teach her to recognize signs and symptoms of infection, such as cloudy urine, burning on urination, and urinary urgency and frequency, especially when accompanied by a low-grade fever and back pain.

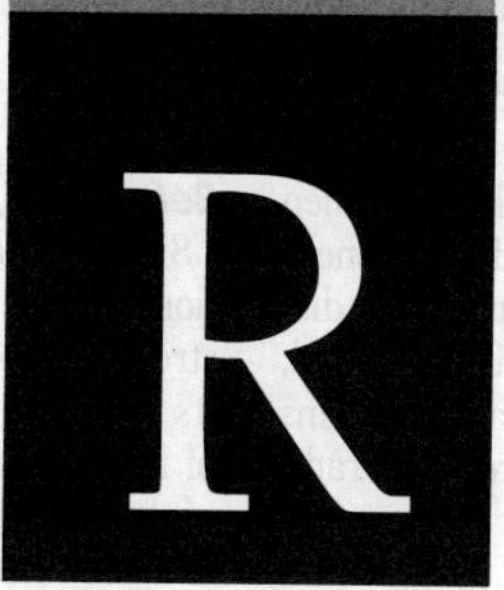

Radiation, external

External radiation therapy, also known as external beam radiation or teletherapy, is used in the treatment of cancer to deliver high levels of radiation externally to a specific area of the body. The goal of this therapy is to destroy malignant cells, which are more sensitive to radiation than normal cells, without permanently damaging adjacent body tissues. Radiation is thought to destroy the cancer cells' ability to grow and multiply by either decreasing the rate of mitosis or impairing the synthesis of deoxyribonucleic acid or ribonucleic acid.

External radiation therapy may be used as part of cancer treatment aimed at curing the patient, or it may be used as a palliative measure in terminal cancer to relieve pain and enhance the patient's quality of life. This therapy is most commonly given on an outpatient basis unless the patient's underlying condition warrants hospitalization.

Curative radiation therapy is generally given 5 days per week for 4 to 8 weeks; palliative radiation therapy is usually given for less time. The dosage and the body areas receiving the beam of rays are determined by the radiation oncologist and marked on the patient's body with tiny tattoos at the beginning of therapy.

Recent advances in external radiation therapy include large-field, large-dose radiation. Half-body treatment – in which half of the body is used as a large field to receive large doses of radiation – is an example of this type of external radiation. It provides an effective, well-tolerated treatment in metastatic disease.

Total skin electron therapy, another advancement, provides radiation to the entire skin surface and has been successful in managing extensive skin disease. Hyperfractionation is an experimental type of radiation therapy that delivers more than one treatment per day in an attempt to achieve better tumor control.

Procedure

The patient is taken to the radiation department of the hospital, where he changes into a patient gown. He is then placed on the treatment table or floor (in the case of large-dose radiation) and told to lie immobile while a large machine, usually overhead, directs radiation at the target site for the prescribed period of time, usually 1 to 2 minutes.

Complications

Because external radiation therapy destroys normal cells in the path of the radiation beam, most patients will experience some degree of skin reaction at the irradiated site. Anorexia, fatigue, and bone marrow suppression, which increase the patient's risk of bleeding or infection, also occur. Other complications are site specific and generally related to dysfunction or change in the structure of body parts within the irradiated area. For example, alopecia may occur when the scalp is irradiated; stomatitis and esophagitis when the head and neck are irradiated; pneumonitis, pericarditis, and upper GI distress when the thoracic area is irradiated; and lower GI and genitourinary problems when the abdominopelvic area is irradiated. (See *Managing adverse effects of radiation therapy.*)

Key nursing diagnoses and patient outcomes

Altered protection related to bone marrow suppression. Based on this nursing diagnosis, you'll establish these patient outcomes. The patient will:

- not have chills, fever, or other signs and symptoms of infection, or excessive bleeding episodes
- demonstrate protective measures, including conserving energy, maintaining a balanced diet, and getting adequate rest
- regain normal bone marrow function when therapy is completed.

Fear related to radiation exposure. Based on this nursing diagnosis, you'll establish these patient outcomes. The patient will:

- identify and express his fears
- obtain correct information about external radiation therapy that will help dispel his fears
- exhibit fewer physical signs and symptoms of fear.

Impaired skin integrity related to adverse effects of external radiation therapy. Based on this nursing diagnosis, you'll establish these patient outcomes. The patient will:

- communicate an understanding of skin-protection measures
- demonstrate skill in caring for areas of impaired skin integrity
- regain skin integrity when therapy is completed.

Nursing interventions

When preparing a patient for external radiation therapy or managing his care afterward, expect to implement these nursing interventions.

Before the procedure

- Since the patient may misinterpret radiation therapy as terminal care, be sure to stress its potentially curative effects and its ability to improve the patient's quality of life. Before treatment, explain the type of therapy, take the patient on a tour of the radiation facilities, and encourage him to ask questions.
- Obtain baseline white blood cell (WBC) and platelet counts. Also obtain a thorough patient history, including any previous radiation treatments and adverse effects.
- Because radiation therapy can reduce the production of sperm, tell the male patient about sperm banking if he intends to start a family later. Inform the female patient undergoing pelvic irradiation that this treatment can decrease hormone levels, which may lead to infertility and amenorrhea.
- Inform the patient that the radiation oncologist may mark the precise areas of treatment on his skin with tiny tattoo "dots."
- Make sure the patient or a responsible family member has signed a consent form.

After the procedure

- Monitor the patient's WBC and platelet counts to help evaluate myelosuppressive effects. Institute bleeding and infection-control measures. Also monitor for other common adverse effects of radiation treatment, such as erythema, nausea, and vomiting.
- Provide comfort measures as indicated by the patient's response to external radiation. Provide supportive care if adverse reactions occur.
- Tell the patient when his next radiation treatment will be, if indicated.

Home care instructions

- Explain that the full benefit of radiation treatment may not occur for up to several months. Instruct the patient to report any long-term adverse effects.

Managing adverse effects of radiation therapy

Radiation therapy can cause both local and systemic effects. Local effects, such as headaches (from cranial tissue irradiation) and erythema, are discussed in the chart below. Systemic effects, which are similar for both radiation therapy and chemotherapy, are discussed in *Managing common adverse effects of chemotherapy*, pages 174 and 175. These effects include GI upset, stomatitis, alopecia, and bone marrow depression.

Adverse effect	Nursing considerations
Headaches, caused by cerebral edema	• Assess for pain. Administer corticosteroids or analgesics, as ordered.
Pneumonitis, pericarditis, or myocarditis caused by irradiation of lung or heart areas	• Auscultate the patient's heart and lungs daily. Monitor his vital signs, as ordered. • Watch for and report coughing, dyspnea, weakness, or pain on inspiration.
Mucositis, pharyngitis, decreased salivation and taste sensation (caused by irradiation of the head and neck area)	• Inspect the oral cavity and evaluate the patient's nutritional status. Tell him to maintain optimal nutrition, emphasizing protein and carbohydrates. • Administer analgesics, such as lidocaine solution or ointment, before meals. • Tell the patient to avoid dry or thick foods, to use artificial saliva, and to drink plenty of fluids with meals. • Instruct the patient to rinse his mouth before meals with equal parts of hydrogen peroxide and water to prevent accumulation of debris and to improve his appetite. • Suggest use of sugarless lemon drops or mints to increase salivation.
Erythema	• Observe reddened areas daily and record any changes. Keep the skin dry and exposed to air.
Desquamation	• If dead surface cells peel off, apply cornstarch to prevent pruritus and irritation from clothing and bed linens. • If desquamation is moist, protect the wound to prevent infection and fluid loss. Apply hydrogel or hydrocolloid dressings to promote comfort and healing. Alternatively, use occlusive dressings, which may be less expensive. Avoid dry dressings because they can damage new epithelium when removed.
Epilation (usually temporary but may be permanent with high doses of radiation)	• If hair loss occurs in the treatment area, be supportive and encourage the use of cosmetic replacements, such as a wig.
Sweat gland destruction	• To maintain skin integrity, instruct the patient to avoid exposure to intense sunlight, wind, or cold. • Apply emollient-based lotions. • Observe for ulceration, telangiectasia, and poor healing after trauma.

• Teach the patient and family how to manage radiation adverse effects at home.
• Stress the importance of keeping follow-up appointments with the doctor.
• Refer the patient to a support group, such as the American Cancer Society.

Radiation, internal

Internal radiation, also known as brachytherapy, involves placing a radiation source into a specific area of the body or onto a body surface. The radiation source may be administered locally or systemically.

If delivered locally, either the interstitial or intracavitary approach may be used. In the interstitial approach, radioactive substances are sealed in applicators, such as molds, needles, beads, seeds, or ribbons, and implanted directly in the tumor or surrounding tissue or placed on top of a body surface. In the intracavitary approach, unsealed radioactive substances are temporarily delivered into a hollow body cavity.

A new method for delivering intracavitary radiation is performed with a machine called a remote afterloader. Radiation is delivered at very high doses to a specific area each day over the course of 3 to 5 days

Several new approaches are being evaluated to determine their effectiveness. One approach is intraoperative radiation in which a large dose of external radiation is directed at the tumor and surrounding tissue during surgery. Another technique is hyperthermia, in which body tissue is exposed to high temperatures. This method may be administered locally, regionally, or to the whole body.

Recently, radiolabeled antibodies have been used to deliver doses of radiation directly to the cancer site. Once injected, the antibodies actively seek out the cancer cells and destroy them by the action of the radiation. This approach may help lessen the risk of radiation damage to healthy cells.

Internal radiation also can be delivered systemically, using radioactive materials in solutions or colloidal suspensions that are given orally or I.V. Systemic applications are used for primary and metastatic thyroid cancer.

Procedure

In the interstitial or intracavitary approach, the doctor usually inserts the applicator for the radioactive source in the operating room with the patient under anesthesia. Then, to minimize exposure of hospital personnel, he places the radioactive source in the applicator after the patient returns to his room.

If the radioactive source isn't permanent, it's usually left in place for 24 to 72 hours and then removed in the patient's room. If a remote afterloader is used, the patient is treated in an inpatient or outpatient department, supplanting the need for hospitalization and isolation because the radioactive source is only in place for a few minutes.

If the patient is having internal radiation involving I.V. or oral administration of a radioactive solution or suspension, or intracavitary instillation of a radioactive suspension (usually by paracentesis or thoracentesis), the radioactive substance is administered in the radiation therapy department. Following intracavitary instillation of a suspension, the patient lies on a flat surface and is rotated every 15 minutes for 2 to 3 hours to distribute the suspension.

Complications

A radiation reaction may occur with any type of internal radiation and cause nausea, vomiting, malaise, diarrhea, anorexia, elevated temperature and, possibly, dehydration. Other complications stem from the death of local healthy cells that are exposed to the radioactive source. They include localized skin burns, hemorrhage due to destruction of bone marrow, and neurologic dysfunction.

Long-term effects of radiation may include a predisposition to leukemia and other cancers and the development of cataracts. When internal radiation is directed toward the gonads, genetic mutations and sterility may occur.

Key nursing diagnoses and patient outcomes

Fear related to having a radioactive substance placed internally. Based on this nursing diagnosis, you'll establish these patient outcomes. The patient will:
- identify and express his fears
- obtain correct information about internal radiation therapy that will help dispel his fears
- demonstrate fewer physical symptoms of fear.

Knowledge deficit related to internal radiation treatment. Based on this nursing diagnosis, you'll establish these patient outcomes. The patient will:
- identify the need to learn about his role in internal radiation treatment
- receive adequate instructions about allowed activities and necessary radiation precautions during treatment
- demonstrate an understanding of the treatment, as evidenced by adhering to radiation safety precautions and performing appropriate self-care activities.

Impaired social interaction related to temporary activity restrictions. Based on this nursing diagnosis, you'll establish these patient outcomes. The patient will:
- communicate an understanding of the reason for social isolation
- seek and use diversional activities, such as reading or watching television
- resume normal social interactions when instructed to do so.

Nursing interventions

When preparing a patient for internal radiation or managing his care after treatment, expect to implement these nursing interventions.

Before the procedure

- Because the patient may misinterpret radiation therapy as terminal care, be sure to stress the potentially curative effects of the treatment and its ability to improve the patient's quality of life. Explain the type of therapy and encourage the patient to ask questions.
- Obtain baseline white blood cell (WBC) and platelet counts. In addition, obtain a thorough patient history, including any previous radiation treatments and adverse effects.
- Tell the female patient undergoing pelvic irradiation that this treatment can decrease hormone levels, which may lead to infertility and amenorrhea.
- Explain the need for temporary isolation after ingestion or instillation because of the patient's radioactivity.
- Explain any possible activity restrictions, such as bed rest, that may be necessary because of the location of the applicator. Evaluate the patient for possible problems in positioning, range of motion, and comfort.
- Prepare the patient for a temporary change in appearance if the implant is placed in a visible area, such as the neck or breast.
- Make sure that the patient or a responsible family member has signed a consent form.

During the procedure

- Monitor the patient's WBC and platelet counts to help evaluate myelosuppressive effects. Also, monitor for other adverse effects that are site specific.
- Take precautions against radiation contamination. (See *Reviewing internal radiation safety precautions,* page 792.) Make sure all hospital personnel and visitors adhere to these precautions.
- Follow your institutions's policy regarding radiation precautions.
- Make sure the patient's call button is always within his reach.
- Provide diversional activities for the patient, such as watching television and reading, during the period of confinement.

Reviewing internal radiation safety precautions

When caring for the patient receiving internal radiation, remember the three main factors in radiation protection: time, distance, and shielding.

- *Time:* the exposure to radiation a patient receives is directly proportional to the time spent within a specific distance from the source.
- *Distance:* as radiation is emitted from a point source, the amount reaching a given area decreases by the square of that distance (law of inverse square)
- *Shielding:* when a sheet of absorbing material is placed between a radiation source and a detector, the amount of radiation that reaches the detector decreases, depending on the energy of the radiation and the nature and thickness of the shield. (The thickness of a shielding material required to reduce the radiation to one-half of its original quantity is referred to as the "half-value layer" [HVL].)

Because shielding is not always possible or practical, time and distance are the two factors that you should incorporate into the patient's plan of care. Thus, the cardinal safety rules of internal radiation therapy using these two factors are highlighted below.

- Wear a radiosensitive badge. Carefully plan the time you spend with the patient to prevent overexposure. (However, don't rush procedures, ignore the patient's psychological needs, or give the impression you can't get out of the room fast enough.)
- Avoid standing where you're in line with the radiation. Radiation loses its intensity with distance.
- Pregnant women should not be assigned to care for these patients.
- Check the position of the source applicator every 4 hours. If it appears dislodged, notify the radiation safety officer or radiation therapist immediately. If it's completely dislodged, remove the patient from the bed, pick up the applicator with long forceps, place it on a lead-shielded transport cart, and notify the radiation safety officer or radiation therapist immediately.
- *Never* pick up the source with your bare hands. Notify the doctor and radiation safety officer whenever there's an accident, and keep a lead-shielded transport cart on the unit as long as the patient has a source in place.

- Notify the radiation safety officer or the radiation therapist immediately if the radiation source is dislodged.
- Ensure that a temporary source of radiation is removed at the designated time in the treatment plan. Inform the patient that the radiation source is gently removed and placed in a sealed lead container and taken to the radiation department. His room will then be checked to ensure that all of the radiation source has been removed.

After the procedure

- Reassure the patient that once the temporary radiation source has been removed or the permanent source of radioactive material has decayed, he can resume his daily activities within the confines of his disease.
- Prepare the patient for follow-up care.

Home care instructions

- Explain that the full benefit of radiation treatment may not occur for several months. Instruct the patient to report any long-term adverse effects.
- Stress the importance of keeping appointments with the doctor.
- Refer the patient to a support group, such as the American Cancer Society.

Radioactive iodine therapy

An alternative to thyroidectomy or drug therapy, administration of the isotope iodine 131 (^{131}I) treats hyperthyroidism and is used adjunctively for thyroid cancer. After oral ingestion, ^{131}I is rapidly absorbed and concentrated in the thyroid as if it were normal iodine. The result is acute radiation thyroiditis and gradual thyroid atrophy that eventually reduces thyroid hormone levels.

When administered in the treatment of hyperthyroidism, ^{131}I causes symptoms to subside after about 3 weeks and exerts its full effect only after 3 months. A patient with acute hyperthyroidism may require ongoing drug therapy during this period. Similarly, a patient who also has cardiac disease must achieve a euthyroid state before the start of ^{131}I therapy, to withstand the initial hypermetabolism.

Although one ^{131}I treatment usually suffices, a second or third treatment may be needed several months later if the patient has severe hyperthyroidism or an unusually large gland.

^{131}I is the treatment of choice for nonpregnant adults who aren't good candidates for spontaneous remission or who weren't treated successfully with thyroid hormone antagonists. This relatively safe procedure exposes only the thyroid to radiation. However, it's contraindicated during pregnancy because ^{131}I does cross the placenta and can adversely affect the fetal thyroid gland. And, despite the fact that no iatrogenic cancers have been documented in the more than 40 years ^{131}I has been in use, this treatment is used cautiously in children and adolescents because of the potential for cancer or leukemia.

Procedure

In the nuclear medicine or radiation therapy department, the patient receives an oral dose of ^{131}I. The amount of ^{131}I given depends on the reason for the treatment. Generally a much larger dose is given when the patient is being treated for thyroid cancer than for hyperthyroidism. When treating hyperthyroidism, the dose depends on the size of the thyroid gland and the degree of radiosensitivity of the gland.

Complications

The most common complication associated with radioactive iodine treatment is the development of hypothyroidism, which may occur up to several years after treatment. Radiation thyroiditis is an occasional immediate complication that may occur within 7 to 10 days of the treatment and causes neck and ear pain, dysphagia, edema of the neck and, possibly, inflammation of the salivary glands. Rarely, it becomes so severe as to cause thyroid crisis (caused by the excessive release of thyroid hormone into the blood).

Key nursing diagnoses and patient outcomes

Fear related to receiving a radioactive substance. Based on this nursing diagnosis, you'll establish these patient outcomes. The patient will:
- identify and express his fears
- obtain correct information about ^{131}I therapy to dispel his fears
- demonstrate fewer physical symptoms of fear.

Knowledge deficit related to radioactive iodine treatment. Based on this nursing diagnosis, you'll establish these patient outcomes. The patient will:
- identify the need to learn about radioactive iodine treatment
- obtain information about the treatment from appropriate sources
- communicate an understanding of the treatment and subsequent care measures.

Impaired social interaction related to temporary activity restrictions required following radioactive iodine treatment. Based on this nursing diagnosis, you'll es-

tablish these patient outcomes. The patient will:

- communicate an understanding of the need to avoid pregnant women and young children for 7 days after treatment
- use diversional activities, such as reading or watching television, to compensate for the temporary decrease in social interaction
- adhere to temporary restrictions related to eating utensils and flushing of bowel and bladder contents.

Nursing interventions

When caring for a patient undergoing radioactive iodine therapy, your chief responsibilities will be to explain the treatment and to teach the patient how to care for himself and avoid exposing others to radiation.

Before the procedure

- Explain the procedure to the patient.
- Instruct the patient to stop thyroid hormone antagonists 4 to 7 days before ^{131}I administration because these drugs reduce the sensitivity of thyroid cells to radiation. Also make sure that the patient isn't taking amiodarone (an antiarrhythmic drug) because it contains a large amount of iodine and will interfere with the uptake of the therapeutic radioiodine by the thyroid.
- Inform the patient that ^{131}I won't be administered if he develops severe vomiting or diarrhea because these decrease absorption.

After the procedure

- Usually the patient is discharged after ^{131}I administration, with appropriate instructions. However, if he received a large dose of radioiodine (30 millicuries or greater), he'll be hospitalized and isolated as mandated by the Nuclear Regulatory Commission. In that case, institute radiation precautions until the hospital's radiation safety officer determines that the patient's radiation level has fallen to a safe level. (If you're pregnant, arrange for another nurse to care for this patient.)
- Encourage the patient to drink plenty of fluids for 48 hours to speed excretion of ^{131}I.
- Instruct the patient to flush the toilet twice after using it for 48 hours after treatment or until he is discharged from the hospital (if hospitalization was required).
- Tell him to use (or give him) disposable eating utensils, and warn him to avoid close contact with young children and pregnant women for 7 days after therapy.

Home care instructions

- Explain to the patient that his urine and saliva will be slightly radioactive for 24 hours and that any vomitus will be highly radioactive for 6 to 8 hours after therapy. Teach him to dispose of these properly.
- Tell the patient he'll start to see improvement in his condition within several weeks but that maximum effects won't occur for up to 3 months.
- Explain that he should take his prescribed thyroid hormone antagonist as ordered, starting 3 to 4 days after ^{131}I therapy and continuing until the doctor determines that his thyroid has become atrophic. If the patient is also taking propranolol, tell him that the doctor may have him continue this temporarily to treat tachycardia, diaphoresis, and tremor.
- Inform the patient that he'll need periodic laboratory tests. If his serum thyroid hormone levels don't fall within 6 to 12 months, the doctor may order another dose of ^{131}I.
- Advise the patient that hypothyroidism may occur 2 to 4 months after therapy. If symptoms become severe, the doctor will prescribe a thyroid hormone replacement. If hypothyroidism persists for 6 to 9 months, the patient may require lifelong therapy for permanent hypothyroidism.
- Tell the patient to notify his doctor if he develops pain, swelling, erythema, or fever (from radiation thyroiditis). Reassure him

that these adverse effects can be treated with anti-inflammatory drugs. Also tell him to notify his doctor if he develops severe exacerbation of hyperthyroidism 3 to 14 days after therapy.
• Advise the female patient of childbearing age to avoid conception for several months after therapy.

Renal calculi

Although they may form anywhere in the urinary tract, renal calculi (sometimes referred to as kidney stones) most commonly develop in the renal pelvis or calyces. Calculi formation occurs when substances that normally are dissolved in the urine (calcium oxalate, calcium phosphate, magnesium ammonium phosphate [struvite] and, occasionally, uric acid or cystine) precipitate. Renal calculi vary in size and may be solitary or multiple.

About 1 in 1,000 Americans develops renal calculi. They're more common in men (especially those ages 30 to 50) than in women and rare in blacks and children.

Causes

Renal calculi are particularly prevalent in certain geographic areas, such as the southeastern United States (called the "stone belt"), possibly because a hot climate promotes dehydration and concentrates calculus-forming substances or because of regional dietary habits. Although the exact cause of renal calculi is unknown, predisposing factors include:
• *Dehydration.* Decreased water excretion concentrates calculus-forming substances.
• *Infection.* Infected, scarred tissue may be a site for calculus development. In addition, infected calculi (usually magnesium ammonium phosphate or staghorn calculi) may develop if bacteria serve as the nucleus in calculus formation. Struvite calculus formation commonly results from *Proteus* infections, which may lead to destruction of renal parenchyma.
• *Changes in urine pH.* Consistently acidic or alkaline urine may provide a favorable medium for calculus formation, especially for magnesium ammonium phosphate or calcium phosphate calculi.
• *Obstruction.* Urinary stasis allows calculus constituents to collect and adhere, forming calculi. Obstruction also encourages infection, which compounds the obstruction.
• *Immobilization.* Immobility from spinal cord injury or other disorders allows calcium to be released into the circulation and, eventually, to be filtered by the kidneys.
• *Metabolic factors.* Hyperparathyroidism, renal tubular acidosis, elevated uric acid (usually with gout), defective metabolism of oxalate, a genetically caused defect in metabolism of cystine, and excessive intake of vitamin D or dietary calcium may predispose a person to renal calculi.

Complications

Calculi may either remain in the renal pelvis and damage or destroy renal parenchyma, or they may enter the ureter; large calculi in the kidneys cause pressure necrosis. In certain locations, calculi cause obstruction, with resultant hydronephrosis, and tend to recur. Intractable pain and serious bleeding also can result from calculi and the damage they cause.

Assessment

Assessment findings vary with the size, location, and cause of the calculi. The key symptom of renal calculi is severe pain, which usually results from obstruction – large, rough calculi occlude the opening to the ureteropelvic junction and increase the frequency and force of peristaltic contractions. The patient usually reports that the pain travels from the costovertebral angle to the flank and then to the suprapubic region and external genitalia (classic renal colic pain). Pain intensity fluctuates and may be excruciating at its peak.

The patient with calculi in the renal pelvis and calyces may complain of more constant, dull pain. He also may report back pain (from calculi causing obstruction within a kidney) and severe abdominal pain (from calculi traveling down a ureter). The patient with severe pain also typically complains of nausea, vomiting and, possibly, fever and chills.

You may note hematuria (when calculi abrade a ureter), abdominal distention and, rarely, anuria (from bilateral obstruction or, in the patient with one kidney, unilateral obstruction).

Diagnostic tests

Diagnosis is based on clinical features and the following tests:

- *Kidney-ureter-bladder (KUB) radiography* reveals most renal calculi.
- *Excretory urography* helps confirm the diagnosis and determine the size and location of calculi.
- *Kidney ultrasonography*—easily performed, noninvasive, and nontoxic—detects obstructive changes, such as unilateral or bilateral hydronephrosis and radiolucent calculi not seen on KUB radiography.
- *Urine culture* of a midstream specimen may indicate pyuria, a sign of urinary tract infection.
- A *24-hour urine collection* is evaluated for calcium oxalate, phosphorus, and uric acid excretion levels. Three separate collections, along with blood samples, are needed for accurate testing.
- *Calculus analysis* shows mineral content.

Other diagnostic test results may suggest the cause of calculus formation.

- *Serial blood calcium and phosphorus levels* detect hyperparathyroidism and show an increased calcium level in proportion to normal serum protein levels.
- *Blood protein levels* determine the level of free calcium unbound to protein.
- If increased, *blood uric acid levels* may indicate gout.

Appendicitis, cholecystitis, peptic ulcer, and pancreatitis must be ruled out as potential sources of pain before the diagnosis can be confirmed.

Treatment

Because 90% of renal calculi are smaller than 5 mm in diameter, treatment usually involves encouraging their natural passage through vigorous hydration (more than 3 liters/day). Other treatment measures include administration of antimicrobial agents for infection (varying with the cultured organism); analgesics, such as meperidine or morphine, for pain; and diuretics to prevent urinary stasis and further calculus formation (thiazides decrease calcium excretion into the urine).

Measures to prevent recurrence include a low-calcium diet, often combined with oxalate-binding cholestyramine, for absorptive hypercalciuria; parathyroidectomy for hyperparathyroidism; administration of allopurinol for uric acid calculi; and daily oral doses of ascorbic acid to acidify the urine.

Calculi too large for natural passage may require removal. A calculus lodged in the ureter may be removed by inserting a cystoscope through the urethra and then manipulating the calculus with catheters or retrieval instruments. Extraction of calculi from other areas, such as the kidney calyx or renal pelvis, may necessitate a flank or lower abdominal approach. Two other methods, percutaneous ultrasonic lithotripsy and extracorporeal shock-wave lithotripsy, shatter the calculus into fragments for removal by suction or natural passage.

Cystine calculi are difficult to treat without surgical intervention or invasive procedure. If electrohydraulic ultrasound isn't effective, the calculi are surgically removed.

Key nursing diagnoses and patient outcomes

Altered urinary elimination related to increased output from high oral fluid intake and potential for calculi to lodge in urinary tract and interfere with urine flow. Based on this nursing diagnosis, you'll establish these patient outcomes. The patient will:
- recognize the need for medical attention and seek it if his oral intake becomes greater than his urine output or anuria occurs
- maintain an oral intake greater than 3 liters/day until calculi have passed
- regain and maintain a normal urinary elimination pattern with eradication of renal calculi.

Risk for infection related to abrasive nature of renal calculi as they pass through the urinary tract. Based on this nursing diagnosis, you'll establish these patient outcomes. The patient will:
- maintain a normal temperature and white blood cell count
- not exhibit signs and symptoms of a urinary tract infection, such as dysuria, hematuria, or cloudy, foul-smelling urine
- remain free of urinary tract infections.

Pain related to presence of renal calculi. Based on this nursing diagnosis, you'll establish these patient outcomes. The patient will:
- verbalize complaints of pain prior to its becoming severe
- express feelings of comfort after analgesic administration
- comply with the prescribed treatment to remove renal calculi and thus alleviate pain
- become pain free with the passage or removal of renal calculi.

Nursing interventions

- To facilitate spontaneous passage of calculi, encourage the patient to walk, if possible. Also force fluids to maintain a urine output of 3 to 4 liters/day (urine should be very dilute and colorless).
- If the patient can't drink the required amount of fluid, give supplemental I.V. fluids.
- To help acidify urine, offer fruit juices, especially cranberry juice.
- Medicate the patient generously for pain when he's passing a calculus.
- Obtain urine culture and sensitivity if infection is suspected.
- Give antibiotics and other medications, as ordered.
- Prepare the patient for surgery, as indicated. If the patient had calculi surgically removed, he'll probably have an indwelling urinary catheter or a nephrostomy tube. Unless one of his kidneys was removed, expect bloody drainage from the catheter. Never irrigate the catheter without a doctor's order. Use sterile technique when changing dressings or providing catheter care.
- Prepare the patient for lithotripsy, as indicated. (See the entry "Lithotripsy.")

Monitoring

- Record intake and output and daily weight to assess fluid status and renal function.
- Monitor the patient's response to pain medication and other administered medications. Also observe for adverse reactions.
- Watch for signs of infection, such as a rising temperature or chills.
- Monitor the patient's urine for evidence of renal calculi. To aid diagnosis, maintain a 24- to 48-hour record of urine pH, using nitrazine pH paper. Strain all urine through gauze or a tea strainer, and save all solid material recovered for analysis.
- If surgery was performed, check dressings regularly for bloody drainage and ask the doctor how much drainage to expect. Immediately report excessive drainage or a rising pulse rate, symptoms of hemorrhage.

Patient teaching

- Encourage increased fluid intake. If appropriate, show the patient how to check his urine pH, and instruct him to keep a daily record. Tell him to immediately report symptoms of acute obstruction, such as pain or an inability to void.

• Urge the patient to follow a prescribed diet and comply with drug therapy to prevent recurrence of calculi. For example, if a hyperuricemic condition caused the patient's calculi, teach him which foods are high in purine.

• If surgery is necessary, supplement and reinforce the doctor's teaching. The patient is apt to be fearful, especially if he needs a kidney removed, so emphasize that the body can adapt well to one kidney. If he's having an abdominal or flank incision, teach deep-breathing and coughing exercises.

Renal failure, acute

About 5% of all hospitalized patients develop acute renal failure – the sudden interruption of renal function resulting from obstruction, reduced circulation, or renal parenchymal disease. This condition is classified as prerenal, intrarenal, or postrenal and normally passes through three distinct phases – oliguric, diuretic, and recovery. It's usually reversible with medical treatment. If not treated, it may progress to end-stage renal disease, uremia, and death.

Causes

The three types of acute renal failure each have separate causes. Prerenal failure results from conditions that diminish blood flow to the kidneys. Between 40% and 80% of all cases of acute renal failure are caused by prerenal azotemia. Intrarenal failure (also called intrinsic or parenchymal renal failure) results from damage to the kidneys themselves, usually from acute tubular necrosis. Postrenal failure results from bilateral obstruction of urine outflow. (See *Causes of acute renal failure.*)

Complications

Ischemic acute tubular necrosis can lead to renal shutdown. Electrolyte imbalance, metabolic acidosis, and other severe effects follow as the patient becomes increasingly uremic and renal dysfunction disrupts other body systems. If left untreated, the patient will die. Even with treatment, the elderly patient is particularly susceptible to volume overload, precipitating acute pulmonary edema, hypertensive crisis, hyperkalemia, and infection.

Assessment

The patient's history may include a disorder that can cause renal failure, and he may have a recent history of fever; chills; GI problems, such as anorexia, nausea, vomiting, diarrhea, and constipation; and central nervous system problems, such as headache.

The patient may appear irritable, drowsy, and confused or demonstrate other alterations in his level of consciousness. In advanced stages, seizures and coma may occur. Depending on the stage of renal failure, his urine output may be oliguric (less than 400 ml/24 hours) or anuric (less than 100 ml/24 hours).

Inspection may uncover evidence of bleeding abnormalities, such as petechiae and ecchymoses. Hematemesis may occur. The skin may be dry and pruritic and, rarely, you may note uremic frost. Mucous membranes may be dry, and the patient's breath may have a uremic odor. If the patient has hyperkalemia, muscle weakness may occur.

Auscultation may detect tachycardia and, possibly, an irregular rhythm. Bibasilar crackles may be heard if the patient has congestive heart failure (CHF).

Palpation and percussion may reveal abdominal pain, if pancreatitis or peritonitis occurs, and peripheral edema, if the patient has CHF.

Causes of acute renal failure

Acute renal failure can be classified as prerenal, intrarenal, or postrenal. All conditions that lead to prerenal failure impair renal perfusion, resulting in decreased glomerular filtration rate and increased proximal tubular reabsorption of sodium and water. Intrarenal failure results from damage to the kidneys themselves; postrenal failure, from obstruction of urine flow.

Prerenal failure

Cardiovascular disorders
- Arrhythmias
- Cardiac tamponade
- Cardiogenic shock
- CHF
- Myocardial infarction

Hypovolemia
- Burns
- Dehydration
- Diuretic abuse
- Hemorrhage
- Hypovolemic shock
- Trauma

Peripheral vasodilation
- Antihypertensive drugs
- Sepsis

Renovascular obstruction
- Arterial embolism
- Arterial or venous thrombosis
- Tumor

Severe vasoconstriction
- Disseminated intravascular coagulation
- Eclampsia
- Malignant hypertension
- Vasculitis

Intrarenal failure

Acute tubular necrosis
- Ischemic damage to renal parenchyma from unrecognized or poorly treated prerenal failure
- Nephrotoxins—analgesics (such as phenacetin), anesthetics (such as methoxyflurane), antibiotics (such as gentamicin), heavy metals (such as lead), radiographic contrast media, organic solvents
- Obstetric complications—eclampsia, postpartum renal failure, septic abortion, uterine hemorrhage
- Pigment release—crush injury, myopathy, sepsis, transfusion reaction

Other parenchymal disorders
- Acute glomerulonephritis
- Acute interstitial nephritis
- Acute pyelonephritis
- Bilateral renal vein thrombosis
- Malignant nephrosclerosis
- Papillary necrosis
- Periarteritis nodosa
- Renal myeloma
- Sickle cell disease
- Systemic lupus erythematosus
- Vasculitis

Postrenal failure

Bladder obstruction
- Anticholinergic drugs
- Autonomic nerve dysfunction
- Infection
- Tumor

Ureteral obstruction
- Blood clots
- Calculi
- Edema or inflammation
- Necrotic renal papillae
- Retroperitoneal fibrosis or hemorrhage
- Surgery (accidental ligation)
- Tumor
- Uric acid crystals

Urethral obstruction
- Prostatic hyperplasia or tumor
- Strictures

Diagnostic tests

Blood test results indicating acute intrarenal failure include elevated blood urea nitrogen, serum creatinine, and potassium levels and low blood pH, bicarbonate, hematocrit, and hemoglobin levels.

Urine specimens show casts, cellular debris, decreased specific gravity and, in glomerular diseases, proteinuria and urine osmolality close to serum osmolality. The urine sodium level is under 20 mEq/liter if oliguria results from decreased perfusion and above 40 mEq/liter if it results from an intrarenal problem. A creatinine clearance test measures the glomerular filtration rate and allows for an estimate of the number of remaining functioning nephrons.

Other studies that help determine the cause of renal failure include kidney ultrasonography, plain films of the abdomen, kidney-ureter-bladder radiography, excretory urography, renal scan, retrograde pyelography, computed tomography scans, and nephrotomography.

An electrocardiogram (ECG) shows tall, peaked T waves, a widening QRS complex, and disappearing P waves if hyperkalemia is present.

Treatment

Supportive measures include a diet high in calories and low in protein, sodium, and potassium, with supplemental vitamins and restricted fluids. Meticulous electrolyte monitoring is essential to detect hyperkalemia. If hyperkalemia occurs, acute therapy may include hypertonic glucose-and-insulin infusions and sodium bicarbonate – all administered I.V. – and sodium polystyrene sulfonate by mouth or enema to remove potassium from the body.

If measures fail to control uremic symptoms, the patient may require hemodialysis or peritoneal dialysis. Early initiation of diuretic therapy during the oliguric phase may benefit the patient.

Key nursing diagnoses and patient outcomes

Fluid volume excess related to decreased ability of the kidneys to excrete water and sodium. Based on this nursing diagnosis, you'll establish these patient outcomes. The patient will:
- adhere to fluid restrictions
- not exhibit signs and symptoms of CHF
- regain and maintain normal fluid volume with alleviation of acute renal failure.

Risk for infection related to renal dysfunction. Based on this nursing diagnosis, you'll establish these patient outcomes. The patient will:
- maintain a normal temperature and white blood cell count
- demonstrate appropriate infection-control measures
- not show signs and symptoms of an infection.

Risk for injury related to potential for hyperkalemia. Based on this nursing diagnosis, you'll establish these patient outcomes. The patient will:
- adhere to a potassium-restricted diet
- maintain a normal serum potassium level
- not show signs and symptoms of hyperkalemia.

Nursing interventions

- Use infection control measures during care because the patient with acute renal failure is highly susceptible to infection. Don't allow staff members or visitors with upper respiratory tract infections to come into contact with the patient. Also use universal precautions when handling all blood and body fluids.
- Replace blood components as ordered. (See *Blood transfusion precaution in acute renal failure.*)
- Maintain proper electrolyte balance. Avoid administering medications that contain potassium.
- Maintain nutritional status. Provide a diet high in calories and low in protein, sodium, and potassium, with vitamin sup-

plements. Give the anorexic patient small, frequent meals.

• Prevent complications of immobility by encouraging frequent coughing and deep breathing and by performing passive range-of-motion exercises. Help the patient walk as soon as possible. Add lubricating lotion to his bath water to combat skin dryness.

• Provide mouth care frequently to lubricate dry mucous membranes. If stomatitis occurs, use an antibiotic solution, if ordered, and have the patient swish it around in his mouth before swallowing.

• Administer medications carefully, especially antacids and stool softeners.

• Provide meticulous perineal care to reduce the risk of ascending urinary tract infection in women and to protect skin integrity caused by frequent loose, irritating stools, particularly when sodium polystyrene sulfonate is used.

• Use appropriate safety measures, such as side rails and restraints, because the patient with central nervous system involvement may become dizzy or confused.

• Prepare the patient for hemodialysis or peritoneal dialysis, as indicated. (See the entries "Hemodialysis" and "Peritoneal dialysis.")

• Administer any prescribed medications after hemodialysis is completed. Many medications are removed from the blood during treatment.

• Provide emotional support to the patient and his family.

Monitoring

• Measure and record intake and output of all fluids, including wound drainage, nasogastric tube output, and diarrhea.

• Weigh the patient daily. You also may need to measure abdominal girth every day. Mark the skin with indelible ink so that measurements can be taken in the same place.

• Monitor renal function studies, electrolytes (especially potassium), and hematocrit and hemoglobin levels regularly, as ordered.

NURSING ALERT

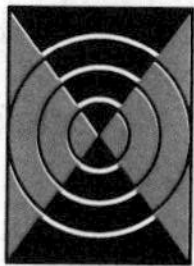

Blood transfusion precaution in acute renal failure

Don't use whole blood for a patient with acute renal failure if he's prone to CHF and can't tolerate extra fluid volume. Packed red blood cells deliver the necessary blood components without added volume.

• Monitor vital signs. Watch for and report signs of pericarditis (pleuritic chest pain, tachycardia, and pericardial friction rub), inadequate renal perfusion (hypotension), and acidosis.

• Watch for symptoms of hyperkalemia (malaise, anorexia, paresthesia, muscle weakness, and ECG changes), and report them immediately.

• Assess the patient frequently, especially during emergency treatment to lower potassium levels. If he receives hypertonic glucose-and-insulin infusions, monitor potassium and glucose levels. If you give sodium polystyrene sulfonate rectally, make sure the patient doesn't retain it and become constipated. This can lead to bowel perforation.

• Monitor for GI bleeding by testing all stools for occult blood, using the guaiac test.

• Evaluate the patient's nutritional status.

• Assess the patient's ability to resume normal activities of daily living, and plan for the gradual resumption of activity.

Patient teaching

• Reassure the patient and his family by clearly explaining all diagnostic tests, treatments, and procedures.

• Tell the patient about his prescribed medications, and stress the importance of complying with the regimen.
• Stress the importance of following the prescribed diet and fluid allowance.
• Instruct the patient to weigh himself daily and report changes of 3 lb or more immediately.
• Advise the patient against overexertion. If he becomes dyspneic or short of breath during normal activity, tell him to report it to his doctor.
• Teach the patient how to recognize edema, and tell him to report this finding to the doctor.

Renal failure, chronic

Usually the end result of a gradually progressive loss of renal function, chronic renal failure also occasionally results from a rapidly progressive disease of sudden onset that gradually destroys the nephrons and eventually causes irreversible renal damage. Few symptoms develop until after more than 75% of glomerular filtration is lost; then, the remaining normal parenchyma deteriorates progressively, and symptoms worsen as renal function decreases.

Chronic renal failure may progress through the following stages:
• reduced renal reserve (glomerular filtration rate [GFR] 35% to 50% of normal)
• renal insufficiency (GFR 20% to 35% of normal)
• renal failure (GFR 20% to 25% of normal)
• end-stage renal disease (GFR less than 20% of normal).

This syndrome is fatal without treatment, but maintenance dialysis or a kidney transplant can sustain life.

Causes

Chronic renal failure may result from:
• *chronic glomerular disease,* such as glomerulonephritis
• *chronic infections,* such as chronic pyelonephritis or tuberculosis
• *congenital anomalies,* such as polycystic kidney disease
• *vascular diseases,* such as renal nephrosclerosis or hypertension
• *obstructive processes,* such as calculi
• *collagen diseases,* such as systemic lupus erythematosus
• *nephrotoxic agents,* such as long-term aminoglycoside therapy
• *endocrine diseases,* such as diabetic neuropathy.

Complications

If this condition continues unchecked, uremic toxins accumulate and produce potentially fatal physiologic changes in all major organ systems.

Even if the patient can tolerate life-sustaining maintenance dialysis or a kidney transplant, he may still have anemia, peripheral neuropathy, cardiopulmonary and GI complications, sexual dysfunction, and skeletal defects.

Assessment

The patient's history may include a disease or condition that can cause renal failure; however, he may not have any symptoms for a long time. Symptoms usually occur by the time the GFR is 20% to 35% of normal, and almost all body systems are affected. (See *Detecting chronic renal failure,* pages 804 and 805.)

Diagnostic tests

These laboratory findings aid in the diagnosis and monitoring of chronic renal failure.
• *Blood studies* show elevated blood urea nitrogen, serum creatinine, sodium, and potassium levels; decreased arterial pH and bicarbonate levels; low hemoglobin and hematocrit; decreased red blood cell

(RBC) survival time; mild thrombocytopenia; platelet defects; and metabolic acidosis. They also show increased aldosterone secretion (related to increased renin production) and increased blood glucose levels similar to those that occur in diabetes mellitus (a sign of impaired carbohydrate metabolism). Hypertriglyceridemia and decreased high-density lipoprotein levels are common.

• *Arterial blood gas analysis* reveals metabolic acidosis.
• *Urine specific gravity* becomes fixed at 1.010; urinalysis may show proteinuria, glycosuria, RBCs, leukocytes, and casts and crystals, depending on the cause.
• *X-ray studies,* including kidney-ureter-bladder radiography, excretory urography, nephrotomography, renal scan, and renal arteriography, show reduced kidney size.
• *Renal biopsy* allows histologic identification of underlying pathology.
• *EEG* shows changes that indicate metabolic encephalopathy.

Treatment

Conservative treatment aims to correct specific symptoms. A low-protein diet reduces the production of end products of protein metabolism that the kidneys can't excrete. (However, a patient receiving continuous peritoneal dialysis should have a high-protein diet.) A high-calorie diet prevents ketoacidosis and the negative nitrogen balance that results in catabolism and tissue atrophy. The diet also should restrict sodium and potassium.

Maintaining fluid balance requires careful monitoring of vital signs, weight changes, and urine volume (if not anuric). Fluid retention can be reduced with loop diuretics such as furosemide (if some renal function remains) and with fluid restriction. Digitalis glycosides in small doses may be used to mobilize the fluids causing the edema; antihypertensives may be used to control blood pressure and associated edema.

Antiemetics taken before meals may relieve nausea and vomiting, and cimetidine or ranitidine may decrease gastric irritation. Methylcellulose or docusate can help prevent constipation.

Anemia necessitates iron and folate supplements; severe anemia requires infusion of fresh frozen packed cells or washed packed cells. Transfusions relieve anemia only temporarily. Synthetic erythropoietin (epoetin alfa) stimulates the division and differentiation of cells within the bone marrow to produce RBCs.

Drug therapy commonly relieves associated symptoms. An antipruritic, such as trimeprazine or diphenhydramine, can relieve itching, and aluminum hydroxide gel can lower serum phosphate levels. The patient also may benefit from supplementary vitamins (particularly B vitamins and vitamin D) and essential amino acids.

Careful monitoring of serum potassium levels is necessary to detect hyperkalemia. Emergency treatment for severe hyperkalemia includes dialysis therapy and administration of 50% hypertonic glucose I.V., regular insulin, calcium gluconate I.V., sodium bicarbonate I.V., and cation exchange resins such as sodium polystyrene sulfonate. Cardiac tamponade resulting from pericardial effusion may require emergency pericardial tap or surgery.

Intensive dialysis and thoracentesis can relieve pulmonary edema and pleural effusion.

Hemodialysis or peritoneal dialysis (particularly the newer techniques – continuous ambulatory peritoneal dialysis and continuous cyclic peritoneal dialysis) can help control most manifestations of end-stage renal disease. Altering the dialysate can correct fluid and electrolyte disturbances. However, maintenance dialysis itself may produce complications, including serum hepatitis (hepatitis B) from numerous blood transfusions, protein wasting, refractory ascites, and dialysis dementia.

Detecting chronic renal failure

These assessment findings reflect the involvement of each body system and, in many cases, the involvement of more than one body system.

Renal

In certain fluid and electrolyte imbalances, the kidneys cannot retain salt and hyponatremias occur. The patient may complain of dry mouth, fatigue, and nausea. You may note hypotension, loss of skin turgor, and listlessness that may progress to somnolence and confusion. Later, as the number of functioning nephrons decreases, so does the kidneys' capacity to excrete sodium and potassium. Urine output decreases, and the urine is very dilute, with casts and crystals present. Accumulation of potassium causes muscle irritability and then muscle weakness, irregular pulses, and life-threatening cardiac arrhythmias as serum potassium levels increase. Sodium retention causes fluid overload, and edema is palpable. Metabolic acidosis also occurs.

Cardiovascular

With cardiovascular involvement, you'll note hypertension and an irregular pulse. Life-threatening cardiac arrhythmias can occur. With pericardial involvement, you may auscultate a pericardial friction rub. Heart sounds may be distant if pericardial effusion is present. Bibasilar crackles may be auscultated, and peripheral edema may be palpated if congestive heart failure occurs.

Respiratory

Pulmonary changes include reduced pulmonary macrophage activity with increased susceptibility to infection. If pneumonia is present, lung sounds may be decreased over areas of consolidation. Bibasilar crackles indicate pulmonary edema. With pleural involvement, the patient may complain of pleuritic pain and you may auscultate a pleural friction rub. Kussmaul's respirations occur with metabolic acidosis.

Gastrointestinal

With inflammation and ulceration of GI mucosa, inspection of the mouth may reveal gum ulceration and bleeding and, possibly, parotitis. The patient may complain of hiccups, a metallic taste in the mouth, anorexia, nausea, and vomiting caused by esophageal, stomach, or

Key nursing diagnoses and patient outcomes

Altered nutrition: Less than body requirements related to adverse GI effects. Based on this nursing diagnosis, you'll establish these patient outcomes. The patient will:

- regain his weight and maintain it within the normal range with no further weight loss
- tolerate oral feedings and obtain an adequate caloric intake
- not develop malnutrition.

Fluid volume excess related to inability of the kidneys to regulate water balance. Based on this nursing diagnosis, you'll establish these patient outcomes. The patient will:

- communicate an understanding of the importance of fluid and sodium restrictions
- adhere to fluid and sodium restrictions
- not exhibit signs and symptoms of excessive fluid retention.

Risk for injury related to adverse effects of chronic renal failure on all major organ systems. Based on this nursing diagnosis, you'll establish these patient outcomes. The patient will:

- recognize and report early signs of organ dysfunction

bowel involvement. You may note a uremic fetor (ammonia smell) to the breath. Abdominal palpation and percussion may elicit pain.

Skin
Inspection of the skin typically reveals a pallid, yellowish-bronze color. The skin is dry and scaly with purpura, ecchymoses, petechiae, uremic frost (most often in critically ill or terminal patients), and thin, brittle fingernails with characteristic lines. The hair is dry and brittle and may change color and fall out easily. The patient usually complains of severe itching.

Neurologic
You may note that the patient has alterations in level of consciousness that may progress from mild behavior changes, shortened memory and attention span, apathy, drowsiness, and irritability to confusion, coma, and seizures. The patient may complain of hiccups, muscle cramps, fasciculations, and twitching, which are caused by muscle irritability. He also may complain of restless leg syndrome. One of the first signs of peripheral neuropathy, this syndrome causes pain, burning, and itching in the legs and feet that may be relieved by voluntarily shaking, moving, or rocking them. This condition eventually progresses to paresthesia, motor nerve dysfunction (usually bilateral footdrop) and, unless dialysis is initiated, flaccid paralysis.

Endocrine
The patient may have a history of infertility, decreased libido, or amenorrhea (in women) or impotence (in men).

Hematologic
Inspection may reveal purpura, GI bleeding and hemorrhage from body orifices, easy bruising, ecchymoses, and petechiae caused by thrombocytopenia and platelet defects.

Musculoskeletal
The patient may have a history of pathologic fractures and complain of bone and muscle pain caused by calcium-phosphorus imbalance and consequent parathyroid hormone imbalances. You may note gait abnormalities or, possibly, that the patient is no longer able to ambulate.

- comply with the prescribed treatment regimen to minimize or prevent complications
- take precautions in daily life to minimize or prevent injury caused by organ dysfunction.

Nursing interventions

- Provide good skin care. Bathe the patient daily, using superfatted soaps, oatmeal baths, and skin lotion to ease pruritus. Give good perineal care, using mild soap and water. Pad side rails to guard against ecchymoses. Turn the patient often, and use a convoluted foam or low-pressure mattress to prevent skin breakdown.
- Prevent pathologic fractures by turning the patient carefully and ensuring his safety. Perform passive range-of-motion exercises for the bedridden patient.
- Provide good oral hygiene. Brush the patient's teeth often with a soft brush or sponge tip to reduce breath odor. Hard candy and mouthwash minimize metallic taste in the mouth and alleviate thirst.
- Offer small, palatable, nutritious meals. Try to provide favorite foods within dietary restrictions, and encourage intake of high-calorie foods.
- Encourage deep breathing and coughing to prevent pulmonary congestion.

• Maintain strict aseptic technique. Use a micropore filter during I.V. therapy. Warn the outpatient to avoid contact with infected people during the cold and flu season.
• Infuse sodium bicarbonate for acidosis and sedatives or anticonvulsants for seizures, as ordered. Keep an oral airway and suction setup at the bedside.
• Schedule medication administration carefully. Give iron before meals, aluminum hydroxide gels after meals, and antiemetics (as necessary) a half hour before meals. Administer antihypertensives at appropriate intervals. If the patient requires a rectal infusion of sodium polystyrene sulfonate for dangerously high potassium levels, apply an emollient to soothe the perianal area. Be sure the sodium polystyrene sulfonate enema is expelled; otherwise, it will cause constipation and won't lower potassium levels. Recommend antacid cookies as an alternative to aluminum hydroxide gels needed to bind GI phosphate. Don't give magnesium products because poor renal excretion can lead to toxic levels.
• Administer loop diuretics and restrict fluid and sodium intake to alleviate excess fluid retention, as ordered.
• Prepare the patient for hemodialysis or peritoneal dialysis, as indicated. (See the entries "Hemodialysis" and "Peritoneal dialysis.")

Monitoring

• Watch for signs of hyperkalemia. Observe for cramping of the legs and abdomen and for diarrhea. As potassium levels rise, watch for muscle irritability and a weak pulse rate. Monitor the electrocardiogram for tall, peaked T waves, a widening QRS complex, a prolonged PR interval, and the disappearance of P waves.
• Carefully assess the patient's hydration status. Check for jugular vein distention, and auscultate the lungs for crackles, rhonchi, and decreased lung sounds. Be alert for clinical signs of pulmonary edema (such as dyspnea and restlessness). Carefully measure daily intake and output, including all drainage, emesis, diarrhea, and blood loss. Record daily weight, presence or absence of thirst, axillary sweat, tongue dryness, hypertension, and peripheral edema.
• Monitor for bone or joint complications.
• Watch for signs of infection (listlessness, high fever, and leukocytosis).
• Carefully observe and document seizure activity. Periodically assess neurologic status, and check for Chvostek's and Trousseau's signs, indicators of low serum calcium levels.
• Observe for signs of bleeding. Watch for prolonged bleeding at puncture sites and at the vascular access site used for hemodialysis. Monitor hemoglobin and hematocrit, and check stool, urine, and vomitus for blood.
• Report signs of pericarditis, such as a pericardial friction rub and chest pain. Also watch for the disappearance of friction rub, with a drop of 15 to 20 mm Hg in blood pressure during inspiration (paradoxical pulse) – an early sign of pericardial tamponade.

Patient teaching

• Teach the patient how to take his medications and what adverse effects to watch for. Suggest that he take diuretics in the morning so that his sleep won't be disturbed.
• Instruct the anemic patient to conserve energy by resting frequently.
• Tell the patient to report leg cramps or excessive muscle twitching. Stress the importance of keeping follow-up appointments to have his electrolyte levels monitored.
• Tell the patient to avoid high-sodium and high-potassium foods. Encourage adherence to fluid and protein restrictions. To prevent constipation, stress the need for exercise and sufficient dietary fiber.
• If the patient is having dialysis, remember that he and his family are under extreme stress. The hospital will probably of-

fer a course on dialysis; if not, you'll need to teach the patient and his family.
• Refer the patient and his family for counseling if they need help coping with chronic renal failure.
• Suggest that the patient wear a medical identification bracelet or carry pertinent information with him.

Renovascular hypertension

When systemic blood pressure rises because of stenosis of the major renal arteries or their branches or because of intrarenal atherosclerosis, renovascular hypertension occurs. This narrowing (sclerosis) may be partial or complete, and the resulting blood pressure elevation may be benign or malignant. About 5% to 10% of patients with high blood pressure display renovascular hypertension.

Causes

In about 95% of patients, renovascular hypertension results from either atherosclerosis (especially in older men) or fibromuscular diseases of the renal artery wall layers (for example, medial fibroplasia and, less commonly, intimal and subadventitial fibroplasia). Other causes include arteritis, anomalies of the renal arteries, embolism, trauma, tumor, and dissecting aneurysm.

Stenosis or a renal artery occlusion stimulates the affected kidney to release renin, an enzyme that converts angiotensinogen (a plasma protein) to angiotensin I. As angiotensin I circulates through the lungs and liver, it converts to angiotensin II, which causes peripheral vasoconstriction, increased arterial pressure and aldosterone secretion and, eventually, hypertension.

Complications

Renovascular hypertension can lead to such significant complications as congestive heart failure, myocardial infarction, cerebrovascular accident and, occasionally, renal failure.

Assessment

In the early stages, the patient may complain of flank pain. During your assessment, you may note reduced urine output, elevated blood pressure, and a systolic bruit over the epigastric vein in the upper abdomen on auscultation.

As the disorder progresses, the patient may report headache, nausea, anorexia, fatigue, palpitations, tachycardia, and anxiety. If renal failure occurs, you may notice alterations in the patient's level of consciousness and pitting edema. Auscultation may reveal bibasilar crackles.

Diagnostic tests

An isotopic renal blood flow scan and rapid-sequence excretory urography are needed to identify renal blood flow abnormalities and discrepancies of kidney size and shape. Renal arteriography reveals the actual arterial stenosis or obstruction.

In addition, samples from the right and left renal veins are obtained for comparison of plasma renin levels with those in the inferior vena cava (split renal vein renins). Increased renin levels from the involved kidney that exceed levels from the uninvolved kidney by a ratio of 1.5:1.0 or greater implicate the affected kidney and determine whether surgery can reverse hypertension.

Laboratory evaluation of serum samples shows hypokalemia, hyponatremia or hypernatremia, and elevated blood volume. Elevated blood urea nitrogen (BUN) and serum creatinine levels signal the onset of renal failure. Urine studies may reveal albuminuria and high specific gravity.

A positive captopril test can differentiate renovascular hypertension from essential hypertension before more invasive tests are done.

Treatment

Surgery, the treatment of choice, is 95% effective in restoring adequate circulation and controlling severe hypertension. It also can improve severely impaired renal function. Surgical techniques include renal artery bypass, endarterectomy, arterioplasty and, as a last resort, nephrectomy.

In selected cases, balloon catheter renal artery dilatation can correct renal artery stenosis without the risks of surgery. Measures to relieve symptoms include antihypertensives, diuretics, and a sodium-restricted diet.

Key nursing diagnoses and patient outcomes

Altered thought processes related to electrolyte imbalance. Based on this nursing diagnosis, you'll establish these patient outcomes. The patient will:
- remain safe in his environment
- regain and maintain orientation to time, person, and place
- have his electrolyte balance restored with appropriate treatment.

Altered urinary elimination related to stenosis of renal arteries or their branches. Based on this nursing diagnosis, you'll establish these patient outcomes. The patient will:
- regain a normal urine output with effective treatment
- not show signs and symptoms of renal failure.

Risk for injury related to potential vascular complications. Based on this nursing diagnosis, you'll establish these patient outcomes. The patient will:
- comply with the prescribed treatment aimed at reducing blood pressure
- have his blood pressure return to normal and remain normal
- show no evidence of vascular complications such as myocardial infarction or cerebrovascular accident.

Nursing interventions

- Prepare the patient for diagnostic tests. For example, adequately hydrate him before tests that use a contrast medium and make sure he's not allergic to the medium used.
- Administer drugs as ordered. Adequately medicate the patient for pain to decrease anxiety and increase comfort.
- Maintain fluid and sodium restrictions.
- If the patient is anorexic, offer appetizing, high-calorie meals to ensure adequate nutrition.
- If a nephrectomy is necessary, reassure the patient that his remaining kidney will be adequate for renal function. Provide appropriate preoperative and postoperative care. (See the entry "Nephrectomy.")
- Provide a quiet, stress-free environment, if possible.
- Encourage cardiovascular fitness, and work with the doctor and patient to develop the most beneficial program.

Monitoring

- Watch for complications after excretory urography or arteriography.
- Accurately monitor and record intake and output and daily weight. Weigh the patient at the same time each day (before a meal) and when he's wearing the same clothing.
- Frequently assess urine specific gravity, BUN, serum creatinine, and protein levels.
- Check blood pressure in both arms regularly, with the patient lying down and standing. A drop of 20 mm Hg or more in either systolic or diastolic pressure on arising may necessitate a dosage adjustment in antihypertensive medications.

Patient teaching

- Help the patient and his family understand renovascular hypertension, and emphasize the importance of following the prescribed treatment regimen.
- Describe the purpose of diagnostic tests, and explain each procedure. If the patient

is scheduled for surgery, explain the procedure and postoperative care.
• Familiarize the patient with his medications, and encourage him to take them as ordered. Suggest taking diuretics in the morning so that sleep patterns won't be disturbed.
• Urge the patient to have regular blood pressure screenings.
• Explain the purpose of a low-sodium diet, and stress the importance of following it. Suggest alternative flavorings and spices to keep the diet palatable. Also stress the need to restrict fluids, if appropriate.

Respiratory acidosis

This acid-base disturbance is characterized by reduced alveolar ventilation and manifested by hypercapnia (partial pressure of carbon dioxide in arterial blood [$PaCO_2$] greater than 45 mm Hg). Respiratory acidosis can be acute (resulting from sudden failure in ventilation) or chronic (resulting from long-term pulmonary disease).

The prognosis depends on the severity of the underlying disturbance and the patient's general clinical condition.

Causes

Factors that predispose a patient to respiratory acidosis include:
• *drugs* such as narcotics, anesthetics, hypnotics, and sedatives, which depress the respiratory control center's sensitivity
• *central nervous system (CNS) trauma,* such as medullary injury, which may impair ventilatory drive
• *chronic metabolic alkalosis,* which may occur when respiratory compensatory mechanisms attempt to normalize pH by decreasing alveolar ventilation
• *neuromuscular diseases,* such as Guillain-Barré syndrome, myasthenia gravis, and poliomyelitis, in which respiratory muscles fail to respond properly to respiratory drive, reducing alveolar ventilation.

In addition, respiratory acidosis can result from an airway obstruction or parenchymal lung disease that interferes with alveolar ventilation or from chronic obstructive pulmonary disease (COPD), asthma, severe adult respiratory distress syndrome, chronic bronchitis, large pneumothorax, extensive pneumonia, and pulmonary edema.

Complications

Acute or chronic respiratory acidosis can produce shock and cardiac arrest.

Assessment

The patient may initially complain of headache and dyspnea. He may also have a predisposing condition for respiratory acidosis. On inspection, you may see that he's dyspneic and diaphoretic. He may report nausea and vomiting.

Palpation may detect bounding pulses. Auscultation may reveal rapid, shallow respirations, tachycardia and, possibly, hypotension.

Ophthalmoscopic examination may uncover papilledema. And neurologic examination may disclose a level of consciousness (LOC) ranging from restlessness, confusion, and apprehension to somnolence, with a fine or flapping tremor (asterixis) and depressed reflexes.

Diagnostic tests

For critical laboratory test results, see *Key abnormal test values in respiratory acidosis,* page 810.

Treatment

Effective treatment aims to correct the source of alveolar hypoventilation. If alveolar ventilation is significantly reduced, the patient may need mechanical ventilation until the underlying condition can be treated. This includes bronchodilators, oxygen, and antibiotics in COPD; drug therapy for conditions such as myasthenia gravis; removal of foreign bodies from the

CHECKLIST

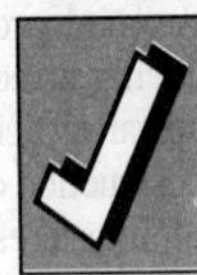

Key abnormal test values in respiratory acidosis

The following ABG values confirm respiratory acidosis:

- ☐ $PaCO_2$ above the normal 45 mm Hg
- ☐ pH typically below the normal range of 7.35 to 7.45
- ☐ normal HCO_3^- levels (22 to 26 mEq/liter) in acute respiratory acidosis but elevated above 26 mEq/liter in chronic respiratory acidosis.

airway in cases of obstruction; antibiotics for pneumonia; dialysis to eliminate toxic drugs; and correction of metabolic alkalosis.

Dangerously low pH levels (less than 7.15) can produce profound CNS and cardiovascular deterioration and may require administration of I.V. sodium bicarbonate. In chronic lung disease, elevated carbon dioxide (CO_2) levels may persist despite treatment.

Key nursing diagnoses and patient outcomes

Fear related to threat of death. Based on this nursing diagnosis, you'll establish these patient outcomes. The patient will:

- identify and express his fear
- use available support systems to help him cope with fear
- show no physical signs or symptoms of fear.

Impaired gas exchange related to alveolar hypoventilation. Based on this nursing diagnosis, you'll establish these patient outcomes. The patient will:

- regain and maintain normal arterial blood gas (ABG) values
- not exhibit signs and symptoms of profound CNS and cardiovascular deterioration
- demonstrate compliance with the prescribed treatment for the underlying cause of respiratory acidosis.

Ineffective breathing pattern related to rapid shallow respirations. Based on this nursing diagnosis, you'll establish these patient outcomes. The patient will:

- reestablish his respiratory rate within normal limits
- express a feeling of comfort with his breathing pattern
- have normal breath sounds on auscultation.

Nursing interventions

- Be prepared to treat or remove the underlying cause, such as an airway obstruction.
- Maintain adequate hydration by administering I.V. fluids.
- Give oxygen (only at low concentrations in patients with COPD) if the level of partial pressure of oxygen in arterial blood drops.
- Give aerosolized or I.V. bronchodilators as prescribed.
- Start mechanical ventilation if hypoventilation cannot be corrected immediately. Maintain a patent airway and provide adequate humidification if acidosis requires mechanical ventilation.
- Perform tracheal suctioning regularly and chest physiotherapy, if ordered.
- Reassure the patient as much as possible, depending on his LOC. Allay the fears and concerns of family members by keeping them informed about the patient's status.

Monitoring

- To detect developing respiratory acidosis, closely monitor patients with COPD and chronic CO_2 retention for signs of acidosis. Also closely monitor all patients who receive narcotics and sedatives.
- Be alert for critical changes in the patient's respiratory, CNS, and cardiovascu-

lar functions. Report any such changes immediately. Also monitor and report variations in ABG levels and electrolyte status.

- Monitor and record the patient's response to administered aerosolized or I.V. bronchodilators.
- Continuously monitor ventilator settings if the patient requires intubation.

Patient teaching

- Instruct the patient who's recovering from a general anesthetic to turn, cough, and perform deep-breathing and coughing exercises frequently to prevent respiratory acidosis.
- If the patient receives home oxygen therapy for COPD, stress the importance of maintaining the dose at the ordered flow rate.
- Instruct the patient and his family in home oxygen therapy use and safety measures.
- Explain the reasons for ABG analysis.
- Alert the patient to possible adverse effects of prescribed medications. Tell him to call the doctor if any occur.

Respiratory alkalosis

Marked by a decrease in the partial pressure of carbon dioxide in arterial blood ($Pa{CO_2}$) to less than 35 mm Hg and a rise in blood pH above 7.45, respiratory alkalosis results from alveolar hyperventilation. Uncomplicated respiratory alkalosis leads to a decrease in hydrogen ion concentration, which raises the blood pH. Hypocapnia occurs when the lungs eliminate more carbon dioxide (CO_2) than the body produces at the cellular level. In the acute stage, respiratory alkalosis is also called hyperventilation syndrome.

Causes

Predisposing conditions to respiratory alkalosis include:

- compensation for metabolic acidosis
- congestive heart failure
- central nervous system (CNS) injury to the respiratory control center
- extreme anxiety
- fever
- overventilation during mechanical ventilation
- pulmonary embolism
- salicylate intoxication (early).

Complications

In extreme respiratory alkalosis, related cardiac arrhythmias may fail to respond to usual treatment. Seizures may also occur.

Assessment

The patient history may reveal a predisposing factor associated with respiratory alkalosis. The patient may complain of light-headedness or paresthesia (numbness and tingling in his arms and legs).

On inspection, he may seem anxious, with visibly rapid breathing. In severe respiratory alkalosis, tetany may be apparent, with visible twitching and flexion of the wrists and ankles. Auscultation may reveal tachycardia and deep, rapid breathing.

Diagnostic tests

For critical arterial blood gas (ABG) values, see *Key abnormal test values in respiratory alkalosis,* page 814, and *Using ABGs to assess respiratory acid-base imbalances.* Serum electrolyte studies may also be performed to detect metabolic acid-base disorders.

Treatment

In respiratory alkalosis, treatment attempts to eradicate the underlying condition – for example, by removing ingested toxins or by treating fever, sepsis, or CNS disease. In severe respiratory alkalosis, the patient may need to breathe into a paper bag, which helps relieve acute anxiety and increase CO_2 levels. If respiratory alkalosis results from anxiety, sedatives and tranquilizers may help the patient.

NURSING PRIORITY

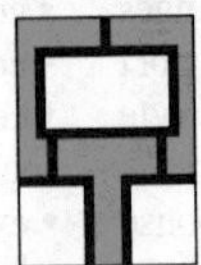

Using ABGs to assess respiratory acid base imbalances

To help determine if a patient is experiencing a respiratory acid-base imbalance, follow the decision tree steps below to interpret the patient's ABGs.

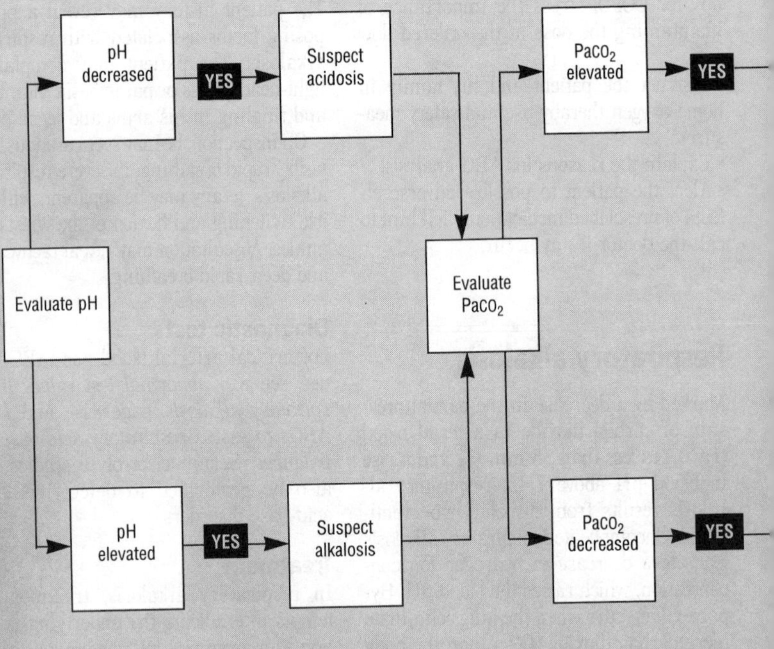

Evaluate pH → pH decreased → YES → Suspect acidosis → Evaluate $PaCO_2$

Evaluate pH → pH elevated → YES → Suspect alkalosis → Evaluate $PaCO_2$

Evaluate $PaCO_2$ → $PaCO_2$ elevated → YES →

Evaluate $PaCO_2$ → $PaCO_2$ decreased → YES →

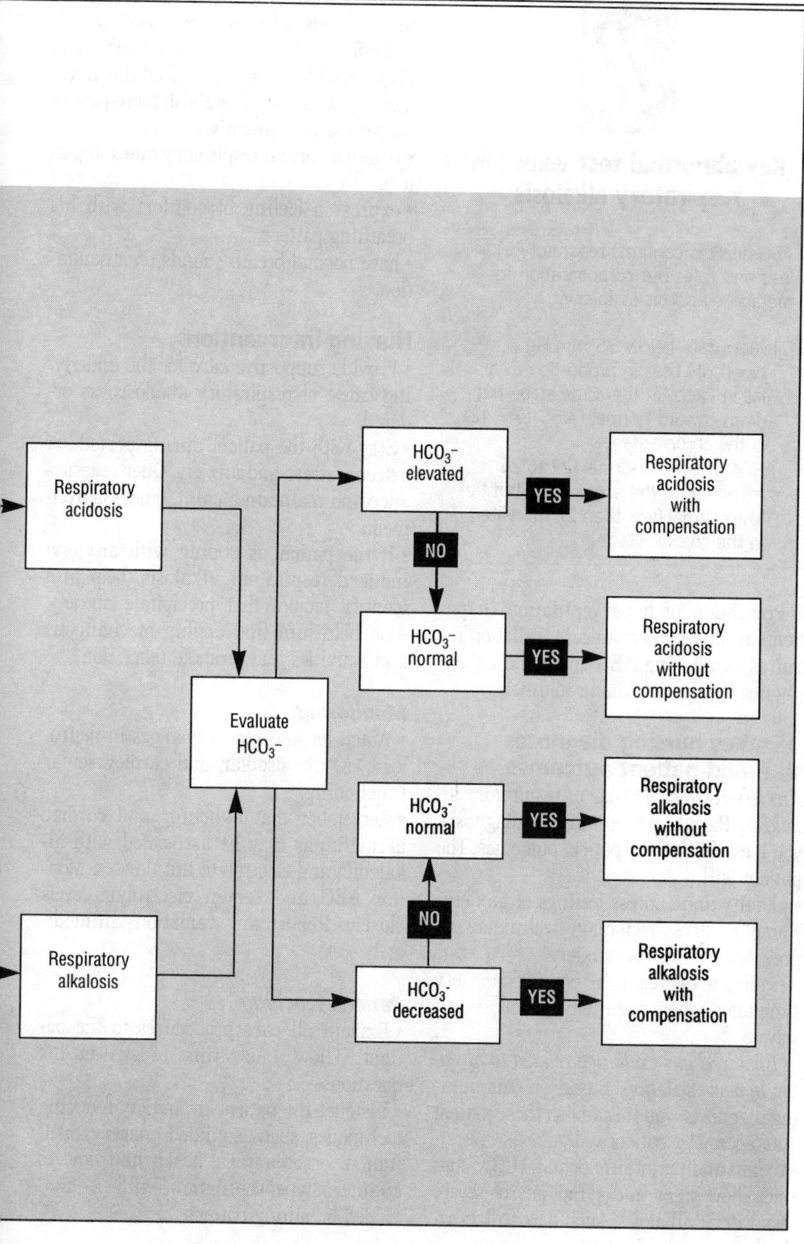
Respiratory acidosis
Respiratory alkalosis
Evaluate HCO_3^-
HCO_3^- elevated
YES
Respiratory acidosis with compensation
NO
HCO_3^- normal
YES
Respiratory acidosis without compensation
HCO_3^- normal
YES
Respiratory alkalosis without compensation
NO
HCO_3^- decreased
YES
Respiratory alkalosis with compensation

CHECKLIST

Key abnormal test values in respiratory alkalosis

ABG analysis confirms respiratory alkalosis and rules out compensation for metabolic acidosis as follows:

- ☐ $PaCO_2$ falls below 35 mm Hg
- ☐ blood pH rises in proportion to a fall in $PaCO_2$ in the acute stage but drops toward normal (7.35 to 7.42) in the chronic stage
- ☐ HCO_3^- level is normal (22 to 26 mEq/liter) in the acute stage but below normal (less than 22 mEq/liter) in the chronic stage.

Prevention of hyperventilation in patients receiving mechanical ventilation requires monitoring ABG levels and adjusting dead-space or minute volume.

Key nursing diagnoses and patient outcomes

Anxiety related to cause of respiratory alkalosis. Based on this nursing diagnosis, you'll establish these patient outcomes. The patient will:
- identify and express feelings of anxiety
- employ stress-reduction techniques to prevent or minimize anxiety
- exhibit a decrease in physical anxiety symptoms when respiratory alkalosis resolves.

Impaired gas exchange related to alveolar hyperventilation. Based on this nursing diagnosis, you'll establish these patient outcomes. The patient will:
- regain and maintain normal ABG values
- not show signs and symptoms of severe respiratory alkalosis, such as cardiac arrhythmias and seizures
- comply with prescribed treatment to correct the cause of respiratory alkalosis.

Ineffective breathing pattern related to deep, rapid breathing. Based on this nursing diagnosis, you'll establish these patient outcomes. The patient will:
- regain a normal respiratory rate and pattern
- express a feeling of comfort with his breathing pattern
- have normal breath sounds on auscultation.

Nursing interventions

- Provide supportive care for the underlying cause of respiratory alkalosis, as ordered.
- Stay with the patient during periods of extreme stress and anxiety. Offer reassurance and maintain a calm, quiet environment.
- If the patient is coping with anxiety-induced respiratory alkalosis, help him identify factors that precipitate anxiety. Also help him find coping mechanisms and activities that promote relaxation.

Monitoring

- Watch for and report changes in neurologic, neuromuscular, and cardiovascular functioning.
- Remember that twitching and cardiac arrhythmias may be associated with alkalemia and electrolyte imbalances. Monitor ABG and serum electrolyte levels closely. Report any variations immediately.

Patient teaching

- Explain all care procedures to the patient. Allow ample time to answer his questions.
- Instruct the patient in anxiety-reducing techniques, such as guided imagery, meditation, or even yoga. Teach him how to counter hyperventilation with a controlled-breathing pattern.

Retinal detachment

In this disorder, separation of the retinal layers creates a subretinal space that fills with fluid. Twice as common in men as in women, retinal detachment may be primary or secondary. The disorder usually involves only one eye but may occur in the other eye later. Rarely healing spontaneously, a detached retina can usually be reattached successfully with surgery. The prognosis depends on the area of the retina affected.

Causes

A retinal detachment may be primary or secondary. A primary detachment occurs spontaneously because of a change in the retina or the vitreous, whereas a secondary detachment results from another problem, such as intraocular inflammation or trauma. The most common cause of retinal detachment is a hole or tear in the retina. This hole allows the liquid vitreous to seep between the retinal layers and separate the sensory retinal layer from its choroidal blood supply. In adults, retinal detachment usually results from degenerative changes related to aging (which cause a spontaneous tear). Predisposing factors include myopia, cataract surgery, and trauma.

Additionally, retinal detachment may result from fluid seeping into the subretinal space as an effect of inflammation, tumors, or systemic disease. Detachment may also result from traction placed on the retina by vitreous bands or membranes (resulting from proliferative diabetic retinopathy, posterior uveitis, or a traumatic intraocular foreign body, for example). Retinal detachment can also be inherited, usually in association with myopia.

Complications

Retinal detachment may result in severe vision impairment and possible blindness.

Assessment

Initially, the patient may complain that he sees floating spots and recurrent light flashes. As detachment progresses, he may report gradual, painless vision loss described as looking through a veil, curtain, or cobweb. He may relate that the "veil" obscures objects in a particular visual field.

Diagnostic tests

- *Direct ophthalmoscopy,* after full pupil dilation, shows folds or discoloration in the usually transparent retina.
- *Indirect ophthalmoscopy* can detect retinal tears.
- *Ocular ultrasonography* may be performed to examine the retina if the patient has an opaque lens.

Treatment

Depending on the detachment's location and severity, treatment may include restricting eye movements to prevent further separation until surgical repair can be made.

A hole in the peripheral retina may be treated with cryotherapy. A hole in the posterior retina may respond to laser therapy.

To reattach the retina, scleral buckling may be performed. In this procedure, the surgeon places a silicone plate or sponge over the reattachment site and secures it in place with an encircling band. The pressure exerted gently pushes the choroid and retina together. Scleral buckling may be followed by replacement of the vitreous with silicone, oil, air, or gas.

Key nursing diagnoses and patient outcomes

Anxiety related to potential for loss of vision in affected eye. Based on this nursing diagnosis, you'll establish these patient outcomes. The patient will:

- identify and express feelings of anxiety
- cope with anxiety by being involved in decisions about his care

• display fewer physical symptoms of anxiety.

Diversional activity deficit related to activity restrictions used to prevent further retinal detachment. Based on this nursing diagnosis, you'll establish these patient outcomes. The patient will:
• identify activities that he can do safely
• express a positive attitude about activity restrictions
• report decreased feelings of boredom.

Sensory or perceptual alterations (visual) related to loss of vision. Based on this nursing diagnosis, you'll establish these patient outcomes. The patient will:
• discuss the impact of visual loss on his life-style
• remain safe in his environment
• compensate for visual loss by using adaptive devices.

Nursing interventions

• Provide encouragement and emotional support to decrease anxiety caused by vision loss.
• Prepare the patient for surgery by cleaning his face with a mild (no-tears) shampoo. Give antibiotics and cycloplegic or mydriatic eyedrops, as ordered.
• Postoperatively, position the patient as directed (the position will vary according to the surgical procedure). To prevent increasing intraocular pressure (IOP), administer antiemetics as indicated. Discourage any activities that would raise IOP.
• In macular involvement, keep the patient on bed rest (with or without bathroom privileges) to prevent further retinal detachment.
• To reduce edema and discomfort following laser therapy, apply ice packs, and administer acetaminophen, as ordered, for headache.
• If the patient receives a retrobulbar injection, apply a protective eye patch because the eyelid will remain partially open.
• After removing the protective patch, give cycloplegic and steroidal or antibiotic eyedrops, as ordered. Apply cold compresses to decrease swelling and pain.
• Give prescribed analgesics as needed.

Monitoring

• Monitor the patient's degree of visual loss.
• Assess the patient for persistent pain and report it if present.
• Observe for slight localized corneal edema and perilimbal congestion, which may follow laser therapy.

Patient teaching

• Explain to the patient undergoing laser therapy that the procedure may be done in same-day surgery. Forewarn him that he may have blurred vision for several days afterward.
• Instruct him to rest and to avoid driving, bending, heavy lifting, or any other activities that increase intraocular pressure for several days after eye surgery. Discourage activities that may cause the patient to bump his eye.
• Encourage leg and deep-breathing exercises to prevent complications of immobility.
• Show the patient having scleral buckling surgery how to instill eyedrops properly. After surgery, remind him to lie in the position recommended by the doctor.
• Advise the patient to wear sunglasses if photosensitivity occurs.
• Instruct the patient to take acetaminophen as needed for headaches and to apply ice packs to his eye to reduce swelling and alleviate discomfort.
• Review the signs of infection, emphasizing those requiring immediate attention.

Rheumatic fever and rheumatic heart disease

A systemic inflammatory disease of childhood, acute rheumatic fever develops after infection of the upper respiratory tract with group A beta-hemolytic streptococci.

Rheumatic fever principally involves the heart, joints, central nervous system, skin, and subcutaneous tissues. It commonly recurs.

The term rheumatic heart disease refers to the cardiac involvement of rheumatic fever–its most destructive effect. Cardiac involvement develops in up to 50% of patients and may affect the endocardium, myocardium, or pericardium during the early acute phase. It may later affect the heart valves, causing chronic valvular disease.

The extent of damage to the heart depends on where the disorder strikes. Myocarditis produces characteristic lesions called Aschoff's bodies (in the acute stages) and cellular swelling and fragmentation of interstitial collagen, leading to formation of a progressively fibrotic nodule and interstitial scars. Endocarditis causes valve leaflet swelling; erosion along the lines of leaflet closure; and blood, platelet, and fibrin deposits, which form beadlike vegetation. It most commonly strikes the mitral valve in females and the aortic valve in males. In both, it affects the tricuspid valves occasionally and the pulmonary valve only rarely.

Long-term antibiotic therapy can minimize the recurrence of rheumatic fever, reducing the risks of permanent cardiac damage and valvular deformity.

Worldwide, 15 to 20 million new cases are reported each year. Although rheumatic fever tends to be familial, this tendency may merely reflect contributing environmental factors. For example, in lower socioeconomic groups, incidence is highest in children between ages 5 and 15, probably as a result of malnutrition and crowded living conditions. This disease strikes most often during cool, damp weather in the winter and early spring. In the United States, it's most common in the northern states.

Causes

Rheumatic fever appears to be a hypersensitivity reaction in which antibodies produced to combat streptococci react and produce characteristic lesions at specific tissue sites. How and why group A streptococcal infection initiates the process are unknown. Because few people infected with *Streptococcus* ever contract rheumatic fever (about 0.3%), altered host resistance probably is involved in its development or recurrence.

Complications

The mitral and aortic valves are often destroyed by rheumatic fever's long-term effects. Their malfunction leads to severe pancarditis and occasionally produces pericardial effusion and fatal heart failure. Of the patients who survive this complication, about 20% die within 10 years.

Assessment

Nearly all affected patients will report having a streptococcal infection a few days to 6 weeks earlier. They usually have a recent history of low-grade fever that spikes to at least 100.4 F° (38 C°) late in the afternoon, unexplained epistaxis, and abdominal pain.

Most patients complain of migratory joint pain (polyarthritis). Swelling, redness, and signs of effusion usually accompany such pain, which most commonly affects the knees, ankles, elbows, and hips.

If the patient has pericarditis, he may complain of sharp, sudden pain that usually starts over the sternum and radiates to the neck, shoulders, back, and arms. The pain commonly is pleuritic, increasing with deep inspiration and decreasing when the patient sits up and leans forward. (This position pulls the heart away from the diaphragmatic pleurae of the lungs.) The pain may mimic that of myocardial infarction.

A patient with heart failure caused by severe rheumatic carditis may complain of dyspnea, right upper quadrant pain, and a hacking, nonproductive cough.

Inspection may reveal skin lesions such as erythema marginatum, a nonpruritic, macular, transient rash. The lesions are red with blanched centers and well-demarcated borders. They typically appear on the trunk and extremities.

Near tendons or the bony prominences of joints, you may notice subcutaneous nodules that are firm, movable, nontender, and about 3 mm to 2 cm in diameter. They occur especially around the elbows, knuckles, wrists, and knees and less often on the scalp and backs of the hands. These nodules persist for a few days to several weeks and, like erythema marginatum, often accompany carditis.

You may notice edema and tachypnea if the patient has left ventricular failure.

Up to 6 months after the original streptococcal infection, you may note transient chorea. Mild chorea may produce hyperirritability, a deterioration in handwriting, or inability to concentrate. Severe chorea causes purposeless, nonrepetitive, involuntary muscle spasms and speech disturbances; poor muscle coordination; and weakness. Chorea resolves with rest and causes no residual neurologic damage.

Auscultation may reveal a pericardial friction rub (a grating sound heard as the heart moves) if the patient has pericarditis. You can hear it best during forced expiration, with the patient leaning forward or on his hands and knees. Murmurs and gallops may also occur. With left ventricular failure, you may hear bibasilar crackles and a ventricular or an atrial gallop. The most common murmurs include the following:

- a systolic murmur of mitral insufficiency (high-pitched, blowing, holosystolic, loudest at apex, possibly radiating to the anterior axillary line)
- a midsystolic murmur caused by stiffening and swelling of the mitral leaflet
- occasionally, a diastolic murmur of aortic insufficiency (low-pitched, rumbling, almost inaudible).

Valvular disease may eventually cause chronic valvular stenosis and insufficiency, including mitral stenosis and insufficiency and aortic insufficiency. In children, mitral insufficiency remains the major sequela of rheumatic heart disease. Palpation may reveal a rapid pulse rate.

Diagnostic tests

No specific laboratory tests can determine the presence of rheumatic fever, but the following test results support the diagnosis.

- *White blood cell count* and *erythrocyte sedimentation rate* may be elevated (during the acute phase); blood studies show slight anemia caused by suppressed erythropoiesis during inflammation.
- *C-reactive protein* is positive (especially during acute phase).
- *Cardiac enzyme levels* may be increased in severe carditis.
- *Antistreptolysin-O titer* is elevated in 95% of patients within 2 months of onset.
- *Throat cultures* may continue to show the presence of group A streptococci; however, they usually occur in small numbers. Isolating them is difficult.
- *Electrocardiography (ECG)* reveals no diagnostic changes, but 20% of patients show a prolonged PR interval.
- *Chest X-rays* show normal heart size (except with myocarditis, heart failure, and pericardial effusion).
- *Echocardiography* helps evaluate valvular damage, chamber size, ventricular function, and the presence of a pericardial effusion.
- *Cardiac catheterization* evaluates valvular damage and left ventricular function in severe cardiac dysfunction.

Treatment

Effective management eradicates the streptococcal infection, relieves symptoms, and prevents recurrence, thus reducing the chance of permanent cardiac damage. During the acute phase, treatment includes penicillin or (for patients with penicillin hypersensitivity) erythromycin. Salicylates, such as aspirin, relieve fever and minimize joint swelling and pain; if the patient has carditis or if salicylates fail to relieve pain and inflammation, the doctor may prescribe corticosteroids.

Supportive treatment requires strict bed rest for about 5 weeks during the acute phase with active carditis, followed by a progressive increase in physical activity. The increase depends on clinical and laboratory findings and the patient's response to treatment.

After the acute phase subsides, a monthly I.M. injection of penicillin G benzathine or daily doses of oral sulfadiazine or penicillin G may be used to prevent recurrence. Such preventive treatment usually continues for at least 5 years or until age 25.

Heart failure requires continued bed rest and diuretics. Severe mitral or aortic valvular dysfunction that causes persistent heart failure will require corrective surgery, such as commissurotomy (separation of the adherent, thickened leaflets of the mitral valve), valvuloplasty (inflation of a balloon within a valve), or valve replacement (with prosthetic valve). Corrective valvular surgery seldom is necessary before late adolescence.

Key nursing diagnoses and patient outcomes

Activity intolerance related to pain and decreased cardiac output. Based on this nursing diagnosis, you'll establish these patient outcomes. The patient will:

- maintain blood pressure and pulse and respiratory rates within normal range during activity
- demonstrate skill in conserving energy while performing daily activities to his tolerance level
- show that he understands the relationship between symptoms of activity intolerance and a deficit in oxygen supply or use.

Decreased cardiac output related to valvular dysfunction. Based on this nursing diagnosis, you'll establish these patient outcomes. The patient will:

- maintain hemodynamic stability, as exhibited by normal vital signs and mental status
- not complain of chest pain and show no arrhythmias on his ECG
- maintain adequate cardiac output.

Risk for infection related to increased susceptibility to group A beta-hemolytic streptococci. Based on this nursing diagnosis, you'll establish these patient outcomes. The patient will:

- communicate an understanding of the need for long-term antibiotic therapy
- incorporate measures to prevent or minimize infection into his daily life
- remain free of the signs and symptoms of infection.

Nursing interventions

- Before giving penicillin, ask the patient (or, if the patient is a child, his parents) if he's ever had a hypersensitivity reaction to it. Even if he hasn't, warn him that such a reaction is possible.
- Administer antibiotics on time to maintain consistent antibiotic blood levels.
- Provide analgesics to relieve pain and oxygen to prevent tissue hypoxia, as needed.
- Stress the importance of bed rest. Assist with bathing, as necessary. Provide a bedside commode because it puts less stress on the heart than using a bedpan. Offer diversional activities that are physically undemanding.
- Place the patient in an upright position to relieve dyspnea and chest pain, if needed.
- If the patient is unstable because of chorea, clear his environment of objects that could make him fall.

- To reduce anxiety, allow the patient to express his concerns about the effects of activity restrictions on his responsibilities and routines. Reassure him that the restrictions are temporary.
- After the acute phase, encourage the patient's family and friends to spend as much time as possible with the patient to minimize his boredom. Advise the parents to secure a tutor to help their child keep up with schoolwork during the long convalescence.
- Help the parents overcome any guilt feelings they may have about their child's illness. Failure to seek treatment for streptococcal infection is common because the illness may seem no worse than a cold.
- Encourage the parents and the child to vent their frustrations during the long, tedious recovery. If the child has severe carditis, help them prepare for permanent changes in the child's life-style.

Monitoring

- Watch the patient closely for a penicillin hypersensitivity reaction.
- Monitor the patient's vital signs and perform frequent cardiopulmonary assessments.
- Observe the patient for signs and symptoms of complications such as pericarditis, heart failure, or recurrent infection. Notify the doctor of any abnormal findings.
- Monitor the patient's ECG for abnormalities. Question him about chest pain.
- Evaluate the patient's physiologic response to activities, and notify the doctor if his tolerance decreases.

Patient teaching

- Explain all tests and treatments to the patient.
- Teach the patient and his family about this disease. Warn the patient or parents to watch for and immediately report signs of recurrent streptococcal infection: sudden sore throat, diffuse throat redness and oropharyngeal exudate, swollen and tender cervical lymph glands, pain on swallowing, temperature of 101° to 104° F (38.3° to 40° C), headache, and nausea. Urge the patient to keep away from people with respiratory tract infections.
- Tell the patient to resume activities of daily living slowly and to schedule rest periods into his routine for a while.
- Tell the parents or patient to stop penicillin therapy and call the doctor immediately if the patient develops a rash, fever, chills, or other signs of allergy.
- Instruct the patient and his family to watch for and report early signs of left ventricular failure, such as dyspnea and a hacking, nonproductive cough.
- Help the patient's family understand the frustrations associated with chorea (nervousness, restlessness, poor coordination, weakness, and inattentiveness). Emphasize that these effects are transient.
- Make sure the patient and his family understand the need to comply with prolonged antibiotic therapy and follow-up care and the need for additional antibiotics during dental surgery. Arrange for a visiting nurse to oversee home care, if necessary.

Rheumatoid arthritis

A chronic, systemic, symmetrical inflammatory disease, rheumatoid arthritis primarily attacks peripheral joints and surrounding muscles, tendons, ligaments, and blood vessels. Spontaneous remissions and unpredictable exacerbations mark the course of this potentially crippling disease.

Rheumatoid arthritis occurs worldwide, affecting more than 6.5 million people in the United States alone. The disease strikes women three times more often than men. Although it can occur at any age, the peak onset period for women is between ages 35 and 50.

Rheumatoid arthritis usually requires lifelong treatment and, sometimes, surgery.

In most patients, the disease follows an intermittent course and allows normal activity, although 10% suffer total disability from severe articular deformity, associated extra-articular symptoms, or both. The prognosis worsens with the development of nodules, vasculitis, and high titers of rheumatoid factor.

Causes

What causes the chronic inflammation characteristic of rheumatoid arthritis isn't known, but various theories point to infectious, genetic, and endocrine factors. A genetically susceptible person may develop abnormal or altered immunoglobulin G (IgG) antibodies when exposed to an antigen. The body doesn't recognize these altered IgG antibodies as "self," and the person forms an antibody known as rheumatoid factor against them. By aggregating into complexes, rheumatoid factor generates inflammation.

Eventually, the cartilage damage that results from the inflammation triggers further immune responses, including complement activation. Complement, in turn, attracts polymorphonuclear leukocytes and stimulates the release of inflammatory mediators, which exacerbates joint destruction.

Much more is known about the pathophysiology of rheumatoid arthritis than about its causes. If unarrested, joint inflammation occurs in four stages. First, synovitis develops from congestion and edema of the synovial membrane and joint capsule. Formation of pannus – thickened layers of granulation tissue – marks the onset of the second stage. Pannus covers and invades cartilage and eventually destroys the joint capsule and bone.

Progression to the third stage is characterized by fibrous ankylosis – fibrous invasion of the pannus and scar formation that occludes the joint space. Bone atrophy and misalignment cause visible deformities and disrupt the articulation of opposing bones, causing muscle atrophy and imbalance and, possibly, partial dislocations or subluxations. In the fourth stage, fibrous tissue calcifies, resulting in bony ankylosis and total immobility.

Complications

Pain associated with movement may restrict active joint use and cause fibrous or bony ankylosis, soft-tissue contractures, and joint deformities.

Between 15% and 20% of patients develop Sjögren's syndrome with keratoconjunctivitis sicca. Rheumatoid arthritis can also destroy the odontoid process, part of the second cervical vertebra. Rarely, spinal cord compression may occur, particularly in patients with longstanding deforming rheumatoid arthritis.

Assessment

The patient's history may reveal an insidious onset of nonspecific symptoms, including fatigue, malaise, anorexia, persistent low-grade fever, weight loss, and vague articular symptoms.

Later, more specific localized articular symptoms develop, frequently in the fingers at the proximal interphalangeal, metacarpophalangeal, and metatarsophalangeal joints. These symptoms usually occur bilaterally and symmetrically and may extend to the wrists, elbows, knees, and ankles.

The patient may report that affected joints stiffen after inactivity, especially on rising in the morning. She may complain that joints are tender and painful, at first only when she moves them, but eventually even at rest. Ultimately, joint function is diminished. She may also experience tingling paresthesia in the fingers, the result of synovial pressure on the median nerve from carpal tunnel syndrome.

Other complaints include stiff, weak, or painful muscles. If the patient has peripheral neuropathy, she may report numbness or tingling in the feet or weakness or loss of sensation in the fingers. If pleuritis develops, she may complain of pain on inspiration (although pleuritis often causes no symptoms). The patient with pulmonary nodules or fibrosis may complain of shortness of breath.

Inspection of the patient's joints may show deformities and contractures, especially if active disease continues. The fingers may appear spindle shaped from marked edema and congestion in the joints. Proximal interphalangeal joints may develop flexion deformities or become hyperextended. Metacarpophalangeal joints may swell dorsally, and volar subluxation and stretching of tendons may pull the fingers to the ulnar side (ulnar drift). The fingers may become fixed in a characteristic swan-neck deformity or in a boutonnière deformity. The hands appear foreshortened, and the wrists boggy. Inspection of pressure areas, such as the elbows, may reveal rheumatoid nodules – subcutaneous, round or oval, nontender masses – the most common extra-articular finding.

If the patient has vasculitis, you may observe such extra-articular signs as lesions, leg ulcers, and multiple systemic complications. If she has scleritis or episcleritis, you may observe redness of the eye.

Palpation may reveal joints that are hot to the touch. If the patient has pericarditis, auscultation may reveal pericardial friction rub (although pericarditis may cause no signs).

If spinal cord compression occurs, your assessment may also reveal signs of upper motor neuron disorder, such as a positive Babinski's sign and weakness. You may also detect signs of other extra-articular findings, including temporomandibular joint disease, infection, osteoporosis, myositis, cardiopulmonary lesions, lymphadenopathy, and peripheral neuritis.

Diagnostic tests

The criteria developed by the American Rheumatism Association can serve as guidelines to establish a diagnosis. But keep in mind that failure to meet these criteria – particularly early in the disease – doesn't exclude the diagnosis. (See *Criteria for classifying rheumatoid arthritis.*)

Although no test definitively diagnoses rheumatoid arthritis, the following are useful:

- *X-rays.* In early stages, X-rays show bone demineralization and soft-tissue swelling. Later, they help determine the extent of cartilage and bone destruction, erosion, subluxations, and deformities. They also show the characteristic pattern of these abnormalities, particularly symmetrical involvement, although no particular pattern is conclusive for rheumatoid arthritis.
- *Rheumatoid factor test.* This test is positive in 75% to 80% of patients, as indicated by a titer of 1:160 or higher. Although the presence of rheumatoid factor doesn't confirm rheumatoid arthritis, it does help determine the prognosis; a patient with a high titer usually has more severe and progressive disease with extra-articular manifestations.
- *Synovial fluid analysis.* Analysis shows increased volume and turbidity, but decreased viscosity and complement (C3 and C4) levels. The white blood cell count often exceeds 10,000/mm³.
- *Serum protein electrophoresis.* This test may show elevated serum globulin levels.
- *Erythrocyte sedimentation rate.* The rate is elevated in 85% to 90% of patients. Because an elevated sedimentation rate frequently parallels disease activity, this test may help monitor the patient's response to therapy (as may a C-reactive protein test).
- *Complete blood count.* This test usually shows moderate anemia and slight leukocytosis.

Treatment

In rheumatoid arthritis, treatment requires a multidisciplinary health care team to reduce the patient's pain and inflammation, preserve functional capacity, resolve pathologic processes, and bring about improvement.

Salicylates, particularly aspirin, are the mainstay of therapy because they decrease inflammation and relieve joint pain. The patient may also receive other nonsteroidal

Criteria for classifying rheumatoid arthritis

The criteria of the American Rheumatism Association allow the classification of rheumatoid arthritis.

Guidelines

A patient who meets four of the seven criteria is classified as having rheumatoid arthritis. She must experience the first four criteria for at least 6 weeks, and a doctor must observe the second through fifth criteria.

A patient with two or more other clinical diagnoses can also be diagnosed with rheumatoid arthritis.

Criteria

- Morning stiffness in and around the joints that lasts 1 hour before full improvement
- Arthritis in three or more joint areas, with at least three joint areas (as observed by a doctor) exhibiting soft-tissue swelling or joint effusions, not just bony overgrowth (the 14 possible areas involved include the right and left proximal interphalangeal, metacarpophalangeal, wrist, elbow, knee, ankle, and metatarsophalangeal joints)
- Arthritis of hand joints, including the wrist, the metacarpophalangeal joint, or the proximal interphalangeal joint
- Arthritis that involves the same joint areas on both sides of the body
- Subcutaneous rheumatoid nodules over bony prominences
- Demonstration of abnormal amounts of serum rheumatoid factor by any method that produces a positive result in less than 5% of patients without rheumatoid arthritis
- Radiographic changes, which usually are seen on posteroanterior hand and wrist radiographs; these must show erosions or unequivocal bony decalcification localized in or most noticeable adjacent to the involved joints

anti-inflammatory agents (such as indomethacin, fenoprofen, and ibuprofen), antimalarials (hydroxychloroquine), gold salts, penicillamine, and corticosteroids (prednisone) – although corticosteroid therapy can cause osteoporosis. Other therapeutic drugs include such immunosuppressants as cyclophosphamide, methotrexate, and azathioprine, which are used in the early stages of the disease. (See *Drug therapy for rheumatoid arthritis,* pages 824 and 825.)

Supportive measures include increased sleep – 8 to 10 hours every night – frequent rest periods between daily activities, and splinting to rest inflamed joints (although, like corticosteroid therapy, immobilization can cause osteoporosis).

A physical therapy program that includes range-of-motion exercises and carefully individualized therapeutic exercises forestalls the loss of joint function; application of heat relaxes muscles and relieves pain. Moist heat (hot soaks, paraffin baths, whirlpools) usually works best for patients with chronic disease. Ice packs help during acute episodes.

Useful surgical procedures include metatarsal head and distal ulnar resectional arthroplasty, and insertion of a Silastic prosthesis between the metacarpophalangeal and proximal interphalangeal joints. Arthrodesis (joint fusion) may bring about stability and relieve pain, but only at the price of decreased joint mobility. Synovectomy (removal of destructive, proliferating synovium, usually in the wrists, fingers, and knees) may halt or delay the course of the disease. Osteotomy (the cutting of bone or excision of a wedge of bone) can realign joint surfaces and redistribute stresses. Tendons that rupture spontaneously need surgical repair. Tendon transfers may prevent deform-

Drug therapy for rheumatoid arthritis

Drug and adverse effects	Nursing interventions
aspirin Prolonged bleeding time; GI disturbances, including nausea, dyspepsia, anorexia, ulcers, and hemorrhage; hypersensitivity reactions ranging from urticaria to anaphylaxis; salicylism (mild toxicity: tinnitus, dizziness; moderate toxicity: restlessness, hyperpnea, delirium, marked lethargy; and severe toxicity: coma, seizures, severe hyperpnea)	• Don't use in patients with GI ulcers, bleeding, or hypersensitivity. • Give with food, milk, an antacid, or a large glass of water to reduce adverse GI effects. • Remember that toxicity can develop rapidly in febrile, dehydrated children. • Monitor salicylate levels. • Teach the patient to reduce the dose, one tablet at a time, if tinnitus occurs. • Teach the patient to watch for signs of bleeding, such as bruising, melena, and petechiae.
fenoprofen, ibuprofen, naproxen, piroxicam, sulindac, and tolmetin Prolonged bleeding time; central nervous system abnormalities (headache, drowsiness, restlessness, dizziness, tremors); GI disturbances, including hemorrhage and peptic ulcer; increased blood urea nitrogen (BUN) and liver enzyme levels	• Don't use in patients with renal disease, in asthmatics with nasal polyps, or in children. • Use cautiously in patients with GI disorders or cardiac disease and in patients allergic to other nonsteroidal anti-inflammatory drugs. • Give with milk or food to reduce adverse GI effects. • Tell the patient that the therapeutic effect may be delayed for 2 to 3 weeks. • Monitor renal, hepatic, and auditory functions in long-term therapy. Stop the drug if abnormalities develop.
gold (oral and parenteral) Dermatitis, pruritus, rash, stomatitis, nephrotoxicity, blood dyscrasias, nitritoid crisis and, with the oral form, GI distress and diarrhea	• Observe for nitritoid crisis (flushing, fainting, sweating). • Check the patient's urine for blood and albumin before each dose. If you get a positive result, withhold the drug and notify the doctor. • Stress the need for regular follow-up examinations, including blood and urine testing. • To avoid local nerve irritation, mix the drug well and give an I.M. injection deep in the buttock. • Advise the patient not to expect an improvement for 3 to 6 months. • Instruct the patient to report rash, bruising, bleeding, hematuria, and oral ulcers.
indomethacin Blood dyscrasias; hemolytic, aplastic, and iron deficiency anemias; headache; blurred vision; corneal and retinal damage; hearing loss; tinnitus; GI disturbances, including GI ulcer and hematuria	• Don't use in children under age 14 or in patients with aspirin intolerance or GI disorders. • Severe headache may occur within 1 hour. Stop the drug if headache persists. • Tell the patient to report any visual changes. Stress the need for regular eye examinations during long-term therapy. • Always give with food or milk. • Administer a single dose at bedtime to alleviate morning stiffness.

Drug therapy for rheumatoid arthritis *(continued)*

Drug and adverse effects	Nursing interventions
methotrexate Bone marrow suppression; stomatitis, nausea, and vomiting; alopecia; tubular necrosis, cirrhosis, hepatic fibrosis, and hyperuricemia; pulmonary infiltrates; diarrhea, possibly leading to hemorrhagic enteritis and intestinal perforation	• If adverse GI reactions occur, you may need to stop the drug as ordered. Administer antiemetics, as ordered, to control nausea and vomiting. • Report rash, redness, or ulcerations in the mouth and pulmonary adverse reactions, which may signal serious complications. • Monitor the patient's serum uric acid, serum creatinine, and BUN levels during therapy. As ordered, reduce the dose if the patient's BUN level reaches 20 to 30 mg/dl or her serum creatinine level reaches 1.2 to 2 mg/dl. Stop the drug, as ordered, if her BUN level rises above 30 mg/dl or her serum creatinine level reaches more than 2 mg/dl.
penicillamine Blood dyscrasias, glomerulonephropathy	• Give on an empty stomach, before meals, and separately from other drugs or milk. • Monitor the patient's urine for protein and blood. Also monitor liver function studies and complete blood count. • Tell the patient to report fever, sore throat, chills, bruising, and bleeding.

ities or relieve contractures. The patient may need joint reconstruction or total joint arthroplasty in advanced disease.

Key nursing diagnoses and patient outcomes

Altered role performance related to crippling effects of rheumatoid arthritis. Based on this nursing diagnosis, you'll establish these patient outcomes. The patient will:
- recognize the limitations imposed by rheumatoid arthritis and express her feelings about them
- help make decisions about the treatment and management of her illness
- function in her usual roles as much as possible.

Impaired physical mobility related to pain and joint deformities. Based on this nursing diagnosis, you'll establish these patient outcomes. The patient will:
- maintain muscle strength and range of motion in unaffected joints
- show no evidence of complications, such as contractures in unaffected joints, skin breakdown, or venous stasis
- achieve the highest level of mobility possible within the confines of the disease.

Pain related to joint inflammation. Based on this nursing diagnosis, you'll establish these patient outcomes. The patient will:
- attain pain relief with salicylates or another prescribed medication regimen
- comply with an exercise program to relieve stiffness and subsequent pain
- avoid overuse of affected joints and other activities that precipitate or increase joint pain.

Nursing interventions

- Administer analgesics as prescribed.
- Give meticulous skin care. Use lotion or cleansing oil – not soap – on dry skin.
- Supply zipper-pull, easy-to-open beverage cartons, lightweight cups, and unpackaged silverware to make it easier for the patient to perform activities of daily liv-

ing, such as dressing and feeding herself. Allow the patient enough time to calmly perform these tasks.
• Be sure that the patient adheres to the prescribed physical therapy program.
• Provide emotional support. Remember that the patient can easily become depressed, discouraged, and irritable. Encourage discussion of her fears concerning dependency, disability, sexuality, body image, and self-esteem. Refer her to appropriate counseling, as needed.
• Prepare the patient for joint replacement, as indicated. (See the entry "Joint replacement.")

Monitoring

• Monitor the patient's vital signs, and note weight changes, sensory disturbances, and level of pain.
• Assess the effectiveness of administered medications and watch for adverse reactions.
• Monitor the patient's compliance with the prescribed treatment regimen.
• Check for rheumatoid nodules. Also monitor for pressure ulcers and skin breakdown, especially if the patient is in traction or wearing splints. These can result from immobility, vascular impairment, corticosteroid treatment, and improper splinting.
• Monitor the duration of morning stiffness. Duration more accurately reflects the severity of the disease than does intensity.

Patient teaching

• Explain the nature of rheumatoid arthritis. Make sure the patient and her family understand that rheumatoid arthritis is a chronic disease that may require major changes in life-style. Be sure they understand that so-called miracle cures don't work.
• Explain all diagnostic tests and procedures.
• Encourage a balanced diet, but make sure the patient understands that special diets won't cure rheumatoid arthritis. Stress the need for weight control because obesity further stresses the joints.
• Teach the patient to maintain erect posture when standing, walking, and sitting. Tell her to sit in chairs with high seats and armrests; she'll find it easier to get up from a chair if her knees are lower than her hips. If she doesn't own a chair with a high seat, recommend putting blocks of wood under the legs of a favorite chair. Suggest that she obtain an elevated toilet seat.
• Instruct the patient to pace daily activities, resting for 5 to 10 minutes out of each hour and alternating sitting and standing tasks. Stress the importance of adequate sleep and correct sleeping posture. Tell her to sleep on her back on a firm mattress and to avoid placing a pillow under her knees, which encourages flexion deformity.
• Teach the patient to avoid putting undue stress on joints and to use the largest joint available for a given task; to support weak or painful joints as much as possible; to avoid flexion and instead use extension; to hold objects parallel to the knuckles as briefly as possible; to always use her hands toward the center of her body; and to slide – not lift – objects whenever possible. Enlist the aid of the occupational therapist to teach the patient how to simplify activities and protect arthritic joints.
• Encourage the patient to take hot showers or baths at bedtime or in the morning to reduce the need for pain medication.
• Stress the importance of wearing shoes with proper support.
• Suggest dressing aids – a long-handled shoehorn, a reacher, elastic shoelaces, a zipper-pull, and a buttonhook – and helpful household items, such as easy-to-open drawers, a hand-held shower nozzle, handrails, and grab bars. The patient who has trouble maneuvering fingers into gloves should wear mittens. Tell her to dress while in a sitting position whenever possible.

• Discuss the patient's sexual concerns. If pain creates problems during intercourse, discuss trying alternative positions, taking analgesics beforehand, and using moist heat to increase mobility.
• Before discharge, make sure the patient knows how and when to take prescribed medication and how to recognize possible adverse effects.
• For more information on coping with rheumatoid arthritis, refer the patient to the Arthritis Foundation.

Rocky Mountain spotted fever

An acute infectious, febrile, and rash-producing illness, Rocky Mountain spotted fever is associated with outdoor activities, such as camping and hiking. Endemic throughout the continental United States, the disease is particularly prevalent in the southeastern, southwestern, southern, and eastern states. As outdoor activities increase in popularity, so does the risk of contracting Rocky Mountain spotted fever – especially in the spring and summer months.

Without early and appropriate treatment, the disease can be fatal (with mortality up to 40%). Appropriate treatment reduces the risk of death to less than 10%. The usual incubation period is 7 days, but it can range from 2 to 12 days. As a rule, the shorter the incubation time, the more severe the infection.

Causes

The *Rickettsia rickettsii* organism causes Rocky Mountain spotted fever. Transmitted by the wood tick (*Dermacentor andersoni*) in the western United States and by the dog tick (*D. variabilis*) in the eastern United States, this rickettsial organism enters humans or small animals with the prolonged bite (4 to 6 hours) of an adult tick. This disease occasionally is acquired through inhalation or through contact of abraded skin with tick excreta or tissue juices. (This explains why people shouldn't crush ticks between their fingers when removing them from others.) In most tick-infested areas, 1% to 5% of the ticks harbor *R. rickettsii.*

Complications

Although uncommon, complications can include lobar pneumonia, pneumonitis, otitis media, parotitis, disseminated intravascular coagulation (DIC), shock, and renal failure.

Assessment

The patient's history may show recent exposure to ticks or tick-infested areas, or a known tick bite, although about 25% of patients with the disease have no history of a tick bite.

The patient typically complains of symptoms that began abruptly, including a persistent fever with temperature ranging between 102° and 104° F (38.9° to 40° C); generalized, excruciating headache; and aching in the bones, muscles, joints, and back. He also may report anorexia, nausea, vomiting, constipation, and abdominal pain.

Inspection may disclose the tongue covered with a thick white coating that gradually turns brown as the fever persists and the patient's temperature rises. The skin initially may appear flushed, but in 2 to 5 days, eruptions begin at the wrists, ankles, or forehead and spread centrally. Within 2 days, the rash covers the entire body (including the scalp, palms, and soles). It consists of erythematous macules 1 to 5 mm in diameter that blanch on pressure. Untreated, the rash may become petechial and maculopapular. By the third week, the skin peels off; sometimes gangrene develops over the elbows, fingers, and toes.

The patient may have a bronchial cough, a rapid respiratory rate (up to 60 breaths/

minute), insomnia, restlessness and, in extreme cases, delirium and circulatory collapse. Urine output decreases considerably, and the urine, which appears dark, contains albumin.

At disease onset, palpation may reveal a strong pulse, which gradually becomes rapid (possibly reaching 150 beats/minute) and thready. The rapid pulse rate and hypotension (less than 90 mm Hg systolic) herald imminent death from vascular collapse. Additionally, you may detect hepatomegaly, splenomegaly, and generalized pitting edema. Postauricular adenopathy may be palpated on one side if the tick bit the patient's head.

Diagnostic tests

Blood cultures to isolate the rickettsial organism can confirm the diagnosis. Some laboratories conduct direct immunofluorescence of cutaneous tissue to detect *R. rickettsii.*

Serologic tests performed during the patient's convalescence can confirm the diagnosis retrospectively. Four tests are performed together (separately, test findings are nonspecific). Diagnostically significant findings include:

- complement fixation titer – 1:16 or more
- indirect hemagglutination titer – 1:128 or more
- indirect immunofluorescence titer – 1:64 or more
- latex agglutination titer – 1:64 or more.

Other laboratory test findings may include a decreased platelet count, white blood cell count, and fibrinogen levels; prolonged prothrombin time and partial thromboplastin time; decreased serum protein levels, especially albumin; hyponatremia and hypochloremia associated with increased aldosterone excretion; and abnormal hepatic function.

Mild mononuclear pleocytosis with slightly elevated protein content in cerebrospinal fluid is common.

Treatment

In Rocky Mountain spotted fever, treatment requires careful removal of the tick and administration of antibiotics, such as tetracycline or chloramphenicol, until 3 days after the fever subsides. Treatment also includes measures to relieve symptoms. If DIC occurs, treatment includes heparin administration and platelet transfusion.

Key nursing diagnoses and patient outcomes

Altered nutrition: Less than body requirements, related to adverse GI effects. Based on this nursing diagnosis, you'll establish these patient outcomes. The patient will:

- regain lost weight and maintain it within the normal range
- tolerate oral feedings following administration of antiemetics
- report alleviation of adverse GI effects with resolution of Rocky Mountain spotted fever.

Hyperthermia related to the inflammatory process caused by Rocky Mountain spotted fever. Based on this nursing diagnosis, you'll establish these patient outcomes. The patient will:

- regain and maintain a normal temperature
- not have signs and symptoms of complications associated with hyperthermia, such as seizures or dehydration.

Impaired skin integrity related to skin eruptions and subsequent peeling of skin. Based on this nursing diagnosis, you'll establish these patient outcomes. The patient will:

- avoid scratching skin lesions
- show no signs or symptoms of complications of impaired skin integrity, such as gangrene or infection
- regain and maintain normal skin integrity.

Nursing interventions

- Administer analgesics, as ordered. Avoid giving aspirin, which increases the patient's risk of bleeding.
- Give antipyretic medications, as ordered, and tepid sponge baths to reduce fever.
- Administer antibiotics at ordered administration times.
- Be prepared to provide oxygen therapy and assisted ventilation for pulmonary complications.
- Adjust the I.V. fluid infusion rate hourly, as prescribed. Deliver enough fluids to prevent dehydration, provided the patient has adequate urine output.
- Provide meticulous mouth and skin care. Offer mentholated lotions to soothe itching resulting from the rash.
- Frequently turn the patient to prevent pressure sores and pneumonia. Encourage incentive spirometry and deep breathing to reduce the patient's risk of atelectasis.
- Plan care to promote adequate rest periods.
- Provide frequent, small, high-protein, high-calorie meals, or administer tube feedings if needed.
- Closely supervise the patient. Use restraining devices only if necessary. Administer sedatives, as ordered. Implement any safety measures needed to prevent patient injury.
- Report condition to local public agencies.

Monitoring

- Monitor vital signs, and watch for profound hypotension and shock.
- Record intake and output. Watch closely for decreased urine output – a possible indicator of renal failure.
- Observe for petechiae.
- Monitor the patient for complications of the disease and for adverse effects of medications.
- Evaluate the patient's daily nutritional intake. Weigh him regularly.

Patient teaching

- Instruct the patient to report any recurrent symptoms to the doctor at once so that treatment can resume promptly.
- To prevent Rocky Mountain spotted fever, advise the patient to avoid tick-infested areas. If he does frequent these areas, instruct him to inspect his entire body (including his scalp) every 3 to 4 hours for attached ticks. Remind him to wear protective clothing, such as a long-sleeved shirt and slacks that are firmly tucked into laced boots. Tell him to apply insect repellant to clothes and exposed skin.
- Teach patients and caregivers how to correctly remove ticks with tweezers or forceps and steady traction. Show them how to avoid leaving mouth parts in skin. Instruct them not to handle the tick or tick fragments.

S

Salmonella infection

One of the most common infections in the United States (more than 2 million new cases appear annually), salmonella infection is caused by gram-negative bacilli of the genus *Salmonella,* a member of the Enterobacteriaceae family. It occurs as enterocolitis, bacteremia, localized infection, typhoid fever, or paratyphoid fever. Nontyphoidal forms of salmonella infection usually produce mild to moderate illness, with low mortality. Enterocolitis and bacteremia are especially common (and more virulent) among infants, elderly people, and people already weakened by other infections, especially human immunodeficiency virus infection. Paratyphoid fever is rare in the United States.

Typhoid fever, the most severe form of salmonella infection, usually lasts from 1 to 4 weeks. Most typhoid patients are under age 30; most carriers are women over age 50. The incidence of typhoid fever in the United States is increasing as a result of travel to endemic areas. Mortality is about 3% in people who are treated and 10% in those who are untreated. An attack of typhoid fever confers lifelong immunity, although the patient may become a carrier.

Causes

The most common species of *Salmonella* include *S. typhi,* which causes typhoid fever; *S. enteritidis,* which usually causes enterocolitis; and *S. choleraesuis,* which commonly causes bacteremia. Of an estimated 1,700 serotypes of *Salmonella,* 10 cause the diseases most common in the United States. All 10 can survive for weeks in water, ice, sewage, and food.

Nontyphoidal salmonella infection usually follows the ingestion of contaminated or inadequately processed foods, especially eggs, chicken, turkey, and duck. Proper cooking reduces the risk of contracting salmonella infection but doesn't eliminate it. Other causes include contact with infected people or animals and ingestion of contaminated dry milk, chocolate bars, or pharmaceuticals of animal origin.

Typhoid fever usually results from drinking water contaminated by excretions of a carrier.

Complications

Salmonella infections may result in complications such as intestinal perforation or hemorrhage, cerebral thrombosis, pneumonia, endocarditis, myocarditis, meningitis, pyelonephritis, osteomyelitis, cholecystitis, hepatitis, septicemia, and acute circulatory failure.

Assessment

Clinical manifestations of salmonella infections vary, depending on the specific clinical syndrome. (See *Assessment findings in salmonella infection.*)

Assessment findings for paratyphoid fever are the same as for typhoid fever, but the clinical course usually is milder. In lo-

Assessment findings in salmonella infection

Depending on the form of salmonella infection, the patient experiences varying signs and symptoms. Typical findings in three forms of salmonella infection – enterocolitis, bacteremia, and typhoid fever – are discussed below.

Enterocolitis

In this form of salmonella infection, the patient may report having eaten contaminated food 6 to 48 hours before the onset of symptoms. He also may report sudden onset of nausea, vomiting (usually self-limiting), myalgia, headache, and a rise in temperature up to 102° F (38.9° C). The cardinal sign, diarrhea, usually persists for less than 7 days and may be accompanied by mild to severe abdominal cramping.

Inspection may reveal signs of dehydration – dry mucous membranes and decreased skin turgor. Auscultation may detect increased bowel sounds; palpation may detect abdominal tenderness.

Bacteremia

The patient's history commonly reveals immunocompromise, especially acquired immunodeficiency syndrome. Typically, the patient complains of anorexia, weight loss (without GI symptoms), joint pain, and chills. The disorder may follow a severe febrile course, lasting for days or weeks. The patient feels profoundly warm, and inspection may reveal dry skin with poor turgor and rapid, shallow breathing.

Auscultation may disclose normoactive or hypoactive bowel sounds and a systolic murmur if tachycardia develops. Palpation may detect a rapid, thready pulse and varying degrees of peripheral edema.

Typhoid fever

In this infection, the patient's history may reveal ingestion of contaminated food or water, typically 1 to 2 weeks before symptoms developed. Symptoms of enterocolitis occasionally arise within hours of ingesting *S. typhi.*

Signs and symptoms follow a typical course. In the 1st week, the patient may report the insidious onset of malaise, anorexia, myalgia, and headache. In the 2nd week, he may complain of chills, weakness, cough, increasing abdominal pain, and diarrhea or, more frequently, constipation. In the 3rd week, he may experience worsening fatigue and weakness (which usually subside by the week's end), although relapses or complications can develop.

The patient's temperature may rise to 104° F (40° C), usually in the evening. The patient looks acutely ill, and rose-colored spots that blanch with pressure may appear on the trunk. Delirium, confusion, and coma may occur. Bowel sounds are typically hypoactive; chest auscultation may reveal crackles. Palpation may disclose abdominal distention and tenderness, the characteristic sensation of displacing air- and fluid-filled loops of bowel, an enlarged liver and spleen and, sometimes, cervical lymphadenopathy.

calized infections, assessment findings depend on the site.

Diagnostic tests

In most cases, diagnosis requires isolating the organism in a culture, particularly blood (in typhoid or paratyphoid fever and bacteremia) or feces (in typhoid or paratyphoid fever and enterocolitis). Other appropriate culture specimens include urine, bone marrow, pus, and vomitus. In endemic areas, clinical symptoms of enterocolitis allow a working diagnosis before the cultures are positive. The presence of *S. typhi* in stools 1 or more years after treatment indicates that the patient is a carrier (about 3% of patients).

Widal's test, an agglutination reaction against somatic and flagellar antigens, may suggest typhoid fever with a fourfold rise in titer. (Drug use or liver disease can increase these titers and invalidate test results.) Other supportive laboratory values may include transient leukocytosis during the 1st week of typhoidal salmonella infection, leukopenia during the 3rd week, and leukocytosis in local infection.

Treatment

The type of antimicrobial agent chosen to treat typhoid fever, paratyphoid fever, or bacteremia depends on organism sensitivity. Possible choices include ampicillin, amoxicillin, chloramphenicol, ciprofloxacin, ceftriaxone, cefotaxime, and, for the severely toxemic patient, co-trimoxazole. Localized abscesses may need surgical drainage. Enterocolitis requires a short antibiotic course only if septicemia or prolonged fever occur.

Symptomatic treatment includes bed rest and, importantly, replacement of fluids and electrolytes. Camphorated opium tincture, kaolin and pectin mixtures, diphenoxylate, codeine, or small doses of morphine may be needed to relieve diarrhea and control cramps for patients who must remain active.

Key nursing diagnoses and patient outcomes

Activity intolerance related to weakened state. Based on this nursing diagnosis, you'll establish these patient outcomes. The patient will:
- perform self-care to his tolerance
- maintain his heart rate, respiratory rate and rhythm, and blood pressure within the normal range during activity
- regain and maintain muscle mass and strength.

Diarrhea related to bowel irritation. Based on this nursing diagnosis, you'll establish these patient outcomes. The patient will:
- report that diarrhea is controlled
- have normal skin integrity in the anal area
- regain and maintain normal elimination patterns with eradication of the infection.

Risk for fluid volume deficit related to adverse GI effects and hyperthermia. Based on this nursing diagnosis, you'll establish these patient outcomes. The patient will:
- exhibit vital signs within the normal range
- have intake equal to or exceeding output
- maintain urine output of 30 ml/hour.

Nursing interventions

- Follow standard precautions. Always wash your hands thoroughly before and after any contact with the patient; advise other hospital personnel to do the same.
- Wear gloves and a gown when disposing of feces or fecally contaminated objects.
- During acute infection, plan your care and activities to allow the patient as much rest as possible. Raise the bed's side rails and use other safety measures because the patient may become delirious. Use a room deodorizer to minimize odor from diarrhea and to provide a comfortable atmosphere for rest.
- Maintain adequate I.V. fluid and electrolyte therapy, as ordered. When the patient can tolerate oral feedings, encourage high-calorie fluids, such as milk shakes.
- Provide good skin and mouth care. Turn the patient frequently, and perform mild passive exercises, as indicated. Apply mild heat to the abdomen to relieve cramps.
- *Don't* administer antipyretics. They mask fever and may lead to hypothermia. Instead, to promote heat loss through the skin without causing shivering, apply tepid, wet towels (don't use alcohol or ice) to the patient's groin and axillae. To promote heat loss by vasodilation of peripheral blood vessels, use additional wet towels on the arms and legs, wiping with long, vigorous strokes.
- Report all salmonella infections to local public health authorities.

Monitoring

- Observe the patient for signs of bowel perforation: sudden pain in the lower right abdomen, possibly after one or more rectal bleeding episodes; sudden fall in tempera-

HEALTH PROMOTION POINTERS

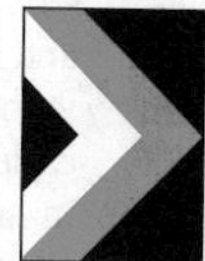

Minimizing the risk of salmonella

To prevent transmission of salmonella, instruct your patient and family to:
• wash hands after using the bathroom and before and after handling food
• cook all foods throughly, especially eggs and chicken
• refrigerate all foods promptly
• avoid cross-contamination of cooked and uncooked foods by cleaning cutting board or food preparation area with hot soapy water and drying thoroughly after use, using a clean surface each time when preparing more than one food, and washing hands before and after handling food
• use a different bathroom than other family members (or thoroughly clean the bathroom after each use) and avoid handling uncooked or prepared foods if he has a positive stool culture.

ture or blood pressure; and rising pulse rate.
• Watch closely for signs and symptoms of dehydration. Assess vital signs regularly and monitor intake and output.
• Monitor for other complications of the disease and evaluate the effectiveness of administered medications.

Patient teaching

• Teach the patient how to prevent infection. (See *Minimizing the risk of salmonella.*)
• Tell the patient to report signs of dehydration or bleeding, or a recurrence of symptoms. Relapse commonly occurs after typhoid or paratyphoid fever.
• Advise the patient's family and close contacts to obtain a medical examination and treatment if cultures are positive.
• Urge those at high risk for contracting typhoid fever (laboratory workers, travelers) to be vaccinated.

Sarcoidosis

A multisystemic, granulomatous disorder, sarcoidosis characteristically produces lymphadenopathy, pulmonary infiltration, and skeletal, liver, eye, or skin lesions.

Sarcoidosis occurs most commonly in young adults ages 20 to 40. In the United States, sarcoidosis occurs predominantly among blacks and affects twice as many women as men. Acute sarcoidosis usually resolves within 2 years. Chronic, progressive sarcoidosis, which is uncommon, is associated with pulmonary fibrosis and progressive pulmonary disability.

Causes

The cause of sarcoidosis is unknown, but several possibilities exist. The disease may result from a hypersensitivity response—possibly from T-cell imbalance—to such agents as atypical mycobacteria, fungi, and pine pollen. The incidence is slightly higher within families, suggesting a genetic predisposition. Or chemicals may trigger the disease (zirconium or beryllium lead to illnesses that resemble sarcoidosis).

Although the exact mechanism of the disease is unknown, research suggests a T-cell problem and, more specifically, a lymphokine production problem. In other granulomatous diseases, such as tuberculosis, granuloma formation occurs from inadequate pathogen clearance by macrophages. These macrophages require the help of T cells that secrete lymphokines, which in turn activate less effective macrophages to become aggressive phagocytes. Lack of lymphokine secretion by T cells may help explain granuloma formation in sarcoidosis.

Complications

Sarcoidosis can eventually lead to pulmonary fibrosis, with resultant pulmonary hypertension and cor pulmonale.

Assessment

The patient may report pain in her wrists, ankles, and elbows; general fatigue and a feeling of malaise; and unexplained weight loss. She may also complain of breathlessness and shortness of breath on exertion and have a nonproductive cough and substernal pain.

On inspection, you may observe erythema nodosum, subcutaneous skin nodules with maculopapular eruptions, and punched-out lesions on the fingers and toes. You may also note weakness and cranial or peripheral nerve palsies. When you inspect the nose, you may see extensive nasal mucosal lesions. Inspection of the eyes commonly reveals anterior uveitis. Glaucoma and blindness occasionally occur in advanced disease.

You may be able to palpate bilateral hilar and right paratracheal lymphadenopathy and splenomegaly, and you may hear such arrhythmias as premature beats on auscultation.

Diagnostic tests

A positive Kveim-Siltzbach skin test points to sarcoidosis. In this test, the patient receives an intradermal injection of an antigen prepared from human sarcoidal spleen or lymph nodes from patients with sarcoidosis. If she has active sarcoidosis, granuloma develops at the injection site in 2 to 6 weeks. When coupled with a skin biopsy at the injection site that shows discrete epithelioid cell granuloma, the test confirms the disease.

Several other tests support the diagnosis.

- *Chest X-rays* demonstrate bilateral hilar and right paratracheal adenopathy, with or without diffuse interstitial infiltrates. Occasionally, they show large nodular lesions in lung parenchyma.
- *Lymph node, skin,* or *lung biopsy* discloses noncaseating granulomas with negative cultures for mycobacteria and fungi.
- *Pulmonary function tests* indicate decreased total lung capacity and compliance, and reduced diffusing capacity.
- *Arterial blood gas (ABG) studies* show decreased partial pressure of oxygen in arterial blood.
- *Tuberculin skin test, fungal serologies, sputum cultures* (for mycobacteria and fungi), and *biopsy cultures* are negative and help rule out infection.

Treatment

An asymptomatic patient with sarcoidosis requires no treatment. However, sarcoidosis that causes ocular, respiratory, central nervous system, cardiac, or systemic symptoms (such as fever and weight loss) requires treatment with systemic or topical corticosteroids. So does sarcoidosis that produces hypercalcemia or destructive skin lesions. Such therapy usually continues for 1 to 2 years, but some patients may need lifelong therapy. A patient with hypercalcemia also requires a low-calcium diet and protection from direct exposure to sunlight.

If the patient has a significant response to the tubercular skin tests, showing tuberculosis reactivation, she'll need isoniazid therapy.

Key nursing diagnoses and patient outcomes

Anxiety related to potential long-term systemic effects caused by sarcoidosis. Based on this nursing diagnosis, you'll establish these patient outcomes. The patient will:
- identify and express feelings of anxiety
- use support systems to assist with coping
- use stress-reduction techniques to avoid anxiety symptoms.

Risk for injury related to neurologic abnormalities. Based on this nursing diagnosis, you'll establish these patient outcomes. The patient will:
• remain safe in her environment
• incorporate safety measures into her daily routine
• remain free of injury from neurologic abnormalities.

Impaired gas exchange related to potential for pulmonary fibrosis. Based on this nursing diagnosis, you'll establish these patient outcomes. The patient will:
• express feelings of comfort with improved air exchange
• perform activities of daily living to her level of tolerance
• maintain normal ABG values.

Nursing interventions

• If the patient has arthralgia, administer analgesics, as ordered.
• Provide a nutritious, high-calorie diet and plenty of fluids. If the patient has hypercalcemia, speak to the dietitian about a low-calcium diet.
• Administer oxygen as needed.
• Institute safety precautions if neurologic abnormalities occur.
• Listen to the patient's fears and concerns, and remain with her during periods of extreme stress and anxiety. Encourage her to identify actions and care measures that will help make her comfortable and relaxed. Then try to perform these measures, and encourage the patient to do so, too.
• Whenever possible, include the patient in care decisions, and include the family in all phases of the patient's care.

Monitoring

• Watch for and report any complications. Also note any abnormal laboratory results (anemia, for example) that could alter patient care.
• Record signs of progressive muscle weakness.
• Monitor the patient's nutritional status. Weigh her regularly to detect weight loss.
• Monitor the patient's respiratory function. Check chest X-rays for the extent of lung involvement, and note and record any bloody or increased sputum. If the patient has pulmonary hypertension or end-stage cor pulmonale, monitor ABG levels and watch for arrhythmias.
• Because corticosteroids may induce or worsen diabetes mellitus, test the patient's blood glucose level at least every 12 hours at the beginning of corticosteroid therapy. Watch for other adverse effects, such as fluid retention, electrolyte imbalance (especially hypokalemia), moon face, hypertension, and personality changes.

During or after corticosteroid withdrawal (particularly if the patient has an infection or another stressor, such as emotional stress or an underlying condition), watch for and report vomiting, orthostatic hypotension, hypoglycemia, restlessness, anorexia, malaise, and fatigue. Remember that the patient on long-term or high-dose therapy is vulnerable to infection.

Patient teaching

• When preparing the patient for discharge, stress the need for compliance with the prescribed steroid therapy. Emphasize the importance of not skipping doses.
• Instruct the patient to take steroids with food.
• Discuss the patient's increased vulnerability to infection, and review ways to minimize exposure to illness.
• Make sure the patient understands the need for regular follow-up examinations and treatment.
• Teach the patient to wear a medical identification bracelet or necklace indicating her corticosteroid therapy.
• Refer the patient with failing vision to community support and resource groups, including the American Foundation for the Blind, if necessary.

Sclerotherapy

Also referred to as endoscopic injection sclerotherapy, this procedure primarily treats bleeding esophageal varices by injecting the swollen veins or surrounding tissue with a sclerosant (a strongly irritating solution). The injection causes thrombosis of the mucosal and submucosal veins. Injection into the tissue beside the distended vein produces a fibrotic area and local edema that compresses the vessel. Eradication of the varix stops the variceal bleeding and prevents rebleeding.

Following the initial treatment to control an acute bleeding episode, the patient is usually scheduled for elective repeat sclerotherapy treatments. These treatments are usually scheduled at intervals of a few weeks, depending on the patient's risk level and healing rate. Prophylactic sclerotherapy aims to prevent rebleeding of the varices.

A similar procedure also successfully treats leg varicosities and hemorrhoids by injecting a sclerosant into the distended vein. The sclerosants generally used in the United States are sodium morrhuate (5%), sodium tetradecyl sulphate (1.5% to 3%), and ethanolamine oleate.

Procedure

After the patient is given I.V. conscious sedation (usually diazepam) and his throat is sprayed with a topical anesthetic, the doctor performs the procedure in conjunction with esophagogastric duodenoscopy. Following oral passage of the endoscope, the doctor locates and identifies the bleeding varix or varices. He then injects about 2 ml of a sclerosing agent through a flexible needle injector into the varix or varices. He withdraws the needle into the sheath and observes the site. Bleeding should stop within 2 to 5 minutes. If bleeding continues, the doctor makes a second injection below the bleeding site. Prophylactic sclerotherapy may then be done on other distended, nonbleeding varices to sclerose potential bleeding sites.

Complications

Transient noncardiac chest pain, dysphagia, and fever are common adverse effects, occurring within the first 24 to 72 hours following sclerotherapy. Other complications include allergic reaction to the sclerosing agent; ulceration at the injection site; pulmonary complications, such as aspiration pneumonia, pleural effusion, pulmonary infiltrates, and adult respiratory distress syndrome; esophageal stricture formation; and bacteremia. Complications attributable to the endoscopic procedure include traumatic esophageal perforation and hemorrhage.

Key nursing diagnoses and patient outcomes

Anxiety related to the need for sclerotherapy. Based on this nursing diagnosis, you'll establish these patient outcomes. The patient will:
- identify and express feelings of anxiety
- use effective coping behaviors
- exhibit fewer physical signs of anxiety.

Risk for injury related to potential complications associated with sclerotherapy. Based on this nursing diagnosis, you'll establish these patient outcomes. The patient will:
- show no signs and symptoms of complications
- maintain baseline cardiopulmonary and GI function following sclerotherapy
- exhibit normal breath sounds and white blood cell count.

Pain related to noncardiac chest discomfort caused by sclerotherapy. Based on this nursing diagnosis, you'll establish these patient outcomes. The patient will:
- express feelings of comfort following analgesic administration
- become pain free within 72 hours following sclerotherapy.

Nursing interventions

To prepare a patient for sclerotherapy or manage his care afterward, expect to implement the following interventions.

Before the procedure

- Explain the procedure to the patient and his family and answer their questions. Inform him that the procedure usually takes about 1 hour and will be performed in his room or in a specially designated hospital area, such as the GI unit or clinic.
- Prepare the patient for perioral endoscopy by having him remove his dentures, put on a patient gown, and empty his bladder.
- Tell the patient to lie still during the procedure to prevent injury to himself.
- Obtain and record baseline vital signs.
- Establish and maintain vascular access for I.V. fluids or blood replacement. Administer the ordered sedation at the prescribed time.

After the procedure

- Observe the patient for signs and symptoms of blood loss, pulmonary complications, fever, perforation, or other complications. Report acute changes to the doctor immediately.
- Monitor the patient's vital signs and auscultate breath sounds frequently until he's fully recovered and his condition has stabilized.
- Discontinue I.V. fluids when ordered to do so.
- Administer pain medication as prescribed.

Home care instructions

- Instruct the patient to report any fever, bleeding, respiratory problems, chest pain, or difficulty swallowing to the doctor immediately.
- Teach the patient how to use analgesics, if ordered, for transient mild chest pain.
- Review any dietary restrictions ordered by the doctor.

Septic arthritis

Also known as infectious arthritis, pyogenic septic arthritis is a medical emergency. It arises when bacteria invade a joint and cause the synovial lining to become inflamed. If the organisms enter the joint cavity, effusion and pyogenesis follow, with eventual destruction of bone and cartilage.

The disorder usually affects a single joint. It most often develops in a large joint but can strike any joint, including the spine and small peripheral joints. Migratory polyarthritis sometimes precedes localization of joint inflammation.

Septic arthritis can lead to ankylosis and even fatal septicemia. However, prompt antibiotic therapy and aspiration or drainage of the joint cure most patients.

Causes

In most cases of septic arthritis, bacteria spread from a primary site of infection, usually in adjacent bone or soft tissue, through the bloodstream to the joint. Common infecting organisms include:

- four strains of gram-positive cocci – *Staphylococcus aureus, Streptococcus pyogenes, S. pneumoniae,* and *S. viridans*
- two strains of gram-negative cocci – *Neisseria gonorrhoeae* and *Haemophilus influenzae*
- various gram-negative bacilli, including *Escherichia coli, Salmonella,* and *Pseudomonas.*

Rarely, fungi or mycobacteria cause the infection. Anaerobic organisms, such as gram-positive cocci, may infect adults and children over age 2. *H. influenzae* most often infects children under age 2.

Various factors can predispose a person to septic arthritis. Any concurrent bacterial infection (of the genitourinary or upper respiratory tract, for example) or serious chronic illness (such as cancer, renal failure, rheumatoid arthritis, septic lupus erythematosus, diabetes, or cirrhosis) heightens susceptibility. Consequently, alcoholics and elderly persons run an increased risk of septic arthritis.

Susceptibility also increases among patients who have immune system depression or a history of immunosuppressant therapy. Abuse of I.V. drugs can also lead to septic arthritis. Other predisposing factors include recent articular trauma, joint surgery, intra-articular injections, and local joint abnormalities.

Complications

Septic arthritis may cause infection of the bone (osteomyelitis) or other adjacent structures and a loss of joint cartilage that leads to joint destruction.

Assessment

The patient may have a history of a known infection outside the involved joint, an immunosuppressive condition, or I.V. drug abuse. He may complain of an abrupt onset of intense pain in the affected joint. He may also have fever and chills if he has a systemic infection. These findings can help differentiate septic arthritis from other types. (See *Other types of arthritis: Characteristics and treatment.*)

Inspection may show that the patient prefers to keep the affected joint flexed. This position eases pain by minimizing intra-articular pressure. You may observe redness and edema over the affected joint and severely reduced range of motion (ROM), both active and passive.

On palpation, you'll usually note warmth and extreme tenderness over the involved joint.

Diagnostic tests

- *Arthrocentesis* allows the collection of a synovial fluid specimen.
- *Synovial fluid analysis* shows gross pus or watery, cloudy fluid of decreased viscosity, typically with 50,000/mm³ or more white blood cells (WBCs) containing primarily neutrophils. It may also show a lower glucose level than a simultaneous 6-hour postprandial blood glucose level.
- *Gram stain* or *culture of the fluid* – or a *biopsy of the synovial membrane* – confirms the diagnosis and identifies the causative organism.
- *Blood cultures* may be positive and confirm the diagnosis even when the synovial culture is negative.
- *X-rays* may be normal for several weeks and usually don't aid the diagnosis; however, radiographic changes may appear as early as a week after infection. These can include distention of the joint capsule, narrowing of the joint space (indicating cartilage damage), and erosion of bone (joint destruction).
- *Radioisotope joint scan* may be used for less accessible joints, such as spinal articulations, and may help detect infection or inflammation. However, the test by itself isn't diagnostic. Joint bone scans are invariably positive but are useful only in occult sepsis (as in vertebral osteomyelitis).
- *Countercurrent immunoelectrophoresis* measures bacterial antigens in body fluids and helps to guide treatment.
- *Gas chromatography,* which defines microorganisms, helps to identify the causative agent.
- *WBC count* may be elevated, with many polymorphonuclear cells.
- *Erythrocyte sedimentation rate* is increased.

Treatment

Parenteral antibiotic therapy should begin right away. Empiric coverage may include a penicillinase-resistant penicillin (such as ticarcillin with clavulanic acid) or a second-generation cephalosporin (such as cefazolin), typically with gentamicin added for gram-negative coverage. Treatment may be modified as needed when sensitivity studies of the infecting organism become available.

I.V. antibiotic therapy continues for 4 to 6 weeks, possibly longer. The patient may need an implantable I.V. device, such as a

Other types of arthritis: Characteristics and treatment

You may care for patients with several other types of arthritis besides septic arthritis. The information below will help you differentiate among those types.

Traumatic arthritis

This disorder results from blunt, penetrating, or repeated trauma or from forced inappropriate motion of a joint or ligament. Clinical effects may include swelling, pain, tenderness, joint instability, and internal bleeding.

Treatment includes analgesics, anti-inflammatory drugs, application of cold followed by heat and, if needed, compression dressings, splints, joint aspiration, casting or, possibly, surgery.

Schönlein-Henoch purpura

A vasculitic syndrome, this condition is marked by palpable purpura, abdominal pain, renal disease, and arthralgia that most commonly affects the knees and ankles. It produces swollen, warm, tender joints without joint erosion or deformity.

Most patients have microscopic hematuria and proteinuria 4 to 8 weeks after onset. Incidence is highest in children and young adults, occurring most often in the spring after a respiratory tract infection. Treatment may include corticosteroids.

Hemophilic arthritis

This disorder may arise when the patient is between ages 1 and 5 and tends to recur until about age 10. It produces transient or permanent joint changes. Attacks typically are precipitated by trauma, but they may be spontaneous.

Hemophilic arthritis usually affects only one joint at a time—most commonly the knee, elbow, or ankle—and tends to recur in the same joint. Initially, the patient may feel only mild discomfort; later, he may experience warmth, swelling, tenderness, and severe pain with adjacent muscle spasms that prompt him to hold the extremity in a flexed position. Mild hemophilic arthritis may cause limited stiffness that subsides within a few days.

Severe hemophilic arthritis may be accompanied by fever and leukocytosis; severe, prolonged, or repeated bleeding may lead to chronic hemophilic joint disease.

Treatment includes I.V. infusion of the deficient clotting factor, bed rest with the affected extremity elevated, application of ice packs, analgesics, and possibly joint aspiration. Physical therapy includes progressive range-of-motion and muscle-strengthening exercises to restore motion and to prevent contractures and muscle atrophy.

Intermittent hydrarthrosis

Benign and very rare, this condition is characterized by regular, recurrent joint effusions. It most commonly affects the knee. The patient may have difficulty moving the affected joint but have no other arthritic symptoms.

The cause of intermittent hydrarthrosis is unknown; it may be linked to familial tendencies, allergies, or menstruation. Onset is usually at or soon after puberty. No effective treatment exists.

Hickman catheter or an implanted infusion port, for home use.

Treatment of septic arthritis requires monitoring of progress through frequent analysis of joint fluid cultures, synovial fluid leukocyte counts, and glucose determinations. Bioassays or bactericidal assays of synovial fluid and bioassays of blood may confirm clearing of the infection.

Codeine or propoxyphene can be given for pain, if needed. (Aspirin causes a misleading reduction in swelling, hindering accurate monitoring of progress.)

The affected joint may be immobilized with a splint or put into traction until the patient can tolerate movement. As the infection resolves, the doctor will add exercise to the treatment regimen to restore strength and mobility.

Needle aspiration (arthrocentesis) to remove grossly purulent joint fluid may be repeated daily until the fluid appears normal. If cultures remain positive or the WBC count remains elevated, the patient may need arthroscopic surgical drainage to remove resistant infection. (Septic arthritis of the hip requires open surgical drainage.)

Reconstructive surgery is warranted only for severe joint damage and only after all signs of active infection have disappeared. This usually takes several months. The patient will most likely undergo arthroplasty or joint fusion. Prosthetic replacement remains controversial because it may exacerbate the infection; however, it has been used successfully when the femoral head or acetabulum has sustained damage.

Key nursing diagnoses and patient outcomes

Anxiety related to long-term effects of septic arthritis on joint use. Based on this nursing diagnosis, you'll establish these patient outcomes. The patient will:
- identify and express feelings of anxiety
- perform stress-reduction techniques to avoid anxiety symptoms
- demonstrate fewer physical symptoms of anxiety.

Impaired physical mobility related to pain and swelling of affected joint. Based on this nursing diagnosis, you'll establish these patient outcomes. The patient will:
- communicate an understanding of the importance of complying with prolonged antibiotic therapy to reduce the risk of permanent joint damage from infection
- regain and maintain joint mobility.

Pain related to inflammation of the affected joint. Based on this nursing diagnosis, you'll establish these patient outcomes. The patient will:
- express feelings of comfort following analgesic administration
- identify factors that intensify pain and modify his behavior accordingly
- describe and carry out appropriate interventions for pain relief.

Nursing interventions

- Practice strict aseptic technique with all procedures. Dispose of soiled linens and dressings properly. Prevent contact between immunosuppressed patients and infected patients.
- Keep the joint in proper alignment, but prevent prolonged immobilization. Start ROM exercises as soon as ordered. Begin with passive ROM and isometric exercises; then add active ROM exercises. Once acute inflammation resolves, the patient may resume weight bearing on the affected joint.
- Provide pain medication as needed, especially before exercise. Administer narcotics and analgesics for acute pain and heat or ice packs for moderate pain.
- Encourage the patient to perform as much self-care as his immobility and pain allow. Give him time to perform these activities at his own pace.
- Throughout therapy, encourage the patient to express his concerns and answer any questions he may have to help reduce his anxiety. Offer support and encouragement when appropriate. Whenever possible, include the patient and his family in care decisions.

Monitoring

- Watch for signs of joint inflammation, such as heat, redness, swelling, pain, and drainage. Monitor the patient's vital signs and fever pattern.
- Check splints or traction regularly.

• Monitor the patient's pain level. (The pain of septic arthritis tends to be underestimated.) Also assess the patient's response to administered pain medications and other pain control measures.
• Evaluate the patient's compliance with antibiotic therapy regularly.
• Carefully evaluate the patient's condition after joint aspiration.

Patient teaching
• Explain all treatments, tests, and procedures to the patient. Warn him that needle aspiration will be extremely painful.
• Discuss all prescribed medications and any adverse reactions they may cause. Tell the patient to call his doctor if he experiences any adverse reactions. Explain why therapy must be closely monitored.
• Instruct the patient and his family about the prescribed exercise regimen. Make sure they understand how to perform each exercise and the importance of rest periods to avoid tiring the patient.
• If the patient needs surgery, explain preoperative and postoperative procedures to him and his family.
• If the patient needs home I.V. therapy, explain the procedure to him and his family.

Septic shock

Low systemic vascular resistance and an elevated cardiac output characterize septic shock. The disorder is thought to occur in response to infections that release microbes or one of the immune mediators.

Septic shock is usually a complication of another disorder or invasive procedure and has a mortality as high as 25%. The incidence of septic shock approaches 500,000 cases annually.

Causes

Any pathogenic organism can cause septic shock. Gram-negative bacteria, such as *Escherichia coli, Klebsiella pneumoniae, Serratia, Enterobacter,* and *Pseudomonas,* rank as the most common causes and account for up to 70% of all cases. Opportunistic fungi cause about 3% of cases. Rare causative organisms include mycobacteria and some viruses and protozoa.

Many organisms that are normal flora on the skin and in the intestines are beneficial and pose no threat. But when they spread throughout the body by way of the bloodstream (gaining entry through any alteration in the body's normal defenses or through artificial devices that penetrate the body, such as I.V., intra-arterial, and urinary catheters and knife or bullet wounds), they can progress to overwhelming infection unless body defenses destroy them.

Initially, these defenses activate chemical mediators in response to the invading organisms. The release of these mediators results in low systemic vascular resistance and increased cardiac output. Blood flow is unevenly distributed in the microcirculation, and plasma leaking from capillaries causes functional hypovolemia. Eventually, cardiac output falls, and poor tissue perfusion and hypotension cause multisystem organ failure and death.

Septic shock can occur in any person with impaired immunity, but elderly people are at greatest risk. About two-thirds of septic shock cases occur in hospitalized patients, most of whom have underlying diseases. Those at high risk include patients with burns; chronic cardiac, hepatic, or renal disorders; diabetes mellitus; immunosuppression; malnutrition; stress; and excessive antibiotic use. Also at risk are patients who have had invasive diagnostic or therapeutic procedures, surgery, or traumatic wounds.

Complications

In septic shock, complications include disseminated intravascular coagulation, renal failure, heart failure, GI ulcers, and abnormal liver function.

Assessment

The patient's history may include a disorder or treatment that can cause immunosuppression. Or it may include a history of invasive tests or treatments, surgery, or trauma. At onset, the patient may have fever and chills, although 20% of patients may be hypothermic.

The patient's signs and symptoms will reflect either the *hyperdynamic* or *warm phase* of septic shock (increased cardiac output, peripheral vasodilation, and decreased systemic vascular resistance) or the *hypodynamic* or *cold phase* (decreased cardiac output, peripheral vasoconstriction, increased systemic vascular resistance, and inadequate tissue perfusion).

In the hyperdynamic phase, the patient's skin may appear pink and flushed. His altered level of consciousness is reflected in agitation, anxiety, irritability, and shortened attention span. Respirations will be rapid and shallow. Urine output is below normal.

Palpation of peripheral pulses may detect a rapid, full, bounding pulse. The skin may feel warm and dry. Blood pressure may be normal or slightly elevated.

In the hypodynamic phase, the patient's skin may appear pale and, possibly, cyanotic. Peripheral areas may be mottled. His level of consciousness may be decreased; obtundation and coma may be present. Respirations may be rapid and shallow, and urine output may be less than 25 ml/hour or absent.

Palpation of peripheral pulses may reveal no pulse or a rapid pulse that's weak or thready. It may also be irregular if arrhythmias are present. The skin may feel cold and clammy.

Auscultation of blood pressure may reveal hypotension, usually with a systolic pressure below 90 mm Hg or 50 to 80 mm Hg below the patient's previous level. Auscultation of the lungs may reveal crackles or rhonchi if pulmonary congestion is present.

If central pressures are being monitored, the pulmonary artery wedge pressure will be reduced or normal and cardiac output will be moderately to severely increased or normal. Rarely, cardiac output will be decreased.

Diagnostic tests

The following are characteristic laboratory findings:

- *Blood cultures* are positive for the offending organism.
- *Complete blood count* shows the presence or absence of anemia and leukopenia, severe or absent neutropenia, and usually the presence of thrombocytopenia.
- *Serum lactate dehydrogenase levels* are elevated with metabolic acidosis.
- *Urine studies* show increased specific gravity (more than 1.020) and osmolality and decreased sodium.
- *Arterial blood gas (ABG) analysis* demonstrates elevated blood pH and partial pressure of oxygen and decreased partial pressure of carbon dioxide with respiratory alkalosis in early stages.

Treatment

Location and treatment of the underlying sepsis is essential to treating septic shock. If any I.V., intra-arterial, or urinary drainage catheters are in place, they should be removed. Aggressive antimicrobial therapy appropriate for the causative organism must be initiated immediately. Culture and sensitivity tests help determine the most effective antimicrobial drug.

In patients who are immunosuppressed because of drug therapy, drugs should be discontinued or reduced. Granulocyte transfusions may be used in patients with severe neutropenia.

Oxygen therapy should be initiated to maintain arterial oxygen saturation greater than 95%. Mechanical ventilation may be required if respiratory failure occurs.

Colloid or crystalloid infusions are given to increase intravascular volume and raise blood pressure. After sufficient fluid volume has been replaced, diuretics such as furosemide can be given to maintain urine output above 20 ml/hour. If fluid resuscitation fails to increase blood pressure, a vasopressor, such as dopamine, can be started. Blood transfusion may be needed if anemia is present.

Key nursing diagnoses and patient outcomes

Decreased cardiac output related to hypodynamic phase of septic shock. Based on this nursing diagnosis, you'll establish these patient outcomes. The patient will:
• regain and maintain adequate cardiac output
• regain and maintain stable vital signs and normal mental status
• remain free of chest pain and arrhythmias.

Fluid volume deficit related to functional hypovolemia. Based on this nursing diagnosis, you'll establish these patient outcomes. The patient will:
• have an oral and I.V. intake equal to or greater than his output
• produce adequate urine volume
• regain and maintain normal fluid and blood volume.

Risk for injury related to potential complications of septic shock. Based on this nursing diagnosis, you'll establish these patient outcomes. The patient will:
• obtain prompt treatment for early signs and symptoms of complications
• maintain normal organ function
• show no permanent adverse effects from septic shock.

Nursing interventions

• Remove any I.V., intra-arterial, or urinary drainage catheters and send them to the laboratory to culture for the presence of the causative organism. New catheters can be reinserted in the intensive care unit.
• Start an I.V. infusion with 0.9% sodium chloride or lactated Ringer's solution, using a large-bore (14G to 18G) catheter, which allows easier administration of later blood transfusions. (See *Infusion precaution in abdominal trauma.*)

NURSING ALERT

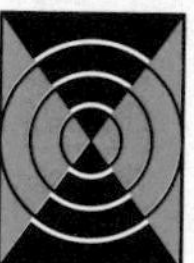

Infusion precaution in abdominal trauma

Don't start an I.V. infusion in the legs of a patient with septic shock who's suffered abdominal trauma. Infused fluid may escape through the ruptured vessel into the abdomen.

• When the patient's blood pressure drops below 80 mm Hg, increase the oxygen flow rate and notify the doctor immediately. A progressive drop in blood pressure accompanied by a thready pulse generally signals inadequate cardiac output from reduced intravascular volume. Notify the doctor and increase the infusion rate.
• Administer appropriate antimicrobial drugs I.V. to achieve effective blood levels rapidly.
• If urine output is less than 30 ml/hour, increase the fluid infusion rate. Notify the doctor if urine output doesn't improve. A diuretic may be ordered to increase renal blood flow and urine output.
• Draw an arterial blood sample to measure ABG levels. Administer oxygen by face mask or airway to ensure adequate tissue oxygenation. Adjust the oxygen flow rate to a higher or lower level, as ABG measurements indicate.
• Provide emotional support to the patient and his family. (See *Nursing care in septic shock,* pages 844 and 845.)
• Document the occurrence of a nosocomial infection and report it to the infection-control nurse. Investigation of all hospital-acquired infections can help identify their sources and prevent future infections.

NURSING PRIORITY

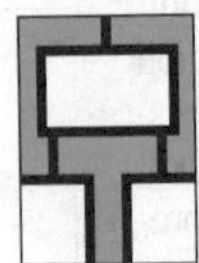

Nursing care in septic shock

Presence of major associated diseases and predisposing factors such as recent surgery, infection, or presence of infection source.
Signs and symptoms, including fever, chills, mental status changes, tachycardia, tachypnea, hypotension, and possible adverse GI effects.
Results of diagnostic tests, including blood cultures, complete blood count (CBC), serum lactate dehydrogenase levels, urine studies, arterial blood gas (ABG) values

Impaired gas exchange related to decreased cardiopulmonary tissue perfusion

↓

Administer oxygen.

↓

- Monitor respiratory function, including breath sounds.
- Monitor ABG values and oxygen (O_2) saturation.
- Check mental status frequently.

↓

Is gas exchange adequate?

YES → Continue O_2 therapy as prescribed.

NO → Expect to intubate patient. → Provide supportive care for mechanical ventilation.

↓

Patient exhibits adequate gas exchange by:
- having normal ABG and O_2 saturation values
- being alert and oriented to time, person, and place
- reporting breathing comfort.

KEY

- Assessment
- Nursing diagnoses
- Interventions
- Evaluation

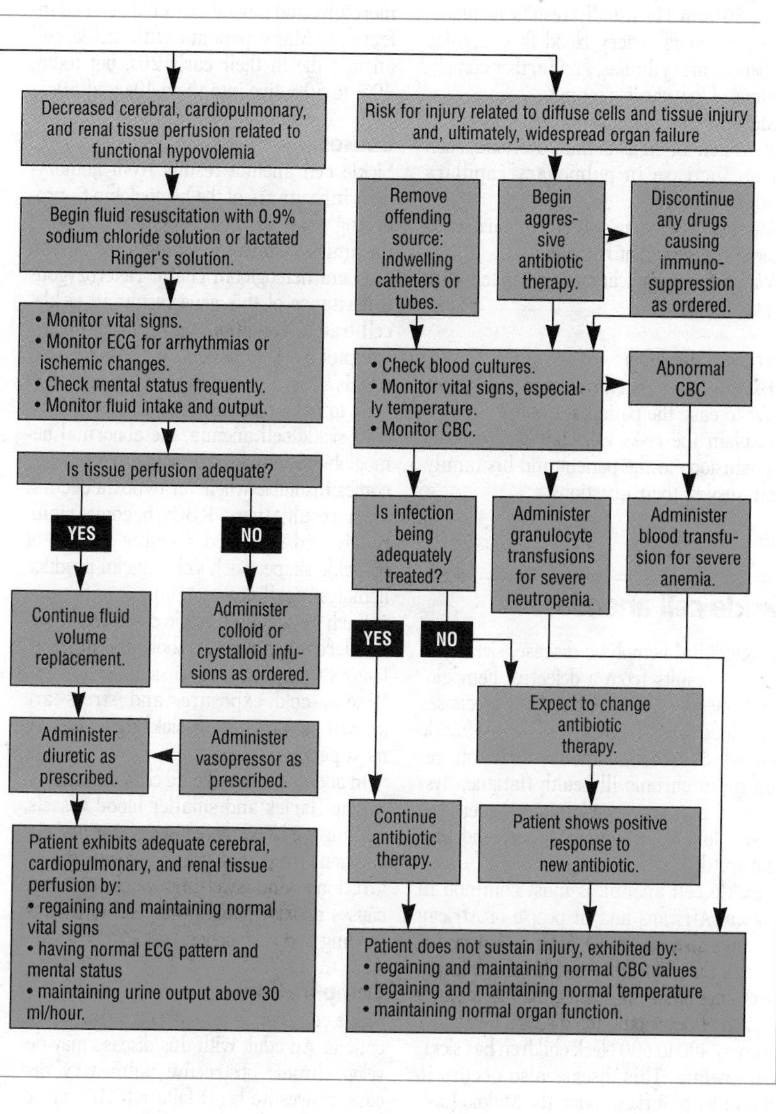
Decreased cerebral, cardiopulmonary, and renal tissue perfusion related to functional hypovolemia
Begin fluid resuscitation with 0.9% sodium chloride solution or lactated Ringer's solution.
• Monitor vital signs.
• Monitor ECG for arrhythmias or ischemic changes.
• Check mental status frequently.
• Monitor fluid intake and output.
Is tissue perfusion adequate?
YES
NO
Continue fluid volume replacement.
Administer colloid or crystalloid infusions as ordered.
Administer diuretic as prescribed.
Administer vasopressor as prescribed.
Patient exhibits adequate cerebral, cardiopulmonary, and renal tissue perfusion by:
• regaining and maintaining normal vital signs
• having normal ECG pattern and mental status
• maintaining urine output above 30 ml/hour.
Risk for injury related to diffuse cells and tissue injury and, ultimately, widespread organ failure
Remove offending source: indwelling catheters or tubes.
Begin aggressive antibiotic therapy.
Discontinue any drugs causing immunosuppression as ordered.
• Check blood cultures.
• Monitor vital signs, especially temperature.
• Monitor CBC.
Abnormal CBC
Is infection being adequately treated?
Administer granulocyte transfusions for severe neutropenia.
Administer blood transfusion for severe anemia.
YES
NO
Expect to change antibiotic therapy.
Continue antibiotic therapy.
Patient shows positive response to new antibiotic.
Patient does not sustain injury, exhibited by:
• regaining and maintaining normal CBC values
• regaining and maintaining normal temperature
• maintaining normal organ function.

Monitoring

- Record the patient's blood pressure, pulse and respiratory rates, and peripheral pulses every 1 to 5 minutes until he is stabilized. Record hemodynamic pressure readings every 15 minutes. Monitor cardiac rhythm continuously. Systolic blood pressure less than 80 mm Hg usually results in inadequate coronary artery blood flow, cardiac ischemia, arrhythmias, and further complications of low cardiac output.
- Measure the patient's hourly urine output. Watch for signs of fluid overload, such as an increase in pulmonary capillary wedge pressure.
- Monitor ABG values. Perform cardiopulmonary assessment frequently.
- Watch for complications associated with septic shock.

Patient teaching

- Explain all procedures and their purpose to ease the patient's anxiety.
- Explain the risks associated with blood transfusions to the patient and his family, and answer their questions.

Sickle cell anemia

A congenital hemolytic disease, sickle cell anemia results from a defective hemoglobin molecule (hemoglobin S) that causes red blood cells (RBCs) to become sickle shaped. Such cells impair circulation, resulting in chronic ill health (fatigue, dyspnea on exertion, swollen joints), periodic crises, long-term complications, and premature death.

Sickle cell anemia is most common in tropical Africans and in people of African descent; about 1 in 10 African-Americans carries the abnormal gene. If two such carriers have offspring, each child has a 1 in 4 chance of developing the disease. Overall, 1 in every 400 to 600 black children has sickle cell anemia. This disease also occurs in Puerto Rico, Turkey, India, the Middle East, and the Mediterranean area. Possibly, the defective hemoglobin S–producing gene has persisted because in areas where malaria is endemic, the heterozygous sickle-cell trait provides resistance to malaria and is actually beneficial.

Penicillin prophylaxis can decrease morbidity and mortality from bacterial infections. Many patients with sickle cell anemia die in their early 20s, but today, 20% to 50% live into their 40s and 50s.

Causes

Sickle cell anemia results from homozygous inheritance of the hemoglobin S–producing gene, which causes substitution of the amino acid valine for glutamic acid in the beta hemoglobin chain. Heterozygous inheritance of this gene results in sickle-cell trait, a condition with minimal or no symptoms. The patient with sickle-cell trait is a carrier; he can pass the sickle cell gene to his offspring.

In sickle cell anemia, the abnormal hemoglobin S found in the patient's RBCs becomes insoluble whenever hypoxia occurs. As a result, these RBCs become rigid, rough, and elongated, forming a crescent or sickle shape. Such sickling can produce hemolysis (cell destruction).

Each person with sickle cell anemia has a different hypoxic threshold and different factors that precipitate a sickle-cell crisis. Illness, cold exposure, and stress are known to precipitate sickling crises in most people.

In addition, these altered cells accumulate in capillaries and smaller blood vessels, making the blood more viscous. Normal circulation is impaired, causing pain, tissue infarctions, and swelling. Such blockage causes anoxic changes that lead to further sickling and obstruction.

Complications

Sickle cell anemia causes long-term complications. An adult with this disease may develop chronic obstructive pulmonary disease, congestive heart failure (CHF), or organ infarction, such as retinopathy and nephropathy. Splenic infarctions are common and often cause significant necrosis early in life, so that splenomegaly leads to a small, nodular, and malfunctioning spleen. Infection or repeated occlusion of small blood vessels and consequent infarction or necrosis of major organs commonly cause premature death. For example, cerebral blood vessel occlusion causes cerebrovascular accident and is the most common cause of death in severe sickle cell disease. Frequent sickling and hyperviscosity can lead to heart murmurs and CHF.

Assessment

Signs and symptoms usually don't develop until after 6 months of age because large amounts of fetal hemoglobin protect infants for the first few months after birth.

Characteristically, the patient history in sickle cell anemia includes chronic fatigue, unexplained dyspnea or dyspnea on exertion, joint swelling, aching bones, chest pain, ischemic leg ulcers (especially around the ankles), and an increased susceptibility to infection. The patient's medical history may include pulmonary infarctions and cardiomegaly.

Inspection may reveal jaundice or pallor. A young child may appear small for his age, whereas an older child may experience delayed growth and puberty. Inspection of an adult usually reveals a spiderlike body build (narrow shoulders and hips, long extremities, curved spine, and barrel chest).

Typically, assessment of the patient's vital signs reveals tachycardia. Palpation may disclose hepatomegaly and, in children, splenomegaly. Splenomegaly usually is absent in adulthood because the spleen shrinks over time. Auscultation may detect systolic and diastolic murmurs.

In sickle-cell crisis, assessment findings may include the following:

- history of recent infection, stress, dehydration, or other conditions that provoke hypoxia, such as strenuous exercise, high altitude, unpressurized aircraft, cold, and vasoconstrictive drugs
- complaints of sleepiness with difficulty awakening, severe pain and, sometimes, hematuria
- pale lips, tongue, palms, and nail beds; lethargy; listlessness; and often irritability
- body temperature over 104° F (40° C) or a temperature of 100° F (37.8° C) that persists for 2 or more days. (See *Differentiating types of sickle-cell crisis,* page 848.)

Diagnostic tests

A positive family history and typical clinical features suggest sickle cell anemia; a stained blood smear showing sickle cells and hemoglobin electrophoresis showing hemoglobin S confirm it. Electrophoresis should be done on umbilical cord blood samples at birth to provide sickle cell disease screening for all neonates at risk. Additional laboratory studies show low RBC counts, elevated white blood cell and platelet counts, decreased erythrocyte sedimentation rate, increased serum iron levels, decreased RBC survival, and reticulocytosis. Hemoglobin levels may be low or normal.

A lateral chest X-ray may be performed to detect the characteristic "Lincoln log" deformity. This spinal abnormality develops in many adults and some adolescents with sickle cell anemia, leaving the vertebrae resembling logs that form the corner of a cabin.

An ophthalmoscopic examination to detect corkscrew or comma-shaped vessels in the conjunctivae, another sign of this disease, may also be performed.

Treatment

Although sickle cell anemia can't be cured, treatments can alleviate symptoms and prevent painful crises. Certain vaccines, such as polyvalent pneumoccocal vaccine and *Haemophilus influenzae* B vaccine; anti-infectives, such as low-dose oral penicillin; and chelating agents, such as de-

Differentiating types of sickle-cell crisis

The following characteristic signs and symptoms help determine the type of sickle-cell crisis the patient is experiencing.

Vaso-occlusive crisis

The most common crisis and the hallmark of this disease, a vaso-occlusive crisis (painful crisis, infarctive crisis) usually appears periodically after age 5. It results from blood vessel obstruction by rigid, tangled sickle cells, which causes tissue anoxia and, possibly, necrosis.

Vaso-occlusive crisis is characterized by severe abdominal, thoracic, muscle, or bone pain and, possibly, increased jaundice, dark urine, or a low-grade fever. Patients with long-term disease may experience autosplenectomy, in which splenic damage and scarring is so extensive that the spleen shrinks and becomes impalpable. This can lead to increased susceptibility to *Streptococcus pneumoniae* sepsis, which can be fatal without prompt treatment. After the crisis subsides (in 4 days to several weeks), infection may develop, producing lethargy, sleepiness, fever, and apathy.

Aplastic crisis

Associated with infection (usually viral), an aplastic crisis (megaloblastic crisis) results from bone marrow depression. It's characterized by pallor, lethargy, sleepiness, dyspnea, possible coma, markedly decreased bone marrow activity, and RBC hemolysis.

Acute sequestration crisis

Occurring in infants between ages 8 months and 2 years, an acute sequestration crisis may cause sudden, massive entrapment of RBCs in the spleen and liver. This rare crisis causes lethargy and pallor and, if untreated, commonly progresses to hypovolemic shock and death.

Hemolytic crisis

This rare type of sickle-cell crisis usually affects patients who have glucose-6-phosphate dehydrogenase deficiency with sickle cell anemia. It probably results from complications of sickle cell anemia, such as infection, rather than from the disorder itself.

In hemolytic crisis, degenerative changes cause liver congestion and hepatomegaly. Chronic jaundice worsens, although increased jaundice doesn't always indicate a hemolytic crisis.

feroxamine, can minimize complications resulting from the disease and from transfusion therapy.

Other medications, such as analgesics, may help to relieve the pain of vaso-occlusive crisis. Iron supplements may be given if folic acid levels are low. A good antisickling agent isn't yet available; the most commonly used drug, sodium cyanate, produces many adverse reactions.

Treatment begins before age 4 months with prophylactic penicillin. If the patient's hemoglobin level drops suddenly or if his condition deteriorates rapidly, hospitalization will be needed for transfusion of packed RBCs.

In an acute sequestration crisis, treatment may include sedation and administration of analgesics, blood transfusion, oxygen therapy, and large amounts of oral or I.V. fluids.

Key nursing diagnoses and patient outcomes

Altered systemic tissue perfusion related to impaired circulation. Based on this nursing diagnosis, you'll establish these patient outcomes. The patient will:

• identify risk factors that exacerbate altered tissue perfusion
• not exhibit signs and symptoms of severe tissue ischemia, such as pain, coldness and color change of affected body part, or organ dysfunction
• regain and maintain tissue perfusion and cellular oxygenation.

Knowledge deficit related to management of sickle cell anemia. Based on this nursing diagnosis, you'll establish these patient outcomes. The patient will:
• express the need to know how to manage sickle cell anemia
• seek and obtain necessary information about sickle cell anemia management from appropriate sources
• demonstrate skill in managing sickle cell anemia, as evidenced by a decrease in the number and severity of sickle-cell crises.

Pain related to tissue ischemia secondary to decreased oxygen-carrying ability of RBCs and impaired circulation. Based on this nursing diagnosis, you'll establish these patient outcomes. The patient will:
• express feelings of comfort following analgesic administration
• identify life-style factors that precipitate a sickle-cell crisis and try to eliminate or decrease them
• become pain free when the sickle-cell crisis is over.

Nursing interventions

• Encourage the patient to talk about his fears and concerns. Try to stay with him during periods of severe crisis and anxiety. Provide reassurance, when possible, but always answer his questions honestly.
• If a male patient develops sudden, painful priapism, reassure him that such episodes are common and have no permanent harmful effects.
• Ensure that the patient receives adequate amounts of folic acid–rich foods, such as leafy green vegetables. Encourage adequate fluid intake to hydrate the patient; give parenteral fluids if necessary. Provide eggnog, ice pops, and milk shakes to meet fluid requirements.
• Apply warm compresses, warmed thermal blankets, and warming pads or mattresses to painful areas of the patient's body. Consider the weight of the warming appliance, to avoid aggravating pain. Never apply cold to a painful area.
• Administer analgesics and antipyretics as necessary. Each patient's level of pain is different; some may require acetaminophen to control the pain; others may have continuous pain during crisis while receiving morphine.
• When cultures demonstrate the presence of infection, administer antibiotics as ordered. Also administer prophylactic antibiotics as ordered. Use strict aseptic technique when performing treatments.
• Administer blood transfusions as ordered. Use strict aseptic technique.
• Encourage bed rest, with the head elevated to decrease tissue oxygen demand. Administer oxygen only if the patient is experiencing severe dyspnea.
• If the patient requires general anesthesia for surgery, help ensure that he receives adequate ventilation to prevent hypoxic crisis. Make sure the surgeon and the anesthesiologist are aware that the patient has sickle cell anemia, and provide a preoperative transfusion of packed RBCs, as needed.

Monitoring

• Monitor the patient's complete blood count regularly.
• Assess the patient's hydration status. Monitor his intake and output, and check for signs of dehydration.
• Monitor for signs and symptoms of sickle-cell crisis and chronic complications.
• Assess the patient's response to administered medication (especially analgesics) and other therapy, such as warm compresses.
• Watch for signs and symptoms of infection, such as fever, chills, or purulent drainage.

• Monitor the patient's respiratory status. Perform a respiratory assessment including auscultation of breath sounds regularly. Monitor arterial blood gases as indicated.

Patient teaching

• To help the patient prevent exacerbation of sickle cell anemia, advise him to avoid tight clothing that restricts circulation.
• Warn against strenuous exercise, vasoconstricting medications, cold temperatures (including drinking large amounts of ice water and swimming), unpressurized aircraft, high altitude, and other conditions that provoke hypoxia.
• Stress the importance of normal childhood immunizations, meticulous wound care, good oral hygiene, regular dental checkups, and a balanced diet as safeguards against infection.
• Emphasize the need for prompt treatment of infection.
• Explain the need to increase fluid intake to prevent dehydration that results from impaired ability to properly concentrate urine. Tell parents to encourage a child with sickle cell anemia to drink more fluids, especially in the summer, by offering milk shakes, ice pops, and eggnog.
• To encourage normal mental and social development, warn parents against being overprotective. Athough the child must avoid strenuous exercise, he can enjoy most everyday activities.
• Refer parents of children with sickle cell anemia for genetic counseling to answer their questions about the risk to future offspring. Recommend screening of other family members to determine if they're heterozygote carriers.
• Because delayed growth and later puberty are common, reassure an adolescent patient that he will grow and mature.
• Review the symptoms of vaso-occlusive crisis so that the patient and his family will recognize and treat it early. As appropriate, explain how to care for this condition at home. Prepare parents for an infant's first vaso-occlusive crisis (called "hand-foot crisis"), during which the infant's hands, feet, or both swell and become painful.
• Inform the patient and his parents that if he must be hospitalized for a vaso-occlusive crisis, I.V. fluids and parenteral analgesics may be administered. He also may receive oxygen therapy and blood transfusions.
• If appropriate, discuss how special conditions, such as surgery and pregnancy, may affect the patient.
• Stress to the patient the need to inform all health care providers that he has this disease before he undergoes any treatment – especially major surgery. Explain that any procedure that involves general anesthesia will require that the patient has adequate ventilation to prevent hypoxic crisis. Urge him to wear medical identification stating that he has sickle cell anemia.
• Warn women with sickle cell anemia that they're poor obstetric risks. However, their use of oral contraceptives is also risky; refer them for birth control counseling. If such women *do* become pregnant, they should maintain a balanced diet during pregnancy and may benefit from a folic acid supplement.
• If necessary, arrange for psychological counseling to help the patient cope. Suggest that he join an appropriate support group, such as the National Association for Sickle Cell Disease.

Silicosis

The most common form of pneumoconiosis, silicosis is a progressive disease characterized by nodular lesions, which frequently progress to fibrosis. It's classified according to the severity of the pulmonary disease and the rapidity of its onset and progression, although it usually occurs as a simple illness without symptoms.

Those who work around silica dust, such as foundry workers, boiler scalers, and stonecutters, have the highest incidence of the disease. Silica in its pure form occurs in the manufacture of ceramics (flint) and building materials (sandstone). It occurs in mixed form in the production of construction materials (cement). It's also found in powder form (silica flour) in paints, porcelain, scouring soaps, and wood fillers, and in the mining of gold, lead, zinc, and iron.

Sand blasters, tunnel workers, and others exposed to high concentrations of respirable silica may develop acute silicosis after 1 to 3 years. Those exposed to lower concentrations of free silica can develop accelerated silicosis, usually after about 10 years of exposure.

The prognosis is good unless the disease progresses to the complicated fibrotic form.

Causes

Silicosis results from the inhalation and pulmonary deposition of respirable crystalline silica dust, mostly from quartz. The risk depends on the concentration of dust in the atmosphere, the percentage of respirable free silica particles in the dust, and the duration of exposure. Although particles up to 10 microns in diameter can be inhaled, the disease-causing particles deposited in the alveolar space usually have a diameter of only 1 to 3 microns.

Nodules result when alveolar macrophages ingest silica particles, which they can't process. As a result, the macrophages die and release proteolytic enzymes into surrounding tissue. The enzymes inflame the tissue, attracting other macrophages and fibroblasts. These produce fibrous tissue to wall off the reaction, resulting in a nodule that has an onionskin appearance.

These nodules develop adjacent to the terminal and respiratory bronchioles. Although frequently accompanied by bullous changes in both lobes, nodules concentrate in upper lung lobes. If the disease doesn't progress, the patient may experience only minimal physiologic disturbances, with no disability. Occasionally, however, the fibrotic response accelerates, engulfing and destroying a large lung area.

Complications

Silicosis may progress to massive areas of pulmonary fibrosis, which may continue to grow even though the patient is no longer exposed to dust. Pulmonary fibrosis in turn may result in cor pulmonale, ventricular or respiratory failure, and pulmonary tuberculosis.

Assessment

The patient has a history of long-term industrial exposure to silica dust. He may complain of dyspnea on exertion, which he's likely to attribute to "being out of shape" or "slowing down." If the disease has progressed to the chronic and complicated state, the patient may report a dry cough, especially in the morning.

When you inspect the patient, you may note decreased chest expansion and tachypnea. If he has advanced disease, he may also act lethargic and look confused. You may percuss areas of increased and decreased resonance. On auscultation, you may hear fine to medium crackles, diminished breath sounds, and an intensified ventricular gallop on inspiration – a hallmark of cor pulmonale.

Diagnostic tests

- *Chest X-rays* in simple silicosis show small, discrete, nodular lesions distributed throughout both lung fields, although they typically concentrate in the upper lung zones. The hilar lung nodes may appear enlarged and show eggshell calcification. In complicated silicosis, X-rays show one or more conglomerate masses of dense tissue.
- *Pulmonary function tests* demonstrate reduced forced vital capacity (FVC) in complicated silicosis. If the patient has obstructive disease (emphysematous silicosis areas), he'll have reduced forced expira-

tory volume in 1 second (FEV_1). A patient with complicated silicosis also has reduced FEV_1 but has a normal or high ratio of FEV_1 to FVC. When fibrosis destroys alveolar walls and obliterates pulmonary capillaries or when it thickens the alveolocapillary membrane, the diffusing capacity for carbon monoxide falls below normal. Both restrictive and obstructive disease reduce maximal voluntary ventilation.

• *Arterial blood gas (ABG) analysis* reveals a normal partial pressure of oxygen in arterial blood in simple silicosis, although it may drop significantly below normal in late stages or complicated disease. The patient has normal partial pressure of carbon dioxide in arterial blood in the early stages of the disease, but hyperventilation may cause it to drop below normal. If restrictive lung disease develops – particularly if the patient is hypoxic and has severe alveolar ventilatory impairment – it may rise above normal.

Treatment

The goal is to relieve respiratory symptoms, manage hypoxia and cor pulmonale, and prevent respiratory tract infections and irritations. Treatment includes careful observation for the development of tuberculosis.

Daily bronchodilating aerosols and increased fluid intake (at least 3 qt [3 liters] daily) relieve respiratory signs and symptoms. Steam inhalation and chest physiotherapy (such as controlled coughing and segmental bronchial drainage) with chest percussion and vibration help clear secretions.

In severe cases, the patient may need oxygen by nasal cannula, mask, or mechanical ventilation (if he can't maintain arterial oxygenation). Respiratory tract infection warrants prompt antibiotic administration.

Key nursing diagnoses and patient outcomes

Fatigue related to chronic hypoxia. Based on this nursing diagnosis, you'll establish these patient outcomes. The patient will:

• identify controllable factors that cause fatigue
• demonstrate skill in conserving energy while carrying out his daily activities to tolerance level
• explain the illness and the relationship between fatigue and deficit in blood oxygenation.

Impaired gas exchange related to changes in pulmonary tissue. Based on this nursing diagnosis, you'll establish these patient outcomes. The patient will:

• express feelings of comfort when air exchange is maintained
• use correct bronchial hygiene
• not show further deterioration in ABG values.

Ineffective breathing pattern related to fatigue. Based on this nursing diagnosis, you'll establish these patient outcomes. The patient will:

• maintain his respiratory rate within a normal range
• achieve maximum lung expansion with adequate ventilation
• not exhibit signs and symptoms of severe hypoxia.

Nursing interventions

• Perform chest physiotherapy, including postural drainage and chest percussion and vibration designed for involved lobes, several times a day.
• Make sure the patient receives enough fluids to loosen secretions.
• Schedule respiratory therapy at least 1 hour before or after meals. Provide mouth care after bronchodilator therapy.
• Provide the patient with a high-calorie, high-protein diet, preferably in small, frequent meals.
• Administer medication as ordered.
• Encourage daily activity, and provide the patient with diversional activities, as ap-

propriate. To conserve his energy, alternate periods of rest and activity.

- Help the patient adjust to the life-style changes associated with a chronic illness. Answer his questions, and encourage him to express his concerns about his illness. Stay with him during periods of extreme stress and anxiety. Include the patient and his family in care decisions whenever possible.

Monitoring

- Assess for changes in baseline respiratory functioning, including changes in sputum quality and quantity, restlessness, increased tachypnea, and changes in breath sounds. Report any changes to the doctor immediately.
- Monitor the patient's ABG values as indicated by the severity of his condition.
- Monitor the patient for desired response and for adverse reactions to any administered medications.
- Watch for complications, such as pulmonary fibrosis, right ventricular hypertrophy, and cor pulmonale.

Patient teaching

- Advise the patient to avoid crowds and people with known infections. He should also receive influenza and pneumococcus immunizations.
- Teach the patient receiving home oxygen therapy the reasons for treatment and the proper use of the equipment. If he needs a transtracheal catheter, teach him catheter care and precautions.
- Show the patient and his family how to perform postural drainage and chest percussion. Also, teach the patient coughing and deep-breathing techniques, explaining that they'll help him breathe and help remove secretions. Tell him to remain in each position for 10 minutes. Percussion and coughing should follow.
- Thoroughly explain all medications.
- Encourage the patient to follow a high-calorie, high-protein diet and to drink plenty of fluids to prevent dehydration and help loosen secretions.
- If the patient smokes, encourage him to quit and, if necessary, refer him to resources that can help.
- Warn the patient of the risk of tuberculosis, and advise him to be tested, as ordered.
- Refer the patient and his family to other support services as appropriate.
- If you have a patient at risk for silicosis, teach him the importance of wearing a mask and using other protective devices to reduce his risk.

Sjögren's syndrome

The next most common autoimmune disorder after rheumatoid arthritis, Sjögren's syndrome results from a chronic exocrine gland dysfunction. The syndrome is marked by diminished lacrimal and salivary gland secretion (sicca complex). The mean age of occurrence is 50 and about 90% of those affected are women.

Sjögren's syndrome may be a primary disorder, or it may be associated with inflammatory connective tissue disorders, such as rheumatoid arthritis (about 50% of patients), scleroderma, systemic lupus erythematosus, primary biliary cirrhosis, Hashimoto's thyroiditis, polyarteritis, and interstitial pulmonary fibrosis.

Nephritis (seldom leading to chronic renal failure) may affect up to 40% of patients with primary Sjögren's syndrome and may result in renal tubular acidosis in about 25% of patients.

Patients with Sjögren's syndrome may also have Raynaud's phenomenon (about 20%) and vasculitis (usually limited to the skin; may be systemic or localized in the legs). Sensory polyneuropathy and biochemical hypothyroidism (resembling Hashimoto's thyroiditis) occur in up to 50% of patients. Rarely, systemic necrotizing vasculi-

Diagnosing Sjögren's syndrome

For a diagnosis of Sjögren's syndrome, the patient must have the following:
- keratoconjunctivitis sicca
- diminished salivary gland flow
- a positive salivary gland biopsy, showing mononuclear cell infiltration
- the presence of autoantibodies in a serum sample, indicating a systemic autoimmune process.

tis develops and involves the skin, peripheral nerves, and GI tract.

Overall, the prognosis for a patient with Sjögren's syndrome is good.

Causes

No one knows what causes Sjögren's syndrome. However, researchers think that genetic and environmental factors may contribute to its development. Viral or bacterial infection – or possibly exposure to pollen – may trigger this disease in a genetically susceptible person. Tissue damage results from infiltration by lymphocytes or deposition of immune complexes. Lymphocytic infiltration may be classified as benign lymphoma, malignant lymphoma, or pseudolymphoma (nonmalignant but tumorlike aggregates of lymphoid cells).

Complications

The disease seldom produces significant complications.

Assessment

The patient typically reports slowly developing dryness affecting the eyes (xerophthalmia), the mouth (xerostomia), and other organs. Initially, she may describe a foreign body sensation in the eye (gritty, sandy eye) along with redness, burning, photosensitivity, eye fatigue, itching, and mucoid discharge. She may also complain of a film across her eyes.

With oral dryness, the patient may report difficulty swallowing and talking; an abnormal taste or smell sensation (or both); thirst; ulcers of the tongue, mouth, and lips (especially at the corners of the mouth); and severe dental caries.

With other dryness – of the respiratory tract, for example – the patient may report epistaxis, hoarseness, chronic nonproductive cough, recurrent otitis media, and frequent respiratory tract infections. With vaginal dryness, the patient may report dyspareunia and pruritus.

Additional complaints include generalized itching, fatigue, recurrent low-grade fever, and arthralgia or myalgia.

Inspection may disclose mouth ulcers, dental caries and, possibly, enlarged salivary glands.

Palpable purpura may be evident if the patient also has vasculitis. Palpable lymph node enlargement may be the first sign of malignant lymphoma or pseudolymphoma.

Diagnostic tests

To be diagnosed as Sjögren's syndrome, symptoms must meet specific criteria. (See *Diagnosing Sjögren's syndrome.*)

Laboratory test values in patients with Sjögren's syndrome include:
- elevated erythrocyte sedimentation rate in more than 90% of patients
- mild anemia and leukopenia in about 30% of patients
- hypergammaglobulinemia in about 50% of patients.

Various autoantibodies are also common, including antisalivary duct antibodies. Typically, 75% to 90% of patients test positive for rheumatoid factor, and 90% of patients test positive for antinuclear antibodies.

Other test findings help support the diagnosis. To measure eye involvement, the patient may undergo Schirmer's test and a slit-lamp examination with rose bengal dye. Labial biopsy (to detect lymphoid foci) is a simple procedure with minimal risk – and the only specific diagnostic technique.

Salivary gland involvement may be evaluated by measuring the volume of parotid saliva, by secretory sialography, and by salivary scintigraphy. Salivary gland biopsy results typically show lymphocytic infiltration in Sjögren's syndrome; lower lip biopsy findings show salivary gland infiltration by lymphocytes.

Diagnosis must rule out other causes of ocular and oral dryness, including sarcoidosis, endocrine disorders, anxiety or depression, and effects of certain therapies, such as radiation to the head and neck. In patients with salivary gland and lymph node enlargement, diagnosis also must rule out cancer.

Treatment

Usually implemented to relieve symptoms, treatment includes conservative measures to moisten the eyes and mouth.

Artificial tears and sustained-release cellulose capsules help to relieve ocular dryness. If eye infection develops, the patient receives antibiotics; topical steroids should be avoided.

Mouth dryness can be relieved by using a methylcellulose swab or spray and by drinking plenty of fluids, especially at mealtime. Meticulous oral hygiene includes regular flossing, brushing, and fluoride treatment at home and frequent dental checkups.

Other treatment measures vary according to extraglandular effects. For parotid gland enlargement, treatment involves local heat and analgesia. For interstitial pulmonary and renal disease, treatment relies on corticosteroids. For cutaneous vasculitis, however, corticosteroids work less effectively.

If the patient has lymphoma, treatment includes a combination of chemotherapy, surgery, and radiation therapy.

Key nursing diagnoses and patient outcomes

Altered oral mucous membrane related to dryness. Based on this nursing diagnosis, you'll establish these patient outcomes. The patient will:
- maintain an adequate fluid intake
- demonstrate skill in performing meticulous oral hygiene
- stop having severe dental caries.

Altered protection related to xerophthalmia. Based on this nursing diagnosis, you'll establish these patient outcomes. The patient will:
- communicate an understanding of the relationship between xerophthalmia and Sjogren's syndrome
- demonstrate skill in the self-administration of eye preparations
- show no evidence of eye damage.

Risk for infection related to frequent respiratory infections. Based on this nursing diagnosis, you'll establish these patient outcomes. The patient will:
- incorporate respiratory infection-control precautions into his daily life
- exhibit no signs and symptoms of respiratory infection
- maintain normal breath sounds and white blood cell count.

Nursing interventions

- Instill artificial tears as often as every 30 minutes to prevent eye damage (corneal ulcerations, corneal opacifications) from insufficient tear secretions. The patient may also benefit from instillation of an eye ointment at bedtime or from using sustained-release cellulose capsules twice daily.
- Administer medications as prescribed.
- Provide plenty of fluids – especially water – for the patient to drink and sugarless chewing gum or candies to promote oral moisture without promoting tooth decay.
- Isolate the patient from people with respiratory infections.

Monitoring

- Regularly inspect the patient's skin, oral cavity, and eyes for cracks or breaks in the skin or mucous membranes and for other effects of dryness.
- Monitor the patient for respiratory infections. Auscultate breath sounds daily.

Patient teaching

- Teach the patient how to instill eyedrops, ointments, or sustained-release capsules.
- Recommend wearing sunglasses to protect eyes from dust, wind, and strong light. Because dry eyes are more susceptible to infection, direct the patient to keep her face clean and to avoid rubbing her eyes.
- Advise the patient to avoid saliva-decreasing drugs, such as atropine derivatives, antihistamines, anticholinergics, and antidepressants. Many nonprescription drugs contain these compounds.
- If mouth lesions make eating painful, suggest high-calorie, protein-rich liquid supplements to prevent malnutrition.
- Instruct the patient to avoid sugar, which contributes to dental caries, and tobacco, alcohol, and spicy, salty, or highly acidic foods, which cause mouth irritation.
- Urge the patient to humidify her home and work environments to help relieve respiratory tract dryness. Suggest using 0.9% sodium chloride solution (in drop or spray form) to relieve nasal dryness.
- Advise the patient to avoid prolonged hot showers and baths and to use moisturizing lotions on dry skin. Suggest using a water-soluble jelly as a vaginal lubricant.
- As appropriate, refer the patient to the Sjögren's Syndrome Foundation for additional information and support.

Sodium imbalance

The major cation (90%) in extracellular fluid (ECF), sodium is the main factor responsible for ECF concentration. Increases or decreases in ECF sodium concentrations greatly affect ECF volume and distribution. Sodium controls the distribution of water throughout the body and regulates ECF volume. It also plays an important role in the transmission of nerve impulses and muscle contraction.

Hyponatremia refers to an excess of body water relative to sodium; it is not synonymous with sodium depletion. Sodium loss is just one state in which hyponatremia may occur. Hypernatremia refers to a deficit of body water relative to sodium. Thirst seems to be the major defense mechanism against hypernatremia.

Although the body requires only 2 to 4 g of sodium daily, most Americans consume 6 to 10 g daily (mostly sodium chloride, as table salt), excreting excess sodium through the kidneys and skin. Under the influence of antidiuretic hormone (ADH) and aldosterone, the kidneys primarily regulate ECF sodium balance.

Causes

Hyponatremia usually results from defective urine dilution, caused by either an excessive loss of sodium or an excessive gain of water. Specific causes of hyponatremia include:

- excessive GI loss of water and electrolytes due to vomiting, suctioning, fistulas, or diarrhea; excessive perspiration; or fever. When such losses decrease circulating fluid volume, increased secretion of ADH promotes maximum water reabsorption, which further dilutes serum sodium. Combined with too much free water intake, these factors are especially likely to cause hyponatremia.
- diuretic therapy, most commonly thiazides
- excessive drinking of water (psychogenic polydipsia); infusion of I.V. dextrose in water without other solutes, particularly during stress
- endocrine disorders, such as adrenal gland insufficiency and moderate to severe hypothyroidism

• chronic illnesses, such as cirrhosis of the liver and congestive heart failure
• syndrome of inappropriate antidiuretic hormone (SIADH) secretion, resulting from central nervous system disorders, such as head injury or cerebrovascular accident; nonmalignant pulmonary diseases, such as tuberculosis; neoplasms with ectopic ADH production, such as oat cell lung tumors; or certain drugs, such as chlorpropamide and clofibrate.

Hypernatremia results from a sodium gain in excess of water or, most commonly, by a water loss in excess of sodium. It may also result from water loss alone. Specific causes of hypernatremia include:
• severe insensible water losses that aren't replaced, such as in patients with fever, hyperventilation, or extensive burns
• severe renal water losses, as in acute diabetes insipidus
• severe vomiting and diarrhea, causing water loss that exceeds sodium loss; serum sodium levels rise, but overall ECF volume decreases
• excess adrenocortical hormones, as in Cushing's syndrome
• water loss in excess of sodium due to diaphoresis, if the patient can't drink
• administration of high-protein feedings without adequate water supplement (due to urea diuresis)
• sodium excess, such as administration of excessive amounts of hypertonic sodium chloride infusions to obtunded patients who can't drink, or inadvertent introduction of hypertonic sodium chloride solution into maternal circulation during therapeutic abortion.

Thirst is such a strong drive that severe, persistent hypernatremia only occurs in persons who can't respond to thirst voluntarily, such as patients with sedative-induced confusion or those who have been restrained. A disturbance of the thirst mechanism is rare.

Complications

States of severe hyponatremia or hypernatremia may result in seizures, coma, and permanent neurologic damage.

Hyponatremia may lead to cerebral edema, as decreased plasma osmolality causes water movement into cells. Increased brain cell volume, in turn, leads to neurologic symptoms.

Increased plasma osmolality associated with hypernatremia causes a water shift out of cells, possibly resulting in cerebral cell dehydration and neurologic symptoms.

Assessment

A patient with hyponatremia may complain initially of anorexia, nausea, abdominal cramping, headache, and exhaustion. When the serum sodium level drops further (between 120 and 125 mEq/liter), neurologic assessment may reveal lethargy, confusion, twitching, and focal weakness, which, if untreated, may progress to seizures and coma.

If hyponatremia is secondary to ECF loss, the patient may complain of dizziness. Palpation may detect dry mucous membranes, and vital signs assessment reflects orthostatic hypotension and tachycardia.

If hyponatremia is secondary to fluid gain, inspection may note edema; palpation may disclose fingerprint edema (with SIADH); further assessment may reveal hypertension and weight gain.

A patient with hypernatremia may complain of fatigue, restlessness, and weakness. When hypernatremia is severe, assessment of level of consciousness may reveal disorientation, which may progress to seizures and coma.

On inspection, the hypernatremic patient may have flushed skin. Palpation may reveal a dry, swollen tongue and sticky mucous membranes. The patient may have a low-grade fever.

Diagnostic tests

Serum sodium levels will be less than 135 mEq/liter with hyponatremia and more than 145 mEq/liter with hypernatremia.

Additional laboratory studies determine the etiology of the imbalance and differentiate between a true deficit and an apparent deficit due to sodium shift or to hypervolemia or hypovolemia.

Treatment

When possible, patients with sodium deficits receive oral sodium supplementation. Therapy for mild hyponatremia associated with hypervolemia usually consists of restricted water intake. If fluid restriction alone fails to normalize serum sodium levels, demeclocycline or lithium, which blocks ADH action in the renal tubules, can be used to promote water excretion.

In extremely rare instances of severe symptomatic hyponatremia, when serum sodium levels fall below 110 mEq/liter, treatment may include infusion of 3% or 5% sodium chloride solution.

Treatment with an infusion of hypertonic saline solution requires careful patient monitoring in an intensive care setting for signs of circulatory overload, which is potentially fatal. (Administration of hypertonic saline solution causes water to shift out of cells, risking intravascular volume overload.) For this reason, furosemide is usually administered concurrently. The hypertonic saline solution is infused slowly, in small volumes.

If indicated, treatment must include correction of the underlying disorder; for example, hormonal therapy may be needed to treat endocrine disorders.

Primary treatment of hypernatremia associated with water deficit aims to stop the water loss with slow, oral replacement of the water deficit. If the patient can't tolerate oral replacement, treatment requires I.V. administration of salt-free solutions (such as dextrose in water) to return serum sodium levels to normal, followed by infusion of 0.45% sodium chloride solution to prevent hyponatremia.

Hypernatremia must be corrected slowly, over about 2 days, to avoid shifting water into brain cells, resulting in cerebral edema. Some clinicians recommend infusion of a hypotonic solution, such as 0.3% sodium chloride, to permit a more gradual lowering of serum sodium levels, reducing the risk of cerebral edema.

Other treatment measures may include restricted sodium intake for patients with sodium gain. Diuretics may be given to increase sodium loss in combination with oral or I.V. water replacement.

Key nursing diagnoses and patient outcomes

Altered thought processes related to neurologic dysfunction. Based on this nursing diagnosis, you'll establish these patient outcomes. The patient will:

- remain safe in his environment
- regain and maintain orientation to time, person, and place.

Risk for injury related to potential for permanent neurologic deficits. Based on this nursing diagnosis, you'll establish these patient outcomes. The patient will:

- identify the early signs and symptoms of sodium imbalance and seek medical treatment promptly
- communicate an understanding of the importance of adhering to prescribed therapy to prevent severe sodium imbalance
- show no evidence of permanent neurologic deficits when his sodium level returns to normal.

Knowledge deficit related to cause and treatment of sodium imbalance. Based on this nursing diagnosis, you'll establish these patient outcomes. The patient will:

- identify the need to learn about the causes and management of his condition
- seek and obtain information about his condition from appropriate sources
- demonstrate skill in managing his condition, as evidenced by maintaining his sodium level within a normal range.

Nursing interventions

For hyponatremia:

- Administer oral potassium supplements, demeclocycline, or lithium as prescribed to treat mild hyponatremia. Have a patent I.V. line in place for administration of sodium chloride solution to treat severe hyponatremia.
- Be sure that the patient adheres to fluid restriction, as ordered.
- Conserve the patient's energy by having him rest and avoid unnecessary fatigue.

For hypernatremia:

- Provide oral and I.V. fluid replacement therapy as ordered. Be aware that fluid replacement therapy must be undertaken slowly because rapid correction of hypernatremia may lead to cerebral edema.
- Be sure that the patient adheres to sodium restriction, as ordered.
- Assist with oral hygiene. Lubricate the patient's lips frequently with a water-based lubricant. Provide mouthwash or gargle if the patient is alert.
- Obtain a drug history to check for drugs that promote sodium retention.

For hyponatremia and hypernatremia:

- Provide a safe environment for the patient with altered thought processes. If seizures are likely, pad the patient's side rails and keep an airway at the bedside. Reorient the patient as needed.

Monitoring

- Watch for and report extreme changes in serum sodium and accompanying serum chloride levels. Monitor urine specific gravity and other laboratory results. Record fluid intake and output accurately, and weigh the patient daily.
- Perform frequent neurologic checks. Report deteriorating level of consciousness.
- During administration of isosmolar or hyperosmolar sodium chloride solution in the treatment of hyponatremia, watch closely for signs of hypervolemia (dyspnea, crackles, engorged neck or hand veins), and report them immediately.
- During fluid replacement therapy in the treatment of hypernatremia, observe for signs and symptoms of cerebral edema, particularly headache, lethargy, nausea, vomiting, widening pulse pressure, decreased pulse rate, and seizures.

Patient teaching

For patients with hyponatremia:

- Refer the patient on maintenance dosage of diuretics to a dietitian for instruction about dietary sodium intake.
- Teach the patient and family the rationale for fluid restriction, if ordered. Inform the patient of ways to minimize thirst, including the use of ice chips, ice pops, or lemon drops.
- Make sure the patient understands his medication regimen, including the drug name, action, dosage, precautions, and potential adverse effects.

For patients with hypernatremia:

- If warranted, explain the importance of sodium restriction, and teach the patient how to plan a low-sodium diet. Refer the patient to a dietitian for additional teaching.

Spinal injuries

Usually the result of trauma to the head or neck, spinal injuries (other than spinal cord damage) include fractures, contusions, and compressions of the vertebral column. Spinal injuries most commonly occur in the twelfth thoracic, first lumbar, and fifth, sixth, and seventh cervical areas. The real danger from such injuries lies in associated damage to the spinal cord.

Causes

Most serious spinal injuries result from motor vehicle accidents, falls, diving into shallow water, and gunshot wounds; less serious injuries, from lifting heavy objects and minor falls. Spinal dysfunction also may result from hyperparathyroidism and neoplastic lesions.

Complications

Spinal injury can be complicated by spinal cord damage, resulting in paralysis and even death. The extent of cord damage depends on the level of injury to the spinal column.

Assessment

The patient's history may reveal trauma, a neoplastic lesion, an infection that could produce a spinal abscess, or an endocrine disorder. The patient typically complains of muscle spasm and back or neck pain that worsens with movement. In cervical fractures, point tenderness may be present; in dorsal and lumbar fractures, pain may radiate to other body areas, such as the legs.

Physical assessment (including a neurologic assessment) helps locate the level of injury and detect any cord damage. General observation of the patient reveals that he limits movement and activities that cause pain. Inspection reveals any surface wounds that occurred with the spinal injury. Palpation can identify pain location and loss of sensation.

If the injury damages the spinal cord, you'll note clinical effects that range from mild paresthesia to quadriplegia and shock.

Diagnostic tests

Spinal X-rays, myelography, and computed tomography and magnetic resonance imaging scans are used to locate the fracture and site of the compression.

Treatment

The primary treatment after spinal injury is immediate immobilization to stabilize the spine and prevent cord damage; other treatment is supportive.

Cervical injuries require immobilization, using sandbags on both sides of the patient's head, a plaster cast, a hard cervical collar, or skeletal traction with skull tongs (Crutchfield, Barton, Vinke) or a halo device. (See *Skeletal traction devices.*)

Treatment of stable lumbar and dorsal fractures consists of bed rest on a firm surface (such as a bed board), analgesics, and muscle relaxants until the fracture stabilizes (usually in 10 to 12 weeks). Later treatment includes exercises to strengthen the back muscles and a back brace or corset to provide support while walking.

An unstable dorsal or lumbar fracture requires a plaster cast, a turning frame and, in severe fracture, laminectomy and spinal fusion.

When the damage results in compression of the spinal column, neurosurgery may relieve the pressure. If the cause of compression is a neoplastic lesion, chemotherapy and radiation may relieve the compression by shrinking the lesion. Surface wounds that accompany the spinal injury require wound care and tetanus prophylaxis unless the patient has recently been immunized.

Key nursing diagnoses and patient outcomes

Fear related to potential for permanent neurologic deficits. Based on this nursing diagnosis, you'll establish these patient outcomes. The patient will:

- identify and express feelings of fear
- use available support systems to cope with fear
- demonstrate healthy coping behaviors in managing fear.

Diversional activity deficit related to potential for prolonged inactivity. Based on this nursing diagnosis, you'll establish these patient outcomes. The patient will:

- express interest in using his leisure time meaningfully
- participate in activities provided
- report a decrease in boredom.

Impaired physical mobility related to neurologic dysfunction. Based on this nursing diagnosis, you'll establish these patient outcomes. The patient will:

Skeletal traction devices

A halo-vest traction device or skull tongs may be used to immobilize the head and neck of a patient with a cervical vertebrae injury.

Halo-vest traction device

Halo devices consist of a metal ring that fits over the patient's head and metal bars that connect the ring to a plastic vest that distributes the weight of the entire apparatus around the chest. This device allows greater mobility than skull tongs and carries less risk of infection because it doesn't require skin incisions and drill holes to position skull pins.

In the low profile (standard) device shown at right, traction and compression are produced by threaded support rods on either side of the halo ring. Flexion and extension are obtained by moving the swivel arm to an anterior or posterior position, depending on the location of the skull pins.

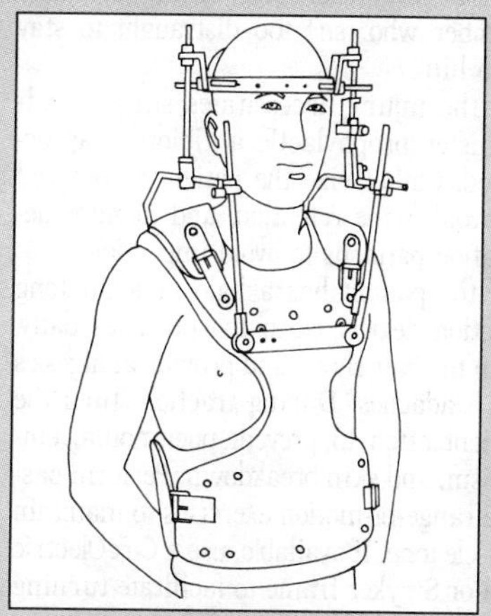

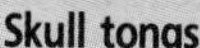

Skull tongs

Skull (or cervical) tongs consist of a stainless steel body with a pin at the end of each arm. Each pin is about ⅛" (0.3 cm) in diameter with a sharp tip. On Crutchfield tongs (shown at right), the pins are placed about 5" (13 cm) apart in line with the long axis of the cervical spine.

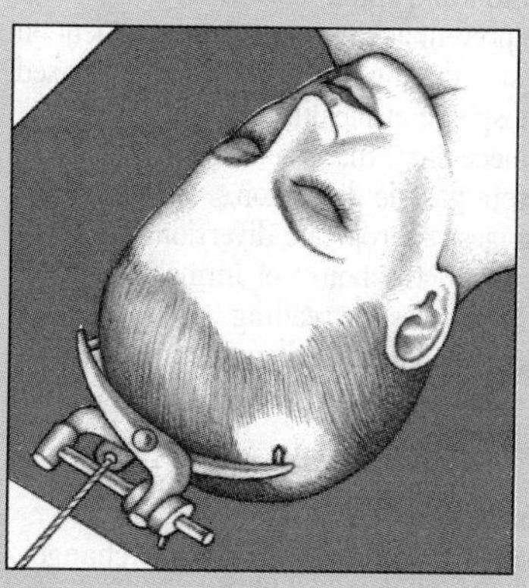

- maintain muscle strength and joint range of motion
- show no evidence of complications, such as contractures, venous stasis, or skin breakdown
- achieve the highest level of mobility possible following spinal injury.

Nursing interventions

- As in all spinal injuries, suspect cord damage until proved otherwise.
- During the initial assessment and X-rays, immobilize the patient on a firm surface, with sandbags on both sides of his head. Tell him not to move. If possible, avoid moving him because hyperflexion can damage the cord. If you must move him, get at least one

other member of the staff to help you logroll him so that you don't disturb his body alignment.

- Offer comfort and reassurance to the patient, talking to him quietly and calmly. Remember, the fear of possible paralysis will be overwhelming. Allow a family member who isn't too distraught to stay with him.
- If the injury necessitates surgery, administer prophylactic antibiotics, as ordered. Catheterize the patient as ordered to avoid urine retention, and monitor defecation patterns to avoid impaction.
- If the patient has a halo or skull tong traction device, clean the pin sites daily, trim his hair short, and provide analgesics for headaches. During traction, turn the patient often to prevent pneumonia, embolism, and skin breakdown. Perform passive range-of-motion exercises to maintain muscle tone. If available, use a CircOlectric bed or Stryker frame to facilitate turning and to avoid spinal cord injury.
- To prevent aspiration, turn the patient on his side during feedings. Create a relaxed atmosphere at mealtimes.
- If necessary, insert a nasogastric tube to prevent gastric distention.
- Suggest appropriate diversionary activities to fill the hours of immobility. Offer prism glasses for reading.
- Help the patient walk as soon as the doctor allows; he'll probably have to wear a back brace.

Monitoring

- Watch closely for neurologic changes. Immediately report changes in skin sensation and loss of muscle strength. Either could point to pressure on the spinal cord, possibly as a result of edema or shifting bone fragments.
- Monitor the patient closely for signs and symptoms of complications associated with spinal injuries or prolonged immobility, such as pneumonia, skin breakdown, and renal calculi.

Patient teaching

- Explain traction methods to the patient and his family, and reassure them that a halo traction device or skull tongs don't penetrate the brain.
- Tell the patient about the prescribed regimen for home care.
- Teach the patient exercises to maintain physical mobility.
- Instruct the patient about his medications, including adverse effects and the duration of treatment.
- Stress the importance of follow-up examinations.

Spinal neoplasms

Similar to intracranial tumors but involving the spinal cord or its roots, untreated spinal neoplasms can eventually cause paralysis. As primary tumors, they originate in the meningeal coverings, the parenchyma of the cord or its roots, the intraspinal vasculature, or the vertebrae. They can also occur as metastatic foci from primary tumors, but death usually results from the primary condition.

Primary tumors of the spinal cord may be extramedullary (occurring outside the spinal cord) or intramedullary (occurring within the cord). Extramedullary tumors may be intradural (meningiomas and schwannomas) and account for about 60% of all primary spinal cord neoplasms. Extramedullary tumors may also be extradural (metastatic tumors from breasts, lungs, prostate, leukemia, or lymphomas) and account for about 25% of these neoplasms.

Intramedullary tumors, or gliomas (astrocytomas or ependymomas), are comparatively rare and account for only about 10% of spinal neoplasms.

Spinal cord tumors are rare compared with intracranial tumors (ratio of 1:4). They occur with equal frequency in men and women, except for meningiomas, which occur more often in women. Spinal cord tumors can grow anywhere along the cord or its roots.

The prognosis depends on tumor control and the extent of residual neurologic deficit.

Causes

Little is known about the cause of spinal cord tumors. They have been associated with central von Recklinghausen's disease, however, and research is ongoing.

Complications

Motor and sensory deficits range from weakness to paralysis as the disease progresses. They may lead to loss of sphincter control and subsequent bladder and bowel dysfunction.

In late stages of disease, especially with paralysis, the complications of immobility, such as skin breakdown, may occur. Other complications depend on the tumor's location. For example, respiratory problems occur in high cervical tumors, whereas chronic urinary tract problems are associated with tumors lower in the spine.

Assessment

Because the spinal cord adjusts to a slow-growing tumor, a tumor may grow for several years and produce minimal neurologic signs. The patient's history, however, may reveal pain described as most severe directly over the tumor and radiating around the trunk or down the limb on the affected side. The patient may report that few measures relieve the pain, not even bed rest. Some patients also complain of constipation.

In the early stages, the patient may express difficulty in emptying the bladder or notice changes in the urinary stream. If you suspect a spinal cord tumor, ask the patient about bladder emptying because many patients overlook or dismiss this sign.

In later stages, urine retention is an inevitable sign of spinal cord compression. If the patient has a cauda equina tumor, he may report bladder and bowel incontinence, usually resulting from flaccid paralysis.

On inspection and palpation, you may find symmetrical spastic weakness, decreased muscle tone, exaggerated reflexes, and a positive Babinski's sign. If the tumor is at the cauda equina level, you may notice muscle wasting. Palpation may reveal muscle flaccidity, wasting, weakness, and progressive diminution in tendon reflexes.

Neurologic examination may disclose contralateral loss of sensation to pain, temperature, and touch (Brown-Séquard syndrome). These losses are less obvious to the patient than functional motor changes. Caudal lesions invariably produce parasthesia in the nerve pathways of the involved roots.

Diagnostic tests

- *Lumbar puncture* reveals clear-yellow cerebrospinal fluid (CSF), resulting from increased protein levels if the flow is completely blocked. If the flow is partially blocked, protein levels rise but the fluid appears only slightly yellow in proportion to the CSF protein level. A Papanicolaou test of the CSF may show malignant cells of metastatic carcinoma.
- *X-rays* show distortions of the intervertebral foramina; changes in the vertebrae or collapsed areas in the vertebral body; and localized enlargement of the spinal canal, indicating an adjacent blockage.
- *Myelography* identifies the lesion's level by outlining the tumor if it causes a partial obstruction. The myelogram shows the anatomic relation to the cord and the dura. If the tumor causes a complete obstruction, the injected contrast agent can't flow past the tumor. This study is dangerous in instances of nearly complete cord compression because withdrawn or escaping CSF will allow the tumor to exert greater pressure against the cord.
- *Radioisotope bone scan* demonstrates metastatic invasion of the vertebrae by de-

tecting a characteristic increase in osteoblastic activity.

• *Computed tomography* and *magnetic resonance imaging scans* show cord compression and tumor location.

• *Frozen section biopsy* performed during surgery identifies the tissue type.

Treatment

Spinal cord tumors are treated with decompression or radiation therapy. Not usually indicated for metastatic tumors, laminectomy may be done for primary tumors that produce spinal cord or cauda equina compression. If the tumor progresses slowly or if it's treated before the cord degenerates from compression, signs and symptoms are likely to subside and function may be restored.

In a patient with metastatic carcinoma or lymphoma who suddenly experiences complete transverse myelitis with spinal shock, functional improvement is unlikely, even with treatment. This patient's prognosis is poor.

If the patient has incomplete paraplegia of rapid onset, emergency surgical decompression may save cord function. Steroid therapy may minimize cord edema until he undergoes surgery.

Partial removal of intramedullary gliomas, followed by radiation therapy, may temporarily ease signs and symptoms. Metastatic extradural tumors can be controlled with radiation therapy, analgesics and, in hormone-mediated tumors (breast and prostate), appropriate hormonal therapy.

Transcutaneous electrical nerve stimulation (TENS) may relieve radicular pain from spinal cord tumors and is a useful alternative to opioid analgesics. TENS works by applying an electrical charge to the skin, thereby stimulating large-diameter nerve fibers and inhibiting the transmission of pain impulses along nerve fibers.

The risk of infection is increased by treatment in many cases, but the risk also increases as the patient's condition deteriorates.

Key nursing diagnoses and patient outcomes

Altered urinary elimination related to spinal cord compression. Based on this nursing diagnosis, you'll establish these patient outcomes. The patient will:

• recognize and report early signs of changes in urinary elimination

• show no complications of changes in urinary elimination, such as urinary tract infection

• demonstrate skill in managing his urinary elimination problem.

Impaired physical mobility related to spinal cord compression. Based on this nursing diagnosis, you'll establish these patient outcomes. The patient will:

• maintain muscle strength and joint range of motion

• show no evidence of complications, such as contractures, venous stasis, or skin breakdown

• maintain the highest level of mobility possible, depending on the severity and extent of spinal cord compression.

Pain related to pressure on spinal cord. Based on this nursing diagnosis, you'll establish these patient outcomes. The patient will:

• report feelings of comfort with the use of nonpharmacologic methods to manage pain, such as TENS

• indicate that pain is decreased or absent after radiation or surgery to relieve pressure.

Nursing interventions

• Set up the patient's care plan to foster emotional support and skilled intervention during acute and chronic disease phases. Aim for early recognition of recurrence, prevention or treatment of complications, and maintenance of the quality of life.

• Use the baseline data from the initial neurologic evaluation to help plan future care and evaluate changes in the patient's clinical status.

• Encourage the patient to voice his concerns about his illness and treatment. Answer any questions. Provide brief, easy-to-understand explanations before performing procedures.

- Recognize that the patient needs emotional support, rehabilitation (including bowel and bladder retraining), and medications and other measures to relieve pain. Prevent infection and skin breakdown.
- If the patient experiences urine retention, provide necessary care, such as intermittent catheterization or indwelling urinary catheter care. If the patient has constipation, administer laxatives and enemas, as ordered.
- Prepare the patient for laminectomy, as indicated. (See the entry "Laminectomy and spinal fusion.")
- Institute safety precautions for the patient with impaired sensation and motor deficits. Use side rails if the patient is bedridden. If he's not, encourage him to wear flat shoes for walking. Remove scatter rugs and clutter to prevent falls.
- Encourage the patient to perform daily activities as independently as possible. To avoid aggravating pain, move the patient slowly, making sure his body is aligned properly when you give personal care.
- If the patient has respiratory problems, provide rest periods between activities. Provide oxygen, as ordered, and assist him into a position that allows maximal chest expansion.
- After radiation therapy, administer steroid and antacid medications, as ordered, for spinal cord edema.
- Enforce bed rest for the patient who has vertebral body involvement until the doctor says he can safely walk. Body weight alone can cause vertebral column collapse and cord laceration from bone fragments.
- Logroll and position the patient on his side every 2 hours to prevent pressure ulcers and other complications of immobility.
- If the patient requires a back brace, make sure he wears it whenever he gets out of bed.
- Help the patient and his family to understand and cope with the spinal tumor diagnosis, treatment, potential disabilities, and necessary changes in life-style.

Monitoring

- Monitor the patient's neurologic status regularly, especially for return of sensory or motor dysfunction, which indicates the need for increased steroid therapy.
- Assess the patient for signs and symptoms of bowel and bladder dysfunction and for the effectiveness of the retraining program, as indicated. Monitor intake and output as needed.
- Evaluate the patient for complications associated with physical immobility, such as contractures, venous stasis, and skin breakdown.
- Assess the patient's pain level and the effectiveness of administered therapy. Alert the doctor if the patient complains of increased pain or if therapy isn't effective.

Patient teaching

- Refer the patient, family, and close friends to support groups, the social service department, and home health care agencies, as appropriate.
- Instruct the patient and family in the care the patient requires, including how to administer medications, maintain skin integrity, reduce discomfort (for example, by using TENS to block radicular pain), prevent infection and injury, and cope with incontinence.

Splenectomy

The surgical removal of the spleen, splenectomy helps treat various hematologic disorders. It's also done as an emergency procedure to stop hemorrhage after traumatic splenic rupture.

The most common reason for splenectomy is hypersplenism – a combination of splenomegaly and cytopenia that occurs in such disorders as hairy cell leukemia, Felty's syndrome, myeloid metaplasia, thalassemia major, and Gaucher's disease. In addition, splenectomy is the treatment of choice for such diseases as hereditary spherocytosis and chronic idiopathic thrombocytopenic purpura. What's more, it may be performed in Hodgkin's disease to establish the stage of the disease and determine the appropriate therapy.

Procedure

After the patient is placed under general anesthesia, the surgeon exposes the peritoneal cavity through a left rectus paramedial or subcostal incision. He ligates the splenic artery and vein and the ligaments that hold the spleen in place. Then he removes the spleen. After carefully checking for any bleeding, he closes the abdomen, often placing a drain in the left subdiaphragmatic space. After the incision site is sutured and dressed, the patient is returned to the postanesthesia room.

Complications

Besides bleeding and infection, splenectomy can cause such complications as pneumonia and atelectasis. The reason: the location of the spleen close to the diaphragm and the need for a high abdominal incision restrict lung expansion after surgery. In addition, splenectomy patients are vulnerable to infection because of the spleen's role in the immune response.

Key nursing diagnoses and patient outcomes

Altered protection related to thrombocytosis. Based on this nursing diagnosis, you'll establish these patient outcomes. The patient will:

- communicate an understanding of the importance of early postoperative ambulation
- demonstrate skill in performing coughing and deep-breathing exercises postoperatively
- show no signs and symptoms of thromboembolic events postoperatively.

Ineffective breathing pattern related to a high abdominal incision. Based on this nursing diagnosis, you'll establish these patient outcomes. The patient will:

- receive adequate postoperative pain sedation to maintain a respiratory rate and depth within the normal range
- maintain adequate ventilation, as demonstrated by normal tissue perfusion
- show no signs and symptoms of respiratory complications, such as pneumonia or atelectasis.

Risk for infection related to the loss of the spleen's role in the immune response. Based on this nursing diagnosis, you'll establish these patient outcomes. The patient will:

- incorporate infection-control measures into everyday living
- show no signs and symptoms of infection
- maintain a normal temperature and white blood cell count.

Nursing interventions

When preparing for or managing a patient with a splenectomy, expect to implement the following nursing interventions.

Before surgery

- Explain to the patient that splenectomy involves removal of his spleen under general anesthesia. Inform him that he'll be able to lead a normal life without it but will be more prone to infection.
- Obtain the results of blood studies, including coagulation tests and a complete blood count, and report them to the doctor. If ordered, transfuse blood to correct anemia or hemorrhagic loss. Similarly, give vitamin K to correct clotting factor deficiencies.
- Take the patient's vital signs and perform a baseline respiratory assessment. Note especially signs of respiratory infection, such as fever, chills, crackles, rhonchi, and a cough. Notify the doctor if you suspect

respiratory infection; he may delay surgery.
- Teach the patient coughing and deep-breathing techniques to help prevent postoperative pulmonary complications.
- Ensure that the patient or a responsible family member has signed a consent form.

After surgery

- During the early postoperative period, watch carefully – especially if the patient has a bleeding disorder – for bleeding from the wound or drain and for signs of internal bleeding, such as hematuria or hematochezia.
- Leukocytosis and thrombocytosis may occur after splenectomy and may persist for years. Because thrombocytosis may predispose the patient to thromboembolism, help the patient exercise and walk as soon as possible after surgery. In addition, encourage him to perform coughing and deep-breathing exercises to reduce the risk of pulmonary complications.
- Administer pain sedation as needed.
- Watch for signs of infection, such as fever and sore throat, and monitor hematologic studies. If infection develops, administer prescribed antibiotics.

Home care instructions

- Inform the patient that he's at an increased risk for infection, and urge him to report any telltale signs and symptoms, such as fever or chills.
- Teach him measures to help prevent infection.

Squamous cell carcinoma

Arising from keratinizing epidermal cells, squamous cell carcinoma of the skin is an invasive tumor with potential for metastasis. It occurs most commonly in fair-skinned white men over age 60. Outdoor employment and residence in a sunny, warm climate (southern United States and Australia, for example) greatly increase the risk of squamous cell carcinoma.

Lesions on sun-damaged skin tend to be less invasive with less tendency to metastasize than lesions on unexposed skin. Notable exceptions are squamous cell lesions on the lower lip and the ears; almost invariably, these are markedly invasive metastastic lesions with a poor prognosis.

Causes

Predisposing factors associated with squamous cell carcinoma include overexposure to the sun's ultraviolet rays, X-ray therapy, ingestion of herbicides containing arsenic, chronic skin irritation and inflammation, exposure to local carcinogens (such as tar and oil), hereditary diseases (such as xeroderma pigmentosum and albinism), and the presence of premalignant lesions (such as actinic keratosis or Bowen's disease).

Rarely, squamous cell carcinoma may develop on the site of smallpox vaccination, psoriasis, or chronic discoid lupus erythematosus.

Transformation from a premalignant lesion to squamous cell carcinoma may begin with induration and inflammation of the preexisting lesion. When squamous cell carcinoma arises from normal skin, the nodule grows slowly on a firm, indurated base. If untreated, this nodule eventually ulcerates and invades underlying tissues.

Complications

Lymph node involvement and visceral metastasis, resulting in respiratory problems, are possible complications from disease progression.

Assessment

The patient history may disclose areas of chronic ulceration, especially on sun-damaged skin.

Inspection may reveal lesions on the face, ears, and dorsa of the hands and forearms and on other sun-damaged skin areas. The lesions may appear scaly and

Staging squamous cell carcinoma

Using the tumor, node, metastasis (TNM) system, the American Joint Committee on Cancer has established the following staging system for squamous cell carcinoma.

Primary tumor
TX—primary tumor can't be assessed
T0—no evidence of primary tumor
Tis—carcinoma in situ
T1—tumor 2 cm or less in greatest dimension
T2—tumor between 2 and 5 cm in greatest dimension
T3—tumor more than 5 cm in greatest dimension
T4—tumor invades deep extradermal structures (such as cartilage, skeletal muscle, or bone)

Regional lymph nodes
NX—regional lymph nodes can't be assessed
N0—no evidence of regional lymph node involvement
N1—regional lymph node involvement

Distant metastasis
MX—distant metastasis can't be assessed
M0—no known distant metastasis
M1—distant metastasis

Staging categories
Squamous cell carcinoma progresses from mild to severe as follows:
Stage 0—Tis, N0, M0
Stage I—T1, N0, M0
Stage II—T2, N0, M0; T3, N0, M0
Stage III—T4, N0, M0; any T, N1, M0
Stage IV—any T, any N, M1

keratotic with raised, irregular borders. In late disease, the lesions grow outward (exophytic), are friable, and tend toward chronic crusting.

As the disease progresses and metastasizes to the regional lymph nodes, the patient may complain of pain and malaise. He may also complain of anorexia and resulting fatigue and weakness.

Diagnostic tests

An excisional biopsy provides definitive diagnosis of squamous cell carcinoma. Appropriate laboratory tests depend on systemic symptoms. (See *Staging squamous cell carcinoma.*)

Treatment

The size, shape, location, and invasiveness of a squamous cell tumor and the condition of the underlying tissue determine the treatment method; a deeply invasive tumor may require a combination of techniques. All the major treatment methods have excellent cure rates. In most cases, the prognosis is better with a well-differentiated lesion than with a poorly differentiated one in an unusual location. Depending on the lesion, treatment may consist of wide surgical excision; curettage and electrodesiccation, which offer good cosmetic results for smaller lesions; radiation therapy, which is generally for older or debilitated patients; chemotherapy; and chemosurgery, which is reserved for resistant or recurrent lesions.

The chemotherapeutic agent fluorouracil is available in various strengths (1%, 2%, and 5%) as a cream or solution. Local application causes immediate stinging and burning. Later effects include erythema, vesiculation, erosion, superficial ulceration, necrosis, and reepithelialization. The 5% solution induces the most severe inflammatory response but provides complete involution of the lesions with little recurrence.

Fluorouracil treatment is continued until the lesions reach the ulcerative and necrotic stages (usually 2, to 4 weeks). Then, a corticosteroid preparation as an anti-inflammatory agent may be applied. Complete healing occurs within 1 to 2 months, with excellent results.

Be careful to keep fluorouracil away from the eyes, scrotum, or mucous membranes. Warn the patient to avoid excessive exposure to the sun during the course of treatment because it intensifies the inflammatory reaction. Possible adverse effects of treatment include postinflammatory hyperpigmentation.

Key nursing diagnoses and patient outcomes

Body image disturbance related to skin lesions. Based on this nursing diagnosis, you'll establish these patient outcomes. The patient will:

- acknowledge and express feelings about his body image change
- participate in decisions about his care
- express positive feelings about himself.

Impaired skin integrity related to skin lesions. Based on this nursing diagnosis, you'll establish these patient outcomes. The patient will:

- demonstrate skill in skin-inspection technique
- exhibit skill in performing his skin-care routine
- regain skin integrity with the eradication of squamous cell carcinoma.

Knowledge deficit related to cause and treatment of squamous cell carcinoma. Based on this nursing diagnosis, you'll establish these patient outcomes. The patient will:

- identify the need to learn how to care for squamous cell carcinoma and prevent a recurrence or new occurrences
- seek and obtain correct information about the management and prevention of squamous cell carcinoma from appropriate sources
- communicate an understanding of the treatment of squamous cell carcinoma and of skin-protection measures.

Nursing interventions

- Although disfiguring lesions are distressing, try to accept the patient as he is to increase his self-esteem and to strengthen a caring relationship.
- Listen to the patient's fears and concerns. Offer reassurance when appropriate. Remain with the patient during periods of severe stress and anxiety.
- Accept the patient's perception of himself. Help the patient and his family set realistic goals and expectations.
- Determine the patient's readiness for decision making; then, involve him in making choices and decisions related to his care. Provide positive reinforcement for the patient's efforts to adapt.
- Coordinate a consistent care plan for changing the patient's dressings. A standard routine helps the patient and his family learn how to care for the wound.
- To promote healing and prevent infection, keep the wound dry and clean.
- Try to control odor with balsam of Peru, yogurt flakes, oil of cloves, or other odor-masking substances, even though they may be ineffective for long-term use. Topical or systemic antibiotics also temporarily control odor and eventually alter the lesion's bacterial flora.
- Provide periods of rest between procedures if the patient fatigues easily.
- Provide supportive care for the adverse effects of chemotherapy and radiation therapy, as indicated.
- Provide small, frequent meals of a high-protein, high-calorie diet if the patient is anorexic. Consult with the dietitian to incorporate foods that the patient enjoys into his diet.

Monitoring

- Monitor the patient for adverse effects of chemotherapy or radiation therapy, such as nausea, vomiting, diarrhea, and alopecia.

• Assess the patient for complications associated with squamous cell carcinoma.
• Evaluate the patient's degree of anxiety and acceptance of changes in body image regularly.

Patient teaching

• Explain all procedures and treatments to the patient and his family. Encourage the patient to ask questions, and then answer them honestly.
• Instruct the patient to avoid excessive sun exposure to prevent recurrence. Direct him to wear protective clothing (hats, long sleeves) whenever he is outdoors.
• Urge the use of a strong sunscreen to protect the skin from ultraviolet rays. Strong sunscreening agents with a skin protection factor of 15 or more are recommended. Apply these agents—as well as lipscreens to protect the lips from sun damage—30 to 60 minutes before sun exposure.
• Advise the patient to relieve local inflammation from topical fluorouracil with cool compresses or with corticosteroid ointment.
• Teach the patient to periodically examine the skin for precancerous lesions and to have any removed promptly.
• If appropriate, direct the patient and his family to hospital and community support services, such as social workers, psychologists, and cancer support groups.

Stomatitis and other oral infections

A common infection, stomatitis may occur alone or as part of a systemic disease. This inflammation of the oral mucosa may also extend to the buccal mucosa, lips, and palate. The two main types are acute herpetic stomatitis and aphthous stomatitis.

Acute herpetic stomatitis is usually self-limiting; however, it may be severe. This type of stomatitis is common in children between ages 1 and 3.

Aphthous stomatitis is common in girls and female adolescents and usually heals spontaneously, without a scar, in 10 to 14 days. Other oral infections include gingivitis, periodontitis, and Vincent's angina. (See *Understanding oral infections.*)

Causes

Acute herpetic stomatitis is caused by the herpes simplex virus. The cause of aphthous stomatitis is unknown, but autoimmune and psychosomatic causes are under investigation. Predisposing factors associated with aphthous stomatitis include stress, fatigue, anxiety, febrile states, trauma, and overexposure to the sun.

Complications

Stomatitis may be complicated by nutritional deficiencies if painful oral lesions cause dysphagia or make chewing difficult.

Assessment

The patient with acute herpetic stomatitis usually reports symptoms of sudden onset, including mouth pain, malaise, lethargy, anorexia, irritability, and a fever that may last 1 to 2 weeks. He may also complain of bleeding gums and extreme tenderness of the oral mucosa.

On inspection, the gums typically appear swollen, with papulovesicular ulcers evident in the mouth and throat. Eventually these ulcers become punched-out lesions with reddened areolae. The pain usually disappears 2 to 4 days before healing of ulcers is complete. Palpation commonly reveals submaxillary lymphadenitis.

In aphthous stomatitis, typical complaints are burning and tingling of the oral mucosa and painful ulcers. Mouth inspection reveals a slight swelling of the mucous membrane and single or multiple shallow ulcers with whitish centers and red borders, measuring about 2 to 5 mm

Understanding oral infections

Diseases and causes	Assessment findings	Treatment
Gingivitis • Early sign of hypovitaminosis, diabetes, blood dyscrasias • Occasionally related to the use of oral contraceptives	• Inflammation with painless swelling, redness, change of normal contours, bleeding, and periodontal pocket (gum detachment from the teeth)	• Removal of irritating factors (calculus, faulty dentures) • Good oral hygiene, dental checkups, vigorous chewing • Oral or topical corticosteroids
Periodontitis • Progression of gingivitis • Early sign of hypovitaminosis, diabetes, blood dyscrasias • Occasionally related to use of oral contraceptives • Dental factors: calculus, poor oral hygiene, malocclusion	• Acute onset of bright-red gum inflammation, painless swelling of interdental papillae, easy bleeding • Loosening of teeth (typically no inflammation) progressing to tooth and alveolar bone loss • Fever, chills	• Scaling, root planing, and curettage for infection control • Periodontal surgery to prevent recurrence • Good oral hygiene, regular dental checkups, vigorous chewing
Vincent's angina • Also called trench mouth and necrotizing ulcerative gingivitis • Fusiform bacillus or spirochete infection • Predisposing factors: stress, poor oral hygiene, insufficient rest, nutritional deficiencies, smoking, immunosuppressant therapy	• Sudden onset of painful, superficial, bleeding gingival ulcers covered with a gray-white membrane • Ulcers become punched-out lesions after slight pressure or irritation • Malaise, fever, excessive salivation, bad breath, pain on swallowing or talking, enlarged submaxillary lymph nodes	• Removal of devitalized tissue with ultrasonic scaler • Antibiotics for infection • Analgesics, as needed • Hourly mouth rinses (with equal amounts of hydrogen peroxide and water) • Soft, nonirritating diet; rest; no smoking • With treatment, improvement common within 24 hours
Glossitis • Streptococcal infection • Irritation or injury, jagged teeth, ill-fitting dentures, biting during seizures, alcohol, spicy foods, smoking, sensitivity to toothpaste or mouthwash • Vitamin B deficiency, anemia • Lichen planus, erythema multiforme, pemphigus vulgaris	• Reddened, ulcerated, or swollen tongue (may obstruct airway) • Painful chewing and swallowing • Speech difficulty • Painful tongue without inflammation	• Treatment of underlying cause • Topical anesthetic mouthwash or systemic analgesics for painful lesions • Good oral hygiene, regular dental checkups, vigorous chewing • Avoidance of hot, cold, or spicy foods and alcohol
Candidiasis • Also called thrush • *Candida albicans* • Predisposing factors: denture use, diabetes mellitus, immunosuppressant therapy	• Cream-colored or bluish white pseudomembranous patches on the tongue, mouth, or pharynx • Pain, fever, lymphadenopathy	• Hydrogen peroxide and saline mouthwashes • Therapy with clotrimazole or nystatin • Varied local or systemic antifungal therapies

in diameter. These ulcers appear and heal at one site but then reappear at another.

Diagnostic tests

Although diagnosis depends on physical examination, these tests may help to identify the type of infection.

- *Smear of ulcer exudate* allows identification of the causative organism in Vincent's angina.
- *Viral cultures* may be performed on fluid and herpetic vesicles in acute herpetic stomatitis.

Treatment

For both acute herpetic and aphthous stomatitis, treatment is conservative, focusing on symptom relief until the infection resolves.

For acute herpetic stomatitis, symptom management includes nonantiseptic warm-water mouth rinses and topical medications to relieve pain and reduce inflammation.

Topical anesthetic solutions that may be used include lidocaine viscous or dyclonine. Topical corticosteroids may also be prescribed. Acyclovir may be ordered to manage herpetic stomatitis. Supplementary treatments to ease symptoms until the infection subsides include a soft, pureed, or liquid diet and, in severe cases of stomatitis, I.V. fluids and bed rest.

For aphthous stomatitis, a topical anesthetic coating agent, such as kaolin and milk of magnesia, is the primary treatment. The coating helps to relieve severe oral pain while preventing further irritation.

Key nursing diagnoses and patient outcomes

Altered nutrition: Less than body requirements, related to oral pain and ulceration. Based on this nursing diagnosis, you'll establish these patient outcomes. The patient will:

- maintain his baseline weight
- be able to ingest a nutritionally balanced diet daily
- show no signs and symptoms of complications, such as dehydration or nutritional deficiencies.

Altered oral mucous membrane related to ulcerations. Based on this nursing diagnosis, you'll establish these patient outcomes. The patient will:

- communicate an understanding of his oral care routine
- demonstrate prescribed oral care routine, as exhibited by healing of the ulcers
- regain and maintain normal oral mucous membrane integrity with eradication of the infection.

Pain related to ulceration of oral mucous membrane. Based on this nursing diagnosis, you'll establish these patient outcomes. The patient will:

- identify foods that increase or precipitate pain and temporarily eliminate them from his diet
- state and carry out appropriate pain-relief measures.

Nursing interventions

- If the patient's mouth hurts, show him how to clean his teeth with sponges instead of a toothbrush. Suggest that he rinse with hydrogen peroxide or saline mouthwash to soothe irritated mucosa, debride oral structures, and prevent superinfection.
- Administer prescribed analgesics to relieve painful stomatitis. If ordered, apply a topical coating or swishing agent to relieve pain.
- If the patient has difficulty chewing or swallowing, contact the dietitian and develop a meal plan based on soft, liquid, or pureed foods. A change in food consistency often eases discomfort while maintaining adequate nutrition. Ice-cold drinks also may be well tolerated. In severe cases, supplement oral foods with I.V. fluid or nasogastric feedings.

Monitoring

- Monitor the patient for signs and symptoms of infection.

• Assess the patient's pain level and the effectiveness of pain-relief measures.
• Monitor the patient's nutritional status. Weigh him regularly.

Patient teaching

• Teach the patient about the infection and its expected course. For the patient with herpetic stomatitis, emphasize the importance of good oral hygiene to prevent the spread of infection.
• Show the patient how to apply ordered topical medications. Discuss recommended dietary changes and adverse effects of prescribed medications.
• Caution the patient to avoid antiseptic mouthwashes while he has stomatitis because these irritate mouth ulcers.
• Advise the patient with aphthous stomatitis to avoid precipitating factors, such as stress and fatigue.

Syndrome of inappropriate antidiuretic hormone secretion

A potentially life-threatening condition, syndrome of inappropriate antidiuretic hormone (SIADH) secretion is marked by excessive release of antidiuretic hormone (ADH), which disturbs fluid and electrolyte balance. SIADH occurs secondary to diseases that affect the osmoreceptors (supraoptic nucleus) of the hypothalamus. The prognosis depends on the underlying disorder and the patient's response to treatment.

Causes

Usually, SIADH results from oat cell carcinoma of the lung, which secretes excessive ADH or vasopressor-like substances. Other neoplastic diseases (such as pancreatic and prostatic cancers, Hodgkin's disease, and thymoma) may also trigger SIADH. Additional causes include:

• central nervous system (CNS) disorders, including brain tumor or abscess, cerebrovascular accident, head injury, and Guillain-Barré syndrome
• pulmonary disorders (such as pneumonia, tuberculosis, lung abscess) and positive-pressure ventilation
• drugs (for example, chlorpropamide, tolbutamide, vincristine, cyclophosphamide, haloperidol, carbamazepine, clofibrate, morphine, and thiazides)
• endocrine disorders, such as adrenal insufficiency, myxedema, and anterior pituitary insufficiency.

Complications

Without prompt treatment, SIADH may lead to water intoxication, cerebral edema, and severe hyponatremia, with resultant coma and death.

Assessment

The patient's medical and medication histories may provide a clue to the cause of SIADH. A history of cerebrovascular disease, cancer, pulmonary disease, or recent head injury is especially significant.

Most commonly, a patient with SIADH complains of anorexia, nausea, and vomiting. Despite these symptoms, the patient may report weight gain. The patient or family also may report CNS symptoms, such as lethargy, headaches, and emotional and behavioral changes.

Inspection usually fails to reveal edema because much of the free water excess is within cellular boundaries. Palpation may detect tachycardia associated with increased fluid volume. Neurologic assessment may detect disorientation, which may progress to seizures and coma. Examination findings may also include sluggish deep tendon reflexes and muscle weakness.

Diagnostic tests

For critical laboratory test values, see *Confirming SIADH,* page 874. Renal function tests are normal with no evidence of dehydration in SIADH.

CHECKLIST

Confirming SIADH

Key abnormal test values in SIADH include:

- ☐ serum osmolality levels less than 280 mOsm/kg of water in conjunction with serum sodium levels less than 123 mEq/liter
- ☐ urine sodium levels more than 20 mEq/liter without the use of diuretics.

Treatment

Based primarily on the patient's symptoms, treatment begins with restricted water intake (500 to 1,000 ml/day). Some patients who continue to have symptoms are given a high-salt, high-protein diet or urea supplements to enhance water excretion. Or, they may receive demeclocycline or lithium to help block the renal response to ADH.

Rarely, with severe water intoxication, administration of 200 to 300 ml of 3% to 5% sodium chloride solution may be necessary to raise the serum sodium level. A loop diuretic may also be prescribed. When possible, treatment should include correction of the underlying cause of SIADH. If SIADH is due to cancer, success in alleviating water retention may be obtained by surgery, irradiation, or chemotherapy. If SIADH is drug-induced, treatment includes withholding the causative drug.

Key nursing diagnoses and patient outcomes

Altered thought processes related to neurologic dysfunction. Based on this nursing diagnosis, you'll establish these patient outcomes. The patient will:

- remain safe within his environment
- regain and maintain his orientation to person, time, and place.

Fluid volume excess related to cellular fluid retention. Based on this nursing diagnosis, you'll establish these patient outcomes. The patient will:

- adhere to fluid restriction
- show no evidence of complications from excess fluid retention
- regain and maintain normal serum osmolality and sodium levels.

Knowledge deficit related to causes and treatment of SIADH. Based on this nursing diagnosis, you'll establish these patient outcomes. The patient will:

- identify and express the need to learn about SIADH
- seek and obtain correct information about the causes and treatment of SIADH
- communicate an understanding of the causes and treatment of SIADH.

Nursing interventions

- Restrict fluids, and provide comfort measures for thirst, including ice chips, mouth care, lozenges, and staggered water intake.
- Reduce unnecessary environmental stimuli and orient the patient, as needed.
- Provide a safe environment for the patient with an altered loss of consciousness (LOC). Take seizure precautions as needed.

Monitoring

- Monitor the patient's serum osmolality and serum and urine sodium levels.
- Closely monitor and record the patient's intake and output, vital signs, and daily weight.
- Perform frequent neurologic checks, depending on the patient's status. Look for and report early changes in LOC.
- Observe for signs and symptoms of heart failure, which may occur due to fluid overload.

Patient teaching

- If SIADH hasn't resolved by the time of discharge, explain to the patient and his family why he *must* restrict his fluid intake. Review ways to decrease his discomfort from thirst.
- If drug therapy is prescribed, teach the patient and family about the regimen, including dosage, action, and possible adverse effects.
- Discuss self-monitoring techniques for fluid retention, including measurement of intake and output and daily weight. Teach the patient to recognize signs and symptoms that require immediate medical intervention.

Syphilis

A chronic, infectious, sexually transmitted disease, syphilis begins in the mucous membranes and quickly becomes systemic, spreading to nearby lymph nodes and the bloodstream. Untreated, the disease progresses in four stages: primary, secondary, latent, and late (formerly called tertiary).

In recent years, incidence has decreased somewhat. In 1994, 20,627 cases of primary and secondary syphilis were reported to the Centers for Disease Control and Prevention. This is the fewest cases reported since 1977. Between 1993 and 1994, the incidence of primary and secondary syphilis in the United States declined from 10.4 to 8.1 cases per 100,000 population.

Untreated syphilis can lead to crippling or death. With early treatment, the prognosis is excellent. The incubation period varies but typically lasts about 3 weeks.

Causes

The spirochete *Treponema pallidum* causes syphilis. Transmission occurs primarily through sexual contact during the primary, secondary, and early latent stages of infection. Prenatal transmission (from an infected mother to the fetus) also is possible. Transmission by way of a fresh blood transfusion is rare. After 96 hours in stored blood, the *T. pallidum* spirochete dies.

Complications

Aortic regurgitation or aneurysm, meningitis, and widespread central nervous system damage can result from advanced syphilis.

Assessment

The typical patient history will point to unprotected sexual contact with an infected person or with multiple or anonymous sexual partners.

In a patient with primary syphilis, you may observe one or more chancres (small, fluid-filled lesions) on the genitalia and others on the anus, fingers, lips, tongue, nipples, tonsils, or eyelids. In female patients, chancres may develop on the cervix or the vaginal wall. These usually painless lesions start as papules and then erode. They have indurated, raised edges and clear bases and typically heal after 3 to 6 weeks, even when untreated. In the primary stage, palpation may reveal enlarged unilateral or bilateral regional lymph nodes (adenopathy).

In secondary syphilis (beginning within a few days or up to 8 weeks after the initial chancres appear), the patient may complain of headache, nausea, vomiting, malaise, anorexia, weight loss, sore throat, and a slight fever.

On inspection, you may see symmetrical mucocutaneous lesions. The rash of secondary syphilis may appear macular, papular, pustular, or nodular. Lesions are uniform, well defined, and generalized. Macules typically erupt between rolls of fat on the trunk and, proximally, on the arms, palms, soles, face, and scalp. In warm, moist body areas (the perineum, scrotum, or vulva, for example), the lesions enlarge and erode, producing highly contagious, pink or grayish white lesions (condylomata lata).

Alopecia, which usually is temporary, may occur with or without treatment. The patient also may complain of brittle, pitted nails.

Palpation may disclose generalized lymphadenopathy.

In latent syphilis, physical signs and symptoms are absent except for possible recurrence of mucocutaneous lesions that resemble those of secondary syphilis.

In late syphilis, the patient's complaints will vary with the involved organ. Late syphilis has three subtypes: neurosyphilis, late benign syphilis, and cardiovascular syphilis.

If neurosyphilis affects meningovascular tissues, the patient may report headache, vertigo, insomnia, hemiplegia, seizures, and psychological difficulties. If neurosyphilis affects parenchymal tissue, he may report paresis, alteration in intellect, paranoia, illusions, and hallucinations. Inspection may reveal Argyll Robertson pupil (a small, irregular pupil that is nonreactive to light but accommodates for vision), ataxia, slurred speech, trophic joint changes, positive Romberg's sign, and a facial tremor.

If the patient has late benign syphilis, he may complain of gummas – lesions that develop between 1 and 10 years after infection. A single gumma may be a chronic, superficial nodule or a deep, granulomatous lesion that's solitary, asymmetrical, painless, indurated, and large or small. Visible on the skin and mucocutaneous tissues, gummas commonly affect bones and can develop in any organ. If they involve the nasal septum or palate, they may cause perforation and disfigurement.

In cardiovascular syphilis, decreased cardiac output may cause decreased urine output and decreased sensorium related to hypoxia. Auscultation may reveal pulmonary congestion.

Diagnostic tests

- *Dark-field microscopy* to identify *T. pallidum* from lesional exudate provides an immediate syphilis diagnosis. This method is most effective when moist lesions are present, as in primary, secondary, and congenital syphilis.
- *Nontreponemal serologic tests* include the Venereal Disease Research Laboratory (VDRL) slide test, the rapid plasma reagin (RPR) test, and the automated reagin test. These tests can detect nonspecific antibodies, which become reactive within 1 to 2 weeks after the primary syphilis lesion appears or 4 to 5 weeks after the infection begins. Rapid and inexpensive, the tests are used for screening patients and blood products.
- *Treponemal serologic studies* include the fluorescent treponemal antibody absorption test, the *Treponema pallidum* hemagglutination assay, and the microhemagglutination assay. These tests detect the specific antitreponemal antibody and can confirm positive screening results. Once reactive, a patient's blood samples will always be reactive.
- *Cerebrospinal fluid examination* identifies neurosyphilis when the total protein level is above 40 mg/dl, the VDRL slide test is reactive, and the white blood cell (WBC) count exceeds 5 WBCs/mm³.

Treatment

Antibiotic therapy – penicillin administered I.M. – is the treatment of choice. For early syphilis, treatment may consist of a single injection of penicillin G benzathine I.M. (2.4 million units). Syphilis of more than 1 year's duration may respond to penicillin G benzathine I.M. (2.4 million units/week for 3 weeks).

Patients who are allergic to penicillin may be successfully treated with tetracycline or erythromycin (in either case, the therapy would be 500 mg by mouth four times a day for 15 days for early syphilis, and for 30 days for late infections). Tetracycline is contraindicated during pregnancy.

Key nursing diagnoses and patient outcomes

Altered sexuality patterns related to abstinence required in syphilis therapy. Based on this nursing diagnosis, you'll establish these expected outcomes. The patient will:
- communicate an understanding of the need for restricted sexual activity during treatment for syphilis
- comply with restricted sexual activity until VDRL and RPR test results are normal.

Impaired skin integrity related to skin lesions. Based on this nursing diagnosis, you'll establish these patient outcomes. The patient will:
- communicate an understanding of skin care measures
- demonstrate skill in performing his skin care routine
- regain skin integrity, as evidenced by eradication of of lesions.

Knowledge deficit related to how syphilis is transmitted and treated. Based on this nursing diagnosis, you'll establish these patient outcomes. The patient will:
- identify and express the need to learn about syphilis
- seek and obtain information about syphilis from appropriate sources
- communicate an understanding of how syphilis is spread and treated.

Nursing interventions

- Follow standard precautions when assessing the patient, collecting specimens, and treating lesions.
- Check for a history of drug sensitivity before administering the first dose of medication.
- Promote rest and adequate nutrition.
- In secondary syphilis, keep lesions clean and dry. If they're draining, dispose of contaminated materials properly.
- In late syphilis, provide care to relieve the patient's symptoms during prolonged treatment.
- As needed, obtain a physical or occupational therapy consultation. Also consult with a social worker to determine home care needs.
- Report all syphilis cases to the appropriate health authorities.

Monitoring

- Check lesions for drainage and healing.
- Assess for complications of late syphilis if the patient's infection is older than 1 year.
- Monitor the patient's compliance to drug therapy.

Patient teaching

- Make sure the patient clearly understands his medication and dosage schedule and knows how to obtain the medication.
- Stress the importance of completing the prescribed course of therapy even after symptoms subside. Evaluate the need for home nursing care.
- Urge the patient to inform sexual partners of his infection and to encourage them to seek testing and treatment.
- Advise the patient to refrain from sexual activity until he completes treatment and follow-up VDRL and RPR test results are normal.
- Counsel the patient and sexual partners about HIV infection, and recommend HIV testing.
- Inform the patient that using condoms may provide protection against sexually transmitted diseases.
- Remind the patient to schedule follow-up tests.

Systemic sclerosis

Also called scleroderma, systemic sclerosis is a diffuse connective tissue disease. It's characterized by fibrotic, degenerative and, occasionally, inflammatory changes in skin, blood vessels, synovial membranes, skeletal muscles, and internal organs (especially the esophagus, intestinal tract, thyroid, heart, lungs, and kidneys).

Systemic sclerosis occurs in two distinct forms: localized (CREST syndrome) and diffuse. CREST syndrome, the more benign form, accounts for 80% of cases. It causes calcinosis cutis, Raynaud's phenomenon, esophageal dysfunction, sclerodactyly, and telangiectasia. Diffuse systemic sclerosis, which accounts for 20% of cases, is marked by generalized skin thickening and invasion of internal organ systems.

Eosinophilic fasciculitis, a rare variant of systemic sclerosis, causes skin changes similar to those of diffuse systemic sclerosis but limited to the fascia. Other differences from systemic sclerosis include eosinophilia, an absence of Raynaud's phenomenon, a good response to prednisone, and an increased risk of aplastic anemia.

Systemic sclerosis is twice as common in women as in men. It usually occurs between ages 30 and 50.

Causes

The cause of systemic sclerosis is unknown.

Complications

In advanced disease, cardiac and pulmonary fibrosis produces arrhythmias and dyspnea. Renal involvement usually causes malignant hypertension, the major cause of death from this disease.

Assessment

Ninety percent of patients complain of symptoms of Raynaud's phenomenon—blanching, cyanosis, and erythema of the fingers and toes in response to stress or exposure to cold. These symptoms may precede diagnosis of systemic sclerosis by months or even years. As the disease progresses, the patient may complain of pain, stiffness, and swelling of fingers and joints.

Eventually, the patient may complain of frequent reflux, heartburn, dysphagia (in 90% of patients), and bloating after meals, all stemming from motility abnormalities, GI fibrosis, and malabsorption. These symptoms may cause her to eat less and lose weight. Other common GI complaints include abdominal distention, diarrhea, constipation, and malodorous floating stools.

In the early stages, inspection may reveal thickened, hidelike skin with loss of normal skin folds. You may also note telangiectasia and areas of pigmentation and depigmentation. The patient's fingers may have shortened because of progressive phalangeal resorption. You may observe slowly healing ulcers on the tips of the fingers or toes—the result of compromised circulation. These ulcers may lead to gangrene.

Later, inspection may disclose taut, shiny skin over the entire hand and forearm from skin thickening. Facial skin may also appear tight and inelastic, causing a wrinkle-free, masklike appearance and a pinched mouth. As tightening progresses, contractures may develop.

With pulmonary involvement, you may observe dyspnea and auscultate decreased breath sounds. With cardiac involvement, you may auscultate an irregular cardiac rhythm, pericardial friction rub, and an atrial gallop. Your assessment may also reveal hypertension if renal involvement occurs.

Diagnostic tests

Typical cutaneous changes provide the first clue to diagnosis. Results of diagnostic tests include the following:

- *Blood studies* show mild anemia, slightly elevated erythrocyte sedimentation rate, hypergammaglobulinemia, positive rheumatoid factor (in 25% to 35% of patients), positive lupus erythematosus preparation, positive antinuclear antibody (low titer, speckled or nucleolar pattern) and, with diffuse systemic sclerosis, scleroderma antibody (in about 35% of patients).
- *Urinalysis* reveals proteinuria, microscopic hematuria, and casts (with renal involvement).

• *Hand X-rays* show terminal phalangeal tuft resorption, subcutaneous calcification, and joint space narrowing and erosion.
• *Chest X-rays* demonstrate bilateral basilar pulmonary fibrosis.
• *GI X-rays* disclose distal esophageal hypomotility and stricture, duodenal loop dilation, small-bowel malabsorption pattern, and large diverticula.
• *Pulmonary function studies* reveal decreased diffusion, vital capacity, and lung compliance.
• *Electrocardiogram* detects possible nonspecific abnormalities related to myocardial fibrosis.
• *Skin biopsy* shows possible changes consistent with the progress of the disease, such as marked thickening of the dermis and occlusive vessel changes.

Treatment

No cure exists for systemic sclerosis. Treatment aims to preserve normal body functions and minimize complications. Immunosuppressants, such as chlorambucil, can help relieve symptoms. Used experimentally, corticosteroids and colchicine seem to stabilize symptoms; D-penicillamine may also be helpful. The patient should have her blood platelet levels monitored throughout immunosuppressant therapy.

Other treatment varies according to symptoms.
• *Raynaud's phenomenon.* Treatment consists of various vasodilators, calcium channel blockers, and antihypertensive agents (such as methyldopa), along with intermittent cervical sympathetic blockade or, rarely, thoracic sympathectomy.
• *Chronic digital ulcerations.* A digital plaster cast immobilizes the affected area, minimizes trauma, and maintains cleanliness; the patient may also need surgical debridement.
• *Esophagitis with stricture.* The patient receives antacids, a histamine-2 antagonist (such as omeprazole, cimetidine, or ranitidine), a soft bland diet, and periodic esophageal dilation.
• *Small-bowel involvement.* The patient receives broad-spectrum antibiotics, such as erythromycin or tetracycline, to counteract bacterial overgrowth in the duodenum and jejunum related to hypomotility.
• *Scleroderma kidney (with malignant hypertension and impending renal failure).* The patient needs dialysis, antihypertensives, and calcium channel blockers; if hypertensive crisis develops, she may receive an angiotensin-converting enzyme inhibitor.
• *Hand debilitation.* Treatment consists of physical therapy to maintain function and promote muscle strength, heat therapy to relieve joint stiffness, and patient teaching to help the patient perform activities of daily living.
• *Pulmonary manifestations.* The patient receives oral or parenteral cyclophosphamide to relieve symptoms of dyspnea, crackles, and constrictive pulmonary function.

Key nursing diagnoses and patient outcomes

Altered peripheral tissue perfusion related to compromised circulation. Based on this nursing diagnosis, you'll establish these patient outcomes. The patient will:
• identify factors that precipitate or increase ischemic tissue changes, such as cold exposure and stress, and try to avoid or minimize them
• report feelings of comfort and the absence of pain in extremities, especially fingers
• show no evidence of severe tissue ischemia and gangrene.

Risk for injury related to potential complications of systemic sclerosis. Based on this nursing diagnosis, you'll establish these patient outcomes. The patient will:
• demonstrate the ability to perform the prescribed care regimen
• identify early signs and symptoms of complications and seek medical attention promptly
• maintain adequate organ function, as evidenced by signs of hemodynamic stability.

Impaired skin integrity related to ulcerations and skin changes. Based on this nursing diagnosis, you'll establish these patient outcomes. The patient will:
• communicate an understanding of skin-protection measures
• demonstrate skill in caring for skin ulcerations
• regain skin integrity.

Nursing interventions

• Because of compromised digital circulation, don't perform any finger-stick blood tests. Provide gloves or sock mittens after warming therapy.
• Use plaster wraps or topical ointments to lessen the painful effects of digital ulcerations.
• If the patient has cardiac and pulmonary fibrosis, provide rest and pulmonary exercises. Coughing, deep breathing, and chest physiotherapy will help keep her lungs clear.
• Provide a high-calorie diet that's smooth, cool, and palatable. Consult the dietitian to ensure the patient has a nutritious, appealing diet. Treat GI disturbances as necessary with antacids and antidiarrheals.
• If the patient suffers from delayed gastric emptying, offer her small, frequent meals and have her remain upright for at least 2 hours after eating. This should help improve her digestion and maintain weight.
• Whenever possible, let the patient participate in treatment by measuring her own intake and output, planning her own diet, assisting in dialysis, giving herself heat therapy, and performing prescribed exercises.
• Help the patient and her family accept the fact that this condition is incurable. Encourage them to express their feelings, and help them cope with their fears and frustrations.

Monitoring

• Regularly assess mobility restrictions, vital signs, level of pain, intake and output, respiratory function, and daily weight.
• Monitor the patient for early signs and symptoms of complications associated with systemic sclerosis, especially cardiopulmonary and renal abnormalities.
• Inspect the skin regularly for evidence of ulcerations. If ulcerations are present, note and record the site, size, and appearance and notify the doctor.

Patient teaching

• Teach the patient and her family about the disease, its treatment, and relevant diagnostic tests.
• Warn the patient to avoid air conditioning, cool showers and baths, and preparing food under cold running water, which may aggravate Raynaud's phenomenon. Also, advise her to wear gloves or mittens outside, even in mild weather; she may want to wear them indoors too.
• Help the patient and her family adjust to her new body image and to the limitations and dependence that these changes cause. To reduce fatigue, teach the patient to pace her activities and organize schedules to include necessary rest and exercise.
• Advise the patient to avoid contact with people who have active infections (especially of the upper respiratory tract).
• Urge the patient to maintain a high-calorie diet. Warn her that supplements may not help her overall condition because they often contribute to diarrhea.
• Advise the patient with GI involvement to avoid late-night meals, to elevate the head of the bed, and to use prescribed antacids and histamine-2 antagonists to reduce the incidence of reflux and resulting scarring.
• If the patient needs dialysis, refer her to the National Kidney Foundation's local support group. Explain that she may have to limit certain foods and liquids for the rest of her life. Reassure her that dialysis can be done close to or in her home.

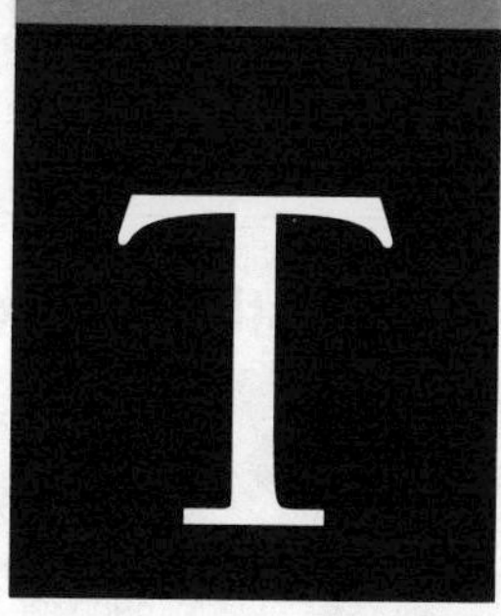

Testicular cancer

Malignant testicular tumors are the most prevalent solid tumors in men ages 20 to 34. Rare in nonwhite men, testicular cancer accounts for less than 1% of all male cancer deaths.

With few exceptions, testicular tumors originate from germ cells. About 40% become seminomas. These tumors, which are characterized by uniform, undifferentiated cells, resemble primitive gonadal cells. Other tumors – nonseminomas – show various degrees of differentiation.

Prognosis in testicular cancer depends on the cell type and stage. When treated with surgery, chemotherapy, and radiation therapy, all of the patients with stage I or stage II seminomas and 90% of those with stage I nonseminomas survive beyond 5 years. The prognosis is poor, however, if the disease advances beyond stage II. Typically, when the cancer extends beyond the testes, it spreads through the lymphatic system to the iliac, para-aortic, and mediastinal nodes. Metastases affect the lungs, liver, viscera, and bone.

Causes

Although researchers don't know the immediate cause of testicular cancer, they suspect that cryptorchidism (even when surgically corrected) plays a role in the developing disease. A history of mumps orchitis, inguinal hernia in childhood, or maternal use of diethylstilbestrol (DES) or other estrogen-progestin combinations during pregnancy also increases the risk for this disease.

Complications

Disease progression may induce back or abdominal pain (from retroperitoneal adenopathy), dyspnea, cough, hemoptysis from lung metastases, and ureteral obstruction.

Assessment

The patient history may disclose previous injuries to the scrotum, viral infections (such as mumps), or the use of DES or other estrogen-progestin drugs by the patient's mother during pregnancy. The patient may describe a feeling of heaviness or a dragging sensation in the scrotum. He may also report swollen testes or a painless lump found while performing testicular self-examination. In late disease stages, the patient may complain of weight loss, a cough, hemoptysis, shortness of breath, lethargy, and fatigue.

On inspection, you may notice that the patient has enlarged testes. Gynecomastia, a sign that the tumor produces chorionic gonadotropins or estrogen, may be obvious also. In later stages of testicular cancer, the patient may appear lethargic, thin, and pallid.

Palpation findings include a firm, smooth testicular mass and enlarged lymph nodes in surrounding areas. In later disease stages, palpation may disclose an abdominal mass as well.

On auscultation you may hear decreased breath sounds.

Staging testicular cancer

Using the tumor, node, metastasis (TNM) system, the American Joint Committee on Cancer has established the following stages for testicular cancer.

Primary tumor
TX—primary tumor can't be assessed (this stage is used in the absence of radical orchiectomy)
T0—histologic scar or no evidence of primary tumor
Tis—intratubular tumor: preinvasive cancer
T1—tumor limited to testicles, including the rete testis
T2—tumor extends beyond tunica albuginea or into epididymis
T3—tumor extends into spermatic cord
T4—tumor invades scrotum

Regional lymph nodes
NX—regional lymph nodes can't be assessed
N0—no evidence of regional lymph node metastasis
N1—metastasis in a single lymph node, 2 cm or less in greatest dimension
N2—metastasis in a single lymph node, between 2 and 5 cm in greatest dimension, or metastases to several lymph nodes, none more than 5 cm in greatest dimension
N3—metastasis in a lymph node more than 5 cm in greatest dimension

Distant metastasis
MX—distant metastasis can't be assessed
M0—no known distant metastasis
M1—distant metastasis

Staging categories
Testicular cancer progresses from mild to severe as follows:
Stage 0—Tis, N0, M0
Stage I—T1, N0, M0; T2, N0, M0
Stage II—T3, N0, M0; T4, N0, M0
Stage III—any T, N1, M0
Stage IV—any T, N2, M0; any T, N3, M0; any T, any N, M1

Diagnostic tests

• *Serum analyses* may be done to evaluate beta-subunit human chorionic gonadotropin (HCG) and alpha-fetoprotein (AFP) levels. Elevated levels of these proteins (tumor markers) suggest testicular cancer and can differentiate a seminoma from a nonseminoma: elevated HCG and AFP levels point to a nonseminoma; elevated HCG and normal AFP levels indicate a seminoma.
• *Computed tomography (CT) scan* can detect metastases.
• *Scrotal ultrasonography* can differentiate between a cyst and solid mass.
• *Chest X-rays* may show pulmonary metastases.
• *CT scan* or *magnetic resonance imaging scan* may reveal additional metastases and evaluate the retroperitoneal lymph nodes.
• *Biopsy* can confirm the diagnosis, help stage the disease, and plan treatment. (See *Staging testicular cancer.*)

Treatment

Treatment includes surgery, radiation therapy, and chemotherapy. Treatment intensity varies with the tumor cell type and stage.

A radical orchiectomy is done to diagnose testicular cancer and is the primary treatment. The amputated testicle can be replaced with a testicular prosthesis. This reconstructive surgery is recommended to help the patient's self-esteem. Many surgeons currently use radical orchiectomy together with diagnostic studies of the retroperitoneal lymph nodes without surgical resection. If retroperitoneal lymph node dissection is performed, impotence is a major complication.

Treatment of seminomas involves postoperative radiation to the retroperitoneal and homolateral iliac nodes. Patients whose disease extends to retroperitoneal structures may be given prophylactic radiation to the mediastinal and supraclavicular nodes. Treatment of nonseminomas includes radiation directed to all cancerous lymph nodes.

Chemotherapy is most effective for late-stage seminomas, and most nonseminomas, when used for recurrent cancer after orchiectomy and removal of the retroperitoneal lymph nodes.

Autologous bone marrow transplantation is usually reserved for patients who don't respond to standard therapy. It involves giving high-dose chemotherapy, removing and treating the patient's bone marrow to kill remaining cancer cells, and returning the processed bone marrow to the patient.

Key nursing diagnoses and patient outcomes

Anxiety related to fear of sexual impairment and disfigurement caused by treatment. Based on this nursing diagnosis, you'll establish these patient outcomes. The patient will:

- identify and express feelings of anxiety
- communicate an understanding of how testicular cancer and its treatment affects sexuality and appearance
- demonstrate healthy coping behaviors to reduce anxiety.

Body image disturbance related to removal of testis or testes and scrotum. Based on this nursing diagnosis, you'll establish these patient outcomes. The patient will:

- acknowledge the change in body image
- use available resources to cope with body image change
- express positive feelings about himself.

Sexual dysfunction related to impotence caused by bilateral testicular cancer treatment. Based on this nursing diagnosis, you'll establish these patient outcomes. The patient will:

- communicate an understanding of the reason for impotence
- express acceptance of impotence
- seek sexual counseling to learn alternative methods for sexual gratification.

Nursing interventions

- Focus on responding to the psychological impact of the disease, preventing postoperative complications, and minimizing and controlling the complications of radiation therapy and chemotherapy.
- Listen to the patient's fears and concerns. Remember that the patient with testicular cancer typically fears sexual impairment and disfigurement. (See *How orchiectomy affects sexual function,* page 884.) When possible, provide reassurance. Stay with the patient during periods of severe anxiety and stress.
- Encourage the patient to ask questions. Base your relationship on trust so that he feels comfortable expressing his concerns.
- Prepare the patient for orchiectomy, as indicated. (See the entry "Orchiopexy.")

During chemotherapy:

- Know what problems to expect and how to prevent or ease them.
- Give antiemetics, as ordered, to prevent severe nausea and vomiting.
- Offer the patient small, frequent feedings to maintain oral intake despite anorexia. Devise a mouth care regimen, making sure to check regularly for stomatitis.
- To prevent renal damage during cisplatin therapy, encourage increased fluid intake. To maximize hydration, give I.V. fluids, as ordered, with a potassium supplement. Provide diuresis, as ordered, by administering furosemide or mannitol.

During radiation therapy:

- Implement appropriate comfort and safety measures. For example, avoid rubbing the skin near radiation target sites. This helps to prevent or alleviate pain, skin breakdown, and infection.

How orchiectomy affects sexual function

Patients with testicular cancer typically are anxious about their future. Besides the usual apprehensions about living with cancer, these patients fear loss of sexual function after surgery (orchiectomy). To help patients face their fear, provide support and a clear explanation of how orchiectomy affects sexual activity.

After unilateral orchiectomy

Unilateral orchiectomy doesn't cause sterility or impotence. And because most surgeons remove only the diseased testicle and leave the scrotum, later reconstructive surgery can be done. This involves implanting a gel-filled testicular prosthesis, which weighs the same as and feels like a normal testicle. The patient can resume sexual activity after the incision heals.

After bilateral orchiectomy

Bilateral testicular cancer is uncommon. However, if the patient loses both testes, he will be sterile. And if nerve or vascular damage (or both) occur with surgery, he will also be impotent.

Be as positive and supportive as possible. Clearly express that a loss of fertility doesn't mean a loss of masculinity. Typically, the patient will take synthetic hormones to replace or supplement depleted male hormone levels.

Monitoring

- Monitor the patient for adverse reactions to chemotherapy and radiation therapy.
- If the patient receives vinblastine, monitor for signs and symptoms of neurotoxicity (peripheral paresthesia, jaw pain, muscle cramps). If he receives cisplatin, check for ototoxicity.

Patient teaching

- Provide reassurance that sterility and impotence usually don't follow unilateral orchiectomy. Explain that synthetic hormones can supplement depleted hormonal levels. Inform the patient that most surgeons don't remove the scrotum. Also explain that a testicular prosthetic implant can correct disfigurement.
- As suitable, review sperm banking procedures before the patient begins treatment, especially if infertility and impotence may result from surgery.
- Explain tests and treatments that the patient will undergo. Make sure he understands each treatment, its purpose, possible complications, and the care required during and after the treatment.
- Teach the patient how to perform testicular self-examination. Tell him that this is the best way to detect a new or recurrent tumor.
- Refer the patient to organizations, such as the American Cancer Society, that offer information and support during and after treatment.

Tetanus

Also referred to as lockjaw, tetanus is an acute exotoxin-mediated infection caused by the anaerobic, spore-forming, gram-positive bacillus *Clostridium tetani.* The infection usually is systemic, but it may be localized. Tetanus is fatal in up to 60% of nonimmunized people, often within 10 days of onset. The disease's incubation period ranges from 3 to 4 weeks in mild tetanus to under 2 days in severe tetanus. When symptoms develop within 3 days of exposure, the prognosis is poor. In North America, about 75% of all cases occur between April and September.

Tetanus occurs worldwide, but it's more prevalent in agricultural regions and developing countries that lack mass immunization programs.

Once *C. tetani* enters the body, it causes local infection and tissue necrosis. It also produces toxins that enter the bloodstream and lymphatics and eventually spread to central nervous system tissue.

Causes

Transmission occurs through a puncture wound that is contaminated by soil, dust, or animal excreta containing *C. tetani,* or by way of burns or minor wounds.

Complications

Atelectasis, pneumonia, pulmonary emboli, acute gastric ulcers, flexion contractures, and cardiac arrhythmias can result from tetanus.

Assessment

The patient's history may reveal inadequate immunization, and the patient may report a recent skin wound or burn. He may complain of pain or paresthesia at the site of injury and recall early complaints of difficulty chewing or swallowing food. He usually has a normal body temperature or a slight fever in the early stages, although his fever may rise as the disease progresses.

If the tetanus remains localized, your assessment may disclose signs of spasm and increased muscle tone near the wound.

If the tetanus becomes systemic, your assessment may reveal an irregular heartbeat, marked muscle hypertonicity, hyperactive deep tendon reflexes, tachycardia, profuse sweating, low-grade fever, and painful, involuntary muscle contractions. Specific findings may include:

- rigid neck and facial muscles (especially cheek muscles), resulting in lockjaw (trismus) and a grotesque, grinning expression called risus sardonicus
- rigid somatic muscles, causing arched-back rigidity (opisthotonos); palpation reveals boardlike abdominal rigidity
- intermittent tonic seizures that last for several minutes and may result in cyanosis and sudden death by asphyxiation.

Despite such pronounced neuromuscular symptoms, assessment shows normal cerebral and sensory function.

Diagnostic tests

Blood cultures and tetanus antibody tests commonly are negative; only a third of patients have a positive wound culture. Cerebrospinal fluid pressure may rise above normal.

Treatment

Within 72 hours after a puncture wound, a patient with no previous history of tetanus immunization first requires tetanus immune globulin or tetanus antitoxin to confer temporary protection. Next, he needs active immunization with tetanus toxoid. A patient who has not received tetanus immunization within 5 years needs a booster injection of tetanus toxoid.

If tetanus develops despite immediate postinjury treatment, the patient will require airway maintenance and a muscle relaxant such as diazepam to decrease muscle rigidity and spasm. If muscle contractions aren't relieved by muscle relaxants, a neuromuscular blocker may be needed.

The patient with tetanus also requires high-dose antibiotics – preferably penicillin (administered I.V.), if he's not allergic to it. If he is allergic to penicillin, tetracycline can be substituted.

Key nursing diagnoses and patient outcomes

Impaired physical mobility related to muscle rigidity and spasms. Based on this nursing diagnosis, you'll establish these patient outcomes. The patient will:

- show no evidence of complications, such as contractures, venous stasis, thrombus

formation, or skin breakdown during the period of immobility
• regain normal physical mobility with eradication of tetanus.

Ineffective airway clearance related to rigid neck muscles. Based on this nursing diagnosis, you'll establish these patient outcomes. The patient will:
• maintain a patent airway
• not have dyspnea or a change in respiratory pattern
• maintain adequate ventilation, as evidenced by clear breath sounds and normal arterial blood gas values.

Pain related to muscle rigidity and spasms. Based on this nursing diagnosis, you'll establish these patient outcomes. The patient will:
• identify activities and body movements that precipitate or increase pain, and make nurses aware of them
• adhere to activity restrictions to decrease or prevent painful muscle spasms
• report pain relief following administration of a muscle relaxant.

Nursing interventions

• Before tetanus develops, thoroughly debride and clean the injury site with 3% hydrogen peroxide and check the patient's immunization history. Record the cause of the injury. If it was caused by an animal bite, report the case to local public health authorities.
• Before giving penicillin and tetanus immune globulin, antitoxin, or toxoid, obtain an accurate history of the patient's allergies to immunizations or penicillin. If the patient has a history of any allergies, keep epinephrine 1:1,000 (for subcutaneous injection) and emergency airway equipment available.
• After tetanus develops, maintain an adequate airway and ventilation to prevent pneumonia and atelectasis. Suction as needed.
• Insert an artificial airway if necessary to prevent tongue injury, and maintain the airway during spasms.
• Keep emergency airway equipment on hand because the patient may require artificial ventilation or oxygen administration. Have endotracheal and tracheotomy equipment on hand. In an emergency, the doctor may perform a tracheotomy if the patient becomes extremely rigid.
• Be prepared to resuscitate the patient and initiate life support.
• Administer I.V. therapy as prescribed.
• Because even minimal external stimulation provokes muscle spasms, keep the patient's room dark and quiet. Warn visitors not to upset or overly stimulate the patient.
• Turn the patient frequently to prevent contractures, pressure ulcers, and pulmonary stasis. Perform range-of-motion exercises to maintain flexibility.
• Place the patient on an air mattress, and use other skin protective measures as warranted.
• Perform all activities of daily living for the sedated patient.
• Give muscle relaxants and sedatives, as ordered, and schedule patient care to coincide with heaviest sedation.
• If urine retention develops, insert an indwelling urinary catheter.
• Provide adequate nutrition to meet the patient's increased metabolic needs. He may need nasogastric feedings or total parenteral nutrition.

Monitoring

• Evaluate the patient's respiratory status continuously, and watch for signs of respiratory distress.
• Monitor intake and output.
• Frequently check the patient's electrocardiogram for arrhythmias. Also monitor vital signs.
• Check the patient's skin for signs of pressure ulcers.
• Monitor the patient's nutritional status. Watch for signs of rapid weight loss and nutritional deficits because of the patient's increased metabolic needs.

• Assess the patient for increased muscle spasms and rigidity and for the effectiveness of administered muscle relaxants.

Patient teaching

• During the patient's convalescence, encourage gradual active exercises.
• Institute a bladder retraining program if the patient was catheterized.
• Stress the importance of maintaining active immunization with a booster dose of tetanus toxoid every 10 years.
• Inform the patient with a skin injury or burn that he should receive tetanus prophylaxis.

Thalassemia

Thalassemia, a group of hereditary hemolytic anemias, is characterized by defective synthesis in one or more of the polypeptide chains (alpha and beta) necessary for hemoglobin production. Because thalessemia affects hemoglobin production, it also impairs red blood cell (RBC) synthesis. This disorder is most common in individuals of Mediterranean ancestry (especially Italians and Greeks), although it also occurs in Blacks and people from southern China, southeast Asia, and India.

In thalassemia, diminished synthesis can affect either pair. Structurally, the chains are normal, but the genetic defect decreases their number. In the most severe form of alpha-thalassemia – hydrops fetalis – severe anemia and congestive heart failure render fetuses hydropic. These fetuses are stillborn or die shortly after birth. Prenatal testing can detect the condition.

Beta-thalassemia is the most common form of this disorder and occurs in three clinical forms: thalassemia major, intermedia, and minor. The severity of the resulting anemia depends on whether the patient is homozygous or heterozygous for the thalassemic trait. The prognosis for beta-thalassemia varies.

Causes

Thalassemia major and intermedia result from homozygous inheritance of the partially dominant autosomal gene responsible for this trait. Thalassemia minor is caused by heterozygous inheritance of the same gene. Total or partial deficiency of beta polypeptide chain production impairs hemoglobin synthesis and results in continual production of fetal hemoglobin, even after the neonatal period has passed.

Complications

As children with thalassemia major grow older, they become prone to pathologic fractures. This occurs because the bone marrow cavities expand as the long bones thin. Other complications include cardiac arrhythmias, heart failure, and conditions resulting from iron deposits in the heart and other tissues caused by repeated blood transfusions.

Assessment

In thalassemia major (also known as Cooley's anemia and erythroblastic anemia), the infant, well at birth, develops severe anemia, bone abnormalities, failure to thrive, and life-threatening complications. Often, the first signs are pallor and yellow skin and scleras in infants between ages 3 and 6 months. Later signs and symptoms are severe anemia, splenomegaly or hepatomegaly with abdominal enlargement, frequent infections, bleeding tendencies, and anorexia.

Children with thalassemia major usually have small bodies and large heads and may also be mentally retarded. Infants may have mongoloid features.

Thalassemia intermedia comprises moderate thalassemic disorders in homozygotes. Patients show some degree of anemia, jaundice, and splenomegaly and may exhibit signs of hemosiderosis caused by increased intestinal absorption of iron.

Thalassemia minor may cause mild anemia but usually produces no signs or symptoms and is often overlooked.

Diagnostic tests

In thalassemia major, laboratory test results show a decreased RBC count and hemoglobin (Hb) level, microcytosis, and increased reticulocyte, bilirubin, and urinary and fecal urobilinogen levels. A low serum folate level suggests increased folate use by hypertrophied bone marrow. A peripheral blood smear reveals target cells, microcytes, pale nucleated RBCs, and marked anisocytosis. X-rays of the skull and long bones show thinning and widening of the marrow space due to overactive bone marrow. The bones of the skull and vertebrae may appear granular. Long bones may show areas of osteoporosis. The phalanges may also be deformed (rectangular or biconvex). Quantitative Hb studies show a significant rise in Hb F and a slight increase in Hb A_2. Diagnosis must rule out iron deficiency anemia, which also produces hypochromia (slightly lower Hb level) and microcytic (notably small) RBCs.

In thalassemia intermedia, laboratory test results show hypochromia and microcytic RBCs, but the anemia is less severe than that in thalassemia major. In thalassemia minor, test results also show hypochromia and microcytic RBCs. Quantitative Hb studies show a significant increase in Hb A_2 levels and a moderate rise in Hb F levels.

Treatment

Treatment of thalassemia major is essentially supportive. For example, infections require prompt treatment with appropriate antibiotics. Folic acid supplements help maintain folic acid levels despite increased requirements. Transfusions of packed RBCs raise Hb levels but must be used judiciously to minimize iron overload. Although splenectomy and bone marrow transplantation have been attempted, their effectiveness has not been confirmed.

Thalassemia intermedia and thalassemia minor usually don't require treatment.

Iron supplements are contraindicated in all forms of thalassemia.

Treatment of children proves more difficult. Regular blood transfusions may minimize physical and mental retardation, but transfusions increase the risk of deadly hemosiderosis and iron overload. Continuous subcutaneous infusion of iron-chelating agents may help produce a negative overall iron balance. If rapid splenic sequestration of transfused RBCs necessitates more transfusions, a splenectomy may be performed.

Key nursing diagnoses and patient outcomes

Altered growth and development related to disease process. Based on this nursing diagnosis, you'll establish these patient outcomes. The patient will:
- show age-appropriate development milestones
- demonstrate adaptations to deficits.

Body image disturbance related to effects of disease on appearance. Based on this nursing diagnosis, you'll establish these patient outcomes. The patient will:
- verbalize a positive self concept
- interact with peers appropriately.

Knowledge deficit related to disease and its treatment. Based on this nursing diagnosis, you'll establish these patient outcomes. The patient or parents will:
- verbalize knowledge of the disease process
- demonstrate appropriate care measures.

Risk for infection related to bone marrow dysfunction and anemia. Based on this nursing diagnosis, you'll establish these patient outcomes. The patient or parents will:
- remain free from infection
- verbalize signs to notify doctor
- exhibit measures to prevent infection.

Nursing interventions

- Watch for adverse reactions – shaking chills, fever, rash, itching, and hives – during and after RBC transfusions.
- Administer antibiotics, as ordered, and watch for adverse reactions.
- Provide an adequate diet and encourage increased consumption of fluids.
- Offer emotional support to help the patient and family cope.

Patient teaching

- Stress measures to prevent infection.
- Discuss with the parents of a young patient options for physical and creative outlets, such as avoiding strenuous activity. Tell them that he may participate in less stressful activities.
- Teach the parents to watch for signs of hepatitis and iron overload.
- Refer the parents for genetic counseling if they have questions about future offspring. Also, refer adult patients with thalassemia minor and intermedia for genetic counseling; they risk transmitting thalassemia major to their children if they marry someone who has thalassemia.
- Be sure to tell patients with thalassemia minor that their condition is benign.

Thoracentesis

Thoracentesis refers to the needle aspiration of fluid or air from the pleural space. Although used primarily to determine the cause of pleural fluid accumulation, this procedure helps treat both transudative and exudative pleural effusions by removing accumulated air or fluid that results from injury or such conditions as tuberculosis or cancer. It improves pulmonary function, relieving dyspnea, tachycardia, and other symptoms. However, unless the underlying cause of the fluid accumulation is identified and corrected, pleural effusion will usually recur. Thoracentesis may also be used to instill medications into the pleural space.

Procedure

Position the patient as ordered. Usually, the patient sits on the edge of the bed, with his legs supported and his head and folded arms resting on a pillow on an overbed table. Or, have him straddle a chair backward and rest his head and folded arms on the back of the chair. If the patient is unable to sit up, turn him on the unaffected side with the arm of the affected side raised above his head. Elevate the head of the bed 30 to 45 degrees if such elevation isn't contraindicated. Proper positioning stretches the back and chest, allowing for easier access to the intercostal spaces. Remind the patient not to move suddenly, cough, or breathe deeply during the procedure to avoid puncture of the visceral pleura or lung.

Using sterile technique, open the thoracentesis tray. After draping the patient, the doctor cleans the site with an antiseptic and injects the local anesthetic into the intercostal space using a small-caliber needle. He then attaches a three-way stopcock with tubing to the aspiration needle and turns the stopcock to prevent air from entering the pleural space through the needle. The other end of the tubing is attached to a drainage bottle.

The doctor then inserts the needle into the pleural space and attaches a 50-ml syringe to the needle's stopcock. A hemostat may be used to hold the needle in place and prevent pleural tear or lung puncture. As an alternative, the doctor may introduce a Teflon catheter into the needle, remove the needle, and attach a stopcock and syringe or drainage tubing to the catheter to reduce the risk for pleural puncture by the needle.

Assist the doctor with fluid drainage, specimen collection, or medication administration, as ordered. After the needle is withdrawn, apply pressure to the puncture site with a sterile 4″ × 4″ gauze pad, followed by the application of a small sterile adhesive bandage.

Complications

Thoracentesis can cause severe complications. These include pneumothorax, tension pneumothorax, fluid reaccumulation, mediastinal shift, and hypovolemic shock. A pyogenic infection can also result if the equipment or puncture site was contaminated during the procedure. Thoracentesis should never be performed on a patient with a bleeding disorder.

Key nursing diagnoses and patient outcomes

Anxiety related to needing thoracentesis. Based on this nursing diagnosis, you'll establish these patient outcomes. The patient will:
- identify and express feelings of anxiety
- demonstrate effective coping behavior during thoracentesis, as evidenced by his ability to remain still
- report alleviation of anxiety following thoracentesis.

Impaired gas exchange related to respiratory complications. Based on this nursing diagnosis, you'll establish these patient outcomes. The patient will:
- maintain arterial blood gas values within normal limits
- have no signs and symptoms of respiratory distress
- maintain adequate ventilation.

Nursing interventions

When caring for a patient undergoing thoracentesis, your primary responsibilities include patient teaching, assisting the doctor with the procedure, and monitoring for complications during and after the procedure.

Before the procedure

- Explain the procedure to the patient. Tell him that he may feel a stinging sensation during injection of the local anesthetic and some pressure during needle insertion and fluid withdrawal. Stress the importance of remaining still during the procedure to reduce the risk of lung injury. Inform him that he'll have a chest X-ray or ultrasonography to locate the fluid.
- Assess the patient's respiratory function and take his vital signs as a baseline. If ordered, administer a sedative.
- Arrange to have a prepackaged sterile thoracentesis tray at the bedside and a chest tube setup and an oxygen source available. Also have laboratory request slips on hand in case the doctor wants specimens sent to the laboratory for analysis.

During the procedure

- Take the patient's vital signs frequently. Be alert for apprehension, cyanosis, sudden breathlessness, and tachycardia, which signal pneumothorax. Mediastinal shift may cause the patient to experience labored breathing, arrhythmias, and sudden hypotension. Sudden pleuritic chest or shoulder pain may indicate that the visceral or diaphragmatic pleurae are being irritated by the needle point.
- Monitor the amount of fluid being removed. No more than 1200 ml should be removed at one time, with no more than 1000 ml during the first 30 minutes. Removing fluids too quickly can cause hypovolemic shock and circulatory collapse.

After the procedure

- Place the patient in a comfortable position. Check his vital signs and assess his respiratory status every 15 minutes for the first hour and then as ordered.
- Tell the patient to call you immediately if he has any difficulty breathing. Watch for a persistent, irritable cough, hemoptysis, and signs of respiratory distress, which may signal pneumothorax or rapid fluid reaccumulation.
- Label the specimens properly and send them to the laboratory.
- Obtain a chest X-ray as ordered.
- Check the puncture site for excessive leakage. Be alert for signs of hypovolemic shock if a large amount of fluid was withdrawn. Notify the doctor immediately if signs occur.

Home care instructions

- Tell the patient to call his doctor if a fever develops. Contamination during thoracentesis can cause infection.
- Instruct the patient to notify his doctor if symptoms recur.

Thoracic aortic aneurysm

Characterized by abnormal widening of the ascending, transverse, or descending part of the aorta, thoracic aortic aneurysm is a potentially life-threatening disorder. This aneurysm may be saccular—an outpouching of the arterial wall with a narrow neck, involving only a portion of the vessel circumference; or fusiform—a spindle-shaped enlargement encompassing the entire aortic circumference.

Dissection of the aneurysm is the circumferential or transverse tear of the aortic wall intima, usually within the medial layer. It occurs in about 60% of patients, is usually an emergency, and has a poor prognosis. (See *Types of aortic dissection,* page 864.)

The ascending thoracic aorta is the most common site for the aneurysm, which occurs predominantly in men under age 60 who have coexisting hypertension. Descending thoracic aortic aneurysms are most common in younger patients who have had chest trauma.

Causes

Commonly, ascending thoracic aortic aneurysm results from atherosclerosis, which weakens the aortic wall and gradually distends the lumen in this area.

Descending thoracic aortic aneurysm usually occurs after blunt chest trauma that shears the aorta transversely (acceleration-deceleration injury), such as in a motor vehicle accident, or a penetrating chest injury, such as a knife wound. It also may be caused by hypertension.

Mycotic aneurysm develops from staphylococcal, streptococcal, or salmonella infections, usually at an atherosclerotic plaque.

Cystic medial necrosis caused by degeneration of the collagen and elastic fibers in the media of the aorta causes aneurysms during pregnancy and in patients with hypertension and Marfan syndrome. However, it can also be the cause without any underlying condition.

Other causes include congenital disorders, such as coarctation of the aorta, syphilis infection, and rheumatic vasculitis.

Complications

Some aneurysms progress to serious and eventually lethal complications, such as rupture of untreated thoracic dissecting aneurysm into the pericardium, with resulting cardiac tamponade.

Assessment

Thoracic aortic aneurysms fail to produce signs and symptoms until they expand and begin to dissect. Pain and other symptoms result from compression of the surrounding structures or from dissection of the aneurysm.

The patient may complain of hoarseness, dyspnea, throat pain, dysphagia, and a dry cough when a transverse aneurysm compresses the surrounding structures. Dissection of the aneurysm causes sudden pain and possibly syncope.

In dissecting ascending aneurysm, the patient may complain of pain with a boring, tearing, or ripping sensation in the thorax or the right anterior chest. It may extend to the neck, shoulders, lower back, and abdomen but seldom radiates to the jaw and arms. The pain is most intense at its onset and is often misdiagnosed as a transmural myocardial infarction (MI).

In dissecting descending aneurysm, the pain is sharp and tearing, is located between the shoulder blades, and often radiates to the chest. In dissecting transverse aneurysm, the pain is sharp, boring, and tearing and radiates to the shoulders.

In a patient with a thoracic aortic aneurysm, you may find pallor, diaphoresis, dyspnea, cyanosis, leg weakness or transient paralysis, and an abrupt onset of intermittent neurologic deficits. Palpation of peripheral pulses in dissecting ascending aneurysm may disclose abrupt loss of radial and femoral pulses and right and left carotid pulses. In dissecting descending

Types of aortic dissection

These drawings illustrate the DeBakey classification of aortic dissections (shaded areas) according to location. Dissections can also be classified by their location in relation to the aortic valve. Thus, Types I and II are proximal; Type III, distal.

Type I
In this, the most common and lethal type of dissection, intimal tearing occurs in the ascending aorta and the dissection extends into the descending aorta.

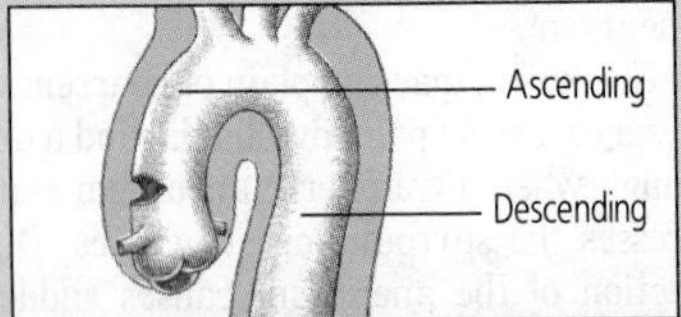

Type II
In this type of dissection, which appears most commonly with Marfan syndrome, dissection is limited to the ascending or the transverse aorta.

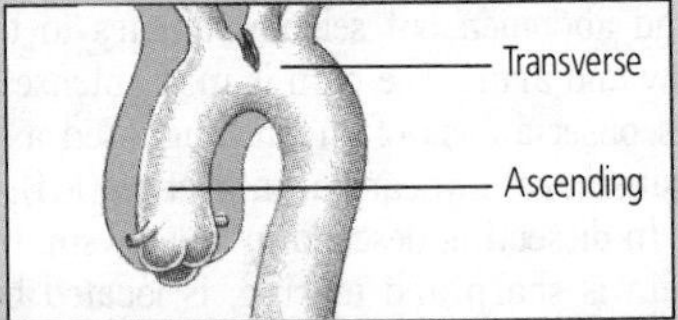

Type III
In Type III, the intimal tear is located in the descending aorta, with distal propagation of the dissection.

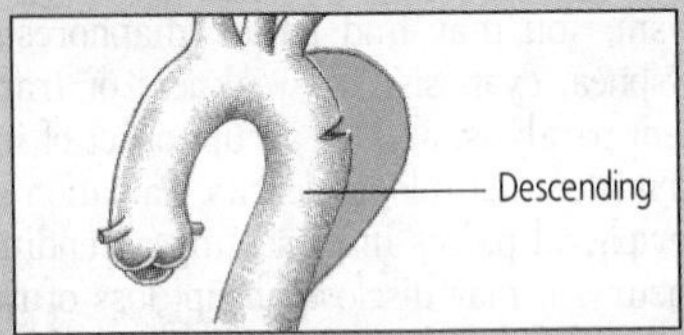

aneurysm, carotid and radial pulses may be present and bilaterally equal.

Percussion of the chest may reveal an increasing area of flatness over the heart, suggesting cardiac tamponade and hemopericardium. Auscultation of the heart in dissecting ascending aneurysm may disclose a murmur of aortic insufficiency, a diastolic murmur, and (if hemopericardium is present) a pericardial friction rub. The blood pressure may be normal or significantly elevated, with a large difference in systolic blood pressure between the right and left arms.

In dissecting descending aneurysm, systolic blood pressure will be bilaterally equal and you'll hear no murmur of aortic insufficiency or pericardial friction rub. You may detect bilateral crackles and rhonchi if pulmonary edema is present.

Diagnostic tests

In an asymptomatic patient, the diagnosis commonly occurs accidentally, through posteroanterior and oblique chest X-rays showing widening of the aorta and mediastinum. These tests help confirm the aneurysm.

- *Aortography,* the most definitive test, shows the lumen of the aneurysm, its size, and its location.
- *Magnetic resonance imaging* and a *computed tomography scan* help confirm and locate the presence of aortic dissection.
- *Electrocardiography (ECG)* helps rule out the presence of MI as the cause of the symptoms.
- *Echocardiography* may help identify dissecting aneurysm of the aortic root.
- *Hemoglobin* levels may be normal or may be decreased, due to blood loss from a leaking aneurysm.

Treatment

For long-term treatment, beta-adrenergic blockers and other agents can control hypertension and cardiac output. In an emergency, antihypertensives, such as nitroprusside; negative inotropic agents, such as labetalol; oxygen for respiratory distress; narcotics for pain; I.V. fluids; and, if needed, whole blood transfusions may be used.

In dissecting ascending aortic aneurysm – an extreme emergency – surgical resection of the aneurysm can restore normal blood flow through a Dacron or Teflon graft replacement. With aortic valve insufficiency, surgery consists of replacing the aortic valve.

Postoperative measures include careful monitoring and continuous assessment in the intensive care unit, antibiotics, insertion of endotracheal and chest tubes, ECG monitoring and, often, pulmonary artery catheterization and monitoring.

Key nursing diagnoses and patient outcomes

Decreased cardiac output related to dissecting thoracic aortic aneurysm. Based on this nursing diagnosis, you'll establish these patient outcomes. The patient will:
• maintain hemodynamic stability, as evidenced by stable vital signs and normal baseline mental status
• show no cardiac arrhythmias, syncope, or other signs and symptoms of a serious alteration in tissue perfusion
• regain normal cardiac output with effective treatment of the aneurysm.

Ineffective breathing pattern related to dissecting thoracic aortic aneurysm. Based on this nursing diagnosis, you'll establish these patient outcomes. The patient will:
• achieve maximum lung expansion with adequate ventilation
• maintain arterial blood gas levels within normal limits
• show no signs and symptoms of severe tissue hypoxia.

Pain related to dissecting thoracic aortic aneurysm. Based on this nursing diagnosis, you'll establish these patient outcomes. The patient will:
• express feelings of comfort following analgesic administration
• become pain free following vascular repair of the aneurysm.

Nursing interventions

• In a nonemergency situation when a patient is diagnosed with a thoracic aneurysm, allow him to express his fears and concerns. Help him identify and use effective coping strategies.
• Offer the patient and family psychological support. Answer all questions honestly and provide reassurance.
• In an acute situation, give analgesics to relieve pain, as ordered. Administer dextrose 5% in water or lactated Ringer's solution, and give antibiotics, as ordered. Administer nitroprusside I.V.; use a separate I.V. line for infusion. Adjust the dose by slowly increasing the infusion rate. With suspected bleeding from an aneurysm, give whole blood transfusions as ordered.
• Prepare the patient for vascular repair of a thoracic aneurysm, as indicated. (See the entry "Vascular repair.")

Monitoring

• In an acute situation, monitor blood pressure, pulmonary capillary wedge pressure, and central venous pressure. Assess pain, breathing, and carotid, radial, and femoral pulses.
• Make sure laboratory tests include a complete blood count with differential, electrolyte measurements, typing and crossmatching for whole blood, arterial blood gas analyses, and urinalysis.
• Insert an indwelling urinary catheter to monitor hourly outputs.
• If nitroprusside is administered, check the patient's blood pressure every 5 minutes until it stabilizes.

Patient teaching

• Explain any diagnostic tests. If surgery is scheduled, explain the procedure and expected postoperative care (I.V. lines, endotracheal and drainage tubes, cardiac monitoring, ventilation).
• Before discharge, ensure compliance with antihypertensive therapy by explaining the need for such drugs, and list their expected adverse effects. Teach the patient

how to monitor his blood pressure. Refer him to community agencies for continued support and assistance as needed.
• Direct the patient to call the doctor immediately if he has any sharp pain in the chest or back of the neck.

Thoracotomy

A surgical incision into the thoracic cavity, a thoracotomy is done to locate and examine abnormalities such as tumors, bleeding sites, or thoracic injuries; to perform a biopsy; or to remove diseased lung tissue. This procedure is most often performed to remove part or all of a lung to spare healthy lung tissue from disease. Lung excision may involve pneumonectomy, lobectomy, segmental resection, or wedge resection.

A pneumonectomy is the excision of an entire lung. It is usually performed to treat bronchogenic cancer but may also be used to treat tuberculosis, bronchiectasis, or lung abscess. It's used only when a less radical approach can't remove all diseased tissue. After pneumonectomy, chest cavity pressures stabilize and, over time, fluid fills the cavity where lung tissue was removed, preventing significant mediastinal shift.

The removal of one of the five long lobes, lobectomy can treat bronchogenic cancer, tuberculosis, lung abscess, emphysematous blebs or bullae, benign tumors, or localized fungal infections. After this surgery, the remaining lobes expand to fill the entire pleural cavity.

Segmental resection is the removal of one or more lung segments and preserves more functional tissue than lobectomy. It's commonly used to treat bronchiectasis. Remaining lung tissue needs to be reexpanded.

The removal of a small portion of the lung without regard to segments, wedge resection preserves the most functional tissue of all the surgeries but can treat only a small, well-circumscribed lesion. Remaining lung tissue needs to be reexpanded. (See *Understanding types of lung excision.*)

Other types of thoracotomy include the following.
• *Exploratory thoracotomy* is done to examine the chest and pleural space in evaluating chest trauma and tumors.
• *Decortication* is used to help reexpand the lung in a patient with empyema. It involves the removal or stripping of the thick, fibrous membrane covering the visceral pleura.
• *Thoracoplasty* is performed to remove part or all of one rib and reduce the size of the chest cavity. It decreases the risk of mediastinal shift when tuberculosis has reduced lung volume.

Procedure

After the patient is anesthetized, the surgeon performs a thoracotomy using one of three approaches. In a posterolateral thoracotomy, the incision starts in the submammary fold of the anterior chest, is drawn below the scapular tip and along the ribs, and then is curved posteriorly and up to the spine of the scapula. Any type of lung excision calls for a posterolateral incision through the fourth, fifth, sixth, or seventh intercostal space.

In an anterolateral thoracotomy, the incision begins below the breast and above the costal margins, extending from the anterior axillary line and then turning downward to avoid the axillary apex. A median sternotomy involves a straight incision from the suprasternal notch to below the xiphoid process and requires the sternum to be transected with an electric or air-driven saw.

Once the incision is made, the surgeon takes a biopsy, locates and ties off sources of bleeding, locates and repairs injuries within the thoracic cavity, or spreads the ribs and exposes the lung area for excision. If he's performing a pneumonectomy, he

Understanding types of lung excision

Pneumonectomy

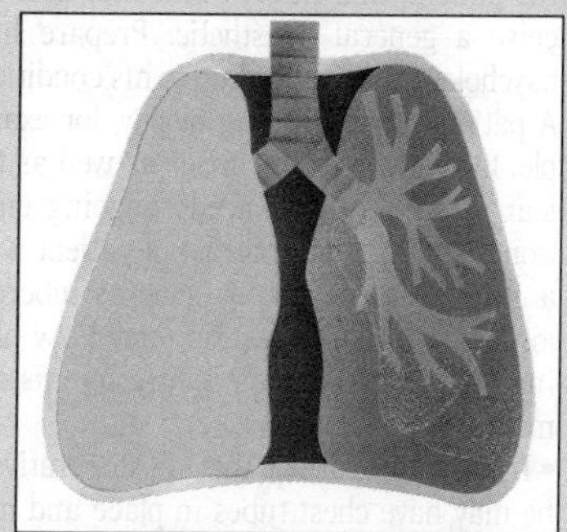

Lobectomy

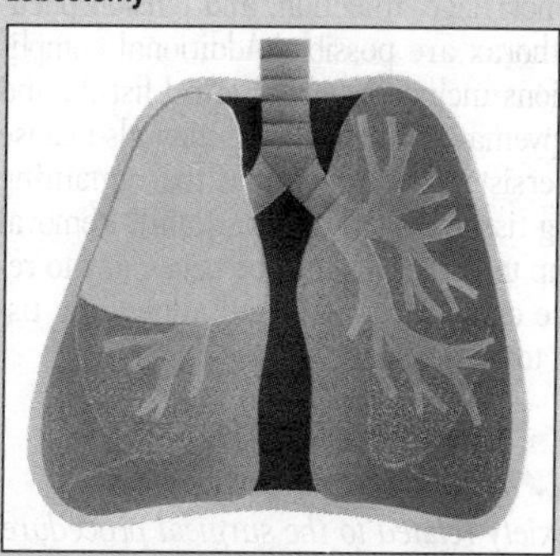

Segmental resection

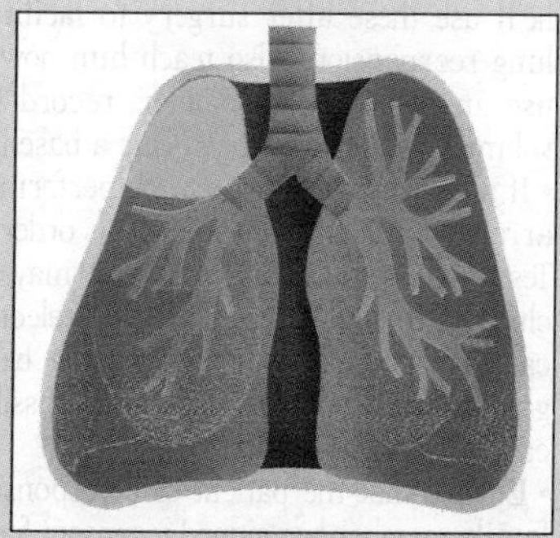

Wedge resection

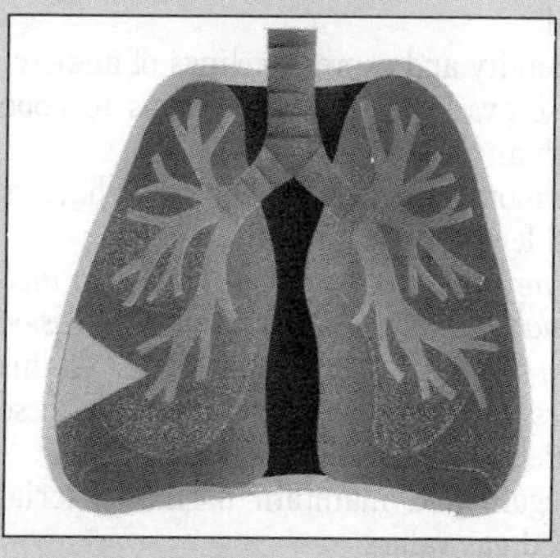

ligates and severs the pulmonary arteries. Next, he clamps the mainstem bronchus leading to the affected lung, divides it, and then closes it with nonabsorbable sutures or staples. He then removes the lung. To ensure airtight closure, he places a pleural flap over the bronchus and closes it. Then, he severs the phrenic nerve on the affected side, allowing it to reduce the size of the pleural cavity. After air pressure in the cavity stabilizes, he closes the chest.

In a lobectomy, the surgeon resects the affected lobe and ligates and severs the appropriate arteries, veins, and bronchial passages. He may insert one or two chest tubes for drainage and to aid lung reexpansion.

In a segmental resection, the surgeon removes the affected segment and ligates and severs the appropriate artery, vein, and bronchus. In a wedge resection, he clamps and excises the affected area and then sutures it. In both resections, he inserts two chest tubes to aid lung reexpansion.

After completing the procedure requiring the thoracotomy, the surgeon closes the chest cavity and applies a dressing.

Complications

Hemorrhage, infection, and tension pneumothorax are possible. Additional complications include bronchopleural fistula and empyema. A lung excision may also cause a persistent air space that the remaining lung tissue doesn't expand to fill. Removal of up to three ribs may be necessary to reduce chest cavity size and allow lung tissue to fit the space.

Key nursing diagnoses and patient outcomes

Anxiety related to the surgical procedure. Based on this nursing diagnosis, you'll establish these patient outcomes. The patient will:
- identify and express feelings of anxiety
- use available support systems to cope with anxiety
- demonstrate healthy coping behaviors and fewer physical signs of anxiety.

Impaired gas exchange related to mismatch between ventilation and perfusion as a result of a thoracotomy. Based on this nursing diagnosis, you'll establish these patient outcomes. The patient will:
- regain and maintain normal arterial blood gas values
- demonstrate maximal lung expansion, as shown on a chest X-ray
- show no signs and symptoms of respiratory distress.

Ineffective airway clearance related to pain caused by thoracotomy. Based on this nursing diagnosis, you'll establish these patient outcomes. The patient will:
- maintain a patent airway
- demonstrate effective deep-breathing and coughing exercises
- be able to expectorate sputum effectively.

Nursing interventions

When caring for a patient undergoing a thoracotomy, your main responsibilities include patient teaching and postoperative care and monitoring.

Before surgery

- Explain the thoracotomy procedure to the patient, and inform him that he'll receive a general anesthetic. Prepare him psychologically, according to his condition. A patient having a lung biopsy, for example, faces the fear of cancer as well as the fear of surgery and needs ongoing emotional support. In contrast, a patient with a chronic lung disorder, such as tuberculosis or a fungal infection, may view having a lung excision as a cure for his ailment.
- Inform the patient that, postoperatively, he may have chest tubes in place and may receive oxygen. Teach him coughing and deep-breathing techniques. Explain that he'll use these after surgery to facilitate lung reexpansion. Also teach him how to use an incentive spirometer; record the volumes he achieves to provide a baseline.
- If a pneumonectomy is to be performed, arrange for laboratory studies, as ordered. Tests to assess cardiac function may include pulmonary function tests, electrocardiography, chest X-ray, arterial blood gas analysis, bronchoscopy and, possibly, cardiac catheterization.
- Ensure that the patient or a responsible family member has signed a consent form.

After surgery

- If the patient had a pneumonectomy, make sure he lies only on his operative side or his back until he's stabilized. This prevents fluid from draining into the unaffected lung if the sutured bronchus opens.
- If the patient has a chest tube in place, make sure it's functioning and monitor him for signs of tension pneumothorax, such as dyspnea, chest pain, an irritating cough, vertigo, syncope, or anxiety. If the patient develops any of these signs or symptoms, pal-

pate his neck, face, and chest wall for subcutaneous emphysema and palpate his trachea for deviation from midline. Auscultate his lungs for decreased or absent breath sounds on the affected side. Then, percuss them for hyperresonance. If you suspect tension pneumothorax, notify the doctor at once and help him to identify the cause.
- Provide analgesics, as ordered.
- Have the patient begin coughing, deep-breathing exercises, and incentive spirometry as soon as he's stabilized. Auscultate his lungs, place him in semi-Fowler's position, and have him splint his incision to facilitate coughing and deep breathing. Have him cough every 2 to 4 hours until his breath sounds clear.
- Perform passive range-of-motion (ROM) exercises the evening of surgery and two or three times daily thereafter. Progress to active ROM exercises.

Home care instructions

- Tell the patient to continue his coughing and deep-breathing exercises to prevent complications. Advise him to report any changes in sputum characteristics to his doctor.
- Instruct the patient to continue performing ROM exercises to maintain mobility of his shoulder and chest wall.
- Tell the patient to avoid contact with people who have upper respiratory tract infections and to refrain from smoking.
- Provide the patient with instructions for wound care and dressing changes and refer to home health care, as needed.

Thrombocytopenia

The most common cause of hemorrhagic disorders, thrombocytopenia is characterized by a deficient number of circulating platelets. Because platelets play a vital role in coagulation, this disease poses a serious threat to hemostasis. The prognosis is excellent in drug-induced thrombocytopenia if the offending drug is withdrawn; in such cases, recovery may be immediate. Otherwise, the prognosis depends on the patient's response to treatment of the underlying cause.

Causes

Thrombocytopenia may be congenital or acquired; the acquired form is more common. In either case, it usually results from decreased or defective production of platelets in the marrow (for example, in leukemia, aplastic anemia, and toxicity with certain drugs) or from increased destruction outside the marrow caused by an underlying disorder (such as cirrhosis of the liver, disseminated intravascular coagulation, and severe infection).

Less commonly, thrombocytopenia results from sequestration (hypersplenism, hypothermia) or platelet loss. Acquired thrombocytopenia may result from the use of certain drugs, such as quinine, quinidine, rifampin, heparin, nonsteroidal anti-inflammatory drugs, histamine blockers, most chemotherapeutic agents, allopurinol, and alcohol.

Thrombocytopenia may also occur transiently after a viral infection (such as Epstein-Barr) or infectious mononucleosis. (See *Causes of decreased circulating platelets,* page 898.) An idiopathic form of thrombocytopenia also occurs. (See the entry "Idiopathic thrombocytopenic purpura.")

Complications

Complications of thrombocytopenia are usually related to bleeding. Severe thrombocytopenia can cause acute hemorrhage, which may be fatal without immediate therapy. The most common sites of severe bleeding include the brain and the GI tract, although intrapulmonary bleeding and cardiac tamponade can also occur.

Assessment

Typically, a patient with thrombocytopenia reports sudden onset of petechiae and ecchymoses from bleeding into mu-

Causes of decreased circulating platelets

Thrombocytopenia usually results from insufficient production or increased peripheral destruction of platelets. Less commonly, it results from sequestration or platelet loss.

Diminished or defective platelet production

Congenital
- Wiskott-Aldrich syndrome
- Maternal ingestion of thiazides
- Neonatal rubella
- Polycythemia

Acquired
- Aplastic anemia
- Marrow infiltration (acute and chronic leukemias, tumor)
- Nutritional deficiency (vitamin B_{12}, folic acid)
- Myelosuppressant agents
- Drugs that directly influence platelet production (thiazides, alcohol, hormones)
- Radiation
- Viral infections (measles, dengue)

Increased peripheral destruction

Congenital
- Nonimmune (prematurity, erythroblastosis fetalis, infection)
- Immune (drug sensitivity, maternal idiopathic thrombocytopenic purpura [ITP])

Acquired
- Nonimmune (infection, disseminated intravascular coagulation, thrombotic thrombocytopenic purpura)
- Immune (drug-induced, especially with quinine and quinidine; posttransfusion purpura; acute and chronic ITP; sepsis; alcohol)
- Invasive lines or devices (intra-aortic balloon pump, prosthetic cardiac valves)

Sequestration of platelets
- Hypersplenism
- Hypothermia

Platelet loss
- Hemorrhage
- Extracorporeal perfusion

cous membranes (GI, urinary, vaginal, or respiratory). He may also complain of malaise, fatigue, and general weakness (with or without accompanying blood loss). In acquired thrombocytopenia, the patient's history may include the use of one or several offending drugs.

Inspection typically reveals evidence of bleeding (petechiae, ecchymoses), along with slow, continuous bleeding from any injuries or wounds. Painless, round, and as tiny as pinpoints (1 to 3 mm in diameter), petechiae usually occur on dependent portions of the body, appearing and fading in crops and sometimes grouping to form ecchymoses. Another form of blood leakage and larger than petechiae, ecchymoses are purple, blue, or yellow-green bruises that vary in size and shape. They can occur anywhere on the body from traumatic injury. In patients with bleeding disorders, they usually appear on the arms and legs. In adults, inspection may reveal large, blood-filled bullae in the mouth. Gentle palpation of edematous ecchymotic areas may cause pain, indicating that these areas are actually hematomas. Superficial hematomas are red; deep hematomas are blue. They typically exceed 1 cm in diameter.

If the patient's platelet count is between 30,000 and 50,000/mm³, expect bruising with minor trauma; if it's between 15,000 and 30,000/mm³, expect spontaneous bruising and petechiae, mostly on the arms and legs. With a platelet count below 15,000/mm³, expect spontaneous bruising or, after minor trauma, mucosal bleeding, generalized purpura, epistaxis, hematuria, and GI or intracranial bleeding. Female patients may report menorrhagia.

Diagnostic tests

The following laboratory findings help establish a diagnosis of thrombocytopenia:
- diminished platelet count (less than 100,000/mm³)
- prolonged bleeding time (although this doesn't always indicate platelet quality)
- normal prothrombin and partial thromboplastin times.

Platelet antibody studies can help determine why the platelet count is low and help direct treatment. Platelet survival studies help differentiate between ineffective platelet production and inappropriate platelet destruction. (Platelet production disorders may occur after radiation exposure, medication ingestion, or an infectious disease. They may also occur idiopathically. Inappropriate platelet destruction may occur with splenic disease and platelet antibody disorders.)

In severe thrombocytopenia, a bone marrow study determines the number, size, and cytoplasmic maturity of the megakaryocytes (the bone marrow cells that release mature platelets). This information may identify ineffective platelet production as the cause of thrombocytopenia and rule out a malignant disease process.

Treatment

Removal of the offending agents in drug-induced thrombocytopenia or proper treatment of the underlying cause (when possible) is essential. Corticosteroids may be used to increase platelet production. Lithium carbonate or folate may also be used to stimulate bone marrow production of platelets. In cases of severe or refractory thrombocytopenia, I.V. gamma globulin has been used experimentally with moderate success.

Platelet transfusions may be used to stop episodic abnormal bleeding caused by a low platelet count. However, if platelet destruction results from an immune disorder, platelet infusions may have only a minimal effect and may be reserved for life-threatening bleeding.

Splenectomy may be necessary to correct thrombocytopenia caused by platelet destruction. A splenectomy should significantly reduce platelet destruction because the spleen acts as the primary site of platelet removal and antibody production.

Key nursing diagnoses and patient outcomes

Altered protection related to decreased platelet count. Based on this nursing diagnosis, you'll establish these patient outcomes. The patient will:
- communicate an understanding of the importance of taking bleeding precautions
- identify bleeding precautions to incorporate into his daily life
- demonstrate skill in carrying out bleeding precautions, as evidenced by a decrease in bleeding episodes or in the number of ecchymoses and hematomas.

Fatigue related to blood loss. Based on this nursing diagnosis, you'll establish these patient outcomes. The patient will:
- explain the relationship between fatigue, thrombocytopenia, and his activity level
- employ measures to prevent and modify fatigue
- express a feeling of increased energy with effective management of thrombocytopenia.

Knowledge deficit related to management of thrombocytopenia. Based on this nursing diagnosis, you'll establish these patient outcomes. The patient will:
- identify the need to learn how to manage thrombocytopenia
- obtain information on thrombocytopenia management from appropriate sources
- communicate an understanding of thrombocytopenia management.

Nursing interventions

- Provide emotional support as necessary. Encourage the patient to discuss his concerns about his condition. Reassure him

that the ecchymoses and petechiae will heal as the disease resolves.
• Provide rest periods between activities if the patient tires easily.
• If the patient has painful hematomas, handle the area gently. Protect all areas of ecchymosis and petechia from further injury.
• Take every possible precaution against bleeding. Protect the patient from trauma. Keep the bed's side rails raised, and pad them if possible. Promote the use of an electric razor and a soft toothbrush. Avoid invasive procedures, such as venipuncture or urinary catheterization, if possible. When venipuncture is unavoidable, exert pressure on the puncture site for at least 20 minutes or until the bleeding stops.
• During active bleeding, maintain the patient on strict bed rest. Keep the head of the bed elevated to prevent gravity-related pressure increases, that may lead to intracranial bleeding.
• When administering platelet concentrate, remember that platelets are extremely fragile; infuse them quickly, using the administration set recommended by the blood bank.
• Be aware that human leukocyte antigen (HLA)-typed platelets may be ordered to prevent febrile reaction. If the patient has a history of minor reactions, he may benefit from acetaminophen and diphenhydramine before the transfusion.

Monitoring

• Monitor platelet count daily.
• Watch for bleeding (petechiae, ecchymoses, surgical or GI bleeding, menorrhagia). Identify the amount of bleeding or the size of ecchymoses at least every 24 hours. Test stool, urine, and emesis for blood.
• During platelet transfusion, monitor for a febrile reaction (flushing, chills, fever, headache, tachycardia, hypertension). Such reactions are common, and a fever will destroy the blood products.
• One to 2 hours after administering platelet concentrate, monitor the patient's platelet count to assess his response to the infusion. A lack of platelet level increase indicates that the patient is making platelet antibodies and should receive HLA-matched platelets.

Patient teaching

• Teach the patient about his disorder and its cause, if known. If appropriate, reassure the patient that thrombocytopenia often resolves spontaneously.
• Teach the patient to recognize and report menorrhagia, gingival or urinary tract bleeding, signs of intracranial bleeding (persistent headache, mood change, nausea, vomiting, and drowsiness), and other signs of bleeding (tarry stools, coffee-ground vomitus, and epistaxis.)
• Teach the patient how to control local bleeding. (See *Agents to control local bleeding.*)
• Advise the patient to avoid straining during defecation or coughing; both can lead to increased intracranial pressure, possibly causing cerebral hemorrhage. Provide a stool softener, if necessary, because constipation and passage of hard stools are likely to tear the rectal mucosa and cause bleeding.
• Discuss the diagnostic tests that may be performed throughout the course of the disease.
• Explain the function of platelets. Warn the patient that the lower his platelet count falls, the more cautious he'll have to be in his activities. Be sure he understands that in severe thrombocytopenia, even minor bumps or scrapes may result in bleeding.
• If thrombocytopenia is drug induced, stress the importance of avoiding the offending drug.
• If the patient must receive long-term steroid therapy, teach him to watch for and report cushingoid symptoms. Emphasize that corticosteroids must be discontinued gradually. While the patient is receiving corticosteroid therapy, monitor his fluid and electrolyte balance and watch for infection, pathologic fractures, and mood changes.

Agents to control local bleeding

The following agents may be used at home and in the hospital to control local bleeding and capillary oozing.

Agents for home use

Let your patient know about preparations that may be used at home, such as absorbable gelatin sponges (Gelfoam) or ice packs.

If the doctor recommends Gelfoam to stop the bleeding from a puncture wound (venipuncture or tooth extraction, for example), tell the patient to saturate this foamlike wafer with an isotonic saline or a thrombin solution. Instruct him to place the sponge on the bleeding site and apply pressure for 10 to 15 seconds. Advise him to keep the sponge in place after the bleeding stops. Explain that this agent, which holds many times its weight in blood, can be systemically absorbed.

If the patient bleeds from a blood vessel or into a joint (hemarthrosis), instruct him to elevate the bleeding part and apply an ice pack to the site until the bleeding subsides.

Inform the patient that Negatan – an astringent and protein denaturant – may be applied to oral ulcers. Tell him first to clean and dry the ulcer and then to apply the preparation for 1 minute. Next, he should neutralize the area with large amounts of water. Because the agent may burn or sting, a topical anesthetic may be applied first.

Agents for hospital use

Inform the surgical patient that bleeding can be controlled with such agents as oxidized cellulose (Surgicel), microfibrillar collagen hemostat (Avitene), or thrombin (Thrombinar).

Surgicel, for instance, helps to control surgical bleeding or external bleeding at open wounds. This agent may remain in place until hemostasis occurs. The caregiver then irrigates it (to prevent fresh bleeding) and removes it with sterile forceps.

Another agent, Thrombinar, may be used during surgery or for GI bleeding. The caregiver mixes Thrombinar with sterile isotonic saline solution or sterile distilled water and applies it to the wound. Or, she mixes the agent with milk, which the patient drinks to control GI bleeding. Some patients react to Thrombinar with hypersensitivity and fever.

- Warn the patient to avoid taking aspirin in any form as well as other drugs that impair coagulation. Teach him how to recognize aspirin compounds and nonsteroidal anti-inflammatory drugs listed on labels of over-the-counter remedies.
- If the patient experiences frequent nosebleeds, recommend that he use a humidifier at night. Also suggest that he moisten his inner nostrils twice a day with an anti-infective ointment.
- Teach the patient to monitor his condition by examining his skin for ecchymoses and petechiae. Instruct him how to test his stools for occult blood.
- Advise the patient to carry medical identification stating that he has thrombocytopenia.

Thrombolytic therapy

The thrombolytic drugs streptokinase, urokinase, alteplase, and anistreplase, along with a promising new investigational drug – single-chain urokinase-type plasminogen activator – provide rapid correction of acute and extensive thrombotic disorders. The Food and Drug Administration has approved these drugs for treating certain thromboembolic disorders, such as acute pulmonary emboli and coronary thrombi. In addition, these drugs may be used to dissolve thrombi in arteriovenous catheters, thereby restoring blood flow. They're the drugs of choice to break down newly formed thrombi.

Except for urokinase, thrombolytic drugs can be given by intracoronary infusion early in acute myocardial infarction to open an occluded coronary artery and prevent primary or secondary thrombus formation in the vessels surrounding the necrotic area, thus minimizing myocardial damage. They seem most effective when given immediately after thrombosis within 6 hours after the onset of symptoms. Streptokinase also helps dissolve acute deep-vein and arterial thrombi.

Thrombolytic drugs work by converting plasminogen to the enzyme plasmin, which lyses thrombi, fibrinogen, and other plasma proteins.

Procedure

Thrombolytic drugs, except for urokinase, can be given by intracoronary infusion. Urokinase must be given by I.V. infusion.

Complications

The major hazards of thrombolytic therapy are bleeding and allergic responses, especially with streptokinase and anistreplase. Resistance to streptokinase may also occur with repeated use. As the myocardium becomes reperfused, arrhythmias may occur.

Key nursing diagnoses and patient outcomes

Anxiety related to therapy and the potential for severe complications. Based on this nursing diagnosis, you'll establish these outcomes. The patient will:
- identify and express feelings of anxiety
- obtain information about thrombolytic therapy from appropriate sources to help allay his fears
- show decreased physical signs of fear.

Decreased cardiac output related to reperfusion arrhythmias. Based on this nursing diagnosis, you'll establish these outcomes. The patient will:
- maintain hemodynamic stability
- show no arrhythmias on an electrocardiogram (ECG)
- regain and maintain an adequate cardiac output.

Risk for fluid volume deficit related to potential for bleeding. Based on this nursing diagnosis, you'll establish these outcomes. The patient will:
- have normal fluid and blood volume, as evidenced by stable vital signs and input that equals or exceeds output
- show no signs and symptoms of bleeding.

Nursing interventions

When caring for a patient undergoing thrombolytic therapy, your main responsibility is monitoring for adverse reactions.

Before therapy

- Before thrombolytic therapy is given, draw serum samples for blood typing and crossmatching and for determination of prothrombin time and partial thromboplastin time. Obtain a baseline ECG and electrolyte, arterial blood gas, blood urea nitrogen, creatinine, and cardiac enzyme levels. Check subsequent findings against these baselines regularly throughout therapy.

During therapy

- At the start of therapy, watch for signs of hypersensitivity: hypotension, shortness of breath, wheezing, a feeling of tightness and pressure in the chest, and angioedema. Keep emergency resuscitation equipment readily available.
- Throughout therapy, continuously monitor the ECG and compare it with baseline readings to detect possible arrhythmias. Inform the doctor of any abnormalities, and be prepared to administer lidocaine or procainamide, as ordered.

• Carefully assess the patient for signs of bleeding. Monitor him every 15 minutes for the first hour, every 30 minutes for the next 7 hours, and then once every 8 hours thereafter. If you detect bleeding, stop therapy and notify the doctor. Ensure that packed red blood cells, whole blood, and aminocaproic acid are readily available to treat possible hemorrhage.
• Check the patient's vital signs frequently, and monitor pulses, color, and sensory function in the extremities every hour.
• Because the patient is prone to bruising during therapy, handle him gently and as little as possible. Keep invasive procedures and venipunctures to a minimum, and pad the side rails of his bed to prevent injury.

After therapy

• Expect to administer anticoagulants to prevent recurrence of thromboses.

Thrombophlebitis

An acute condition characterized by inflammation and thrombus formation, thrombophlebitis may occur in deep or superficial veins. It typically occurs at the valve cusps because venous stasis encourages the accumulation and adherence of platelets and fibrin. Thrombophlebitis usually begins with localized inflammation alone (phlebitis), but such inflammation rapidly provokes thrombus formation. Rarely, venous thrombosis develops without associated inflammation of the vein (phlebothrombosis).

Deep vein thrombophlebitis affects small veins, such as the lesser saphenous vein, or large veins, such as the iliac, femoral, and popliteal veins and the vena cava. It is more serious than superficial vein thrombophlebitis because it affects the veins deep in the leg musculature that carry 90% of the venous outflow from the leg. The incidence of deep vein thrombophlebitis involving the subclavian vein is rising with the increased use of subclavian vein catheters.

Some studies indicate that up to 35% of hospitalized patients develop deep vein thrombophlebitis. Some hospitalized patients are more at risk than others; however, the risk of developing deep vein thrombophlebitis increases dramatically after age 40 and triples with each additional 20 years.

Superficial vein thrombophlebitis is usually self-limiting and, because these veins have fewer valves than the deep veins, is less likely to cause complications.

Causes

Virchow, in 1846, identified three major factors that promote development of venous thrombosis. Known as Virchow's triad, they are hypercoagulability, venous stasis, and intimal damage.

Deep vein thrombophlebitis may be idiopathic, but it is more likely to occur in the presence of certain diseases, treatments, injuries, or other factors, such as the following:
• hypercoagulable states – cigarette smoking; circulating lupus anticoagulant; deficiencies of antithrombin III, protein C, or protein S; disseminated intravascular coagulation; estrogen use; dysfibrinogenemia; myeloproliferative diseases; systemic infection
• intimal damage – infection, infusion of irritating I.V. solutions, trauma, venipuncture
• neoplasms – lung, ovary, pancreas, stomach, testicles, urinary tract
• surgery – abdominal, genitourinary, orthopedic, thoracic
• fracture – spine, pelvis, femur, or tibia
• venous stasis – acute myocardial infarction, congestive heart failure, dehydration, immobility, incompetent vein valves, postoperative convalescence, cerebrovascular accident
• venulitis – Behçet's disease, homocystinuria, thromboangiitis obliterans
• other – pregnancy, previous deep vein thrombosis.

EXPERT GERIATRIC CARE

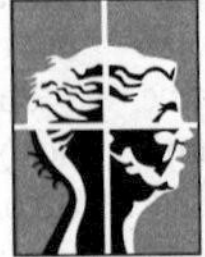

Managing chronic venous insufficiency

Chronic venous insufficiency results from the valvular destruction of deep vein thrombophlebitis, usually in the iliac and femoral veins and sometimes in the saphenous veins. It often occurs with incompetence of the communicating veins of the ankle, causing increased venous pressure and fluid migration into the interstitial tissue. Because of age-related changes in the vasculature, the elderly are at high risk for developing chronic venous insufficiency.

Signs and symptoms

Chronic swelling of the affected leg occurs from edema, leading to tissue fibrosis and induration; skin discoloration from extravasation of blood in subcutaneous tissue; and stasis ulcers around the ankle. Because the skin is very friable and can easily break down, ulcers in the elderly may take longer to heal.

Treatment

Therapy for small stasis ulcers consists of bed rest, elevation of the legs, warm soaks, and antibiotics for infection.

Increased venous pressure, due to reflux from the deep venous system to superficial veins, may be treated with compression dressings, such as a sponge rubber pressure dressing or a zinc gelatin boot (Unna's boot), after massive swelling subsides.

Large stasis ulcers unresponsive to conservative treatment may require excision and skin grafting.

Complications

The major complications of thrombophlebitis are pulmonary embolism and chronic venous insufficiency. (See *Managing chronic venous insufficiency.*)

Assessment

Clinical features vary with the site of inflammation and length of the affected vein. Patients with deep vein thrombophlebitis may be asymptomatic or may complain of some tenderness, aching, or severe pain in the affected leg or arm; fever; chills; and malaise. Complete your physical examination carefully because much of the patient's subsequent care will depend on your findings.

Inspection may reveal redness, swelling, and cyanosis of the affected leg or arm. Some patients with deep vein thrombophlebitis of a leg vein may have a positive Homans' sign (pain on dorsiflexion of the foot), but this is unreliable. A positive cuff sign (elicited by inflating a blood pressure cuff until pain occurs) may be present in deep vein thrombophlebitis of the arm or leg. When palpated, the affected leg or arm may feel warm.

Patients with superficial vein thrombophlebitis may also be asymptomatic or complain of pain localized to the thrombus site. Inspection may disclose redness and swelling at the site and surrounding area. When palpated, the area feels warm, and a tender, hard cord extends over the affected vein's length.

Diagnostic tests

Diagnosis must rule out arterial occlusive disease, lymphangitis, cellulitis, and myositis. Diagnosis of superficial vein thrombophlebitis is based on physical findings; diagnosis of deep vein thrombophlebitis is based on these characteristic test findings.

• *Doppler ultrasonography* identifies reduced blood flow to a specific area and any

obstruction to venous flow, particularly in iliofemoral deep vein thrombophlebitis.
• *Plethysmography* shows decreased circulation distal to the affected area; it's more sensitive than ultrasonography in detecting deep vein thrombophlebitis.
• *Phlebography* usually confirms the diagnosis and shows filling defects and diverted blood flow.

Treatment

In deep vein thrombophlebitis, treatment includes bed rest, with elevation of the affected arm or leg; application of warm, moist compresses to the affected area; and analgesics. After the acute episode subsides, the patient may begin to ambulate while wearing antiembolism stockings (applied before he gets out of bed).

Treatment may include anticoagulants (initially, heparin; later, warfarin) to prolong clotting time. However, the full anticoagulant dose must be discontinued during any surgery to avoid the risk of hemorrhage. After some types of surgery, especially major abdominal or pelvic operations, prophylactic doses of anticoagulants may reduce the risk of deep vein thrombophlebitis.

For lysis of acute, extensive deep vein thrombophlebitis, treatment should include streptokinase or urokinase if the risk of bleeding doesn't outweigh the potential benefits of thrombolytic treatment.

Rarely, deep vein thrombophlebitis may cause complete venous occlusion, which necessitates venous interruption through simple ligation to vein plication, or clipping. Embolectomy may be done if clots are being shed to the pulmonary and systemic vasculature and other treatment is unsuccessful. Caval interruption with transvenous placement of an umbrella filter can trap emboli, preventing them from traveling to the pulmonary vasculature.

Therapy for severe superficial vein thrombophlebitis may include an anti-inflammatory drug, such as indomethacin, along with antiembolism stockings, warm compresses, and elevation of the patient's leg.

Key nursing diagnoses and patient outcomes

Altered protection related to increased risk of bleeding caused by anticoagulant therapy. Based on this nursing diagnosis, you'll establish these patient outcomes. The patient will:
• communicate an understanding of bleeding precautions
• incorporate bleeding precautions into daily living
• show no signs and symptoms suggestive of bleeding.

Risk for injury related to potential for pulmonary emboli. Based on this nursing diagnosis, you'll establish these patient outcomes. The patient will:
• identify the signs and symptoms of pulmonary emboli and report any occurrence immediately
• maintain adequate ventilation
• not develop a pulmonary emboli.

Pain related to inflammation of vessel wall. Based on this nursing diagnosis, you'll establish these patient outcomes. The patient will:
• express feelings of comfort following analgesic administration
• use bed rest and the application of warm compresses to reduce inflammation and, thus, pain
• report the alleviation of pain when thrombophlebitis is eradicated.

Nursing interventions

• Enforce bed rest, as ordered, and elevate the patient's affected arm or leg. If you plan to use pillows for elevating the leg, place them so they support its entire length to avoid compressing the popliteal space.
• Apply warm compresses or a covered aquamatic K pad to increase circulation to the affected area and to relieve pain and inflammation. Give analgesics to relieve pain, as ordered.
• Administer heparin I.V., as ordered, with an infusion monitor or pump to control the flow rate, if necessary.

• To prevent thrombophlebitis in high-risk patients, perform range-of-motion exercises while the patient is on bed rest, use intermittent pneumatic calf massage during lengthy surgical or diagnostic procedures, apply antiembolism stockings postoperatively, and encourage early ambulation.

Monitoring

• Mark, measure, and record the circumference of the affected arm or leg daily, and compare this measurement with that of the other arm or leg. To ensure accuracy and consistency of serial measurements, mark the skin over the area and measure at the same spot daily.
• Measure partial thromboplastin time regularly for the patient on heparin therapy. Measure prothrombin time for the patient on warfarin (therapeutic anticoagulation values for both are one and one-half to two times control values).
• Watch for signs and symptoms of bleeding, such as tarry stools, coffee-ground vomitus, and ecchymoses. Watch for oozing of blood at I.V. sites, and assess gums for excessive bleeding.
• Be alert for signs of pulmonary emboli (crackles, dyspnea, hemoptysis, sudden changes in mental status, restlessness, and hypotension).

Patient teaching

• Before discharge, emphasize the importance of follow-up blood studies to monitor anticoagulant therapy.
• If the patient is being discharged on heparin therapy, teach him or his family how to give subcutaneous injections. If he requires further assistance, arrange for a home health care nurse.
• Tell the patient to avoid prolonged sitting or standing to help prevent a recurrence.
• Teach the patient how to properly apply and use antiembolism stockings. Tell him to report any complications, such as cold, blue toes.
• To prevent bleeding, encourage the patient to use an electric razor and to avoid medications that contain aspirin.

Thyroid cancer

Although thyroid cancer occurs in all age groups, patients who have had radiation therapy in the neck area are especially susceptible. Before the 1950s, radiation therapy was commonly given to children to shrink enlarged thymus glands, tonsils, or adenoids and to treat acne and other skin disorders. About 25% of those who had these treatments later developed thyroid nodules; 25% of those nodules became malignant.

The risk of developing a malignant tumor after radiation correlates with the dose (a threshold dose has not been defined) and the patient's age (a malignant tumor is rare in patients who begin radiation therapy after age 21). Papillary and follicular carcinomas are the most common forms of thyroid cancers and are usually associated with the longest survival times.

Papillary carcinoma accounts for about 60% of thyroid cancer cases in adults. It can occur at any age but is most common in women of childbearing age. Usually multifocal and bilateral, it metastasizes slowly into regional nodes of the neck, mediastinum, lungs, and other distant organs. It is the least virulent form of thyroid cancer.

Less common (about 20% of all cases), follicular carcinoma is more likely to recur and metastasize to the regional lymph nodes and spread through blood vessels into the bones, liver, and lungs.

Medullary (solid) carcinoma originates in the parafollicular cells derived from the last branchial pouch and contains amyloid and calcium deposits. It can produce calcitonin, histaminase, corticotropin (producing Cushing's syndrome), and prostaglandin E_2 and F_3 (producing diarrhea). This form of thyroid cancer is familial, possibly inherited as an autosomal dominant trait, and usually associated with pheochromocytoma. A rare (5%) form of thyroid cancer, it typically occurs in women over age 40. It is curable when detected before it causes symptoms. Untreated, it grows rapidly, frequently metastasizing to bones, liver, and kidneys.

Anaplastic carcinoma resists radiation and is almost never curable by resection. Tumors usually occur in older patients with a long history of goiter. This cancer metastasizes rapidly, causing death by invading the trachea and compressing adjacent structures. It accounts for between 10% and 15% of thyroid cancers.

Causes

Besides exposure to radiation, suspected causes of thyroid cancer include prolonged secretion of thyroid-stimulating hormone (TSH) (through radiation or heredity), familial predisposition, and chronic goiter.

Complications

Dysphagia and stridor are typical complications of thyroid cancer – especially in untreated disease. They usually result from pressure caused by a space-occupying lesion that extends into neck structures. Additional complications include hormone alterations and distant metastases.

Assessment

The first indication of disease may be a painless nodule discovered incidentally or detected during physical examination.

If the tumor grows large enough to destroy the thyroid gland, the patient's history may include sensitivity to cold and mental apathy (hypothyroidism). If the tumor triggers excess thyroid hormone production, the patient may report sensitivity to heat, restlessness, and overactivity (hyperthyroidism). The patient may also complain of diarrhea, dysphagia, anorexia, irritability, and ear pain. When speaking with the patient, you may hear hoarseness and vocal stridor.

On inspection, you may detect a disfiguring thyroid mass, especially if the patient is in the later stages of anaplastic thyroid cancer.

Palpation may disclose a hard nodule in an enlarged thyroid gland or palpable lymph nodes with thyroid enlargement.

By auscultation, you may discover bruits if thyroid enlargement results from an increase in TSH, which increases thyroid vascularity.

Diagnostic tests

- *Fine-needle aspiration biopsy* may help to differentiate benign from malignant thyroid nodules. *Histologic analysis* will help to stage the disease and guide treatment. (See *Staging thyroid cancer,* page 908.)
- *Thyroid scan* may differentiate functional nodes (rarely malignant) from hypofunctional nodes (commonly malignant) by measuring how readily nodules trap isotopes compared with the rest of the thyroid gland. In thyroid cancer, *scintigraphy* findings may demonstrate a cold, nonfunctioning nodule.
- *Ultrasonography* evaluates changes in the size of thyroid nodules after thyroxine suppression therapy, guides fine-needle aspiration, and detects recurrent disease.
- *Magnetic resonance imaging* and *computed tomography scans* provide information for treatment planning because they establish the extent of the disease within the thyroid and in surrounding structures.
- *Calcitonin assay* is a reliable clue to silent medullary carcinoma. An elevated fasting calcitonin level and an abnormal response to calcium stimulation – a high release of calcitonin from the node in comparison with the rest of the gland – are indicative of medullary cancer. Carcinoembryonic antigen (CEA) is also a useful marker for diagnosis and follow-up with medullary carcinoma.

Staging thyroid cancer

Thyroid cancer classifications signify the tumor's (T) size and extent at its origin, its invasion of regional (cervical and upper mediastinal) lymph nodes (N), and the disease's spread or metastasis (M) to other structures. After accumulating data about the tumor and its spread, staging further defines the disease process.

The following summarizes the classification and staging systems adopted by the American Joint Committee on Cancer.

Primary tumor

TX—primary tumor can't be assessed
T0—no evidence of primary tumor
T1—tumor 1 cm or less in greatest dimension and limited to the thyroid
T2—tumor more than 1 cm but less than 4 cm in greatest dimension and limited to the thyroid
T3—tumor more than 4 cm and limited to the thyroid
T4—tumor (any size) extends beyond the thyroid

Regional lymph nodes

NX—regional lymph nodes can't be assessed
N0—no evidence of regional lymph node metastasis
N1—regional lymph node metastasis
N1a—metastasis in ipsilateral cervical nodes
N1b—metastasis in bilateral, midline, or contralateral cervical or mediastinal lymph nodes

Distant metastasis

MX—distant metastasis can't be assessed
M0—no evidence of distant metastasis
M1—distant metastasis

Staging categories for papillary or follicular cancer

Papillary or follicular cancer progresses from mild to severe as follows:
Stage I—any T, any N, M0 (patient under age 45); T1, N0, M0 (patient age 45 or over)
Stage II—any T, any N, M1 (patient under age 45); T2, N0, M0; T3, N0, M0 (patient age 45 or over)
Stage III—T4, N0, M0; any T, N1, M0 (patient age 45 or over)
Stage IV—any T, any N, M1 (patient age 45 or over)

Staging categories for medullary cancer

Medullary cancer progresses from mild to severe as follows:
Stage I—T1, N0, M0
Stage II—T2, N0, M0; T3, N0, M0; T4, N0, M0
Stage III—any T, N1, M0
Stage IV—any T, any N, M1

Staging categories for undifferentiated cancer

(All cases are Stage IV)
Stage IV—any T, any N, any M

Treatment

Surgery is recommended initially for all forms of thyroid cancer, but the extent of surgery and the postoperative treatments vary. Ideally, the patient should have normal thyroid function (euthyroid) before surgery, as demonstrated by normal thyroid function tests, pulse rate, and electrocardiogram.

Treatment may include one or a combination of the following:

- total or subtotal thyroidectomy with modified node dissection (bilateral or homolateral) on the side of the primary cancer (for papillary or follicular cancer)
- total thyroidectomy and radical neck excision (for medullary or anaplastic cancer)

• radioisotope (iodine 131) therapy with external radiation (sometimes postoperatively in lieu of radical neck excision) or alone (for metastasis)
• Levothyroxine (T_4) therapy replacement with follow up blood levels of free T_4 iodide or free T_4 and TSH levels.
• adjunctive thyroid suppression (with exogenous thyroid hormones suppressing TSH production) and simultaneous administration of an adrenergic blocking agent, such as propranolol, to increase tolerance to surgery and radiation therapy
• chemotherapy limited to treating symptoms of widespread metastasis, as a palliative measure; not effective for treating medullary and anaplastic carcinoma.

Key nursing diagnoses and patient outcomes

Altered nutrition: Less than body requirements) related to dysphagia. Based on this nursing diagnosis, you'll establish these patient outcomes. The patient will:
• maintain his weight within baseline range
• consume a nutritionally balanced diet daily
• show no signs and symptoms of nutritional deficits.

Impaired swallowing related to presence of tumor. Based on this nursing diagnosis, you'll establish these patient outcomes. The patient will:
• adjust his eating habits to compensate for swallowing impairment
• show no evidence of complications, such as aspiration pneumonia or malnutrition
• regain normal swallowing ability with eradication of the thyroid tumor.

Impaired verbal communication related to presence of tumor. Based on this nursing diagnosis, you'll establish these patient outcomes. The patient will:
• communicate his needs and desires without undue frustration
• use alternate means of communication
• regain normal speaking ability with eradication of the thyroid tumor.

Nursing interventions

• Prepare the patient for scheduled surgery. (See the entry "Thyroidectomy.")
• If radioactive iodine therapy is prescribed, prepare the patient accordingly. (See the entry "Radioactive iodine therapy.")
• Provide supportive care, such as nutritional supplements and analgesic administration for pain, as needed.
• Encourage the patient to voice his concerns, and offer reassurance.

Monitoring

• Monitor the patient for signs and symptoms of complications, such as dysphagia and hormonal imbalances.
• Regularly monitor the patient's thyroid function studies, as ordered, to determine when he's reached a euthyroid state and is ready for surgery.
• If dysphagia is present, monitor the patient's nutritional status. Weigh him regularly.

Patient teaching

• Preoperatively, advise the patient to expect temporary voice loss or hoarseness for several days after surgery. Also, explain the operation and postoperative procedures and positioning.
• Before discharge, ensure that the patient knows the date and time of his next appointment. Answer his questions about his treatment and home care. Be sure he understands the purpose of his medications and their dosage, administration times, and possible adverse effects.
• Refer the patient to resource and support services, such as the social service department, home health care agencies, hospices, and the American Cancer Society.

Thyroidectomy

The surgical removal of part or all of the thyroid gland, thyroidectomy allows treatment of hyperthyroidism, respiratory obstruction from goiter, and thyroid cancer. Subtotal thyroidectomy, used to correct hyperthyroidism when drug therapy fails or radiation therapy is contraindicated, reduces secretion of thyroid hormone. It also effectively treats diffuse goiter. After surgery, the remaining thyroid tissue usually supplies enough thyroid hormone for normal function.

Total thyroidectomy may be performed for certain types of thyroid cancers, such as papillary, follicular, medullary, or anaplastic neoplasms. After this surgery, the patient requires life-long thyroid hormone replacement therapy.

Procedure

After the patient is anesthetized, the surgeon extends the neck fully and determines the incision line by measuring bilaterally from each clavicle. Then he cuts through the skin, fascia, and muscle and raises skin flaps from the strap muscles. He separates these muscles midline, revealing the thyroid's isthmus, and ligates the thyroid artery and veins to help prevent bleeding. Next, he locates and visualizes the laryngeal nerves and parathyroid glands and then begins dissection and removal of thyroid tissue, trying not to injure these nearby structures.

Before the surgeon sutures the incision, he may insert a Penrose drain or a closed wound drainage device, such as a Hemovac drain.

Complications

Most often performed under general anesthesia, thyroidectomy has a low incidence of complications if the patient is properly prepared with thyroid hormone antagonists preoperatively. Potential complications include hemorrhage; parathyroid damage, causing postoperative hypocalcemia, which can lead to tetany; and laryngeal nerve damage, causing vocal cord paralysis. This last complication can result in hoarseness if only one vocal cord is damaged and respiratory distress (necessitating a tracheotomy) if both cords are affected. Thyroid storm is a potential complication when a thyroidectomy is performed as treatment for hyperthyroidism. It can be prevented if the patient is properly prepared with antithyroid drugs preoperatively.

Key nursing diagnoses and patient outcomes

Risk for injury related to potential complications associated with thyroidectomy. Based on this nursing diagnosis, you'll establish these patient outcomes. The patient will:

- recognize and report early signs and symptoms of a postoperative complication
- show no signs and symptoms of complications, such as neuromuscular irritability, respiratory distress, bleeding, or unstable vital signs
- maintain a normal serum calcium level.

Ineffective airway clearance related to neck pain and swelling. Based on this nursing diagnosis, you'll establish these patient outcomes. The patient will:

- demonstrate controlled coughing techniques
- expectorate sputum effectively
- maintain a patent airway.

Knowledge deficit related to drug therapy used in hyperthyroidism to achieve a euthyroid state preoperatively. Based on this nursing diagnosis, you'll establish these patient outcomes. The patient will:

- identify the need to learn about preoperative drug therapy
- obtain the necessary instructions about his prescribed drug therapy
- communicate an understanding of the importance of achieving a euthyroid state before thyroidectomy.

Nursing interventions

When caring for a patient undergoing a thyroidectomy, your primary responsibilities are patient teaching and monitoring for postoperative complications.

Before surgery

• Explain to the patient that thyroidectomy will remove diseased thyroid tissue or, if necessary, the entire gland. Tell him that he'll have an incision in his neck; that he'll have a dressing, and possibly, a drain in place after surgery; and that he may experience some hoarseness and a sore throat from intubation and anesthesia. Reassure him that he'll receive analgesics to relieve his discomfort.

• If thyroidectomy is being performed to treat hyperthyroidism, ensure that the patient has followed his preoperative drug regimen, which will render the gland euthyroid to prevent thyroid storm during surgery. He probably will have received either propylthiouracil or methimazole, usually starting 4 to 6 weeks before surgery. Expect him to be receiving iodine as well for 10 to 14 days before surgery to reduce the gland's vascularity and thus prevent excess bleeding. He may also be receiving propranolol to block adrenergic effects. Notify the doctor immediately if the patient has failed to follow his medication regimen.

• Collect samples for serum thyroid hormone determinations to check for euthyroidism. If necessary, arrange for an electrocardiogram to evaluate cardiac status.

• Ensure that the patient or a responsible family member has signed a consent form.

After surgery

• Keep the patient in high Fowler's position to promote venous return from the head and neck and to decrease oozing into the incision. Check for laryngeal nerve damage by asking the patient to speak as soon as he awakens from anesthesia.

• Watch for signs of respiratory distress. Tracheal collapse, tracheal mucus accumulation, laryngeal edema, and vocal cord paralysis can all cause respiratory obstruction, with sudden stridor and restlessness. Keep a tracheotomy tray at the patient's bedside for 24 hours after surgery, and be prepared to assist with emergency tracheotomy, if necessary.

• Assess for signs of hemorrhage, which may cause shock, tracheal compression, and respiratory distress. Check the patient's dressing and palpate the back of his neck, where drainage tends to flow. Expect about 50 ml of drainage in the first 24 hours; if you find no drainage, check for drain kinking or the need to reestablish suction. Expect only scant drainage after 24 hours.

• Assess for hypocalcemia, which may occur when the parathyroid glands are damaged. Test for Chvostek's and Trousseau's signs, indicators of neuromuscular irritability from hypocalcemia. Keep calcium gluconate available for emergency I.V. administration.

• Be alert for signs of thyroid storm, a rare but serious complication.

• As ordered, administer a mild analgesic to relieve a sore neck or throat. Reassure the patient that his discomfort should resolve within a few days.

• If the patient doesn't have a drain in place, prepare him for discharge the day following surgery, as indicated. However, if a drain is in place, the doctor will usually remove it, along with half of the surgical clips, on the second day after surgery; the remaining clips, the following day, before discharge.

Home care instructions

• If the patient is discharged the day after surgery, teach him to report any signs of respiratory distress or bleeding.

• If the patient has had a total thyroidectomy, explain the importance of regularly taking his prescribed thyroid hormone replacement. Teach him to recognize and report signs of hypothyroidism and hyperthyroidism.

• If parathyroid damage occurred during surgery, explain to the patient that he'll need to take calcium supplements. Teach him to recognize the warning signs of hypocalcemia.

• Tell the patient to keep the incision site clean and dry. Help him cope with concerns about its appearance. Suggest loosely buttoned collars, high-necked blouses, jewelry, or scarves, which can hide the incision until it has healed. The doctor may recommend using a mild body lotion to soften the healing scar and improve its appearance.
• Arrange follow-up appointments, as necessary, and explain to the patient that the doctor needs to check the incision and serum thyroid hormone levels.

Toxic shock syndrome

An acute bacterial infection, toxic shock syndrome most commonly is associated with continuous use of tampons, especially the superabsorbent type, during menstruation. Of the reported cases, 96% involve women, and 92% of these cases begin during menstruation. The incidence of this infection continues to rise, and the recurrence rate is about 30%. Most patients recover fully.

Causes

Toxic shock syndrome is caused by penicillin-resistant *Staphylococcus aureus.* Although tampons are clearly implicated in this infection, their exact role is uncertain. They may contribute to the infection by:
• introducing *S. aureus* into the vagina during insertion
• absorbing toxin from the vagina
• traumatizing the vaginal mucosa during insertion, thus leading to infection
• providing a favorable environment for growth of *S. aureus.*

When toxic shock syndrome is unrelated to menstruation, it seems to be linked to *S. aureus* infections such as abscesses, osteomyelitis, and postoperative infections.

Complications

Toxic shock syndrome can lead to persistent neurologic and psychological abnormalities, renal failure, rash, dehydration, and peripheral cyanosis.

Assessment

The patient commonly reports that she consistently uses tampons – especially the superabsorbent type – throughout menstruation and changes tampons infrequently. She may complain of intense myalgia, vomiting, diarrhea, and headache. Her temperature may be over 104° F (40° C).

Inspection may reveal rigors, conjunctival hyperemia, vaginal hyperemia, and vaginal discharge. A deep-red rash also may develop, especially on the palms and soles. The rash appears within a few hours of the onset of infection and later desquamates. The patient may seem listless and confused.

Palpation may disclose signs of shock – a rapid, thready pulse and hypotension.

Diagnostic tests

Isolation of *S. aureus* from vaginal discharge or lesions helps support the diagnosis, but a confirmed diagnosis must follow the criteria set by the Centers for Disease Control and Prevention. (See *Diagnosing toxic shock syndrome.*) Negative results on blood tests for Rocky Mountain spotted fever, leptospirosis, and measles help rule out these disorders.

Treatment

Appropriate treatment may consist of I.V. antistaphylococcal antibiotics that are beta-lactamase resistant, such as oxacillin, nafcillin, and methicillin. To reverse shock, the patient will need fluid replacement with saline solution and colloids. Other measures may include supportive treatment for diarrhea, nausea, and vomiting.

Key nursing diagnoses and patient outcomes

Altered thought processes related to neurologic dysfunction. Based on this nursing

diagnosis, you'll establish these patient outcomes. The patient will:
• remain safe in her environment
• regain normal thought processes with eradication of toxic shock syndrome.

Diarrhea related to infectious process. Based on this nursing diagnosis, you'll establish these patient outcomes. The patient will:
• achieve control of diarrhea with medication
• show no signs and symptoms of complications associated with diarrhea, such as skin breakdown or electrolyte imbalance.

Fluid volume deficit related to diarrhea and shock. Based on this nursing diagnosis, you'll establish these patient outcomes. The patient will:
• regain and maintain normal vital signs
• regain and maintain normal fluid balance
• produce an adequate urine volume.

Nursing interventions

• Administer I.V. antibiotics over a 15-minute period to ensure peak levels that destroy microorganisms.
• Replace fluids I.V., as ordered.
• Obtain specimens of vaginal and cervical secretions for culture of *S. aureus.*
• Reorient the patient as needed. Use appropriate safety measures to prevent injury.
• Use standard precautions for any vaginal discharge and lesion drainage.
• Administer analgesics cautiously because of the risk of hypotension and liver failure.
• Report case to public health authorities.

Monitoring

• Frequently monitor the patient's vital signs.
• Watch for signs of penicillin allergy.
• Monitor intake, output, and weight daily to assess fluid balance and to prevent dehydration and renal failure.
• Check neurologic status and vital signs every 4 to 8 hours.

Diagnosing toxic shock syndrome

According to the Centers for Disease Control and Prevention, a diagnosis of toxic shock syndrome can't be made unless a physical assessment and diagnostic tests reveal at least three of the following:
• GI effects, including vomiting and profuse diarrhea
• muscular effects, with severe myalgia or a fivefold or greater increase in serum creatine phosphokinase levels
• mucous membrane effects, such as frank hyperemia
• renal involvement, with blood urea nitrogen or serum creatinine levels at least double the norm
• hepatocellular damage, with levels of serum bilirubin, alanine aminotransferase (formerly SGPT), and aspartate aminotransferase (formerly SGOT) at least double the norm
• blood involvement, with signs of thrombocytopenia and a platelet count of less than 100,000/mm^3
• central nervous system effects, such as disorientation without focal signs.

Patient teaching

• Advise the patient to avoid using tampons, particularly the superabsorbent type, because of the risk of recurrence.

Toxoplasmosis

Depending on their environment and eating habits, up to 70% of people in North America are infected with *Toxoplasma gondii*—making toxoplasmosis one of the most common infectious diseases. Occurring worldwide, it's less common in cold or in hot, arid climates and at high elevations.

The disease usually causes localized infection. However, it may produce significant generalized infection, especially in immunodeficient patients, such as acquired immunodeficiency syndrome (AIDS) patients, patients who've recently had an organ transplant, those with lymphoma, and those receiving immunosuppressant therapy.

Once infected, the patient may carry the organism for life. Reactivation of the acute infection can occur. Congenital toxoplasmosis, characterized by lesions in the central nervous system (CNS), may result in stillbirth or serious birth defects.

Causes

Toxoplasmosis is caused by the protozoan *T. gondii,* which exists in trophozoite forms in the acute stages of infection and in cystic forms (tissue cysts and oocysts) in the latent stages. The infection is transmitted by ingestion of tissue cysts in raw or undercooked meat (heating, drying, or freezing destroys these cysts) or by fecal-oral contamination from infected cats. Because toxoplasmosis has also struck vegetarians who aren't exposed to cats, other means of transmission may exist.

Congenital toxoplasmosis follows transplacental transmission from a mother who acquires primary toxoplasmosis shortly before or during pregnancy. Congenital infection is more severe when acquired early in the pregnancy.

Complications

Toxoplasmosis may cause encephalitis, myocarditis, pneumonitis, hepatitis, or polymyositis. If the disease is acquired in the first trimester of pregnancy, it commonly results in stillbirth. About one-third of infants who survive have congenital toxoplasmosis with CNS involvement and chorioretinitis.

Assessment

The patient's history may reveal an immunocompromised state, exposure to cat feces, or frequent ingestion of poorly cooked meat.

A patient with localized (mild, lymphatic) toxoplasmosis may complain of mononucleosis-like symptoms: malaise, myalgia, headache, fatigue, and sore throat. He'll also have a fever. A patient with generalized (fulminating, disseminated) infection may complain of headache, vomiting, cough, and dyspnea. His temperature may run as high as 106° F (41.1° C).

Inspection of the patient with generalized disease reveals delirium and seizures – signs of encephalitis. You also may note a diffuse maculopapular rash (except on the palms, soles, and scalp) and cyanosis.

Auscultation of a patient with toxoplasmosis may reveal coarse crackles.

Diagnostic tests

Isolation of *T. gondii* in mice after their inoculation with specimens of body fluids, blood, and tissue, or *T. gondii* antibodies in such specimens, confirms toxoplasmosis.

Treatment

Most effective during the acute stage, treatment consists of sulfonamides and pyrimethamine for 4 to 6 weeks. The patient also may receive folinic acid to control pyrimethamine's adverse effects.

These drugs act synergistically against the trophozoites but don't eliminate already developed tissue cysts. For this reason, and because they don't alleviate the underlying immune system defect in AIDS, an AIDS patient should receive toxoplasmosis treatment for life.

An AIDS patient who can't tolerate sulfonamides may receive clindamycin instead. This drug also is the primary treatment in ocular toxoplasmosis.

Key nursing diagnoses and patient outcomes

Risk for injury related to neurologic dysfunction. Based on this nursing diagnosis,

you'll establish these patient outcomes. The patient will:
• remain safe in his environment
• not sustain injury as a result of a neurologic impairment
• regain normal neurological function with resolution of toxoplasmosis.

Hyperthermia related to infectious process. Based on this nursing diagnosis, you'll establish these patient outcomes. The patient will:
• regain and maintain a normal body temperature following antipyretic administration and resolution of toxoplasmosis
• show no signs and symptoms of complications associated with hyperthermia, such as seizures.

Risk for fluid volume deficit related to hyperthermia, vomiting, and sore throat. Based on this nursing diagnosis, you'll establish these patient outcomes. The patient will:
• have normal blood pressure and pulse and respiratory rates
• have an intake that equals or exceeds output
• maintain normal fluid balance.

Nursing interventions

• Give antipyretics and, possibly, tepid sponge baths to decrease fever.
• Make sure the patient with a high fever, vomiting, and sore throat receives sufficient fluid intake. Provide nutritionally adequate foods and, if needed, small, frequent feedings.
• Promote bed rest during the acute stage. Later, help the patient gradually increase his level of activity.
• Don't palpate the patient's abdomen vigorously; this could lead to a ruptured spleen. For the same reason, discourage vigorous activity.
• Modify the environment as needed to protect a patient with neurologic manifestations or chorioretinitis. Refer him for rehabilitation or counseling, as needed.
• Report all cases of toxoplasmosis to the local public health department.

Monitoring

• Monitor the patient's vital signs, especially temperature.
• Frequently assess respiratory status, especially in the immunocompromised patient. Provide chest physiotherapy and administer oxygen, as needed. Assist ventilation if needed.
• Assess the patient for signs of neurologic involvement.
• Carefully monitor the patient's drug therapy.
• Because sulfonamides cause blood dyscrasias and pyrimethamine depresses bone marrow, closely monitor the patient's hematologic values.

Patient teaching

• Teach the patient about necessary medications, including the need for frequent blood tests.
• Emphasize the importance of regularly scheduled follow-up care.
• Advise all people to wash their hands after working with soil because it may be contaminated with cat oocysts; to cook meat thoroughly and to freeze it promptly if it's not for immediate use; to change cat litter daily (cat oocysts don't become infective until 1 to 4 days after excretion); to cover children's sandboxes; and to keep flies away from food because flies transport oocysts.

Tracheotomy

The surgical creation of an opening into the trachea through the neck, tracheotomy is most commonly performed to provide an airway for the intubated patient who needs prolonged mechanical ventilation. It may also be performed to prevent an unconscious or paralyzed patient from aspirating food or secretions; to bypass upper airway obstruction caused by trauma, burns, epiglottitis, or a tumor; or to help remove lower tracheobronchial secretions in a patient who can't clear them.

Although endotracheal intubation is the treatment of choice in an emergency, tracheotomy may be used if intubation is impossible. For the laryngectomy patient, a permanent tracheotomy in which the skin and the trachea are sutured together provides the necessary stoma.

After creation of the surgical opening, a tracheostomy tube is inserted to permit access to the airway. Selection of a specific tube depends on the patient's condition and the doctor's preference. (See *Comparing tracheostomy tubes.*)

Procedure

If the patient doesn't have an endotracheal tube in place, the doctor inserts this tube with the patient under general anesthesia. Then the doctor makes a horizontal incision in the skin below the cricoid cartilage and vertical incisions in the trachea. He places a tracheostomy tube between the second and third tracheal rings, and he may also place retraction sutures in the stomal margins to stabilize the opening. Finally, he inflates the tube cuff (if present), provides ventilation, suctions the airways, and provides oxygen by mist.

Complications

Tracheotomy can cause serious complications. Within 48 hours after surgery, the patient may develop hemorrhage at the site, bleeding or edema within the tracheal tissue, aspiration of secretions, pneumothorax, or subcutaneous emphysema. After 48 hours, continued attention to sterile suctioning, careful cuff monitoring, and meticulous stoma care can reduce the risk of subsequent complications, such as stoma or pulmonary infection, ischemia and hemorrhage, airway obstruction, hypoxia, and arrhythmias.

Key nursing diagnoses and patient outcomes

Risk for infection related to removal of normal protective barrier with insertion of tracheostomy tube. Based on this nursing diagnosis, you'll establish these patient outcomes. The patient will:
- maintain his body temperature and white blood cell count and differential within a normal range
- have a tracheostomy site that is clean, pink, and free of purulent secretions
- remain free of all other signs and symptoms of infection.

Impaired verbal communication related to inability to speak. Based on this nursing diagnosis, you'll establish these patient outcomes. The patient will:
- communicate his needs and desires without undue frustration
- use alternate means of communication
- regain normal verbal ability when a temporary tracheostomy is removed or demonstrate the correct use of adaptive equipment if the tracheostomy is permanent.

Ineffective airway clearance related to accumulation of tracheobronchial secretions and inability to mobilize secretions. Based on this nursing diagnosis, you'll establish these patient outcomes. The patient will:
- have secretions removed regularly
- maintain a patent airway
- demonstrate equal bilateral breath sounds and clear lung fields on a chest X-ray.

Nursing interventions

When caring for a patient who has undergone tracheotomy, your primary responsibilities are instructing the patient, monitoring for postoperative complications, and performing postoperative care, including suctioning and changing dressings.

Before surgery

- For an emergency tracheotomy, briefly explain the procedure to the patient (if possible), and quickly obtain supplies or a tracheotomy tray.
- For a scheduled tracheotomy, explain the procedure and the need for general anesthesia to the patient and his family. If pos-

Comparing tracheostomy tubes

Tracheostomy tubes, made of plastic or metal, come in cuffed, uncuffed, or fenestrated varieties. Tube selection depends on the patient's condition and the doctor's preference. Make sure you're familiar with the advantages and disadvantages of these commonly used tracheostomy tubes.

Tube type	Advantages	Disadvantages
Uncuffed (plastic or metal) 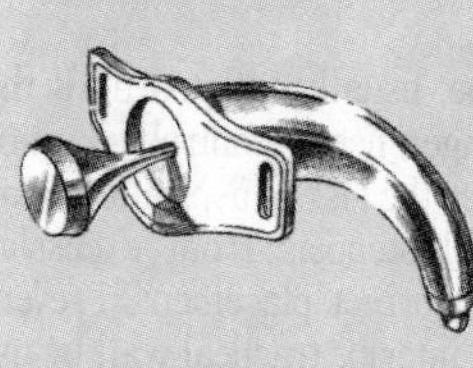	• Permits free flow of air around tube and through larynx • Reduces risk of tracheal damage • Recommended for children because these tubes don't require a cuff • Allows mechanical ventilation in patient with neuromuscular disease	• In adults, lack of cuff increases the risk of aspiration. • An adapter may be necessary for ventilation.
Plastic cuffed (low pressure and high volume) 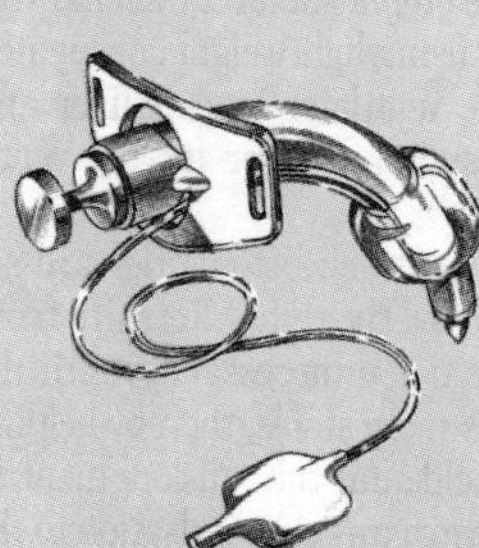	• Disposable • Cuff bonded to tube; won't detach accidentally inside trachea • Cuff pressure is low and evenly distributed against tracheal wall; no need to deflate periodically to lower pressure • Reduces risk of tracheal damage	• This tube may be costlier than other tubes.
Fenestrated 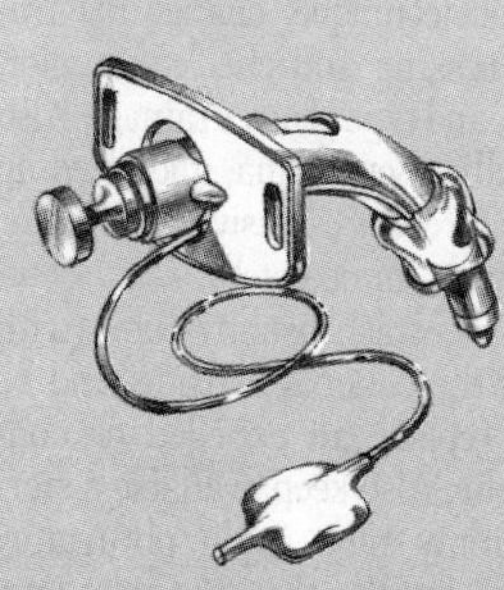	• Permits speech through upper airway when external opening is capped and cuff is deflated • Allows breathing by mechanical ventilation with inner cannula in place and cuff inflated • Inner cannula can be easily removed for cleaning	• Fenestration may become occluded. • Inner cannula can become dislodged.

sible, mention whether the tracheostomy will be temporary or permanent. As needed, discuss a communication system with the patient, such as a letter board, a magic slate, or flash cards, and have him practice using it so he can communicate comfortably while his speech is limited. If the patient will have a long-term or permanent tracheostomy, introduce him to someone who has undergone a similar procedure and has adjusted well to tube and stoma care.

• Ensure that samples for arterial blood gas (ABG) analysis and other diagnostic tests required by your hospital have been collected and that the patient or a responsible family member has signed a consent form.

After surgery

• Auscultate breath sounds every 2 hours after tracheotomy, noting crackles, rhonchi, or diminished sounds. Turn the patient every 2 hours to prevent pooling of tracheal secretions. Note the amount, consistency, color, and odor of secretions. As ordered, provide chest physiotherapy to help mobilize secretions. (See *Combating complications of tracheotomy.*)

• Provide humidification to reduce the drying effects of oxygen on mucous membranes and to thin secretions. Expect to deliver oxygen through a T-piece connected to a nebulizer or heated cascade humidifier. Monitor ABG results and compare them with baseline values, to help determine if oxygenation and carbon dioxide removal is adequate. As ordered, also monitor the patient's oximetry values.

• Using sterile equipment and technique, suction the tracheostomy, as ordered, to remove excess secretions. Use a suction catheter no larger than half the diameter of the tracheostomy tube, and minimize oxygen deprivation and tracheal trauma by keeping the bypass port open while inserting the catheter. Once the catheter is in as far as it can be advanced, do not apply suction. Withdraw the catheter 3 to 5 cm and then apply suction using a gentle, twisting motion as you withdraw it to help minimize tracheal and bronchial mucosal irritation. Apply suction for no longer than 10 seconds at a time, and discontinue suctioning if the patient develops respiratory distress. Monitor for arrhythmias, which can occur if suctioning decreases partial pressure of oxygen in arterial blood levels below 50 mm Hg. Allow oxygen saturation to rise to 92% to 94% before further suctioning is continued. Evaluate the effectiveness of suctioning by auscultating for breath sounds.

• A cuffed tube, usually inflated until the patient no longer needs controlled ventilation or is over the risk of aspiration, may cause tracheal stenosis from excessive pressure or incorrect placement. Prevent trauma to the interior tracheal wall by using pressures less than 25 cm H_2O (18 mm Hg) and minimal leak technique when inflating the cuff. Reduce the risk of trauma to the stoma site and internal tracheal wall by using lightweight corrugated tubing for the ventilator or nebulizer and providing a swivel adapter for the ventilator circuit.

• Make sure the tracheostomy ties are secure but not overly tight. Refrain from changing the ties unnecessarily until the stoma track is more stable, thereby helping to prevent accidental tube dislodgment or expulsion. Report any tube pulsation to the doctor, since this may indicate its proximity to the innominate artery, predisposing the patient to hemorrhage.

• Using aseptic technique, change the tracheostomy dressing and check the color, odor, amount, and type of any drainage. Also check for swelling, erythema, and bleeding at the site, and report excessive bleeding or unusual drainage immediately.

• Keep a sterile tracheostomy tube (with obturator) at the patient's bedside, and be prepared to replace an expelled or contaminated tube. Also keep available a sterile tracheostomy tube (with obturator) that's one size smaller than the tube currently being used, since the trachea begins

Combating complications of tracheotomy

Complication	Prevention	Detection	Treatment
Aspiration	• Evaluate patient's ability to swallow. • Elevate his head and inflate cuff during feeding and for 30 minutes afterward.	• Assess for dyspnea, tachypnea, rhonchi, crackles, excessive secretions, and fever.	• Obtain chest X-ray, if ordered. • Suction excessive secretions. • Give antibiotics if necessary.
Bleeding at tracheotomy site	• Don't pull on the tracheostomy tube; don't allow ventilator tubing to do so. • If dressing adheres to wound, wet it with hydrogen peroxide and remove gently.	• Check dressing regularly; slight bleeding is normal, especially if patient has a bleeding disorder.	• Keep cuff inflated to prevent edema and blood aspiration. Give humidified oxygen. • Document character of bleeding. Check for prolonged clotting time. • As ordered, assist with Gelfoam application or ligation of a small bleeder.
Infection at tracheotomy site	• Always use strict aseptic technique. • Thoroughly clean all tubing. • Change nebulizer or humidifier jar and all tubing daily. • Collect sputum and wound drainage specimens for culture.	• Check for purulent, foul-smelling drainage from stoma. • Be alert for other signs of infection: fever, malaise, increased white blood cell count, and local pain.	• As ordered, obtain culture specimens and administer antibiotics. • Inflate tracheostomy cuff to prevent aspiration. • Suction the patient frequently; avoid cross-contamination. • Change dressing whenever soiled.
Pneumothorax	• Assess for subcutaneous emphysema, which may indicate pneumothorax. Notify doctor if this occurs.	• Auscultate for decreased or absent breath sounds. • Check for tachypnea, pain, and subcutaneous emphysema.	• If ordered, prepare for chest tube insertion. • Obtain chest X-ray, as ordered, to evaluate pneumothorax or to check placement of chest tube.
Subcutaneous emphysema	• Make sure cuffed tube is patent and properly inflated. • Avoid displacement by securing ties and using lightweight ventilator tubing and swivel valves.	• Most common in mechanically ventilated patients. • Palpate neck for crepitus; listen for air leakage around cuff; check site for unusual swelling.	• Inflate cuff correctly or use a larger tube. • Suction patient and clean tube to remove any blockage. • Document extent of crepitus.
Tracheal malacia	• Avoid excessive cuff pressures. • Avoid suctioning beyond end of tube.	• Dry, hacking cough and blood-streaked sputum when tube is being manipulated.	• Minimize trauma from tube movement. • Keep cuff pressure below 18 mm Hg.

to close after tube expulsion, making insertion of the same size tube difficult.

Home care instructions

- Tell the patient to notify his doctor if he experiences any breathing problems, chest or stoma pain, or change in the amount or color of his secretions.
- Ensure that the patient can effectively care for his stoma and tracheostomy tube. Instruct him to wash the skin around his stoma with a moist cloth. Emphasize the importance of not getting water in his stoma. He should, of course, avoid swimming. When he showers, he should wear a stoma shield or direct the water below his stoma.
- Tell the patient to place a foam filter over his stoma in winter, thereby warming inspired air, and to wear a bib over the filter.
- Teach the patient to bend at his waist during coughing to help expel secretions. Tell him to keep a tissue handy to catch expelled secretions.

Traction

Mechanical traction exerts a pulling force on a part of the body—usually the spine, pelvis, or long bones of the arms and legs. It's used to reduce fractures, treat dislocations, correct or prevent deformities, improve or correct contractures, or decrease muscle spasms. The type of traction used is determined by the doctor and is based on the patient's condition, age, and weight, the condition of his skin, the length of time he'll be maintained in traction, and the purpose for which it is used.

Skin traction is applied directly to the skin and thus indirectly to the bone. It's ordered when a light, temporary, or noncontinuous pulling force is required. In skeletal traction, an orthopedist inserts a device through the bone and attaches the traction equipment to the device to exert a direct, constant, longitudinal pulling force. This type of traction is most often used for fractures of the femur, humerus, tibia, or cervical spine. (See *Comparing traction types.*)

Procedure

Skin traction can be applied at the patient's bedside. The doctor uses adhesive or nonadhesive traction tape or another skin traction device to exert a pulling force—usually 5 to 8 lb (2.3 to 3.6 kg)—on the patient's skin. Types of skin traction include Buck's, pelvic with pelvic belt, and cervical with cervical halter.

Skeletal traction is done under local, general, or spinal anesthesia in aseptic surroundings. The doctor inserts pins, wires, or tongs into or through the bones; he then attaches weighted equipment to these pins, wires, or tongs. The usual amount of weight is 25 to 40 lb (11.3 to 18.1 kg). Types of skeletal traction include balanced skeletal, overhead arm, and cervical with tongs. Pads, slings, or pushers may be used along with the traction to reduce the fracture.

Complications

Immobility during traction may result in pressure ulcers, muscle atrophy, weakness, contractures, and osteoporosis. Immobility can also cause GI disturbances, such as constipation; urinary problems, including stasis and calculi; respiratory problems, such as stasis of secretions and hypostatic pneumonia; and circulatory disturbances, including stasis and thrombophlebitis. Prolonged immobility, especially after traumatic injury, may promote depression or other emotional disturbances. Skeletal traction may cause osteomyelitis originating at the pin or wire sites. Nonunion or delayed union of the bone, pin breakage, or both may also occur.

Key nursing diagnoses and patient outcomes

Constipation related to immobility. Based on this nursing diagnosis, you'll establish

these patient outcomes. The patient will:
• identify measures to prevent constipation
• participate in a bowel program to prevent or minimize constipation
• maintain a normal bowel pattern while in traction

Impaired physical mobility. Based on this nursing diagnosis, you'll establish these patient outcomes. The patient will:
• maintain muscle strength and joint range of motion
• show no evidence of complications, such as contractures, venous stasis, thrombus formation, or skin breakdown
• regain baseline mobility when traction is discontinued.

Impaired tissue integrity related to immobility. Based on this nursing diagnosis, you'll establish these patient outcomes. The patient will:
• demonstrate correct methods of movement to ease pressure on bony prominences
• identify and take precautions to prevent skin breakdown, such as maintaining adequate fluid and nutritional intake and alleviating dry skin
• maintain normal skin integrity.

Nursing interventions

When caring for a patient in traction, your main responsibilities include patient teaching, maintaining the traction apparatus, assessing for complications of immobility and, for patients with skeletal traction, caring for and assessing the pin insertion sites.

Before the procedure

• Explain the purpose of traction to the patient and his family. Emphasize the importance of maintaining proper body alignment.
• Teach the patient how to use the overhead trapeze to assist with position changes.
• Have all appropriate traction equipment transported to the patient's room on a traction cart.
• Set up the traction frame according to established hospital policy.

Comparing traction types

Traction therapy restricts movement of a patient's affected limb or body part and may confine the patient to bed rest for an extended period. The limb is immobilized by pulling with equal force on each end of the injured area—an equal mix of traction and countertraction. Weights provide the pulling force. Countertraction is produced by using other weights or by positioning the patient's body weight against the traction pull.

Skin traction

This procedure immobilizes a body part intermittently over an extended period through direct application of a pulling force to the patient's skin. The force may be applied using adhesive or nonadhesive traction tape or skin traction devices such as a boot, belt, or halter.

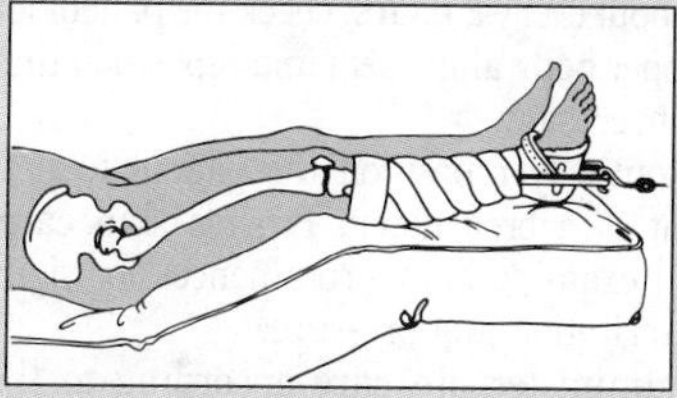

Adhesive attachment allows more continuous traction, whereas nonadhesive attachment allows easier removal for care.

Skeletal traction

This technique immobilizes a body part for prolonged periods by attaching weighted equipment directly to the patient's bones with pins, screws, wires, or tongs. Skeletal traction allows more prolonged traction with heavier weight than skin traction.

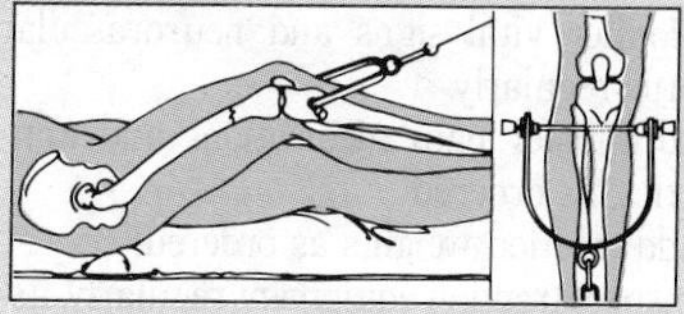

During the procedure
- Assist the doctor with the skeletal traction procedure as needed. Apply skin traction if appropriately trained. Apply ordered weights slowly and carefully to avoid jerking the affected extremity.
- Offer emotional support to the patient.

After the procedure
- Show the patient how much movement he's allowed, and instruct him not to readjust the equipment. Tell him to report any pain or pressure from the traction equipment.
- Assess for signs and symptoms of immobility complications.
- Monitor patients with skeletal traction for signs of infection, such as elevated temperature or an increase in redness, drainage, or swelling at pin sites.
- Unwrap skin traction every shift to assess for redness, warmth, blisters, and other signs of skin breakdown.
- About every 2 hours, check the patient for proper body alignment and reposition him as necessary.
- Routinely reposition the patient to prevent skin breakdown. Provide skin care, and examine bony prominences for signs of irritation and pressure.
- Administer pin care according to the doctor's order.
- Encourage coughing and deep-breathing exercises, and assist the patient with ordered range-of-motion exercises for his unaffected extremities. Apply elastic support stockings, as ordered.
- Monitor the patient's elimination pattern, and provide dietary fiber and sufficient fluids to prevent constipation. If necessary, administer stool softeners, laxatives, or enemas, as ordered.
- Monitor vital signs and neurovascular status regularly.
- Administer pain medications and antibiotics, as ordered.
- Add traction weights as ordered.
- Inspect traction equipment regularly. Assess for kinks, knots, or frays in ropes, and make sure weights hang freely and don't touch the floor. Traction must be continuous to be effective.
- Encourage the patient to do as much for himself as possible to reestablish a positive self-concept.

Tricuspid insufficiency

In this disorder, also known as tricuspid regurgitation, an incompetent tricuspid valve allows blood to flow back into the right atrium during systole, decreasing blood flow to the lungs and the left side of the heart. Cardiac output also decreases.

Causes
Tricuspid insufficiency results from marked dilation of the right ventricle and tricuspid valve ring. It most commonly occurs in the late stages of heart failure because of rheumatic or congenital heart disease.

Less commonly, it results from congenitally deformed tricuspid valves, atrioventricular canal defects, or Ebstein's anomaly of the tricuspid valve. Other causes include infarction of the right ventricular papillary muscles, tricuspid valve prolapse, carcinoid heart disease, endomyocardial fibrosis, infective endocarditis, and trauma.

Complications
Fluid overload in the right side of the heart can lead to right ventricular failure.

Assessment
The patient may have a history of a disorder that can cause tricuspid insufficiency.

The patient may complain of dyspnea, fatigue, weakness, and syncope. Peripheral edema may cause him discomfort.

Inspection may reveal jugular vein distention with prominent *v* waves in a patient with normal sinus rhythm. In severe tricuspid insufficiency that has progressed to right ventricular failure, the patient may appear jaundiced, with severe peripheral edema and ascites. He may also appear malnourished.

Auscultation may disclose a blowing holosystolic murmur at the lower left sternal border that increases with inspiration and decreases with expiration and Valsalva's maneuver.

Palpation may reveal hepatomegaly (when the patient has right ventricular failure), systolic pulsations of the liver, and a positive hepatojugular reflex. You also may feel a prominent right ventricular pulsation along the left parasternal region.

Diagnostic tests

- *Cardiac catheterization* demonstrates markedly decreased cardiac output. The right atrial pressure pulse may exhibit no *x* descent during early systole, but instead a prominent *c-v* wave with a rapid *y* descent. The mean right atrial and right ventricular end-diastolic pressures typically are elevated.
- *Chest X-rays* show right atrial and ventricular enlargement.
- *Echocardiography* reveals right ventricular dilation and prolapse or flailing of the tricuspid leaflets.
- *Electrocardiography* discloses right atrial hypertrophy, right or left ventricular hypertrophy, atrial fibrillation, and incomplete right bundle-branch heart block.

Treatment

A sodium-restricted diet and diuretics help reduce hepatic congestion before surgery. When rheumatic fever has deformed the tricuspid valve and resulted in severe insufficiency, the patient usually will need open-heart surgery for tricuspid annuloplasty or tricuspid valve replacement.

Key nursing diagnoses and patient outcomes

Decreased cardiac output related to reduced blood flow to left ventricle. Based on this nursing diagnosis, you'll establish these patient outcomes. The patient will:

- maintain hemodynamic stability, as exhibited by stable vital signs and orientation to time, person, and place
- show no evidence of organ dysfunction caused by inadequate tissue perfusion
- regain normal cardiac output with valve replacement.

Fatigue related to decreased tissue oxygenation caused by decreased cardiac output. Based on this nursing diagnosis, you'll establish these patient outcomes. The patient will:

- identify activities that increase fatigue and obtain help with these activities
- incorporate measures that modify fatigue into his daily routine
- demonstrate skill in conserving energy while carrying out activities of daily living to his tolerance level.

Fluid volume excess related to backflow of blood into systemic circulation. Based on this nursing diagnosis, you'll establish these patient outcomes. The patient will:

- comply with fluid and sodium restrictions
- have an output greater than his intake
- show no signs and symptoms of right ventricular heart failure.

Nursing interventions

- Alternate periods of activity and rest to prevent extreme fatigue and dyspnea.
- Keep the patient's legs elevated while he's sitting in a chair to improve venous return to his heart.
- Elevate the head of his bed to improve ventilation.
- Maintain a low-sodium diet. Consult with a dietitian to ensure that the patient receives foods that he likes while adhering to the diet restrictions.
- To reduce anxiety, allow the patient to express his concerns about the effects of activity restrictions on his responsibilities and routines. Reassure him that the restrictions are temporary.
- Prepare the patient for surgery, as indicated. (See the entry "Heart valve replacement.")

Monitoring

- Be alert for signs of heart failure, pulmonary edema, and adverse reactions to drug therapy.
- Monitor the patient's vital signs and mental status for changes suggestive of decreased cardiac output, such as hypotension, tachycardia, and confusion.

Patient teaching

- Teach the patient about diet restrictions, medications, signs and symptoms that should be reported, and the importance of consistent follow-up care.
- Tell the patient to elevate his legs whenever he's sitting.

Tricuspid stenosis

This relatively uncommon disorder obstructs blood flow from the right atrium to the right ventricle, which causes the right atrium to dilate and hypertrophy. Eventually, this leads to right ventricular failure and increases pressure in the vena cava.

Tricuspid stenosis seldom occurs alone and most often is associated with mitral stenosis. It's most common in women.

Causes

Although this disorder is usually caused by rheumatic fever, it also may be congenital.

Complications

Patients with untreated tricuspid stenosis may develop right ventricular failure.

Assessment

The patient with tricuspid stenosis may complain of dyspnea, fatigue, weakness, and syncope. Peripheral edema may cause her discomfort.

Inspection may reveal jugular vein distention with giant *a* waves in a patient who has normal sinus rhythm. The patient with severe tricuspid stenosis that has progressed to right ventricular failure may appear jaundiced, with severe peripheral edema and ascites. She also may appear malnourished.

Auscultation may reveal a diastolic murmur at the lower left sternal border and over the xiphoid process. It's most prominent during presystole in sinus rhythm. The murmur increases with inspiration and decreases with expiration and during Valsalva's maneuver.

Palpation may discover hepatomegaly when the patient has right ventricular failure.

Diagnostic tests

- *Cardiac catheterization* shows an increased pressure gradient across the valve, increased right atrial pressure, and decreased cardiac output.
- *Chest X-rays* demonstrate right atrial and superior vena cava enlargement.
- *Echocardiography* indicates thick tricuspid valve and right atrial enlargement.
- *Electrocardiography* reveals right atrial hypertrophy, right or left ventricular hypertrophy, and atrial fibrillation. Tall, peaked P waves appear in lead II, and prominent, upright P waves appear in lead V_1.

Treatment

In tricuspid stenosis, treatment is based on the patient's symptoms. A sodium-restricted diet and diuretics can help to reduce hepatic congestion before surgery.

A patient with moderate to severe stenosis probably will require open-heart surgery for valvulotomy or valve replacement. Valvuloplasty may be performed on elderly patients with end-stage disease in the cardiac catheterization laboratory.

Key nursing diagnoses and patient outcomes

Decreased cardiac output related to reduced blood flow to left ventricle. Based on this nursing diagnosis, you'll establish these patient outcomes. The patient will:

• maintain hemodynamic stability, as exhibited by stable vital signs and orientation to time, person, and place
• show no evidence of organ dysfunction caused by inadequate tissue perfusion
• regain normal cardiac output with valve replacement or valvuloplasty.

Fatigue related to decreased tissue oxygenation caused by decreased cardiac output. Based on this nursing diagnosis, you'll establish these patient outcomes. The patient will:
• identify activities that increase fatigue and obtain help with these activities
• incorporate measures that modify fatigue into her daily routine
• demonstrate skill in conserving energy while carrying out activities of daily living to her tolerance level.

Fluid volume excess related to backflow of blood into systemic circulation. Based on this nursing diagnosis, you'll establish these patient outcomes. The patient will:
• comply with fluid and sodium restrictions
• have an output greater than her intake
• show no signs and symptoms of right ventricular heart failure.

Nursing interventions

• Alternate periods of activity and rest to prevent extreme fatigue and dyspnea.
• When the patient sits in a chair, elevate her legs to improve venous return to the heart.
• Elevate the head of the bed to improve ventilation.
• Keep the patient on a low-sodium diet. Consult with a dietitian to ensure that the patient receives foods that she likes while adhering to the diet restrictions.
• Allow the patient to express her fears and concerns about the disorder, its impact on her life, and any impending surgery. Reassure her as needed.
• Prepare the patient for surgery, as indicated. (See the entries "Heart valve replacement" and "Valvuloplasty, balloon.")

Monitoring

• Watch for signs of heart failure, pulmonary edema, and adverse reactions to drug therapy.
• Monitor the patient's vital signs and mental status for changes suggestive of decreased cardiac output, such as hypotension, tachycardia, and confusion.

Patient teaching

• Teach the patient about diet restrictions, medications, signs and symptoms that should be reported, and the importance of consistent follow-up care.
• Urge the patient to elevate her legs whenever she sits down.

Tuberculosis

An acute or chronic infection, tuberculosis is characterized by pulmonary infiltrates and by formation of granulomas with caseation, fibrosis, and cavitation. The American Lung Association estimates that active disease afflicts nearly 14 of every 100,000 persons.

The disease is twice as common in men as in women and four times as common in nonwhites as in whites. But incidence is highest in people who live in crowded, poorly ventilated, unsanitary conditions, such as those in some prisons, tenement houses, and homeless shelters. The typical newly diagnosed tuberculosis patient is a single, homeless, nonwhite man. With proper treatment, the prognosis is usually excellent. (See *Who's at risk for TB?* page 926.)

Causes

Tuberculosis results from exposure to *Mycobacterium tuberculosis* and sometimes other strains of mycobacteria. Transmission occurs when an infected person coughs or sneezes, spreading infected droplets.

When a person without immunity inhales these droplets, the bacilli lodge in the

Who's at risk for TB?

The risk of tuberculosis is higher in the following:
- Black and Hispanic men between ages 25 and 44
- those in close contact with a newly diagnosed tuberculosis patient
- those who have had tuberculosis before
- people with multiple sexual partners
- recent immigrants from Africa, Asia, Mexico, and South America
- gastrectomy patients
- people affected with silicosis, diabetes, malnutrition, cancer, Hodgkin's disease, or leukemia
- drug and alcohol abusers
- patients in mental institutions
- nursing home residents, who are 10 times more likely to contract tuberculosis than anyone in the general population
- those receiving treatment with immunosuppressants or corticosteroids
- people with weak immune systems or diseases that affect the immune system, especially those with acquired immunodeficiency syndrome.

alveoli, causing irritation. The immune system responds by sending leukocytes, lymphocytes, and macrophages to surround the bacilli, and the local lymph nodes swell and become inflamed. If the encapsulated bacilli (tubercles) and the inflamed nodes rupture, the infection contaminates the surrounding tissue and may spread through the blood and lymphatic circulation to distant sites – a process called hematogenous dissemination. This same phagocytic cycle occurs whenever the bacilli spread.

After exposure to *M. tuberculosis,* roughly 5% of infected people develop active tuberculosis within 1 year; in the remainder, microorganisms cause a latent infection. The host's immunologic defense system usually destroys the bacillus or walls it up in a tubercle. But the live, encapsulated bacilli may lie dormant within the tubercle for years, reactivating later to cause active infection.

Complications

Tuberculosis can cause massive pulmonary tissue damage, with inflammation and tissue necrosis eventually leading to respiratory failure. Bronchopleural fistulas can develop from lung tissue damage, resulting in pneumothorax. The disease can also lead to hemorrhage, pleural effusion, and pneumonia. Small mycobacterial foci can infect other body organs, including the kidneys and the central nervous and skeletal systems.

Assessment

The patient with a primary infection may complain of weakness and fatigue, anorexia and weight loss, and night sweats. The patient with reactivated tuberculosis may report chest pain and a cough that produces blood or mucopurulent or blood-tinged sputum. He may also have a low-grade fever.

When you percuss, you may note dullness over the affected area, a sign of consolidation or the presence of pleural fluid. On auscultation, you may hear crepitant crackles, bronchial breath sounds, wheezes, and whispered pectoriloquy.

Diagnostic tests

- *Chest X-rays* show nodular lesions, patchy infiltrates (mainly in upper lobes), cavity formation, scar tissue, and calcium deposits. However, they may not help distinguish between active and inactive tuberculosis.
- A *tuberculin skin test* reveals that the patient has been infected with tuberculosis at some point, but it doesn't indicate active disease. In this test, intermediate-strength purified protein derivative or 5 tuberculin units (0.1 ml) are injected intradermally on the forearm and read in 48 to 72 hours. A positive reaction (equal to or more than a 10-mm induration) develops within 2 to 10 weeks after infection with the tubercle

bacillus in both active and inactive tuberculosis.

• *Stains* and *cultures* – of sputum, cerebrospinal fluid, urine, drainage from abscess, or pleural fluid – show heat-sensitive, nonmotile, aerobic, acid-fast bacilli.

• *Computed tomography* or *magnetic resonance imaging scans* allow the evaluation of lung damage or confirm a difficult diagnosis.

• *Bronchoscopy* may be performed if the patient can't produce an adequate sputum specimen.

Several of these tests may need to be performed to distinguish tuberculosis from other diseases that may mimic it (such as lung cancer, lung abscess, pneumoconiosis, and bronchiectasis).

Treatment

Antitubercular therapy with daily oral doses of isoniazid or rifampin (with ethambutol added in some cases) for at least 9 months usually cures tuberculosis. After 2 to 4 weeks, the disease is no longer infectious and the patient can resume his normal activities while continuing to take medication.

The patient with atypical mycobacterial disease or drug-resistant tuberculosis may require second-line drugs, such as capreomycin, streptomycin, para-aminosalicylic acid, pyrazinamide, and cycloserine.

Key nursing diagnoses and patient outcomes

Altered protection related to potential for recurrence and possible transmission of mycobacterial foci to other areas of the body. Based on this nursing diagnosis, you'll establish these patient outcomes. The patient will:

• show no signs and symptoms of organ dysfunction outside of the lungs

• comply with the prescribed tuberculosis treatment to eradicate the infection and minimize the risk of other organs becoming infected

• identify and promptly report early signs and symptoms of organ dysfunction.

Impaired gas exchange related to changes in pulmonary tissue. Based on this nursing diagnosis, you'll establish these patient outcomes. The patient will:

• regain and maintain adequate ventilation

• show no signs and symptoms of hypoxia

• regain and maintain normal arterial blood gas values.

Knowledge deficit related to tuberculosis. Based on this nursing diagnosis, you'll establish these patient outcomes. The patient will:

• identify the need to learn about tuberculosis

• obtain correct information about tuberculosis

• communicate an understanding about how tuberculosis is contracted and managed, and how a recurrence can be prevented.

Nursing interventions

• Administer ordered antibiotics and antitubercular agents. Give isoniazid and ethambutol with food.

• Institute standard and airborne precautions. Isolate the infectious patient in a quiet, well-ventilated room until he's no longer contagious. Provide diversional activities, and check on him frequently. Make sure the call button is nearby.

• Place a covered trash can nearby or tape a waxed bag to the bedside for used tissues. Tell the patient to wear a mask when outside his room. Visitors and hospital personnel should also wear masks in the patient's room.

• Make sure the patient gets plenty of rest. Provide for alternating periods of rest and activity to promote health as well as conserve energy and reduce oxygen demand.

• Provide the patient with well-balanced, high-calorie foods, preferably in small, frequent meals to conserve energy. (Small, frequent meals may also encourage the anorexic patient to eat more.) If the patient needs oral supplements, consult with the dietitian.

• Perform chest physiotherapy, including postural drainage and chest percussion, several times a day.
• Give the patient supportive care, and help him adjust to the changes he may have to make during his illness. Include the patient in care decisions, and let the family take part in the patient's care whenever possible.

Monitoring

• Monitor the patient's respiratory status. Auscultate breath sounds frequently.
• Weigh the patient weekly, and report significant weight loss (greater than 2 lb [about 1 kg] per week).
• Because isoniazid can cause hepatitis or peripheral neuritis, monitor levels of aspartate aminotransferase (formerly SGOT) and alanine aminotransferase (formerly SGPT).
• If the patient receives ethambutol, watch for signs of optic neuritis; report them to the doctor, who will probably discontinue the drug. Assess the patient's vision monthly.
• If the patient receives rifampin, watch for signs of hepatitis, purpura, and a flulike syndrome as well as other complications, such as hemoptysis. Monitor liver and kidney function tests throughout therapy.
• Monitor the patient's compliance with treatment.

Patient teaching

• Show the patient and his family how to perform postural drainage and chest percussion. Also, teach the patient coughing and deep-breathing techniques. Instruct him to maintain each position for 10 minutes and then to perform percussion and cough.
• Teach the patient the adverse effects of his medication, and tell him to report reactions immediately. Emphasize the importance of regular follow-up examinations, and instruct the patient and his family concerning the signs and symptoms of recurring tuberculosis. Stress the need to follow long-term treatment faithfully.
• Warn the patient taking rifampin that the drug will temporarily make his body secretions appear orange; reassure him that this effect is harmless. If the patient is a woman, warn her that oral contraceptives may be less effective while she's taking rifampin.
• Teach the patient the signs and symptoms that require medical assessment: increased cough, hemoptysis, unexplained weight loss, fever, and night sweats.
• Stress the importance of eating high-calorie, high-protein, balanced meals.
• Explain standard and airborne precautions to the hospitalized patient. Before discharge, tell him that he must take precautions to prevent spreading the disease – such as wearing a mask around others – until his doctor tells him he's no longer contagious. He should tell all health care providers he sees, including his dentist and eye doctor, that he has tuberculosis so that they can institute infection-control precautions.
• Teach the patient other specific precautions to avoid spreading the infection. Tell him to cough and sneeze into tissues and to dispose of the tissues properly. Stress the importance of washing his hands thoroughly in hot, soapy water after handling his own secretions. Also, instruct him to wash his eating utensils separately in hot, soapy water.
• Advise anyone exposed to an infected patient to receive tuberculin tests and, if ordered, chest X-rays and prophylactic isoniazid.
• Assess for need of home oxygen; teach oxygen administration and safety.
• Emphasize the importance of scheduling and keeping follow-up appointments.
• Refer the patient to such support groups as the American Lung Association.

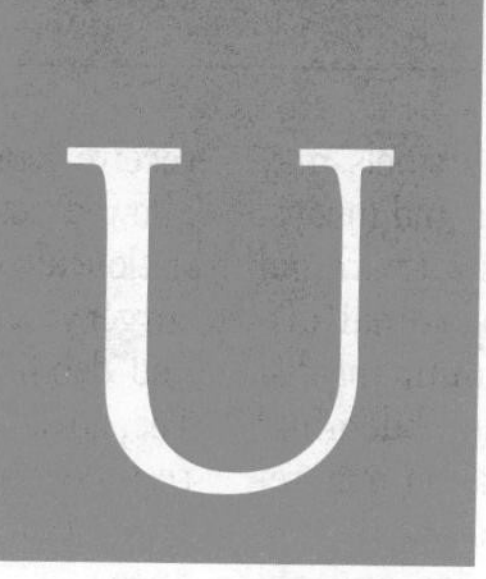

Ulcerative colitis

An inflammatory, commonly chronic disease, ulcerative colitis affects the mucosa of the colon. It usually begins in the rectum and sigmoid colon and may extend upward into the entire colon; it rarely affects the small intestine, except for the terminal ileum. Ulcerative colitis produces congestion, edema (leading to mucosal friability), and ulcerations. Severity ranges from a mild, localized disorder to a fulminant disease that can cause many complications.

Ulcerative colitis occurs primarily in young adults, especially women; it is also more prevalent among Jews and higher socioeconomic groups. The incidence of the disease is unknown; however, some studies indicate that as many as 1 out of 1,000 persons are affected. Onset of symptoms seems to peak between ages 15 and 20 and again between ages 55 and 60.

Causes

Although the etiology of ulcerative colitis is unknown, it may be related to an abnormal immune response in the GI tract, possibly associated with food or bacteria. Stress was once thought to be a cause of ulcerative colitis. Studies show that, although it's not a cause, stress can increase the severity of an attack.

Complications

Ulcerative colitis may lead to a variety of complications, depending on the severity and site of inflammation. Nutritional deficiencies are the most common complication, but the disease can also lead to perineal sepsis with anal fissure, anal fistula, perirectal abscess, hemorrhage, and toxic megacolon. A patient with ulcerative colitis has an increased risk of various arthritis types (forty times more prevalent in this group than in the general population) and cancer (if the disease has persisted more than 10 years since childhood).

Other complications include coagulation defects resulting from vitamin K deficiency, erythema nodosum on the face and arms, pyoderma gangrenosum on the legs and ankles, uveitis, pericholangitis, sclerosing cholangitis, cirrhosis, possible cholangiocarcinoma, ankylosing spondylitis, loss of muscle mass, strictures, pseudopolyps, stenosis, and perforated colon, leading to peritonitis and toxemia.

Assessment

Usually, the patient's history will reveal periods of remission and exacerbation of symptoms. During an exacerbation, the patient generally reports mild cramping, lower abdominal pain, and recurrent bloody diarrhea – as often as 10 to 25 times daily. She may also experience nocturnal diarrhea. During these periods, she may complain of fatigue, weakness, anorexia, weight loss, nausea, and vomiting.

On inspection, the patient's stools may appear liquid, with visible pus and mucus. Check for blood in the stools – a cardinal sign of ulcerative colitis. Abdominal distention may be present in fulminant disease. Palpation may disclose abdominal tenderness. A rectal examination may reveal perianal irritation, hemorrhoids, and fissures. Rarely, rectal fistulas and abscesses may be evident.

Diagnostic tests

- *Sigmoidoscopy* confirms rectal involvement in most cases by showing increased mucosal friability, decreased mucosal detail, and thick inflammatory exudate.
- *Colonoscopy* may determine the extent of the disease and also evaluate the strictured areas and pseudopolyps. This test is not performed when the patient has active signs and symptoms.
- *Biopsy,* performed during colonoscopy, can help confirm the diagnosis.
- *Barium enema* evaluates the extent of the disease and detects complications, such as strictures and carcinoma. This study is not performed in a patient with active signs and symptoms.
- *Stool specimen analysis* reveals blood, pus, and mucus, but no pathogenic organisms.
- *Other supportive laboratory tests* show decreased serum levels of potassium, magnesium, hemoglobin, and albumin, as well as leukocytosis and increased prothrombin time. Erythrocyte sedimentation rate elevation correlates with the severity of the attack.

Treatment

The goals of treatment are to control inflammation, replace nutritional losses and blood volume, and prevent complications. Supportive treatment includes dietary therapy, bed rest, I.V. fluid replacement, and medications. Blood transfusions or iron supplements may be needed to correct anemia.

Dietary measures depend on disease severity. Patients with severe disease usually receive total parenteral nutrition and are allowed nothing by mouth. Parenteral nutrition also is used for patients awaiting surgery or showing signs of dehydration and debilitation from excessive diarrhea. The goals of parenteral nutrition are to rest the intestinal tract, decrease stool volume, and restore positive nitrogen balance.

The patient with moderate signs and symptoms may receive an elemental feeding source, such as Ensure, to provide adequate nutrition with minimal bowel stimulation. A low-residue diet may be ordered for the patient with mild signs and symptoms. As signs and symptoms subside, the diet may gradually advance to include a greater variety of foods.

Drug therapy to control inflammation includes corticotropin and adrenal corticosteroids, such as prednisone, prednisolone, and hydrocortisone; sulfasalazine, which has anti-inflammatory and antimicrobial properties, may also be used. Antispasmodics, such as tincture of belladonna, and antidiarrheals, such as diphenoxylate and atropine, are used only for the patient with frequent, troublesome diarrhea whose ulcerative colitis is otherwise under control. These drugs may precipitate massive dilation of the colon (toxic megacolon) and are generally contraindicated.

Surgery, considered the cure for ulcerative colitis, is performed if the patient has toxic megacolon, if she fails to respond to drugs and supportive measures, or if she finds signs and symptoms unbearable.

The most common surgical technique is proctocolectomy with ileostomy. Total colectomy and ileorectal anastomosis is done less often because of its mortality rate (2% to 5%). This procedure removes the entire colon and anastomoses the rectum and the terminal ileum. It requires observation of the remaining rectal stump for any signs of cancer or colitis.

Pouch ileostomy, in which a pouch is created from a small loop of the terminal ileum and a nipple valve is formed from the distal ileum, is gaining popularity. The resulting stoma opens just above the pubic hairline; the pouch empties through a catheter inserted in the stoma several times a day. In ulcerative colitis, colectomy to prevent colon cancer is controversial.

Ileoanal reservoir is a newer surgical technique that preserves the anal sphincter and provides the patient with a reservoir made from the ileum and attached to the anal opening. First, the rectal mucosa is excised, then an abdominal colectomy is performed, and a reservoir is constructed and attached. Next, a temporary loop ileostomy is made to allow the new rectal reservoir to heal. Finally, the loop ileostomy is closed after a 3- or 4-month waiting period. Stools from the reservoir are similar to the stools from an ileostomy.

Key nursing diagnoses and patient outcomes

Altered nutrition: Less than body requirements related to inflammation of lower GI tract. Based on this nursing diagnosis, you'll establish these patient outcomes. The patient will:

- show no further evidence of weight loss
- tolerate oral, tube, or I.V. feedings without adverse effects
- regain and maintain a normal nutritional state.

Diarrhea related to inflammation of lower GI tract. Based on this nursing diagnosis, you'll establish these patient outcomes. The patient will:

- be able to control diarrhea with medication
- show no signs of skin breakdown in the anal area
- report that her elimination pattern has returned to normal.

Risk for fluid volume deficit related to loss of fluid and electrolytes from diarrhea. Based on this nursing diagnosis, you'll establish these patient outcomes. The patient will:

- maintain electrolyte values within normal limits
- show no evidence of fluid volume deficit
- maintain stable vital signs and a normal urine output.

Nursing interventions

- Support the patient emotionally. Stay with her when she's acutely distressed. Spend a few minutes with her several times a day and listen to her concerns. Offer reassurance when appropriate.
- Provide diet therapy as ordered.
- Provide frequent mouth care for the patient who is allowed nothing by mouth.
- Administer medications as prescribed.
- Give blood transfusions as ordered.
- Schedule care to allow for frequent rest periods. These patients are often very tired and weak.
- After each bowel movement, thoroughly clean the skin around the rectum and apply a soothing and protective agent, such as petroleum jelly, to the irritated area. Provide an air mattress to help prevent skin breakdown.
- Prepare the patient for bowel surgery, as indicated. (See the entries "Bowel resection with anastomosis" and "Bowel resection with ostomy.")

Monitoring

- Regardless of the prescribed diet, monitor intake and calorie count. Record intake and output, noting the frequency and volume of stools.
- Monitor the fluid and electrolyte status of the patient on total parenteral nutrition. Assess the insertion site for inflammation. Check blood glucose and urine acetone levels every 6 hours.
- Monitor hemoglobin and hematocrit levels.
- Assess the patient regularly for desired effects of administered medication. Note any adverse reactions, such as those from prolonged corticosteroid therapy (moon face, edema, gastric irritation). Be aware that such therapy may mask infection.

• Watch for signs of dehydration (poor skin turgor, furrowed tongue) and electrolyte imbalances, especially signs of hypokalemia (muscle weakness, paresthesia) and hypernatremia (tachycardia, fever, dry tongue).
• Watch closely for signs of complications, such as a perforated colon and peritonitis (fever, severe abdominal pain, abdominal rigidity and tenderness, cool clammy skin), and toxic megacolon (abdominal distention, decreased bowel sounds).

Patient teaching

• Teach the patient about the disorder and review its signs and symptoms. Explain diagnostic tests and ordered treatments.
• Discuss all prescribed dietary changes and help the patient understand how these measures will decrease her symptoms. If she's placed on parenteral nutrition or a very restricted diet, reassure her that she will be able to progress to a more advanced diet as her symptoms resolve. In general, caution the patient to avoid GI stimulants, such as caffeine, alcohol, and tobacco products.
• Review the patient's medications with her. Explain the desired actions, dosage, and adverse effects.
• If the patient is scheduled for surgery, reinforce the doctor's explanation of the procedure and its possible complications. As part of preoperative teaching, describe the stoma and explain how it differs from normal anatomy. Provide additional patient information as needed (available from the United Ostomy Association). Arrange for a visit by an enterostomal therapist and, ideally, a recovered ileostomate.
• After a proctocolectomy and ileostomy, teach stoma care. After a pouch ileostomy, demonstrate procedures to insert the catheter and care for the stoma.
• Emphasize the need for regular physical examinations because of the increased risk for colorectal cancer (unless an ileostomy has been done).

Urinary diversion surgery

A urinary diversion provides an alternative route for urine excretion when pathology impedes normal flow through the bladder. Most commonly performed in patients who've undergone a cystectomy, diversion surgery also may be performed in patients with a congenital urinary tract defect; a severe, unmanageable urinary tract infection that threatens renal function; an injury to the ureters, bladder, or urethra; an obstructive malignancy; or a neurogenic bladder.

There are several ways that urinary diversion surgery can be performed. Possible procedures include ileal conduit (also known as ureteroileal urinary conduit, ileal bladder, ileal loop, Bricker's procedure, and ureteroileostomy), continent internal ileal reservoir (also known as a Kock pouch), and orthotopic bladder replacement. (See *Reviewing selected types of urinary diversion.*)

Urinary diversions may be categorized as incontinent or continent. Incontinent diversions include the ileal conduit, ureterosigmoidostomy, and nephrostomy. With these types, urine flow is constant and an external collection device is required permanently. Continent diversions include the Kock pouch, Indiana pouch, Mainze reservoir, and Camey procedure (also known as the orthotopic bladder replacement). The advantage of these procedures is that an external collection bag is not needed. However, there is the possibility of urine leakage.

Ileal conduit, the most common urinary diversion, involves anastomosis of the ureters to a small portion of the ileum excised especially for the procedure, followed by the creation of a stoma from one end of the ileal segment. This resulting stoma is called a urostomy. It drains urine continuously and requires the patient to wear an external pouch at all times.

Reviewing selected types of urinary diversion

Types of urinary diversion include ileal conduit, continent internal ileal reservoir (Kock pouch or Indiana pouch), and orthotopic bladder replacement.

Ileal conduit
Both ureters are anastomosed to a small segment of ileum, one end of which is brought to the surface of the lower abdomen to form a stoma.

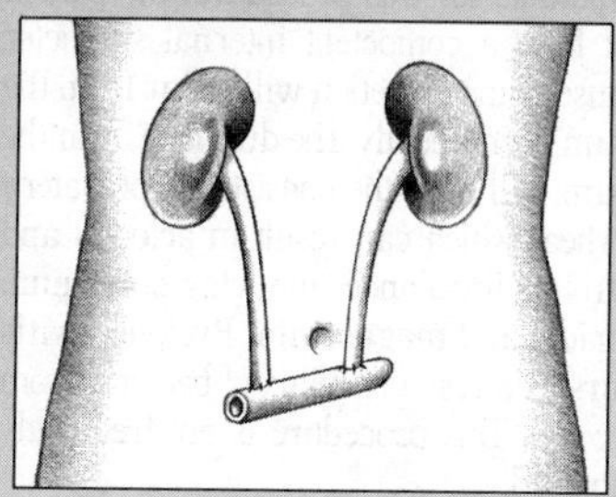

Orthotopic bladder replacement
An internal pouch is created from the small bowel or small and large bowel. The urethral stump is anastomosed to the pouch. The patient voids through the urethra. This procedure is performed in men only. The patient commonly experiences nocturnal incontinence.

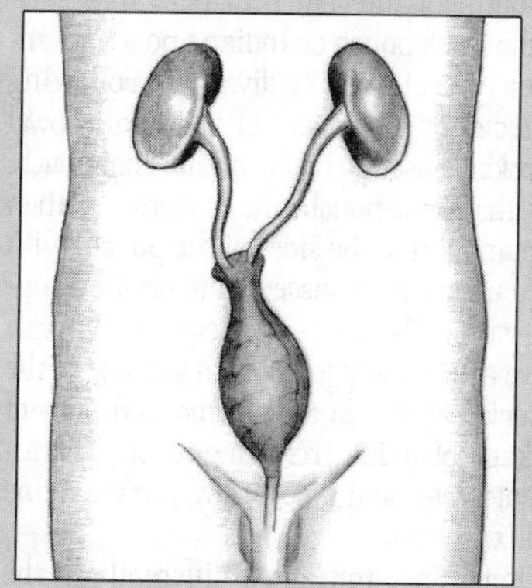

Continent internal ileal reservoir (Kock pouch)
An internal pouch is created from a segment of ileum. The ureters are implanted into the pouch's sides, and nipple valves are intussuscepted to them. One valve prevents urine backflow; the other valve is used to form a stoma.

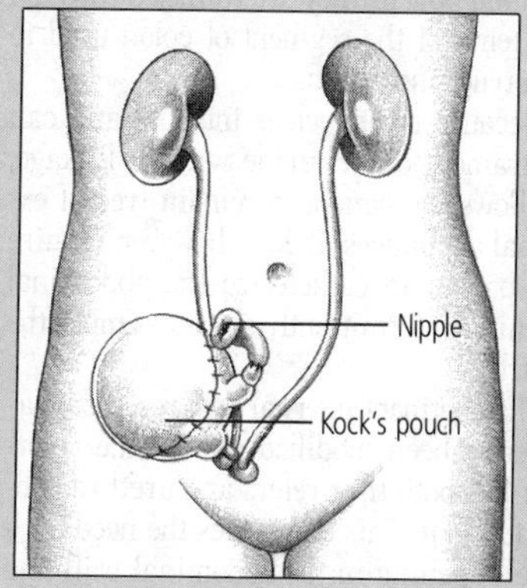

A ureterosigmoidostomy is an internal urinary diversion that redirects urine through the colon and then out the rectum. This detour into the colon causes two major complications: metabolic disorders (hyperchloremic acidosis) and pyelonephritis. To be a candidate for this procedure, the patient must have a competent internal sphincter because urine excretion will occur from the rectum permanently. The drainage from the rectum will have the consistency of watery diarrhea, which can result in acidosis and electrolyte imbalances involving potassium, chloride, and magnesium. Pyelonephritis occurs as a result of reflux of bacteria from the colon. This procedure is not frequently performed.

Continent internal ileal reservoir, such as the Kock pouch or Indiana pouch, is another type of urinary diversion. Following cystectomy, a segment of the small bowel or colon is used to create an internal pouch. For the Kock pouch, the ureters are then implanted into the sides of the pouch, with each ureter intussuscepted to create a nipple valve. The efferent ureter and nipple valve are brought to the skin surface of the anterior abdomen as a stoma and prevent leakage of urine from the pouch. The afferent ureter and nipple valve prevent urine reflux.

Ureters are implanted differently in the Indiana pouch. They are tunneled through the tenia of the segment of colon used to construct the pouch.

Because the pouch is internal and can be trained to hold urine without leakage, it allows the patient to remain free of external appliances. It does, however, require the patient to catheterize the abdominal opening intermittently so as to empty the pouch.

The continent internal ileal reservoir has recently been modified so that the reservoir has both the ureters and urethra connected to it. This eliminates the need for a small opening in the abdominal wall and helps preserve the patient's body image. However, unless the lower portion of the bladder can be spared, continence depends solely on the urethra and external sphincter. Consequently, total bladder substitution is usually limited to men. Drainage of the internal pouch relies on passive emptying when the external sphincter is relaxed and on abdominal straining. If these techniques aren't sufficient, the patient must learn intermittent self-catheterization. Complications, such as tumor recurrence in the urethra and frequent nocturnal enuresis, can affect up to 50% of patients and are major drawbacks of the procedure.

Another possible procedure is a nephrostomy, which is a short-term technique that diverts urine away from an obstruction or lesion below the level of the renal pelvis.

Procedure

After the patient is anesthetized, the surgeon makes a midline or paramedial abdominal incision.

To construct an ileal conduit, the surgeon excises a 6″ to 8″ (15- to 20-cm) segment of the ileum (also taking its mesentery to help preserve tissue viability) and then anastomoses the remaining ileal ends to maintain intestinal integrity. Next, he dissects the ureters from the bladder and implants them in the ileal segment. The surgeon then sutures one end of the ileal segment closed and brings the other end through the abdominal wall to form a stoma.

To create a nephrostomy, the surgeon inserts a catheter into the renal pelvis either percutaneously or through a flank incision. This procedure is usually palliative because it carries a high risk of infection and stone formation.

The surgeon may create any one of a number of different types of continent internal ileal reservoirs (such as the Kock pouch or the Indiana pouch) using segments of the small bowel and colon. For example, if he decides to make a Kock pouch, he excises 24″ to 32″ (60 to 80 cm) of ileum and anastomoses the remaining ileal ends to maintain intestinal integrity. After shaping the isolated ileum segment into a pocket to serve as a bladder, he connects the Kock pouch to the urethra or uses an intussuscepted nipple valve to connect the pouch to the external skin of the anterior abdominal wall. He then constructs a second nipple valve at the other end of the pouch to prevent urine from flowing backward into the ureters. Finally, he implants the ureters at the site of the second nipple valve along with ureteral stents. The ureteral stents, which originate in the pelvis of the kidneys and extend through the ureter into the reservoir and out through the abdominal opening or separate stab wounds, are used to keep the ureters patent until they are no longer needed (usually 7 to 10 days postoperatively).

Depending on the length, type of tubing used, and exit site, the stents may be placed to dependent drainage or may be contained with a pouching system. One or two drainage tubes are then inserted into the reservoir to maintain unobstructed drainage from the reservoir until healing has occurred and pouch integrity is confirmed.

To construct an orthotopic bladder replacement, the surgeon creates a pouch from the small bowel or small and large bowel and connects it to the urethral stump. An indwelling catheter is inserted for about 3 weeks. After the catheter is removed, the patient voids through the urethra. Voiding is accomplished by abdominal straining.

Complications

Postoperative complications of urinary diversion surgery include skin breakdown around the stoma site, wound infection or wound dehiscence, urinary extravasation, ureteral obstruction, small-bowel obstruction, peritonitis, hydronephrosis, and stomal gangrene. Delayed complications include ureteral obstruction, stomal stenosis, pyelonephritis, renal calculi, and electrolyte disturbances. If chronic pyelonephritis occurs over a period of years, end-stage renal disease is possible. Also, the patient with a continent internal ileal reservoir may experience incontinence and, if the reservoir is connected to the urethra, frequent UTIs and tumor recurrence (if cystectomy was done due to bladder cancer).

Patients also commonly suffer psychological problems, such as depression and anxiety, related to altered body image and concern about life-style changes associated with the stoma and urine drainage. Even patients with a continent urinary reservoir attached to the urethra may still have a grief reaction to the loss of their natural bladder.

Key nursing diagnoses and patient outcomes

Body image disturbance related to presence of stoma. Based on this nursing diagnosis, you'll establish these patient outcomes. The patient will:
- acknowledge the change in body image
- be able to perform self-care on his stoma without showing negative behavior
- express positive feelings about himself.

Risk for infection related to potential for intraperitoneal leakage and greater exposure of the renal system to bacteria. Based on this nursing diagnosis, you'll establish these patient outcomes. The patient will:
- maintain a normal body temperature and white blood cell count
- know the signs and symptoms of infection
- communicate an understanding of how to prevent or reduce the risk of infection.

Impaired skin integrity related to urinary drainage from stoma. Based on this nursing diagnosis, you'll establish these patient outcomes. The patient will:
- communicate an understanding of how to manage his type of urinary diversion
- demonstrate correct stoma care
- maintain skin integrity.

Nursing interventions

When preparing a patient for surgery or managing his care afterward, your responsibilities include instructing the patient and monitoring for complications.

Before surgery

• Review the planned surgery with the patient, reinforcing the doctor's explanations as necessary. Try using a simple anatomic diagram to enhance your discussion, and provide printed information from the United Ostomy Association or other sources, if possible and appropriate. Explain to the patient that he'll receive a general anesthetic and have a nasogastric (NG) tube in place after surgery.

• If appropriate, prepare the patient for the appearance and general location of the stoma. For example, if he's scheduled for an ileal conduit, explain that the stoma will be located somewhere in the lower abdomen, probably below the waistline.

• Ensure that the patient having a continent internal ileal reservoir understands that his "new bladder" will not function identically to the natural bladder. If the reservoir will be attached to the external skin, explain that the stoma will be flush with the skin of the anterior abdominal wall, and that the exact location of the stoma is often decided during surgery.

• Review the enterostomal therapist's explanation of the urine collection device or catheterization procedure to be used after surgery. Reassure the patient that he'll receive complete training on how to manage urine drainage after he returns from surgery.

• If possible, arrange for a visit by a well-adjusted patient who's undergone the same type of urinary diversion as your patient. He can provide a firsthand account of the operation and offer some insight into the realities of ongoing care of urinary drainage. And, as appropriate, be sure to include the patient's family in all aspects of preoperative teaching – especially if they'll be providing much of the routine care after discharge. Ensure that the patient or a responsible family member has signed a consent form.

• Before surgery, prepare the bowel to reduce the risk of postoperative infection from intestinal flora. As ordered, maintain the patient on a low-residue or clear liquid diet and administer a cleansing enema and an antimicrobial drug, such as erythromycin or neomycin. Other possible measures may include total parenteral nutrition or fluid replacement therapy for debilitated patients and prophylactic I.V. antibiotics.

After surgery

• After the patient returns from surgery, monitor his vital signs every hour until they're stable. Carefully check and record urine output; report any decrease, which could indicate obstruction from postoperative edema or ureteral stenosis. Observe urine drainage for pus and blood; keep in mind that urine is often blood-tinged initially but should rapidly clear.

• Record the amount, color, and consistency of drainage from the incisional or stoma drain, ureteral stents (if present), and NG tube. Notify the doctor of any urine leakage from the drain or suture line; such leakage may point to developing complications, such as hydronephrosis. Watch for signs of peritonitis (fever, abdominal distention and pain), which can develop from intraperitoneal urine leakage.

• Check dressings frequently and change them at least once each shift. (The doctor will probably perform the first dressing change.) When changing dressings, check the suture line for redness, swelling, and drainage.

• Maintain fluid and electrolyte balance and continue I.V. replacement therapy, as ordered. Provide total parenteral nutrition, if necessary, to ensure adequate nutrition.

• Perform routine ostomy maintenance, as indicated. Make sure the collection device fits tightly around the stoma; allow no more than a 1/8" (0.3-cm) margin of skin between the stoma and the device's faceplate. Regularly check the appearance of the stoma and peristomal skin. The stoma should appear bright red; if it becomes deep red or bluish, suspect a problem with blood flow and notify the doctor. It should also be smooth; report any dimpling or retraction, which may point to stenosis. Check the peristomal skin for irritation or breakdown. Remember that the main cause of irritation is urine leakage around the edges of the collection device's faceplate. If you detect leakage, change the device, taking care to properly apply the skin sealer to ensure a tight fit.

- If the patient has a continent internal ileal reservoir, irrigate the drainage tube as ordered (usually every 2 to 8 hours) with about 60 ml of 0.9% sodium chloride solution to maintain its patency. To avoid abdominal distention during the postoperative period and allow suture lines to heal, perform irrigations gently.
- If skin breakdown occurs, clean the area with warm water and pat it dry; then apply a light dusting of karaya powder and a thin layer of protective dressing. If you detect severe excoriation, notify the doctor promptly.
- Provide emotional support throughout the recovery period to help the patient adjust to the stoma and collection pouch or to self-catheterization, as indicated. Assure him that the pouch shouldn't interfere with his life-style and that he can eventually resume all of his former activities.

Home care instructions

- Make sure the patient and his family understand and can properly perform stoma care and change the ostomy pouch. With a continent internal ileal reservoir, be sure they can care for the pouch drainage tube until it's removed (usually 3 weeks postoperatively), empty the pouch correctly (using either passive emptying or intermittent self-catheterization), and irrigate the pouch as necessary.
- Instruct the patient and his family to watch for and report signs of complications, such as fever, chills, flank or abdominal pain, and pus or blood in the urine.
- Tell the patient that he should be able to return to work soon after discharge; however, if his job requires heavy lifting, tell him to talk to his doctor before resuming work. Explain that he can safely participate in most sports, even such strenuous ones as skiing, skydiving, and scuba diving. Do, however, suggest that he avoid contact sports, such as football and wrestling.
- If the patient expresses doubts or insecurities about his sexuality related to the stoma and collection device, refer him for sexual counseling. Assure the female ostomate that pregnancy should cause her no special problems. But urge her to consult with her doctor before she becomes pregnant.
- Stress the importance of keeping scheduled follow-up appointments with the doctor and enterostomal therapist to evaluate reservoir function and stoma care and make any necessary changes in equipment. For instance, stoma shrinkage, which normally occurs within 8 weeks after surgery, may require a change in pouch size to ensure a tight fit.
- Refer the patient to a support group, such as the United Ostomy Association.

Urinary tract infection, lower

The two forms of lower urinary tract infection (UTI) are cystitis (infection of the bladder) and urethritis (infection of the urethra). They're nearly 10 times more common in females than in males (except in elderly males) and affect 10% to 20% of all females at least once.

In males, lower UTIs typically are associated with anatomic or physiologic abnormalities and therefore need close evaluation. Most UTIs respond readily to treatment, but recurrence and resistant bacterial flare-up during therapy are possible.

Causes

Most lower UTIs result from ascending infection by a single gram-negative, enteric bacterium, such as *Escherichia coli, Klebsiella, Proteus, Enterobacter, Pseudomonas,* and *Serratia.* In a patient with neurogenic bladder, an indwelling urinary catheter, or a fistula between the intestine and bladder, a lower UTI may result from simultaneous infection with multiple pathogens.

Studies suggest that infection results from a breakdown in local defense mechanisms in the bladder that allows bacteria to invade the bladder mucosa and multiply. These bacteria can't be readily eliminated by normal urination.

Bacterial flare-up during treatment usually is caused by the pathogen's resistance to the prescribed antimicrobial therapy. Even a small number of bacteria (fewer than 10,000/ml) in a midstream urine specimen obtained during treatment casts doubt on the effectiveness of treatment.

In almost all patients, recurrent lower UTIs result from reinfection by the same organism or by some new pathogen. In the remaining patients, recurrence reflects persistent infection, usually from renal calculi, chronic bacterial prostatitis, or a structural anomaly that's a source of infection. The high incidence of lower UTI among females probably occurs because natural anatomic features facilitate infection. (See *UTI risk factors.*)

Complications

If untreated, chronic UTI can seriously damage the urinary tract lining. Infection of adjacent organs and structures (for example, pyelonephritis) also may occur. When this happens, the prognosis is poor.

Assessment

The patient may complain of urinary urgency and frequency, dysuria, bladder cramps or spasms, itching, a feeling of warmth during urination, nocturia, and urethral discharge (in men). Other complaints include low back pain, malaise, nausea, vomiting, pain or tenderness over the bladder, chills, and flank pain. Inflammation of the bladder wall also causes hematuria and fever.

Diagnostic tests

The following tests are used to diagnose lower UTI:

- *Microscopic urinalysis* showing red blood cell and white blood cell counts greater than 10 per high-power field suggests lower UTI.
- *Clean-catch urinalysis* revealing a bacterial count of more than 100,000/ml confirms UTI. Lower counts don't necessarily rule out infection, especially if the patient is urinating frequently, because bacteria require 30 to 45 minutes to reproduce in urine. Clean-catch collection is preferred to catheterization, which can reinfect the bladder with urethral bacteria.
- *Sensitivity testing* determines the appropriate antimicrobial drug. If the patient history and physical examination warrant, a blood test or a stained smear of uretheral discharge can rule out venereal disease.
- *Voiding cystoureterography* or *excretory urography* may detect congenital anomalies that predispose the patient to recurrent UTI.

Treatment

Appropriate antimicrobials are the treatment of choice for most initial lower UTIs. A 7- to 10-day course of antibiotics is standard, but studies suggest that a single dose or a 3- to 5-day regimen may be sufficient to render the urine sterile. (Elderly patients may still need 7 to 10 days of antibiotics to fully benefit from treatment.) If a culture shows that urine still isn't sterile after 3 days of antibiotic therapy, bacterial resistance probably has occurred, and a different antimicrobial will be prescribed.

A single dose of amoxicillin or co-trimoxazole may be effective for females with acute, uncomplicated UTI. A urine culture taken 1 to 2 weeks later will indicate whether the infection has been eradicated. Recurrent infections from infected renal calculi,

UTI risk factors

Certain factors increase the risk of UTI. They include natural anatomic variations, trauma or invasive procedures, urinary tract obstructions, and urine reflux.

Natural anatomic variations
Females are more prone to UTI than males because the female urethra is shorter than the male urethra (about 1" to 2" [2.5 to 5 cm] compared with 7" to 8" [18 to 20 cm]). It's also closer to the anus than the male urethra. This proximity facilitates bacterial entry into the urethra from the vagina, perineum, or rectum or from a sexual partner.

Pregnant women are especially prone to UTIs because of hormonal changes and because the enlarged uterus exerts greater pressure on the ureters. This restricts urine flow, allowing bacteria to linger longer in the urinary tract.

In men, release of prostatic fluid serves as an antibacterial shield. Men lose this protection around age 50 when the prostate gland begins to enlarge. This enlargement, in turn, may promote urine retention.

Trauma or invasive procedures
Fecal matter, sexual intercourse, and instruments, such as catheters and cystoscopes, can introduce bacteria into the urinary tract to trigger infection.

Obstructions
A narrowed ureter or calculi lodged in the ureters or the bladder can obstruct urine flow. Slowed urine flow allows bacteria to remain and multiply, risking damage to the kidneys.

Reflux
Vesicourethral reflux results when pressure inside the bladder (caused by coughing or sneezing) pushes a small amount of urine from the bladder into the urethra. When the pressure returns to normal, the urine flows back into the bladder, bringing bacteria from the urethra with it.

In vesicoureteral reflux, urine flows from the bladder back into one or both ureters. The vesicoureteral valve normally shuts off reflux. However, damage can prevent the valve from doing its job.

Other risk factors
Urinary stasis can promote infection, which, if undetected, can spread to the entire urinary system. And because urinary tract bacteria thrive on sugars, diabetes also is a risk factor.

chronic prostatitis, or structural abnormalities may necessitate surgery. Prostatitis also requires long-term antibiotic therapy. In patients without these predisposing conditions, long-term, low-dose antibiotic therapy is the treatment of choice.

Key nursing diagnoses and patient outcomes

Altered urinary elimination related to inflammation of the lower urinary tract. Based on this nursing diagnosis, you'll establish these patient outcomes. The patient will:

- comply with antibiotic therapy
- report that signs and symptoms of abnormal urinary elimination are diminishing
- regain and maintain normal urinary elimination.

Risk for infection related to high incidence of recurrence of UTI. Based on this nursing diagnosis, you'll establish these patient outcomes. The patient will:

- take precautions to prevent recurrence of UTI

• communicate an understanding of the early signs and symptoms of UTI that should be reported
• remain free of recurrent UTIs, as exhibited by a normal urinalysis and the absence of signs and symptoms of UTI.

Pain related to bladder spasms and cramps. Based on this nursing diagnosis, you'll establish these patient outcomes. The patient will:
• report less perineal discomfort after taking sitz baths or applying warm compresses
• describe when and how to use a topical antiseptic correctly for pain relief
• become pain free when the UTI is eliminated.

Nursing interventions

• If ordered, administer nitrofurantoin macrocrystals with milk or meals, to prevent GI distress.
• If sitz baths don't relieve perineal discomfort, apply warm compresses sparingly to the perineum, but be careful not to burn the patient. Apply topical antiseptics on the urethral meatus, as necessary.
• Collect all urine specimens for culture and sensitivity testing carefully and promptly.

Monitoring

• Monitor the patient for GI disturbances from antimicrobial therapy and for other possible adverse reactions.
• Assess the patient for complications of UTI.
• Evaluate the patient's voiding pattern.

Patient teaching

• Explain the nature and purpose of antimicrobial therapy. Emphasize the importance of completing the prescribed course of therapy or, with long-term prophylaxis, of strictly adhering to the ordered dosage.
• Familiarize the patient with prescribed medications and their possible adverse effects. If antibiotics cause GI distress, explain that taking nitrofurantoin macrocrystals with milk or a meal can help prevent such problems. If therapy includes phenazopyridine, warn the patient that this drug turns urine red-orange.
• Explain that an uncontaminated midstream urine specimen is essential for accurate diagnosis. Before collection, teach the female patient to clean the perineum properly and to keep the labia separated during urination.
• Suggest warm sitz baths for relief of perineal discomfort.
• To prevent recurrent lower UTIs, teach a female patient to carefully wipe the perineum from front to back and to thoroughly clean it with soap and water after bowel movements. If she's infection-prone, she should urinate immediately after sexual intercourse. Tell her never to postpone urination and to empty her bladder completely.
• Tell the male patient that prompt treatment of predisposing conditions, such as chronic prostatitis, will help prevent recurrent UTIs.
• Urge the patient to drink about 2,000 ml (at least eight glasses) of fluids a day during treatment. More or less than this amount may alter the antimicrobial's effect. Be aware that the elderly patient may resist this suggestion because it causes him to make frequent trips, possibly up and down the stairs, to urinate.
• Explain that fruit juices, especially cranberry juice, and oral doses of vitamin C may help acidify urine and enhance the medication's action.

Urticaria and angioedema

Also known as hives, urticaria and angioedema are common allergic reactions. Urticaria is an episodic, rapidly occurring, usually self-limiting skin reaction. It involves only the superficial portion of the dermis, which erupts with local wheals surrounded by an erythematous flare. Angioedema, another dermal eruption, involves additional skin layers (including the subcutaneous tissue) and produces deeper, larger wheals (usually on the hands, feet, lips, genitalia, and eyelids). Angioedema causes diffuse swelling of loose subcutaneous tissue and also may affect the upper respiratory and GI tracts.

Urticaria and angioedema can occur separately or simultaneously, but angioedema may persist longer. Urticaria and angioedema affect about 20% of the general population at some time. Episodes tend to occur more often after adolescence, with the highest incidence in people in their 30s. Recurrent acute episodes last less than 6 weeks; episodes that persist longer than 6 weeks are considered chronic.

Causes

Urticaria and angioedema may result from allergy to drugs, foods, insect stings, and, occasionally, inhalant allergens (animal danders, cosmetics) that provoke an IgE-mediated response to protein allergens. However, certain drugs may cause urticaria without an IgE response. When urticaria and angioedema are part of an anaphylactic reaction, they almost always persist long after the systemic response subsides because circulation to the skin is restored last after an allergic reaction. This slows histamine reabsorption at the reaction site.

Urticaria and angioedema not triggered by an allergen are probably also related to histamine release. External physical stimuli, such as cold (usually in young adults), heat, water, and sunlight, may also provoke urticaria and angioedema. Dermatographism, which develops after stroking or scratching the skin, may affect as much as 20% of the population. Such urticaria develops with varying pressure, most often under tight clothing, and is aggravated by scratching.

Several mechanisms and disorders may provoke urticaria and angioedema. These include IgE-induced release of mediators from cutaneous mast cells; binding of IgG or IgM to antigen, resulting in complement activation; and disorders such as localized or secondary infection (respiratory infection), neoplastic disease (Hodgkin's disease), connective tissue diseases (systemic lupus erythematosus), collagen vascular disease, and psychogenic disease.

Angioedema without urticaria occurs with C1 inhibitor deficiency, which can occur as an autosomal dominant characteristic (hereditary angioedema) or be acquired with lymphoproliferative disorders.

Complications

Skin abrasion and secondary infection may result from scratching. Angioedema that involves the upper respiratory tract may cause life-threatening laryngeal edema. GI involvement may cause severe abdominal colic that may lead to unnecessary surgery.

Assessment

The patient's history may or may not reveal the source of the offending substance. Check the drug history, including nonprescription preparations, such as vitamins, aspirin, and antacids.

Investigate frequently troublesome foods, such as strawberries, milk products, and seafood. Environmental allergens may include pets, clothing (wool or down), soap, inhalants (hair sprays), cosmetics, hair dyes, and insect bites or stings. Remember to inquire about exposure to physical factors, such as cold, sunlight, exercise, and trauma (dermatographism).

Skin inspection typically discloses distinct, raised, evanescent dermal wheals surrounded by a reddened flare (urticaria). Varied in size, these lesions typically erupt on the extremities, external genitalia, and face, particularly around the eyes and lips. In cholinergic urticaria, the wheals may appear tiny and blanched with an erythematous rim.

Angioedema characteristically produces nonpitted swelling of deep subcutaneous tissue on the eyelids, lips, genitalia, and mucous membranes. Usually, these swellings don't itch but may burn and tingle.

With upper respiratory tract involvement, auscultation may detect respiratory stridor caused by laryngeal obstruction. The patient may appear anxious and gasping for breath. With GI involvement, he may complain of abdominal colic with or without nausea and vomiting.

Diagnostic tests

Careful skin testing with the suspected offending substance to see if a local wheal and flare result can confirm diagnosis. Diagnosis may also be confirmed by injecting the patient's serum into a skin site of a normal recipient, resulting in a wheal and flare reaction to the antigen (Prausnitz-Küstner reaction). Total IgE elevation or peripheral eosinophilia may be present.

An elimination diet and a food diary documenting foods eaten and times, amounts, and circumstances may help to pinpoint provoking allergens. Or the food diary may suggest other allergies. For instance, a patient allergic to fish may also be allergic to an iodine-based radiographic contrast medium.

Laboratory tests (complete blood count, urinalysis, and erythrocyte sedimentation rate) and chest X-rays may be done to rule out infections.

Recurrent angioedema without urticaria, along with a family history of angioedema, points to hereditary angioedema. Decreased serum levels of C1, C4, and C2 inhibitors confirm the diagnosis.

Treatment

Appropriate treatment aims to prevent or limit contact with triggering factors. Once the triggering stimulus has been removed, urticaria usually subsides in a few days – unless it results from a drug reaction. Then it may persist as long as the drug remains in the tissues.

Treatment may involve desensitization to the triggering antigen. During desensitization, progressively larger doses of specific antigens (identified by skin testing) are injected intradermally. Diphenhydramine or another antihistamine can ease itching and swelling.

Key nursing diagnoses and patient outcomes

Altered protection related to presence of allergens that can induce urticaria and angioedema when triggered. Based on this nursing diagnosis, you'll establish these patient outcomes. The patient will:
• seek to identify the triggering antigens and take steps to avoid them if possible
• participate in a desensitization program, as indicated
• report fewer or no episodes of urticaria and angioedema.

Risk for suffocation related to potential for laryngeal edema. Based on this nursing diagnosis, you'll establish these patient outcomes. The patient will:
• identify early warning signs and symptoms of laryngeal edema
• communicate an understanding of the need to seek emergency help immediately if he suspects laryngeal edema
• keep an anaphylaxis kit in his home, at work, and in his car.

Impaired skin integrity related to scratching caused by pruritus. Based on this nursing diagnosis, you'll establish these patient outcomes. The patient will:
• refrain from scratching during episodes of urticaria and angioedema
• use antihistamine therapy to reduce itching, as prescribed
• regain and maintain skin integrity.

Nursing interventions

• Reduce or minimize environmental exposure to offending allergens and irritants, such as wools and harsh detergents. This may be easier if the offending substance is known. If it isn't, gradually eliminate suspected substances.
• If food is a suspected cause, gradually eliminate foods from the diet.
• Administer antihistamines, as prescribed, to make the patient more comfortable.

• Keep emergency equipment nearby in case of life-threatening complications, such as laryngeal edema.

Monitoring

• Watch for an improvement of the patient's condition with the removal of offending substances.
• Inspect the patient's skin for surface breaks and signs of secondary infection caused by scratching.
• Monitor the patient for signs and symptoms of serious respiratory compromise.

Patient teaching

• To help identify the cause of urticaria and angioedema, teach the patient how to keep a diary. Information to record includes exposure to suspected offending substances and signs and symptoms that appear after exposure.
• If the patient modifies his diet to exclude food allergens, teach him to monitor his nutritional status. Provide him with a list of food replacements for nutrients lost by excluding allergy-provoking foods and beverages.
• Instruct him to keep his fingernails short to avoid abrading the skin when scratching.
• Review signs and symptoms that indicate a skin infection. Explain hygiene measures for managing minor infection, and direct the patient to seek medical attention as needed.

Uterine cancer

The most common gynecologic cancer, uterine cancer (cancer of the endometrium) typically afflicts postmenopausal women between ages 50 and 60. It's uncommon between ages 30 and 40 and rare before age 30. Most premenopausal women who develop uterine cancer have a history of anovulatory menstrual cycles or other hormonal imbalance. About 34,000 new cases of uterine cancer are reported annually; of these, approximately 6,000 are eventually fatal.

Causes

Uterine cancer appears linked to several predisposing factors:
• low fertility index and anovulation
• history of infertility or failure of ovulation
• obesity, hypertension, diabetes, or nulliparity
• familial tendency
• history of uterine polyps or endometrial hyperplasia
• prolonged estrogen therapy without use of progesterone.

In most patients, uterine cancer is an adenocarcinoma that metastasizes late, usually from the endometrium to the cervix, ovaries, fallopian tubes, and other peritoneal structures. It may spread to distant organs, such as the lungs and the brain, by way of the blood or the lymphatic system. Lymph node involvement can also occur. Less common uterine tumors include adenoacanthoma, endometrial stromal sarcoma, lymphosarcoma, mixed mesodermal tumors (including carcinosarcoma), and leiomyosarcoma.

Complications

Intestinal obstruction, ascites, increasing pain, and hemorrhage can result from disease progression.

Assessment

The patient history may reflect one or more predisposing factors. In the younger patient, it may also reveal spotting and protracted, heavy menstrual periods. The postmenopausal woman may report that bleeding began 12 or more months after menses had stopped. In either case, the patient may describe the discharge as watery at first, then blood-streaked, and gradually becoming bloodier.

In more advanced stages, palpation may disclose an enlarged uterus.

Staging uterine cancer

The International Federation of Gynecology and Obstetrics defines uterine (endometrial) cancer stages as follows:

Stage 0
Carcinoma is in situ.

Stage I
Carcinoma is confined to the corpus.

Stage IA
Length of the uterine cavity is 8 cm or less.

Stage IB
Length of the uterine cavity is more than 8 cm.

Stage I cases are subgrouped by the following histologic grades of the adenocarcinoma:

G1—Highly differentiated adenomatous carcinoma
G2—Moderately differentiated adenomatous carcinoma with partly solid areas
G3—Predominantly solid or entirely undifferentiated carcinoma

Stage II
Carcinoma has involved the corpus and the cervix but has not extended outside the uterus.

Stage III
Carcinoma has extended outside the uterus but not outside the true pelvis.

Stage IV
Carcinoma has extended outside the true pelvis or has obviously involved the mucosa of the bladder or rectum.

Stage IVA
Carcinoma has spread to adjacent organs.

Stage IVB
Carcinoma has spread to distant organs.

Diagnostic tests

• *Endometrial, cervical,* or *endocervical biopsy* confirms cancer cells.
• *Fractional dilatation and curettage* identifies the problem when the disease is suspected but the endometrial biopsy is negative.

Positive diagnosis requires the following tests to provide baseline data and permit staging:
• *multiple cervical biopsies* and *endocervical curettage* to pinpoint cervical involvement
• *Schiller's test,* the staining of the cervix and vagina with an iodine solution that turns healthy tissues brown (cancerous tissues resist the stain)
• *computed tomography scan* or *magnetic resonance imaging* to detect metastasis to the myometrium, cervix, lymph nodes, and other organs
• *excretory urography* and, possibly, *cystoscopy* to evaluate the urinary system
• *proctoscopy* or *barium enema studies,* which may be performed if bowel and rectal involvement are suspected
• *blood studies, urinalysis,* and *electrocardiography* may also help in staging the disease. (See *Staging uterine cancer.*)

Treatment

Depending on the cancer's extent, treatment may include one or more of the following measures.
• *Surgery* usually involves total abdominal hysterectomy, bilateral salpingo-oophorectomy or, possibly, omentectomy with or without pelvic or para-aortic lymphadenectomy.

Total pelvic exenteration removes all pelvic organs, including the rectum, bladder, and vagina, and is only performed when the disease is sufficiently contained to allow surgical removal of diseased parts. This surgery seldom is curative, especially in nodal involvement.
• *Radiation therapy* is used when the tumor isn't well differentiated. Intracavitary radiation, external radiation, or both may be given 6 weeks before surgery to inhibit recurrence and lengthen survival time.
• *Hormonal therapy,* using tamoxifen, shows a response rate of 20% to 40%.
• *Chemotherapy,* including both cisplatin and doxorubicin, is usually tried when other treatments have failed.

Key nursing diagnoses and patient outcomes

Fear related to possible metastasis. Based on this nursing diagnosis, you'll establish these patient outcomes. The patient will:
• express fears related to uterine cancer
• use available support systems to assist in coping with fear
• report reduced feelings of fear.

Risk for infection related to immunosuppression caused by radiation therapy or chemotherapy. Based on this nursing diagnosis, you'll establish these patient outcomes. The patient will:
• maintain a normal body temperature and white blood cell count
• show no signs and symptoms of infection
• incorporate infection-control measures into everyday life.

Sexual dysfunction related to surgical procedure. Based on this nursing diagnosis, you'll establish these patient outcomes. The patient will:
• express feelings about changes in sexuality
• use available support systems to cope with changes in sexual function
• reestablish sexual activity at her preillness level.

Nursing interventions

• Listen to the patient's fears and concerns. She may be fearful for her survival and concerned that treatment will alter her life-style or prevent sexual intimacy. Encourage her to use available support systems to cope with loss of fertility, if applicable. Remain with the patient during periods of severe stress and anxiety.
• Administer ordered pain medications as necessary. Patients who require pain medications for this disease are often in the later stages. Encourage the patient to identify actions that promote comfort and then be sure to perform them as often as possible. Provide distractions and help her perform relaxation techniques that may ease her discomfort.
• Prepare the patient for surgery, as indicated. (See the entry "Hysterectomy.")
• Find out whether the patient will have internal or external radiation or both. Usually, internal radiation therapy is used first. (See the entries "Radiation, internal" and "Radiation, external.")
• Provide supportive care for adverse effects of radiation therapy or chemotherapy.

Monitoring

• Monitor the patient's complete blood count (including differential) regularly for signs of immunosuppression caused by radiation therapy and chemotherapy. Also assess for signs and symptoms of infection, bleeding, and anemia regularly, and monitor vital signs.
• Assess the patient for other adverse effects of uterine cancer or its treatments.
• Evaluate the effectiveness of administered analgesics.

Patient teaching

• Emphasize that prompt treatment significantly improves a patient's likelihood of survival. Discuss tests to diagnose and stage the disease, and explain treatments, which may include radiation therapy, surgery, hormonal therapy, chemotherapy, or a combination of these.

• If the patient is premenopausal, explain that removal of her ovaries will induce menopause.
• As appropriate, explain that except in total pelvic exenteration, the vagina remains intact and that once she recovers, sexual intercourse is possible.
• Describe the procedure for radiation therapy to the patient. Answer the patient's questions and counsel her about radiation's adverse effects. Advise her to rest frequently and to maintain a well-balanced diet.
• To minimize skin breakdown and reduce the risk of skin infection, tell the patient to keep the treatment area dry, to avoid wearing clothes that rub against the area, and to avoid using heating pads, alcohol rubs, or irritating skin creams. Because radiation therapy increases susceptibility to infection (possibly by lowering the white blood cell [WBC] count), encourage the patient to avoid people with colds or other infections.
• Explain chemotherapy or immunotherapy to the patient and her family and be sure they understand what adverse effects to expect and how to alleviate them. If the patient is receiving a synthetic form of progesterone, such as hydroxyprogesterone, medroxyprogesterone, or megestrol, tell her to watch for depression, dizziness, backache, swelling, breast tenderness, irritability, and abdominal cramps. Instruct her to report signs of thrombophlebitis, such as pain in the calves, numbness, tingling, or loss of leg function.
• Advise the patient receiving chemotherapy that WBC counts must be checked weekly, and reinforce the importance of preventing infection. Assure her that hair loss is temporary.
• If the patient is employed and is undergoing chemotherapy, point out that continuing to work during this period may offer an important diversion. Advise her to talk with her employer about a flexible work schedule.
• Refer the patient to the social service department and to community services that offer psychological support and information, such as the American Cancer Society.

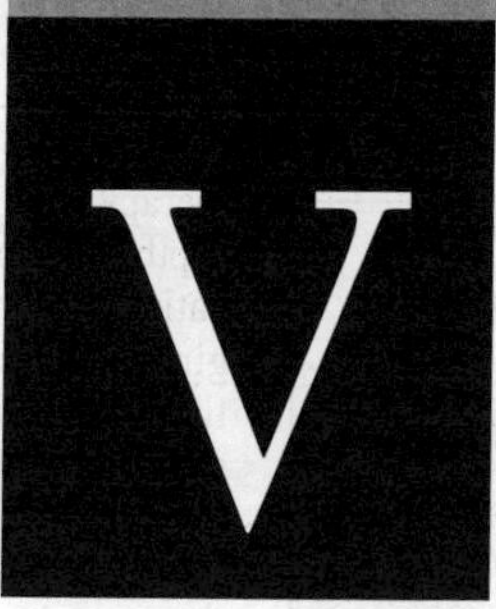

Vaginal cancer

The rarest gynecologic cancer, vaginal cancer usually appears as squamous cell carcinoma, but occasionally as melanoma, sarcoma, or adenocarcinoma. Vaginal cancer usually occurs in women at about age 60, but some rarer types do appear in younger women.

Causes

Although the relation is unclear, certain factors predispose the patient to the development of squamous cell carcinoma of the vagina. These include advancing age, trauma, chronic pessary use, and the use of chemical carcinogens, such as those in some sprays and douches. There is also a possible causative association between vaginal cancer and the human papillomavirus.

Cancer in this area may also be an extension of a previous cancer of the endometrium, vulva, or cervix. Vaginal adenocarcinoma has also been associated with the use of diethylstilbestrol (DES) by the patient's mother during pregnancy.

Because the vagina is a thin-walled structure with rich lymphatic drainage, cancer here varies in severity, depending on its exact location and effect on lymphatic drainage. Vaginal cancer resembles cervical cancer in that it may progress from an intraepithelial tumor to an invasive cancer. It spreads more slowly than cervical cancer, however.

A lesion in the upper third of the vagina, the most common site, usually metastasizes to the groin nodes; a lesion in the lower third, the second most common site, usually metastasizes to the hypogastric and iliac nodes. A lesion in the middle third metastasizes erratically. A posterior lesion displaces and distends the vaginal posterior wall before spreading to deep layers. By contrast, an anterior lesion spreads more rapidly into other structures and deep layers because unlike the posterior wall, the anterior vaginal wall is not flexible.

Complications

Metastasis may affect the cervix, uterus, and rectum.

Assessment

The history may reveal one or more risk factors and the most frequent presenting signs – bloody vaginal discharge and irregular or postmenopausal bleeding. The patient may also complain of urine retention or urinary frequency if the lesion is close to the neck of the bladder. Vaginal examination may reveal a small or large ulcerated lesion in any area of the vagina.

Diagnostic tests

Several tests help identify and stage vaginal cancer.

• *Papanicolaou test* shows abnormal cells.
• *Biopsy of the lesion* is performed to identify cancerous cells. Biopsy of the cervix

Staging vaginal cancer

The International Federation of Gynecology and Obstetrics has established this staging system as a guide to the treatment and the prognosis of vaginal cancer.

Stage 0
Carcinoma in situ, intraepithelial carcinoma.

Stage I
The carcinoma is limited to the vaginal wall.

Stage II
The carcinoma has involved the subvaginal tissue but has not extended to the pelvic wall.

Stage III
The carcinoma has extended to the pelvic wall.

Stage IV
The carcinoma has extended beyond the true pelvis or has involved the mucosa of the bladder or rectum.

and vulva may also be performed to rule out these areas as primary cancer sites.

- *Colposcopy* may be used to locate lesions that may have been missed during the pelvic examination.
- *Lugol's solution* painted on the suspected area helps identify malignant areas by staining glycogen-containing normal tissue; abnormal tissue resists staining.
- *Barium enema* is performed to rule out gastrointestinal pathophysiology. (See *Staging vaginal cancer*.)

Treatment

Early-stage treatment aims to treat the malignant area and preserve the vagina. Topical chemotherapy with fluorouracil and laser surgery can be used for stages 0 and I. Recommendations for radiation therapy and surgery vary with the size, depth, and location of the lesion, and the patient's desire to preserve a functional vagina. Such preservation is possible only in the early stages. Survival rates are the same for patients treated with radiation as for those who undergo surgery.

Surgery may be recommended only when the tumor is so extensive that exenteration is needed because the vagina's close proximity to the bladder and rectum allows only minimal tissue margins around resected vaginal tissue. Radiation therapy is the preferred treatment for all stages of vaginal cancer. Most patients need preliminary external radiation treatment to shrink the tumor before internal radiation can begin. Then, if the tumor is localized to the vault and the cervix is present, radiation (radium or cesium) can be given with an intrauterine tandem and colpostats (ovoids); if the cervix is absent, then a specially designed vaginal applicator is used instead. To minimize complications, radioactive sources and filters are carefully placed away from radiosensitive tissues, such as the bladder and rectum. Such treatment lasts 48 to 72 hours, depending on the dosage.

Key nursing diagnoses and patient outcomes

Altered sexuality patterns related to presence of vaginal cancer. Based on this nursing diagnosis, you'll establish these patient outcomes. The patient will:

- express feelings about changes in sexuality patterns
- obtain help from an appropriate counselor or support group.

Risk for infection related to ulceration of vaginal tissue from radiation or chemotherapy. Based on this nursing diagnosis, you'll establish these patient outcomes. The patient will:

- maintain a normal body temperature and white blood cell count
- not have purulent vaginal discharge
- not show signs and symptoms of systemic infection.

Impaired tissue integrity related to ulceration of vaginal tissue caused by vaginal cancer or internal radiation. Based on this nursing diagnosis, you'll establish these patient outcomes. The patient will:
• adhere to activity restrictions during internal radiation to prevent or minimize irritation and breakdown of irradiated areas
• exhibit healing of ulcerated areas
• regain tissue integrity.

Nursing interventions

• Listen to the patient's fears and concerns and offer psychological support. The patient may fear both the disease and its impact on her sexual behavior.
• When appropriate, administer ordered analgesics and provide comfort measures and distractions that help minimize pain.
• Prepare the patient for radiation therapy, as indicated. (See the entries "Radiation, internal" and "Radiation, external.")
• Perform measures that help prevent or alleviate complications of radiation therapy and chemotherapy.

Monitoring

• Watch for complications of prescribed treatments.
• Monitor the patient for local vaginal infection and systemic infection if immunosuppression occurs with radiation or chemotherapy.

Patient teaching

• Explain all treatments to the patient and, as appropriate, her family.
• Before external radiation therapy, stress the importance of providing good skin care to the target site after treatment to maintain skin integrity. Tell the patient to avoid constrictive clothing over the area, to avoid extremes of hot or cold, and to avoid vigorously rubbing the area. Also stress the need to take measures to prevent infection, such as avoiding crowds and washing her hands.
• Before internal radiation therapy, explain the necessity of immobilization during therapy, and tell the patient what this therapy entails (such as no linen changes and the use of an indwelling urinary catheter).
• After internal radiation therapy, instruct the patient to use a stent or prescribed dilator exercises to prevent vaginal stenosis. Coitus also helps prevent such stenosis.
• Refer the patient for psychological counseling, if necessary, or to the social service department and support groups, such as the American Cancer Society.

Valvuloplasty, balloon

Balloon valvuloplasty is used to enlarge the orifice of a heart valve that's stenotic because of a congenital defect, calcification, rheumatic fever, or aging. A doctor performs valvuloplasty in a cardiac catheterization laboratory by inserting a balloon-tipped catheter through the femoral vein or artery, threading it into the heart, and repeatedly inflating it against the leaflets of the diseased valve.

Despite valvuloplasty's benefits, the treatment of choice for valvular heart disease remains surgery–either valve replacement or commissurotomy. But for those who are considered poor candidates for surgery, valvuloplasty offers an alternative.

Procedure

After preparing and anesthetizing the catheter insertion site, the doctor inserts a catheter into the femoral artery (for left-heart valves) or femoral vein (for right-heart valves). He then passes the balloon-tipped catheter through this catheter and, guided by fluoroscopy, slowly threads it into the heart.

Next, he positions the deflated balloon in the valve opening and repeatedly inflates it with a solution containing 0.9% sodium chloride and a contrast medium. As the balloon inflates, the valve leaflets split free of one another, permitting them to open and close properly and increasing the valvular orifice.

Valvuloplasty is considered a success if hemodynamic pressure decreases across the valve after balloon inflation. If it does, the doctor removes the balloon-tipped catheter. However, he'll leave the other catheter in place in case the patient needs to return to the laboratory for a repeat procedure.

Complications

Balloon valvuloplasty can worsen valvular insufficiency by misshaping the valve so that it doesn't close completely. Another serious complication is embolism caused by pieces of the calcified valve breaking off and traveling to the brain or lungs. In addition, valvuloplasty can cause severe damage to the delicate valve leaflets, requiring immediate surgery to replace the valve. Other complications include bleeding and hematoma at the arterial puncture site, arrhythmias, myocardial ischemia, myocardial infarction (MI), and circulatory defects distal to the catheter entry site.

Elderly patients with aortic disease frequently experience restenosis 1 to 2 years after undergoing valvuloplasty. Fortunately, the most serious complications of valvuloplasty – valvular destruction, MI, and calcium emboli – rarely occur.

Key nursing diagnoses and patient outcomes

Anxiety related to valvuloplasty. Based on this nursing diagnosis, you'll establish these patient outcomes. The patient will:

- identify and express feelings of anxiety
- exhibit healthy behaviors to cope with anxiety
- be able to cooperate during valvuloplasty.

Risk for injury related to complications of valvuloplasty. Based on this nursing diagnosis, you'll establish these patient outcomes. The patient will:

- maintain hemodynamic stability during and after valvuloplasty
- not show signs and symptoms of complications associated with valvuloplasty during or after the procedure
- not sustain an injury as a result of valvuloplasty.

Risk for fluid volume deficit related to bleeding from insertion site during and after valvuloplasty. Based on this nursing diagnosis, you'll establish these patient outcomes. The patient will:

- not show signs of bleeding from groin sites
- maintain baseline hemoglobin, hematocrit, and coagulation values after the procedure
- maintain normal vital signs and urine output.

Nursing interventions

When caring for a patient undergoing balloon valvuloplasty, your primary responsibilities include monitoring for complications after the procedure and patient teaching.

Before the procedure

- Reinforce the doctor's explanation of the procedure, including its risks and alternatives, to the patient. Restrict food and fluid intake for at least 6 hours before valvuloplasty, or as ordered.
- Explain that the patient will have an I.V. line inserted to provide access for any medications. Mention that the patient's groin area will be shaved and cleaned with an antiseptic and that he'll feel a brief stinging sensation when a local anesthetic is injected.
- In simple and reassuring terms, explain that the doctor will insert a catheter into an artery or vein in the groin area and that the patient may feel pressure as the catheter moves along the vessel. Also explain to the patient that he needs to be awake because the doctor may need him to take deep breaths (to allow visualization of the catheter) and to answer questions about how he's feeling. Warn him that the

procedure lasts up to 4 hours and that he may feel discomfort from lying flat on a hard table during that time.

• Ensure that the patient has signed a consent form.

• Make sure that results of routine laboratory studies and blood typing and crossmatching are available. Just before the procedure, palpate the bilateral distal pulses (usually the dorsalis pedis or posteriortibial pulses) and mark them with indelible ink. Take vital signs and assess color, temperature, and sensation in the patient's extremities to serve as a baseline for posttreatment assessment. Administer a sedative, as ordered.

• Once you've prepared the patient, place a 5-lb (2.3-kg) sandbag on his bed to be used later for applying pressure over the puncture site.

After the procedure

• When the patient returns to the critical care unit or postanesthesia area, he may be receiving I.V. heparin or nitroglycerin. He'll also have the sandbag placed over the cannulation site to minimize bleeding until the arterial catheter is removed, and will require continuous arterial and electrocardiogram monitoring.

• To prevent excessive hip flexion and migration of the catheter, keep the affected leg straight and elevate the head of the bed no more than 15 degrees. (At mealtime, you can elevate the head of the bed 15 to 30 degrees.) For the first hour, monitor vital signs every 15 minutes, then every 30 minutes for 2 hours, and then hourly for the next 5 hours. If vital signs are unstable, notify the doctor and continue to check them every 5 minutes.

• When you take vital signs, assess peripheral pulses distal to the insertion site and the color, temperature, and capillary refill time of the extremity. If pulses are difficult to palpate because of the size of the arterial catheter, use a Doppler stethoscope. Notify the doctor if pulses are absent.

• Observe the catheter insertion site for hematoma formation, ecchymosis, or hemorrhage. If an expanding ecchymotic area appears, mark the area to help determine the pace of expansion. If bleeding occurs, apply direct pressure and notify the doctor.

• Following the doctor's orders or your hospital's protocol, auscultate regularly for murmurs, which may indicate worsening valvular insufficiency. Notify the doctor if you detect a new or worsening murmur.

• Provide I.V. fluids at a rate of at least 100 ml/hour, or as ordered, to help the kidneys excrete the contrast medium. But be sure to assess for signs of fluid overload: distended neck veins, atrial and ventricular gallops, dyspnea, pulmonary congestion, tachycardia, hypertension, and hypoxemia.

• The doctor will remove the catheter 6 to 12 hours after valvuloplasty. Afterward, apply a pressure dressing and assess vital signs according to the same schedule you used when the patient first returned to the unit.

Home care instructions

• Tell the patient that he can resume normal activity. Most patients with successful valvuloplasties experience increased exercise tolerance.

• Instruct the patient to call his doctor if he experiences any bleeding or increased bruising at the puncture site or any recurrence of symptoms of valvular insufficiency, such as breathlessness or decreased exercise tolerance.

• Stress the need for regular follow-up visits with his doctor.

Varicose veins

Resulting from improper venous valve function, varicose veins are dilated, tortuous veins, engorged with blood. They can be either primary or secondary. Primary varicose veins originate in the superficial veins – the saphenous veins and their branches – whereas secondary varicose veins occur in the deep and perforating veins.

Primary varicose veins tend to run in families, affect both legs, and are twice as common in women as in men. Usually, secondary varicose veins only occur in one leg. Both types are more common in middle adulthood.

Causes

Primary varicose veins can result from congenital weakness of the valves or venous wall; from conditions that produce prolonged venous stasis, such as pregnancy or wearing tight clothing; or from occupations that necessitate standing for an extended period.

Secondary varicose veins result from disorders of the venous system, such as deep vein thrombophlebitis, trauma, and occlusion.

Complications

Long-standing varicose veins produce venous insufficiency and venous stasis ulcers, particularly around the ankles.

Assessment

The patient with varicose veins may be asymptomatic or complain of mild to severe leg symptoms, including a feeling of heaviness that worsens in the evening and in warm weather; cramps at night; diffuse, dull aching after prolonged standing or walking; aching during menses; and fatigue. Exercise may relieve symptoms because venous return improves.

Inspection of the affected leg reveals dilated, purplish, ropelike veins, particularly in the calf. Deep vein incompetence causes orthostatic edema and stasis of the calves and ankles. Palpation may reveal nodules along affected veins and valve incompetence, which can be checked by the manual compression test and Trendelenburg's test.

To do the *manual compression test,* palpate the dilated vein with the fingertips of one hand. With the other hand, firmly compress the vein at a point at least 8" (20 cm) higher. Feel for an impulse transmitted to your lower hand. With competent saphenous valves, you won't detect any impulse. A palpable impulse indicates incompetent valves in a vein segment between your hands.

To do *Trendelenburg's test (retrograde filling test),* mark the distended veins with a pen while the patient stands. Then have her lie on the examination table and elevate her leg for about a minute to drain the veins. Next, have her stand while you measure venous filling time. Competent valves take at least 30 seconds to fill. If the veins fill in less than 30 seconds, have the patient lie on the examination table again and elevate her leg for 1 minute. Then apply a tourniquet around her upper thigh. Next, have her stand. If leg veins still fill in less than 30 seconds, suspect incompetent perforating vein and deep vein valves (functioning valves block retrograde flow).

Next, remove the tourniquet. If the veins fill again in less than 30 seconds, suspect incompetent superficial vein valves that allow backward blood flow.

To pinpoint incompetent valve location, repeat this procedure by applying the tourniquet just below the knee and then around the upper calf.

Diagnostic tests

- *Photoplethysmography,* a noninvasive test, characterizes venous blood flow by noting changes in the skin's circulation.
- *Doppler ultrasonography* quickly and accurately detects the presence or absence of venous backflow in deep or superficial veins.
- *Venous outflow* and *reflux plethysmography* can detect deep venous occlusion.
- *Ascending* and *descending venography* can demonstrate venous occlusion and pat-

terns of collateral flow. It's an invasive test and not routinely used.

Treatment

In mild varicose veins, treatment involves wearing elastic stockings, avoiding tight clothing and prolonged standing, exercising, and elevating the legs. Treatment in moderate varicose veins consists of wearing antiembolism stockings or elastic bandages. Severe varicose veins may require custom-fitted, surgical-weight stockings with graduated pressure (highest at the ankle, lowest at the top). An exercise program, such as walking, promotes muscle contraction and forces blood through the veins, thereby minimizing venous pooling.

Severe varicose veins may require stripping and ligation or, in patients who are poor surgical risks, injection of a sclerosing agent into small segments of affected veins.

Key nursing diagnoses and patient outcomes

Fatigue related to varicose veins. Based on this nursing diagnosis, you'll establish these patient outcomes. The patient will:
- identify activities that increase fatigue
- articulate a plan to resolve fatigue problems
- employ measures to prevent and modify fatigue.

Knowledge deficit related to lack of information about varicose veins. Based on this nursing diagnosis, you'll establish these patient outcomes. The patient will:
- identify the need to learn about varicose veins
- obtain correct information about varicose veins from appropriate sources
- communicate an understanding of daily measures to minimize or prevent further development of varicose veins.

Pain related to engorged veins. Based on this nursing diagnosis, you'll establish these patient outcomes. The patient will:
- identify activities that cause or increase leg discomfort
- incorporate measures into everyday life that will prevent or minimize pain
- report increased comfort following stripping and ligation or after injection of a sclerosing agent.

Nursing interventions

- After stripping and ligation or after injection of a sclerosing agent, administer analgesics, as ordered, to relieve pain.
- When ordered, rewrap bandages at least once a shift, wrapping from toe to thigh, with the leg elevated.

Monitoring

- Following stripping and ligation or after injection of a sclerosing agent, frequently check circulation in toes (color and temperature), and observe elastic bandages for bleeding.
- Watch for signs and symptoms of complications, such as sensory loss in the leg (which could indicate saphenous nerve damage), calf pain (thrombophlebitis), and fever (infection).

Patient teaching

- To promote comfort and minimize worsening of varicose veins, tell the patient to avoid wearing constrictive clothing.
- Tell the patient to elevate her legs above heart level when possible and to avoid prolonged standing or sitting.
- Teach the patient to put on the elastic, antiembolism, or compression stockings before getting out of bed in the morning. If she can't do that, tell her to lie with her legs raised for 1 minute and then to put on the stockings.
- Teach the patient to avoid injury to the lower legs, ankles, and feet and to observe for altered skin integrity of those areas. Have her report any problems to the doctor as soon as possible. Impaired tissue perfusion will reduce the leg's healing ability and predispose it to infection and further tissue damage.

Vascular repair

Surgical repair often represents the treatment of choice for vessels damaged by arteriosclerotic or thromboembolic disorders (such as aortic aneurysm or arterial occlusive disease), trauma, infections, or congenital defects. It may also be used for patients with obstructions that severely compromise circulation or for patients with vascular disease that doesn't respond to drug therapy or nonsurgical treatments, such as balloon angioplasty. Emergency surgery is typically required for life-threatening dissecting or ruptured aortic aneurysms or limb-threatening acute arterial occlusion.

Vascular repair includes aneurysm resection, bypass grafting, embolectomy, and vein stripping. The specific surgery used depends on the type, location, and extent of vascular occlusion or damage.

Procedure

Vascular repair surgeries are usually performed under general anesthesia. See *Understanding types of vascular repair,* for a description of the different surgeries.

Complications

All vascular surgeries carry the potential for serious complications, such as vessel trauma, emboli, hemorrhage, and infection. Bypass grafting carries added risks: The graft may occlude, narrow, dilate, or rupture.

Key nursing diagnoses and patient outcomes

Anxiety related to vascular repair and potential for complications. Based on this nursing diagnosis, you'll establish these patient outcomes. The patient will:
• identify and express feelings of anxiety
• use available support systems to cope with anxiety
• exhibit healthy coping behaviors for dealing with anxiety.

Risk for injury related to complications associated with vascular repair. Based on this nursing diagnosis, you'll establish these patient outcomes. The patient will:
• not have signs and symptoms of organ dysfunction postoperatively
• regain and maintain adequate tissue perfusion, demonstrated by strong, palpable pulses and warm skin with no evidence of cyanosis
• not complain of discomfort suggestive of tissue ischemia, such as chest pain or sensory changes in his extremities.

Activity intolerance related to location of surgical incision. Based on this nursing diagnosis, you'll establish these patient outcomes. The patient will:
• communicate an understanding of the need to maximize his activity level and show a willingness to do so
• not have signs and symptoms of inactivity-related complications, such as thrombus formation or skin breakdown
• regain and maintain his normal activity level.

Nursing interventions

When caring for a patient undergoing vascular repair surgery, your main responsibilities include instructing the patient and monitoring for preoperative and postoperative complications.

Before surgery

• If the patient needs to undergo emergency surgery, briefly explain the procedure to him, if possible. If he doesn't require immediate surgery, make sure that he and his family understand the doctor's explanation of the surgery and its possible complications.
• Inform the patient that he'll receive a general anesthetic. Mention that he'll awaken from the anesthetic in the intensive care or postanesthesia unit. Explain that he'll have an I.V. line in place to provide access for fluids and drugs. He may also have an indwelling urinary catheter in place to allow accurate output mea-

Understanding types of vascular repair

The following information summarizes the purpose for and the procedure involved in various types of vascular repair.

Aortic aneurysm repair

This procedure reinforces the wall of the aorta or removes an aneurysmal segment of the aorta.

The surgeon first makes an incision to expose the aneurysm site. If necessary, he places the patient on a cardiopulmonary bypass machine; then he clamps the aorta just above and below the aneurysm. Depending on the severity of the aneurysm—and on whether it's ruptured—he wraps the weakened arterial wall with Dacron to reinforce it (right) or replaces the damaged portion with a Dacron graft.

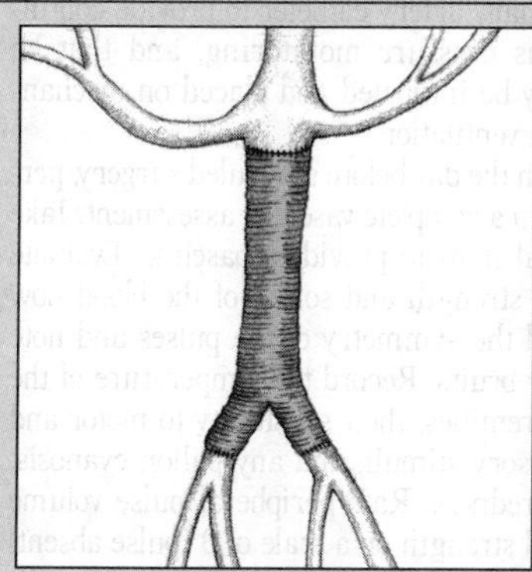

Bypass grafting

This procedure is done to bypass an arterial obstruction resulting from arteriosclerosis. The surgeon first exposes the affected artery. He then anastomoses a synthetic or autogenous graft to divert blood flow around the occluded arterial segment. The graft may be synthetic, or it may be a vein harvested from elsewhere in the patient's body.

The illustration here shows a femoropopliteal bypass.

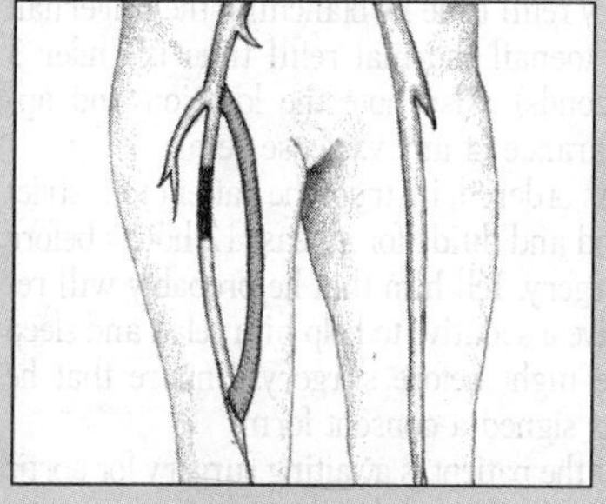

Embolectomy

To remove an embolism from an artery, the surgeon inserts a balloon-tipped catheter into the artery and passes it through the thrombus (top). He then inflates the balloon and withdraws the catheter to remove the thrombus (bottom).

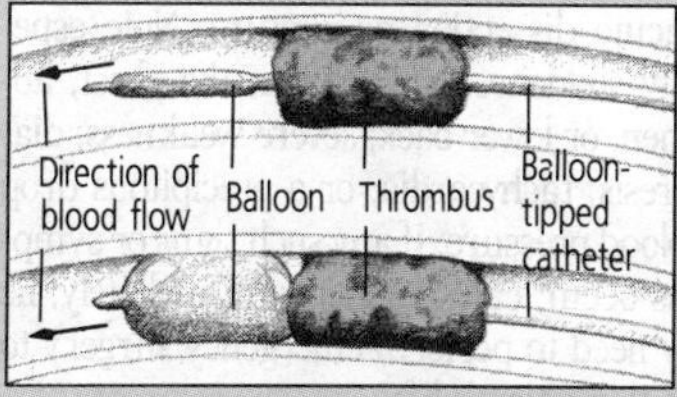

Vein stripping

In this procedure, the surgeon removes the saphenous vein and its branches to treat varicosities. He first ligates the saphenous vein. Then he threads the stripper into the vein, secures it, and pulls it out, bringing the vein with it.

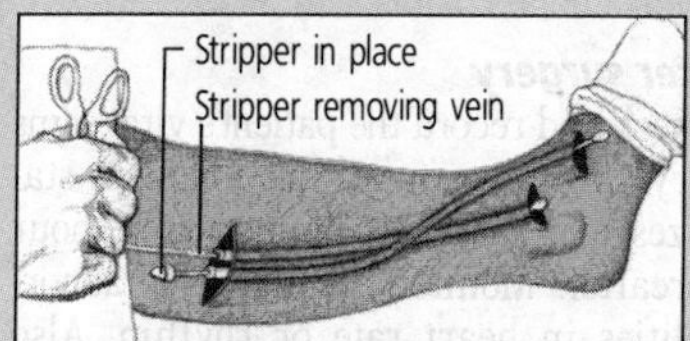

surement. Also explain that his vital signs and incision site will be checked regularly. If appropriate, explain that he'll have electrocardiogram (ECG) electrodes on his chest for continuous cardiac monitoring, that he'll have an arterial line or a pulmonary artery catheter to provide continuous pressure monitoring, and that he may be intubated and placed on mechanical ventilation.

• On the day before scheduled surgery, perform a complete vascular assessment. Take vital signs to provide a baseline. Evaluate the strength and sound of the blood flow and the symmetry of the pulses and note any bruits. Record the temperature of the extremities, their sensitivity to motor and sensory stimuli, and any pallor, cyanosis, or redness. Rate peripheral pulse volume and strength on a scale of 0 (pulse absent) to 4 (bounding, strong) and check capillary refill time by blanching the fingernail or toenail (normal refill time is under 3 seconds). Also note the location and appearance of any varicose veins.

• As ordered, instruct the patient to restrict food and fluids for at least 12 hours before surgery. Tell him that he probably will receive a sedative to help him relax and sleep the night before surgery. Ensure that he has signed a consent form.

• If the patient is awaiting surgery for aortic aneurysm repair, be on guard for symptoms of acute dissection or rupture. Note especially sudden severe pain in the chest, abdomen, or lower back; severe weakness; diaphoresis; tachycardia; or a precipitous drop in blood pressure. If any such signs or symptoms occur, call the doctor immediately; he may need to perform emergency surgery to save the patient's life.

After surgery

• Check and record the patient's vital signs every 15 minutes until his condition stabilizes and every 30 minutes to 1 hour thereafter. Monitor the ECG for abnormalities in heart rate or rhythm. Also monitor other pressure readings and carefully record intake and output. Check the patient's dressing regularly for excessive bleeding. Position the patient as ordered, and instruct him on recommended levels of activity during early stages of recovery. Provide analgesics, as ordered, for the patient's incisional pain.

• Frequently assess peripheral pulses, using Doppler ultrasonography if palpation proves difficult. Check all extremities for muscle strength and movement, color, temperature, and capillary refill time.

• Throughout the patient's recovery period, assess him often for signs of complications. Fever, cough, congestion, or dyspnea may indicate pulmonary infection. Low urine output and elevated blood urea nitrogen and serum creatinine levels may point to renal dysfunction. Severe pain and cyanosis in a limb may indicate occlusion. Hypotension, tachycardia, restlessness and confusion, shallow respirations, abdominal pain, and increased abdominal girth may signal hemorrhage; report any of these signs or symptoms immediately. In addition, frequently check the incision site for drainage and signs of infection.

• As the patient's condition improves, help wean him from the ventilator, if appropriate. To promote good pulmonary hygiene, encourage him to cough, turn, and deep-breathe frequently. As ordered, assist him with range-of-motion exercises in his legs to help prevent thrombus formation.

Home care instructions

• If appropriate, instruct the patient to check his pulse in the affected extremity before rising from bed each morning. If the patient can't check his own pulse, teach a family member to do it for him. Tell the patient to notify the doctor if he can't palpate his pulse or if he develops coldness, pallor, or pain in the extremity.

• Teach the patient how to care for his incision. Tell him to notify the doctor if he sees any signs of redness, swelling, or purulent drainage at the incision site.

• Explain the importance of strict compliance with any prescribed medication regimen. Make sure the patient understands the schedule and the expected adverse effects of all prescribed medications.
• Also stress the importance of regular checkups to monitor his condition.

Vasculitis

An autoimmune condition, vasculitis includes a broad spectrum of disorders characterized by blood vessel inflammation and necrosis. Clinical effects depend on the vessels involved and reflect tissue ischemia caused by blood flow obstruction.

The prognosis varies with the disease form. For example, hypersensitivity vasculitis is usually benign and limited to the skin, whereas the more extensive polyarteritis nodosa can be rapidly fatal.

Except for the mucocutaneous lymph node syndrome, which affects only children, vasculitis can affect a person at any age. Vasculitis may be a primary disorder or secondary to other disorders, such as rheumatoid arthritis and systemic lupus erythematosus.

Causes

Exactly how vascular damage develops in vasculitis isn't well understood. Some think that vasculitis may follow serious infectious disease, such as hepatitis B and bacterial endocarditis, and may be related to high doses of antibiotics.

Current theory holds that vasculitis is initiated by excessive circulating antigen, which triggers the formation of soluble antigen-antibody complexes. Then, because the reticuloendothelial system cannot effectively clear these complexes, they're deposited in blood vessel walls (Type III hypersensitivity). Theorists think that increased vascular permeability (associated with release of vasoactive amines by platelets and basophils) enhances this deposition. The deposited complexes activate the complement cascade. The result: chemotaxis of neutrophils, which release lysosomal enzymes which, in turn, cause vessel damage and necrosis. These effects may precipitate thrombosis, occlusion, hemorrhage, and tissue ischemia.

Another mechanism that may contribute to vascular damage is the cell-mediated (T-cell) immune response, whereby circulating antigen triggers sensitized lymphocytes to release soluble mediators. This attracts macrophages, which release intracellular enzymes, causing vascular damage. They can also transform into the epithelioid and multinucleated giant cells that typify the granulomatous vasculitides. Macrophagic phagocytosis of immune complexes enhances granuloma formation.

Complications

Renal, cardiac, and hepatic involvement can be fatal if vasculitis isn't treated. Renal failure, renal hypertension, glomerulitis, fibrous scarring of the lung tissue, cerebrovascular accident, and GI bleeding are a few of the severe complications associated with vasculitis.

Assessment

The patient's history and the physical assessment findings will vary, depending on the blood vessels involved. (See *Assessment and test findings in vasculitis,* pages 958 to 961.)

Diagnostic tests

Not all vasculitis disorders can be diagnosed definitively by specific tests. The most useful general diagnostic procedure is biopsy of the affected vessel. In some disorders, arteriography may be informative.

Treatment

Appropriate treatment aims to minimize irreversible tissue damage associated with ischemia. In primary vasculitis, treatment may involve removal of an offending antigen or use of anti-inflammatory or im-

(Text continues on page 961.)

Assessment and test findings in vasculitis

Vasculitis is a diverse group of inflammatory conditions, all of which cause vascular necrosis. Notable types are listed here, together with typical assessment and diagnostic findings.

Type	Assessment findings	Diagnostic test findings
Polyarteritis nodosa • This disorder affects small to medium arteries throughout the body. Lesions, which tend to be segmental and located at arterial bifurcations and branchings, spread distally to arterioles. In patients with severe disease, lesions circumferentially involve adjacent veins. • Aneurysms, hemorrhage, thrombosis, and fibrosis occur. Although any vessel can be affected, commonly involved ones are in the kidneys, heart, liver, GI tract, muscle, and testes. • The disorder affects males twice as frequently as females. Average onset is at age 45.	• Abdominal pain, myalgia, headache, hypertension, joint pain, weakness, weight loss, and malaise may occur. • The patient may also report signs and symptoms of specific organ dysfunction, such as chest pain, seizures, altered mental status, and edema.	• Laboratory findings include elevated erythrocyte sedimentation rate (ESR), leukocytosis, anemia, thrombocytosis, hypergammaglobulinemia, depressed C3 complement levels, rheumatoid factor (RF) titer greater than 1:60, and circulating immune complexes. • Tissue biopsy reveals the disease's hallmark: acute necrotizing inflammation of the arterial media with fibrinoid necrosis and extensive inflammatory cell infiltration of all coats of the vessel and surrounding tissue. • Arteriography demonstrates characteristic abnormalities, such as aneurysms in the small and medium arteries of the kidneys and abdominal viscera.
Allergic angiitis and granulomatosis (Churg-Strauss syndrome) • These disorders affect small to medium arteries and arterioles, capillaries, and venules, mainly in the lungs but also in other organs. The disorders resemble polyarteritis nodosa but include intravascular and extravascular granuloma formation, eosinophilic tissue infiltration, and associated severe asthma and peripheral eosinophilia. • The disorders strike men more commonly than women. Average age at onset is 44, but the disorders can occur at any age.	• The patient usually reports symptoms similar to those of polyarteritis nodosa and severe pulmonary involvement (asthma).	• Typical laboratory results are similar to those in polyarteritis nodosa. Eosinophilia (greater than 1,000 cells/ml) may also be seen. • Tissue biopsy shows granulomatous inflammation with eosinophilic infiltration. • X-ray studies show pulmonary infiltrates.

Assessment and test findings in vasculitis *(continued)*

Type	Assessment findings	Diagnostic test findings
Polyangiitis overlap syndrome • This syndrome affects small to medium arteries and other vessels in the lungs and other organs.	• The patient usually complains of symptoms of polyarteritis nodosa and allergic angiitis and granulomatosis.	• Laboratory findings are the same as those in polyarteritis nodosa and allergic angiitis and granulomatosis. • Tissue biopsy shows granulomatous inflammation with eosinophilic infiltration. • X-rays show pulmonary infiltrates.
Wegener's granulomatosis • This type of vasculitis involves small to medium vessels of the respiratory tract and the kidneys (causing glomerulonephritis). • The patient may be any age, but the average age at onset is 40. • The incidence is only slightly higher in men than in women.	• The patient usually reports fever, paranasal sinus pain and drainage, pulmonary congestion, cough, dyspnea, malaise, anorexia, and weight loss. Serous otitis media may occur. • Inspection may reveal saddle nose deformity, skin lesions, and purulent or bloody nasal discharge with or without nasal mucosal ulceration. You may also detect eye involvement, such as conjunctivitis, episcleritis, scleritis, granulomatous sclerouveitis, ciliary vessel vasculitis, and proptosis (bulging) from lesions of the retro-orbital mass. • Clinical findings may include pericarditis and, rarely, cardiomyopathy. Renal involvement may cause glomerulitis, possibly leading to renal failure.	• Laboratory tests may detect anemia and leukocytosis; mild hypergammaglobulinemia (particularly IgA); elevated ESR; mildly elevated RF levels; circulating immune complexes; and antineutrophil cytoplasmic autoantibodies. • Tissue biopsy may demonstrate necrotizing vasculitis with granulomatous inflammation.
Temporal arteritis (giant cell arteritis) • This disorder occurs in medium to large arteries, usually the branches of the carotid artery and particularly the temporal artery. • The typical patient is a woman over age 55. (The disorder seldom occurs in blacks.)	• The patient may complain of fever, myalgia, malaise, fatigue, anorexia, weight loss, sweats, arthralgia, jaw and tongue claudication, headache, and stiffness, aching, and pain in the muscles of the neck, shoulders, lower back, hips, and thighs associated with polymyalgia rheumatica. • The patient may also report sudden blindness (caused by ischemic optic neuritis).	• Laboratory results show monochromic or slightly hypochromic anemia, elevated ESR, and increased levels of alkaline phosphatase, IgG, complement, and circulating immune complexes. • Tissue biopsy shows panarteritis with infiltration of mononuclear cells, giant cells within the vessel wall, fragmentation of internal elastic lamina, and proliferation of intima.

(continued)

Assessment and test findings in vasculitis *(continued)*

Type	Assessment findings	Diagnostic test findings
Takayasu's arteritis (aortic arch syndrome) • This syndrome affects medium to large arteries, especially the aortic arch and its branches and, possibly, the pulmonary artery. Inflammatory mononuclear cell infiltrates and giant cells appear in the vessel wall, resulting in marked proliferation and fibrosis, scarring and vascularization of the media, and disruption and degeneration of the elastic lamina. Cardiomegaly and cardiac failure secondary to aortic or pulmonary hypertension occur and may progress to cerebrovascular accident. • Most patients are adolescents and young women.	• The patient may report malaise, fever, nausea, night sweats, arthralgia, anorexia, weight loss, pain or paresthesia distal to affected areas, syncope, and – if the carotid artery is involved – diplopia and transient blindness. • On inspection, you may notice pallor. On palpation, you may not find a distal pulse. Auscultation may disclose bruits and aortic regurgitation.	• Laboratory reports may indicate anemia, leukocytosis, positive lupus erythematosus cell findings, elevated immunoglobulin levels, and elevated ESR. • Tissue biopsy findings include inflammation of vascular adventitia and intima and thickening of vessel walls. • Arteriography may disclose irregular vessel walls, stenosis, poststenotic dilation, aneurysms, and calcified, obstructed vessels.
Hypersensitivity vasculitis • A heterogenous group of disorders thought to be caused by a hypersensitivity reaction, this vasculitis type involves small vessels, especially those of the skin. • The disorders affect both sexes and all age-groups.	• The patient typically reports such symptoms as fever, malaise, myalgia, and anorexia. • Inspection may reveal palpable purpura, papules, nodules, vesicles, bullae, ulcers, or chronic or recurrent urticaria.	• Laboratory results show mild leukocytosis with or without eosinophilia and elevated ESR. • Tissue biopsy shows leukocytoblastic angiitis, usually in postcapillary venules, with infiltration of polymorphonuclear leukocytes, fibrinoid necrosis, and extravasation of erythrocytes.
Mucocutaneous lymph node syndrome (Kawasaki disease) • Small to medium vessels, primarily of the lymph nodes, are affected. Lesions may progress to involve coronary arteries. Intimal proliferation and infiltration of the vessel wall with mononuclear cells may occur. Beadlike aneurysms and thromboses may form along the artery. • This syndrome may progress to myocarditis, pericarditis, myocardial infarction, and cardiomegaly. Although usually benign and self-limiting, it can be fatal if coronary artery aneurysms develop.	• The patient usually reports fever and other signs, such as inflamed neck glands (nonsuppurative cervical adenitis), edema, and conjunctival congestion. • Inspection findings may include erythema of the mouth, lips, and palms and desquamation of the fingertips.	• Tissue biopsy shows intimal proliferation and vessel walls infiltrated with mononuclear cells.

Assessment and test findings in vasculitis *(continued)*

Type	Assessment findings	Diagnostic test findings
Behçet's syndrome • This syndrome involves small vessels, primarily of the mouth and genitalia but also of the eyes, skin, joints, GI tract, and central nervous system. The underlying cause is leukocytoblastic venulitis. • The syndrome most commonly strikes young adults and proves more severe in men than women.	• The patient commonly reports recurrent aphthous ulcers and eye pain (from lesions caused by iritis, posterior uveitis, retinal vessel occlusions, and optic neuritis). • Inspection findings may include genital lesions and cutaneous lesions (folliculitis, erythema nodosum, and an acnelike exanthem). Nonspecific inflammatory skin reactions may also be seen.	• Laboratory tests may reveal leukocytosis, elevated ESR and C-reactive protein levels, and antibodies to human oral mucosa.

munosuppressant drugs. Antigenic drugs, food, and other offending environmental substances should be identified and eliminated, if possible.

Drug therapy in primary vasculitis typically involves daily administration of low-dose oral cyclophosphamide and corticosteroids.

In rapidly fulminant vasculitis, the daily cyclophosphamide dose may be increased significantly for the first 2 to 3 days and then returned to the regular dose. In addition, the patient usually receives prednisone in daily divided doses for 7 to 10 days, with consolidation to a single morning dose by 2 to 3 weeks. When the vasculitis appears to be in remission, or when prescribed cytotoxic drugs take full effect, corticosteroid therapy is tapered to a single daily dose and then to an alternate-day schedule that may continue for 3 to 6 months.

In secondary vasculitis, treatment focuses on the underlying disorder.

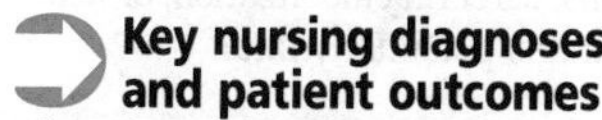

Key nursing diagnoses and patient outcomes

Altered peripheral tissue perfusion related to vasculitis. Based on this nursing diagnosis, you'll establish these patient outcomes. The patient will:

- express feelings of comfort or an absence of pain with activity
- maintain strong peripheral pulses
- not have evidence of severe ischemia.

Risk for injury related to potential complications of vasculitis. Based on this nursing diagnosis, you'll establish these patient outcomes. The patient will:

- comply with the prescribed therapy to minimize or prevent injury
- not show signs of organ dysfunction.

Sensory alteration related to tissue ischemia. Based on this nursing diagnosis, you'll establish these patient outcomes. The patient will:

- remain safe in his environment
- incorporate safety precautions into his daily life to compensate for sensory changes
- not have further sensory changes.

Nursing interventions

- For the patient with Wegener's granulomatosis, instill nose drops to lubricate the mucosa and to minimize crusting. Or irrigate the nasal passages with warm 0.9% sodium chloride solution.

• Keep the patient well hydrated (about 3 liters of fluid daily) to reduce the risk of hemorrhagic cystitis associated with cyclophosphamide therapy.
• To prevent falls, ensure that the patient with decreased visual acuity has a safe environment.
• Regulate environmental temperature to prevent additional vasoconstriction caused by cold.
• Provide supportive care for organ dysfunction, as indicated and prescribed.
• Provide emotional support to help the patient and his family cope with an altered body image – the result of the disorder or its therapy. (For example, with Wegener's granulomatosis, saddle nose may develop. Corticosteroid therapy may cause weight gain, and cyclophosphamide therapy may cause alopecia.)

Monitoring

• Assess for dry nasal mucosa in patients with Wegener's granulomatosis.
• Monitor vital signs. Use a Doppler ultrasonic flowmeter, if available, to auscultate blood pressure in patients who have Takayasu's arteritis and whose peripheral pulses are difficult to palpate.
• Measure intake and output. Check daily for edema.
• Monitor the patient's white blood cell and platelet counts during cyclophosphamide therapy to avoid severe leukopenia and thrombocytopenia. Also assess for GI disturbances.
• Watch for signs and symptoms of organ involvement.

Patient teaching

• Teach the patient and his family to recognize adverse effects of drug therapy (for example, with corticosteroids) and to watch for signs of bleeding: black tarry stools, hemoptysis, epistaxis, and multiple ecchymoses. Instruct them to report any of these findings to the doctor.
• Advise the patient to wear warm clothes and gloves when going outside in cold weather.

Ventricular aneurysm

This potentially life-threatening condition involves an outpouching – almost always of the left ventricle – that produces ventricular wall dysfunction in about 20% of patients after myocardial infarction (MI). Ventricular aneurysm may develop within days to weeks after MI or may be delayed for years. Resection improves the prognosis in patients with ventricular failure or ventricular arrhythmias.

Causes

MI causes ventricular aneurysm. When MI destroys a large muscular section of the left ventricle, necrosis reduces the ventricular wall to a thin sheath of fibrous tissue. Under intracardiac pressure, this thin layer stretches and forms a separate noncontractile sac (aneurysm). Abnormal muscle wall movement accompanies ventricular aneurysm. (See *Aneurysm effects on the ventricular wall.*)

During systolic ejection, the abnormal muscle wall movements associated with the aneurysm cause the remaining normally functioning myocardial fibers to increase the force of contraction to maintain stroke volume and cardiac output. At the same time, a portion of the stroke volume is lost to passive distention of the noncontractile sac.

Complications

Ventricular aneurysms enlarge but seldom rupture. However, an untreated ventricular aneurysm can lead to ventricular arrhythmias, cerebral embolization, or heart failure and is potentially fatal.

Aneurysm effects on the ventricular wall

A ventricular aneurysm can cause the ventricular wall to contract in abnormal ways. In the sketches below, the arrows represent motions from end diastole to end systole.

Normal contraction
Change of 25% to 30% in outside wall diameter

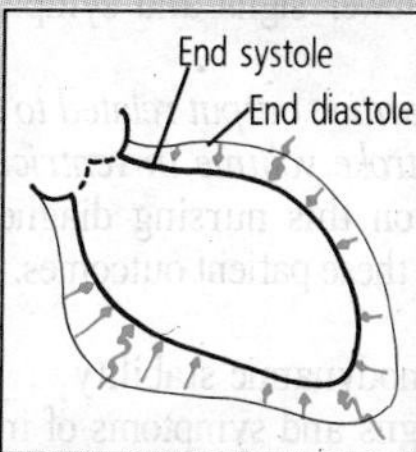

Hypokinesia
Decreased mobility

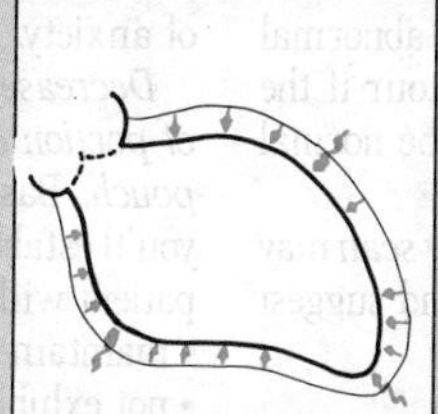

Asynergia
Decreased, inadequate movement

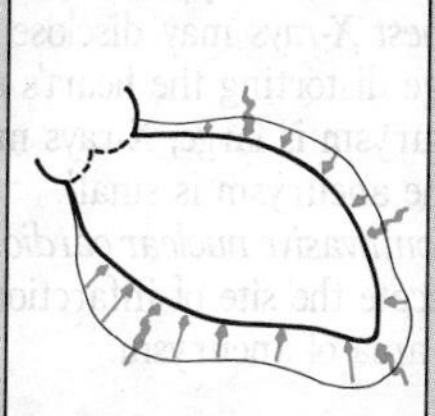

Akinesia
Lack of movement

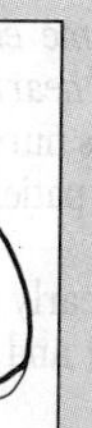

Dyskinesia
Paradoxical systolic expansion

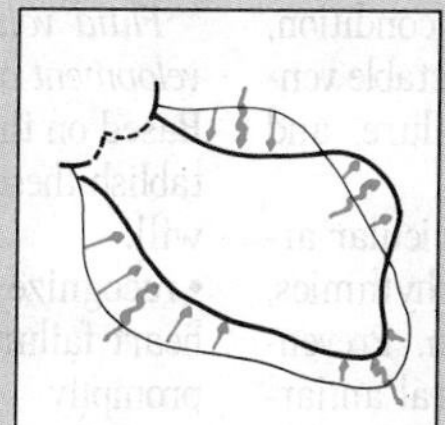

Asynchrony
Uncoordinated movement

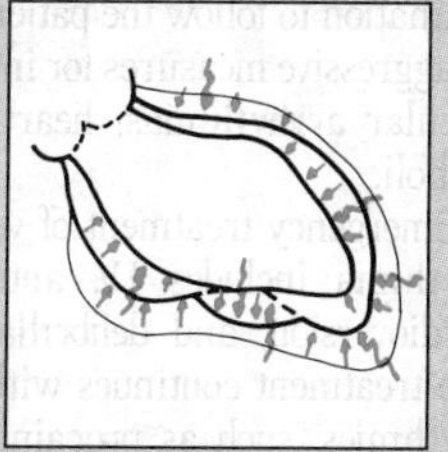

Assessment

The patient may have a history of a previous MI. However, sometimes MI is silent, and the patient may be unaware of having had one. He may complain of palpitations and anginal pain.

If the patient has developed heart failure as a result of the aneurysm, he may complain of dyspnea, fatigue, and edema.

Inspection of the chest may reveal a visible or palpable systolic precordial bulge. Distended neck veins may appear if heart failure is present.

Palpation of peripheral pulses may reveal an irregular rhythm caused by arrhythmias (such as premature ventricular contractions or ventricular tachycardia). A pulsus alternans may be felt. Palpation of the chest usually detects a double, diffuse, or displaced apical impulse.

Auscultation of the heart may detect an irregular rhythm and a gallop rhythm. Crackles and rhonchi may be present in the lung if heart failure is present.

Diagnostic tests

The following tests may determine the presence of a ventricular aneurysm:

• *Two-dimensional echocardiography* demonstrates abnormal motion in the left ventricular wall.
• *Left ventriculography* reveals left ventricular enlargement, with an area of akinesia or dyskinesia (during cineangiography) and diminished cardiac function.
• *Electrocardiography* may show persistent ST-T wave elevations at rest. ST-segment elevation over the aneurysm creates an elevated rounded appearance.
• *Chest X-rays* may disclose an abnormal bulge distorting the heart's contour if the aneurysm is large; X-rays may be normal if the aneurysm is small.
• *Noninvasive nuclear cardiology scan* may indicate the site of infarction and suggest the area of aneurysm.

Treatment

Depending on the size of the aneurysm and the presence of complications, treatment may require only routine medical examination to follow the patient's condition, or aggressive measures for intractable ventricular arrhythmias, heart failure, and emboli.

Emergency treatment of ventricular arrhythmia includes I.V. antiarrhythmics, cardioversion, and defibrillation. Preventive treatment continues with oral antiarrhythmics, such as procainamide, quinidine, or disopyramide.

Emergency treatment for heart failure with pulmonary edema includes oxygen, digitalis I.V., furosemide I.V., potassium replacement, morphine sulfate I.V. and, when necessary, nitroprusside I.V. and endotracheal intubation. Maintenance therapy may include oral nitrates, prazosin, and hydralazine.

Systemic embolization requires anticoagulation therapy or embolectomy. Refractory ventricular tachycardia, heart failure, recurrent arterial embolization, and persistent angina with coronary artery occlusion may require surgery. The most effective surgery is aneurysmectomy with myocardial revascularization.

Key nursing diagnoses and patient outcomes

Anxiety related to increased risk of complications. Based on this nursing diagnosis, you'll establish these patient outcomes. The patient will:
• express feelings of anxiety and identify their source
• use available support systems to cope with anxiety
• demonstrate fewer signs and symptoms of anxiety.

Decreased cardiac output related to loss of portion of stroke volume in ventricular pouch. Based on this nursing diagnosis, you'll establish these patient outcomes. The patient will:
• maintain hemodynamic stability
• not exhibit signs and symptoms of inadequate tissue perfusion
• comply with the prescribed treatment to minimize the severity of decreased cardiac output.

Fluid volume excess related to the development of heart failure, a complication. Based on this nursing diagnosis, you'll establish these patient outcomes. The patient will:
• recognize early signs and symptoms of heart failure and seek medical treatment promptly
• regain normal fluid balance with effective treatment of heart failure.

Nursing interventions

• Arrhythmias require elective cardioversion. If the patient is conscious, give diazepam I.V., as ordered, before cardioversion.
• Provide psychological support for the patient and his family to reduce anxiety.
• If the patient is scheduled to undergo resection, explain expected postoperative care in the intensive care unit (such as an endotracheal tube, a ventilator, hemodynamic monitoring, and chest tubes).

Monitoring

• In a patient with heart failure, closely monitor vital signs, heart sounds, intake

and output, fluid and electrolyte balance, and blood urea nitrogen and serum creatinine levels.
• Be alert for sudden changes in sensorium that indicate cerebral embolization and for any signs that suggest renal failure or MI.
• Monitor the electrocardiogram for arrhythmias. If the patient is receiving antiarrhythmics, check appropriate laboratory tests. For instance, if the patient takes procainamide, check antinuclear antibodies because the drug may induce signs and symptoms that mimic lupus erythematosus.
• After surgery, monitor vital signs, intake and output, heart sounds, and the pulmonary artery catheter. Watch for signs of infection, such as fever and drainage.

Patient teaching
• Teach the patient how to check for pulse irregularity and rate changes. Encourage him to follow his prescribed medication regimen – even during the night – and to watch for adverse reactions.
• Because arrhythmias can cause sudden death, refer the family to a community-based cardiopulmonary resuscitation training program.

Volvulus

Marked by sudden onset of severe abdominal pain, volvulus is a twisting of the intestine at least 180 degrees on itself. Volvulus results in blood vessel compression and causes obstruction both proximal and distal to the twisted loop. (See *What happens in volvulus.*)

Volvulus occurs in a bowel segment long enough to twist. The most common area, particularly in adults, is the sigmoid colon. Other common sites include the stomach and cecum.

Causes
In volvulus, twisting may result from an anomaly of bowel rotation in utero, an ingested foreign body, or an adhesion. Volvulus secondary to meconium ileus may occur in patients with cystic fibrosis. In some patients, however, the cause is unknown.

Complications
Without immediate treatment, volvulus can lead to strangulation of the twisted bowel loop, ischemia, infarction, perforation, and fatal peritonitis.

What happens in volvulus

Although volvulus may occur anywhere in a bowel segment long enough to twist, the most common site, as this illustration depicts, is the sigmoid colon. Here, a counterclockwise twist has occluded the colon, causing edema within the closed loop and obstruction at both its proximal and distal ends.

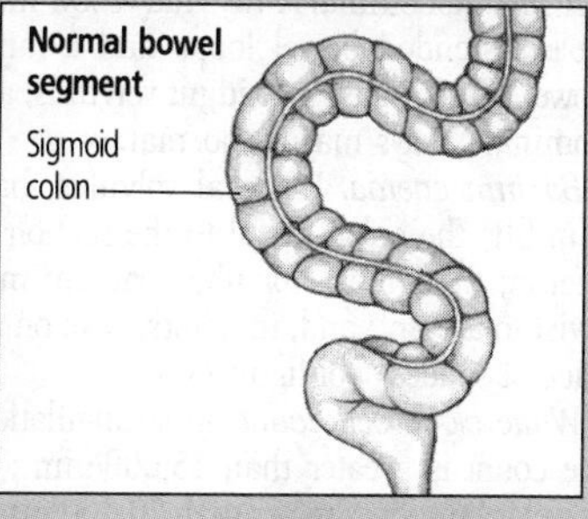

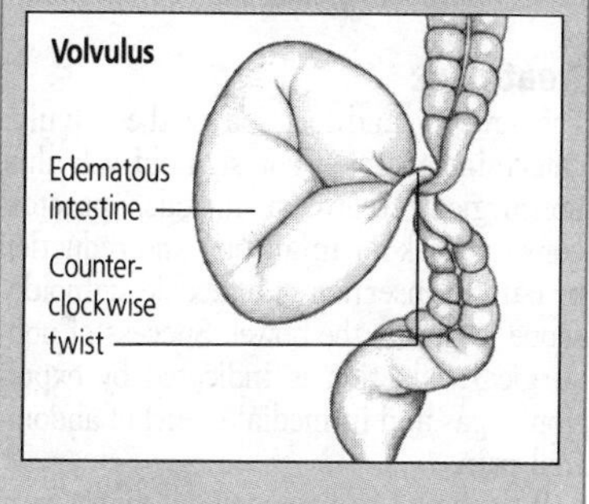

Assessment

The patient with volvulus complains of severe abdominal pain and may report bilious vomiting. The history may also reveal the passage of bloody stools.

On inspection, the patient appears to be in pain. Abdominal inspection and palpation may reveal distention and a palpable mass.

Diagnostic tests

- *X-rays.* Abdominal X-rays may show multiple distended bowel loops and a large bowel without gas; in midgut volvulus, abdominal X-rays may be normal.
- *Barium enema.* In cecal volvulus, barium fills the colon distal to the section of cecum; in sigmoid volvulus, barium may twist to a point; and, in adults, take on an "ace of spades" configuration.
- *White blood cell count.* In strangulation, the count is greater than 15,000/mm³; in bowel infarction, greater than 20,000/mm³.

Treatment

The severity and location of the volvulus determine therapy. For sigmoid volvulus, nonsurgical treatment includes proctoscopy to check for infarction and reduction by careful insertion of a flexible sigmoidoscope to deflate the bowel. Success of nonsurgical reduction is indicated by expulsion of gas and immediate relief of abdominal pain.

If the bowel is distended but viable, surgery consists of detorsion (untwisting); if the bowel is necrotic, surgery includes resection and anastomosis. Prolonged total parenteral nutrition and I.V. administration of antibiotics are usually necessary. Sedatives may be needed.

Key nursing diagnoses and patient outcomes

Altered gastrointestinal tissue perfusion related to blood vessel compression. Based on this nursing diagnosis, you'll establish these patient outcomes. The patient will:

- seek emergency care at the onset of symptoms to minimize the risk of ischemia causing permanent damage to gastrointestinal tissue
- not develop bowel necrosis
- regain adequate gastrointestinal tissue perfusion with treatment.

Risk for infection related to potential for peritonitis to develop. Based on this nursing diagnosis, you'll establish these patient outcomes. The patient will:

- maintain a normal temperature and white blood count
- not show signs and symptoms of peritonitis.

Pain related to twisted bowel and obstruction. Based on this nursing diagnosis, you'll establish these patient outcomes. The patient will:

- express feelings of comfort following analgesic administration
- become pain free when volvulus is resolved.

Nursing interventions

- Provide psychological support. Listen to the patient's concerns, and offer reassurance; take time to answer his questions.
- Administer analgesics and broad-spectrum antibiotics, as ordered.
- Administer I.V. fluids, as ordered.
- Insert a nasogastric tube and connect to low-pressure intermittent suction, if ordered, to relieve abdominal distention.
- Prepare the patient for proctoscopy, as indicated.
- If the patient is scheduled for detorsion surgery, provide appropriate preoperative and postoperative care, as for any patient undergoing abdominal surgery. If the patient requires bowel resection and anastomosis, see the entry "Bowel resection with anastomosis."

Monitoring

- Monitor the patient for the desired effects and potential adverse reactions to administered analgesics and antibiotics.

• Routinely monitor vital signs, intake and output, and fluid and electrolyte balance.

Patient teaching

• Explain what happens in volvulus, using teaching aids, if available. Review its signs and symptoms and possible complications. Discuss necessary diagnostic procedures and treatments.

• Reinforce the doctor's explanation of scheduled surgery and its possible complications. Provide preoperative teaching.

• If surgery was extensive, or if the patient's condition requires it, refer him and his family to the social service department and a local home health care agency.

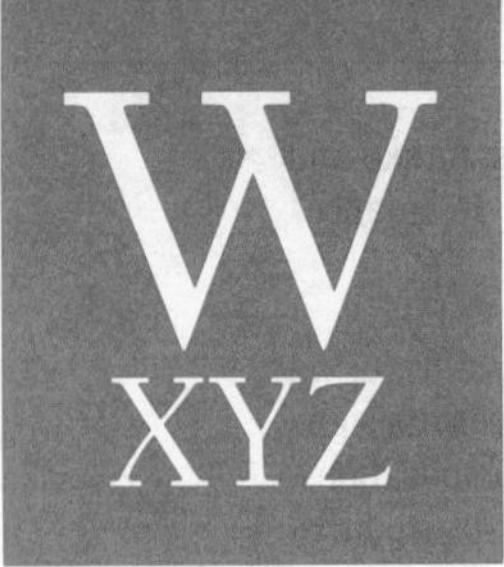

Whiplash

Also known as acceleration-deceleration cervical injury, whiplash results from sharp hyperextension and flexion of the neck that damages muscles, ligaments, disks, and nerve tissue. The prognosis is excellent; symptoms usually subside with treatment.

Causes

Any injury that forcibly causes hyperextension and flexion of the neck can result in whiplash. Common causes include motor vehicle accidents, sports accidents, and falls. For example, in a motor vehicle accident, a rear-end collision propels the patient's trunk forward on the pelvis, throwing the head into hyperextension and stretching the anterior structure of the neck; a head-on impact initially produces acute flexion and subsequently a reflex hyperextension.

Complications

Although rare, a possible complication of acceleration-deceleration injuries is nerve damage that results in numbness, tingling, or weakness.

Assessment

The patient's history reveals an acceleration-deceleration injury. He usually reports that symptoms first appeared 12 to 24 hours after the injury. If the injury is mild, symptoms may not appear for another 12 to 24 hours.

The patient typically complains of moderate to severe pain in the anterior and posterior neck. Within several days, the anterior pain diminishes but posterior pain persists or even intensifies. (You may not see the patient until he has reached this point because many patients don't seek medical attention at first.) He also may report dizziness, headache, and vomiting.

During inspection of the neck, you may note neck muscle asymmetry. Neurologic examination may reveal gait disturbances, rigidity or numbness in the arms, and spacial instability that affects balance. Palpation reveals pain at the exact location of the injury.

Diagnostic tests

Full cervical spine X-rays rule out cervical fracture.

Treatment

Until X-rays rule out cervical fracture, treatment focuses on protecting the cervical spine. Initial treatment includes bed rest, the use of a soft cervical collar, and ice packs. Oral analgesics provide pain relief, and oral corticosteroids help reduce inflammation and relieve chronic discomfort. To restore flexibility, physical therapy, including mobilization exercises, is started at 72 hours after the injury. It is combined with application of moist heat and a gradually decreased use of the soft collar.

If the patient experiences persistent ligamentous or articular pain, he may benefit from cervical traction and diathermy treatment.

Key nursing diagnoses and patient outcomes

Anxiety related to cervical injury. Based on this nursing diagnosis, you'll establish these patient outcomes. The patient will:
- express feelings of anxiety and identify their source
- become educated about whiplash injuries
- have decreased physical symptoms of anxiety.

Impaired physical mobility related to pain. Based on this nursing diagnosis, you'll establish these patient outcomes. The patient will:
- comply with the prescribed therapy, especially physical therapy
- regain his former physical mobility.

Pain related to inflammation at the site of injury. Based on this nursing diagnosis, you'll establish these patient outcomes. The patient will:
- express feelings of comfort following analgesic administration
- use nonpharmacologic measures, such as cold therapy, to help minimize pain
- not develop chronic pain.

Nursing interventions

- As in all suspected spinal injuries, assume that the patient has an injured spine until proved otherwise. If you're at the scene of the accident, make sure a patient with suspected whiplash or other injuries receives careful transportation to the hospital. To do this, place him in a supine position on a spine board, and immobilize his neck with tape and a hard cervical collar or sandbags.
- Until an X-ray rules out cervical fracture, move the patient as little as possible. Before X-rays are taken, carefully remove any neck jewelry the patient is wearing. Warn him against movements that could injure his spine.
- Administer medications for pain as ordered.
- Apply a soft cervical collar as directed.

Monitoring

- Monitor the effectiveness of administered analgesics and nonpharmacologic measures, such as cold therapy, to relieve pain.
- Observe the patient for complications, such as gait disturbances, rigidity or numbness in arms, and spatial disturbances.

Patient teaching

- The patient with whiplash is likely to be discharged immediately. To help decrease his anxiety, reassure him that uncomplicated whiplash has an excellent prognosis. Be sure he fully understands the treatment and why he must restrict his activity.
- Stress the importance of limiting activity during the first 72 hours after the injury. Tell the patient to rest for a few days and not to lift heavy objects.
- If the patient needs a soft cervical collar, teach him how to put it on.
- If a narcotic has been prescribed for pain relief, emphasize the need for safety in the home. Tell the patient not to drive and to avoid the use of alcohol while taking the medication.
- Warn the patient to return to the hospital or to call the doctor immediately if he develops persistent pain or numbness, tingling, or weakness on one side.

Selected references

American Hospital Formulary Service, *Drug Information 97.* Bethesda, Md.: American Society of Hospital Pharmacists, 1997.

Beare, P.G., et al. *Journal of Adult Health Nursing,* 2nd ed. St. Louis: Mosby-Year Book, Inc., 1994.

Berek, J., et al. *Novak's Gynecology,* 12th ed. Baltimore: Williams & Wilkins, 1996.

Brozenec, S. "Medications in the Treatment of Peptic Ulcer Disease," *RN* 59(9):48-53, 1996.

Brunsted, J., and Riddick, D. "Menstruation and Disorders of Menstrual Function," in *Danforth's Obstetrics and Gynecology,* 7th ed. Edited by Scott, J., et al. Philadelphia: J.B. Lippincott Co., 1994.

Bullock, B.L. *Pathophysiology: Adaptations and Alterations in Function,* 4th ed. Philadelphia: J.B. Lippincott Co., 1996.

Cave, D.R., and Hoffman, J.S. "Management of *Helicobacter pylori* Infection in Ulcer Disease," *Hospital Practice* 31(1):63-75, 1996.

Centers for Disease Control and Prevention. *Hantavirus Illness.* In the U.S. Hantavirus Report. March 9, 1995.

Chandrasoma, P., and Taylor, C. *Concise Pathology.* Norwalk, Conn.: Appleton & Lange, 1995.

DeVita, V.T., et al., eds. *Cancer: Principles and Practice,* 4th ed. Philadelphia: J.B. Lippincott Co., 1993.

Diagnostics Test Cards. Springhouse, Pa.: Springhouse Corp., 1996.

Diseases, 2nd ed. Springhouse, Pa.: Springhouse Corp., 1997.

Division of STD Prevention. *Sexually Transmitted Disease Surveillance.* 1994 U.S. Department of Health and Human Services, Public Health Service. Atlanta: Centers for Disease Control and Prevention, September 1995.

Fischbach, F. *A Manual of Laboratory and Diagnostic Tests,* 5th ed. Philadelphia: J.B. Lippincott Co., 1996.

Greenspan, F., and Baxter, J. *Basic and Clinical Endocrinology.* Norwalk, Conn.: Appleton & Lange, 1994.

Groenwald, S.L., et al., eds. *Cancer Symptom Management.* Sudbury, MA: Jones & Bartlett, 1996.

Gulanick, M., et al. *Nursing Care Plans: Nursing Diagnosis and Intervention,* 3rd ed. St. Louis: Mosby-Year Book, Inc., 1994.

Harwood, K. "Straight Talk about Breast Cancer," *Nursing96* 26(10):39-46, October 1996.

Hepatitis Branch, Centers for Disease Control and Prevention. *Epidemiology and Prevention of Viral Hepatitis A to E. An Overview.* U.S. Department of Health and Human Services. Atlanta: Centers for Disease Control, 1996.

Hoffman, R., et al., eds. *Hematology: Basic Principles and Practice.* New York: Churchill Livingstone Inc., 1995.

Ignatavicius, D., and Bayne, M.V. *Medical-Surgical Nursing,* 2nd ed. Philadelphia: W.B. Saunders Co., 1995.

Illustrated Manual of Nursing Practice, 2nd ed. Springhouse, Pa.: Springhouse Corp., 1994.

Isselbacher, K.J., et al. *Harrison's Principles of Internal Medicine,* 13th ed. New York: McGraw-Hill Book Co., 1994.

Karlowicz, K.A. *Urologic Nursing: Principles and Practice.* Philadelphia: W.B. Saunders Co., 1995.

Lewis, S., et. al. *Medical Surgical Nursing.* St. Louis: Mosby-Year Book, Inc., 1996.

McCance, K., and Huether, S. *Understanding Pathophysiology.* St. Louis: Mosby-Year Book, Inc., 1996.

McGovren, J.P. "Pharmacologic Principles," in *Cancer Chemotherapy Handbook,* 2nd ed. Edited by Dorr, R.T., and Von Hoff, D.D. Norwalk, Conn.: Appleton & Lange, 1994.

Metheny, N.H. *Fluid and Electrolyte Balance,* 3rd ed. Philadelphia: J.B. Lippincott Co., 1996.

Monahan, F.D., et al. *Nursing Care of Adults.* Philadelphia: W.B. Saunders Co., 1994.

National Instituties of Health. *Diabetes in America,* 2nd ed. National Institutes of Diabetes and Digestive and Kidney Disease, NIH Publication No. 95-1468, 1995.

Nettina, S. *The Lippincott Manual of Nursing Practice,* 6th ed. Philadelphia: J.B. Lippincott Co., 1996.

Norton, R.A. "Diabetes 2000. The Right Mix of Diet and Exercise." *RN* 58(4):20-25, April 1995.

Occupational Safety and Health Association. *Controlling Occupational Exposure to Hazardous Drugs,* (OSHA Instruction CPL 2-2.20B CH-4). Directorate of Technical Support, 1995.

Ondrusek, R.S. "Spotting an MI before It's an MI," *RN* 59(4):26-30, April 1996.

Parker, S.L., et al. "Cancer Statistics," *Cancer* 46(1):5-28, 1996.

Phipps, W.J., et al. *Medical-Surgical Nursing: Concepts and Clinical Practice,* 5th ed. St. Louis: Mosby-Year Book, Inc., 1995.

Polaski, A.L., and Tatro, S.E. *Luckman's Core Principles and Practice of Medical Surgical Nursing.* Philadelphia: W.B. Saunders Co., 1996.

Professional Guide to Signs and Symptoms, 2nd ed. Springhouse, Pa.: Springhouse Corp., 1997.

Reilly, N.J. "Advances in Quality of Life After Cystectomy: Urinary Diversions," *Innovations in Urology Nursing* 5(2):17-33, 1994.

Smeltzer, S.C., and Bare, B.G. *Brunner and Suddarth's Textbook of Medical-Surgical Nursing,* 8th ed. Philadelphia: J.B. Lippincott Co., 1996.

Sparks, S.M., and Taylor, C.M. *Nursing Diagnosis Reference Manual,* 3rd ed. Springhouse, Pa.: Springhouse Corp., 1995.

Swearingen, P. *Manual of Medical-Surgical Nursing Care.* St. Louis: Mosby-Year Book. Inc., 1994.

Thompson, S.D., et al. "When Ovarian Cancer Strikes," *Nursing96* 26(10):33-38, October 1996.

Whaley, L.F., and Wong D.L. *Nursing Care of Infants and Children,* 5th ed. St. Louis: Mosby-Year Book, Inc., 1995.

Yamada, D.T. *Textbook of Gastroenterology.* Philadelphia: J.B. Lippincott Co., 1995.

Index

Boldface page numbers indicate major entries; i refers to an illustration; t refers to a table

Boldface page numbers indicate major entries; i refers to an illustration; t refers to a table

Boldface page numbers indicate major entries; i refers to an illustration; t refers to a table

Boldface page numbers indicate major entries; i refers to an illustration; t refers to a table